COMPREHENSIVE
Hospital Medicine:
An Evidence-Based Approach

Mark V. Williams, M.D., F.A.C.P.
Professor of Medicine
Chief, Division of Hospital Medicine
Northwestern University Feinberg School of Medicine
Chicago, Illinois

Scott A. Flanders, M.D.
Associate Professor of Internal Medicine
University of Michigan
Director, Hospitalist Program
Associate Director, Inpatient Programs
University of Michigan Health System
Ann Arbor, Michigan

Winthrop F. Whitcomb, M.D.
Assistant Professor of Medicine
University of Massachusetts Medical School
Worcester, Massachusetts
Director, Clinical Performance Improvement
Mercy Medical Center
Springfield, Massachusetts

Steven L. Cohn, M.D., F.A.C.P.
Clinical Professor of Medicine
State University of New York–Downstate
Chief, Division of General Internal Medicine
Director, Medical Consultation Service
Kings County Hospital
Brooklyn, New York

Franklin A. Michota, M.D.
Head, Section of Hospital Medicine
Department of General Internal Medicine
The Cleveland Clinic Foundation
Cleveland, Ohio

Russell Holman, M.D.
Chief Operating Officer
National Medical Director
Cogent Healthcare
Nashville, Tennessee

Richard Gross, M.D., F.A.C.P.
Professor of Medicine
Departments of Medicine and Interdisciplinary Oncology
University of South Florida College of Medicine
Chief, Division of Internal and Hospital Medicine
H. Lee Moffitt Cancer Center and Research Institute
Tampa, Florida

Geno J. Merli, M.D., F.A.C.P.
Senior Vice President, Chief Medical Officer
Director, Jefferson Center for Vascular Disease
Thomas Jefferson University Hospital
Jefferson Medical College
Philadelphia, Pennsylvania

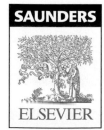

SAUNDERS

ELSEVIER

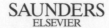

SAUNDERS
ELSEVIER

1600 John F. Kennedy Blvd.
Ste 1800
Philadelphia, PA 19103-2899

COMPREHENSIVE HOSPITAL MEDICINE:
AN EVIDENCE-BASED APPROACH

Expert Consult: Online and Print: ISBN: 978-1-4160-0223-9
Expert Consult Premium Edition Enhanced Online Features and Print: ISBN: 978-1-4160-0297-0

Notice

Knowledge and best practice in this field are constantly changing. As new research and experience broaden our knowledge, changes in practice, treatment, and drug therapy may become necessary or appropriate. Readers are advised to check the most current information provided (i) on procedures featured or (ii) by the manufacturer of each product to be administered, to verify the recommended dose or formula, the method and duration of administration, and contraindications. It is the responsibility of the practitioner, relying on their own experience and knowledge of the patient, to make diagnoses, to determine dosages and the best treatment for each individual patient, and to take all appropriate safety precautions. To the fullest extent of the law, neither the Publisher nor the Author assumes any liability for any injury and/or damage to persons or property arising out of or related to any use of the material contained in this book.

The Publisher

Library of Congress Cataloging-in-Publication Data

Comprehensive hospital medicine: an evidence-based approach / [edited by]
    Mark V. Williams.—1st ed.
        p. ; cm.
    Includes bibliographical references.
    ISBN 1-4160-0223-5
    1. Hospital care.   2. Evidence-based medicine.   3. Internal medicine.   I. Williams, Mark, 1959 Nov. 7-[DNLM: 1. Inpatients.   2. Patient Care.   3. Evidence-Based Medicine.   4. Hospitalization. WX 162 C7375 2007]
    RA972.C662 2007
    362.11—dc22

                                                                                    2006046170

Senior Acquisition Editor: Rolla Couchman
Project Manager: Mary Stermel
Design Direction: Steve Stave
Multi-Media Producer: David Wisner
Marketing Manager: Laura Meiskey

Printed in China

Last digit is the print number: 9   8   7   6   5   4   3   2   1

To Mom and Dad for helping me believe that becoming a doctor was possible. Heartfelt love and gratitude to my patient, supportive wife, Karee, and my considerate children, Caroline, Stephen, and Jason. Not so many more hours away from you at the computer.

Mark V. Williams

To Juliet, Tessana, Colin, and Malia Flanders, for your unwavering love and support.

Scott A. Flanders

To my two finest teachers, my wife and my father, both consummate physicians and healers.

Winthrop F. Whitcomb

To my wife, Deborah, and children, Alison and Jeffrey, for your patience, understanding, and support during this project. Hopefully, I will now have more time to spend with my family.

Steven L. Cohn

To my wife, Niki, and my children, Michael, Ryan, and Olivia.

Franklin A. Michota

To my family, past and present, with love and gratitude.

Richard Gross

To my wife, Charlotte, for all her support.

Geno J. Merli

Editors of Manual of Evidence-Based Admitting Orders and Therapeutics, 5th Edition: PocketConsult Handheld Software

Karen A. McDonaugh, M.D.
Assistant Professor of Medicine
Director, Inpatient Hospitalist Service
University of Washington Medical Center
Consultative & Hospital Medicine Program
Seattle, Washington

Eric B. Larson, M.D., M.P.H., F.A.C.P.
Executive Director
Group Health Cooperative
Center for Health Studies
Seattle, Washington

CONTRIBUTORS

Alpesh N. Amin, M.D., M.B.A.
Professor of Medicine
Executive Director, Hospitalist Program
Vice Chair for Clinical Affairs and Quality
Department of Medicine
University of California–Irvine
Irvine, California

Frank A. Anania, M.D., F.A.C.P.
Associate Professor of Medicine
Emory University School of Medicine
Director of Hepatology
Emory Clinic and Emory University Hospital
Emory Healthcare
Atlanta, Georgia

Ashish Aneja, M.D.
Associate Staff
Section of Hospital and Perioperative Medicine
The Cleveland Clinic Foundation
Cleveland, Ohio

Rendell W. Ashton, M.D.
Assistant Professor of Pulmonary and Critical
　Care Medicine
Upstate Medical University
Syracuse, New York

David J. Axelrod, M.D., J.D.
Instructor of Medicine
Jefferson Medical College
Co-Medical Director
Palliative Care Consultation Service
Associate, Jefferson Internal Medicine Associates
Thomas Jefferson University
Philadelphia, Pennsylvania

Vanitha Bala, M.D.
Instructor in Hospital Medicine
Emory Healthcare
Emory University School of Medicine
Atlanta, Georgia

John R. Bartholomew, M.D.
Head, Section of Vascular Medicine
Departments of Cardiovascular Medicine and
　Hematology/Oncology
The Cleveland Clinic Foundation
Cleveland, Ohio

Darrin Beaupre, M.D., Ph.D.
Associate Director
Medical Sciences Early Development
Amgen
Thousands Oaks, California

Rodney Bell, M.D.
Professor of Neurology
Thomas Jefferson Medical College
Vice Chairman, Department of Neurology for
　Hospital Affairs
Chief, Division of Neurocritical Care and
　Cerebrovascular Disease
Thomas Jefferson University
Philadelphia, Pennsylvania

**Glen Bergman, M.M.Sc., R.D., L.D.,
　C.N.S.D.**
Clinical Preceptor, Dietetic Internship Program
Clinical Nutritionist
Nutrition and Metabolic Support Service
Emory University Hospital
Atlanta, Georgia

Lisa Bernstein M.D.
Assistant Professor of Medicine
Director, Clinical Methods Course
Emory University School of Medicine
Atlanta, Georgia

Suzanne F. Bradley, M.D.
Associate Professor of Internal Medicine
University of Michigan Medical School
Staff Physician
Geriatric Research Education and Clinical Center
Veterans Affairs Ann Arbor Healthcare System
Ann Arbor, Michigan

William T. Branch, M.D.
Carter Smith, Sr., Professor of Medicine
Director, Division of General Internal Medicine
Emory University School of Medicine
Chief, General Internal Medicine
Grady Memorial Hospital
Atlanta, Georgia

William F. Bria II, M.D.
Adjunct Clinical Associate Professor of Medicine
University of Michigan
Ann Arbor, Michigan
Clinical Associate Professor of Medicine
University of South Florida
Chief Medical Information Officer
Shriners Hospitals for Children System
Tampa, Florida

Erica Brownfield, M.D., F.A.C.P.
Associate Professor of Medicine
Clerkship Director, Internal Medicine
Emory University School of Medicine
Staff Physician
Grady Health System
Atlanta, Georgia

Debora Bruno, M.D.
Hematologist/Medical Oncologist
Nebraska Cancer Care
Hastings, Nebraska

Gregory M. Bump, M.D.
Assistant Professor
Division of General Medicine
University of Pittsburgh School of Medicine
Pittsburgh, Pennsylvania

Jada Bussey-Jones, M.D.
Assistant Professor
Emory University School of Medicine
Director, Primary Care Center
Grady Memorial Hospital
Atlanta, Georgia

Joan Cain, M.D.
Fellow, Hematology/Oncology
Emory University School of Medicine
Atlanta, Georgia

Paul Cantey, M.D., M.P.H.
Assistant Professor of Medicine
Emory University School of Medicine
Atlanta, Georgia

Kulsum K. Casey, D.O.
Clinical Instructor of Medicine
Mayo Clinic College of Medicine
Rochester, Minnesota

Murtaza Cassoobhoy, M.D.
Hospitalist
Gwinnett Medical Center
Atlanta, Georgia

Robert M. Centor, M.D.
Professor, Division of General Internal Medicine
University of Alabama at Birmingham
Birmingham, Alabama
Associate Dean
University of Alabama at Birmingham School of
     Medicine
Huntsville Regional Medical Campus
Huntsville, Alabama

Hubert Chen, M.D., M.P.H.
Clinical Instructor
University of California–San Francisco
San Francisco, California

Carol E. Chenoweth, M.D.
Associate Professor, Clinical Track
Medical Director
Infection Control and Epidemiology
University of Michigan Hospitals and Health
     Centers
Ann Arbor, Michigan

Cuckoo Choudhary, M.D.
Assistant Professor of Medicine
Thomas Jefferson University
Philadelphia, Pennsylvania

Mina K. Chung, M.D.
Associate Professor of Medicine
Cleveland Clinic Lerner College of Medicine
Case Western Reserve University
Staff, Department of Cardiovascular Medicine
Section of Cardiac Electrophysiology and Pacing
The Cleveland Clinic Foundation
Cleveland, Ohio

Steven L. Cohn, M.D., F.A.C.P.
Clinical Professor of Medicine
State University of New York–Downstate
Chief, Division of General Internal Medicine
Director, Medical Consultation Service
Kings County Hospital
Brooklyn, New York

Eric A. Coleman, M.D., M.P.H.
Associate Professor
Division of Health Care Policy and Research
University of Colorado at Denver and Health
     Sciences Center
Denver, Colorado

Nicole M. Daignault, R.D., C.N.S.D.
Nutrition Support Dietitian
Nutrition and Metabolic Support Service
Emory University Hospital
Atlanta, Georgia

**Steven B. Deitelzweig, M.D., R.V.T.,
     C.M.D., F.A.C.P., F.S.V.M.B.**
Clinical Associate Professor of Medicine
Tulane University Medical College
Chairman, Hospital Medicine
President, Medical Staff
Ochsner Clinic Foundation
New Orleans, Louisiana

Sheetal Desai, Pharm.D., B.C.O.P.
Clinical Assistant Professor
University of Florida, College of Pharmacy
Gainesville, Florida
Clinical Pharmacy Specialist
H. Lee Moffitt Cancer and Research Institute
Tampa, Florida

Gretchen Diemer, M.D.
Instructor of Internal Medicine
Assistant Program Director
Internal Medicine
Thomas Jefferson University
Philadelphia, Pennsylvania

Lorenzo Di Francesco, M.D., F.A.C.P.
Associate Professor of Medicine
Associate Program Director
J. Willis Hurst Internal Medicine Residency
Emory University School of Medicine
Atlanta, Georgia

Vesselin Dimov, M.D.
Section of Hospital Medicine
Department of General Internal Medicine
The Cleveland Clinic Foundation
Cleveland, Ohio

Joseph L. Dorsey, M.D., M.P.H.
Clinical Professor of Medicine
Harvard Medical School
Senior Physician, Brigham and Women's Hospital
Medical Director for Inpatient Programs
Harvard Vanguard Medical Associates
Boston, Massachusetts

Maged Doss, M.D.
Assistant Professor of Medicine
Emory University School of Medicine
Hospitalist, Internal Medicine
Emory Crawford Long Hospital
Atlanta, Georgia

Daniel D. Dressler, M.D., M.Sc.
Assistant Professor of Medicine
Director of Hospital Medicine
Emory University Hospital
Emory University School of Medicine
Atlanta, Georgia

**M. Tray Dunaway, M.D., F.A.C.S., C.S.P.,
     C.H.C.O., C.H.C.C.**
Certified Healthcare Compliance Officer and
     Consultant
President & CEO, Healthcare Value, Inc.
Camden, South Carolina

James R. Eckman, M.D.
Professor of Hematology, Oncology, and Medicine
Adjunct Professor of Pediatrics
Winship Cancer Institute
Director, Georgia Comprehensive Sickle Cell
     Center
Emory University School of Medicine
Atlanta, Georgia

Norman Egger, M.D., M.S.
Assistant Professor
Mayo Clinic College of Medicine
Rochester, Minnesota

Mark D. Eisner, M.D., M.P.H.
Associate Professor of Medicine and Anesthesia
Division of Occupational and Environmental
     Medicine
Division of Pulmonary and Critical Care
     Medicine
Department of Medicine
University of California, San Francisco
San Francisco, California

Woodruff English, M.D., M.M.M.
Clinical Assistant Professor
Department of Public Health and Preventive
     Medicine
Oregon Health and Science University
Lead Hospitalist
Providence St. Vincent Medical Center
Portland, Oregon

Mark Enzler, M.D.
Clinical Assistant Professor of Medicine
Department of Internal Medicine and Hospital
     Internal Medicine
Consultant, Division of Hospital Internal Medicine
Mayo College of Medicine, Mayo Clinic
Rochester, Minnesota

Kenneth R. Epstein, M.D., M.B.A., F.A.C.P.
Clinical Instructor, University of Colorado
Denver, Colorado
Director of Medical Affairs
IPC, The Hospitalist Company
North Hollywood, California

Wassim H. Fares, M.D.
Assistant Professor of Medicine
Department of General Internal Medicine
Cleveland Clinic Lerner College of Medicine
Associate Staff
The Cleveland Clinic Foundation
Cleveland, Ohio

David R. Farley, M.D.
Professor of Surgery
Mayo Clinic College of Medicine
Program Director
General Surgery Residency Program
Mayo Clinic
Rochester, Minnesota

W. Bradley Fields, M.D., M.S.
Fellow, Pulmonary and Critical Care Medicine
University of Michigan Health System
Ann Arbor, Michigan

Rachel Fissell, M.D., M.S.
Department of Internal Medicine
Division of Nephrology
University of Michigan Medical Center
University of Michigan
Ann Arbor, Michigan

William Fissell, M.D.
Associate Staff
Nephrology and Hypertension
The Cleveland Clinic Foundation
Cleveland, Ohio

Jonathan M. Flacker, M.D.
Assistant Professor of Medicine
Division of Geriatric Medicine and Gerontology
Emory University School of Medicine
Medical Director, Emma I. Darnell Geriatrics
    Center
Grady Health System
Atlanta, Georgia

Kevin R. Flaherty, M.D., M.S.
Assistant Professor
Department of Internal Medicine
Associate Director
Fellowship in Pulmonary and Critical Care
    Medicine
University of Michigan Health System
Ann Arbor, Michigan

Scott A. Flanders, M.D.
Associate Professor of Internal Medicine
University of Michigan
Director, Hospitalist Program
Associate Director, Inpatient Programs
University of Michigan Health System
Ann Arbor, Michigan

Eric Flenaugh, M.D.
Associate Professor of Medicine
Section Chief
Division of Pulmonary and Critical Care
    Medicine
Morehouse School of Medicine
Co-Director, Medical Intensive Care Unit
Grady Memorial Hospital
Atlanta, Georgia

Leslie Flores, M.H.A.
Partner
Nelson/Flores Associates, LLC
Upland, California

Shaun Frost, M.D., F.A.C.P.
Regional Medical Director
Cogent Healthcare
Irvine, California

Ognjen Gajic, M.D., M.Sc., F.C.C.P.
Assistant Professor of Medicine
Mayo Clinic College of Medicine
Senior Associate Consultant
Division of Pulmonary and Critical Care
    Medicine
Mayo Clinic
Rochester, Minnesota

Steven E. Gay, M.D.
Assistant Professor
Assistant Dean of Admissions
Medical Director, Critical Care Support Services
Department of IM Pulmonary and Critical Care
    Medicine
University of Michigan Health System
Ann Arbor, Michigan

Inginia Genao, M.D.
Assistant Professor of Medicine
Division of General Internal Medicine
Yale University School of Medicine
Medical Director, Primary Care Center
Yale New Haven Hospital
New Haven, Connecticut

Jody Hoffer Gittell, Ph.D.
Associate Professor of Management
The Heller School for Social Policy and
    Management
Brandeis University
Waltham, Massachusetts

Jeffrey Glasheen, M.D.
Associate Professor of Medicine
Director, Hospital Medicine Program
Director, Inpatient Clinical Services
Associate Program Director
Internal Medicine Residency Training Program
Program Director, Hospitalist Training Program
Department of Medicine
University of Colorado at Denver and Health
    Sciences Center
Denver, Colorado

Beth B. Golden, C.P.C.
Director, Compliance Analysis
Emory Healthcare
Atlanta, Georgia

Norbert Goldfield, M.D.
Medical Director
3M Health Information Systems, Inc.
Attending Physician
Brightwood Riverview Health
Wallingford, Connecticut

Mark G. Graham, M.D., F.A.C.P.
Associate Professor of Medicine
Jefferson Medical College of Thomas Jefferson
    University
Director, Jefferson Hospital Ambulatory Practice
Associate Director, Internal Medicine Residency
Thomas Jefferson University Hospital
Philadelphia, Pennsylvania

Paul Grant, M.D.
Clinical Instructor
University of Michigan
Ann Arbor, Michigan

Ron Greeno, M.D., F.A.C.P.
Chief Medical Officer
Cogent Healthcare
CMO and Senior Consultant
The Cogent Group
Nashville, Tennessee

Jeffrey L. Greenwald, M.D.
Associate Professor of Medicine
Boston University School of Medicine
Director, Hospital Medicine Unit
Boston Medical Center
Boston, Massachusetts

Brian P. Griffin, M.D., F.A.C.C.
Director
Cardiovascular Disease Training Program
The Cleveland Clinic Foundation
Cleveland, Ohio

Richard Gross, M.D., F.A.C.P.
Professor of Medicine
Departments of Medicine and Interdisciplinary
    Oncology
University of South Florida College of Medicine
Chief, Division of Internal and Hospital Medicine
H. Lee Moffitt Cancer Center and Research
    Institute
Tampa, Florida

Stephanie Grossman, M.D.
Assistant Professor, Emory University
Hospitalist, Emory Crawford Long Hospital
Palliative Care Consultant
Emory University Hospital and Emory Crawford
    Long Hospital
Emory Clinic
Atlanta, Georgia

David V. Gugliotti, M.D.
Clinical Assistant Professor of Medicine
Cleveland Clinic Lerner College of Medicine
Case Western Reserve University
Associate Staff, Department of General Internal
    Medicine
Section of Hospital and Perioperative Medicine
The Cleveland Clinic Foundation
Cleveland, Ohio

Lakshmi K. Halasyamani, M.D.
Vice-Chair
Department of Internal Medicine
Saint Joseph Mercy Hospital
Ann Arbor, Michigan

Robert Hayward, M.D., M.P.H.
Associate Professor, Medicine and Dentistry
Assistant Dean, Faculty of Medicine and
    Dentistry
Director, Centre for Health Evidence
Director, Health Information Management
University of Alberta
Edmonton, Alberta, Canada

Michael Heisler, M.D., M.P.H.
Associate Professor of Medicine
Interim Director, Section of Hospital Medicine
Emory University School of Medicine
Atlanta, Georgia
Medical Director, Emory Eastside Medical Center
Snellville, Georgia

Jay H. Herman, M.D.
Professor
Departments of Medicine and Pathology,
    Anatomy and Cell Biology
Jefferson Medical College
Thomas Jefferson University
Director, Transfusion Medicine
Thomas Jefferson University Hospital
Philadelphia, Pennsylvania

Stacy M. Higgins, M.D., F.A.C.P.
Assistant Professor of Medicine
Program Director
Primary Care Residency Program
Associate Program Director, Ambulatory
    Education
Emory University School of Medicine
Atlanta, Georgia

Russell Holman, M.D.
Chief Operating Officer
National Medical Director
Cogent Healthcare
Nashville, Tennessee

Björn Hölmstrom, M.D.
Assistant Professor of Medicine
University of South Florida College of Medicine
Assistant Professor of Medicine
Internal and Hospital Medicine
H. Lee Moffitt Cancer Center and Research
    Institute
Tampa, Florida

Jeanne M. Huddleston, M.D., F.A.C.P.
Assistant Professor of Medicine
Mayo Clinic College of Medicine
Consultant, General Internal Medicine
Mayo Clinic
Rochester, Minnesota

Darrin R. Hursey, M.D.
Clinical Lecturer in Internal Medicine
Division of General Medicine
University of Michigan Medical School
Ann Arbor, Michigan

Robert C. Hyzy, M.D.
Assistant Professor of Internal Medicine
Division of Pulmonary and Critical Care
    Medicine
Medical Director, Critical Care Medicine Unit
University of Michigan
Ann Arbor, Michigan

Nurcan Ilksoy, M.D.
Assistant Professor of Medicine
Emory University School of Medicine
Hospitalist, Hospital Medicine Unit
Grady Memorial Hospital
Atlanta, Georgia

Amir K. Jaffer, M.D.
Associate Professor of Medicine
Lerner College of Medicine of Case Western
    Reserve University
Medical Director, IMPACT (Internal Medicine
    Preoperative Assessment Consultation and
    Treatment) Center
Medical Director, The Anticoagulation Clinic
The Cleveland Clinic Foundation
Cleveland, Ohio

Christopher J. Jankowski, M.D.
Assistant Professor of Anesthesiology
Mayo Clinic College of Medicine
Consultant, Mayo Clinic
Rochester, Minnesota

Henna Kalsi, M.D., R.V.T., R.P.V.I.
Staff, Mayo Clinic
Rochester, Minnesota

Kanchan Kamath, M.D.
Assistant Professor
Department of Internal Medicine
University of South Florida College of Medicine
Tampa, Florida

Tyler Kang, M.D.
Division of Hematology/Oncology
The Cleveland Clinic Foundation
Cleveland, Ohio

Daniel R. Kaul, M.D.
Assistant Professor, Division of Infectious Diseases
Department of Internal Medicine
University of Michigan Medical School
Ann Arbor, Michigan

Kris Kaulback, M.D.
Assistant Professor of Surgery
Thomas Jefferson University Hospital
Philadelphia, Pennsylvania

Powel Kazanjian, M.D.
Professor of Internal Medicine
Chief, Division of Infectious Diseases
University of Michigan Medical School
Ann Arbor, Michigan

Burke T. Kealey, M.D.
Assistant Professor of Internal Medicine
University of Minnesota Department of Internal
    Medicine
Minneapolis, Minnesota
Assistant Medical Director, Hospital Medicine
HealthPartners Medical Group
Bloomington, Minnesota

A. Scott Keller, M.D., M.S.
Instructor in Medicine, Mayo Clinic College of
    Medicine
Consultant, Mayo Clinic
Rochester, Minnesota

Arthur C. Kendig, M.D.
Clinical Associate, Section of Hospital Medicine
Department of General Internal Medicine
The Cleveland Clinic Foundation
Cleveland, Ohio

Mahsheed Khajavi, M.D.
Assistant Professor of Medicine
Emory University School of Medicine
Hospitalist
Cartersville Medical Center
Cartersville, Georgia

Anna Kho, M.D.
Assistant Professor of Medicine
Emory University School of Medicine
Atlanta, Georgia

Chong-Sang Kim, M.D.
Clinical Professor
University of California School of Medicine
Irvine, California
Neurologist
Kaiser-Permanente Medical Center
Anaheim, California

Christopher Kim, M.D., M.B.A.
Clinical Instructor
University of Michigan Medical School
Ann Arbor, Michigan

Lisa Kirkland, M.D., F.A.C.P., C.N.S.P., M.S.H.A.
Assistant Professor of Medicine
Mayo Clinic College of Medicine
Rochester, Minnesota

Jennifer Kleinbart, M.D.
Associate Professor of Medicine
Emory University School of Medicine
Hospitalist
Grady Memorial Hospital
Atlanta, Georgia

Thomas Klockgether, M.D.
Professor of Neurology
University of Bonn
Clinical Director, Department of Neurology
University Hospital Bonn
Bonn, Germany

Andrew M. Knoll, M.D., J.D., F.A.C.P., F.C.L.M.
Clinical Associate Professor of Medicine
State University of New York Upstate Medical University
Associate Attorney
Scolaro, Shulman, Cohen, Fetter & Burstein, P.C.
Syracuse, New York

Sunil Kripalani, M.D., M.Sc.
Associate Professor
Emory University School of Medicine
Assistant Director for Research
Grady Hospitalist Program
Atlanta, Georgia

Irene Krokos, M.D.
Clinical Instructor
University of Michigan Medical Center
Ann Arbor, Michigan
Hospitalist, Presbyterian Hospital
Albuquerque, New Mexico

David Lawson, M.D.
Professor of Hematology-Oncology
Chief, Section of Medical Oncology
Winship Cancer Institute
Emory University School of Medicine
Atlanta, Georgia

Solomon Liao, M.D.
Associate Professor of Medicine
University of California–Irvine
Geriatric Hospitalist
University of California at Irvine Medical Center
Orange, California

Alan Lichtin, M.D.
Associate Professor, Department of Medicine
Cleveland Clinic, Lerner College of Medicine
Case Western Reserve University
Staff Physician
Department of Hematologic Oncology and Blood Disorders
The Cleveland Clinic Foundation
Cleveland, Ohio

Steven T. Liu, M.D.
Assistant Professor of Medicine
Hospitalist, Emory University School of Medicine
CEO, Ingenious Med, Incorporated
Atlanta, Georgia

Joseph Locala, M.D.
Associate Professor, Department of Psychiatry
Case Western Reserve University
Director, Consultation Psychiatry and Emergency Services
University Hospitals of Cleveland
Cleveland, Ohio

Michael P. Lukela, M.D.
Assistant Professor, Internal Medicine, Pediatrics
Associate Director
Internal Medicine-Pediatrics Program
Director, M2 Clinical Comprehensive Assessment
University of Michigan
Ann Arbor, Michigan

S. Melissa Mahoney, M.D.
Assistant Professor of Medicine
Emory University School of Medicine
Co-Director, Palliative Care Consult Service
Emory Healthcare
Atlanta, Georgia

Brian F. Mandell, M.D., Ph.D, F.A.C.R.
Professor of Medicine
Cleveland Clinic Lerner College of Medicine
Case Western Reserve University
Vice Chairman of Medicine
Center for Vasculitis Care and Research
Rheumatic and Immunologic Disease
The Cleveland Clinic Foundation
Cleveland, Ohio

Dennis M. Manning, M.D., F.A.C.P., F.A.C.C.
Assistant Professor
Mayo Clinic College of Medicine
Director, Quality and Patient Safety,
Department of Medicine, Mayo Clinic
Rochester, Minnesota

Laura J. Martin, M.D.
Assistant Professor of Medicine
Emory University School of Medicine
Atlanta, Georgia

Greg Maynard, M.D., M.Sc.
Associate Clinical Professor of Medicine
Chief, Division of Hospital Medicine
Department of Medicine
University of California at San Diego
San Diego, California

Calvin McCall, M.D.
Associate Professor of Dermatology
Emory University School of Medicine
Chief of Service, Dermatology
Grady Health System
Atlanta, Georgia

Geno J. Merli, M.D., F.A.C.P.
Senior Vice President, Chief Medical Officer
Director, Jefferson Center for Vascular Disease
Thomas Jefferson University Hospital
Jefferson Medical College
Philadelphia, Pennsylvania

Joseph M. Messana, M.D.
Associate Professor of Internal Medicine
Clinical Service Chief
Division of Nephrology
University of Michigan Health System
Ann Arbor, Michigan

Barbara J. Messinger-Rapport, M.D., Ph.D.
Assistant Professor of Medicine
Cleveland Clinic, Lerner College of Medicine
Case Western Reserve University
Staff, Section of Geriatric Medicine
The Cleveland Clinic Foundation
Cleveland, Ohio

Jordan Messler, M.D.
Medical Director, Morton Plant Hospitalist Group
Clearwater, Florida

Franklin A. Michota, M.D.
Head, Section of Hospital Medicine
Department of General Internal Medicine
The Cleveland Clinic Foundation
Cleveland, Ohio

Joseph A. Miller, M.S.
Senior Vice President
Society of Hospital Medicine
Philadelphia, Pennsylvania
Principal, Northeast Hospitalist Consultants
Needham, Massachusetts

Lesley Miller, M.D.
Assistant Professor of Medicine
Emory University School of Medicine
Atlanta, Georgia

Bipinchandra Mistry, M.D., M.R.C.P. (Ireland)
Faculty, Internal Medicine Residency Program
Medical Director, Metrowest Medical Center
Framingham, Massachusetts

Brent W. Morgan, M.D.
Associate Professor, Emergency Medicine
Director, Medical Toxicology Fellowship
Department of Emergency Medicine
Emory University School of Medicine
Atlanta, Georgia

Douglas C. Morris, M.D.
J. Willis Hurst Professor of Medicine
Vice Chair for Clinical Affairs
Department of Medicine
Emory University School of Medicine
Director, The Emory Heart and Vascular Center
Emory Healthcare
Atlanta, Georgia

Mandakolathur Murali, M.D.
Director, Clinical Immunology Laboratory
Division of Allergy, Immunology and
    Rheumatology
Massachusetts General Hospital
Harvard Medical School
Boston, Massachusetts

Deirdre E. Mylod, Ph.D.
Vice President, Public Policy
Press Ganey Associates, Incorporated
South Bend, Indiana

Rangadham Nagarakanti, M.D.
Clinical Research Fellow
Lankenau Institute for Medical Research
Wynnewood, Pennsylvania

Bradly J. Narr, M.D.
Chair and Associate Professor
Department of Anesthesiology
Mayo College of Medicine
Rochester, Minnesota

John R. Nelson, M.D., F.A.C.P.
Medical Director, Hospitalist Practice
Overlake Hospital Medical Center
Partner, Nelson/Flores Associates, LLC
Bellevue, Washington

Saira Noor, M.D.
Hospitalist, Section of Hospital Medicine
Department of Internal Medicine
The Cleveland Clinic Foundation
Cleveland, Ohio

Armando Paez, M.D.
Assistant Professor
Tufts University School of Medicine
Staff, Infectious Disease Division
Hospital Medicine Program
Woundcare & Hyperbaric Medicine Program
Baystate Medical Center
Springfield, Massachusetts

Robert M. Palmer, M.D., M.P.H.
Professor of Medicine
Cleveland Clinic Lerner College of Medicine
Case Western Reserve University
Head, Section of Geriatric Medicine
Department of General Internal Medicine
The Cleveland Clinic Foundation
Cleveland, Ohio

Vikas I. Parekh, M.D.
Assistant Professor of Internal Medicine
University of Michigan Medical Center
Associate Director, Hospitalist Program
Associate Director
Internal Residency Program
University of Michigan Health System
Ann Arbor, Michigan

Uptal D. Patel, M.D.
Assistant Professor of Medicine and Pediatrics
Divisions of Nephrology and Pediatric
    Nephrology
Duke University School of Medicine
Staff Physician, Section of Nephrology
Durham Veterans Affairs Medical Center
Duke University Medical Center
Duke Children's Hospital and Health Center
Durham, North Carolina

Stephen G. Patterson, M.D.
Assistant Professor
University of South Florida College of Medicine
Department of Interdisciplinary Oncology
H. Lee Moffitt Cancer Center and Research
    Institute
Tampa, Florida

Michael P. Phy, D.O., M.Sc.
Assistant Professor
Associate Program Director
Department of Internal Medicine
Texas Tech University Health Sciences Center
Lubbock, Texas

James C. Pile, M.D., F.A.C.P.
Assistant Professor of Medicine
Case Western Reserve University School of
    Medicine
Acting Director, Division of Hospital Medicine
MetroHealth Medical Center
Cleveland, Ohio

Allan F. Platt, Jr., M.S., PA-C
Faculty, Physician Assistant Program
Emory University School of Medicine
Atlanta, Georgia

Leopoldo Pozuelo, M.D., F.A.C.P.
Discipline Leader Psychiatry
Cleveland Clinic Lerner College of Medicine
Head, Section of Consultation-Liaison Psychiatry
Program Director, Adult Psychiatry
The Cleveland Clinic Foundation
Cleveland, Ohio

Anitha Rajamanickam, M.D.
Clinical Assistant Professor
Associate Staff
Cleveland Clinic Lerner College of Medicine
Case Western Reserve University
Cleveland, Ohio

Allan Ramirez, M.D.
Assistant Professor of Medicine
McKelvey Lung Transplantation Center
Emory University
Atlanta, Georgia

Antonio Ramos-De la Medina, M.D.
Gastrointestinal Surgical Scholar
Mayo College of Medicine
Rochester, Minnesota
Chief of Education and Research
Veracruz Regional Hospital
Universidad Autónoma de Veracruz
Universidad Cristóbal Colon
Veracruz, Mexico

Asha Ramsakal, D.O.
Assistant Clinical Professor of Medicine
University of South Florida College of Medicine
Coordinator of Internal Medicine Resident
    Education
Hospitalist, H. Lee Moffitt Cancer Center
Tampa, Florida

James Riddell IV, M.D.
Assistant Professor
University of Michigan
Ann Arbor, Michigan

Leonardo Rodriguez, M.D., F.A.C.C.
Department of Cardiovascular Medicine
The Cleveland Clinic Foundation
Cleveland, Ohio

Richard Rohr, M.D., M.M.M.
Director, Hospitalist Service
Milford Hospital
Milford, Connecticut

Marc D. Rosenberg, M.S., M.D.
Clinical Assistant Professor of Medicine
Emory University School of Medicine
Partner, Atlanta Gastroenterology Associates
Atlanta, Georgia

David J. Rosenman, M.D.
Instructor of Medicine
Mayo Clinic College of Medicine
Senior Associate Consultant
Department of Internal Medicine
Mayo Clinic
Rochester, Minnesota

Robert Rosenwasser, M.D., F.A.C.S.
Professor and Chairman, Department of
   Neurological Surgery
Professor of Radiology
Cerebrovascular Surgery and Interventional
   Neuroradiology
Thomas Jefferson University
Jefferson Medical College
Jefferson Hospital for Neuroscience
Philadelphia, Pennsylvania

Sanjay Saint, M.D., M.P.H.
Professor of Medicine
University of Michigan Medical School
Research Investigator
Director, VA/UM Patient Safety Enhancement
   Program
Senior Associate Chief, Division of General
   Medicine
Ann Arbor VA Medical Center
Ann Arbor, Michigan

Jeffrey Samet, M.D., M.A., M.P.H.
Professor of Medicine and Social and Behavioral
   Sciences
Boston University Schools of Medicine and Public
   Health
Chief, General Internal Medicine
Boston Medical Center
Boston, Massachusetts

S. Sandy Sanbar, M.D., Ph.D., J.D., F.C.L.M.
Past President, American College of Legal
   Medicine
Medical Consultant
Department of Disability Services, Social Security
   Administration
Cardiologist, Royal Oaks Cardiovascular Clinic
Clinical Sub-Investigator
The Oklahoma Hypertension and Cardiovascular
   Center
Oklahoma City, Oklahoma

Hasan F. Shabbir, M.D.
Assistant Professor of Medicine
Emory University School of Medicine
Hospitalist
Emory Johns Creek Hospital
Atlanta, Georgia

Pratima Sharma, M.D.
GI Fellow, Division of Gastroenterology
Department of Medicine
University of Michigan Health System
Ann Arbor, Michigan

Bradley A. Sharpe, M.D.
Assistant Clinical Professor
Assistant Chief of the Medical Service
Moffit-Long Hospital
University of California–San Francisco School of
   Medicine
San Francisco, California

Eric M. Siegal, M.D.
Regional Medical Director
Cogent Healthcare
Madison, Wisconsin

Jamie Siegel, M.D.
Clinical Associate Professor of Medicine
Cardeza Foundation for Hematologic Research
   and Division of Hematology
Director, Hemophilia and Thrombosis Center
Medical Director, Cardeza Foundation
Special Hemostasis Laboratory
Thomas Jefferson University
Philadelphia, Pennsylvania

Vaishali Singh, M.D., M.P.H., M.B.A.
Clinical Assistant Professor of Medicine
Cleveland Clinic Lerner College of Medicine
Case Western Reserve University
Hospitalist, Department of General Internal
   Medicine
The Cleveland Clinic Foundation
Cleveland, Ohio

Thomas H. Sisson, M.D.
Assistant Professor
University of Michigan Medical School
Ann Arbor, Michigan

Gerald W. Smetana, M.D.
Associate Professor of Medicine
Division of General Medicine and Primary Care
Beth Israel Deaconess Medical Center
Harvard Medical School
Boston, Massachusetts

G. Randy Smith, Jr., M.D.
Instructor, Emory Hospital Medicine Unit
Department of Medicine
Emory University School of Medicine
Atlanta, Georgia

Nathan O. Spell, M.D., F.A.C.P.
Assistant Professor of Medicine
Emory University School of Medicine
Chief Quality Officer, Emory University Hospital
Atlanta, Georgia

Gerald Staton, M.D.
Professor of Medicine
Emory University School of Medicine
Medical Director
Wesley Woods Long Term Acute Care Hospital
Atlanta, Georgia

Brian D. Stein, M.D.
Fellow
Section of Pulmonary and Critical Care Medicine
University of Chicago Hospital
Chicago, Illinois

Jason Stein, M.D.
Assistant Professor of Medicine
Emory University School of Medicine
Hospitalist
Emory University Hospital
Atlanta, Georgia

James Steinberg, M.D.
Professor of Medicine
Emory University School of Medicine
Chief Medical Officer
Emory Crawford Long Hospital
Atlanta, Georgia

James Stone, M.D.
Assistant Professor of Medicine
Emory University School of Medicine
Hospitalist
Emory Johns Creek Hospital
Atlanta, Georgia

Sheri Chernetsky Tejedor, M.D.
Assistant Professor, Department of Medicine
Emory University School of Medicine
Hospitalist
Emory University Hospital
Atlanta, Georgia

Nomi L. Traub, M.D.
Assistant Professor of Medicine
Emory University School of Medicine
Atlanta, Georgia

Amy K. Trobaugh, Pharm.D.
Clinical Pharmacist
Emory Crawford Long Hospital
Atlanta, Georgia

**Guillermo E. Umpierrez, M.D., F.A.C.P.,
   F.A.C.E.**
Associate Professor of Medicine
Associate Director, General Clinical Research
   Center
Emory University School of Medicine
Director, Diabetes and Endocrinology Section
Grady Health System
Atlanta, Georgia

Alexandra Villa-Forte, M.D., M.P.H.
Head, Vasculitis Clinic
Universidade do Estado do Rio de Janeiro
Rio de Janeiro, Brazil

Michael D. Wang, M.D.
Assistant Clinical Professor of Medicine
University of California at Irvine School of
   Medicine
Attending Physician
University of California–Irvine Medical Center
Irvine, California

Clyde Watkins, Jr., M.D.
Assistant Professor of Medicine
Emory University School of Medicine
Atlanta, Georgia

Saul N. Weingart, M.D., Ph.D.
Associate Professor
Harvard Medical School
Vice President for Patient Safety
Director, Center for Patient Safety
Dana-Farber Cancer Institute
Boston, Massachusetts

Scott Weingarten, M.D., M.P.H.
Clinical Professor of Medicine
David Geffen School of Medicine
University of California at Los Angeles
Chief Executive Officer, Zynx Health,
   Incorporated
Director of Health Services Research
Cedars-Sinai Health System
Los Angeles, California

Martin C. Were, M.D.
NLM Medical Informatics Fellow
Indiana University School of Medicine
Regenstrief Institute, Inc.
Indianapolis, Indiana

David H. Wesorick, M.D.
Clinical Assistant Professor
University of Michigan
Ann Arbor, Michigan

Ursula Whalen, M.D.
Clinical Instructor
Emory University School of Medicine
Atlanta, Georgia

Christopher M. Whinney, M.D.
Director, Hospital Medicine Fellowship
Section of Hospital Medicine
Department of General Internal Medicine
The Cleveland Clinic Foundation
Cleveland, Ohio

Winthrop F. Whitcomb, M.D.
Assistant Professor of Medicine
University of Massachusetts Medical School
Worcester, Massachusetts
Director, Clinical Performance Improvement
Mercy Medical Center
Springfield, Massachusetts

Kevin Whitford, M.D.
Instructor
Mayo Clinic Medical School
Rochester, Minnesota

Mark V. Williams, M.D., F.A.C.P.
Professor of Medicine
Chief, Division of Hospital Medicine
Northwestern University Feinberg School of
   Medicine
Chicago, Illinois

Neil Winawer, M.D.
Associate Professor of Medicine
Director, Hospital Medicine Unit
Grady Memorial Hospital
Emory University School of Medicine
Atlanta, Georgia

Thomas R. Ziegler, M.D.
Associate Professor of Medicine
Division of Endocrinology, Metabolism and Lipids
Emory University School of Medicine
Associate Program Director
Emory Center for Clinical and Molecular
   Nutrition
Co-Director, Nutrition and Metabolic Support
   Service
Emory University Hospital
Atlanta, Georgia

FOREWORD

By now hospital medicine is no longer an interesting sideline in medical practice but an established part of health care. The Society of Hospital Medicine (SHM), as the professional medical society for hospitalists, has been involved in defining hospital medicine. There is enormous promise for what this new specialty can do as part of the evolution of health care.

At the forefront of the change is a reordering of medical practice to a system that is patient centered and emphasizes measurable quality delivered by true teams. The themes of *Comprehensive Hospital Medicine* further define the elements that will be crucial to this transition.

Hospitalists have been portrayed by some as simply replacing internists, family practitioners, and pediatricians in the inpatient setting. While this is true on the face of it, hospitalists bring much more to the table. Certainly, hospitalists need to be experts in the common medical conditions that acutely ill patients bring to the hospital. These illnesses (e.g., heart failure, pneumonia, stroke, deep vein thrombosis) are delineated in the table of contents of this book, and the thorough chapters in this reference provide content to the SHM's Core Competences for Hospital Medicine.[1]

Because hospitalists devote most if not all of their professional focus to inpatient care, they will certainly be called upon to see greater numbers of all of these clinical conditions. Practice does make perfect, but more to the point, hospitalists can and must be experts in the nuances of acute care.

In my medical career as a busy internist in the "old days" it was enough to make the right diagnosis and order the correct therapy. Today's hospitalists must be aware of disease-specific performance standards and must even participate locally in implementation strategies to define what will be measured. The third part of *Comprehensive Hospital Medicine*, System Issues, covers essential nonclinical aspects of the hospitalist's role and provides tools for their measurement. In addition to helping measure the effectiveness of current hospital care, hospitalists are critical team members who will work with nurses, pharmacists, case managers, and other physicians, as well as the hospital administration, to develop changes in health care work flow to improve performance.

Hospitalists will also need to be prepared to look at how the hospital functions. When is the antibiotic actually received by the patient? How can we improve the way patients move through the emergency department (ED) to allow the ED physicians to do their job more efficiently? How can we work with the intensivists and the ICU staff to transition patients out of crowded ICUs when there is so much demand to create available ICU capacity? Providing comprehensive information and guidance, *Comprehensive Hospital Medicine* can be a resource for hospitalists wanting to know how best to manage patient flow.

Because hospitals are concerned with both effectiveness and efficiency, hospitalists need to maximize the skills of the entire inpatient team. Working with pharmacists, hospitalists need to be well versed in pharmacoeconomics, using not necessarily the least expensive therapeutic agent, but the one that has the best chance of getting the patient better quicker and keeping them out of the hospital. Working with the nurses and the case managers, hospitalists need to fashion the ideal hospitalization for each inpatient they see. Where do diagnosis and therapy intersect with patient education and the important transition from inpatient to outpatient, especially in today's health care world where patients are often discharged not fully cured, but well enough to leave the hospital and the expense of inpatient care?

Hospitalists are also bringing their new and improved vision of health care to many other parts of the hospital. Surgeons and medical subspecialists now routinely rely on hospitalists to comanage their patients, freeing them up to concentrate on their specialty expertise. Hospitalists need to be experts in perioperative care and palliative and end-of-life care as well as certain aspects of critical care.

We have moved from the lone-ranger physician, operating individually to cure his or her patients, to health care delivered by teams, as well described in *Comprehensive Hospital Medicine*'s chapter on teamwork. Because of this, hospitalists need information and training to manage groups of hospitalists and provide leadership for other health professionals. Unfortunately, most of these skills are not taught in medical schools or residency programs. Yet they are essential if hospital medicine is to realize the promise of this new specialty.

This textbook takes a giant step toward bringing together the current body of knowledge to help hospitalists succeed in this challenging environment. It complements web-based tools developed by SHM for education and to improve quality as well as SHM courses on practice management and leadership to train the next generation of physician leaders. This combination of a comprehensive reference textbook written by leaders in hospital medicine and interactive resources developed by SHM can allow us to close the knowledge gap.

We are entering a new day in health care where there are increased expectations for better quality outcomes, delivered in an efficient hospital setting. We want more for our health care dollar. No physician specialty has ever been asked both to improve measurable quality *and* save the system money while they do it.

Soon there will be hospitalists at most if not all hospitals. They will be called upon to play a significant role in improving the health of their patients and leading their institutions into the future. Hospitalists bring the enthusiasm and energy to take this on. Hospitalists need to rely on textbooks like this one for comprehensive information designed to help them succeed. SHM will do our part to provide additional resources specific to hospitalists.

Together we will meet the challenge and take health care to a new level.

Laurence D. Wellikson, M.D., F.A.C.P.
Chief Executive Officer
Society of Hospital Medicine

[1] Core Competencies for Hospital Medicine. *Journal of Hospital Medicine 2006;S1.*

PREFACE

More than 20,000 physicians now practice as hospitalists across the United States. The specialty of hospital medicine is also spreading through Europe, Canada, Australia, New Zealand, and South America. Hospitalists are caring for patients 24 hours a day, every day of the year. While delivering individualized hospital care with increasingly sophisticated diagnostic and treatment regimens, hospitalists are also partnering with other members of the hospital team—nurses, pharmacists, dieticians, physical and occupational therapists, administrators, non-hospitalist physicians, and nurse-practitioners and physicians' assistants—to improve the system of care delivery. This reference, *Comprehensive Hospital Medicine*, was developed for both hospitalists and members of the inpatient care team. Recognizing that about one third of all U.S. health care expenditures go to the care of hospitalized patients, we need evidence-based recommendations and guidance on optimizing hospital care delivery.

Comprehensive Hospital Medicine represents a major step in the journey to provide hospital-based practitioners with an inclusive, practical reference that covers all the diverse aspects of hospital medicine. The desire for a *comprehensive* resource for the field of hospital medicine drove the contributors to generate what we hope is a useful, frequently utilized tool.

Comprehensive Hospital Medicine is separated into three major parts. The first part (General Hospital Medicine Care) addresses common clinical issues that hospitalists encounter in the care of hospitalized patients, while the second (Consultative Hospital Medicine) focuses on the increasingly important role of hospitalists in perioperative care and providing consultative services. This reference text finishes with an entire part (System Issues) of 20 chapters devoted to explaining how best to organize and operate hospitalist programs, conduct hospital performance improvement projects, and address legal and ethical concerns.

We begin the approach to general hospital medicine care with chapters on applying evidence-based principles, communication and cultural competence, nutritional assessment and support, optimizing care of the frail elderly (typically our most frequent patients), and hospital discharge. Following a section devoted to preventive care in the hospital, subsequent chapters cover medical conditions and situations hospitalists commonly encounter, ranging from cardiovascular disorders to infectious, oncologic, and critical-care conditions. Chapters employ liberal use of tables, diagrams, algorithms, and pictures to distill information into readily accessible formats. We standardized chapters on common medical conditions so you can access the information when you need it. A *Background* section includes basics of epidemiology and pathophysiology when appropriate, but the primary focus is on *Assessment* of patients' clinical presentation and *Management*. Chapters in this part typically finish with discharge and follow-up plans with primary care providers. This structure will assist clinicians in quickly finding relevant information for diagnosis and treatment.

The second major part, Consultative Hospital Medicine, covers both preoperative evaluation and care of postoperative complications. The part is complemented with chapters on management of the medical complications of pregnancy and medical consultation for patients with psychiatric disorders necessitating hospitalization. The third and final part, System Issues, emphasizes the importance of attending to nonclinical issues to optimize the operations of a hospitalist program and the system of hospital care delivery. Topics covered include scheduling, compensation, coding and billing, leadership, managing patient transitions of care, staff performance improvement, establishing a teamwork model with hospital staff, patient safety, and quality improvement.

All of the authors and editors sought to make *Comprehensive Hospital Medicine* useful to clinicians caring for hospitalized patients. In undertaking such a complex endeavor, we recognize that improvements in subsequent editions will be made. The patient-safety movement sweeping the medical world accepts that humans are not infallible, and though we tried our best to ensure the accuracy of the content of this reference, we certainly accept this axiom. Additionally, new scientific advances in diagnosis and treatment are reported every day. So we encourage and appreciate your feedback on how we may improve *Comprehensive Hospital Medicine*. The entire content of the book will also be on the web (hospitalisttext.com), and all the footnoted references are located there. We placed only suggested readings in the textbook version. The web-based version of *Comprehensive Hospital Medicine* will be updated regularly, so we can respond quickly to your feedback and new advances in hospital care.

We hope this reference will serve as an authoritative resource for hospitalists and members of the hospital team seeking to improve the overall delivery of hospital care. It was developed for you, and we look forward to continuing to enhance it so you can optimize care for your patients needing hospital care.

ACKNOWLEDGMENTS

The editors are forever grateful to everyone who assisted us in completing this monumental project. In particular, it never would have been finished without the supportive, steady encouragement of our publisher, Rolla Couchman. We are indebted to your persistence, tolerance, and help rounding up the authors' contributions and editors' input. We don't know how you maintain your cheery outlook, but we certainly appreciate your unrelenting optimism. We also wish to thank Thom Moore for stimulating us to undertake this task so many years ago. Marla Sussman was phenomenal in her editing and formatting skills. Bruce Siebert and Mary Stermel superbly polished the final product. This was a team effort and every editor contributed in his or her unique way. We especially appreciate the remarkable contributions by the authors; with no previous editions as a measure, they entrusted us to create a valuable reference for hospital medicine.

CONTENTS

Contributors   v

Foreword   xiii

Preface   xv

Acknowledgments   xvii

PART ONE   **GENERAL HOSPITAL MEDICINE CARE**

Section 1   *General Approach to a Hospitalized Patient*   *1*

1   Evidence-Based Clinical Practice • *Robert Hayward*   3

2   A Patient-Centered Approach • *Mark V. Williams*   7

3   Cultural Competence in Hospital Settings: Communication and Culture   15
Jada Bussey-Jones, Inginia Genao, William T. Branch

4   Nutritional Assessment and Support   21
G. Randy Smith, Jr., Nicole M. Daignault, Glen Bergman, Thomas R. Ziegler

5   Approach to the Geriatric Patient • *Robert M. Palmer*   29

6   Functional Assessment of the Elderly Hospitalized Patient   37
Barbara J. Messinger-Rapport

7   Skin Integrity and Pressure Ulcers: Assessment and Management   43
Jonathan M. Flacker

8   Constipation • *Sheri Chernetsky Tejedor*   53

9   Symptom Management: Nausea • *Sheri Chernetsky Tejedor*   61

10   Diarrhea • *Sheri Chernetsky Tejedor*   69

11   Hospital Discharge • *Sunil Kripalani, Amy K. Trobaugh, Eric A. Coleman*   77

Section 2   *Preventive Services in the Hospitalized Patient*   *83*

12   Vaccination • *Vaishali Singh*   85

13   Smoking Cessation in Hospitalized Patients • *Ursula Whalen, Sunil Kripalani*   93

14   Prophylaxis for Venous Thromboembolism (VTE) in the Hospitalized
Medical Patient • *Greg Maynard, Jason Stein*   99

15   Osteoporosis • *Laura J. Martin*   105

16   Substance Abuse and Dependence in the Hospitalized Patient   111
Jeffrey L. Greenwald, Jeffrey Samet

17   Preventing Nosocomial Infections • *Armando Paez, James C. Pile*   119

Section 3   *Cardiovascular*   *125*

18   Chest Pain • *Ashish Aneja, Vesselin Dimov, Paul Grant*   127

19   Acute Coronary Syndromes: Acute MI • *Jennifer Kleinbart, Douglas C. Morris*   135

20   Acute Coronary Syndromes: Unstable Angina and Non-ST Segment
Elevation Acute Myocardial Infarction • *Jennifer Kleinbart*   149

21   Heart Failure • *Wassim H. Fares, Franklin A. Michota*   159

22   Bradyarrhythmias • *Arthur C. Kendig, Mina K. Chung*   167

23   Tachyarrhythmias • *Arthur C. Kendig, Mina K. Chung*   173

24   Cardiac Arrest • *David V. Gugliotti*   189

25   Syncope • *Anitha Rajamanickam, Saira Noor, Franklin A. Michota*   197

26   Deep Vein Thrombosis • *Amir K. Jaffer*   207

27   Pulmonary Embolism • *Steven B. Deitelzweig*   217

28   Acute Aortic Dissection • *Eric M. Siegal*   227

29   Valvular Heart Disease • *Leonardo Rodriguez, Brian P. Griffin*   235

30   Acute Pericarditis • *Lorenzo Di Francesco*   247

31   Peripheral Arterial Disease (PAD) • *Henna Kalsi, John R. Bartholomew*   255

32   Hypertensive Crises • *Erica Brownfield*   263

Section 4   *Infectious Diseases*   *269*

33   Community-Acquired Pneumonia (CAP) • *Bradley A. Sharpe, Scott A. Flanders*   271

34   Nosocomial Pneumonia • *Scott A. Flanders*   279

35   Urinary Tract Infections • *Carol E. Chenoweth, Sanjay Saint*   285

36   Skin and Soft Tissue Infections • *Lakshmi K. Halasyamani*   291

37   Acute Bacterial Meningitis • *Christopher Kim, James C. Pile*   299

38   Infective Endocarditis • *Suzanne F. Bradley*   307

39   Vascular Catheter-Related Infections • *Carol E. Chenoweth, Sanjay Saint*   317

40   Septic Arthritis • *Vikas I. Parekh, James Riddell IV*   323

41   HIV and AIDS • *Daniel R. Kaul, Powel Kazanjian*   331

42   Bioterrorism • *James C. Pile*   337

43   Fever in the Hospitalized Patient • *Daniel R. Kaul*   343

Section 5   *Pulmonary*   *349*

44   Chronic Obstructive Pulmonary Disease   351
Daniel D. Dressler, Alpesh N. Amin, Gerald Staton

45   Asthma • *Michael P. Lukela, William F. Bria II*   361

46   Pleural Disease: Pleural Effusion and Pneumothorax   369
Irene Krokos, Steven E. Gay

47   Interstitial Lung Disease • *W. Bradley Fields, Kevin R. Flaherty*   375

48   Pulmonary Hypertension • *Jordan Messler, Allan Ramirez*   383

Section 6   *Nephrology*   *389*

49   Acute Renal Failure • *Gregory M. Bump, Rachel Fissell, William Fissell*   391

50   Chronic Renal Failure and Dialysis • *Uptal D. Patel, Joseph M. Messana*   399

51 Hyponatremia and Hypernatremia • *David H. Wesorick, Robert M. Centor*   407

52 Other Electrolyte Disorders • *David H. Wesorick*   419

53 Acid-Base Disorders • *David H. Wesorick, Robert M. Centor*   429

Section 7   *Gastroenterology*   *439*

54 Upper Gastrointestinal Bleeding • *Erica Brownfield, Marc D. Rosenberg*   441

55 Acute Hepatitis • *Nomi L. Traub*   445

56 Cirrhosis and Its Complications   451
Vanitha Bala, Pratima Sharma, Frank A. Anania

57 Spontaneous Bacterial Peritonitis • *Rangadham Nagarakanti*   459

58 Acute Abdominal Emergencies • *Mark G. Graham, Kris Kaulback*   463

59 Inflammatory Bowel Disease • *Cuckoo Choudhary*   471

60 Gastroenteritis • *Gretchen Diemer*   477

61 Diarrhea and *Clostridium difficile* Colitis • *Jeffrey Glasheen*   485

Section 8   *Endocrinology*   *493*

62a Diabetic Ketoacidosis • *Paul Cantey, Guillermo E. Umpierrez*   495

62b Managing Diabetes Mellitus and Hyperglycemia in Hospitalized Patients   503
Paul Cantey, Guillermo E. Umpierrez

63 Thyroid Disorders • *Martin C. Were*   509

64 Adrenal Insufficiency in Hospitalized Patients • *Mahsheed Khajavi*   517

65 Central Diabetes Insipdus Following Craniotomy • *Kanchan Kamath*   523

Section 9   *Oncology*   *527*

66 Acute Complications of Therapeutic Agents Used in the Management
of Cancer • *Björn Holmström, Sheetal Desai*   529

67 Anticoagulation in Cancer Patients • *Kanchan Kamath*   541

68 Cancer Emergencies: Fever and Neutropenia • *Joan Cain, David Lawson*   545

69 Cancer Emergencies: Hypercalcemia • *Joan Cain, David Lawson*   549

70 Cancer Emergencies: Hyperviscosity Syndromes   553
Asha Ramsakal, Darrin Beaupre

71 Cancer Emergency: Elevated Intracranial Pressure   555
Asha Ramsakal, Stephen G. Patterson

72 Cancer Emergencies: Spinal Cord Compression   557
Asha Ramsakal, Stephen G. Patterson

73 Cancer Emergencies: Tumor Lysis Syndrome   559
Asha Ramsakal, Stephen G. Patterson

74 Cancer Emergencies: Paraneoplastic Neurologic Syndromes   563
Kanchan Kamath

Section 10   *Hematology*   *567*

75 Transfusion Medicine • *Debora Bruno, Jay H. Herman*   569

76 Anemia • *Tyler Kang, Alan Lichtin*   577

77 Sickle Cell Crises • *James R. Eckman, Allan F. Platt, Jr.*   **583**

78 Hemorrhagic and Thrombotic Disorders • *Jamie Siegel*   591

Section 11   Rheumatology, Immunology, and Dermatology   601

79   Acute Arthritis in the Hospitalized Patient • *Brian F. Mandell*   603

80   Systemic Vasculitis • *Alexandra Villa-Forte, Brian F. Mandell*   609

81   Allergic Reactions and Angioedema • *Neil Winawer, Mandakolathur Murali*   615

82   Dermatology in Hospitalized Patients   621
         Calvin McCall, Murtaza Cassoobhoy, Lesley Miller

Section 12   Critical Care   639

83   Sepsis and Shock • *W. Bradley Fields, Robert C. Hyzy*   641

84   Acute Respiratory Failure • *Hubert Chen, Mark D. Eisner*   649

85   Sedation and Pain Management in the Critically Ill • *Kenneth R. Epstein*   655

86   Noninvasive Ventilation • *Darrin R. Hursey, Thomas H. Sisson*   663

87   Basic Mechanical Ventilation • *Eric Flenaugh, Michael Heisler*   669

88   Poisoning and Drug Overdose • *Brian D. Stein, Brent W. Morgan*   677

89   Alcohol Withdrawal Syndromes   687
         Hasan F. Shabbir, Nurcan Ilksoy, Jeffrey L. Greenwald

Section 13   Neurology   695

90   Ischemic Stroke • *Geno J. Merli, Rodney Bell*   697

91   Intracerebral Hemorrhage • *Geno J. Merli, Robert Rosenwasser, Mark V. Williams*   705

92   Coma • *Chong-Sang Kim, Alpesh N. Amin*   711

93   Altered Mental Status: Delirium • *Michael D. Wang, Solomon Liao, Alpesh N. Amin* 719

94   Pain Management of the Hospitalized Patient • *David J. Axelrod*   725

95   Palliative Care in the Hospital • *Stephanie Grossman, S. Melissa Mahoney*   733

PART TWO   CONSULTATIVE HOSPITAL MEDICINE

Section 14   Consultative Hospital Medicine   739

96   The Hospitalist as Consultant • *David J. Rosenman, Geno J. Merli*   741

97   Anesthesia Effects and Complications • *A. Scott Keller, Christopher J. Jankowski* 745

Section 15   Preoperative Assessments and Preparation   753

98   Preoperative Evaluation and Testing • *Mark Enzler, Bradly J. Narr*   755

99   Perioperative Medication Management • *Nathan O. Spell, Steven L. Cohn*   761

100 Perioperative Anticoagulation: Prophylaxis for Venous Thromboembolism
         (VTE) • *Jason Stein, Michael P. Phy, Amir K. Jaffer*   765

101 Management of Long-term Warfarin for Surgery   771
         Jason Stein, Michael P. Phy, Amir K. Jaffer

102 Cardiovascular Preoperative Risk Assessment and Evaluation   775
         Steven L. Cohn, Dennis M. Manning

103 Pulmonary Preoperative Risk Assessment and Evaluation   783
         Rendell W. Ashton, Ognjen Gajic, Gerald W. Smetana

104 Perioperative Management of Diabetic Patients   789
         Maged Doss, Guillermo E. Umpierrez

105 Nutrition in the Perioperative Period • *Lisa Kirkland*   795

Section 16   Postoperative Evaluation and Care   803

106   Routine Postoperative Assessment and Management   805
       Norman Egger, Kevin Whitford

107   Perioperative Pain Management • Kevin Whitford, Norman Egger   809

108   General Wound Care, Postoperative Evaluation and Care   811
       Antonio Ramos-De la Medina, David R. Farley

109   Postoperative Abnormal Signs and Symptoms   817
       Kulsum K. Casey, Jeanne M. Huddleston

110   Postoperative Cardiac Complications   821
       Michael P. Phy, Jeanne M. Huddleston

111   Non-cardiac Postoperative Complications   827
       Kulsum K. Casey, Jeanne M. Huddleston

112   Surgical Site Infection Prophylaxis   833
       James Stone, Jason Stein, James Steinberg

Section 17   Medical Complications of Pregnancy   837

113   Medical Complications of Pregnancy   839
       Lisa Bernstein, Stacy M. Higgins, Anna Kho, Guillermo E. Umpierrez, Clyde Watkins, Jr.

Section 18   Consultation for the Psychiatric Patient   849

114   Evaluation and Management of Medical Patients with Psychiatric Disorders   851
       Christopher M. Whinney, Leopoldo Pozuelo, Joseph Locala

115   Preoperative Psychiatric Evaluation and Perioperative Management of
       Patients with Psychiatric Disorders   863
       Leopoldo Pozuelo, Christopher M. Whinney, Joseph Locala

PART THREE   SYSTEM ISSUES

Section 19   Hospitalist Program Operations   871

116   Developing the Financial Plan and Establishing Workforce Needs for a
       Hospital Medicine Program   873
       Leslie Flores, Winthrop F. Whitcomb, John R. Nelson

117   Structuring a Hospital Medicine Program: An Overview of Contracting
       Options, Operating Procedures, and Recruitment Strategies   881
       Leslie Flores, John R. Nelson

118   Scheduling and Staff Deployment for Hospital Medicine Programs   887
       Bipinchandra Mistry, Winthrop F. Whitcomb

119   Communication in Hospitalist Systems   893
       Winthrop F. Whitcomb, Russell Holman, John R. Nelson

120   Compensation Principles and Practices   899
       Russell Holman, Winthrop F. Whitcomb, John R. Nelson

121   Documentation, Coding, Billing, and Compliance in Hospital Medicine   905
       M. Tray Dunaway, Beth B. Golden, Steven T. Liu

122   Measuring Value of a Hospital Medicine Program • Ron Greeno   911

Section 20   Hospital Performance Improvement   917

123   Managing Physician Performance in Hospital Medicine   919
       Russell Holman

124   Leadership in Hospital Medicine • Russell Holman   927

125 Quality Improvement in the Hospital: Theory, Tools, and Trends 933
Norbert Goldfield

126 Quality Improvement in the Hospital • *Jason Stein, Greg Maynard* 939

127 An Overview of Patient Safety for the Hospitalist 947
Lakshmi K. Halasyamani, Saul N. Weingart

128 Establishing a Teamwork Model of Care for Inpatient Medicine 955
Joseph A. Miller, Joseph L. Dorsey, Jody Hoffer Gittell

129 Patient Flow and Hospital Throughput • *Burke T. Kealey* 961

130 Strategies for Standardizing Care and Applying Evidence to Practice 967
Scott Weingarten

131 Assessing Patient Satisfaction in the Hospital Setting 971
Woodruff English, Deirdre E. Mylod

Section 21 *Legal and Ethical Issues* 977

132 Ethics in Hospital Medicine • *Shaun Frost* 979

133 Medical Malpractice • *S. Sandy Sanbar* 989

134 Legal Issues in Hospitalist-Hospital Relationships • *Andrew M. Knoll* 993

135 Developing and Maintaining the Physician-Hospital Relationship 999
Richard Rohr

Appendix One: NIH Stroke Scale 1003

Appendix Two: Eligibility Criteria Indications for tPA Administration/ 1005
Treatment

Appendix Three: RASS and CAM-ICU Worksheet 1007

Index 1009

Section

One

General Approach to a Hospitalized Patient

1   Evidence-Based Clinical Practice
    Robert Hayward

2   A Patient-Centered Approach
    Mark V. Williams

3   Cultural Competence in Hospital Settings:
    Communication and Culture
    Jada Bussey-Jones, Inginia Genao, William T. Branch

4   Nutritional Assessment and Support
    G. Randy Smith, Jr., Nicole M. Daignault, Glen Bergman,
    Thomas R. Ziegler

5   Approach to the Geriatric Patient
    Robert M. Palmer

6   Functional Assessment of the Elderly Hospitalized Patient
    Barbara J. Messinger-Rapport

7   Skin Integrity and Pressure Ulcers: Assessment
    and Management
    Jonathan M. Flacker

8   Constipation
    Sheri Chernetsky Tejedor

9   Symptom Management: Nausea
    Sheri Chernetsky Tejedor

10 Diarrhea
    Sheri Chernetsky Tejedor

11 Hospital Discharge
    Sunil Kripalani, Amy K. Trobaugh, Eric A. Coleman

CHAPTER ONE

Evidence-Based Clinical Practice

Robert Hayward, MD, MPH

"It's an incredibly simple idea and one that is blindingly obvious to most lay people . . . assess the existing evidence and concentrate on the reliable stuff." Iain Chalmers, 1996

The emerging health policy agenda is preoccupied with evidence. From federal agencies to integrated health networks, and from tertiary care facilities to primary health centres, every participant in the health care endeavor is aware of evidence: the need for it, the lack of it, and the various definitions of it. How is it that physician practices vary so much, that solid information takes so long to find its way to practice, and that expensive clinical trials often do not connect with common concerns? That the best evidence should always inform health choices is blindingly obvious to most lay people.

A health informatics agenda is emerging that is preoccupied with technology. After years of underinvestment in information systems, large-scale health infostructure initiatives consume substantive portions of health care budgets in Western economies. The governments of the United States, Britain, and Canada all commit to widespread deployment of electronic health records. These, together with "evidence-based information systems," should ensure that decision-makers at all levels have easy access to relevant and timely information. That the best evidence will be beamed to the bedside is promised by most health informaticians.

In reality, more bedside evidence may only worsen the informational plight of busy clinicians. They experience information hunger in the midst of plenty. Each year hundreds of thousands of new clinical trials are added to millions of existing trials in tens of thousands of journals. To keep up with relevant developments, clinicians would have to track hundreds of articles per day, 365 days per year, with the number increasing yearly. Even if all important new evidence could be tracked by clinicians, they will continue to encounter challenges for which evidence is unavailable or exists but is confusing, conflicting, or impractical. The last thing busy clinicians want is disorganized knowledge dumped at the bedside while they remain ill equipped to deal with it. That evidence and practice work together is not obvious to many physicians.

For better information to beget better health, at least three things must happen. First, health care decision-makers must be able to tell better from worse information. Second, changes in knowledge must lead to changes in health practices. Finally, improved outcomes must relate to altered practices. In short, better information begets better health through the medium of informed decision-making.

For physicians to make more informed decisions, they need to:

- **Know what to do** because best information supporting best practices is used at the point of decision-making
- **Do what is known** because they recognize problems, formulate questions, seek evidence, and apply new knowledge appropriately
- **Understand what is done** because health care choices and outcomes are tracked

Evidence-based practice (EBP) is a particular conceptualization about what it means to know what to do. It calls for a paradigm shift in medical thinking to de-emphasize personal intuition in favor of the judicious integration of best available clinical research evidence with clinical experience and patient values. The focus is on being more aware of the type and strength of any link between what we do and why we do it. Accordingly, the evidence-based practitioner greets new information with questions about:

- **Validity** (Is the information likely to be true?)
- **Importance** (If true, will the information make a difference that patients will care about?)
- **Applicability** (Can the information be used?)

These considerations are not restricted to assessing results from clinical trials; they pertain as much to consultants' recommendations as to primary research reports.

How we articulate considerations of validity, importance, and applicability depends on the type of clinical problem we address. Individual patients hope that physicians will anticipate (prevent) and detect (diagnose) health problems, identify benefits and risks (harms) associated with management options, predict outcomes (prognosis), and promote patient goals (therapy, rehabilitation, palliation, etc.). Groups of patients hope that practitioners will work to prevent, detect, and treat health problems in a way that maximizes the opportunity of all patients to avail themselves of high-quality health care (economics, health utilization, practice guidelines, etc.). Users' guides to the medical literature offer straightforward tests of validity, importance, and applicability that physicians can apply to these different domains of care (Table 1-1).

Thankfully, an increasing number of evidence-based information resources use validity guides to preappraise evidence and

Table 1-1 Examples of Guides for Selecting Articles Most Likely to Provide Valid Results

Therapy	Were patients randomized? Was follow-up complete?
Diagnosis	Was the patient sample representative of those with the disorder? Was the diagnosis verified using credible criteria that were independent of the clinical manifestations under study?
Harm	Did the investigators demonstrate similarity in all known determinants of outcome or adjust for differences in the analysis? Was follow-up sufficiently complete?
Prognosis	Was there a representative and well-defined sample of patients at a similar point in the course of disease? Was follow-up sufficiently complete?
Economic	Did the investigators consider all relevant patient groups, management options, and possible outcomes? Did the investigators consider the timing of costs and consequences?
Guidelines	Is there a systematic review of evidence linking options to outcomes for each relevant question? Is there an appropriate specification of values or preferences associated with outcomes?

summarize it in ways that clinicians can easily access and use. Indeed, all hospitalists should expect rapid access to "filtered" evidence, including research synopses, systematic reviews, clinical practice guidelines, and clinical decision support tools at the point of care. Unfortunately, widespread availability of such databases, while ensuring that clinicians can "know what to do," has exposed a more fundamental need: busy physicians have difficulty applying new knowledge to patient care.[1]

For physicians to better connect evidence with action, they need complementary skills in "doing what is known." In addition to cultivating good taste in evidence, the evidence-based practitioner must integrate best evidence into day-to-day practice. The requisite information management skills can be summarized with the 5 A's of an evidence-based information cycle: Assess, Ask, Acquire, Appraise, and Apply. Using the cycle repeatedly to tackle complex problems improves the clinician's capacity for:

- **Assessing** an initially disorganized information mix in order to recognize and detect important patient problems
- **Asking** questions that are directly relevant to patient care and specific enough to facilitate an efficient search for evidence
- **Acquiring** the most important and convincing evidence from appropriate resources
- **Appraising** retrieved information to expose bias and variability
- **Applying** useful evidence while monitoring outcomes to see whether patient goals are achieved

By way of example, a hospitalist may be alerted to a 54-year-old woman with ovarian cancer, dyspnea, pleuritic chest pain, unilateral leg swelling, and a negative contrast computed tomography (CT) angiogram. This scenario could expose a wide range of information needs. In **assessing** the scenario, the clinician implicitly or explicitly identifies a priority issue by seeking a central concern, identifying decisions to be made, or highlighting areas of uncertainty. If the referring physician were to ask for advice about what to do "now that pulmonary embolism has been ruled out," the hospitalist may choose to focus on the performance characteristics of CT angiography.

The next step is to **ask** an appropriate clinical question. The most obvious question might be: "How well does CT angiography detect pulmonary emboli?"

However, this will net a deluge of information from health information repositories. To better connect the patient's issue with what may be known by a study of similar patients, a well-built question will contain specifics about the **population** of interest, the diagnostic **test,** a "gold standard" **comparison** test that detects a specific **condition,** and whether the **intent** is to rule in or rule out the condition: "When compared with pulmonary angiography, how well does a negative CT angiography result rule out pulmonary embolism in a patient with a high pretest probability (>75%) for pulmonary embolism?"

This question leads us to a smaller set of information repositories and more focused searching within those resources. Different question structures may be used for other clinical issues. The patient, intervention, comparison, outcome (PICO) format, for example, works well for questions about the effects of therapies.

There are many types of clinical questions and many information resources that could yield answers. Before deciding where to **acquire** evidence, the clinician considers what types of evidence could exist, what levels of evidence quality might prevail, and where such evidence is likely to be found. There are many questions for which randomized controlled trials may be inappropriate, impractical, or unethical study designs. In the case of the CT angiogram, it is reasonable to expect studies to compare the test performance with an appropriate gold standard among patients about which clinicians experienced genuine diagnostic uncertainty. Because the health condition is well studied, it is also reasonable to seek secondary literature, starting with disease guidance systems, practice guidelines, systematic reviews, or research syntheses in filtered evidence repositories. Should this prove unrewarding, then evidence-based search strategies can improve the yield of high-quality citations from unfiltered databases, such as PubMed.

Hopefully, an efficient search will produce an evidence-based synthesis closely matched to the original question. The evidence repository may have a selection and synthesis protocol that qualifies it as a source of preappraised evidence, sparing the clinician the task of **appraising** the study results. Instead, reassured that key validity guides were applied (*see* Table 1-1), the clinician can focus on the importance and applicability of the evidence for the patient in question. In our example, syntheses of multiple high-quality studies and the PIOPED II study indicate that CT angiography has a sensitivity of about 83%, with a negative likelihood ratio of 0.18.[2,3] Given an estimated pretest probability of PE as high as 75%, a likelihood ratio calculator[4] can be used to determine that the post-test likelihood of pulmonary embolus remains as high as 35%. This may well be above the "treatment threshold" for many physicians and patients, even though the CT angiogram is reported as negative.

Even when good, pertinent evidence is readily available, clinicians must apply it in a fuzzy context that implicitly or explicitly includes consideration of costs, patient preferences, comorbidity, and a broad range of health outcomes, many of which do not figure in controlled trials. When **applying** the evidence to clinical decision-making, the physician may compare available equipment and how CT angiograms are performed locally with the protocols, expertise, and equipment used in the research studies. In addition, there will be some threshold probability of pulmonary embolism that will justify treatment, and the test result is significant if, when added to the clinician's assessment, the probability of disease crosses that threshold, which may not be the same for all patients.

PRACTICE-BASED EVIDENCE

By starting with the messy phenomena of everyday practice and focusing on the information needs of busy clinicians, practice-based evidence can offer a practical approach to implementing evidence-based practice. Whereas evidence-based practice highlights research reports as the unit of information, evidence appraisal as a core skill, and knowledge transfer as a primary goal, practice-based evidence promotes prioritized questions as the unit of information, evidence application as a core skill, and knowledge use as the overarching goal.

Practice-based evidence is facilitated by evidence-based information systems. These help decision-makers:

- Know how to know by helping them voice meaningful questions; direct the questions to the right type of knowledge; and then search, select, and synthesize information
- Use what is known by highlighting the settings, patients, and practitioners to which the knowledge pertains

Information tools can make it easier for decision-makers to find and use high quality information when conferring with colleagues, consultants, and clients. To support practice-based evidence, health information systems must deliver:

- **Information convenience** because all the right information is available in the right place at the right time
- **Information discrimination** because relevant, valid, and important information is sifted from that which is misleading and distracting
- **Information integration** because meaningful relationships between clinical observations and evidence are highlighted

Information convenience is the first and most pressing need for busy practitioners. They seek uncluttered, straightforward, and consistent presentation of information through an intuitive interface that requires minimum effort and training. Convenience is also characterized by information accessibility. The point of clinical questioning and point of reflection are often separated in time and place, often outside the time-space "borders" of institutional information services. Even single-sign-on access to a drug information system, a limited collection of high-quality evidence syntheses, and key clinical records—whenever and wherever decisions are made or reviewed—would represent a leap forward in most physicians' access to information.

Given information convenience, clinicians' next priority is information discrimination. More evidence does not, by itself, enable evidence-based practice. Instead, busy clinicians need highly refined distillates of valid, important, and applicable patient-reported, clinician-observed, and research-derived evidence—all presented in a way that is tightly linked to patient priorities. The level of evidence selection and distillation can be represented with five categories of point-of-care information resources:

- **Systems** explicitly connect evidence with action and include clinical decision support tools, clinical practice guidelines, clinical algorithms and prediction rules, drug information databases, and disease guidance systems.
- **Synopses** provide brief, refereed, standardized summaries of high-quality studies and reviews, often emphasizing the clinical utility of evidence.
- **Syntheses** integrate results from multiple studies, usually in the form of systematic reviews or meta-analyses.
- **Summaries** provide background information about health conditions or interventions and include electronic textbooks (e.g., Comprehensive Hospital Medicine) and atlases.
- **Studies** include electronic journals and bibliographic databases, often providing access to the full text of original health care research.

Brevity begets value at the point of care. When high-quality evidence is no more than 5 seconds or 5 clicks from clinical information, clinicians favor brief (<3 minute) visits to Systems and Synopses.[5] These have been shown to help improve quality of care and reduce medical errors.[6] References such as this textbook, especially the online version, provide potential access at the point of care.

Integration of information systems can occur at a number of levels:

- **Combined** systems unite one or more components under a common interface. A combined drug prescription system, for example, may include menus that allow the clinician to search for dosing details or patient-advice handouts before generating prescriptions.
- **Clustered** systems use information about the provider to predetermine which information tools to present to the user. Presentation of a relevant drug database, for example, can be automated upon recognizing that a particular specialist physician is logged on.
- **Context**-sensitive systems are "aware" of the clinical context. The decision-making context is defined by one or more of five elements: patient, practitioner, problem, procedure, and policy. A context-sensitive drug prescription support system, for example, would allow the user to view a laboratory result in one software application, then switch to a drug information database, where a search for drug dosing modifications is automatically tuned to the patient's age and primary medical problems.
- **Coupled** systems automatically link knowledge to observations, given a specific clinical event. A coupled drug prescription system, for example, would alert the clinician to alternative, potentially cheaper, interventions just before a prescription is generated.
- **Cognizant** systems use artificial intelligence to respond to clinical events, detect patterns, and determine which knowledge resources are most appropriate for problem solving.

The most advanced clinical information environments present physicians with their own unique mix of software, communications tools, educational resources, and feedback. The user's information "personae" becomes part of a computing context that all software applications can access.

The clinicians' need for information convenience, discrimination, and integration informs both the content and presentation of comprehensive hospital medicine. Issues of direct relevance to hospitalists are prioritized by considerations of urgency (**critical** diagnoses or interventions, even if low probability), opportunity (**correctable** problems, even if low probability), prevalence (**common** issues), context (some problems become more important given the clinical **context** and patient types seen by hospitalists), and competence (that **comprehensive** list of problems within the clinical scope of hospitalist practice). Evidence is anchored to recognizable clinical presentations and patient management problems. For each clinical challenge, practice recommendations are sequenced by clinical workflow (background, assessment with both diagnosis and prognosis when feasible, and management including discharge planning). As much as possible, readers are provided with strategies for linking evidence with patient circumstances. In this way, comprehensive hospital medicine is made "practice-based evidence ready," "caremap ready," and "order-set ready," with the electronic version optimized for serving point-of-care clinical decision support.

CONCLUSION

Evidence-based practice portends a change in what it means to be an effective clinician. Proficiency with just-in-time knowledge requires more than good information retrieval skills. Rapid access must be paired with rapid assessment. The core tenet of evidence-based practice is that the *way* one knows is as important as *what* one knows. Practice-Based Evidence emphasizes the behaviors and skills required to integrate evidence access and reflection with clinical workflow at the point of care.

Key Points

- The best evidence should always inform medical decisions and health choices.

- Unfiltered bedside evidence may only worsen the informational plight of busy clinicians.

- For physicians to make more informed decisions, they need to:
  a. Know what to do
  b. Do what is known
  c. Understand what is done

- Evidence-based practice calls for a paradigm shift in medical thinking to de-emphasize personal intuition in favor of the judicious integration of best available clinical research evidence with clinical experience and patient values.

- The evidence-based practitioner greets new information with questions about validity, importance, and applicability.

- The requisite information management skills can be summarized with the 5 A's of an evidence-based information cycle: Assess, Ask, Acquire, Appraise, and Apply.

SUGGESTED READING

Dawes M, Sampson U. Knowledge management in clinical practice: a systematic review of information seeking behavior in physicians. Int J Med Inform 2003; 71(1):9–15.

Guyatt G, Rennie D, eds. Users' Guides to the Medical Literature: A Manual for Evidence-based Clinical Practice. Chicago: American Medical Association Press, 2002. (http://www.usersguides.org).

Harris JM, Jr., Salasche SJ, Harris RB. The internet and the globalisation of medical education. BMJ 2001; 323(7321):1106.

Haynes RB. Of studies, syntheses, synopses, and systems: the "4S" evolution of services for finding current best evidence. ACP J Club 2001; 134(2):A11–A13.

Smith R. What clinical information do doctors need? BMJ 1996; 313(7064):1062–1068.

CHAPTER TWO

A Patient-Centered Approach

Mark V. Williams, MD, FACP

"The good physician knows his patient through and through, and his knowledge is bought dearly. Time, sympathy, and understanding must be lavishly dispensed, but the reward is to be found in the personal bond which forms the greatest satisfaction of the practice of medicine. One of the essential qualities of the clinician is interest in humanity, for the secret of the care of the patient is in caring for the patient."[1]

Francis W. Peabody, MD
October 21, 1925

INTRODUCTION

In one year, a hospitalist may have thousands of contacts with patients and care for hundreds of new ones admitted to the hospital. While each interaction will have its unique aspects, preparation and certain communication skills can optimize the outcomes of these encounters. Dr. Peabody's famous quote encapsulates a seminal component of a physician's approach to any patient in the hospital—caring for the patient. In general, society and patients provide special privileges and status to the medical profession. In response, physicians are expected to conduct themselves in a manner exemplifying professionalism.[2]

The hospital is a foreign place for patients and their families,[3] unfortunately yielding an experience often perceived as degrading by the public.[4] Through both verbal and nonverbal communication, physicians can allay patients' fears and provide a more hospitable environment of care. The importance of such interpersonal skills is reflected in surveys that document that people may place more importance on these skills than on physicians' medical judgment or experience. A nationwide cross-sectional poll of 2,267 adults found that 85% consider treating a patient with dignity and respect and listening carefully as extremely important qualities, compared to 58% believing medical judgment and experience were this valuable.[5] This chapter reviews important aspects of the interaction between the physician and patient, focusing on a patient-centered approach that seeks to establish trust and build a patient's confidence in the diagnostic and therapeutic effectiveness of the health care provider. After defining patient-centered care, the chapter describes the vital role of professionalism in physicians' contract with society, and then delineates the roles of appearance and communication in delivering patient-centered care. These basic skills allow a physician to elucidate a hospitalized patient's concerns, complaints, and findings while seeking to manage symptoms, specific diseases, and situations addressed in detail in the remaining chapters of this reference.

PATIENT-CENTERED CARE

Balint initially described patient-centered medicine with the goal that each patient should "be understood as a unique human being."[6] Lipkin et al. subsequently proposed training for a patient-centered approach to the medical interview.[7] This approach provides a framework for physicians' interactions and communications with patients, aiming to gain an understanding of the patient as well as the disease; that is, assessing the psychosocial as well as biologic aspects of the patient's illness. Historically, the disease, instead of the entire patient, has been the focus of the physician's diagnostic and therapeutic efforts. Ideally, a physician should seek to "see the illness through the patient's eyes."[8] Accomplishing this goal can be achieved through understanding and utilizing multiple dimensions of patient-centered care (Box 2-1). Physicians must also consider cultural factors which are reviewed in detail in Chapter 3.

The move toward patient-centered care advocates that patients play a more active role in their care, including engagement in medical decision making.[9,10] Of note, physicians must assess the degree to which patients actually want to participate. Although almost all patients prefer to be asked their opinions (up to 96%), about half may wish to leave final decisions to their physicians; the elderly and non-Caucasians appear more likely to prefer that physicians make decisions.[11] Physicians should ask which style a patient prefers, and they can balance the extremes of a paternalistic approach versus forcing completely independent patient choice by following an "enhanced autonomy" model that encourages active exchange of ideas and discussion of differences.[12] Such an approach allows patients to make choices which are informed by medical evidence and the physician's experience. The topic of autonomy is reviewed in more depth in Chapter 132.

Hospitalists should be mindful that illness severity and the hospital setting certainly contribute to shifting the balance toward a more authoritarian role for health care providers. People tend to be more passive when sick, and they may be content to allow health care workers to take care of them and make decisions.

Box 2-1 Principles of Patient-Centered Care[13,16,42]

- Adopt the biopsychosocial perspective.
- View the patient as a person and not just a disease or body with illness.
  - Respect the patient's values and preferences
  - Provide relief from pain and discomfort
  - Provide emotional support and allay anxiety and fears
  - Involve family and friends
- Share power and responsibility between the doctor and patient with input from both.
- Build an effective relationship or alliance to achieve management goals.
- Recognize the physician as a person and not just a technician.

Adapted from: Beach MC, Saha S, Cooper LA. The role and relationship of cultural competence and patient-centeredness in health care quality. New York City: The Commonwealth Fund, 2006; and Mead N, Bower P. Patient-centredness: a conceptual framework and review of the empirical literature. Social Science & Medicine. 2000; 51:1087–1110; and Allshouse KD. Treating patients as individuals. In: Gerteis M, Edgman-Levitan S, Daley J, DelBanco TL, eds. Through the Patient's Eyes: Understanding and Promoting Patient-Centered Care. San Francisco: Jossey-Bass Publishers, 1993.

Box 2-2 STEEEP Aims for Health Care System Improvement[15]

- **S**afe—avoiding injuries to patients from the care that is intended to help them
- **T**imely—reducing waits and sometimes harmful delays for both those who receive and those who give care
- **E**ffective—providing services based on scientific knowledge to all who could benefit and refraining from providing services to those not likely to benefit (avoiding underuse and overuse, respectively)
- **E**fficient—avoiding waste, including waste of equipment, supplies, ideas, and energy
- **E**quitable—providing care that does not vary in quality because of personal characteristics such as gender, ethnicity, geographic location, and socioeconomic status
- **P**atient-centered—providing care that is respectful of and responsive to individual patient preferences, needs, and values and ensuring that patient values guide all clinical decisions

From: The Committee on Quality of Health Care in America, Institute of Medicine. Crossing the Quality Chasm: A new health system for the 21st century. Washington, D.C.: National Academy Press, 2001. 3–4.

Moreover, technologically advanced tests (e.g., MRI or angiography) commonly require passive participation. Attempts at assertiveness or control by patients may even seem disruptive. In the hospital, physicians should strive to provide honest, accurate information about their assessments and plans as well as the prognosis. Provision of such informed medical knowledge while soliciting patient opinion ensures that the patient is able to communicate what he or she considers to be acceptable risks and side effects.[13]

In addition to its ethical basis, research from more than 20 years ago demonstrated that expanded patient involvement in care yields improved health outcomes.[14] The Institute of Medicine (IoM) endorsed this approach in its report *Crossing the Quality Chasm* depicting patient-centered care as one of its six domains for health system improvement (Box 2-2).[15] The model of patient-centered care has evolved from a focus on the interpersonal interaction between patient and provider to include the patient's treatment by the health care system as a whole.[16] With their ability to influence overall care delivery by the hospital and their direct interactions with patients, hospitalists can lead the members of the hospital team to focus on patient-centered care delivery.

The national recognition of the importance of a patient-centered approach that yields greater satisfaction is apparent with the roll-out in 2007 of the Hospital Consumer Assessment of Healthcare Providers and Systems (HCAHPS) survey.[17] Developed through a partnership of the Centers for Medicare & Medicaid Services (CMS) and the Agency for Healthcare Research and Quality (AHRQ), this survey provides a national standard for collecting and publicly reporting patients' perspective on the hospital care they received. It has been formally endorsed by the National Quality Forum (NQF). Some of the critical aspects of the hospital experience assessed by the HCAHPS survey include communication with doctors, pain control, communication about medicines, and discharge information. Additionally, the HCAHPS survey will allow comparisons among hospitals while enhancing public accountability, and it will generate incentives for hospitals and hospitalists to improve their quality of care.[18] By pursuing a patient-centered approach to care and quality improvement initiatives, hospitalists can have a profoundly positive impact on a hospital's survey results.

PROFESSIONALISM

Physicians practice in the midst of an upheaval in health care with dramatic changes in technology, consistent cost increases exceeding inflation, and a reimbursement system that primarily rewards quantity and not quality in the U.S. Given that the "conditions of medical practice are tempting physicians to abandon their commitment to the primacy of patient welfare," leadership from internal medicine organizations in the U.S. and Europe (ABIM Foundation, ACP Foundation, and European Federation of Internal Medicine) proposed the Charter on Medical Professionalism.[2] Table 2-1 lists the three principles and ten commitments composing the Charter, providing guidelines for the medical profession's fundamental values needed for service to others.

As members of a profession, physicians have a contract with society that assigns them unique roles and responsibilities. The integrity of individual physicians and the entire profession establishes a trust that we will place the interests of the patient above those of the physician while maintaining standards of competence. Such medical professionalism represents ideals that physicians can pursue to improve the welfare of patients. While some have raised concerns that a physician at the bedside cannot also be concerned about distribution of finite resources, such an altruistic commitment to the patient should not conflict with efforts in

Table 2-1 Charter on Medical Professionalism[2]

Fundamental Principles

1) Primacy of Patient Welfare
   – dedication to serving the interest of the patient
2) Patient Autonomy
   – through honest communication empower patients to make informed decisions
3) Social Justice
   – promote fair distribution of health care resources

Set of Professional Responsibilities
Commitments to:

1) Professional Competence
   • Pursuit of lifelong learning with responsibility to maintain adequate medical knowledge and clinical and team skills necessary for quality care
2) Honesty with Patients
   • Ensure that patients are completely and honestly informed about their care with the goal of empowering them to decide on the course of therapy
3) Patient Confidentiality
   • Apply appropriate confidentiality safeguards to disclosure of patient information.
4) Maintaining Appropriate Relations with Patients
   • Never exploit patients for sexual, financial, or private gain.
5) Improving Quality of Care
   • Dedication to continuous quality improvement with the goals of reducing medical error, increasing patient safety, minimizing overuse of resources, and optimizing outcomes
6) Improving Access to Care
   • Reduce barriers to health care with the goal of providing a uniform and adequate standard of care
7) Just Distribution of Finite Resources
   • Cost-effectively manage limited clinical resources through development of guidelines for cost-effective care
8) Scientific Knowledge
   • Uphold scientific standards, promote research, create new knowledge, and ensure its appropriate use.
9) Maintaining Trust by Managing Conflicts of Interest
   • Recognize, disclose to the public, and deal with conflicts of interest.
10) Professional Responsibilities
   • Work collaboratively while respecting one another to optimize patient care, and set standards for education and professional performance. This includes participation in the processes of self-regulation, and the remediation and disciplinary process for members failing to meet professional standards.

Adapted from: ABIM Foundation, ACP-ASIM Foundation, European Federation of Internal Medicine. Medical professionalism in the new millennium: A physician charter. Ann Intern Med 2002; 136:243–246.

administrative and political contexts to allocate health care fairly.[19] To accomplish this goal, physicians cannot operate independently, but must partner with other disciplines such as nursing and pharmacy to achieve a teamwork approach to care delivery.[20] With a backbone of medical professionalism, physicians can interact with patients, effectively communicate with them, and collaboratively deliver health care.

Appearance

A first step in medical professionalism may be to convey respect and a professional identity through a well-groomed mode of dress.[21] The patient's first impression of the physician will usually be visual, and a doctor's attributes of clothing and grooming can have a profound impact upon subsequent communication and interaction. Even Hippocrates recognized the significance of appearance, stating that the physician "must be clean in person, well dressed, and anointed with sweet-smelling unguents."[22] More than 30 studies have evaluated the influence of physician dress on patients, showing that dressing well has salutary effects, though two older studies indicated that dress had no effect on patient attitudes.[23,24]

However, more recent research demonstrates that a physician's dress has a profound effect on patients' trust and confidence. A study of 400 patients in South Carolina found that 76% preferred professional clothing with a white coat.[25] While about 10% favored surgical scrubs and 9% coat and tie (i.e., business dress), only 5% preferred casual clothes. Of note, surgical scrubs were preferred by 32% in an "emergency" situation versus 62% favoring professional dress with a white coat. Figure 2-1 displays the various options shown to the study participants. Importantly, surveyed individuals reported they would be more willing to share social, sexual, and psychological problems with a professionally dressed doctor. Professional attire generated more trust and the belief that the physician was more knowledgeable, competent, caring, compassionate, responsible, and authoritative. Elderly and African-American patients seemed particularly impressed by the valuable effect of well-dressed physicians.

An even larger study of 451 patients, of whom 202 were hospitalized, from New Zealand demonstrated that patients preferred doctors dressed in semi-formal clothes (male wearing long-sleeved shirt with tie or female wearing blouse with a dark-colored skirt or trousers).[26] Wearing a white coat was rated close to this semi-formal outfit while a formal suit was rated lower, and

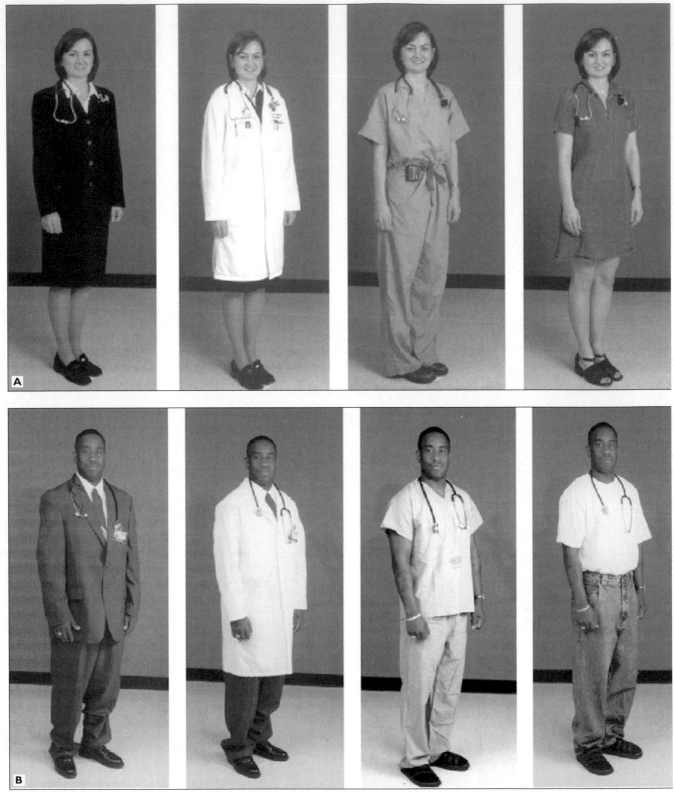

Figure 2-1 • Physician Attire—Business, professional with white coat, surgical scrubs, and casual. From: Rehman SU, Nietert PJ, Cope DW, et al. What to wear today? Effect of doctor's attire on the trust and confidence of patients. Am J Med 2005; 118:1279–1286.

informal clothes (jeans) were least preferred. Beyond considering just clothes, physicians should also recognize the impact of accessories such as facial piercings. A study conducted with emergency department patrons and medical school faculty documented the potentially negative impact of nose and eyebrow piercings. Less than one fourth of patients felt piercings were appropriate, negatively affecting perceived competency and trustworthiness. The majority of medical faculty was also "bothered" by them.

While a physician's dress may contribute only a small, though potentially substantive, component toward a trusting patient–physician relationship, it certainly can enhance initial impressions. Without question, communication skills are most important in developing a relationship, and the next section addresses how to optimize communication with patients.

HISTORY

Typically, a physician first interacts with a hospitalized patient through the process of performing the admission history and physical examination. Physicians are comfortable "taking" a history from patients using structured disease-oriented queries about symptoms that yield short answers or yes/no responses. They usually strive to focus their efforts toward development of a short list of possible diagnoses.[27] After establishing a diagnosis or differential diagnoses, physicians then formulate their evaluation and treatment plans. Our reimbursement system reinforces this approach by requiring documentation in a structured format. It is not surprising that patients voice complaints that the doctor is not listening, given the combination of time pressures and need for specific documentation of aspects of the chief complaint, past medical history, family history, social history, and comprehensive review of systems.[28] By eliciting the patient's entire agenda, the physician can ensure that critical issues are not ignored and that the patient feels he or she was "heard."[29]

Pursuing an alternative approach of "building" a history can accomplish both tasks of documenting essential biomedical information and appreciating the patient's perspective on his or her illness.[27] Once medical stabilization has occurred for the hospitalized patient, the physician can then focus on identifying the patient's agenda through open-ended questions and then assess how that agenda relates to the proposed therapeutic plan.[29]

- How may I help you? Why did you come to the hospital?
- What are your main concerns?
- What concerns does the clinician have? How do these match those of the patient?
- What needs to be addressed immediately versus later?
- What else? What other problems are bothering you?

Answering these questions will allow the physician to prioritize the patient's concerns and negotiate how and when they will be addressed. Initiating the patient–doctor interaction by setting the agenda demonstrates respect for the patient and lessens the likelihood of last-second requests for consideration of unmet patient needs. Concomitantly, the patient will appreciate the attention of the doctor to his or her expressed needs, instead of just to those of documentation in the too-common effort to admit and dispatch with the patient.

Specific statements, questions, words, or actions can be used to facilitate bringing forth needed information while demonstrating empathy to patients.[27,28,30] Table 2-2 provides examples. Though physicians commonly fear that this approach takes too much time, research indicates it does not. Moreover, a better relationship with the patient certainly reduces the likelihood of malpractice suits,[31–33] while possibly saving time over the course of a hospitalization. Importantly, the entire process of the patient interview should be accomplished in a facilitative manner. This includes sitting down so as not to appear rushed, and attempting to listen without interrupting the patient.

COMMUNICATION AND EDUCATION

A critical component of a physician's duties is to communicate information to hospitalized patients and to educate them, particularly at the time of discharge (*see* Chapter 11). Concomitant with the marked expansion in pharmaceuticals and medical technology, there has been a dramatic increase in learning demands on patients. Thirty years ago, there were fewer than 1,000 prescription medications, while today there are >10,000. Hospitalization for an acute myocardial infarction 30 years ago resulted in a multi-week stay versus 4–5 days now. Additionally, hospitalization commonly involves sophisticated tests that can be invasive and/or imposing and require informed consent. Explaining the

Table 2-2 Facilitating Empathy—Actions, Words, Statements, and Queries[27,28]

Words or Action	Effect
Silence	Indicates receptivity and attention to listening
Head nod; "Uh-huh"; "Go on . . ."; "Could you tell me a little more about that?"	Facilitates continued dialog
Patient—"I have a headache." Physician—"A headache?"	Reflection through repeating what the patient states as a question to elicit more information
"Let me make sure I have this right, you said . . ."	Paraphrasing to ensure understanding
"Help me understand what you were feeling." "Tell me how that felt."	Clarification
"That sounds difficult." "That must have been painful." "I can't imagine how hard that must have been."	Empathic statements
"I only have a couple more minutes to talk. What else should I know?"	Time management

Adapted from: Coulehan JL, Platt FW, Egener B, et al. "Let me see if I have this right . . .": Words that help build empathy. Ann Intern Med 2001; 135:221–227; and Haidet P, Paterniti DA. Building a history rather than taking one: A perspective on information sharing during the medical interview. Arch Intern Med 2003; 163:1134–11140.

evidence for testing and treatment so that patients are more likely to participate in decision-making can be accomplished through specific steps: (1) appreciating the patient's experience and expectations, (2) partnering with the patient, (3) sharing the evidence along with uncertainties, (4) providing recommendations, and (5) checking for understanding and agreement.[34]

Expectations of hospital care include ensuring that patients understand their diagnosis, treatment, and tests; and obtaining informed consent. Discharge from the hospital includes the learning needs of follow-up plans and medications as well as warning signs and symptoms that should provoke seeking urgent medical care. Patients may also be required to perform a daunting myriad of tasks, including self-assessment of their illness (e.g., weigh themselves, check their blood pressure), adjustment of their medications, and monitoring of their diet while undertaking exercise programs. Preparing patients and educating them is fraught with barriers that afflict attempts at communication (Table 2-3). However, solutions can be employed to overcome these barriers (Table 2-4).

Successful communication of vital information requires that patients comprehend what they have been told. Regrettably, physicians may obfuscate the message with their facile use of medical terms. Compounding this, many patients have inadequate health literacy[35,36] and even patients with adequate literacy skills may not understand commonly used medical terminology.[37] To ensure comprehension, physicians need to assess patients' understanding and not assume that accurate communication has occurred.

Unfortunately, physicians rarely assess patients' understanding (<5% of the time in one study).[38] Even if they do, simply asking patients "Do you understand?" or "Do you have any questions?" is insufficient. Many patients, especially those with low literacy skills and poor education, will acquiesce and nod their head in assent, even when they do not understand, for fear of revealing their ignorance or challenging the physician. Instead, physicians should assess a patient's comprehension by asking him or her to repeat or "teach-back" what he or she is supposed to know or do. Taking this universal approach[39] to all patients is endorsed by the NQF as a patient safety standard—"Ask each patient or legal surrogate to recount what he or she has been told during the informed consent discussion"[40]—and is one of 11 top patient safety practices based on strength of scientific evidence.[41] Box 2-3 lists simple steps that a physician can follow to optimize communication and education for hospitalized patients.

CONCLUSION

Hospitalists care for patients when they are at their most vulnerable, sick enough to be hospitalized and sometimes near death. Utilizing a patient-centered approach, hospitalists can optimize care delivery and facilitate a teamwork approach to hospital care delivery. Identifying a hospitalized patient's agenda and using open-ended, empathetic queries can facilitate patients' participation in their care and engender respect and cooperation. Attempts at education should be sensitive to a patients' health literacy,

Table 2-3 Barriers to Communication and Understanding

Patient	Physician
Fund of health care knowledge	Use of medical jargon and technical terms
Trust	Lack of respect
Impact of illness	Stereotyping
Language	Language
Inadequate health literacy	Failure to assess comprehension
Fear and lack of assertiveness	Lack of cultural competence
Shame	Failure to assess patient preferences

Box 2-3 Steps to Enhance Patient Understanding

1. Sit down and slow down.
2. Use "living room" (i.e., plain) language.
3. Show, draw pictures.
4. Limit information at each interaction; repeat instructions.
5. Use a "teach-back" or "show me" approach to confirm understanding.
6. Be respectful, caring, sensitive.

Table 2-4 Problems and Solutions in Physician Communication with Patients[37,39]

Problems	Solutions
Use of medical jargon and technical terms	Use plain language with all patients.
Communication of a large amount of information in a short time	Provide small amounts of information at each encounter and repeatedly.
Not distinguishing major from minor points	Identify major issues first.
Failure to use pictures, patient education handouts, or audiovisual materials	Utilize pictures, educational materials, and patient educators for assistance.
Inadequate time for questions and clarification	Schedule discrete time for patient and family questions, and encourage them.
No confirmation of patient comprehension or demonstration of the skills being taught	Utilize "teach back" and assess patients' comprehension.

and comprehension must be confirmed using a "teach-back" approach. Finally, the tenets of medical professionalism should guide all of a physician's activities.

"Knowing is not enough; we must apply. Willing is not enough; we must do."

—Goethe

Key Points

- The hospital is a foreign place for patients and their families, and hospitalization can be a degrading experience for patients.

- Physicians should take a patient-centered approach to delivering care and attempt to involve patients in medical decision-making.

- Hospitalized patients across the nation are being surveyed about their hospital experience, and the results will be reported publicly so hospitals can be compared.

- Physicians should adhere to principles of medical professionalism.

- By wearing semi-formal clothes or a white coat and eschewing facial piercings, physicians can improve first impressions and enhance patients' trust.

- Use of open-ended interviewing skills, empathetic methods, and determining the patient's agenda facilitates communication and diminishes the risk of malpractice suits.

- Cognizant of a patient's health literacy, the physician should confirm patient understanding by using a "teach-back" approach

SUGGESTED READINGS

Mead N, Bower P. Patient-centredness: a conceptual framework and review of the empirical literature. Soc Sci Med 2000; 51:1087–1110.

Levinson W, Kao A, Kuby A, et al. Not all patients want to participate in decision making: A national study of public preferences. J Gen Intern Med 2005; 20:531–535.

Goldstein E, Farquhar M, Crofton C, et al. Measuring hospital care from the patients' perspective: an overview of the CAHPS Hospital Survey development process. Health Serv Res 2005; 40:1977–1995.

Rehman SU, Nietert PJ, Cope DW, et al. What to wear today? Effect of doctor's attire on the trust and confidence of patients. Am J Med 2005; 118:1279–1286.

ABIM Foundation, ACP-ASIM Foundation, European Federation of Internal Medicine. Medical professionalism in the new millennium: a physician charter. Ann Intern Med 2002; 136:243–246.

Haidet P, Paterniti DA. Building a history rather than taking one: A perspective on information sharing during the medical interview. Arch Intern Med 2003; 163:1134–1140.

Coulehan JL, Platt FW, Egener B, et al. "Let me see if I have this right . . .": Words that help build empathy. Ann Intern Med 2001; 135:221–227.

Baker LH, O'Connell D, Platt FW. "What else?": Setting the agenda for the clinical interview. Ann Intern Med 2005; 143:766–770.

Platt FW, Gaspar DL, Coulehan JL, et al. "Tell me about yourself": The patient-centered interview. Ann Intern Med 2001; 134:1079–1085.

Sage WM. Putting the patient in patient safety: linking patient complaints and malpractice risk. JAMA 2002; 287:3003–3005.

Williams MV, Davis T, Parker RM, et al. The role of health literacy in patient-physician communication. Fam Med 2002; 34:383–389.

Paasche-Orlow MK, Schillinger D, Greene SM, et al. How health care systems can begin to address the challenge of limited literacy. J Gen Intern Med 2006; 21:884–887.

Epstein RM, Alper BS, Quill TE. Communicating evidence for participatory decision making. JAMA 2004; 291:2359–2366.

CHAPTER THREE

Cultural Competence in Hospital Settings: Communication and Culture

Jada Bussey-Jones, MD, Inginia Genao, MD, and William T. Branch, MD

BACKGROUND

Health care professionals are increasingly expected to be culturally competent. Cultural competence has been defined as congruent behaviors, attitudes, and policies that come together in a system, agency, or among professionals that enable the organization or individuals to work effectively in cross-cultural situations.[1] An Institute of Medicine report highlighted the need for training in navigating cross-cultural interactions.[2] Additionally, several governing bodies, including the Joint Commission of Accreditation of Hospital Organizations, the Liaison Committee on Medical Education, and the Accreditation Council on Graduate Medical Education (JCAHO, LCME, ACGME, respectively), specifically mandate implementation of cultural competence training and practices in clinical care. In part, this reflects demographic shifts in the United States, with substantial and continued growth in minority populations. However, the lack of concurrent change in the demographic composition of the health care provider workforce leads to an ethnic and cultural discordance between patients and most of their health care providers.

The increasingly acknowledged impact of culture on health provides additional support for the emphasis on cultural competence training. Culture affects the health of patients in ways not easily recognized. For example, beliefs about causes and cures of illness may delay the pursuit of Western medicine interventions and interfere with needed treatment. Religious attitudes and beliefs about death and the afterlife also influence a patient's decision on treatment and interaction with health care providers. The use of non-Western methods for symptom relief might not be shared with the provider and can adversely affect disease management. Patient expectations of the provider and the health care system based on cultural background and previous experiences may influence health outcomes both positively and negatively, depending on the degree of communication. Culture also plays a role in patients' behavior in response to an illness. Health care providers must be aware and knowledgeable of how culture may influence behaviors.

Achieving competence in culturally appropriate communication may help avoid contributing to common health disparities in minority populations already documented by a large body of literature. Much of this research has been done in hospital based settings. For example, authors have reported that minorities have lower rates of coronary artery bypass,[3] less analgesia for long bone fractures,[4] and lower quality of care for pneumonia and congestive heart failure.[5] Health care providers are likely to narrow the health disparity gap by debunking ethnocentric and stereotypical beliefs; by changing attitudes; and by encouraging greater awareness, experiences, education, and exposure to alternative ideas. Many teaching hospitals serve a high proportion of patients from minority and lower socioeconomic status. Yet, in these settings there is often very little ethnic or cultural overlap among patients and health care providers. A recent systematic review of outcomes in cultural competence education suggests that this training shows promise as a strategy for improving the knowledge, attitudes, and skills of health professionals.[6] While clinical outcomes were not confirmed, it is likely that establishing cultural competence of in-training and staff physicians will likely improve doctor–patient communication and increase patients' satisfaction, while enhancing doctor–patient collaboration, diagnosis, patient compliance and cooperation, and proper use of resources.

Utilizing inpatient vignettes to highlight clinical relevance, this chapter will focus on:

1. Language/appropriate use of interpreter services
2. Explorations of patient's explanatory model (Box 3-1) and use of complementary and alternative medicine
3. Cultural influences on patient autonomy and end-of-life care
4. Trust and communication

These case examples describe the differences that may exist between the patient's and the clinician's understanding and explanation of disease and illness. Recognizing that language is an integral part of culture and that language barriers play a very significant role in access and quality of care, we will also focus on effective use of a medically trained interpreter. We will also identify modes for eliciting the patient's illness experience, health beliefs, and complementary/alternative medicine (CAM) usage, and we will discuss the impact of trust and communication. Finally, we will review the importance of cultural influences on autonomy and end-of-life care, and the interaction of trust and communication.

LANGUAGE/APPROPRIATE USE OF INTERPRETER SERVICES

"Mrs. B" is a 43-year-old female who emigrated from Mexico 2 years ago. She works at a small cafeteria in the area and only

Box 3-1 Eliciting a Patient's Explanatory Model: Kleinman's Questions

1. What do you think has caused your problem?

2. Why do you think it started when it did?

3. What do you think your sickness does to you? How does it work?

4. How severe is your sickness? Will it have a short or long course?

5. What kind of treatment do you think you should receive?

6. What are the most important results you hope to receive from this treatment?

7. What are the chief problems your sickness has caused for you?

8. What do you fear most about your sickness?

Kleinman AK, Eisenberg L, Good B. Culture, illness and care: clinical lessons from anthropologic and cross-cultural research. Ann Intern Med 1978; 88:251–58.

Box 3-2 Guidelines for Choosing an Appropriate Interpreter and Strategies to Increase Effective Communication During Use of an Interpreter

Selecting an interpreter

- A trained interpreter is **ALWAYS** preferred.

- Never use a child to interpret because this may disrupt social roles and put undue stress on a child.

- Do not ask a stranger from the waiting room to interpret because of potential confidentiality breech.

- It may occasionally (in emergent situations) be appropriate to use an adult whom the patient brings to the visit for this purpose. However, be aware of potential problems of medical terminology and revelation of personal information/questions. Additionally, both your comments and those of the patients may be edited (saving face, not asking "sensitive" questions, etc.).

- Ask the patient if the designated interpreter is acceptable to him or her.

During encounter

- Introduce the interpreter formally at the beginning of the interview.

- Direct questions to the patient, not to the interpreter unless they are meant for the interpreter.

- Maintain visual contact with the patient during interpretation. You may pick up important nonverbal clues.

- Avoid technical terms, abbreviations, professional jargon, and idioms.

- Ask the interpreter to interpret as literally as possible rather than paraphrasing or omitting information.

- Use nonlanguage aids (e.g., charts, diagrams) whenever possible.

- To check the patient's understanding and accuracy of the interpretation, ask the patient to repeat instructions/advice in his or her own words, with the interpreter facilitating.

- Expect the interpreter to be a cultural bridge to explain cultural-bound syndromes.

- Be patient; an interpreted interview takes longer.

speaks Spanish. She complains of headaches and generalized weakness. She has been seen several times in the emergency department and ambulatory clinic with similar concerns over the last 2 months. Her 23-year-old son is concerned and has accompanied her on each visit, serving as her interpreter. Efforts to diagnose her condition have been unsuccessful. Other doctors conclude that she is imagining her symptoms and have suggested a psychiatric and social services consultations. At this emergency room visit, she has become increasingly agitated, tearful, and uneasy. Her son expresses desperation. She is admitted for observation and psychiatric evaluation. Her son must leave early to return to work, and the patient speaks and motions frantically after he has left the room. You request an interpreter and find that at each visit, the patient has been attempting to discuss cervical pain during intercourse and irregular vaginal bleeding that has progressed. The patient is subsequently diagnosed with uterine malignancy.

Discussion

This case demonstrates the importance of language as a key component of culture and communication. Using a relative as an interpreter can limit or even distort the history obtained, sometimes becoming an obstacle in providing good medical care. Health care providers may fail to utilize reliable interpretation because of unavailability or time constraints. In this case, this Spanish-speaking patient had no medically trained interpreter on several occasions. The lack of a medically trained interpreter resulted in the physician's decreased understanding of symptoms and delayed the diagnosis, while prolonging the patient's suffering and increasing her frustration.

Approximately 32 million people, nearly 14% of the US population, speak a language other than English in their homes.[7] The federal government, as a major purchaser of health care and enforcer of civil rights laws, plays a large role in mandating linguistic competence. In fact, the United States Department of Health and Human Services Office for Civil Rights views inadequate interpretation in health care as a form of discrimination.[8]

In spite of this, many health care facilities do not have salaried, professional interpreters available.[8,9]

Health care providers who see patients with limited English proficiency (LEP) rely heavily on ad hoc interpreters, family members, hospital staff, other patients, or no interpreter at all. Some who speak enough of the patient's language to "get by" rely on this approach. Each of these situations is obviously imperfect and often results in errors in interpretation. One investigator found that 23–52% of physicians' questions were misinterpreted or not interpreted at all.[10] The author lists several examples of interpreter errors, including "chest" for "ribs," "neck" for "tonsil," "teeth" for "jaw," "fat" for "swelling," and "laxative" for "diarrhea." Family dynamics also influence interpretation—in one example, a child was embarrassed to ask questions regarding menses and bowel movements. It is easy to predict that these errors will have adverse clinical ramifications. Box 3-2 shows general guidelines for selection and use of medical interpreters.

Explorations of Patient's Explanatory Model and Use of Complementary and Alternative Medicine

"Mrs. L" is a 60-year-old woman admitted for a thrombus in her deep femoral vein. She is Chinese and does not speak English but is accompanied by a bilingual nurse hired to care for her. You review her past history and find that she has osteoporosis and a prior proximal deep vein thrombosis complicated by pulmonary embolism. At the time of her last hospital discharge, she was prescribed Coumadin, and her estrogen was discontinued. After extensive inquiry, she tells you that she is seeing a doctor in Chinatown for her Fung Sui Bing, and she is drinking the ginseng tea that he has given her so that "I can walk." Mrs. L drinks this tea three or four times a day, especially when it rains. After more investigation, you find that the brand of ginseng tea that Mrs. L is drinking increases the level of estrogen and/or estrogen-like substances in the body. You discuss the implications of estrogen therapy on thrombosis and suggest that Mrs. L discontinue her tea. She responds by explaining her lengthy relationship with her Chinese doctor, who has "never been wrong."

Discussion

This case highlights several issues, including the importance of explanatory models of disease, cultural aspects of health care–seeking behaviors, and use of complementary and alternative medicines (CAM). A nonjudgmental inquiry of patients' perceptions of their illness and treatment can be revealing (Fig. 3-1). In this case, it led to the revelation of Mrs. L's perceptions of her disease and the therapeutic approaches sought.

CAM has been defined as practices used to prevent or treat illnesses that are not widely taught in medical schools and are not typically available in hospitals.[11] It has been estimated that 60 million Americans used CAM in 1990.[11] The authors of this report conducted telephone interviews of over 1,500 adults in a national sample and found that >70% of the patients who reported using CAM never told their physicians. While physicians are increasingly aware of CAM, its use continues to increase, and this frequently unspoken issue has many important implications for patient care.

Although data are limited on the safety and efficacy of many CAM modalities, it is important to explore their use. Patients may rely on marketing campaigns and anecdotes for justification to try these new therapies. Physicians must be concerned about possible risks related to CAM use. These therapies may be toxic alone or in combination with other medications. For example, there are cases of overdoses and death related to the use of Herba ephedra (herbal ephedrine), also known as *ma huang*.[11] This and other examples make the case for having the discussion with your patients, if only to safeguard them.

Additionally, physician knowledge of patients' use of these therapies can facilitate responsible use and build partnerships with patients. Over 80% of patients who reported using CAM combined these with conventional medicine.[12] Several authors have found that use of CAM is not confined to patients of any particular social class or to patients who seem to be dissatisfied or mistrusting of conventional medicine.[13,14] Health care providers'

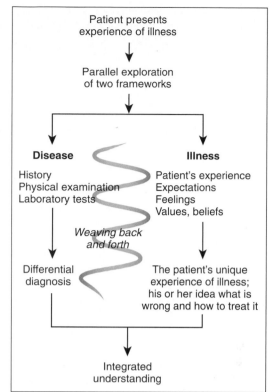

Figure 3-1 • The Patient-Centered Clinical Method. Adapted from Stewart M. Patient-Centered Medicine: Transforming the Clinical Method. Thousand Oaks: Sage Publications, 1995.

discussion of CAM practices may build trust and facilitate future negotiations. In Mrs. L's case, use of an estrogen-containing substance clearly has clinical relevance. Equally important is creating an environment in which the patient feels comfortable discussing with the heath care provider the use of specific therapies, healers, and CAM practices.

This case also demonstrates that seeking care at a physician's office or a hospital may be viewed as a last option by patients. Patients may seek advice from several sources, including family members, friends, and, as in this case, a Chinese doctor. Additionally, many medical symptoms are self-diagnosed and self-treated.[15] Inquiring about and addressing previous attempts at treatment can help demonstrate the course of the disease, identify potentially harmful or helpful interventions taken, and build therapeutic alliances. In this case, rather than disregarding the practices and beliefs of the patient, the physician contacted her Chinese doctor, who was instrumental in maintaining the patient's compliance with the therapeutic regimen. He agreed to replace her tea with one that had no estrogen. Understanding the patient's explanatory model, recognizing her strong beliefs, acknowledging these beliefs, and incorporating them improved patient satisfaction and trust.

CULTURAL INFLUENCES ON PATIENT AUTONOMY AND END-OF-LIFE

"Mr. K" is a 60-year-old Japanese man who has been admitted for evaluation of progressive dysphagia, weight loss, and dehydration. After you see the patient on his second hospital day, his son follows you to the hall and confides that he fears his father is seriously ill and feels very strongly that the patient should not be told of a terminal diagnosis. This, he states, would sound like a death sentence to his father, causing him to lose hope and decline more rapidly. He also explains that he will feel that he is a burden on his son and daughter-in-law if he is made aware of the diagnosis, and that these requests would be honored if the patient were in his home country. His test results have just shown evidence of advanced stomach cancer, and you are unsure how to proceed.

Discussion

In the United States, decision-making at the end of life is focused primarily on the individual, with a high value placed on the patient's right to know. American providers have generally advocated full disclosure of the facts of disease, diagnosis, and treatment.[16,17] The evolution of medical decision-making in this country has patient autonomy at its core. This assumes that the individual patient will want to make his/her own health care decisions. Patient autonomy is so highly valued that efforts now exist to allow patient control over decision-making, even in the face of diminished mental capacity, via advanced care directives.

Many non-Western cultures, however, do not share this view. For example, studies of physician practices and attitudes in Spain, Japan, France, and Eastern Europe show that they rarely tell patients of a cancer diagnosis.[18–20] These cultures may emphasize the family-centered model. Informed consent is not mandated, and families may prefer to receive information first and filter what is given to the patient.[21,16] Reasons often cited by family members include the fear that truth-telling will lead to loss of hope, and a desire to protect the patient from bad news.[16,17]

Ethical conflicts may arise when providers, patients, and their families have different beliefs about patient autonomy. Excluding a patient from discussion about a life-threatening illness may conflict with a provider's values, beliefs, and medical training. In this case, several valuable points should be made. First, respecting patients' autonomy does not necessarily mean that they have to be informed of their diagnosis or that they have to make all medical decisions. Patients may prefer to relinquish those rights to designated family members. Not acknowledging and accepting these preferences when they exist may be disrespectful and verges on a paternalism that, in fact, counters patient autonomy principles. Second, it is important to establish the way the patient and the family prefer to receive medical information and make medical decisions. This discussion is best conducted prior to initiation of diagnostic workup so that expectations are clear. Thus, health care providers should discuss preferences clearly with patients and document this in the medical record. The patient in this case preferred to have his son receive medical information and make decisions. The physician and medical team respected these wishes and had regular family meetings to discuss information and treatment plans with the patient's son.

TRUST AND COMMUNICATION

"Ms. P" is a 65-year-old African American woman admitted to the hospital with chest pain. Laboratory results reveal liver enzyme elevation, and she is diagnosed with hepatitis. She has been very healthy, and her interactions with the health system were related to four uncomplicated vaginal deliveries. She is very perplexed by the diagnosis of hepatitis and asks that blood tests be repeated; they confirm the diagnosis. She says, "You know, I have been a very healthy person, clean, sex with one man in my whole life. I should have had my babies at home." The health care provider, intrigued by her comment, says, "Please tell me more about that." The patient goes on to say, "You doctors want to know too much—experiment on people, especially poor people like me. Who knows . . ." In spite of multiple attempts, this patient refuses further hepatic or cardiac evaluation. She continues to have more chest pain consistent with unstable angina.

Discussion

Several studies have demonstrated that even when the larger social and institutional issues such as insurance coverage, socioeconomic status, and health status are similar, differences in treatment exist when comparing whites to minority populations.[22,23] One multi-hospital study found lapses in the most basic levels of clinical care when comparing African American and white Medicare beneficiaries.[5] These reports suggest that minority patients may not be receiving medically indicated treatments. Is the issue patient preference? Do minority patients trust the health care system? Were the procedures not explained in a culturally competent way?

Several reports have documented racial differences in perceptions of patients regarding their health care. For example, African Americans and Hispanics were more likely to report knowledge of a friend, family member, or acquaintance who received unfair medical treatment because of race.[24] Another study found that minority patients had less positive perceptions and ratings of their physicians' style and less trust in their physicians.[25] Additionally, the issue of trust in the medical setting should be contextualized by minority patients' personal experiences with societal discrimination. This personal history is underscored by historical precedents such as the Tuskegee study—a US Public Health Service Study of untreated syphilis in African Americans—which has left many African Americans wary of the health care system.

In addition to diminished patient trust, communication may also play a significant role in this case. In one study, both low income and African American race were found to be predictive of physicians using a communication pattern characterized by low psychosocial talk, low patient control of communication, and high levels of closed-ended question-asking.[26] Moreover, independent observers coded 150 physician–patient encounters and found that patient characteristics (ethnicity, sex, age, appearance) significantly influenced physician interpersonal behaviors such as nonverbal attention, empathy, courtesy, and information giving.[27] Minority patients received less positive forms of communication. There is also a substantial body of evidence supporting a relationship between encounter characteristics and patient satisfaction, compliance, and outcomes.[26,28,29]

The medical profession will need to examine closely the influences of trust, patient preferences, and communication to understand better the extent to which they may compromise health outcomes. As this case demonstrates, when trust and communication are at issue, there are some interventions that may improve patients' care. First, rather than simply labeling as "noncompliant," it is important to explore causes of medical non-

Box 3-3 Recommendations for Negotiations in Cross-Cultural Encounters

- Use good manners. Many patients of minority populations have often been denied the basic symbols of civility and courtesy. Be prompt when possible; introduce yourself, and do not use first names unless the patient has requested this.

- Develop an increased self-awareness and recognize that there are few people who are free from all prejudice. If we first are able to recognize these attitudes, we can then do something to effect personal growth and change.

- Do not stereotype and label people. There is tremendous heterogeneity within any group, race, culture, or class.

- Bring the patient's feelings of distrust, resentment, and anger out in the open. This acknowledgement can increase communication and rapport.

- Appreciate social limitations. Excessive demands on a patient with limited resources can result in disappointment and frustration for the physician and the patient.

- Learn more about the life experiences and culture of the patients that you treat.

health organization leadership to educate culturally and linguistically competent providers. This is an ongoing, interactive, and complex process, given the constantly changing demographics, the processes of acculturation, and the interethnic variation and social change of both patients and health care providers. Cultural competence is clearly broader than the issues discussed in these cases. It must go beyond cultural sensitivity and knowledge. It must include the ability to navigate effectively these cross-cultural encounters. We must be willing to participate in lifelong learning that helps integrate the principles of biomedicine with the many beliefs and values of our patients—by improving communication, knowledge, and negotiations to reach an agreement for the best medical care possible.

Key Points

- Language is a key component of culture and communication. Proper use of medically trained interpreters can minimize misunderstandings and breeches of confidentiality.

- Nonjudgmental explorations of patients' perceptions of their illness and the use of complementary and alternative medicine and treatment can assist in diagnostic and treatment plans.

- There are often cultural influences on decision-making and end-of-life care. An assessment of patient preferences regarding medical decision-making is often helpful.

- The medical profession will need to examine the influences of trust, patient preferences, and communication to understand better the extent to which they may compromise health outcomes.

adherence. For example, the patient may have differing beliefs about his or her illness (and therefore treatment), poor health literacy, prior negative health care experiences, or financial barriers to obtaining treatments, as well as mistrust of physicians and medicine. Secondly, when mistrust, fears, and concerns are discovered (as in this case, the patient had concerns regarding experimentation and bias), they should not be belittled or dismissed. In this context, cross-cultural communication and negotiation skills (Box 3-3) become more relevant. When a personal relationship with a provider is perceived as compassionate and trustworthy, this may supersede a general mistrust of medicine. Finally, negotiation involves understanding patients' concerns and desires, explaining your perspective, and having the flexibility to find creative ways to meet their needs while aiming for the best possible outcomes.

This patient's input was heard without judgment or pressure from the medical team. The physician offered continued reassurance of the patient's rights and role in the decisions affecting her health care and, via participatory style in communication, negotiated a partnership in the treatment. While she refused a surgical intervention, she did agree to take medications. Her chest pain symptoms resolved, and she remains stable.

CONCLUSION

Plans to care for an ever more ethnically and racially diverse population must include strong community ties and buy-in from

SUGGESTED READING

Astin J. Why patients use alternative medicine: results of a national study. JAMA 1998; 279(19):1548–1553.

Blackhall LJ, Murphy ST, Frank G, et al. Ethnicity and attitudes toward patient autonomy. JAMA 1995; 274(10):820–825.

Doescher MP, Saver BG, Franks P, et al. Racial and ethnic disparities in perceptions of physician style and trust. Arch Fam Med 2000; 9(10):1156–1163.

Institute of Medicine. Unequal Treatment: Confronting Racial and Ethnic Disparities in Healthcare. Washington, DC: National Academy of Sciences, 2003.

Woloshin S, Bickell NA, Schwartz LM, et al. Language barriers in medicine in the United States. JAMA 1995; 273(9):724–728.

CHAPTER FOUR

Nutritional Assessment and Support

G. Randy Smith, Jr., MD, Nicole M. Daignault, RD, CNSD, Glen Bergman, MMSc, RD, LD, CNSD, and Thomas R. Ziegler, MD

BACKGROUND

Malnutrition is one of the most common conditions present in the hospital setting.[1-3] As a comorbid condition in patients hospitalized for acute illness, malnutrition is associated with increased mortality via infectious complications, increased length of hospital stay, increased hospital costs, and increased rehabilitation costs. Despite the high prevalence of malnutrition in hospitalized patients, recognition of it and subsequent use of nutritional support modalities by physicians remains low.[1] The main goal for provision of nutritional support in the hospitalized patient is provision of adequate macronutrients and micronutrients for basic metabolism, tissue repair, maintenance of lean body mass (LBM) or attenuation of LBM loss, and support of the immune system and organ function. This chapter will focus on nutritional assessment and on prevention and treatment of macronutrient and micronutrient malnutrition in adult hospitalized patients.

ASSESSMENT

Clinical Presentation

Prevalence and Presenting Signs and Symptoms

Malnutrition is defined as a physiologic state resulting from an inappropriate supply of nutrients to the patient, from an inability to make use of nutrients metabolically, or from a combination of both factors. A deficiency in protein, total calories, or both, as well as depletion of specific micronutrients, can result in a malnourished state. Previous studies in both developed and developing countries, including societies with a high prevalence of obesity, indicate that between 30% and 50% of hospitalized patients may suffer from some degree of protein-energy malnutrition.[1]

A clinically applicable, uniform, quantitative definition of malnutrition has proved elusive. Nearly all measurements used to quantify malnutrition are either nonspecific due to effects of comorbid conditions on body habitus and laboratory values, too cumbersome or expensive for routine clinical use, or are only applicable to select patient populations. Generalized weakness, weight loss, and difficulty with oral intake are the most common presenting complaints in malnourished patients. On physical examination, patients may present with loss of subcutaneous tissue, as evidenced by loosening of the skin on the triceps, the midaxillary line of the costal margin, or the interosseous areas of the hands. Loss of skeletal muscle mass is most easily identified by symmetric loss of tone or bulk in the quadriceps (a neurologic lesion should always be considered if loss is asymmetric); loss in other muscle groups can be masked if the patient is obese.

Peripheral edema can occur in severe protein or total calorie malnutrition and is usually present in dependent areas such as the ankles or sacrum. Edema from malnutrition may be of such significant degree that patients appear to be at their normal body weight clinically, thereby masking true body mass loss.[2] While a considerable number of malnourished patients do present with a low body-mass index (<18), height and weight may be difficult to accurately obtain in severely debilitated or critically ill individuals due to multiple functional and logistical factors. Edema from intravenous resuscitative efforts or disease processes may further affect body weight, making these measurements unreliable for excluding malnutrition in many patients.[3]

Differential Diagnosis

The specific goals of nutritional support depend on the cause of the patient's malnourished state and the underlying clinical conditions. In general, patients who are malnourished due to inadequate provision, absorption, or utilization of nutrients can exhibit an anabolic response to nutritional supplementation and repletion of deficient micronutrients.

In the more common scenario, hospital patients are malnourished due to sickness associated anorexia and decreased food intake, coupled with increased nutrient losses and/or increased nutrient requirements due to an ongoing catabolic condition such as chronic infection or inflammation, sepsis, or trauma. These individuals have an impaired ability to exhibit protein anabolism regardless of provision of nutritional support, and they have increased micronutrient needs. Impaired anabolism is likely mediated indirectly by cytokines such as tumor necrosis factor (TNF-alpha) and interleukins (e.g., IL-6 and -8) and induction of catabolic counter-regulatory hormones (glucocorticoid, glucagons, catecholamines). Catabolic states are also associated with increased expression of intramuscular transcriptional and translational pathways that result in up-regulation of the ubiquitin proteasome pathway (UPP), the degradation pathway primarily responsible for catabolism in skeletal muscle.[4] Acidosis, in the presence of glucocorticoids, also up-regulates the UPP.[46]

Stress-induced protein catabolism can continue for several weeks after resolution of acute illness.[47] Anabolism is not possible in the setting of the above factors. Therefore, the primary goal of nutritional support in patients with severe acute illness is adequate provision of metabolic substrates to support body function.

Diagnosis

All patients admitted to the hospital should be screened for nutritional risk within 24 hours.[6] All patients who are determined to be at nutrition risk should undergo a nutrition assessment by a practitioner with specialized expertise in the area of nutrition. Patients are deemed to be at nutrition risk if they have evidence of malnutrition at baseline or have the potential for developing malnutrition. Patients who are currently receiving specialized enteral nutrition (EN) or parenteral nutrition (PN) support, and postoperative, trauma, or chronically ill patients can also be considered to be at nutrition risk. Each institution should have established criteria to determine patients' level of nutrition risk.[7]

No clinically applicable single test, laboratory value, or clinical finding exists that accurately assesses nutritional status in all clinical situations. When single physical examination measurements (e.g., triceps skin fold thickness) are used alone, variations in body mass distribution can result in misclassification of nutritional status in 30% of patients.[8] Multiple algorithms exist that combine history, physical examination findings, and/or laboratory markers to screen for malnutrition. However, many of these nutrition assessment parameters have related shortcomings when applied to use in the clinical setting.

The Subjective Global Assessment (SGA) employs a combination of history and physical examination, is widely adopted, and is the most thoroughly scrutinized tool for nutrition assessment (see Table 4-1). The factors have no numerical weighting scheme and are instead combined subjectively into an overall global assessment. Patients are then assigned one of three classes: class A, well-nourished or low risk of developing further malnutrition; class B, moderately malnourished or at risk of severe malnutrition; or class C, severely malnourished. Of note, patients who give a history of recent weight gain after prolonged or severe weight loss are considered well nourished, and patients who report an increased caloric intake after a prolonged period (≥6 months) of decreased intake are considered to be less at risk for continued malnutrition.[2] The SGA has been validated to accurately predict

risk of increased inpatient mortality, complications, and length of hospitalization[1] including inpatients with critical illness and concomitant renal failure.[47] The SGA has the added advantage of ease of applicability; however, a high level of training and expertise in the clinician is required. Limitations in completing the assessment tool due to patient's sedation or altered mental status may render it an unreliable tool in select certain clinical settings.

Biochemical Markers

Serum Albumin

In healthy individuals, approximately 200 mg/kg is produced via hepatic synthesis, which is matched by degradation and loss.[9] The half-life of albumin is 21 days, and its plasma concentration is also influenced by vascular permeability and total body water distribution between the intravascular and extravascular compartments.[9,10] Approximately one third of total body albumin normally resides in the intravascular compartment. Protein-calorie malnutrition results in decreased synthesis of albumin and subsequent decrease in the serum concentration during the first 8–12 weeks. In malnourished states lasting longer than approximately 12 weeks, degradation of albumin decreases, and changes in total body water distribution may result in normalization of the serum albumin concentration.[10,11] Serum concentrations of albumin, a negative acute phase reactant, rapidly decrease in acute episodes of infection or inflammation, as well as with hepatic disease or syndromes of increased protein loss, such as with peritoneal dialysis, nephrotic syndrome, or abdominal fistulae.[3,11] Thus, in the acute care setting, albumin is an extremely poor indicator of nutritional status, but, as an index of illness severity, it is an excellent predictor of clinical outcome.[10]

Other Serum Proteins

Transferrin and prealbumin (transthyretin) have the advantage of a shorter half-life of 8–10 days and 3 days, respectively, and therefore may reflect more acute changes in nutritional status. However, as with albumin, both transferrin and prealbumin are negative acute phase reactants.[9,11] These levels are therefore poor indicators for nutritional assessment in the hospitalized setting.[11]

C-Reactive Protein

C-Reactive protein is a positive acute phase reactant that increases during times of acute or catabolic illness. Hence, it may

Table 4-1 Subjective Global Assessment		
History	**Physical Examination***	**Classification**
Weight loss in last 6 months? In last 2 weeks?	Subcutaneous fat loss? (triceps, chest)	**Class A** <5% weight loss or >5% total weight loss with recent weight gain and/or improvement in appetite
Change in dietary intake? Duration of change?	Muscle wasting? (quadriceps, deltoids)	
Type of diet change (suboptimal solid, full liquid, hypocaloric liquid, starvation)	Edema? Ankle edema?	**Class B** 5%–10% weight loss, poor dietary intake, 1+ subcutaneous tissue loss
GI symptoms? (nausea, vomiting, diarrhea, dysphagia, anorexia)	Sacral edema? Ascites?	**Class C** >10% weight loss, 2– 3+ subcutaneous tissue loss, edema
Decreased functional capacity? Duration? Degree? (ambulatory, bedridden)		

* = Each category rated 0 to 3+.

Detsky AS, et al. Is this patient malnourished? JAMA 1994; 271(1):54–58.

Box 4-1 Major Components of Baseline and Serial Nutritional Assessment

1. Review past medical-surgical history and history of current illness and pre- and postsurgical course
   - Degree of catabolic stress
   - Organ function
   - Medications that may affect nutrient absorption, metabolism, or excretion
   - Medical/surgical procedures that are likely in the near-term

2. Perform detailed physical examination
   - Skeletal muscle wasting
   - Loss of fat stores
   - Skin/hair/tongue/conjunctival lesions suggestive of micronutrient deficiency
   - Evidence of organ dysfunction (e.g., gastrointestinal, liver, renal, cardiopulmonary)
   - Fluid status (e.g., normal, dehydrated, fluid overloaded, capillary leak)

3. Obtain body weight history
   - Current body weight (in light of fluid status)
   - Usual body weight, dry body weight
   - % Weight loss past several weeks, past several months
   - Current weight as % of ideal body weight

4. Determine dietary intake pattern
   - General food intake pattern, unusual consumption of specific foods
   - Previous enteral or parenteral nutritional support
   - Use of nutritional supplements

5. Evaluate gastrointestinal tract function
   - Swallowing difficulties, intestinal ileus, obstruction
   - Diarrhea, nausea, vomiting
   - Gastrointestinal bleeding

6. Evaluate selected biochemical tests relevant to nutritional status and organ function
   - Standard organ function indices and triglyceride levels
   - Electrolytes, including calcium, magnesium, and phosphorus

7. Estimate energy (calorie), protein and micronutrient needs
   - Harris-Benedict × 1.3 (use dry weight and adjusted weight if obese)
   - Protein/amino acid at goal 1.5 g/kg/day; adjust dose per usual criteria based on organ function

8. Evaluate enteral and parenteral access for nutrient delivery
   - Ability to take oral diet and/or liquid supplements
   - Central venous access, peripheral line access
   - Nasogastric, nasoenteric tube access

be a good means to evaluate the severity of patient physiologic stress, so as to better determine the usefulness in relying on other serum protein levels as a nutrition assessment parameter.

Nitrogen Balance

Nitrogen balance is calculated as follows:

$$= \frac{24 \text{ hour protein intake}}{6.25} - 24 \text{ hour urine urea nitrogen (UUN)} - k$$

k = estimated skin and stool daily nitrogen losses
≈ 2.5 g/day in healthy individuals

In theory, nitrogen balance is measured to assess ongoing adequacy of nutritional support, and therefore nutritional status, with positive values deemed to be indicative of lean mass anabolism. The value of the constant, k, can increase considerably in the setting of acute illness and, if uncorrected, can lead to falsely positive values. The 24-hour urine specimen requires accurate timing, and values may be influenced by glomerular filtration rate, renal disease, or presence of microbes in the genitourinary system or collecting receptacle. As a consequence, 24-hour UUN values are often prone to error.[11]

Prognosis

A loss of 10% of body weight in the setting of malignancy is associated with higher morbidity and mortality.[12] Weight loss greater than one third of body weight is associated with extremely high mortality within a few weeks of assessment.[13] Loss of lean body mass is associated with increased infection rates and prolonged recovery.[14] Malnutrition severity by SGA class is directly associated with risk of overall inpatient mortality.[1]

Biochemical markers influenced by physiologic stressors, such as those described in the preceding section, may serve as a reflection of clinical status and outcome. Low serum concentrations of albumin, total cholesterol, and HDL cholesterol are associated with increased surgical mortality, stroke mortality, and incidence of nosocomial infections, respectively.[15–17] It is unclear how provision of nutritional support affects morbidity and mortality as predicted by these laboratory values. Subsequent inappropriate provision of nutritional support based on biochemical markers may cause complications without achievement of any benefit.

Treatment

Initiation of Parenteral or Enteral Feeding: Specialized Nutritional Support (SNS)

In patients who are assessed to be well nourished at baseline, expert recommendations state that initiation of SNS may be delayed for up to 5–7 days after the clinical insult or initiation of hospitalization, unless the duration of insufficient intake is anticipated to exceed this period.[5,6] Few objective, clinical data are available to guide the timing of nutrient administration in critically ill patients. For patients in shock, adequate restoration of organ oxygenation and perfusion to peripheral tissues should be accomplished before SNS is initiated.[18] Prior to initiation of SNS, it is important that the risks versus benefits of this intervention be examined and the wishes of the patient or primary caregiver be discussed. Specific indications for initiation of SNS are listed in Box 4-2.

Box 4-2 Some Clinical Indications for Specialized Enteral or Parenteral Nutrition Support in Critically Ill Patients

- Food intake not possible for >5–7 days due to underlying illness
- Severe catabolic stress (e.g., burns, trauma, sepsis)
- Major gastrointestinal operations (PN)
- Medical illness associated with prolonged gastrointestinal dysfunction (diarrhea, nausea/vomiting) and/or in which oral food intake is contraindicated:
  – Bone marrow transplantation
  – Inflammatory bowel disease
  – Pancreatitis
  – High-output enterocutaneous fistula
  – Ileus or bowel obstruction
- Short bowel syndrome
- Preexisting moderate-to-severe protein-energy malnutrition and inability to maintain adequate enteral feeding to promote anabolism (PN)

PN = parenteral nutrition.

Table 4-2 Guidelines for Amino Acid/Protein Administration in Adult Hospital Patients

Condition	Amino Acid/Protein Intake Goal* (g protein/kg body weight per day)
Malnourished, clinically stable	1.5–2.0
Mild-to-moderate catabolic stress	1.5
Critically ill	1.5
Encephalopathy	0.6
Hepatic failure	0.6–1.0
Renal failure, not dialyzed	0.6–0.8
Renal failure, dialyzed	1.2

*Intake is adjusted proportional to hepatic and renal function indices.

Estimation of Energy Requirements

There is insufficient evidence to support the use of any one predictive equation for caloric requirements in hospitalized patients. Indirect calorimetry remains the gold standard and should be relied on when possible.[19–21] This technique is particularly useful in certain patient populations when estimation of requirements is challenging (i.e., patients who are very thin or very obese, with large wounds, severe critical illness, or on prolonged mechanical ventilation).[19] When indirect calorimetry is unavailable, the Harris-Benedict equation may be used to determine basal energy expenditure (BEE) in kcal/day.[21]

The Harris-Benedict Equation:

$$BEE\ for\ Men = 66 + (13.8 \times kg) + (5 \times cm\ height) - (6.76 \times age)$$
$$BEE\ for\ Women = 655 + (9.6 \times kg) + (1.85 \times cm\ height) - (4.7 \times age)$$

Predictive equations for energy expenditure in the hospitalized patient, including the Harris-Benedict equation, have many limitations. The presence of edema often makes body weight an unreliable variable for estimation of LBM. Metabolic alterations, numerous pharmacologic agents, level of physical activity, and comorbidities all play a vital role in influencing caloric and protein requirements. Predictive equations serve only as a general guideline to aid the clinician in determining patient requirements; clinical judgment should play a primary role in formulating the nutrition assessment, and reassessment should be performed at routine intervals. With this in mind, as general rule, a factor ranging from 1.2–1.5 times the BEE derived from the Harris-Benedict equation may be used for most hemodynamically stable hospitalized patients, with higher ranges used for patients in higher states of catabolic stress or those classified at increased nutritional risk based upon a higher SGA score.[5,6] Likewise, the lower end of the range should satisfy maintenance requirements. For intentional weight loss, a deficit of no more than 500 kcal/day should be applied.

Assessment of energy expenditure in the critically ill patient may present even more of a challenge. Cytokine and glucocorticoid-mediated glucose utilization is up-regulated in the central nervous system, immune system, and gastrointestinal tract, but down-regulated in nearly all other tissues by insulin resistance present after the glucose cell-wall transporter.[22] Increases in glucose production far exceed increases in glucose utilization in the setting of shock or other severe stress, resulting in hyperglycemia.[4,23] Uncontrolled hyperglycemia has been shown to increase mortality considerably, both in medical and surgical ICU populations, possibly due to the deleterious effects of hyperglycemia on hepatocyte mitochondrial function and circulating lipid composition.[24–27] Overfeeding of calories in the setting of stress-induced insulin resistance predisposes to hyperglycemia, without benefit of increased utilization of metabolic substrate.[22] Therefore, hypocaloric feeding goals are suggested during critical illness (e.g., <20 kcal/kg/day),[28] with maintenance of blood glucose control between 80–110 mg/dL and adequate amino acid/protein, micronutrient, and electrolyte provision (see below) as the primary emphasis until resolution of critical illness. Additional research is required to further delineate precise caloric needs in diverse critical care populations and the response to differing levels of energy intake.

Estimation of Amino Acid/Protein Requirements

The recommended daily allowance (RDA) for protein intake in healthy individuals is 0.8 g/kg/day. However, protein requirements in physiologically stressed hospitalized patients may vary considerably, dependent upon clinical circumstances, as outlined in Table 4-2. The optimal protein dose for physiologically stressed adult patients in the presence of normal renal and hepatic function appears to be approximately 1.5 g/kg/day, based on currently available data.[29–31] In patients with renal failure or insufficiency, the protein intake may need to be restricted to 0.6–0.8 g/kg/day, while patients receiving dialysis are typically able to tolerate 1.2–1.3 g/kg/day.[32] Some advocate early initiation of dialysis in renal failure patients, as opposed to a protein restricted regimen.[33]

Patients with hepatic failure with evidence of encephalopathy should be protein restricted ($\leq$ 0.6 g/kg/day).[34] Patients who suffer from chronic hepatitis or cirrhosis without encephalopathy may tolerate a somewhat higher intake of protein at approximately 1.2 g/kg.[34] Estimation of protein requirements by using a dry weight is preferred in patients with renal or hepatic disease. It is important to note that adequate total caloric intake is necessary for utilization of protein for anabolism; with insufficient energy, protein will be oxidized for energy and not used in protein synthetic reactions.[14]

Route of Specialized Natritional Support

In the setting of a functional gastrointestinal tract, enteral nutrition (EN) is the preferred route of nutrition support. Compared to parenteral nutrition (PN), EN support has been associated with such benefits as modulation of the immune response,[35] enhanced nitrogen balance,[36] improved glycemic control,[37,38] increased gastrointestinal morphology, integrity of barrier function,[39,40] and reduced cost.[41,42] PN support is associated with an increased incidence of infectious complications and a higher prevalence of steatosis, cholestasis, and hyperglycemia, often due to improper delivery of nutrients and overfeeding.[6,34,43] However, in conditions rendering the gastrointestinal tract nonfunctional (such as GI fluid loss, malabsorptive syndromes, ileus/obstruction), PN support is indicated. Feeding patients via the parenteral route may also serve to provide a more consistent delivery of nutrients and energy and a more rapid progression to the goal regimen.[37,42]

Administration of Parenteral Nutrition

The initial delivery of PN support should be gradual enough to establish tolerance to the prescribed feeding regimen. Patients who are nutritionally compromised at baseline are likely to undergo a refeeding response, as evidenced by a rapid fall in potassium, phosphorus, and magnesium levels in the blood during the first few days after initiation of nutrition support.[44,45] This is particularly evident with the introduction of a high dextrose-containing parenteral nutrition solution; however, it may also be seen following the provision of enteral feedings—in both cases mediated by an insulin-induced intracellular shift in potassium, magnesium, and phosphorus.[44,45] Initial parenteral solutions should thus be conservative with regard to the dextrose content, in order to better manage the refeeding response and promote better blood glucose control, particularly in patients who are deemed to be highly malnourished or hyperglycemic at baseline. An initial dextrose content of 100–150 g/day has been suggested for patients at high risk for refeeding. This may be titrated upward, as tolerated, over a period of several days in order to meet caloric goals, providing the final dextrose concentration does not exceed the maximum glucose oxidation rate of 5 mg/kg/minute.

Excessive carbohydrate loads are associated with such adverse effects as hyperglycemia, hepatic steatosis, and cholestasis.[5,6,34] The minimum requirement for carbohydrate has not been established; however, as a general recommendation, an estimate of 1 mg/kg/minute is suggested.[44,45] Protein requirements may often be met on the first day, unless the PN solution is limited due to volume restrictions. The exact requirement for fat intake in catabolic states has not been established. It is estimated that 2% to 4% of the caloric intake should be derived from linoleic and linolenic acid in order to prevent essential fatty acid deficiency.

Table 4-3 Macronutrient Table

Macronutrient	Estimated kilocalories/gram	Recommended source of kilocalories/day by percentage
Protein	4	15–25
Carbohydrate	3.4	45–65
Lipid	9	20–30

From Klein, S. A primer of nutritional support for gastroenterologists. Gastroenterol 2002; 122: 1677–1687.

This requirement can be satisfied with as little as 10% of the total calories from standard soy or safflower-based intravenous lipid emulsions.

There are potential immunosuppressive and proinflammatory effects from current soybean-based and omega-6 fatty acid-rich lipid emulsions by way of serving as a precursor to dienoic prostaglandins, specifically PGE_2. Thus, guidelines recommend limiting intravenous lipid emulsion to provide no more than 30% of the total calories or 1 g/kg/day. A further restriction in the lipid concentration may need to be applied if lipid clearance is determined to be compromised, based upon elevated triglyceride levels.[48] The amount of calories per macronutrient gram is provided in Table 4-3.

The initial provision of electrolytes may need to be increased in accordance with the anticipated severity of the refeeding response and serum levels upon initiation of nutrition therapy.[5,6,44,45] Further adjustments in the electrolyte content of the PN solution are based upon renal function, fluid and gastrointestinal losses, and various pharmacologic agents that may impact levels. Patients who are assessed to be malnourished at baseline and are at a high risk for refeeding syndrome and/or patients who have other high water-soluble nutrient losses (including diuresis) should receive thiamine supplementation at 100–200 mg/day for approximately 3 days, which may ameliorate refeeding syndrome electrolyte disturbances.[44]

The dosage of electrolytes required to maintain normal plasma levels is directly related to the dose of administered dextrose in patients with normal renal function. Table 4-4 shows typical dosage ranges for daily PN electrolyte concentrations in central venous PN formulas (which generally contain 10% to 25% dextrose) and peripheral vein PN solutions, which generally provide 5–7% dextrose. It is critical to serially monitor plasma glucose, electrolytes, and triglycerides and to adjust the PN prescription accordingly. The metabolic response to PN should be assessed clinically during periods of clinical instability by indirect calorimetry when available.[19–21] When the patient is extremely unstable, it may be necessary to provide a lowered amount or even discontinue specialized feeding until organ function stabilizes.

Therapy for intravenous trace elements and vitamins is directed at meeting the recommended dietary allowances (RDA) for micronutrients, with adjustments based on IV delivery.[6] Zinc is an important nutrient for immune function, wound healing, protein synthesis, and gastrointestinal mucosal regeneration. Supplemental zinc (and possibly other trace elements such as selenium) should be provided in patients with burns, large wounds, severe

Table 4-4 Guidelines for Electrolyte and Micronutrient Administration in Parenteral Nutrient (PN) Solutions

Element	Peripheral PN	Central PN
Potassium (mEq/L)	20–40	40–60
Sodium (mEq/L)	30–75	50–75
Phosphorus (mEq/L)	5–8	10–15
Calcium (mEq/L)	5	5
Magnesium (mEq/L)	5–8	10–15
Multivitamins	Standard products available to admix	
Trace elements	Standard products available to admix	
Vitamin K (mg/day)	1	1

Electrolytes are adjusted as indicated to maintain serially measured serum levels within the normal range; the percentage of sodium and potassium salts as chloride is increased to correct metabolic alkalosis, and the percentage of salts as acetate is increased to correct metabolic acidosis.

pancreatitis, and/or significant gastrointestinal fluid losses. Approximately 12 mg of zinc are lost per liter of small bowel fluid, and urinary excretion of zinc increases dramatically as a function of the degree of catabolic stress. Administration of 5–10 mg per day of additional zinc intravenously (or 200–400 mg of zinc sulfate per day enterally) during severe catabolic illness reduces the risk of continued total body zinc depletion. Recent data also suggest that depletion of thiamine is not uncommon in patients receiving chronic diuretic therapy, as noted previously.[6]

Initiation and Administration of Enteral Nutrition Support

The decision on EN access should be based upon the anticipated duration of nutrition therapy. For shorter-term EN support, a nasoenteric feeding tube is advised, or an oroenteric tube when the nasal route is contraindicated. For patients for whom a longer course of EN support is indicated, placement of a more permanent feeding tube such as a percutaneous gastrostomy tube (G-tube or PEG) or jejunostomy tube (J-tube) is advised. In patients with normal gastric function, a nasogastric or G-tube/ PEG is preferred. Patients with delayed gastric emptying, those who have undergone gastric resection, or patients at a high risk for aspiration may benefit from feeding tube placement in the small bowel.[6]

The determination of the most appropriate enteral formula may vary, based upon the patient's specific disease requirements, fluid status, and gastrointestinal function. Specialty enteral feeding products are available to meet the specific needs for patients with many specific diseases. Specific fiber, protein, and immunomodulatory nutrient supplemented formulas exist (their description is beyond the scope of this chapter). Enteral feedings are typically initiated via a slow continuous infusion and may be slowly titrated up to the goal infusion rate via set increments, dependent upon patient tolerance as determined clinically. Measurement of enteral residual content of feedings alone should not supplant clinical judgment in determining patient tolerance of EN. In patients who require a more prolonged course of EN support, a transition to an evening cyclic feeding regimen or bolus/gravity flow feedings for patients with gastric feeding tube access may be indicated.

Key Points

- Between 30% and 50% of hospitalized patients may suffer from some degree of protein-energy malnutrition, and it has a significant effect on morbidity and mortality in a variety of clinical situations.

- All hospitalized patients should undergo assessment of nutritional status.

- The Subjective Global Assessment (SGA) is superior to individual clinical or biochemical markers for accurate assessment of nutritional status.

- Albumin is an extremely poor indicator of nutritional status, but, as an index of illness severity, it is an excellent predictor of clinical outcome.

- Anabolism is not possible in the setting of critical illness; the goal of nutritional support in critical illness is to support bodily functions, and overfeeding to attempt anabolism in the setting of critical illness may be harmful.

- Once resuscitation is accomplished, specialized nutritional support should be instituted earlier as the risk of present or developing nutritional compromise increases.

SUGGESTED READING

Waitzberg DL, et al. Nutritional assessment in the hospitalized patient. Curr Opin Clin Nutr Metab Care 2003; 6:531–538.

ASPEN Board of Directors and the Clinical Guidelines Task Force. Guidelines for the use of parenteral and enteral nutrition in adult and pediatric patients. JPEN J Parenter Enteral Nutr 2002; 26(Suppl 1): 1SA–138SA.

Russell MK, Andrews MR, Brewer CK, et al. Standards for specialized nutrition support: adult hospitalized patients. Nutr Clin Prac 2002; 17:384–391.

Covinsky KE, Covinsky MH, Palmer RM, et al. Serum albumin concentration and clinical assessments of nutritional status in hospitalized older people: different sides of different coins? J Am Geriatr Soc 2002; 50:631–637.

Canturk NZ, Canturk N, Okay E, et al. Risk of nosocomial infections and effects of total cholesterol, HDL cholesterol in surgical patients. Clin Nutr 2002; 21:431–436.

Jacobs DG, Jacobs DO, Kudsk KA, et al. Practice management guidelines for nutritional support of the trauma patient. J Trauma 2004; 57:660–679.

MacDonald A, Hildebrandt L. Comparison of formulaic equations to determine energy expenditure in the critically ill patient. Nutrition 2003; 19:233–239.

Frankenfield DC, Muth ER, Rowe WA. The Harris-Benedict studies of human basal metabolism: history and limitations. J Am Diet Assoc 1998; 98:970–971.

Mesotten D, Swinnen JV, Vanderhoydone F, et al. Contribution of circulating lipids to the improved outcome of critical illness by glycemic control with intensive insulin therapy. J Clin Endocrinol Metab 2004; 89:219–226.

Jeejeebhoy KN. Permissive underfeeding of the critically ill patient. NCP 2004; 19:477–480.

Jeejeebhoy KN. Enteral and parenteral nutrition: evidence-based approach. Proc Nutr Soc 2001; 60:399–402.

Braga M, Gianotti L, Gentilini O, et al. Early postoperative enteral nutrition improves gut oxygenation and reduces costs compared with total parenteral nutrition. Crit Care Med 2001; 29:242–248.

Crook MA, Haliy V, Panteli JV. The importance of the refeeding syndrome. Nutr 2001; 17:632–637.

CHAPTER FIVE

Approach to the Geriatric Patient

Robert M. Palmer, MD, MPH

BACKGROUND

Although they comprise only 13% of the American population, patients aged 65 years and older account for more than 38% of discharges from nonfederal acute hospitals and 46% of days of care.[1] Compared to younger adults, elderly patients have longer lengths of stay and greater costs of care. Rates of hospitalization are more than twice as great for the age group 85 years and older compared with those age 65–74 years.[1] Aging of the population and the high prevalence of chronic diseases help explain the growing recognition that hospital care is mostly geriatric care, whether clinical practice is in general medicine or surgery.

The diagnostic evaluation, management, and posthospital care of hospitalized patients are often very different for the oldest patients compared to younger adults. The oldest patients frequently present to the hospital with multiple chronic diseases, functional impairments or disability, nonspecific presentations of disease, cognitive impairment, and social dysfunction. Their hospital course is often complicated by a loss of self-care ability that ultimately increases their risk of placement in a skilled nursing facility or nursing home. Not uncommonly, the acute medical illness resolves promptly with appropriate medical treatment, but the patients get worse as they become more physically dysfunctional. This "dysfunctional syndrome" is attributable to characteristics of the patients and to elements of hospitalizations that are potentially amenable to interventions of comprehensive assessment and interdisciplinary team collaboration.[2] A systematic evaluation of the older patient enables the hospitalist to detect patients at risk for adverse outcomes of hospitalization that are most commonly associated with "geriatric syndromes"—complexes of common medical problems with multiple causes (Table 5-1). Chapter 6 explores functional assessment of the hospitalized geriatric patient in more detail.

ASSESSMENT: GERIATRIC SYNDROMES

Functional Dependency (Disability)

Even prior to an acute illness that requires hospitalization, more than one third of medically ill patients with a mean age of 80 years require personal assistance for the performance of five basic activities of daily living (ADL): bathing, dressing, transferring from bed to chair, toileting, and eating. By the time of hospital discharge, a third of these patients will lose independence in one or more of these ADL.[3] Advanced age is associated with the failure to recover ADL function during hospitalization in patients who declined before admission and who experience new losses of ADL function during hospitalization. Patients 90 years of age or older are less likely to recover ADL function lost before admission and more likely to develop new functional deficits during hospitalization.[4] About 40% of elderly medical patients lose independence in one or more instrumental ADL (IADL: using a telephone, shopping for groceries, using public transportation, preparing meals, taking medications, handling finances) 90 days after discharge compared to their pre-illness. Functional decline in elderly hospitalized patients is associated with advanced age, cognitive impairment (especially delirium) at hospital admission, dependence prior to admission in performance of IADL, depressive symptoms, and subjective reports of unsteadiness at admission.[5]

Dependence in basic ADL and IADL has major significance for elderly patients. Functional dependency is associated with a longer length of hospital stay, greater risk of nursing home transfer, and death. The importance of functional measures as predictors of 1-year mortality was demonstrated in a study of hospitalized patients with a mean age of 80 years. Independent risk factors for mortality included male sex, number of dependent activities of daily living (ADL) at discharge, congestive heart failure, cancer, creatinine level >3.0 mg/dL, and serum albumin <3.5 g/dL.[6] Dependence in baseline IADL is also a predictor of 2-year mortality.

Interventions designed to reduce the risks of functional decline in elderly hospitalized patients have shown modest benefits in functional status, length of hospital stay, and skilled nursing home admissions, although mortality has not been reduced.[3,7] Many of the interventions used in clinical trials can be easily adapted by hospitalists working with an interdisciplinary team. Together with the patient's nurses, the hospitalist can observe the patient's ability to perform ADL. Steps can be taken to prevent functional decline or to restore function that was lost with the acute illness (see Table 5-1). Close collaboration with advanced practice nurses during transitional care of hospitalized patients with heart failure can also help to prevent unplanned hospital readmission.[8]

Table 5-1 Geriatric Syndromes in Hospitalized Patients

Syndrome	Clinical Features	Management
Functional disability	Need for personal assistance in the performance of basic activities of daily living (BADL): bathing, dressing, transferring from bed to chair, using toilet, and eating. Detected by physician and nurse observing patient perform BADL in hospital.	Encourage independent self-care and ambulation: Avoid physical restraints. Avoid "bed rest" orders. Keep patient out of bed. Order bedside commode. Consult occupational therapy for more formal ADL assessment if ADL decline/impairment is present. Consult physical therapy if patient has mobility, transfer, or gait impairments. Prescribe assistive devices and aids to enable patient self-care. Avoid prescribing hypnotics or sedatives.
Cognitive impairment: *Delirium*	Change in mental status from baseline; inattentive; fluctuating level of alertness; inappropriate behavior or thought processes; altered level of consciousness and motor activity (the confusion assessment method criteria).	Create supportive environment: For patient with risk factors for delirium, "reality orientation": introduce yourself each visit, remind patient of day, reason for hospitalization, upcoming diagnostic studies and consultants, plans for follow-up visit. Correction and prevention of dehydration
Dementia	Progressive decline over months to years in cognition; patient is alert and attentive; memory, language skills, and self-care are impaired	Optimize vision (corrective lenses, diffuse lighting in room) and hearing (aids, amplifying devices, face-to-face conversations with door of patient's room closed). Encourage family visits and social interactions or assign sitter for demented patients.
Malnutrition	Low body mass index; generalized muscle atrophy or weakness (sarcopenia); history of unintentional weight loss; anemia, low serum albumin, low serum cholesterol	Choose enteral over parenteral alimentation; order modified barium swallow when oropharyngeal dysphagia is suspected; add nutritional supplements, calorie-dense foods (Figure 5-1).
Immobility	Patient unable to transfer from bed to chair, bear weight or walk without assistance; common causes are physical deconditioning, neurologic diseases, medications, and physical restraints.	Prescribe graded aerobic and low-intensity resistive exercises: range-of-motion (passive or active), resistance of feet and legs against hands during bedside rounds, assisted ambulation; avoid physical restraints and psychotropic drugs; treat orthostatic hypotension; obtain physical therapy consultation; prescribe assistive devices, walkers, lifts.
Urinary incontinence	Involuntary loss of urine; suspect in patients who are immobile, cognitively impaired, restrained, or are receiving drugs with anticholinergic effects.	Evaluate for overflow incontinence due to bladder outlet obstruction or an acontractile bladder: suprapubic fullness, large postvoid residual (>150 mL) after catheterization. Use indwelling catheter or intermittent straight catheterization for overflow incontinence. Begin toileting schedule, bedside commode or urinal for stress or urge incontinence.
Pressure ulcers	Patients often immobile, cognitively impaired, malnourished. Pressure ulcer, stages I-IV: nonblanching erythema; blisters or open ulcers to dermis; or through dermis; or through subcutaneous structures.	Reduce pressure on bony prominences, shearing forces, friction, and skin moisture; turn frequently; use air support mattresses, consider skin emollients; skin care nurse consult; surgical consult for stage IV ulcers.
Constipation	Immobile, dehydrated patients; treatment with medications that interfere with colonic motility: narcotics, drugs with anticholinergic effects; low-fiber diet	Ensure adequate oral or intravenous hydration; evacuate fecal impactions, then begin water-soluble fiber supplements plus osmolar laxatives; progressive physical activity: up in chair, assisted ambulation, walking.
Depression	Depressive symptoms or history of major affective disorder; "failure-to-thrive"; uncooperative, poorly motivated; dysphoric mood, anxiety, or impaired concentration	Supportive environment: encourage family visits, occupational therapies; consultation by nurse specialist or psychiatrist; review of medications (discontinue central nervous system depressants).

Cognitive Impairment

Impaired cognition, usually due to dementia or delirium (*see* Table 5-1), is present in approximately one third of hospitalized elderly patients admitted to general medical services. Delirium is more common in elderly patients with baseline cognitive and sensory impairments, and dehydration. Medications, especially those with psychotropic properties (e.g., anticholinergic agents, antihistamines), are associated with delirium. Detection of cognitive impairment due to either dementia or delirium includes a mental status examination at admission and an interview with family caregivers to determine the patient's baseline level of cognition. Progress notes from physicians, nurses, and other health care professionals can also reveal evidence of possible delirium, suggested by the notation of a "change in mental status." Certain behaviors (agitation, restlessness, inappropriate verbalizations) are often suggestive of the diagnosis of delirium. Delirium can be diagnosed with confidence when the patient's symptoms meet the criteria of the confusion assessment method (*see* Table 5-1). A quick method of detecting delirium during bedside rounds is the digit span test (Box 5-1). Patients with impaired attention are often unable to repeat up to five consecutive digits, whereas normal or only mildly demented patients usually can.

Delirium in at-risk medically ill, hospitalized elderly patients can be reduced by 40% with a multicomponent targeted risk factor intervention. The intervention is multidisciplinary and targeted at patients age 70 years and older who have one or more risk factors for delirium (cognitive impairment, sleep deprivation, immobility, dehydration, vision or hearing impairment). The interventions include daily visitors and reality orientation, therapeutic activities, early mobilization, visual protocols (visual aids), hearing amplification, oral volume repletion and/or feeding assistance, and sleep enhancement with a nondrug protocol.[9] The incidence of postoperative delirium is reduced in elderly hip fracture patients through attention to the patient's oxygenation, fluid and electrolyte balance, treatment of severe pain, elimination of unnecessary medications, adequate nutritional intake, early mobilization and rehabilitation, and appropriate environment stimuli.[10] These simple steps to prevent delirium are also appropriate care for dementia patients.

The severity of cognitive impairment can be documented with the use of standardized and validated measures, such as the Mini-Mental State Examination, a 30-item measure, a clock drawing test, or elements of both combined in the Mini-Cog screen.[11] Repeat administration of these instruments provides objective evidence of changes in mental status throughout the hospitalization. This information helps to guide estimates of patient prognosis and discharge disposition.

Malnutrition

Undernutrition, especially protein–energy malnutrition (PEM), and specific nutrient deficiencies are common in chronically ill elderly patients who are hospitalized for treatment of acute exacerbations of chronic diseases. However, nutritional needs are frequently unrecognized or unaddressed early in the patient's hospital course, often delaying recovery from an acute illness or the healing of wounds and pressure ulcers.[12] PEM also contributes to the excess risk of death from various chronic diseases, such as congestive heart failure. PEM can be suspected in patients with unintentional weight loss, physical evidence of muscle atrophy, and low levels of serum proteins (e.g., serum albumin <3.5 g/dL). Assessment of nutritional status considers the presence of sarcopenia (loss of muscle mass with aging), the effects of chronic diseases (e.g., chronic lung and heart diseases, cancer), and the effects of inflammation on the common nutritional markers (e.g., increasing serum transferrin, declining serum albumin). Although no single parameter is diagnostic of malnutrition, PEM is likely in elderly patients who have a documented history of weight loss, low body weight, muscle atrophy, and generalized muscle weakness.[13]

Studies suggest that nutritional supplements containing balanced mixtures of amino acids, fat, carbohydrate, vitamins, and minerals improve the prognosis of elderly patients with specific illnesses. The strongest evidence for the effectiveness of nutritional supplementation exists for meeting the oral protein and energy requirements for treatment of hip fractures.[14] Frequent calorie-dense, nutritious, and palatable food supplements or snacks are recommended for malnourished and weak patients who may be unable to consume a standard meal. Patients at risk for aspiration pneumonia due to generalized weakness or oropharyngeal dysphagia should undergo formal evaluation of swallowing conducted by a speech therapist, usually followed by a modified barium swallow. A pureed diet or thickened liquids for patients with dysphagia for liquids may enable them to swallow safely, and can provide sufficient calories and hydration. In general, the oral tract is the preferred route for feeding patients. Because dysphagia is common in elderly ill patients, alternative methods of nutritional support are often employed until the patient can safely eat and drink fluids. The common routes of nutritional interventions are summarized in Figure 5-1. Percutaneous endoscopic gastrostomy (PEG) tubes have been used to provide nutrition to demented patients. In prospective studies of hospitalized patients with advanced dementia, high 6-month median mortality occurs, and tube feeding is not associated with survival.[15] There is no evidence that PEG tubes prevent aspiration pneumonia or other infections. Consequently, in the absence of clinical trials, a PEG tube is best considered for treatment of patients with acute illnesses whose prognosis for improvement is good, but their ability to take food by mouth is predicted to be delayed for weeks to months.

Practical issues arise when using intravenous lines or feeding tubes. Cognitively impaired patients might inadvertently pull out

Box 5-1 Digit Span Test

1. Gain the patient's attention, eliminate extraneous noise.

2. Instruct the patient, "I am going to ask you to repeat some numbers after me. First I will say them. Then you say them." (e.g., "If I say '3, 8', you would say _____?").

3. Once patient appears to understand the instructions, begin by asking him to repeat three random single numbers, spoken in a monotone at one-second intervals (e.g., 3, 8, 2).

4. Repeat the task by increasing the repetition from three to four, then five random numbers.

Patients with delirium are usually unable to repeat five random numbers correctly.

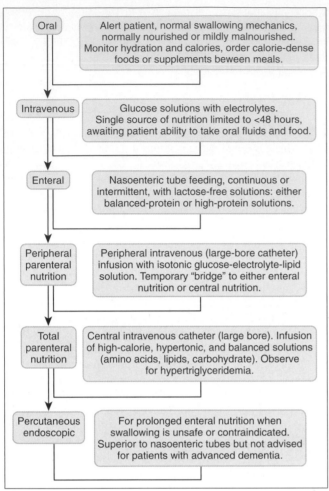

Oral	Alert patient, normal swallowing mechanics, normally nourished or mildly malnourished. Monitor hydration and calories, order calorie-dense foods or supplements beween meals.
Intravenous	Glucose solutions with electrolytes. Single source of nutrition limited to <48 hours, awaiting patient ability to take oral fluids and food.
Enteral	Nasoenteric tube feeding, continuous or intermittent, with lactose-free solutions: either balanced-protein or high-protein solutions.
Peripheral parenteral nutrition	Peripheral intravenous (large-bore catheter) infusion with isotonic glucose-electrolyte-lipid solution. Temporary "bridge" to either enteral nutrition or central nutrition.
Total parenteral nutrition	Central intravenous catheter (large bore). Infusion of high-calorie, hypertonic, and balanced solutions (amino acids, lipids, carbohydrate). Observe for hypertriglyceridemia.
Percutaneous endoscopic	For prolonged enteral nutrition when swallowing is unsafe or contraindicated. Superior to nasoenteric tubes but not advised for patients with advanced dementia.

Figure 5-1 • Nutritional routes: clinical considerations.

these lines or disconnect them from the infusion line. Rather than restraining these patients, nurses often attempt to hide the line, cover it with gauze or large pads, or place the nasogastric tube out of patient view or reach (e.g., above forehead). Many restraint reduction programs in hospitals with multidisciplinary teams have developed alternatives to physical restraint that appear to be acceptable to patients and do not increase the risk of disruption of needed therapies.[16]

Immobility

Acute illness often leads to loss of mobility, free movement, and walking. Elderly patients are predisposed to immobility as a result of impaired homeostatic reserves (organ system dysfunction), reduced muscle mass and strength, disuse atrophy, the catabolic effects of severe disease, and various tethers such as physical restraints that prevent free movement. Furthermore, prolonged bed rest reduces the patient's ability to transfer from bed to chair or to stand without assistance. Immobility is also associated with postural hypotension, falls, skin tears, pressure ulcers, and venous thromboses.[17] Prolonged immobility often causes hypoxemia, constipation, reduced cardiac output, and bone demineralization.

Mobility can be achieved by encouraging patients to get out of bed and to walk in hallway corridors with or without personal assistance or mobility aids such as walkers or canes, and with

physical therapy consultation. With supervision, patients can perform low-impact aerobic and low-intensity resistive exercises and range-of-motion (passive or active) exercises.[18] During hospital rounds, the hospitalist can observe the patient's efforts to transfer and walk. At the bedside, patients can be asked to resist feet and legs against hands as they are observed for signs of weakness or pain. Mobility is further encouraged by avoiding orders for physical restraints and psychotropic drugs and by treating orthostatic hypotension with fluids and compression stockings. Impaired patients are further evaluated for causes of immobility.

Other Geriatric Syndromes

Urinary and bowel incontinence, constipation, and pressure sores are common occurrences in hospitalized elderly patients (*see* Table 5-1). Acute onset of urinary incontinence should always raise the possibility of overflow incontinence, especially in males. A check of postvoid residual will help to sort out the cause of incontinence: a high postvoid residual (e.g., >150 mL) suggests either bladder outlet obstruction or an acontractile bladder, and implies the need for placement of an indwelling urinary catheter pending further evaluation or resolution. Constipation is easier to prevent or treat if patients are allowed to be mobile, to consume foods high in fiber and fluids, and stopped from receiving medications that have anticholinergic effects (e.g., Benadryl). Pressure ulcers are a complication of immobility. See Chapter 27 for a detailed review. Prevention is often difficult but achievable through recognition of patients at risk, frequent turning of immobile patients, and reduction of pressure on bony prominences. Treatment of pressure ulcers depends on the stage of the ulcer but is usually medical for superficial ulcers (stages 1–3) and surgical for deeper ulcers (stage 4).

Clinical depression is found in about 25% of medically ill hospitalized elderly patients. Depression can be detected through a careful medical history of treatment for a mood disorder and the use of screening instruments. Patients with adjustment disorders due to acute or chronic diseases may present with depressive symptoms that improve with treatment of their medical conditions. Depression predicts functional decline and increases the risk of subsequent mortality.[19] Major depression will require psychologic and/or pharmacologic therapy. In the absence of clinical trials, an effort to detect and treat depression in the hospital is warranted, given its adverse effects on clinical outcomes.

Iatrogenic Illness

Iatrogenic illness is any illness that results from a diagnostic procedure or therapeutic intervention and that is not a natural consequence of the patient's disease. Iatrogenic illness arises from either medications, diagnostic and therapeutic procedures, nosocomial infections, or environmental hazards. Prevention of illness resulting from medications begins with an appreciation of age-related changes in drug disposition and sensitivity; a knowledge of the pharmacology of drugs in relation to aging; the use of lower than usual doses when the geriatric dose in unknown; the avoidance of psychoactive drugs when alternatives such as behavioral or environmental alternatives are available; and the cautious monitoring of patients receiving two or more drugs that are inducers or inhibitors of phase I hepatic metabolism (cytochrome P450), or are highly protein bound.[20] The risk of

Table 5-2 Medications of Risk and Their Alternatives

Medications of Risk	Recommendations	Alternatives
Antihistamines: Confusion, oversedation, orthostatic hypotension, falls, constipation and urinary retention due to anticholinergic effects		
Diphenhydramine Hydroxyzine	Avoid use as hypnotic. Avoid use as opioid adjunct. Use lowest effective dose for allergic reactions. Use a nonsedating antihistamine for seasonal allergy.	Hypnotics: Temazepam 7.5 mg hs Zolpidem 5 mg hs Trazodone 50 mg hs (off-label indication) Nonsedating antihistamines: Loratadine 10 mg daily Fexofenadine 60 mg daily or BID
Narcotic Analgesics: Meperidine—confusion, oversedation, orthostatic hypotension, falls, constipation, and urinary retention due to anticholinergic effects; metabolite may produce agitation and seizures; short duration of analgesia. Propoxyphene—poor analgesic effect with usual opioid anticholinergic effects		
Meperidine Propoxyphene	Use alternative pain medication.	Acetaminophen—provides analgesia equivalent to propoxyphene; add codeine or oxycodone if pain relief inadequate: oxycodone 2.5 mg q4–6 h Morphine: initially low doses (e.g., 2–4 mg q3–4 h) suffice
Benzodiazepines: Confusion, sedation, and falls		
Diazepam Chlordiazepoxide	Use shorter acting agent for anxiety, and for alcohol or benzodiazepine withdrawal. Use a low dose antipsychotic to treat agitation and psychosis.	Anxiety or withdrawal: Lorazepam 0.5–1 mg q6 h prn Oxazepam 10 mg q6 h prn Agitation/psychosis: Haloperidol 0.5–2 mg BID or TID Risperidone 0.5 mg BID
Tricyclic Antidepressants: Confusion, oversedation, orthostatic hypotension, falls, constipation, and urinary retention due to anticholinergic effects		
Amitriptyline Imipramine Doxepin	Use less anticholinergic TCA for neuropathic pain; use alternative agents (e.g., SSRI) for depression	Neuropathic pain: Desipramine 10–20 mg daily Nortriptyline 10–25 mg daily
Antiemetics: Confusion, oversedation, orthostatic hypotension, falls, constipation, and urinary retention due to anticholinergic effects. Trimethobenzamide—low potency antiemetic, highly anticholinergic		
Promethazine Prochlorperazine Trimethobenzamide	Use lowest effective dose. Avoid use as opioid adjunct.	Promethazine 12.5 mg q6 h prn Prochlorperazine 5 mg q6 h prn
Histamine–2 Receptor Blocker: Confusion, depression, and headache due to decreased renal elimination		
Famotidine	Reduce usual dose by 50%	Famotidine 10–20 mg daily or 20 mg every other day Consider proton pump inhibitor as alternative.

TCA—tricyclic antidepressants; SSRI—selective seratonin reuptake inhibitor

adverse drug events can be reduced by avoiding use of medications with anticholinergic or psychotropic effects, avoiding use of meperidine; and judiciously using opioids, nonsteroidal anti-inflammatory agents and histamine-2 antagonists (Table 5-2).[21] Elderly patients are often prescribed multiple, evidence-based, medications that are recommended in disease-specific guidelines. The guidelines largely ignore the issue of tradeoffs between the marginal benefits of multiple medications and the risks of adverse effects on physical, social, and cognitive functioning in older patients.[22] Caution is needed before adding more guideline-driven medications to the hospitalized patient's regimen.

PERSONAL PREFERENCES FOR CARE

The optimal care of seriously ill patients is often best understood by taking into account their treatment preferences.[23] A review of the patient's advance directives, either a living will or a durable power of attorney for health care, will help guide clinical decision making when the patient is unable to make informed decisions. When discussing advance directives with capable patients, hospi-

talists should also seek their wishes for end-of-life care, including cardiopulmonary resuscitation, intensive care, or nutritional support during acute or end-stage illness. When decisions need to be made under emergent conditions, it may be unclear what course of action to take for a patient facing critical illness. Frequent discussions with the patient and family will inform decision-making by identifying the patients' personal values about health and their expectations of hospitalization. For the most challenging patients and their families, this may be best accomplished in a "family conference" (Box 5-2).

DISCHARGE PLANNING

Discharge planning is facilitated by an interdisciplinary process that identifies patients who will need nursing home placement or home care services. It also serves to estimate the patient's hospital length of stay; to review with the patient and family the patient's diagnosis, prognosis, and choices for discharge location; and to review medications, home safety and the promotion of self-care. The site of discharge is largely based on the patient's functional

Box 5-2 The Family Conference

A family conference is helpful when:

- Patient has complex illness: unclear or multiple concurrent diseases.
- Need exists to clarify goals of therapy: patient's wishes and values, likely outcomes of hospitalization.
- Need exists to review advance directives: CPR (code status), ICU transfers, life support, artificial nutrition.
- Need exists to resolve conflicts in care management between health professionals, patients, family members ("adjudication" of differences).

Process of Family Conference

Through interdisciplinary team collaboration, identify patients with indications for family conference.

With cognitively intact patients:

- Review the presumed diagnoses
- Review advance directives
- Review diagnostic and therapeutic plans and their alternatives
- Ascertain their goals of therapy and expectations of the outcome of the current hospitalization

With patient consent: review the above with the patient's next of kin, power of attorney for health care, and family members designated by the patient.

With cognitively impaired patients:

- Review advance directives
- Meet or call power of attorney for health care (or, if none, the next of kin)
- Review presumed diagnoses
- Review advance directives
- Review diagnostic and therapeutic plans and their alternatives
- Ascertain their goals of therapy and expectations of the outcome of the current hospitalization ("substituted judgment")

Overcome any barriers to communication and agreement among team members, family, and patient: consider

- Second opinion from another specialist
- Ethics consultation when ethical dilemma is identified
- Second family conference when all family members are available for mediation
- Additional support services (family counseling)
- Clergy consultation and assistance

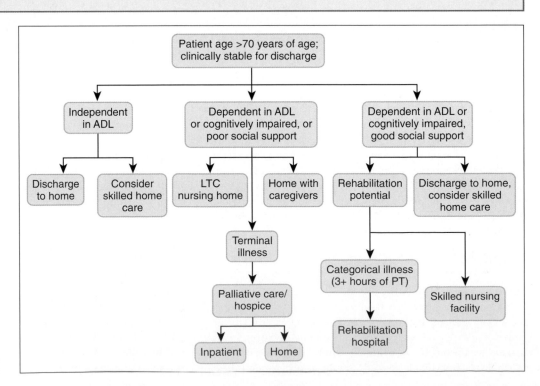

Figure 5-2 • Discharge sites.

ADL—activities of daily living; LTC—long-term care; PT—physical therapy

status and the availability of family and paid caregivers (Fig. 5-2). For patients with limited rehabilitation potential, a long-term care nursing home can provide personal care and ensure the patient's safety. Patients with an educational disadvantage appear to be at greater risk of functional decline.[23] Patients with low education (less than high school) compared to those with greater level of education have poorer functional recovery. Patients with cognitive dysfunction at the time of hospital admission are also less likely to recover in the short term and will be more likely to need an alternative site at discharge.[24] The patient's baseline level of ADL functioning can be used at the time of hospitalization to project functional recovery, although the oldest patients will have the slowest rate of recovery.[4, 25] Ideally, patients should be discharged when clinically stable; when there is no new finding on the planned day of discharge of incontinence (e.g., chest pain, dyspnea, delirium, tachycardia, or hypotension; a temperature >38.3°C; or a diastolic blood pressure is ≥105 mmHg).

Key Points

- About 40% of elderly medical patients lose independence in one or more instrumental ADL after discharge compared to prior to the illness that precipitated hospitalization.

- Interventions designed to reduce the risks of functional decline in elderly hospitalized patients have shown modest benefits on functional status, length of hospital stay, and skilled nursing home admissions, although mortality has not been reduced.

- A quick method of detecting delirium during bedside rounds is the digit span test.

- Delirium in at-risk, medically ill, hospitalized elderly patients can be reduced by 40% with a multicomponent targeted risk factor intervention.

- The incidence of postoperative delirium is reduced in elderly hip fracture patients through attention to the patient's oxygenation, fluid and electrolyte balance, treatment of severe pain, elimination of unnecessary medications, adequate nutritional intake, early mobilization and rehabilitation, and appropriate environment stimuli.

- Protein–energy malnutrition (PEM) is common in chronically ill elderly patients who are hospitalized for treatment of acute exacerbations of chronic diseases, but frequently unrecognized or unaddressed early in the patient's hospital course, often delaying recovery from an acute illness or the healing of wounds and pressure ulcers.

- PEG tube is best considered for treatment of patients with acute illnesses whose prognosis for improvement is good, but their ability to take food by mouth is predicted to be delayed for weeks to months. It does not reduce mortality among patients with advanced dementia.

- Prolonged bed rest or immobility reduces a patient's ability to transfer from bed to chair or to stand without assistance, and is associated with postural hypotension, falls, skin tears, pressure ulcers, and venous thromboses.

SUGGESTED READING

Counsell SR, Holder CM, Liebenauer LL, et al. Effects of a multicomponent intervention on functional outcomes and process of care in hospitalized older patients: a randomized controlled trial of acute care for elders (ACE) in a community hospital. J Am Geriatr Soc 2000; 48:1572–1581.

Covinsky KE, Palmer RM, Fortinsky RH, et al. Loss of independence in activities of daily living in older adults hospitalized with medical illnesses: increased vulnerability with age. J Am Geriatr Soc 2003; 51:451–458.

Lindenberger EC, Landefeld CS, Sands LP, et al. Unsteadiness reported by older hospitalized patients predicts functional decline. J Am Geriatr Soc 2003; 51:621–626.

Walter LC, Brand RJ, Counsell SR, et al. Development and validation of a prognostic index for 1-year mortality in older adults after hospitalization. JAMA 2001; 285:2987–2994.

Naylor MD, Brooten DA, Campbell RL, et al. Transitional care of older adults hospitalized with heart failure: a randomized controlled trial. J Am Geriatr Soc 2004; 52:675–684.

Marcantonio ER, Flacker JM, Wright RJ, et al. Reducing delirium after hip fracture: a randomized trial. J Am Geriatr Soc 2001; 49:516–522.

Borson S, Scanlan JM, Chen P, et al. The Mini-Cog as a screen for dementia: validation in a population-based sample. J Am Geriatr Soc 2003; 51:1451–1454.

Avenell A, Handoll HH. Nutritional supplementation for hip fracture aftercare in the elderly. Cochrane Database Syst Rev 2005; (1).

Meier DE, Ahronheim JC, Morris J, et al. High short-term mortality in hospitalized patients with advanced dementia: lack of benefit of tube feeding. Arch Intern Med 2001; 161:594–599.

Mion LC, Fogel J, Sandhu S, et al. Outcomes following implementation of a physical restraint reduction program in two acute care settings. Joint Commission Journal on Quality Improvement 2001; 27:605–618.

Fick DM, Cooper JW, Wade WE, et al. Updating the Beers criteria for potentially inappropriate medication use in older adults: results of a US consensus panel of experts. Arch Intern Med 2003; 163:2716–2724.

Chaudry SI, Friedkin RJ, Horwitz RI, Inouye SK. Educational disadvantage impairs functional decline after hospitalization in older patients. Am J Med 2004; 117:650–656.

CHAPTER SIX

Functional Assessment of the Elderly Hospitalized Patient

Barbara J. Messinger-Rapport, MD, PhD

INTRODUCTION

Functional impairment in the older adult is common and has many potential causes, including age-related changes, social factors, and disease. At baseline, 20% of persons older than 65 years and living in the community are chronically disabled, with higher prevalence in advancing years.[1] Poor functional status is a predictor for lower health quality, higher health costs,[2] and increased mortality.[3] Organized geriatric interventions in a variety of settings—home, hospital, long-term care institution, office—have demonstrated improved functional status, suggesting that at least some disability is preventable.

Baseline and ongoing functional assessment in the hospital setting is important to establish goals of treatment; to identify functional change during hospitalization; and to guide discharge planning for rehabilitation, placement, or support services after hospitalization. Approximately 17% of older adults suffer decline in functional ability between admission and discharge during a medical hospitalization, not including the 18% who declined shortly prior to admission and did not recover function.[4] Functional decline in elderly hospitalized patients is associated with advanced age, cognitive impairment at baseline admission, dependence in complex activities of daily living prior to admission, depressive symptoms, and history of imbalance at baseline.[4,5] The old-old cohort is also at the greatest risk of not recovering from functional deficits acquired prior to or during hospitalization.[4] Ongoing functional assessment during hospitalization is important to identify deconditioning, delirium, adverse medication effects, and other hazards of hospitalization.

Functional assessment and optimization are cornerstones of geriatric medicine, involving a multidisciplinary team with medical, nursing, social services, nutritional, and therapy expertise. Specialized units involving such teams have demonstrated improvement in functional outcomes in hospitalized patients. For example, the Acute Care for the Elderly (ACE) intervention demonstrated improved processes of care and a composite outcome of function or nursing home placement at discharge and at a year after discharge.[6] The Hospital Elder Life Program (HELP) model reduced the incidence of delirium and functional decline.[7] The functional assessments described in this chapter are screening tools that can be performed by a physician, nurse, or physician extender and can be used directly by the hospitalist in caring for the patient. These assessments are intended to be used in the context of a problem-focused evaluation of a patient's functional status as it applies to the reason for hospitalization and the goals of care. An ACE team, if supported by the hospital, may elaborate on the functional assessments and make further recommendations. If the patient is at high risk for decline, co-management with or consultation by a geriatrician may be considered.

IMPLICATION OF ADL IMPAIRMENTS

The Katz index of the basic ADLs[8] is used primarily to measure physical functioning (Box 6-1). It is used by state long-term care programs to determine eligibility for nursing home waiver programs, by insurers who offer private long-term care insurance policies, by federal legislation, and by research protocols assessing hospital outcomes. Although basic ADL query was intended as a proxy for physical ability, ADL impairment may implicate other problems. For example, the person needing prompting or cueing to complete his or her basic ADLs may have a geriatric syndrome such as a sensory (e.g., visual) deficit, polypharmacy (causing sedation or balance problems), or cognitive impairment (from dementia).

The Lawton and Brody scale of Instrumental Activities of Daily Living (IADLs) was developed to capture more complex life activities (Box 6-2).[9] In some cases, the inability to do an IADL is social rather than physical or cognitive; that is, a person may have never performed the IADL. For instance, the husband never managed the shopping or meal preparation, or the wife never learned to drive. In such cases, the IADL impairment is not treated as a disability for clinical or service eligibility requirements. Although physical ability is needed for most of the IADLs, certain IADLs can be used to identify individuals with cognitive impairments. Specifically, those IADLs considered to be most closely associated with cognitive impairment are limitations in a person's ability to manage medications, manage finances, and use the telephone.[10] Identification of cognitive impairment early is important in terms of directing the patient's care in the hospital. Among hospitalized medical patients, 31–40% may lack capacity to make important decisions regarding their care, and this deficiency is usually missed by both clinicians and close family members.[11]

In an elder who is highly functional and independent prior to admission, identification of functional impairment may be difficult. A brief, guided discussion with the patient, supplemented by a knowledgeable informant, about target activities such as par-

---

Box 6-1 Basic Activities of Daily Living (ADLs)

Bathing

Dressing

Eating

Transferring

Continence

Toileting

Box 6-2 Instrumental Activities of Daily Living (ADLs)

Transportation

Shopping

Cooking

Using the telephone

Managing money

Taking medications

Cleaning

Laundry

---

ticipation in book club, bridge leagues, golf or other hobbies, or employment if not retired will often identify a subtle loss. If an elder has dropped or is struggling to maintain a target activity, an early impairment may be present. Causes of impairment include worsening of a specific medical condition such as angina; a sensory deficit such as hearing loss; a geriatric syndrome such as imbalance, urinary incontinence, executive dysfunction from depression, or cognitive impairment from early dementia.

Impairments in instrumental and basic ADLs may have somewhat different implications regarding disposition after discharge. For example, persons who need assistance with IADLs can often have services brought to the home once or twice weekly. Persons dependent in basic ADLs such as transfer and continence may require round-the-clock assistance. If the impairments are severe or coupled with cognitive impairment, the level of assistance required may exceed the availability of the home support network.

ROLE OF THE CAREGIVER OR INFORMANT

Identifying the primary caregiver of a physically or cognitively impaired elder early in the hospitalization facilitates completion of the medical history and provides baseline functional information. Living arrangements (nursing facility, assisted living, or private residence), relationships of others occupying the home, community or private services employed for managing ADLs and IADLs, and details of the support network can be clarified. The content of the caregiver interview also includes the identity of other family caregivers, completion of advance directives, and identification of the possible existence of a Durable Power of Attorney for Health Care (DPOA-HC) and/or guardian.

Even when caring for an apparently cognitively intact elder, it is desirable to confirm at least portions of the history with an informant. For instance, a pattern of impaired driving skills or evolving difficulty with medication management may emerge from such a discussion. Informants are usually the spouse or local adult child or sibling. Alternatively, the informant can be a friend, neighbor, or out-of-town relative. Permission to speak with the informant should be sought from the cognitively intact patient.

Interacting with the patient and primary caregiver(s) provides an opportunity to screen for abuse, neglect, and exploitation. Abuse occurs less often than neglect or exploitation. Patients are more likely to be abused, neglected, or exploited if they have cognitive or physical impairment, if the caregiver lives in the home and is financially dependent upon the patient, and when there is alcohol abuse by the caregiver.[12] Abuse or neglect of an older patient with dementia may occur in the setting of caregiver strain, where the caregiver is poorly educated about the disease process, anxious, and/or isolated from his or her own support network. Abuse of a demented elder is also more likely when the premorbid relationship between the caregiver and dependent was poor, when the dependent is himself or herself verbally or physically abusive, or when the dependent displays problem behavior.[13] Examples of caregiver actions that may harm the patient include: physically restraining a patient who wanders by tying him or her to the bed or chair, emotionally or physically abusing a demented elder who displays agitated behavior, or leaving a person with poor mobility and judgment unattended at home or in a car while the caregiver runs errands. Evidence for caregiver strain can be assessed by asking the caregiver directly, or by offering a self-administered test such as the modified Caregiver Strain Index.[14,15] Social Services can be helpful in referring the caregiver to the proper agencies. Caregivers often require treatment for their own emotional and physical conditions neglected under the strain of caregiving. Occasionally, it may be necessary to arrange a different site of discharge to separate the patient from the caregiver, or to plan for Adult Protective Services to see the patient at home after discharge.

FUNCTIONAL STATUS AT BASELINE AND DURING HOSPITALIZATION

Baseline functioning during the month prior to admission to identify impairments in any of the ADLs and IADLs listed in Boxes 6-1 and 6-2 can be provided by the patient, but should be corroborated by an informant, preferably a caregiver. Determination of services currently utilized by the patient (bill-paying, homemaking, home-health aide) helps identify baseline functional deficits in basic and instrumental ADLs, and helps substantiate the patient and caregiver information. Box 6-3 provides a sample of functional assessments that can be performed on admission.

Cognitive Deficits

Cognitive deficits, revealed by impairments in ADL and IADL or medical history or caregiver interview, are common in elders admitted to the hospital. Problems underlying cognitive dysfunction include dementia, affective disorders, and delirium. Delirium (in patients without dementia)[16] and depression[17] are both independent predictors for mortality after discharge. Among hospitalized older medical patients, 10–40% are delirious upon admission; during hospitalization, an additional 25–50% develop

Box 6-3 Screens for Baseline Function at Hospital Admission

1. <u>ADLs</u>: "X" through those not doing on admission. Circle if was able to do it 2–4 weeks prior to admission:

   Bathing   Dressing   Transferring   Toileting   Grooming   Feeding

2. <u>IADLs</u>: "X" through those not doing on admission. Circle if was able to do it 2–4 weeks prior to admission:

   Telephone   Meal   Cleaning   Laundry   Shopping   Transportation   Medication   Finances

3. <u>Vision screen</u>: (If wears glasses, state, "When you are wearing your glasses") do you have difficulty with any activities (driving, watching TV, reading, etc) because of your vision? Y N

   If Yes, consider Snellen Eye Chart and visual fields.

4. <u>Hearing screen</u>: (If uses a hearing aid, state, "When you are wearing your hearing aids") do you have difficulty hearing conversations or listening to the TV or radio? Y N

   If Yes, consider cerumen impaction

5. <u>Cognitive screen</u>:

   <u>Orientation</u>: "Please tell me the date" (Day Season Date Month Year).

   <u>Three item registration</u>: "Please repeat these items for me now, and I will ask you again in a few minutes." *Apple Table Penny*

   <u>Attention</u>: Request performance of serial sevens. Alternatively, "Please spell *WORLD* backwards"; "Tell me the days of the week backwards"; or "Tell me the months of the year backwards."

   <u>Recall</u>: "Please repeat those three items I asked you to remember." *Apple Table Penny*

   <u>Clock Drawing Test</u>: You may draw the circle (optionally let the patient draw it) and ask the patient to place the numbers of the clock inside. Then, ask the patient to draw the hands and set it to 2:35.

   Numbers in right order?   Y N

   Numbers in correct quadrants?   Y N

   Hands on correct time?   Y N

6. <u>Mood</u>: (If abnormal, consider 15- or 30-point Geriatric Depression Scale. If depressive symptoms interfere with care in the hospital, appear to limit ability to care for himself or herself after discharge, or if there is an expressed death wish, consider a psychiatric consultation.)

   "During the past 2 weeks, have you often felt sad (or hopeless, unhappy, discouraged, miserable, helpless, worthless, or blue)?" Y or N

7. <u>Strength and Gait</u> (Consider therapy consultation for any abnormal finding):

   <u>Query</u>: Do you feel unsteady with walking? Y N

   <u>Mobility</u>

Full ROM shoulders:	Right Y N	Left Y N
Hip flexion	Right Y N	Left Y N
Hip extension	Right Y N	Left Y N
Knee flexion	Right Y N	Left Y N
Knee extension	Right Y N	Left Y N

   c) <u>Timed Up and Go</u>: Rise from chair, walk 10 feet away, turn, return to chair.

   Abnormal >20 sec.

8. <u>Caregiver assessment if living at home</u> (consider Social Worker consult for any bold "No" answer):

   Is there a support person or family member? Y N

   Name and relationship to patient: _____

   Does support network appear adequate? Y N

   Circle community resources used at this time:

   Meal-on-Wheels homemaker service home health aide lifeline button other (If currently utilizing services, may need case manager to re-instate when patient returns home.)

   Is the patient safe at home (for example, abnormal cognitive screen and living alone with inadequate support)? Y N

   Do you anticipate inability to return home after hospitalization? Y N

Table 6-1 Differentiating Characteristics of Dementia, Delirium, and Depression[39]

	Dementia	Delirium	Depression
Onset of Symptoms	Typically gradual (e.g., Alzheimer's disease) over weeks, months, or years	Acute over a period of hours to days	Gradual over weeks to months
Reversibility	No	Yes	Yes
Predominant deficits	Memory	Attention	Mood
Associated features	Does not appreciate memory deficit and may not be concerned. Impaired orientation as disease progresses. Urinary and fecal incontinence not seen until moderate-to-severe stage. Psychotic symptoms (visual hallucinations, paranoid delusions) may be seen in moderately advanced dementia.	Impaired immediate and short-term memory. Disoriented. 40–70% hallucinate, some only at night. Hallucinations typically visual and frightening. In hypoactive delirium, hallucinations less likely, and elders may be apathetic. Urinary and fecal incontinence common.	Selective disorientation. May have mild memory deficit and be concerned about it. Psychomotor retardation, apathy, difficulty with concentration, and/or psychotic features (usually delusions) can be present. Psychotic features occur in 20–45% of hospitalized depressed elderly and 3.6% of community-dwelling elderly depressives.
Course	Usually progressive over months to years.	Fluctuates in hospital. Typically resolves with treatment of precipitating condition. Resolution may take days to weeks.	Improvement occurs over 4–6 week period with antidepressants; resolution over 6–12 months or longer.
EEG	May have slowing of dominant background activity.	Bilateral, diffuse slowing. Delirium tremens and delirium induced by benzodiazepine withdrawal have low-voltage fast activity.	N/A

delirium.[18] Rates are higher in intensive care units and in terminally ill patients before death. Dementia is found in at least 20% of hospitalized medical patients.[19] About 20% of medically ill hospitalized elders have major depression, and another 20–30% have minor depression.[20,21] Some general guidelines to differentiate delirium, dementia, and depression are given in Table 6-1. Caution regarding interpretation is needed, however, since two or even three of these conditions may coexist in the hospitalized geriatric patient. Additionally, a new diagnosis of dementia is difficult in the acute setting, since metabolic, inflammatory, and infectious causes of cognitive dysfunction may cloud the picture.

Delirium

Delirium is associated with prolonged hospitalization, increased risk of complications such as fall and injury, worsening functional decline, and nursing home placement. The medical geriatric patient is more likely to develop delirium during his or her hospitalization if he or she is cognitively impaired at baseline, sensory deprived, has a severe illness, or has poor hydration (elevated BUN/Cr ratio).[22] During a medical hospitalization, delirium is more likely to ensue following implementation of physical restraints, development of malnutrition, addition of more than three medications, use of a bladder catheter, or experience of any iatrogenic event.[23] Postoperative delirium following noncardiac surgery is more likely with postoperative anemia and with certain

procedures, particularly intrathoracic surgery and abdominal aneurysm surgery. Other factors associated with postoperative delirium include age ≥70 years, cognitive impairment, limited physical function, history of alcohol abuse, and electrolyte abnormalities. Type of anesthesia and intraoperative hypotension, bradycardia, and tachycardia are *not* independently associated with delirium.[24] Data demonstrate that multidisciplinary preventive efforts reduce the incidence and duration of delirium, but not the severity or the recurrence rate, suggesting that prevention of delirium is the best approach.[25]

Measures and Screening

Screens for delirium usually include a test of attention, such as subtracting serial sevens, spelling "world" backward, digit span, or reciting the days of the week or the months of the year backward. These tests have low sensitivity compared with more involved tests such as the research-oriented Delirium Rating Scale. However, these tests are useful because of their brevity and because acute decline in ability during hospitalization suggests delirium. Baseline deficits in attention can be seen in either delirium or dementia. Persons with depression may have difficulties with concentration as well. Physicians and nurses are sensitive to agitation and hallucinations as evidence for delirium. Hypoactive delirium is often mistaken for depression when lethargy, malaise, and somnolence are present.[31] Delirium is also more likely to be missed in elders 80 years and over, in the visually impaired, and in those with baseline dementia.

Mental State Examination

The Folstein Mini-Mental State Examination (MMSE) is a 30-point test of several areas of cognition: orientation, attention and calculation, registration and recall, naming, visuospatial function, and executive function.[26] It has been validated widely in different clinical populations and age-groups. When adjusted for education,[27] it offers insight into cognitive deficits but cannot be used independently of history, physical findings, and other testing to diagnose dementia or differentiate between dementia and delirium. In lieu of the entire test, portions of the MMSE may be helpful to identify cognitive deficits. The date, three-item recall, and design copy can be used as a short screen, with the option to complete the Folstein if any of the responses are abnormal. The Clock Draw Test involves visuospatial, attention, and executive skills. It can be used alone[28] or with the three-item recall as a "Mini-Cog."[29] The Mini-Cog may be more accurate than the MMSE in multiethnic elderly and is less biased by low literacy.[30]

Depression Assessment

The Geriatric Depression Scale (GDS) has been validated as a screening measure for major depression in the older hospitalized patient.[32] A shorter version has been shown to detect depression and predict function and mortality after discharge.[17,33] A score of ≥6 out of 15 on the short GDS suggests depression, and further testing or consultation can be considered. Given that less than a quarter of hospitalized older adults are likely to have major depression,[34] a one-question test of affect may be helpful to screen for depression prior to utilizing even the shorter GDS. A sample question might be: "Do you ever feel sad or depressed?" (see Box 6-3), and this can be followed by a longer interview or the short form GDS if appropriate. The sensitivity and specificity of the GDS are lower with dementia. The test is also affected by impairments in ability to perform ADLs.[35] There are ethnic differences as well. Older African American males are less likely to admit to depressive symptoms, so self-rated scales are relatively insensitive in this cohort.[34]

Sensory and Mobility Assessment

Baseline sensory deficits in vision and hearing will make it difficult to communicate with the patient during hospitalization, may increase the risk for falls, and may predispose to delirium. Sensory deficits identified early can be addressed by urging patients with glasses or hearing aids to use them during the hospitalization.

Large muscle groups involved with ADLs and mobility may be tested and sense of balance queried to direct therapy if needed. The Timed Up and Go (TUG) is helpful. The majority of community-dwelling individuals can rise from a chair, walk 3 meters, turn, and return to the chair within 12 seconds, and nearly all in under 20 seconds. More than half of institutionalized elderly women are unable to complete the TUG in less than 20 seconds.[36] Although performing the TUG in >12 seconds is considered abnormal, the ability to live at home is probably not threatened by mobility until the TUG is 20 seconds or higher. In elders, the TUG may be influenced by the nature of the chair. For

instance, a lower chair or a chair without armrests may increase the TUG score by 1–2 seconds.[37]

Direct observation of function is the most accurate method of changes in functional assessment during hospitalization. The physician can couple his or her observations of the patient performing the basic ADLs in the hospital with those of the nurses and physician extenders (nurse practitioner or physician assistant). The Confusion Assessment Method[38] is available as well as a tool based on nursing observations and documentation to improve the accuracy of diagnosis of delirium.

Box 6-4 provides a sample functional assessment that can be performed daily during hospitalization.

DISCHARGE DETERMINATION

Discharge plans reflect the functional status and goals of care of the older patient. It is as important to recognize the *absence* of functional impairment in the older adult as to recognize its *presence*. For example, an independent, functionally intact elder may undergo curative treatment in the hospital and aggressive rehabilitation in an acute or subacute rehabilitation unit. But frail patients functionally impaired at baseline may be better served by treatment goals that offer prolonged survival, relief of specific symptoms, maintaining or regaining ability to live independently, or obtaining comfort while dying. Discharge plan goals are more likely to be home with family, perhaps with a brief course of therapy and skilled nursing; skilled nursing facility (SNF); or nursing home placement, depending upon function and treatment goals. Elders may also be discharged from the acute-care setting prior to resolution of delirium. These persons often require a brief nursing facility stay with rehabilitation prior to returning to the community. In a complex situation, or if the parties involved cannot agree on treatment goals or a discharge date or site, a comprehensive and interdisciplinary approach to discharge planning may offer the optimal plan acceptable to attending physicians, patients, and their families.

Box 6-4 Daily Query for Change in Function During Hospitalization

1. Any loss of an ADL present at admission? Which? _____

2. Any decline in cognition (i.e., development of delirium)? Circle correct responses

   (Orientation) *Month Date Year Day of Week*

   (Attention): *Sun Sat Fri Thurs Wed Tues Mon*

3. Decline in strength or alteration in gait? Which muscle group involved? _____

   For any change in above, evaluate for cause (new metabolic or infectious cause, adverse drug effect, restraint, neurologic event, nutritional deficit, etc.), consider a treatment (therapy, assist device, change in nutrition) and readdress the discharge plan.

4. New discharge plan: *Home Home with skilled nursing/therapy services Rehab* (example: Subacute if anticipate 1–2 weeks, Skilled Nursing Facility [SNF] if anticipate >2 weeks) *Nursing Facility*

Key Points

- Functional assessment of the older patient is done at baseline and portions of the assessment should be repeated daily.

- Basic and instrumental ADLs may provide complementary information.

- Goals of treatment are related to function.

- Establishing the support network is needed for discharge planning.

- Interacting with the patient and primary caregiver(s) provides an opportunity to screen for abuse, neglect, and exploitation. Abuse occurs less often than neglect or exploitation.

- The patient's support network may need to accommodate, at least temporarily, complex medical and surgical regimens and more assistance with basic and instrumental ADLs than needed prior to admission. Inability of the support network to accommodate this need may signal placement, at least temporarily.

SUGGESTED READING

Covinsky KE, Palmer RM, Fortinsky RH, et al. Loss of independence in activities of daily living in older adults hospitalized with medical illnesses: increased vulnerability with age. J Am Geriatr Soc 2003; 51:451–458.

Lindenberger EC, Landefeld CS, Sands LP, et al. Unsteadiness reported by older hospitalized patients predicts functional decline. J Am Geriatr Soc 2003; 51(5):621–626.

Counsell SR, Holder CM, Liebenauer LL, et al. Effects of a multicomponent intervention on functional outcomes and process of care in hospitalized older patients: a randomized controlled trial of Acute Care for Elders (ACE) in a community hospital. J Am Geriatr Soc 2000; 48(12):1572–1581.

Inouye SK, Bogardus ST, Jr., Baker DI, et al. The hospital elder life program:a model of care to prevent cognitive and functional decline in older hospitalized patients. J Am Geriatr Soc 2000; 48:1697–1706.

Raymont V, Bingley W, Buchanan A, et al. Prevalence of mental incapacity in medical inpatients and associated risk factors: cross-sectional study. Lancet 2004; 364:1421–1427.

Marcantonio ER, Goldman L, Orav EJ, et al. The association of intraoperative factors with the development of postoperative delirium. Am J Med 1998; 105:380–384.

Inouye SK, Bogardus ST, Jr., Charpentier PA, et al. A multicomponent intervention to prevent delirium in hospitalized older patients. N Engl J Med 1999; 340:669–676.

Borson S, Scanlan JM, Watanabe J, et al. Simplifying detection of cognitive impairment: comparison of the Mini-Cog and Mini-Mental State Examination in a multiethnic sample. J Am Geriatr Soc 2005; 53(5):871–874.

Inouye SK, Foreman MD, Mion LC, et al. Nurses' recognition of delirium and its symptoms: comparison of nurse and researcher ratings. Arch Intern Med 2001; 161:2467–2473.

Siggeirsdottir K, Jonsson BY, Jonsson H, et al. The timed "up & go" is dependent on chair type. Clin Rehabil 2002; 16(6):609–616.

CHAPTER SEVEN

Skin Integrity and Pressure Ulcers: Assessment and Management

Jonathan M. Flacker, MD

BACKGROUND

The skin is the first line of defense against the environmental threats of the outside world. Compromised integrity puts patients at risk for discomfort and infection. Anything that breaches the skin barrier, including lacerations, burns, dermatitis, skin tears, and pressure ulcers, can compromise its integrity. This chapter will focus on skin tears and pressure ulcers that are both commonly encountered and often avoidable in the hospital setting.

Pressure ulcers are "any lesion caused by unrelieved pressure resulting in damage of underlying tissue."[1] Pressure ulcers are associated with four underlying causes: pressure, shear, friction, and moisture. Pressure, usually on a bony prominence, is the primary cause of such ulcers. Shear, or the interaction of gravity and friction on the skin, contributes to pressure ulcers by causing twisting or kinking of blood vessels. Friction damages the skin at the epidermal/dermal interface (the basement membrane). Moisture contributes to pressure ulcer development by weakening the cell wall of individual skin cells. Taken alone, or more commonly in combination, these four factors place patients at high risk for breakdown of skin integrity.

ASSESSMENT

Clinical Presentation

Prevalence and Presenting Signs and Symptoms

The prevalence of pressure ulcers is difficult to pinpoint in the acute-care setting due to the various methodologies used in published studies; the prevalence, however, seems to be 10.1–17.0% with an incidence of 0.4–38%.[2] One recent large survey found overall hospital pressure ulcer prevalence was 14.8%, with a nosocomial pressure ulcer prevalence of 7.1%.[3] Thus, about half of hospitalized patients with pressure ulcers develop them in the hospital. Staging of pressure ulcers is standardized using a I–IV scale (Table 7-1) ranging from superficial redness being stage I to a stage IV ulcer extending into muscle, bone, or supporting structures (Fig. 7-1).

Pressure ulcers have important characteristics that should be examined and documented (Box 7-1). Using the "black, yellow, red" system to describe ulcer bed color gives a sense of the viabil-

ity of the exposed tissue. "Red" corresponds to the presence of muscle or granulation tissue in wound bed. "Yellow" indicates necrotic tissue or slough in wound bed and/or presence of subcutaneous tissue, fascia, or support structures like ligaments/tendons. "Black" wounds have necrotic eschar within or obscuring the wound.

The presence of dead space, such as undermining or tunneling must be assessed and managed to prevent complications such as premature wound closure and/or abscess formation. Ulcer margins also have implications for wound healing. When intact, this indicates that the skin surrounding the wound is attached to the edge of the ulcer bed, and epithelialization of the ulcer can occur more readily. Complete circumferential undermining means the ulcer margins are not attached.

Skin tears, often a precursor to pressure ulcers, are classified separately from pressure ulcers. Their true prevelance is unknown. The Payne-Martin Classification system is commonly used to stage skin tears.[4] Category I is a skin tear without tissue loss. Category II denotes a skin tear with partial tissue loss. Category III indicates a skin tear with complete tissue loss and absent epidermal flap.

Differential Diagnosis

Pressure ulcers most commonly occur over area of bony prominences. When they occur elsewhere on the body, an external source of frequent, constant pressure must be present. This external pressure source may be the patient's own limb, as in the case of contractures or orthopedic abnormalities. At other times, the external pressure may come from the patient's environment, such as broken or ill-fitting wheelchair parts, bed frames, or chairs. Tight or ill-fitting clothing, shoes, bra straps, and orthopedic splints may also be a source of external pressure. An ulcer appearing on a part of the body that does not have a source of frequent constant pressure is probably not a pressure ulcer, but rather has another etiology such as vascular insufficiency, infection, or local trauma.

Note that so-called stage I ulcers are not yet ulcerated. Stage I ulcers may be more difficult to detect in patients with darker skin, but are often evidenced by a purple discoloration (especially under halogen light) and/or bogginess/induration of the skin. Stage I ulcers may thus be confused with simple bruising. Any new bruise over a bony prominence or an area of frequent pressure should be suspected to be a stage I pressure ulcer.

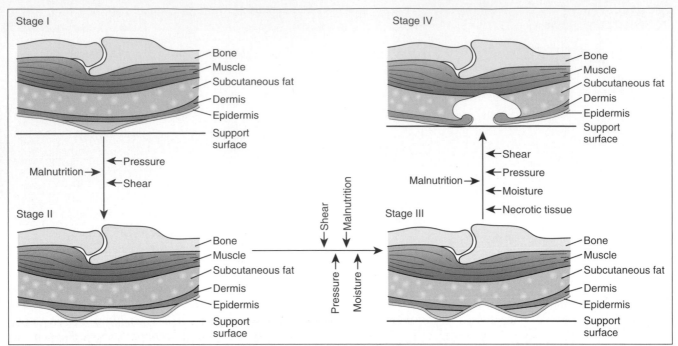

Figure 7-1 ● Progression of Pressure Ulcer.

Table 7-1 Pressure Ulcer Staging	
Stage I	An area of pressure at risk for ulcer development. Can be identified as a defined area of erythema that does not blanch. In dark-skinned persons may be purple or blue. Also area may be warmer or cooler than surrounding skin, feel firm or boggy, and/or be painful or itchy.
Stage II	Shallow ulceration through the epidermis and/or dermis. May also look like a blister.
Stage III	Deeper ulceration down to the fascia, but not penetrating the pascia.
Stage IV	Very deep ulceration that penetrates through the fascia into the deep tissue layers such as muscle and bone.

NOTE: Eschar must be removed in order to stage a pressure ulcer. An ulcer covered whole or in part by eschar in **unstagable**.

Diagnosis

Preferred Studies

The diagnosis of a pressure ulcer is a clinical one. Laboratory studies are focused on a good nutritional assessment. Prealbumin is the most sensitive indicator of nutritional status in hospitalized patients. It has a 2 to 3-day half-life, whereas albumin has a 21-day half-life and can be affected by hydration status.[5]

When quantification of bacterial levels in the ulcer is desired, a correctly done swab, tissue biopsy, and needle aspiration each have similar accuracy, sensitivity, and specificity.[15] To properly swab culture a pressure ulcer, clean the wound thoroughly with normal saline, then debride down to the base of the wound. Roll the swab a full rotation on the deepest part of the wound with the most visible signs of infection. Eschar should never be cultured.

With stage IV ulcers, the question of osteomyelitis often arises. Clinical examination is highly inaccurate for determining if osteomyelitis is present, and x-rays are typically unhelpful. Bone biopsy remains the gold standard for determining the presence of osteomyelitis. Jamshidi core needle bone biopsy has been shown to have reasonable test characteristics for osteomyelitis (sensitivity of 73%; specificity of 96%) and may be especially useful for guiding therapy prior to surgical closure of a pressure ulcer.[7] CT scans exhibit poor sensitivity for osteomyelitis in patients with pressure sores, while technicium and gallium bone scans have poor specificity. Indium-labeled WBC scans have not been adequately studied in the setting of pressure ulcers. MRI seems to perform significantly better, but clear data on accuracy and cost-effectiveness are not yet available.

Prognosis

During Hospitalization

Recent information on the implications of pressure ulcers for patient prognosis is lacking. One older study found that 67% of patients who develop a pressure ulcer during a hospitalization died as compared with 15% of at-risk patients without pressure ulcers.[8]

Postdischarge

Many factors such as nutrition, mobility, and comorbidities affect healing rates of pressure ulcers. The healing of pressure ulcers requires attention to care and patience for a considerable period of time. Individualized protocols to predict pressure ulcer healing rates have also been developed.[9] In general, a stage II pressure ulcer should heal within 1–2 months in a healthy, mobile, well-

Key Elements of Assessing the Physical State of the Pressure Ulcer:

____ Size including depth

____ Location

____ Stage

____ Necrotic tissue

____ Slough

____ Exudate

____ Infection

____ Granulation tissue

____ Undermining

____ Tunneling

____ Abscess formation

____ Visible subcutaneous tissue/fascia/ligaments/tendons/ bone

____ Pain

____ Odor

____ Intact margins

Assessment should be supported by photography (calibrated with a ruler) where possible.

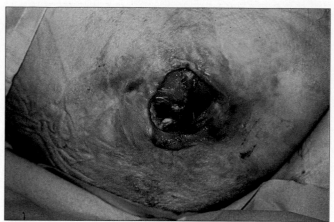

Figure 7-2 • With good care, even a stage IV pressure ulcer will usually heal. From Tallis RC, Fillet HM. Brocklehurst's Textbook of Geriatric Medicine and Gerontology, 6th Edition. Churchill Livingstone, 2003.

nourished older person. Deeper stage II and stage III ulcers may take several months to heal. Most stage IV ulcers take more than 6 months to heal. Importantly, pressure ulcers that develop during acute hospitalization are not associated with reduced 1-year survival among high-risk older persons after adjusting for important confounders.[10]

MANAGEMENT

Treatment

The principles of pressure ulcer healing center around three key areas of intervention: pressure management, nutrition optimization, and direct ulcer management. Pressure management includes interventions ranging from improving mobility to special beds that relieve pressure on the area of the wound, while avoiding placing additional areas at risk. Nutrition optimization involves determining and implementing a feeding regimen the patient can tolerate and that meets their goals of care. Direct ulcer management covers the choices of debridement techniques and wound-care products appropriate for the patient's particular ulcer. Although care must be individualized to the patients, general guidelines for ulcer management are indicated in Table 7-2 (Fig. 7-2).

Initial

Support Surface or Bed

The initial step in pressure management is to provide an appropriate support surface. There are three basic types of support surfaces: mattress overlays, mattress replacements, and full spe-

cialty beds. Mattress overlays may be foam, air, or gel. Mattress replacements may be foam, air, gel, or water. They may be static, alternating air, low air loss, or immersion. Specialty replacement beds are integrated bed systems that can function as do the mattress replacements, and they sometimes provide an integrated rotation feature. While the choices may seem complex, for patients who have a single small stage II ulcer, a static mattress may suffice. However, for those with multiple stage II ulcers, or stage III or IV ulcers, a mattress overlay or specialty mattress is usually required. The alternating pressure feature is especially useful for patients who have little or no healthy turning surfaces such as those with sacral and ischial ulcers. General guidelines for specialty support surface use are indicated in Table 7-3 (Fig. 7-3).

Mobility

Improving mobility helps to minimize continuous pressure on a single area of the body. Attention must be paid to how long such patients are left on stretchers awaiting tests or on hard operating room tables. Physical or occupational therapists can be very helpful in this regard. Even if patients are bed bound, a bed trapeze may allow patients to reposition themselves without having to wait for nursing staff to do so.

Nutrition Management

Nutrition management begins with the determination of whether the patient can take oral feeding. If so, he or she should be fed orally; but if not, discussion of nasogastric or gastrostomy tubes should take place. It is important to note that a recent Cochrane review found that "it was not possible to draw any firm conclusions on the effect of enteral and parenteral nutrition on the prevention and treatment of pressure ulcers."[11] Vitamin C is usually recommended at a dose of 500 mg BID to help collagen synthesis and tensile strength. Zinc is given at a dose of 220 mg daily to help with protein synthesis, though higher doses may impair healing. There are fewer data to support the routine use of other vitamins and micronutrients such as copper, manganese, and vitamins A and E. A dietician should be consulted for all patients with pressure ulcers.

Table 7-2 Management of Pressure Ulcers by Stage

Ulcer Stage	Nutrition Interventions	Pressure Interventions	Wound Care Interventions	Wound Products to Consider

Stage I	• Dietitian consult to evaluate intake of:
	  • Protein
	  • Calories
	  • Vitamin C
	  • Zinc
		• OT/PT consult for positioning
		• Static pressure reduction
		• Mattress/wheelchair pad
			• Cleanse with mild soap and water
			• Carefully, gently pat dry
				• Wound covering products:
				  • Transparent film dressing
				  • Hydrocolloid sheet

Stage II	• Dietitian consult as above	• As above	• Cleanse as above	• Wound covering products as above

Stage III	• Dietitian consult as above	• As above
		• If progressive ulcer or ulcers on multiple turning surfaces use low air loss/alternating pressure mattress overlay/bed
			• Debride any eschar for nonheel ulcers	• Wound packing products:
				  • Saline-dampened gauze
				  • Hydrogel
				  • Alginate

Stage IV	• Dietitian consult as above	• Low air loss/alternating pressure mattress overlay/bed	• Debride any eschar for nonheel ulcers
			• Evalute for osteomyelitis
			• Systemic antibiotics if infection source
			• Surgical consult if extensive debridement or bone biopsy needed
				• Wound packing products
				  • Saline-dampened gauze
				  • Hydrogel
				  • Alginate
				• Wound V.A.C. System®

Table 7-3 Special Support Surface Use

Patient Characteristic	Intervention
Individuals at risk for pressure ulcers	Use static pressure reduction mattress or 4–6″ thick foam overlay

Patient can assume multiple positions
  – Can avoid putting weight directly on the pressure ulcer
  – Does not bottom out
	Use static pressure reduction mattress or 4–6″ thick foam overlay

Patient can assume multiple positions
  – Can NOT avoid putting weight directly on the pressure ulcer
  – Bottoms out on a static device
	Use a dynamic support surface

Patient has multiple stage III or IV pressure ulcers on multiple turning surfaces, OR excess moisture is a significant contributing factor to the ulcer	Use a low air-loss or air-fluidized bed

Adapted from: Panel for Pressure Ulcer Treatment, Clinical Practice Guideline No. 15. Rockville, Md: US Department of Health and Human Services, Public Health Service. Agency for Health Care Policy and Research; 1994, AHCPR Publication No. 95-0652 (pp 39–41).

Wound Management

The key aspects of direct wound management increase with increasing stage of the ulcer.

Ulcers need a clean base to allow epithelial cells to grow and heal the ulcer, so all necrotic tissue must be removed. Appropriate moisture control is key here. Too much moisture leads to maceration of the wound. Excessive dryness leads to chafing. Both can result in further injury and poor epithelia cell growth.

The goal of cleaning or debridement is to remove the unwanted dead tissue, while preserving the granulation tissue that will heal the wound. If cleaning with gauze or sponges, only slight pressure should be applied to avoid disturbing the wound bed. If irrigating, a syringe and 19-guage angiocath with gentle pulsatile lavage can achieve acceptable low pressures of 4–15 psi, or a commercial system may be used. Ulcers should generally be cleaned only with normal saline; do not use the long list of skin cleansers and antiseptic agents ranging from iodine to sodium hypochlorite solution (Dakin's solution). Although topical growth factors may speed healing, their role and the most cost-effective approach to use is unclear.[12] A description of common products used for wound care is indicated in Table 7-4 (Fig. 7-4).

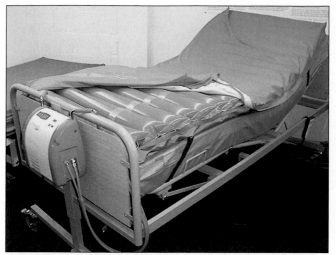

Figure 7-3 • An alternating pressure mattress overlay. From Tallis RC, Fillet HM. Brocklehurst's Textbook of Geriatric Medicine and Gerontology, 6th Edition. Churchill Livingstone, 2003.

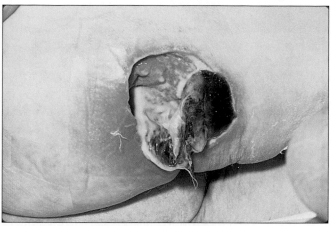

Figure 7-4 • A stage IV pressure ulcer in need of debridement. From Tallis RC, Fillet HM. Brocklehurst's Textbook of Geriatric Medicine and Gerontology, 6th Edition. Churchill Livingstone, 2003.

Table 7-4 Wound Products

Product Type	Cover Ulcer	Pack Ulcer	Absorb Exudate	Debride	Comments	Sample Products
Transparent adhesive films	Yes	No	Light	Light	Good to reduce friction May cause further damage in "thin skin" patients	Derma Film, OpSite, Polyskin, Tegaderm Adaptic, Exu-Dry, Telfa, Vaseline Gauze
Nonadherent dressing	Yes	No	Light	No	Good for patients with "thin skin"	
Gauze rolls and sponges	Yes	Yes	Moderate to heavy	Yes	Allow gauze to dry if debridement desired, otherwise keep damp between changes	Various
Foam sheets	Yes	No	Moderate to heavy	No		Allevyn, Curafoam, Flexzan, Lyofoam, Mitraflex, Polymem
Hydrocolloid Sheets	Yes	No	Light to moderate	Yes	Occlusive. Do not use if anerobic infection. Monitor closely if diabetic or imunocompromised	CarraSmart, Combiderm, Comfeel Plus, Cutinova, DermaCol, DuoDerm, Exuderm, Replicare, Restore, Sorbex, Tegasorb, Ultec
Hydrogel sheet	Yes	No	Light to moderate	Yes	Soothes minor burns; has "cooling" effect	Aquaflo, CarraDress, Elastogel, NuGel, Vigilon
Hydrogel amorphous gel	No	Yes	Light	Yes	Needs cover dressing May macerate intact skin	Biolex Gel, Carrasyn Gel, Curafil, Curasol Gel, Intrasite, Saf-Gel, Tegagel, Wound' Dres
Alginate	No	Yes (Pads)	Moderate to heavy	No	Needs cover dressing Comes in pads and ropes May dessicate wound with light or no exudates Hemostatic properties	AlgiSite, Calcicare, Curasorb, FyBron, Kalginate, Kaltostat, Seasorb, Sorbsan, Tegagen
Hydrofiber	No	Yes (Rope only)	Moderate to heavy	Some	Vertical wicking reduces maceration	Aquacel
Enzymatic debrider	No	No	No	Yes	May take 1–2 weeks to achieve debridement	Accuzyme

Table 7-5 Debridement Techniques

Debridement Type	Technique for Removal of Devitalized Tissue	Indications	Contraindications	Relevant Wound Care Products
Autolytic	Natural	• Necrotic tissue • Dry eschar	• Dry gangrene • Dry ischemic wounds	Include, but not limited to: • Transparent films • Hydrocolloids • Hydrogels • Alginates • Gauze
Mechanical	Outside force	• Necrotic wounds	• Foul odor • Devitalized tissue • Macerated tissue	Include, but not limited to: • Wet to dry dressings • Whirlpool • Wound irrigation
Enzymatic	Topical application of specialized protein	• Necrotic wounds	• Clean wounds • Dry gangrene Dry ischemic Wounds • Hypersensitivity	Include, but not limited to: • Accuzyme • Panafil • Santyl
Sharp	Sharp instruments	• Necrotic wounds • Sepsis • Progressive cellulitis • Callus formation	• Arterial insufficiency • Gangrene • Stable heel ulcers • Inability to identify structures in wound	

Unless the need for sharp debridement is urgent, mechanical, autolytic, and enzymatic debridement are equally acceptable (Table 7-5). If progressive cellulitis or sepsis is present, sharp debridement should be used and should usually take place within 12 hours, along with a tissue biopsy for culture and sensitivity if systemic infection is suspected. Ulcer cleansing and debridement may also reduce bacterial colonization in stage II–IV ulcers. Some stage III or IV ulcers can take a long time to be fully debrided, and frequent treatments may be needed in the presence of purulent drainage or foul odor. Enzymatic products like Accuzyme (papain–urea) are effective debridement agents, but they take longer than sharp debridement. Often, they are used with Iodosorb gel or Iodoflex pads (small hydrophilic beads with 0.9% cadexomer iodine) that adsorb bacteria and cellular debris by capillary action, leading to less inflammation and odor. Whirlpool treatment is best for ulcers with heavy slough, exudate, or necrotic tissue and should be stopped when the ulcer is clean. If debridement is associated with bleeding, apply a dry dressing initially, followed by a moist dressing after 8 to 24 hours.[1] Based on expert opinion, stable heel eschar without erythema, edema, or drainage should not be debrided, but needs to be assessed daily for complications that may necessitate debridement.[1]

A wide range of products can be applied to ulcers (*see* Table 7-3). For a typical stage I ulcer, one should protect the skin; and reduce pressure, shear, and friction. For a stage II ulcer, one should additionally protect and hydrate the wound. A stage III ulcer further requires debridement as necessary. A stage IV ulcer requires all of the above, as well as obliteration of dead space. In grade III or IV pressure ulcers, treatment using first alginate and then hydrocolloid dressing yields more rapid improvement than hydrocolloid alone.[13] Pain control is also critical, and patients with pressure ulcers report pain and tend to receive inadequate analgesia,[14] perhaps due to the false belief that stage III–IV pressure ulcers are painless due to nerve fiber destruction.

The treatment of skin tears is a bit more straightforward, but follows the principles of pressure ulcer management. The size of the tear shoud be documented along with a drawing if helpful. In general, the area should be gently cleaned with normal saline and allowed to air dry or dry by gentle patting. The skin flap should be approximated and held in place with either Steri-Strips or a moist nonadherent dressing. Clear film dressings are acceptable, but care must be taken when removing the dressing to avoid further skin injury or reinjury. An arrow drawn on the dresssing that identifies the direction of the skin tear can help in this regard.

Although it is important for the hospital physician to understand the basic tenets of pressure ulcer management, it is equally important that physicians understand the components of a Skin Integrity team. Such teams are typically composed of a nurse who has advanced training in wound care (Skin Clinical Nurse Specialist), a nutritionist, and a therapist. The nurse will typically advise on local wound care measures and assist in selecting from the hundreds of available skin products according to the patient's need and hospital formulary. A nutritionist is important to ensure that negative nitrogen balance is avoided, and to advise on the type, route, and composition of feeding. Finally, a therapist (in some places this will be a Physical Therapist and in others an Occupational Therapist) is essential to advise on positioning techniques, pressure reduction devices, and optimization of mobility.

Subsequent Care

One should expect to see signs of healing in a clean ulcer by 2–4 weeks. An accurate skin assessment must be performed and documented when patients are transferred to other health care facilities. For patients being discharged to home, visiting nurse services skilled in pressure ulcer management should be arranged, along with any special equipment, including hospital bed, special support mattresses, and lifts. Caregivers should be instructed on wound care and turning procedures prior to discharge of the patient.

If a clean ulcer on an inpatient has persistent exudate and/or shows no signs of healing despite optimal care for 2–4 weeks, then a 2-week trial of topical antibiotics should be considered. A culture is usually not needed, as culture results are not likely to alter the treatment since these infections typically do not involve deep tissue invasion. Vacuum-assisted closure is a reasonable intervention for large chronic pressure ulcers. Color photos taken on initial assessment and reevaluation are helpful in monitoring changes in the ulcer as long as the photo accurately depicts the appearance of the ulcer. The appropriate role of various growth factors in speeding healing is the subject of active investigation.

Operative intervention is a last resort and should take place after a careful analysis of risks and benefits. Important factors to consider are medical stability, prognosis, nutritional status, risks of blood loss, postoperative immobility, quality of life, treatment goals, patient preferences, and risk of recurrence. Because smoking, spasticity, bacterial colonization of wound, and incontinence may impair wound healing, these should be addressed before surgical intervention.

PREVENTION

Pressure ulcer prevention shares similarities with pressure ulcer treatment. Important keys to pressure ulcer prevention can be found in Box 7-2. Important aspects include staff education. This includes proper use, documentation, and implementation of protocols based on assessment tools such as the Braden or Norton Scales. For example, factors assessed by the Braden Scale

---

Box 7-2 Keys to Pressure Ulcer Prevention

1. Staff Education
   A. Focus on nurses and nursing assistants.
      i. Clear Assessment Expectations
         a. Complete skin assessment on admission
         b. Complete skin assessment every 48 hours
         c. Complete skin assessment whenever the patient's condition significantly changes
      ii. Clear Documentation Expectations
         a. Assessment with reliable and standardized tool such as Braden or Norton Scales
      iii. Clear Action Expectations
         a. Triggered prevention protocols implemented within 12 hours
         b. Communication with physician regarding assesment and protocol implementation
         c. Home caregiver instruction

2. Pressure management
   A. Patient-Centered
      i. Keeping the patient as active as possible
      ii. Instruction patient to perform small weight shifts every 15 minutes when able
      iii. Limit head of bed elevation to no more than 30 degrees
      iv. Trapeze to assist with self-mobility
   B. Caregiver Centered
      i. Turn every 2 hours if consistent with overall care goals
      ii. Hourly repositioning of chair or wheelchair bound patients
      iii. Always use transfer sheet to move the patient
   C. Material-Centered
      i. Special support surface such as thick foam or static pressure mattress

      ii. Cushions to keep bony prominences from direct contact with each other
      iii. Cushions or devices to raise heels of bedbound patients off the bed
      iv. Protect the patient's elbows, heels, sacrum, and back of the head if he where exposed to friction
      v. Heel and elbow protectors
      vi. No Massage of reddened bony prominences
      vii. No donut devices

3. Moisture Management
   A. Treat Excess moisture
      i. Identify source
      ii. Regular use of a bedpan or urinal
      iii. Cleaning the skin quickly after any soiling
      iv. Absorbent pads that wick moisture
      v. Barrier dressings or creams
   B. Treat excess dryness
      i. Lotion use after bathing
      ii. No hot water
      iii. No drying soaps

4. Nutrition management
   A. Assure adequate nutrition
      i. Dietitian consultation if at risk
      ii. Increase protein, calorie, and/or vitamin intake as needed
      iii. Give a cup of water given with the turning schedule to maintain hydration
      iv. Monitor NPO status due to multiple tests
      v. Peripheral parenteral nutrition (PPN) if NPO over several days

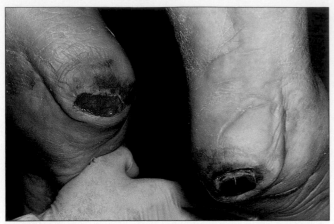 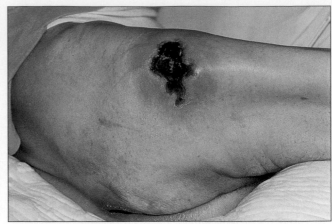

Figures 7-5, 7-6 • The heels and greater trochanter are common sites for the development of pressure ulcers. From Tallis RC, Fillet HM. Brocklehurst's Textbook of Geriatric Medicine and Gerontology, 6th Edition. Churchill Livingstone, 2003.

include sensory perception, moisture, activity, mobilty, nutrition, friction, and shear. Braden scale scores range from 0–23, with increased risk indicated by a score of 18 or below for elderly and persons with darkly pigmented skin, and 16 or below for other adults.

Other helpful prevention techniques indicated in the Agency for Healthcare Research and Quality (AHRQ) prevention recommendations[1] target the key areas of pressure management, moisture management, nutrition management, and friction/shear minimization (Figs. 7-5, 7-6).

The heels are an area of special risk. Preventive heel precautions include assessment of the feet twice daily. Use of a transparent film, hydrocolloid dressing, or even socks can minimize friction. Heel pressure can be removed through the use of pillows, blanket rolls, or heel lift devices. Active and/or passive range of motion of the ankle can be achieved through ankle movements twice daily. For patients not able to place the ankle in neutral position easily, occupational or physical therapy consultation is helpful.

For skin tears, prevention consists of the basic principles of pressure ulcer prevention. In addition, high-risk patients can wear long sleeves or pants to protect their extremities. Adequate lighting reduces the risk of bumping into furniture or equipment. A safe area for wandering should be provided if possible. Nursing assistants need to understand how to protect patients from self-injury or injury during routine care and turning. Dangling arms and legs should be supported with pillows or blankets. Padding equipment, such as wheelchair arm and leg supports, offers additional protection from accidental injury. Elderly, frail skin should have only nonadherent dressings, and only paper tape should be used on the skin. Gauze wraps, stockinettes, or other wraps that can be taped to themselves to secure dressings are useful in frail patients.

CLINICAL ALGORITHM(S)

There are many studies and protocols suggested for use in long-term care facilities, and algorithms specific to the inpatient setting appear to be based on these. The AHRQ guidelines on pressure ulcer prevention and treatemnt of pressur ulcers are available online at www.ahrq.gov/clinic/cpgonline.htm.

DISCHARGE/FOLLOW-UP PLANS

For patients returning home, appropriate support surface should be arranged, and Visiting Nurse referral made. For complicated ulcers, a Skin Clinical Nurse Specialist should be specifically requested. A wound clinic referral, when available, is a useful adjuvant for difficult ulcers. For patients being transferred to another facility, pressure ulcer location, depth, size, stage, and treatment should always be documented in the transfer records.

Patient Education

Patient educational should address basic information such as the etiology and risk factors for pressure ulcers, and the basics of skin assessment. If a special support surface is needed, home caregivers should be instructed on its use as well as positioning techniques. The use of lifts, transfer sheets, and wound-care techniques also must be clearly explained.

Outpatient Physician Communication

It is best if the outpatient physician contact information be provided to the home health agency and wound clinic so the primary care provider can assume management of the ulcer after discharge. The Primary Care provider, however, must be provided information regarding the stage, size, and treatment plan for the ulcer, as well as contact information for the home health agency and wound clinic that will be providing assistance with ulcer management.

Key Points

- Stage I pressure ulcers identify at risk areas that have not broken down yet.

- Pressure ulcers most commonly occur over areas of bony prominences.

- An ulcer appearing on a part of the body that does not have a source of frequent constant pressure is probably not a pressure ulcer.

- The principles of pressure ulcer healing center around three key areas of intervention: pressure management, nutrition optimization, and direct ulcer management.

- The Hospital's Skin Integrity Team should be utilized early on as collaborators in the care and management of patients with pressure ulcers.

- Standardized assessment tools should be routinely used to identify patients at increased risk for pressure ulcers.

SUGGESTED READING

Amlung SR, Miller WL, Bosley LM. The 1999 national pressure ulcer prevalence survey: a benchmarking approach. Adv Skin Wound Care 2001; 14(6):297–301.

Livesley NJ, Chow AW. Infected pressure ulcers in elderly individuals. Clin Infect Dis 2002; 35(11):1390–1396. Epub 2002.

Wallenstein S, Brem H. Statistical analysis of wound-healing rates for pressure ulcers. Am J Surg 2004; 188(1A Suppl):73–78.

Thomas DR, Goode PS, Tarquine PH, et al. Hospital-acquired pressure ulcers and risk of death. J Am Geriatr Soc 1996; 44(12):1435–1440.

Langer G, Schloemer G, Knerr A, et al. Nutritional interventions for preventing and treating pressure ulcer. Coch Database Syst Rev 2003; (4):CD003216.

Thomas DR. The promise of topical growth factors in healing pressure ulcers. Ann Intern Med 2003; 139(8):694–695.

Belmin J, Meaume S, Rabus M, et al. Sequential treatment with calcium alginate dressings and hydrocolloid dressings accelerates pressure ulcer healing in older subjects: a multicenter randomized trial of sequential versus nonsequential treatment with hydrocolloid dressings alone. J Am Geriatr Soc 2002; 50:269–274.

Cullum N, Deeks J, Sheldon TA, et al. Beds, mattresses & cushions for pressure sore prevention & treatment (Cochrane Review). The Cochrane Library, 2, Oxford Update Software; 2001.

Dow G. Bacterial swabs and the chronic wound: When, how, and what do they mean. Ostomy Wound Mgt 2001; 49(5A, suppl):8–13.

Argenta LC, Morykwas M. Vacuum-assisted closure: A new method for wound control and treatment: clinical experience. Ann Plast Surg 1997; 38(6): 563–576.

Bergstrom N, Braden BJ, Laguzza A, et al. The Braden Scale for predicting pressure sore risk. Nurs Res 1987; 36(4):205–210.

CHAPTER EIGHT

Constipation

Sheri Chernetsky Tejedor, MD

BACKGROUND

Hospital care is typically focused on treatment and resolution of a patient's underlying disease. Symptoms such as constipation, nausea and vomiting, or diarrhea are often part of the constellation of symptoms associated with a particular condition or are a consequence of treatment. "PRN" medications, typically ordered on admission or during the hospitalization, are often the only response to such symptoms. However, hospitalists must not ignore these symptoms and should elicit, assess, and respond to such symptomatic complaints. In a prospective cohort study of more than 2,000 hospitalized medical patients, the persistence of symptoms at the time of hospital discharge was predicted by a shorter length of hospital stay and the severity of symptoms on admission. Patient dissatisfaction with hospital care was linked to residual symptoms at discharge, emphasizing the importance of symptomatic relief in patient-centered care.[1] This chapter and the next two on nausea and diarrhea, respectively, focus on the evaluation and management of these important and common symptoms among hospitalized patients.

When defined broadly, constipation is a common problem affecting 12–19% of the general population. Constipation can be subdivided into two physiologic subgroups: slow transit constipation and impaired anorectal expulsion. Infrequent defecation (fewer than 3 stools per week), straining on stools, hard stools, and the sensation of incomplete evacuation are all part of the definition of constipation.[2]

ASSESSMENT

Clinical Presentation

Prevalence and Presenting Signs and Symptoms

Constipation commonly complicates multiple systemic diseases. Twenty to 30% of diabetics experience constipation.[26] Gastrointestinal dysmotility is also well described in Parkinson's disease, scleroderma, and multiple sclerosis. Advanced age, inactivity, certain medications (Box 8-1), non-Caucasian race, low socioeconomic class, low caloric intake, female gender, and depression have all been associated with self-reported constipation.[4–6]

The history and physical examination should be focused to exclude critical diagnoses and guide additional investigations and therapy (Table 8-1, Fig. 8-1). Elderly patients, bed-bound patients, and those with fecal or urinary incontinence should be evaluated for fecal impaction. Patients who are empirically treated with fiber or laxatives should be reevaluated for impaction if there is no bowel movement after 3 days, before additional laxatives are given. Anorectal examination should focus on sphincter tone and evidence of fissures or hemorrhoids. High-pitched bowel sounds, abdominal tenderness, surgical scars, rebound, and guarding may suggest obstruction.

Differential Diagnosis

A few important diagnoses must be excluded in the patient with constipation. So-called "alarm symptoms," such as blood in the stool, nausea, vomiting, abdominal pain, or weight loss in a patient with advanced age, should prompt early imaging with tests as described below to evaluate for malignancy or obstruction. A history of inflammatory bowel disease or radiation may predispose to stricture and support a decision to pursue early imaging. Constipation in the postoperative patient, especially when accompanied by nausea or vomiting, should raise the question of ileus, intestinal ischemia, or obstruction. Metabolic derangements (uremia), underlying conditions (pregnancy), and diseases (Parkinson's) may contribute to constipation in the hospitalized patient (Table 8-1).

Constipation presenting as a new complaint in the hospitalized patient should prompt a thorough review of medications. Multiple medications are known to cause constipation through different mechanisms—some alter colonic motility; some desiccate stool. Box 8-1 lists common offenders.

Diagnosis

Preferred Studies

If a patient's constipation is not believed to be a side effect from medication, then an initial trial of medical and dietary therapy is appropriate before pursuing diagnostic testing. A review of serum chemistry results is worthwhile. Serum TSH is reasonable for patients with appropriate symptoms and chronic constipation but may be difficult to interpret in the acutely ill patient (see Chapter 10).

Most stable patients without vomiting or abdominal pain will not require early imaging in the evaluation of constipation. Imaging is most useful in cases of suspected obstruction from

Box 8-1 Medications That Cause Constipation

Opioids

SSRIs

TCAs

Anticholinergics

Antispasmodics

Chemotherapuetic agents

Calcium channel blockers

Phenothiazines

Diuretics

Antihistamines

Antiparkinsonian drugs (Amantadine)

Antacids with calcium or aluminum, calcium supplements

Antidiarrheal agents

Previous laxative use

NSAIDs

Iron

NSAIDs—Nonsteroidal anti-inflammatory drugs

stricture, adhesions or tumor, patients with a suspected ileus, or those with abdominal pain in which perforation must be excluded. Early imaging may be considered in demented patients with severe constipation, as the history and physical may not be adequate to rule out obstruction. Patients who fail a trial of medical therapy and diet may need further evaluation, including radiographs or colonoscopy. Plain radiographs may show megacolon or megarectum in patients with stricture or obstructing mass and can delineate the extent of fecal impaction. Evidence of bowel obstruction and perforation may be obvious on plain films. A water-soluble contrast enema (Gastrografin [meglumine diatrizoate] or Hypaque [diatrizoate sodium]) can pass an impacted area and evaluate for a more proximal mass, stricture, or perforation. It can also be therapeutic in cases of fecal impaction.[7,8] In contrast, barium requires a bowel prep and can worsen fecal impaction. Additional testing for patients with chronic, refractory constipation, including manometry and colonic transit studies, most often is performed in the outpatient setting.

MANAGEMENT

Treatment

Many of the trials evaluating interventions to prevent and treat constipation in adults are in healthy outpatients with chronic constipation. Indeed, constipation is not, by definition, an acute

Table 8-1 Causes of Constipation

Cause	Associated Features
Irritable bowel syndrome	Alternating constipation and diarrhea, small-volume stools, bloating, pain
Amyloidosis	Nephropathy, cardiac disease, hepatomegaly
Scleroderma	Cutaneous disease, Raynaud's
Pregnancy	
Autonomic neuropathy	DM, HIV, postural hypotension, gastroparesis
Heavy metal ingestion	Occupational exposure, renal failure, abdominal pain
Hyponatremia	Encephalopathy, seizure
Hypercalcemia	Shortened QT interval, weakness, renal insufficiency, cognitive dysfunction
Uremia	Anorexia, edema, vomiting
Multiple sclerosis	Visual disturbance, paresthesias, pain
Stricture	History of IBD or diverticular disease
Colonic pseudoobstruction (Ogilvie's)	Abdominal distention, pain, dilated colon
Tumor	Weight loss, blood in stools, anemia
Spinal cord injury	Paraplegia
Parkinson's disease	Rigidity, gait abnormalities
DM	Poor glycemic control, peripheral neuropathy
Hypothyroidism	Weight gain, fatigue, depression, edema, cold intolerance
Intestinal ischemia	Weight loss, abdominal angina, nausea
Condyloma	Painful defecation, burning
Proctitis	Painful defecation
Fissures	Painful defecation, straining on stool, Crohn's
Inflamed hemorrhoids	Painful defecation, rectal bleeding, straining on stool
Ileus, obstruction	Abdominal distention and pain, nausea
Rectocele	Vaginal prolapse
Adult Hirschsprung's	Abdominal distention, chronic constipation

DM—Diabetes mellitus

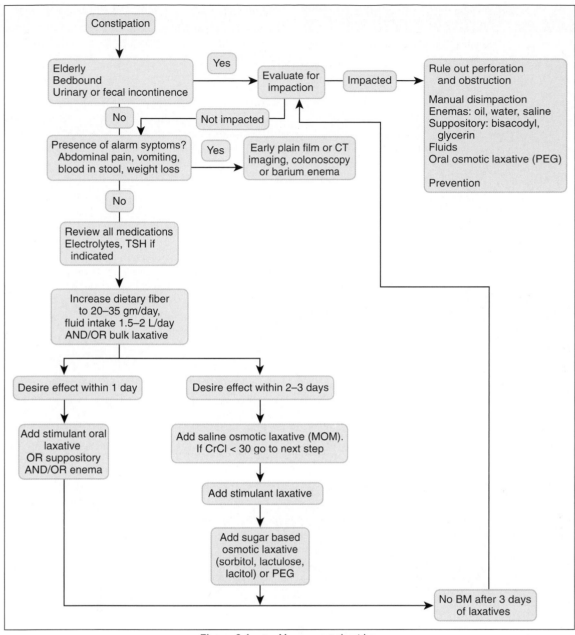

Figure 8-1 • Management algorithm.

problem. In a 1997 review by Tramonte[6] of 36 randomized trials involving almost 1,815 patients (60% were under age 60, and 70% were female) evaluating interventions for constipation, only 8% of study participants were hospitalized. A variety of laxatives and fiber supplements consistently increased bowel movement frequency when compared to placebo, by approximately 1.5 bowel movements per week. It was not clear if they decreased the likelihood of impaction. Fiber and bulk laxatives also appear to diminish abdominal pain and improve stool consistency. There are few good-quality head-to-head comparisons of specific laxatives.

In contrast, institutionalized and hospitalized patients made up the majority of study participants in a more recent review by Petticrew et al.[9] of randomized trials (n = 7) of laxative therapies in the elderly population. Osmotic and stimulant laxatives increased bowel movement frequency in most trials, but small sample size and nonsignificant trends favoring treatment limit the interpretation of these trials.

Preferred

Initial

Diet and Physical Activity The effects of increased physical activity and fluid intake are unclear in the management of constipation. One study of young patients with functional constipation found that increasing water intake to 2 L per day in addition to a diet with 25 g of fiber per day increased stool frequency and reduced laxative use, compared to patients drinking 1 L of water per day.[10] Fluid therapy is a rational choice for patients who are clinically dehydrated, but its added benefit in euvolemic patients with constipation is not clear.[5] Inactivity has been identified as a risk factor for the development of constipation, but increasing physical activity has not been clearly shown to improve constipation.[3] Unfortunately, physical activity is limited in most medical inpatients.

There are few randomized trials of dietary fiber therapy for treatment and prevention of constipation. Observational studies

Table 8-2 Therapy

	Dosing/Renal dosing	Notes	Onset	Cost per Dose ($)
Bulking Agents		Not advised for those who cannot take in enough water, works best in patients with normal colonic transit	$\frac{1}{2}$ to 3 days or longer	
Psyllium (Metamucil)	Each dose contains 2–2.4 g of soluble fiber. 2–6 capsules with 8 oz of water, can increase to 3 doses per day	Causes flatus, Metamucil wafers contain 20 mg sodium and 120 kcal per dose, sugar-free product contains phenylalanine (warning for PKU), risk of allergic reactions/asthma with powder inhalation		0.23
Methylcellulose (Citrucel)	2–4 capsules, 1–3 times daily	Semisynthetic fiber, somewhat resists bacterial degradation, less flatus		0.30
Polycarbophil (Fibercon)	1–2 tabs up to QID with 8 oz of liquid	Synthetic fiber, resists bacterial degradation (less flatus)		0.12
Stool Softeners				
Docusate sodium (Colace)	50–500 mg per day, divided doses	Low sodium, only 5 mg per capsule, increases the amount of water and fat in stool, can prepare as an enema with saline	12–72 hours	0.23
Docusate calcium (Surfak)	50–500 mg/day			0.14
Mineral oil—not recommended	15–45 mL/day	Interferes with intestinal absorpition of fat-soluble vitamins, warfarin, OCP, danger of lipid pneumonia, systemic absorption	6–8 hours	0.38
Osmotic Laxatives *Salt Based*				
Magnesium hydroxide (Milk of Magnesia)	30–60 mL/day, single or divided doses	Avoid in renal insufficiency CrCl <30 mL/min, may cause	0.5–3 hours	0.21
Magnesium sulfate (Epsom Salt)	10–30 g/day single or divided doses	hypermagnesemia, hypernatremia,		0.05
Magnesium citrate	120–300 mL (up to 1 bottle)	hyperphospatemia, metabolic acidosis, hypokalemia,		0.81
Sodium phosphate (Fleets Phospho-Soda)	20–30 mL, no more than 45 mL/day, take with 12 oz water	hypocalcemia, volume overload	1–3 hours	2.52
Carbohydrate Based		Not used in anuria	2–3 days	
Sugar alcohols (Sorbitol)	30–150 mL of 70% solution	May cause flatus Often given with activated charcoal for treatment of unintended drug ingestion or overdose		0.22
Synthetic dissacharides (Lactulose)	Syrup contains 10 g/15 mL, 10–20 g per day up to 60 mL/day	Use with caution in diabetes mellitus Milder laxative effect Synthetic sugar not absorbed in small intestine, fermented in colon, causes gas and bloating; not for patients with galactosemia		1.01
Polyethylene glycol with electrolytes (GoLYTELY, NuLYTELY)	Consumed at a rate of 1.5 L/hr for bowel cleansing, 100 mL/hr for impaction	May cause less bloating and cramping than other sugars; not metabolized by colonic bacteria	1 hour	13.89–18.98

Table 8-2 Therapy—Cont'd

	Dosing/Renal dosing	Notes	Onset	Cost per Dose ($)
Polyethylene glycol 3350 (Miralax)	Dissolve 1 teaspoon (17 g powder) in 8 oz of liquid, daily	Not fermented into hydrogen or methane gas; may still cause gas, does not contain electrolytes, small packages for more frequent use, use <14 days	2–4 days	1.07
Stimulant Laxatives		Can cause cramps, melanosis coli; chronic use may cause hypokalemia, salt overload, protein-losing enteropathy		
Cascara sagrada	2–5 mL, 100 mg up to 3 capsules per day	Use no more than 2 days	6–12 hours	0.12
Sennosides (Senna, Senokot)	8.6 mg sennosides, take 2 tablets daily, max 4 tablets BID, 15–100 mg per day divided BID	Allergic reactions	6–12 hours	3.06
Bisacodyl (Dulcolax, Correctol)	5–15 mg PO single dose	Not taken within 1 hour of dairy or antacids	6–10 hours	0.02
Enemas, Suppository				
Mineral oil: (Fleets)	60–150 mL enema	Relieves fecal impaction; evacuates the rectum, sigmoid, part of the descending colon; electrolyte abnormalities if retained	2–5 min	1.48
Phosphate enema	4.5 oz, may repeat once			0.85
Tap water enema				
Soapsuds enema				
Glycerin suppository	3 g, retain for 15 minutes, 1–2 times daily		15–60 min	0.03
Bisacodyl	10 mg		15–60 min	0.08

suggest that fiber therapy is effective for prevention.[9] Dietary modification is a reasonable first step for patients with mild complaints and should accompany most laxatives. Dietary fiber appears to increase stool weight, shorten colonic transit time, and decrease abdominal pain and fullness when compared to placebo. A high-fiber diet will typically benefit most patients with normal colonic transit; however, patients with slow transit constipation or outlet obstruction may not benefit from fiber therapy alone. Nonetheless, treatment with dietary fiber is an important part of constipation management, except for patients at risk of impaction, certainly a preferred initial treatment compared to Colace.

Fiber intake should be increased to 20–35 g per day. High-fiber foods available in most hospitals include: whole wheat bread, prunes, dates, peas, spinach, baked beans, bran muffins, and oatmeal. Patient compliance with dietary modification may be limited due to poor dietary intake or NPO status related to testing. Patients may experience flatus and bloating from increased dietary fiber due to fiber degradation in the colon. Fluid intake must be increased concomitantly to prevent intestinal obstruction from the increased stool bulk. Patients who cannot adequately increase their dietary intake may benefit from commercially available bulk laxatives (e.g., psyllium).

Bulk-Producing Agents Bulk laxatives appear to have the same effects on stool consistency, abdominal pain, and fullness as increased dietary fiber. Bulking laxatives, like dietary fiber, take advantage of the water-holding effect of undigested fiber in the intestine. Bacterial mass increases following partial fiber diges-

tion, which enlarges the lumen of the colon. Ultimately, this leads to softened stool, decreased intraluminal pressure, and increased colonic transit. Like dietary fiber therapy, bulking agents work best in patients with normal colon transit and should be avoided in patients with outlet obstruction.

Fluid intake must match the fiber intake to prevent intestinal obstruction. At least 8 oz of liquid should be taken with each dose. This is especially important for patients taking a diuretic. For this reason, bulking agents are often not advised in palliative care, because these patients are often unable to remain adequately hydrated. Dosing should be avoided prior to meals, as it can impair gastric emptying and reduce appetite. Bowel movement results are typically seen in 12–72 hours. Fiber degradation and fermentation in the colon can cause flatus and bloating, but this can be reduced with synthetic agents (e.g., methylcellulose, polycarbophil).

Osmotic Laxative Patients who fail or are unable to tolerate dietary or supplemental fiber should be offered an osmotic laxative. These are typically hypertonic agents composed of poorly absorbed salts or disaccharides that facilitate water retention in the intestinal lumen and increase stool bulk. The laxative effect depends on the metabolism and mucosal absorption of the drug and the amount of time it remains in the intestinal lumen. Osmotic laxatives can take several hours to days to work.

An inexpensive salt-based osmotic laxative such as magnesium hydroxide is an appropriate choice for patients who have not responded to dietary or synthetic fiber therapy alone. Other magnesium salts (sulfate and citrate) and sodium phosphate are often used as bowel preparations for endoscopy. All of these agents can lead to electrolyte disturbances (hyperphosphatemia, hypophosphatemia, hypocalcemia, hypermagnesemia) and volume overload and patients with renal failure should avoid them.

Sugar-based osmotic laxatives (sorbitol, lactuose, lactitol) tend to work more slowly than saline laxatives. The safety and efficacy of lactulose were established in elderly patients in the 1960s and 1970s.[6] Like fiber and bulk laxatives, lactulose may improve stool consistency. Sorbitol is often used as a cathartic in combination with charcoal for decontamination of the poisoned patient. One small study of 30 nondiabetic elderly men with chronic constipation found that a 70% sorbitol syrup (containing 30 mL/21 g) was as effective as the same dose of lactulose (30 mL/20 g) at approximately one-tenth the cost.[11] Carbohydrate-based agents can cause flatus and bloating due to degradation of sugars in the colon. They should be used with caution in diabetics, though there are few reported cases of hyperglycemia (Micromedex).

PEG (polyethylene glycol) is not metabolized by colonic bacteria and causes fewer side effects of bloating. PEG electrolyte lavage solutions (GoLYTELY, NuLYETLY) are often used in preparation for colonoscopy and typically produce prompt and dramatic results. These preparations require ingestion of a large volume of fluid, but when ingested rapidly there is little risk of electrolyte disturbances. However, if ingested slowly, there is a risk of absorption of the salt component. A single 500-mL dose could provide a 3-g sodium load. A PEG electrolyte solution combined with disimpaction and suppositories or enemas resulted in complete resolution in the majority of patients and no serious side effects in studies of several small groups of patients with fecal impaction. Many of these patients had significant underlying comorbidities.[7,9,12,13]

PEG 3350 (Miralax) is a tasteless powder that can be mixed with an assortment of beverages. It does not contain a salt component and therefore does not appear to carry the same risk as the PEG electrolyte lavage solutions. PEG 3350 still requires fluid consumption, approximately 250 mL per 17 g. The efficacy of PEG for the short-term treatment of constipation was established in a trial of outpatients without significant co-morbidities such as renal or cardiac disease. PEG 3350 resulted in 1.3–1.8 more bowel movements per week than placebo, and there was no increase in cramping or flatus; in fact, there was less in the treatment group.[14] PEG 3350 can take 2–4 days to work.

Because of their high cost, PEG 3350 and lactulose should be reserved for patients who cannot tolerate a salt-based osmotic laxative and those who fail or cannot take a stimulant laxative. PEG 3350, in spite of its cost, may be a good early option for palliative care patients.[15]

Stimulant Laxatives Stimulant laxatives (typically combined with fiber) are appropriate for patients who have failed a trial of fiber and an osmotic laxative, those with slow transit constipation, or those who desire an effect within hours.[25] Several small trials have demonstrated the superiority of the combination of a stimulant laxative and a bulking agent to traditional osmotic agents.[6,16] Orally administered stimulant laxatives often work within 6–12 hours and are typically prescribed at bedtime.

Anthraquinones, including senna, cascara sagrada, and aloe (casanthranol), alter water and electrolyte transport in the colon and increase colonic motility by stimulating intestinal formation of prostaglandins. Senna also softens stools and increases stool weight and frequency. Diphenylmethanes (Bisacodyl) inhibit water absorption in the small intestine, alter fluid and electrolyte transport in the colon, and stimulate the smooth muscles of the intestine. They also appear to cause reversible changes in intestinal epithelial cells.[17]

Stimulant laxative use is limited by concerns of adverse drug effects. All of these agents can cause abdominal cramping. Pseudomelanosis coli has been attributed to anthraquinones. It is characterized by brown pigment in the colonic mucosa, typically developing after months of regular use. The clinical significance of pseudomelanosis coli is unknown, and it appears to be reversible. No prospective human trials have established that these agents can cause damage to enteric neural cells or smooth muscle cells, though concerns have been raised by prospective animal studies and observations. Cases of cathartic colon are rare now, and it has been proposed that an outdated stimulant laxative no longer in use caused these historical cases. Stimulant laxatives have also been postulated to contribute to colon cancer, but this connection is still unproven in humans. Short-term use of these drugs appears to be safe and effective.[17,18]

Castor oil (ricinoleic acid) exerts its action as a secretogogue in the small and large intestines. The action is similar to the actions of unabsorbed fatty acids in some malabsorption disorders. It can cause mucosal damage, which may be the mechanism of action for water and electrolyte secretion. This drug is now nearly obsolete because it can cause severe cramping and diarrhea.[17,18]

Stimulant agents should not be used in patients with fecal impaction until after the colon has been cleansed with disimpaction, enemas, and suppositories because of the risk of colonic perforation.

Lubricants, Emollients, Enemas, and Suppositories Enemas and suppositories have a role in the treatment of patients with fecal impaction and spinal cord lesions as well as patients with pelvic floor dysfunction. Enemas work by distending the colon, resulting in reflex evacuation. Tap water and saline washout enemas are the first choice in this category because they cause no direct effect to the colonic mucosa. However, water enemas carry the risk of hyponatremia if they are retained. Phosphate enemas exert a local osmotic effect, drawing water into the colon. Systemic absorption leading to hyperphosphatemia and hypocalcemia can develop in patients unable to evacuate the enema promptly.[19] Hypertonic enemas can cause superficial injury to rectal mucosa, which typically promptly reverses.[20] Soap enemas are rarely used because of bowel injury and hyperkalemia with potassium-based soaps.[19] Docusate mini-enemas may have some efficacy in patients with spinal cord injury.

Lubricating agents are most often used for palliative care and patients with impaction. Mineral oil enemas act as a lubricant for hard stool and can be useful for patients with impaction and for those who must avoid straining on stool. Glycerin is not absorbed by the colon and can therefore be safely used as a lubricating suppository. Bisacodyl suppositories work locally on the enteric nervous system, resulting in vigorous but brief peristalsis, typically acting within 1 hour. Regular use is not advised.

Oral mineral oil has a long history in the treatment of constipation, but the risk of aspiration and development of lipoid pneumonia and malabsorption of fat-soluble vitamins probably contraindicates its use in most clinical scenarios except palliative care.[15]

Stool softeners such as docusate sodium (Colace) and dioctyl sodium act as detergents, lowering the surface tension of the stool and allowing water and fat to enter; they also may have some stimulant effects. Commonly used for the prevention and treatment of constipation in elderly, bed-bound, and chronically ill patients, this practice is supported by very little experimental evidence.[18,21] Some small studies have shown a slight trend toward increased stool frequency with docusate. Unfortunately, most of these trials have had either extremely small sample sizes (n = 15), high dropout rates, or poor design.[3,21,22] Given the frequent use of these drugs, a well-designed randomized, controlled trial would be useful.

Miscellaneous Interventions

Other drugs that may increase stool output but are not commonly used because of side effects, unproven benefit, or limited availability in the United States include: metoclopramide, erythromycin, cisapride (restricted availability in the United States), tegaserod (FDA advisory issued), urecholine, colchicine, misoprostol, neurotrophin-3, and neostigmine.

Surgery has been used in some refractory cases with total colectomy reserved for patients with intractable slow-transit constipation or rectal surgery for patients with significant rectoceles.[5]

Fecal Impaction

Fecal impaction deserves special mention, as it is an unfortunate consequence of severe constipation seen often in the geriatric population. Patients are unable to pass a compacted, hard mass of stool. Predisposing factors include decreased rectal sensation, poor diet, inadequate toilet access, spinal cord injury, opiate and anticholinergic use, renal failure, and decreased colonic motility.[8,23] Complications of impaction include pain, colonic ulceration, perforation, dehydration, decubitus ulcers, rectal bleeding, and urinary infection. The mortality of patients with impaction and obstruction is reported to be as high as 16%.[8]

Presenting symptoms include new diarrhea or fecal incontinence, urinary frequency or incontinence, nausea, tachypnea, dysrthymias, and rectal pain. Associated features include a history of impaction and the presence of hemorrhoids. Symptoms including abdominal pain, nausea and vomiting, fever, and leukocytosis can be seen with impaction; and a complete obstruction and perforation must be ruled out if these symptoms are present. Plain films will demonstrate excessive stool and can show dilated loops of bowel. Meglumine diatrizoate enemas can be diagnostic and therapeutic, ruling out a perforation. Perforation and obstruction should be ruled out before enemas or laxatives are administered.

Initial therapy includes manual removal of the stool mass with lidocaine lubricant jelly. Oil or tap water enemas and glycerin suppositories may facilitate stool passage. Oral laxatives may be given when perforation and obstruction have been ruled out and after disimpaction. PEG electrolyte solutions given at a slow rate (100 mL/hr) have shown promise and safety in several small studies.[7,9,12,23] Surgery may be required in refractory cases with obstruction. Consider the possibility of an underlying neoplasm, especially in more proximal obstructions. Prevention is the best strategy.[8]

Alternative Options

Prevention

Prevention of constipation is appropriate in at-risk patients. Those with inactivity, inadequate caloric intake, opioid or other offending medication use, and certain medical conditions such as Parkinson's disease and spinal cord injury may benefit from preventive interventions beginning with dietary fiber. Observational studies support the use of fiber as a first choice for constipation prevention.[9] Patients with severe hypertension, myocardial ischemia or infarction, elevated intracranial pressure, or recent perineal surgery are occasionally prescribed stool softeners, suppositories, or oral laxatives because of the presumed risks of straining on stool.

Patients receiving chronic opioid therapy rarely develop tolerance to the constipating effects, and more than 50% of them experience constipation. Thus, essentially all patients should be given scheduled laxative therapy; approximately 58% will require more than two types of treatments, and one third will require a rectal treatment. One algorithm is scheduled dosing of a stimulant laxative with a suppository if there is no bowel movement for over 24 hours.[24] Refractory constipation may be relieved with low-dose oral naloxone or other opiate antagonists (starting at 1 mg, up to 10–20% of the daily morphine dose). Naloxone has limited bioavalability, acts at the enteric opioid receptors, and carries little of a risk of systemic opioid reversal.[24] Opiate rotation is another option. There is some evidence that fentanyl and methadone may cause less constipation than morphine.[24]

Patients receiving palliative care experience constipation at a rate of at least 32%. These patients may have inactivity, predisposing medical conditions, and depression contributing to their constipation. Adequate fiber and fluid intake, indeed minimal caloric intake, may be difficult to achieve. Bulk laxatives can precipitate obstruction without adequate fluid intake. Sugar-based osmotic laxatives may cause unpleasant side effects, and stimulant laxatives may cause cramping. PEG 3350, lubricating agents, and suppositories may be reasonable options in these patients.[15]

Patients with fecal impaction should be maintained on a bowel regimen after disimpaction, with a goal of a bowel movement every 24–48 hours. Oral laxatives and glycerin suppositories or occasional bisacodyl suppositories or enemas should be used to ensure frequent bowel movements. Time for defecation and assistive devices including toilet handrails should be provided to elderly and disabled patients. Patients who are capable of adequate fluid intake can be safely given fiber therapy.[23]

DISCHARGE/FOLLOW-UP PLANS

Patient Education

Scheduled toileting after meals capitalizes on the gastrocolic reflex and should be encouraged. Increased physical activity, adequate fluid intake, and a high-fiber diet should be recommended at the time of discharge for patients with a normal colon. Chronic laxative use should be discouraged.

Outpatient Physician Communication

Constipation without impaction will rarely require prolongation of the hospital stay. A bowel regimen should be prepared for patients who continue to have constipation at discharge. Patients with normal colonic transit are likely to respond ultimately to medical and dietary interventions. Referral for colonoscopy is appropriate in those patients with alarm symptoms and patients with refractory constipation.

Patients with suspected pelvic floor dysfunction or slow transit constipation may require further diagnostics and interventions after discharge, including colonic transit testing and manometry.

Key Points

- A few critical diagnoses must be excluded in the patient with constipation. Stricture, malignancy, and spinal cord lesion are typically suggested by the history or physical examination. So called "alarm symptoms," such as blood in the stool, nausea, vomiting, abdominal pain, or weight loss in a patient with advanced age, should prompt early imaging. Most stable patients without vomiting or abdominal pain will not require early imaging in the evaluation of constipation.

- The first step in managing constipation is to increase dietary fiber and add a bulking laxative, provided the patient is able to increase fluid intake. Patients receiving palliative care are often unable to increase fluid intake and can develop fecal impaction from supplemental fiber. Saline osmotic laxatives should be tried first (if renal function is normal) followed by stimulant laxatives and sugar-based osmotic laxatives. Enemas and suppositories can be used if more prompt results are desired. Patients who have not had a bowel movement after 3 days of laxative therapy should be evaluated for fecal impaction prior to additional laxative or fiber therapy.

- Elderly patients, bed bound patients, and those with fecal or urinary incontinence should be evaluated for fecal impaction. Other presenting symptoms include new diarrhea, urinary frequency, nausea, tachypnea, dysrthymias, and rectal pain. The treatment of fecal impaction involves manual disimpaction, enemas, suppositories, increased fluid intake, and oral osmotic laxatives such as polyethylene glycol once obstruction has been ruled out.

- A majority of patients receiving chronic opioid therapy experience constipation. Most patients require scheduled laxative therapy. Scheduled dosing of a stimulant laxative with a suppository if there is no bowel movement for over 24 hours is one option. Refractory constipation may be relieved with low-dose oral naloxone or other opiate antagonists. Opiate rotation is another option.

- Constipation presenting as a new complaint in the hospitalized patient should prompt a thorough review of medications. Multiple medications are known to cause constipation through different mechanisms—some alter colonic motility; some desiccate stool. Common offenders include opioids, calcium channel blockers, SSRIs, antidiarrheals, and iron.

SUGGESTED READING

Kroenke K, Stump T, Clark DO, et al. Symptoms in hospitalized patients: outcome and satisfaction with care. Am J Med 1999; 107(5):425–431.

Locke GR, Pemberton JH, Phillips SF. American Gastroenterological Association medical position statement: guidelines on constipation. Gastroenterology 2000; 119:1761–1778.

Petticrew M, Watt I, Sheldon T. Systematic review of the effectiveness of laxatives in the elderly. Health Technol Assess 1997; 1(13):1–66.

Rao SS. Constipation: evaluation and treatment. Gastroenterol Clin North Am 2003; 32:659–683.

Schiller LR. Review article: the therapy of constipation. Aliment Pharmacol Ther 2001; 15:749–763.

Tramonte SM, Brand MB, Mulrow CD, et al. The treatment of chronic constipation in adults: a systematic review. J Gen Intern Med 1997; 12:15–24.

CHAPTER NINE

Symptom Management: Nausea

Sheri Chernetsky Tejedor, MD

BACKGROUND

Patients complain of nausea and vomiting as part of the presenting symptomatology in up to 43% of general medical admissions to the hospital.[1,2] Nausea and vomiting can lead to metabolic derangements, dehydration, esophageal tearing, aspiration, and patient distress. This chapter will focus on the general approach to evaluating and treating these symptoms in the hospitalized patient, including determination of the underlying etiology, assessment of the physical consequences of emesis, and treatment for symptomatic relief.

The majority of the data on the treatment of nausea and vomiting is from studies of prevention and therapy for postoperative patients, patients receiving chemotherapy, and pregnant women. Hospitalists can draw inferences for other patient groups from this data.

Postoperative nausea and emesis are commonly managed in the recovery room, but will often be encountered by the consulting hospitalist on the floor. Chemotherapy-related nausea and emesis are seen less frequently, as most chemotherapeutic regimens are given on an outpatient basis. Exceptions include patients receiving highly emetogenic chemotherapeutic drugs, those at risk for tumor lysis, patients with acute leukemia, and those with severe underlying comorbidities.[3]

ASSESSMENT

Clinical Presentation

Prevalence and Presenting Signs and Symptoms

Nausea and vomiting are common, occurring in 5–22% of diabetics and up to 50% of patients with HIV infection.[4–6] Acute gastroenteritis with nausea and vomiting occurs at a rate of 0.8 episodes per person per year.[7] Up to 30% of unselected and 80% of high-risk postoperative patients will experience nausea and/or vomiting.[8] Cancer patients using opiods experience nausea at a rate of 40–70%, and particular chemotherapeutic regimens carry a risk over 90%.[9]

The history should focus on new medications, presence of neurologic symptoms, change in stools, and any evidence of gastrointestinal bleeding. In assessing the severity of the emesis, there unfortunately are no physical examination findings that combine adequate sensitivity and specificity in the assessment of nonhem-

orrhagic hypovolemia. Dry mucous membranes and furrows on the tongue are sensitive but lack specificity (i.e., if absent, dehydration is unlikely; but if present, do not rule in hypovolemia from vomiting). Dry axilla, postural hypotension, sunken eyes, and weakness are specific but lack sensitivity (i.e., rule in hypovolemia when present, but are not always found among patients with hypovolemia from vomiting).[10,11] In the hospital setting, serum electrolytes are readily available and should be used as part of the assessment of volume status. The physical examination should include examination of the teeth for evidence of enamel erosion suggesting frequent vomiting, neurologic and fudoscopic examination if indicated by the history, abdominal examination including ascultation for bruits, and inspection for abdominal scars as well as examination of the stool for occult blood.

Differential Diagnosis

The history and physical examination will suggest the most critical diagnoses that must be considered as possible causes for nausea and vomiting (Table 9-1). Increased intracranial pressure from a mass lesion, blood, or meningoencephalitis will be suggested by headache, focal neurologic findings, a history of head trauma, or fever. Textbook "projectile vomiting" in adult patients is not often seen and may still be due to abdominal pathology.

Small bowel obstruction should be considered and ruled out in patients with a history of abdominal surgery, colicky abdominal pain, bilious vomiting, abdominal distention, and inability to pass flatus or stool, although these may be late findings (Fig. 9-1). Paralytic ileus should be considered, especially in postoperative patients and those with pancreatitis or cholelithiasis. Vomiting may relieve the discomfort of patients with a small bowel obstruction (SBO) or an ulcer, but will typically not lessen the abdominal pain of hepatitis or pancreatitis.

Acute coronary syndromes (ACS) can present with nausea and/or vomiting, and the lack of chest pain makes the diagnosis elusive. In a review of presenting symptoms of over 430,000 patients with an acute myocardial infarction, 33% did not have chest pain. Patients with diabetes, females, and older patients with ACS were more likely to present in an atypical fashion.[12] Women with an ACS experience nausea and vomiting, alone or in combination with other symptoms, more often than men (30% of women compared to 16% of men).[13] Patients presenting with nausea and vomiting with cardiac risk factors and additional

Table 9-1 Causes of Nausea and Vomiting

Cause	Associated Findings
Small bowel obstruction, gastric outlet obstruction	Bilious vomiting, colicky pain, obstipation or diarrhea
Gastroenteritis	Diarrhea, headache, myalgias, fever
Tumor	Weight loss
Gastric outlet obstruction	History of ulcer disease
Mucosal disease, ulcer, gastritis	Heme-positive stool, anemia
Hepatitis	Elevated AST and ALT
Ileus	Abdominal distention
Cholecystitis, cholelithiasis,	Abdominal pain
Appendicitis	Abdominal pain
Eosinophilic gastroenteritis	Eosinophillia, allergies
Gastroparesis	Delayed 1 hour after meals, early satiety
Mesenteric ischemia	Postprandial abdominal pain
Pancreatitis	Alcohol use, postprandial pain
Esopahgeal (achalasia, stricture, Zencker's diverticulum)	Vomiting undigested food
Functional dyspepsia	Normal upper endoscopy, no organic cause
Irritable bowel syndrome	Constipation, diarrhea
Inflammatory bowel disease	Bloody stool, abdominal pain, weight loss
Medications	New medication
Pyelonephritis	Fever, flank pain
Nephrolithiasis	Flank pain, groin pain
Starvation	Ketonemia
Alcohol, alcoholic ketosis	Ingestion
Toxins	Ingestion, suicidality
Increased intracranial pressure	Headache with straining, morning headache, positional headache
Migraine	Headache, aura
HELLP syndrome	Thrombocytopenia, LFT abnormalities
Acute fatty liver of pregnancy	Abnormal LFTs, leukocytosis
Hyperemeis gravidarum	Missed menses, abnormal LFTs
Adrenal insufficiency	Hyperkalemia, hyponatremia
Bulemia, anorexia nervosa	Vomiting immediately after meals
Labrynthine disorders	Vertigo
GVHD	Maculopapular rash, abnormal LFTs, hematopoietic cell transplant
Hypercalcemia, parathyroid disease	Weakness, constipation, short QT interval
Uremia	Edema, pulmonary edema, delirium
Diabetics ketoacidosis	Hyperglycemia, fruity breath
Hyperthyroidism	Tachycardia, weight loss
CHF	Dyspnea, abdominal distention
Acute coronary syndrome	Chest pain
Radiation	Exposure history

CHF, congestive heart failure; *GVHD*, graft versus host disease; *LFT*, liver function tests

symptoms such as dyspnea or fatigue warrant evaluation for ACS.[12]

Nausea and vomiting in the cancer patient cannot be immediately attributed to chemotherapy. Central nervous system (CNS) metastases, hypercalcemia, gastrointestinal (GI) obstruction from tumor or graft-versus-host disease need to be considered.

When patients with HIV/AIDS present with vomiting and a headache, cryptococcal meningoencephalitis and toxoplasmic encephalitis should be considered.

Nausea that develops in the hospitalized patient after admission should prompt a detailed review of medications. Table 9-2 lists the most common offending drugs.[14,15] Medication-induced nausea and vomiting is, typically an acute phenomenon unless it is due to the development of gastritis. Additionally, pancreatitis-associated nausea and vomiting can be caused by commonly used medications such as diuretics, metronidazole, or salicylates.

The possibility of esophageal tearing (Mallory-Weiss tears) or rupture (Boerhaave's syndrome) should be considered in patients

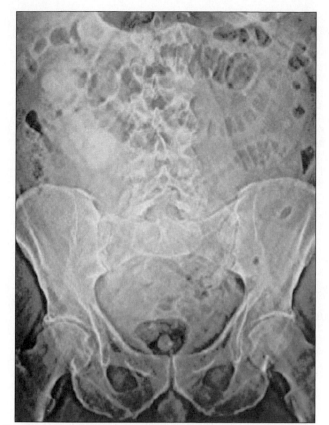

Figure 9-1 • Partial small bowel obstruction. From Frager D. Intestinal obstruction: role of CT. Gastroenterol Clin North Am 2002; 31:777–799.

Table 9-2 Medications That Cause Nausea	
NSAIDs	Digoxin
Gout medications	Gold compounds
Aspirin, sulfasalazine	Azathioprine
Chemotherapuetic agents	Oral diabetic agents
Iron, prenatal vitamins	Diuretics
Antibiotics (erythromicin, sulfonamides)	Antihypertensives
Narcotics	Antiepileptics
Antiparkinsonian drugs	Oral contraceptives
Theophylline	Nicotine

NSAIDs, non-steroidal anti-inflammatory drugs

who develop gastrointestinal bleeding after vomiting or retrosternal chest pain occurring after vomiting or retching, respectively. Fever is often present. Chest x-ray may demonstrate free air in the peritoneum or mediastinum in esophageal rupture. CT scan or gastrograffin swallow should be considered for anyone with possible Boerhaave's syndrome, as plain films may be normal in the initial hours. Endoscopy can be used to visualize an esophageal tear. Though Boerhaave's is rare, it can be lethal, and hospitalists need to realize that up to 21% of patients with this condition do not have a history of emesis.[16] Prompt recognition and surgery are critical.[17]

Diagnosis

Preferred Studies

Initial Studies

In patients with a history or examination suggestive of increased intracranial pressure, stroke, or hypertensive encephalopathy, neuroimaging with computed tomography (CT) or magnetic resonance imaging (MRI), retinal examination, and possibly lumbar puncture are indicated. Basic laboratory tests guide the remainder of the investigation and assist with determination of volume status. A basic metabolic panel, calcium, liver function tests, CBC, amylase and lipase are reasonable initial tests. In appropriate patients, drug levels of digoxin, theophylline, and salicylates as well as serum hCG or thyroid function tests may be warranted (Fig. 9-2).

Abdominal imaging (initially, plain films followed by CT scanning with oral and IV contrast) should be considered for patients with abdominal pain, constipation, risk factors for SBO, and no clear cause for nausea. Plain films may be normal in up to 22% patients with partial small bowel obstruction.[18] Upper endoscopy may be useful for patients with blood in the stool or a suspicion of gastritis or ulcer. A solid phase gastric emptying study may be useful in patients with findings suspicious for gastroparesis; however, empiric treatment with a prokinetic is a reasonable first step.[18]

Alternative Options

Prediction Rule

Nausea and vomiting have been extensively studied in patients receiving chemotherapy and in postoperative patients, and prediction rules have been established for these patients.

Postoperative Nausea and Vomiting (PONV) The preoperative assessment can identify risk factors for nausea and emesis postoperatively and help plan appropriate prophylaxis. Apfel et al. developed a risk score based on the presence of four risk factors for PONV: history of PONV or motion sickness, female gender, nonsmoker, and the need for opiods. When 0, 1, 2, 3, or 4 of these factors are present, the risk of PONV is approximately 10%, 20%, 40%, 60% or 80%, respectively. Prophylaxis is generally recommended for patients with a risk score of 2 or above. Other suspected risk factors for PONV include: use of volatile anesthetics, prolonged surgery, and the type of surgery (laparoscopy, breast, ENT, and neurosurgery are higher risk).[19]

Prediction of Chemotherapy–Related Nausea Chemotherapy-related nausea and emesis is strongly correlated with the type of agent used. For example, cisplatin has a high risk (>90%), while bleomycin has little risk (<10%) of nausea and emesis. Patient factors such as female sex, nausea and vomiting with prior chemotherapy, younger age, and little chronic alcohol use predict chemotherapy-related nausea and emesis.[9]

MANAGEMENT

Treatment

Treat the Effects of Vomiting

Vomiting, depending on the duration, can lead to various metabolic consequences, including hypokalemia and metabolic alkalosis. Volume depletion is of particular concern in the elderly. In

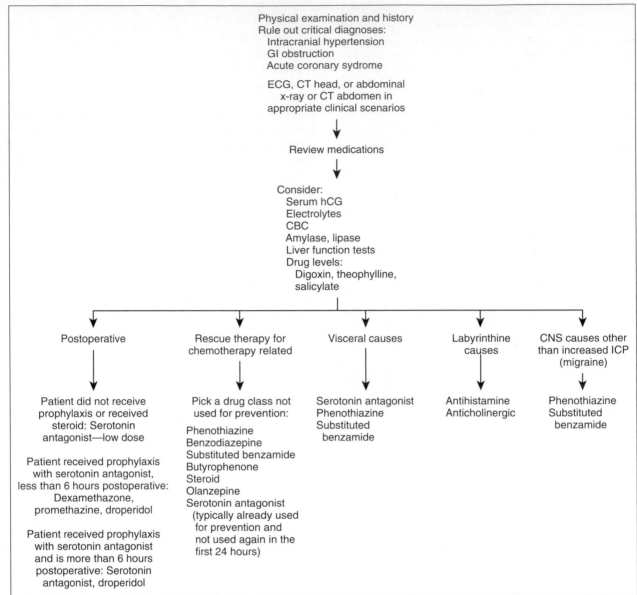

Figure 9-2 • Evaluation and Treatment of Nausea and Vomiting.

CNS, central nervous system; *CT*, computed tomography; *ECG*, electro cardiogram; *HCG*, human chorionic gonadotropin; *ICP*, intracranial pressure

patients with a small bowel obstruction, nasogastric tube output should be monitored to help guide volume replacement. Volume resuscitation can be achieved with normal saline with or without dextrose and potassium.

Preferred

Vomiting appears to be more responsive to treatment than nausea. Several neurotransmitters are involved in nausea and vomiting, including histamine (H_1), acetylcholine, dopamine (D2), serotonin (5-HT-3), and substance P, and they are the focus of most pharmacologic interventions. The clinical use of antiemetics is guided in large part by data from trials of patients with specific factors predisposing to nausea and emesis, including chemotherapy, radiation, or surgery. For other causes of nausea and vomiting, the suggested therapy is based on the mechanism of action of the drug, and there is little clinical data.

For nausea from central origin (medication induced, metabolic), antidopaminergic agents may be most effective. Therapy

for nausea from labrynthine origin (vertigo, motion sickness, and Meniere disease) involves antihistamines and anticholinergics. Nausea related to visceral stimulation from gastric irritation, chemotherapy, or abdominal radiation may respond best to serotonin antagonists and dopamine antqagonists[20] (Table 9-3).

Table 9-3 General Treatment Guidelines	
Etiology of Nausea and Vomiting	**Drugs to Consider**
Central origin (migraine, medications, metabolic)	Antidopaminergic agents
Labrynthine origin (motion sickness, Meniere disease)	Antihistamines Anticholinergics
Visceral stimulation (gastroenteritis, billiary disease, pancreatitis)	Serotonin antagonists Dopamine antagonists

In general, adding antiemetics has an additive rather than synergistic effect. When a drug from one class has been used for prevention of emesis (e.g., chemotherapy), a different drug class should be used for treatment failures. Table 9-4 details specific drugs in each class, including indications and dosing regimens.

Antihistamines

Drugs with histamine (H_1) receptor antagonistic properties have central antiemetic effects which are modest. These drugs are traditionally used for nausea and emesis of labyrinthine origin, including motion sickness and vertigo, as well as migraine headache. Their use is limited by central side effects including sedation.[18]

Anticholinergics

Cholinergic muscarinic M_1 receptor antagonists are typically used for prevention and treatment of motion sickness and other labrynthine disorders. Their unfavorable side effect profile limits their use.[18]

Dopamine Antagonists

Phenothiazines

Phenothiazines and butyrophenones have antiemetic action through their dopaminergic action in the area postrema in the base of the fourth ventricle. Phenothiazines also appear to act at the muscarinic and histamine receptors. These drugs have significant antiemetic effects and are used for a variety of causes, including nausea from central and visceral stimulation. A recent randomized trial of young emergency department patients with uncomplicated gastroenteritis found 10 mg of IV prochlorperazine (Compazine) to be more effective than 25 mg of IV promethazine (Phenergan), with no difference in extrapyramidal side effects.[21]

The phenothiazines additionally have efficacy in the setting of migraine headache.[20,22] Prochloperazine is an appropriate choice for rescue therapy in patients who have failed a serotonin antagonist in the prevention of chemotherapy-related emesis.

Side effects occur frequently and include sedation, orthostatic hypotension, extrapyramidal symptoms such as dystonia, and tardive dyskinesia. Rarely, blood dyscrasias and jaundice as well as neuroleptic malignant syndrome have occurred. These drugs may also lower the seizure threshold. Coadministration with other QT prolonging drugs including quinolones should be undertaken with caution.[15,18,23]

Butyrophenones

The butyrophenones, including droperidol and haloperidol, have a moderate antiemetic effect. Droperidol combined with dexamethasone is useful for postoperative nausea and is appealing because of its low cost (compared to ondansetron); however, its use has been limited because of several cases of QT prolongation and fatal torsades.[24] A black box warning has been issued for this drug. The quality and quantity of evidence supporting this conclusion have been questioned.[25,26]

Coadministration of butyrophenones with other QT-prolonging medications is not advised.[15,23]

Substituted Benzamides

These drugs exert antiemetic effects largely via central and peripheral antidopaminergic effects and prokinetic effects on the esophagus, stomach, and small intestine. Both agents in this class are moderately effective as antiemetics. Metoclopramide (Reglan) may also be useful in the setting of migraine headache with pain control and reduction in nausea seen in several trials.[22] It is not FDA approved for this indication, however, and it may be less efficacious than other antiemetics (phenothiazines).

Metoclopramide often requires high doses for effectiveness in the setting of chemotherapy. Ondansetron (Zofran) has been shown to be superior to metoclopramide for chemotherapy-related emesis; but in low-risk patients, metoclopramide may be used for prevention and for treatment if prevention with a serotonin antagonist has failed.[18]

Metoclopramide appears to increase the tone of the esophageal sphincter and is often used for patients with gastroparesis and gastroesophageal reflux, given its prokinetic effects. Central nervous system side effects occur frequently and include drowsiness, hyperprolactinemia and galactorrhea, and extrapyramidal symptoms

Because domperidone (Motilium®) does not cross the blood–brain barrier, the neurologic side effects common with metoclopramide are not seen. This drug is not yet available in the United States. It may be a good choice for patients with Parkinson's disease suffering from nausea exacerbated by their dopaminergic agents.[18]

Serotonin Antagonists

Serotonin receptors (5-HT3) are present both peripherally on the vagus nerve (innervating the small bowel) and centrally in the area postrema. Efficacy of these medications has been established mostly in cancer and postoperative patients. Cytotoxic chemotherapy appears to stimulate the release of serotonin from the enterochromaffin cells in the small intestine, which may stimulate vagal afferents and cause vomiting. The serotonin antagonists appear to have more of an antiemetic than an antinausea effect.

The serotonin antagonists are used as first-line therapy for the prevention of chemotherapy-related and PONV in high- and moderate-risk patients. Because of their long half-life, another drug class should be selected for rescue therapy if they fail, unless it is more than 6 hours postoperative.

With one exception, there appears to be no difference in efficacy among these medications (in the prophylaxis and treatment of postoperative and chemotherapy-related nausea). Palonosetron (Aloxi) has a much higher affinity for the 5-HT3 receptor and a 40-hour half-life. It appears to be more effective in preventing delayed emesis than the other drugs in this class. It is FDA approved for prevention only, not for treatment.

At least one randomized trial has shown superiority of ondansetron compared to placebo in the treatment of children with acute gastroenteritis; however, there are very little data supporting the use of serotonin antagonists in adults with gastroenteritis.[27]

Dosing of the serotonin antagonists is typically one-time dosing, coincident with the inciting event (chemotherapy or surgery). One exception is Zofran, which can be given every 4 hours for a three-dose regimen with chemotherapy. Dosing regimens involving the other 5HT3 blockers with multiple daily doses are not supported by clinical evidence and are expensive.

Severe side effects are uncommon with these drugs. Headache is most common, occurring in up to 30% of patients; dizziness, sedation, constipation, and diarrhea have also been reported. Rare cases of QT prolongation, arrhythmia, seizure, extrapyra-

Table 9-4 Medical Treatment of Nausea

	Dose	Dose Adjustments	Indications	Major Side Effects	Cost ($)
Antihistamines			For labyrinth disorders (motion sickness, vertigo) and migraine Can be combined with Reglan for chemotherapy-related emesis prevention	Drowsiness	
Meclizine (Antivert)	25–50 mg PO qd-BID				0.06
Diphenhydramine (Benadryl)	25–50 mg PO or IV q4–6 hr				0.05 (PO) 0.30 (IV)
Other agents: Buclizine (Bucladin-S)					
Cyclizine (Marezine)					0.43
Dimenhydrinate (Dramamine)					5.94
Anticholinergics Scopolamine (Transderm Scop)			Prevention of PONV motion sickness		5.95
Dopamine antagonists			PONV, motion sickness, second line for chemotherapy-related	Extrapyramidal effects, orthostatic hypotension, seizure, marrow toxicity, glaucoma, urinary retention, galactorrhea, arrhythmias, prolonged QT, anitcholinergic effects, lowers seizure threshold	
Phenothiazines Promethazine (Phenergan)	12.5–25 mg q4–6 hr	Liver disease, avoid or reduce dose in elderly, not dialyzed, not used in Parkinson's or myasthenia gravis	Gastroenteritis		0.41 (PO) 1.84 (IV)
Prochlorperazine (Compazine)	5–10 mg PO q6–8 hr, 2.5–10 mg IM/IV q6–8 hr maximum of 40 mg daily		Gastroenteritis, migraine		0.16 (PO) 7.41 (IV)
Chlorpromazine (Thorazine)			Migraine		0.29 (PO) 4.02 (IV)
Butyrophenones Droperidol (Inapsine)	2.5 mg IM or slow IV, additional 1.25 mg doses prn		Anticipatory and chemotherapy-related nausea, PONV	Prolonged QT, fatal torsades, limited availability, black box warning, continuous ECG monitoring	1.64
Haloperidol (Haldol)	1–2 mg PO q4–6 hr or 1–3 mg IV q4–6 hr				0.23 (PO) 9.22 (IV)
Substituted benzamides Metoclopramide (Reglan)	Chemo related: 20-40 mg PO q4–6 hr or 1–2 mg/kg IV q3–4 hr Other: 5–10 mg IV q6–8 hr	Renal Dosing: CrCl > 51 mL/min no adjustment, Cr-Cl 10–50 mL/min 75% of dose, Cr-Cl < 10 mL/min 50% of dose, not used for elderly	Migraine (not FDA approved), gastroparesis, second line for chemotherapy related	Crosses blood-brain barrier, CNS/ extrapyramidal effects (>10%): restlessness, drowsiness, tardive dyskinesia	0.07 (PO) 0.94 (IV)
Trimethobenzamide (Tigan) Domperidone (Motilium)	200–300 mg PO/IM tid-qid			Parkinsonism, sedation, jaundice cardiac arrhythmia, sudden death; neurologic side effects are rare, Motiliun does not cross blood-brain barrier Not in the United States	1.35 (PO) 20.97 (IV)

Table 9-4 Medical Treatment of Nausea—cont'd

	Dose	Dose Adjustments	Indications	Major Side Effects	Cost ($)
Serotonin antagonists		Not needed for elderly, renal, hepatic disease	First line for cancer chemotherapy and postoperative nausea and vomiting	QT prolongation, headache (24.3%), diarrhea (12.4%)	
Dolasetron (Anzemet)	1.8 mg/kg or 100 mg IV or 100 mg PO 30 min prior to chemotherapy 12.5 mg for prevention and treatment of PONV				19.52
Granisetron (Kytril)	1 mg PO bid or 0.01 mg/kg up to 1 mg IV, treatment: 0.1 mg				47.05
Ondansetron (Zofran)	Chemo related: single 32 mg dose or three doses of 0.15 mg/kg q4 hr PONV: 4 mg given a the end of surgery, treatment of PONV: 1 mg (1/4 dose)	In liver disease Child-Pugh ≥10, single max daily dose 8 mg			38.25
Palonosetron	0.25 mg IV		FDA approved for prevention of nausea with chemotherapy only, preferred agent for prevention		288.46
Steroids Dexamethasone	2.5 mg may be effective for PONV, 8 to 20 mg PO or IV daily most effective, no more often than q8 hr		Given before induction for prevention of PONV, with Reglan or ondansetron, prevention and treatment of chemotherapy related emesis		0.94–4.04
Benzodiazepines Lorazepam	0.5–2 mg PO q4–6 hr		Adjunctive treatment of chemotherapy related anticipatory nausea		0.47
Substance P/Neurokinin 1 Receptor Antagonist Aprepitant	FDA approved as a 3 day regimen of 125 mg on day 1 (prechemo) and 80 mg on days 2 and 3 (post chemo).	No adjustment	Complementary mechanism of action to all other commercially available available antiemetics	Multiple drug interactions, including certain chemotherapuetic agents	83.43
Other Erythromycin	3 mg/kg or 200 mg IV q 8 hr then 250 mg PO qac for 5–7 days		Prokinetic	QT prolongation, cramping, diarrhea	3.30
Dronabinol	5–10 mg po q3–6 hr		Refractory chemotherapy related nausea and emesis	Active substance in marijuanna, abuse potential	none
Olanzepine	2.5–5 mg PO BID		Cancer related (not an FDA approved indication)	Hyperglycemia and ketosis	4.70

midal effects, and LFT abnormalities have been associated with serotonin antagonist use.[20]

Steroids

The addition of dexamethasone improves the antiemetic effect of the 5-HT3 antagonists when used for chemotherapy-related emesis. It is typically used for prevention, but can be combined with a 5-HT3 antagonist or high-dose metoclopramide for treatment.

Dosing regimens vary. For the prevention of postoperative nausea and vomiting, 2.5 mg may be effective; but doses up to 8 to 20 mg, typically with metoclopramide or ondansetron, are superior for chemotherapy-related emesis. Steroids have been studied in pregnant women with hyperemesis gravidarum with mixed results. The utility of steroids in other patient populations has not been established.

NK-1-Receptor Antagonist

Aprepitant (Emend) is a newly approved agent which blocks the binding of substance P at the NK-1 receptor in the central nervous system. It is used in combination with 5-HT3 antagonists and dexamethasone for the prevention of chemotherapy-related nausea and emesis. It is not approved for rescue treatment and is less effective than ondansetron when used as monotherapy.

Benzodiazepines

Benzodiazepines are used as adjunctive treatment for chemotherapy related nausea. They are low-potency antiemetics and are not typically used as monotherapy. They may be useful for anticipatory nausea in large part because of their anxiolytic effect.

Cannabinoids

Dronabinol (Marinol) contains the psychoactive ingredient of marijuana. It can be used for anorexia in AIDS patients and refractory nausea in patients receiving chemotherapy. It has not been shown to be effective for PONV. Side effects include sedation, hypotension, ataxia, dizziness, and euphoria.

Prokinetics

Many antiemetics have prokinetic effects; however, their cardiac and neurologic side effects have limited their effectiveness. Cholinergic agents appear to have prokinetic effects but are rarely used because of frequent side effects. Metoclopramide and domperidone have prokinetic action and have demonstrated efficacy in gastroesophageal reflux and gastroparesis. Cisapride appears to act through a serotonin mediated effect. It has been removed from the US market because of proarrhythmic effects, but is still available from the manufacturer in a limited access program. Erythromycin inhibits pyloric tone and directly stimulates foregut motility and has been used off label for its prokinetic effects. Ventricular tachycardia and QT prolongation have been reported. Side effects can include nausea and diarrhea.

PREVENTION

Prevention of nausea and vomiting appears to have been studied only in the postoperative and chemotherapy settings. There are several interventions that may reduce the risk of postoperative nausea and vomiting, including the use of propofol, avoidance of volatile anesthetics, adequate hydration, and regional instead of general anesthesia. Prophylaxis is cost effective in high-risk but not low-risk patients.

Prevention of chemotherapy-related nausea and emesis is based on the emetogenic potential of the agent given. The NCCN (http://www.nccn.org/professionals/physician_gls/PDF/antiemesis.pdf) has specific guidelines for prophylactic therapy. Anticipatory nausea and emesis (a conditioned response) are treated with behavioral therapy, aggressive control of emesis with each cycle of chemotherapy, and benzodiazepines.

Key Points

- The clinical use of antiemetics is guided in large part by data from trials of patients with specific factors predisposing to nausea and emesis, including chemotherapy, radiation, surgery, or pregnancy. For other causes of nausea and vomiting, the suggested therapy is based on the mechanism of action of the drug, and there is little clinical outcomes-based data available. Hospitalists must draw inferences for other patient groups from this data.

- The possibility of esophageal tearing (Mallory-Weiss tears) or rupture (Boerhaave's syndrome) should be considered in patients who develop gastrointestinal bleeding or retrosternal chest pain after vomiting or retching, respectively.

- Nausea that develops in the hospitalized patient after admission should prompt a detailed review of medications.

- For nausea from central origin (medication induced, metabolic), antidopaminergic agents may be most effective. Therapy for nausea from labrynthine origin (vertigo, motion sickness, and Meniere disease) involves antihistamines and anticholinergics. Nausea related to visceral stimulation from gastric irritation, chemotherapy, or abdominal radiation may respond best to serotonin antagonists and dopamine antagonists.

- Multiple antiemetics capable of prolonging the QT interval include: serotonin antagonists, butyrophenones, and phenothiazines.

SUGGESTED READING

Feldman, Friedman and Sleisenger, eds. Gastrointestinal and liver disease online: comprehensive hospital medicine. CITY??: Elsevier, 2005.

Flake ZA, Scalley RD, Bailey AG. Practical Selection of Antiemetics. Am Fam Physician 2004; 69:1169–74.

Gan TJ, Meyer T, Apfel CC, et al. Consensus guidelines for managing Postoperative nausea and vomiting. Anesth Analg 2003; 97:62–71.

Quigley EM, Hasler WL, Parkman HP. AGA technical review on nausea and vomiting. Gastroenterology 2001; 120:261–286.

Spiller RC. ABC of the upper gastrointestinal tract, anorexia, nausea, vomiting, and pain. BMJ 2001; 323:1354–7.

Townes JM. Acute infectious gastroenteritis in adults: seven steps to management and prevention. Postgraduate Medicine 2004; 115 (5): 11.

CHAPTER TEN

Diarrhea

Sheri Chernetsky Tejedor, MD

BACKGROUND

Diarrhea causes significant morbidity and mortality worldwide, predominantly in children and elderly adults, with an estimated 8,400 deaths from diarrhea per day.[1] In developed nations, the incidence is less; approximately one episode occurs per person per year.[2] Averaging data from the National Hospital Ambulatory Medical Care Survey and the National Hospital Discharge Survey, a CDC report from 1999 estimated that nearly 1 million US hospitalizations annually result from gastroenteritis, with 3.5 hospitalizations per 1,000 person-years. They estimated that gastroenteritis contributed to the deaths of 6,402 people in the United States in 1997.[1,3] In the United States, the elderly bear a disproportionate share of the deaths from gastroenteritis. Although the elderly (age > 60) comprised only a quarter of the admissions for diarrhea, the majority of deaths due to diarrhea (85%) occurred in this age group.[4,1,5]

Even when patients are admitted for other diagnoses, diarrhea is often encountered. One survey of admission and discharge symptoms found that 16% of patients admitted to the hospital complained of diarrhea as part of their symptomatology. Diarrhea persisted at discharge in 27% of those patients.[6] Given the rising incidence of antibiotic-associated diarrhea and *Clostridium difficile* colitis, these are reviewed separately in Chapter 20.

ASSESSMENT

Clinical Presentation

Prevalence and Presenting Signs and Symptoms

Diarrhea is defined as three or more watery stools or one or more bloody stools in 24 hours and is acute if present fewer than 14 days. Community-acquired diarrhea is defined as diarrhea presenting at the time of admission or within 3 days of admission to the hospital; nosocomial diarrhea occurs after 3 days of hospitalization.[5,7]

Stool character and presenting signs and symptoms should help to distinguish noninflammatory from inflammatory diarrhea. Large volumes of watery stool without blood, pus, or mucous in an afebrile patient suggest a noninflammatory diarrheal disease. The presence of tenesmus, frequent small-volume stools with blood or pus (dysentery), in a patient with fever or abdominal pain suggests an invasive enteric pathogen and an inflammatory diarrhea.[5] Patient factors including exposures and comorbidities will influence the evaluation and treatment.

Differential Diagnosis

A focused history and physical examination will exclude most critical diagnoses requiring specific interventions and will guide a cost-effective evaluation (Table 10-1). Assessment of stool quality and quantity will also assist in diagnosis. Steatorrhea should be ruled out in the patient complaining of a change in stool character. Gastrointestinal bleeding, ischemic colitis, inflammatory bowel disease, and dysentery are critical diagnoses to consider.

Acute infectious diarrhea is most often viral. Viral pathogens including adenoviruses, calciviruses such as Norwalk virus, and rotaviruses represent approximately 50–70% of all cases of infectious diarrhea. Bacterial pathogens, including *Campylobacter jejuni*, *Salmonella*, *E. coli*, and *Shigella* represent 15–20% of cases, and parasites such as *Giardia lamblia* and *E. histolytica* comprise only 10–15% of cases.[7]

For patients presenting with community-acquired diarrhea, the history will often suggest the etiology. Recent travel, diet, exposures and contacts (including day-care centers), new medications, duration of symptoms, and the presence of nausea and vomiting are all important clues. Hospital-acquired diarrhea in an otherwise healthy patient, in the absence of an obvious outbreak, necessitates scrutiny of the medication list and evaluation for *C. difficile*.

Antibiotic-associated diarrhea, including *C. difficile* infection, occurs at a rate of 5–25%, depending on the medication. *C. difficile* infection (discussed in detail in Chapter 61) accounts for only 10–20% of antibiotic-associated diarrhea but accounts for the majority of cases of colitis. Other causes of antibiotic-associated diarrhea include direct mucosal effects and occasionally other enteric pathogens (*Salmonella*, *Staphylococcus aureus*, *Clostridium perfringens* type A).[8] Antibiotics are responsible for only 25% of drug-induced diarrhea, and there are multiple other causes of hospital-acquired diarrhea. Particular medications can lead to diarrhea (Table 10-2) through multiple mechanisms, including osmotic effects, malabsorption, and shortened transit time.[9] Additives to medications in liquid form (sorbitol, mannitol, or lactose) can lead to an osmotic diarrhea (Table 10-3).[10] Tube feeds can also be associated with an osmotic diarrhea with an

Table 10-1 Differential Diagnosis of Diarrhea

Present at Admission	Developing in the Hospital
Inflammatory bowel disease	Medication-induced diarrhea
Community-acquired infectious diarrhea	Hospital-acquired infectious diarrhea: C. difficile, salmonella, Staphylococcus aureus, C. perfringens type A
GI bleeding	Diarrhea secondary to tube feeds
Intestinal ischemia	
Malabsorption	
Radiation enteritis	
Thyrotoxicosis	
Appendicitis	
Irritable bowel syndrome	
Medication effect	
Pancreatitis	
Diverticulitis	

incidence of 25–68%; however, these patients also frequently receive liquid medications, which may also contribute to loose stool.[11,12] In a series of 29 patients experiencing diarrhea while on tube feeds, only 21% of these episodes (5% of the total population on tube feeds) were caused by the tube feeding. The remainder of cases were caused by liquid medications (62%) and pseudomembranous colitis (17%).[12,13]

Preferred Studies

The majority of patients with hospital-acquired diarrhea should have only a cytotoxin assay for *C. difficile* on diarrheal stool sent to the laboratory. Enzyme immunoassays are an alternative when the tissue culture cytotoxin assay is not available, but they require larger amounts of stool and have a false negative rate up to 20%. Repeating the test on two to three stools increases the diagnostic yield by 10%.[5,8]

The utility of routine testing for inflammatory markers in the stool (fecal leukocytes, lactoferrin, and occult blood) in hospitalized patients is questionable. The presence or absence of fecal leukocytes alone does not appear to predict a positive stool culture or *C. difficile* toxin assay among hospitalized patients and should not necessarily be used to guide further testing.[14] Stool cultures in patients hospitalized >3 days are rarely positive, and clinical criteria rather than fecal leukocytes should guide further evaluation (see below). For stable patients with hospital-acquired diarrhea, *C. difficile* testing alone is most often sufficient.

Patients with additional risk factors and those with persistent community-acquired or hospital-acquired diarrhea will need stool cultures, and inflammatory markers may add additional supporting evidence. Combined with the clinical presentation, the presence of fecal leukocytes and occult blood will support the diagnosis of an invasive bacterial diarrheal illness and may add additional support to the use of empiric antibiotics.[2,7] Fecal leukocytes may not be present in enterotoxin producing *E. coli*, emphasizing that the clinical picture rather than the presence or absence of fecal leukocytes should guide further evaluation.[1,15,16]

A retrospective review of stool culture results of nearly 14,000 specimens found that the culture positivity rate was only 1.4%

among patients hospitalized more than 3 days, and the cost per positive culture was approximately $1,000.[17] The "3-day rule" in which patients hospitalized longer than this are only tested for *C. difficile* infection, is not appropriate for all patients. Exceptions to this rule include immunocompromised patients, elderly patients (over age 65), and patients with inflammatory bowel disease or other comorbid conditions such as diabetes or renal failure. Patients with atypical presentations and nonenteric manifestations including rash or polyarthritis should also have stool cultures. Suspicion of a nosocomial outbreak warrants stool cultures, regardless of hospital day. This modified 3-day rule appears to be safe and still results in significant cost savings[18]

Testing of patients diagnosed with community-acquired diarrhea should be guided by the clinical presentation, risk factors, and past medical history (Fig. 10-1). Young patients with gastroenteritis and less than 1 day of a watery diarrheal illness, no comorbidities, and no evidence of severe dehydration do not need initial stool testing and can receive symptomatic therapy. Diarrhea persisting for >3 days should prompt stool testing. Patients with bloody stool, fever, abdominal pain, or comorbidities warrant stool studies. Testing for ova and parasites should be limited to patients with HIV infection, male homosexuals, those with persistent diarrhea, a pertinent travel history (Nepal, mountainous regions, Russia, Mexico), exposure to day-care center attendees, or in cases of suspected water-borne outbreak. Routine testing for ova and parasites is not cost effective.[19] Patients with bloody diarrhea, even in the absence of fever, should be tested for *E. coli* O157 : H7 and Shiga toxin.[1,5] The identification of a pathogen such as *Campylobacter, E. coli* O157 : H7 or *E. histolytica* may prevent potentially harmful evaluations and treatments such as colonoscopy, steroids, or surgery in a patient with bloody stool and cramping who may be suspected of having inflammatory bowel disease.[1]

Additional testing of serum chemistries including magnesium and complete blood count (CBC) are appropriate for patients with moderate to severe diarrhea. Blood cultures may be considered in the febrile patient, especially if there is concern for *Salmonella*, as bacteremia occurs in 2–14% of patients infected with it (especially the elderly and immunosupressed).[7] Abdominal imaging and sigmoidoscopy may be necessary for patients who do not improve despite empiric therapy.

MANAGEMENT

Rehydration and Diet

The initial management of diarrhea involves fluid resuscitation in dehydrated patients and electrolyte replacement. Oral rehydration therapy is the mainstay of rehydration therapy in patients who are able to tolerate it because the patient is more able to regulate volume status based on thirst, and it may be all that is needed for the stable patient. A standard approach of NPO and IV fluids is not appropriate if the patient can also take fluids by mouth. Stable adults without comorbidities can drink diluted juices, broths, and sports drinks with saltine crackers. Oral rehydration solutions containing sodium and glucose (pedialyte, Rehydralyte, Resol, WHO formula, Rice-lyte) often used in children may be used for elderly and immunocompromised patients. IV fluids (normal saline or lactated Ringer's, which has 4 mEq/L potassium) are often necessary to correct severe volume depletion and for patients with vomiting.

Table 10-2 Medications That Can Cause Diarrhea

Class	Example (Frequency)
Laxatives	Lactulose, sorbitol, magnesium salts
Antacids	Magnesium salts (36–46%)
Cardiac glycosides	Digoxin
Antigout	Colchicine (up to 80%)
NSAIDs	Ibuprofen
Antibiotics	Clindamycin (3.5–10%) Aminopenicillins (5–10%) Cephalosporins (3.5%)
Antineoplastics	Idarubicin (9–22%), epirubicin (13%), pentostatin (10%), mitoguazone (30%), mitoxantrone (up to 16%) docetaxel (8 to 25%), teniposide, flucytosine Fluorouracil
Promotility	Reglan (>10%) Erythromycin (7%)
Gold salts	Auranofin (40–50%)
Statins	Simvastatin (<5%)
Anticonvulsants	Carbamazepine
Biguanides	Metformin (10–53%)
Calcium regulator	Calcitonin (>10%)
5-Aminosalicylic acid derivative	Olsalazine (12–25%)
Prostaglandins	Misoprostol (15%)
Antiplatelet	Ticlopidine
Thyroid hormone	Synthroid
Bile acid sequestrants	Cholestyramine
Antihypertensives	Methyldopa Propranolol
Lipase inhibitor	Orlistat (60–95%)
Somatostatin analogs	Octreotide (5–13%) (34% to 61% when treating acromegaly)
Anti-Parkinson's agents	Levodopa/carbidopa Levodopa/benserazide
Antiarrhythmics	Quinidine (8%)
Histamine-2 blockers	Ranitidine
Interleukin-1 Inhibitor	Diacerein (37%)
Bisphosphonates	Etidronate (3–20%)
Acetylcholinesterase inhibitor	Tacrine (>10%) Donepezil (>10%)
Bile acid	Chenodeoxycholic acid (40–50%)

Antiretroviral agents
  Nucleoside reverse transcriptase inhibitors
  Protease inhibitors
	
	Didanosine (17–34%)
	Ritonavir (>10%)
	Nelfinavir (>10%)
	Amprenavir (39–60%)

SSRI	Sertraline (>10%)
Methylxanthine	Theophylline
α-Glucosidase inhibitors	Acarbose (10–33%)

Bowel rest is typically unnecessary; early feeding has not been shown to prolong the course of diarrheal illnesses.[20] Adequate calories should be provided to assist enterocyte renewal.[7,2,20] A study comparing dietary restriction with a clear liquid diet, advanced to a bland, nondairy diet without red meat versus an unrestricted diet in a small randomized trial of young adults with traveler's diarrhea receiving antibiotics, showed no difference in outcomes.[20] Additional, larger studies are needed to make more formal recommendations. A low-fat, lactose-, alcohol- and caffeine-free diet is typically recommended because of concerns for transient lactase deficiency and the promotility effects of caffeine and alcohol. Avoidance of undiluted simple sugars (apple juice) is typically advised because of osmotic effects on the intestine.[2]

Table 10-3 Liquid Medications That May Contain Sorbitol

Acetaminophen	Furosemide
Amantadine	Lithium
Cimetidine	Metoclopramide
Theophyline	Valproic acid
Codeine, hydrocodone	Sucralfate
Isoniazid	Perphenazine
Trimethoprim-sulfamethoxasole	Ranitidine
Carbamazepine	Dexamethasone

Symptomatic Therapy: Antidiarrheals

Antidiarrheal agents are appropriate in selected patients with acute diarrhea, as they can shorten the clinical illness and improve quality of life.[7] Patients with a noninflammatory, community-acquired, watery diarrhea, without additional risk factors, may safely receive antimotility agents. Most patients with traveler's diarrhea can safely receive bismuth or loperamide, combined with antibacterials. Patients with suspected *C. difficile* infection, dysentery, or comorbidities should have additional testing before antidiarrheals are initiated. *See* Table 10-4 for specific therapies.

Table 10-4 Symptomatic Treatment of Diarrhea

	Dosing	Hepatic/Renal Dosing	Side Effects	Contraindications	Cost
Antisecretory					
Bismuth subsalicylate (Pepto-Bismol, Kaopectate)	2 tablets or 30 mL every 30 minutes to 1 hour as needed up to 8 doses/24 hours. Each tablespoon contains 130 mg of aspirin; extra-strength liquid has 236 mg.	Avoid in renal failure.	Rarely bismuth encephalopathy; black tongue and stools, tinnitus	HIV, immunocompromised patients, aspirin allergy, fecal impaction	0.44
Antimotility agents					
Loperamide (Immodium)	4 mg (2 tablets) initially, then 2 mg after unformed stool, <16 mg/day, <2 days	Use caution in liver disease.	Sedation, delirium, nausea, dry mouth	Not used if high fever, bloody diarrhea, psuedomembranous colitis	0.11
Diphenoxylate with atropine (Lomotil)	2 tablets, 4 mg QID, <2 days	Use with caution in hepatic or renal disease.	Toxic megacolon, addiction, respiratory depression, tachycardia, urinary retention, blurred vision	Severe liver disease, narrow-angle glaucoma	0.39
Antiperistaltics Anticholinergics Hyoscyamine (Levsin)	0.125–0.25 mg PO q4 hr to max of 1.5 mg/day		Urinary retention, ileus, worsening of glaucoma, dry mouth, tachycardia, dizziness, apnea, psychosis	Narrow-angle glaucoma, myasthenia gravis, obstructive uropathy, caution in cardiac disease and the elderly	0.07
Dicyclomine (Bentyl)	Not FDA approved for diarrhea 20–40 mg qid start with 10 mg in elderly, up to 160 mg/day	Use caution in hepatic and renal disease.	Urinary retention, ileus, worsening of glaucoma, dry mouth, tachycardia, dizziness, apnea, psychosis	Narrow-angle glaucoma, myasthenia gravis, obstructive uropathy, caution in cardiac disease and the elderly	0.33
Oral enkephalinase inhibitor (Racecadotril)	Not yet FDA approved 100 mg TID/qac, up to 300 mg TID in HIV		Nausea, abdominal distention, constipation are rare		0.07
Octreotide	50–100 mcg subcutaneously TID, used for VIPomas, carcinoid, refractory AIDS associated diarrhea (off label)	Adjust in renal failure.			11.50

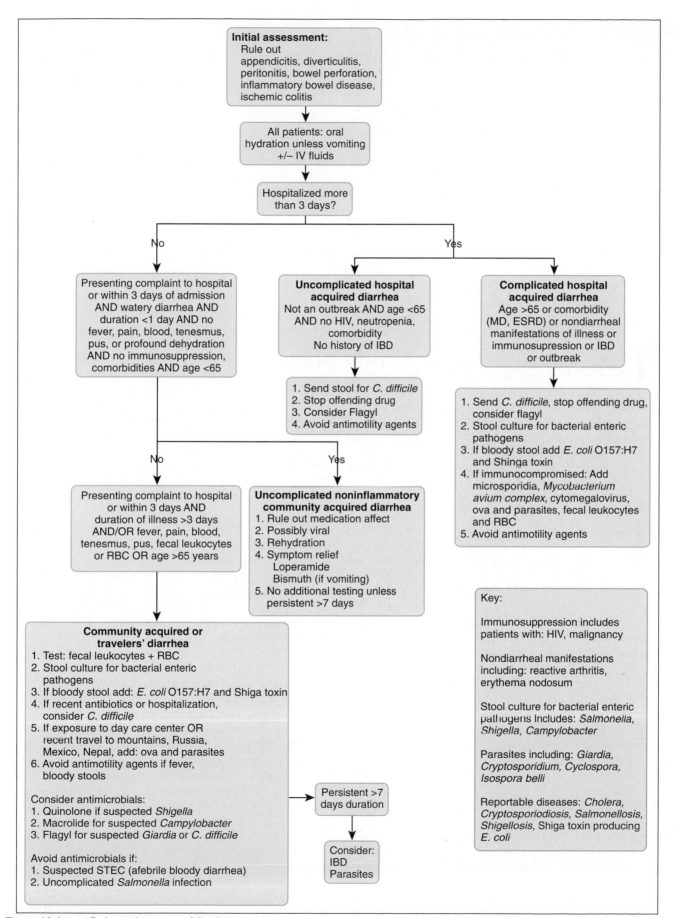

Figure 10-1 • Evaluation/treatment of diarrhea.

RBC—red blood cells; ESRD—end stage renal disease; MD—modical disease (including diabetes mellitus, stroke, pulmonary disease, cirrhosis); IBD—inflammatory bowel disease; STEC—Shiga toxin–producing E. coli

Antisecretory/Adsorbents

Adsorbent agents increase stool consistency but may not decrease fluid or electrolyte losses and may actually mask ongoing stool losses; these agents are not used in febrile, bloody diarrhea.[5] Continued rehydration is imperative when these drugs are used.

Bismuth subsalicylate (Pepto-Bismol) is the primary drug in this category. It is the preferred drug for patients with viral gastroenteritis with vomiting as a prominent feature accompanying their diarrhea.[2,5] It has antisecretory effects, stimulating intestinal sodium and water reabsorption, which reduces the number of loose stools by up to 50% compared to placebo.[2,7] Bismuth may have some antimicrobial effects and has been shown to inhibit enterotoxin activity in animal models.[21] In direct comparisons with loperamide, bismuth was less effective at reducing the number of unformed stools.[22]

Bismuth therapy often requires high doses for symptomatic improvement and must be used with caution because of its salicylate content. Each tablespoon of bismuth subsalicylate contains an equivalent of 130 mg aspirin; extra-strength liquid has 236 mg. For this reason, it should not be used in patients with renal disease. Bismuth encephalopathy is a rare and often reversible complication of chronic bismuth ingestion. It typically requires several years of ingestion, but in some cases has developed after weeks of therapy. It typically presents with lethargy, mental status changes, myoclonus, tremor, and ataxia. Bismuth is not recommended by the American College of Gastroenterology in patients with HIV infection and chronic diarrhea because of concerns for bismuth encephalopathy. Loperamide is the preferred agent in these patients.

Antimotility and Antiperistaltic Agents

These drugs inhibit peristalsis often with some antisecretory properties. They can lead to pooling of fluid in the intestine and therefore mask fluid losses as stool frequency decreases. Loperamide (Imodium) is the drug of choice in this category. Other agents (diphenoxylate—Lomotil, paregoric, tincture of opium, codeine) have central opiate effects as well as some anticholinergic effects. Loperamide does not have CNS action and is therefore not addictive. The efficacy has been established mostly in patients with traveler's diarrhea, typically combined with antibiotics (trimethoprim-sulfamethoxazole [TMP-SMZ] or ciprofloxacin) and may reduce the duration of diarrhea by approximately 1 day. Loperamide appears to be most useful in the first 24 hours of a diarrheal illness. It generally reduces stool frequency by 80%.[2]

Antimotility agents are traditionally not used in patients with inflammatory diarrhea. The risk of toxic megacolon in patients with psuedomembranous colitis, hernolytic uremic syndrome (HUS) in patients (mostly children) with Shiga toxin producing E. coli, and prolongation of fever in patients with Shigella infections may contraindicate their use.[23] This is not commonly seen in clinical practice, and at least one study has demonstrated safety in patients with dysentery (mostly shigellosis) given loperamide with antibiotics; however, larger studies are needed to address these safety concerns.[24]

The antispasmodics are anticholinergic agents that may reduce pain and cramping. They do not reduce the volume or frequency of stools.[5] Because of their anticholinergic effects and uncertain efficacy, these drugs are not generally recommended. They should be avoided in the elderly.[25] Dicyclomine (Bentyl) is FDA approved for the treatment of irritable bowel syndrome, but not for diarrhea; however, hyoscyamine (Levsin) is FDA approved for symptomatic treatment of acute enterocolitis.

Somatostatin Analogs

Somatostatin slows gastric motility and reduces intestinal fluid volume. Octreotide has been used successfully in different types of secretory diarrhea, including refractory AIDS-associated diarrhea, radiation enteritis, excessive ileostomy output, and diarrhea associated with chemotherapy. It is FDA approved only for diarrhea from carcinoid tumors and VIPomas. Because of its expense and need for subcutaneous administration, it should be considered only after traditional therapies have failed.[2,5]

Alternative Options

The oral enkephalinase inhibitor racecadotril (Acetorphan), has been found to be equivalent to loperamide for acute, presumed infectious diarrhea and appears to reduce rehydration requirements; it has not yet received FDA approval. Efficacy has also been established in HIV patients with chronic diarrhea. It may be a less toxic choice because it does not have an antimotility effect and has few CNS effects. Racecadotril acts by preventing the degradation of endogenous opioids, reducing the secretion of water and electrolytes into the intestines. Side effects, including constipation, nausea, and abdominal distention, have rarely occurred.[5,26,27] Other drugs under investigation as antisecretory agents include chloride channel blockers, calmodulin inhibitors, and drugs that interfere with prostaglandin-mediated pathways.[23]

Antimicrobial Therapy

Acute watery diarrhea that is often viral or a side effect of medications does not warrant antimicrobial therapy. Antimicrobial therapy for C. difficile infection is reviewed in detail in Chapter 10. Antimicrobial therapy in severe community-acquired diarrhea appears to reduce the duration of illness by 1–2 days.[23]

The current IDSA guidelines recommend antimicrobials for moderate-to-severe traveler's diarrhea, suspected giardiasis, and febrile patients with a suspected inflammatory diarrhea. Empiric therapy can be with a fluoroquinolone (metronidazole is used for Giardia and C. difficile). Erythromycin or azithromycin for fluoroquinolone resistant Campylobacter should be considered in certain clinical settings, including in those who are immunocompromised, are severely ill, or are travelers to southern Asia.[23,1] An important exception is suspected or confirmed cases of Shiga toxin producing enterohemorrhagic E. coli (Shiga toxin–producing E. coli [STEC]; including E. coli O157:H7), as antimicrobials do not appear to improve the clinical course and are suspected of increasing the risk of hemolytic uremic syndrome. STEC should be considered in patients who are afebrile with bloody diarrhea and abdominal pain. Exposure clues include rare hamburger or seed sprout ingestion. Antibiotics may also prolong shedding and increase the risk of relapse in patients with Salmonella and are reserved for patients with extremes of age, valvular heart disease, atherosclerosis, uremia, or cancer. The risks of antimicrobial therapy include prolonged shedding of some pathogens, increased risk of relapse, and development of resistance.[1,23]

PATIENT EDUCATION

Patients should be educated to continue oral rehydration therapy until stools are formed and they have fully recovered. Diuretics and antihypertensives may need to be adjusted in patients who are recovering from a diarrheal illness. Dietary modification with avoidance of caffeine and dairy is prudent, though data supporting this practice is limited.

Outpatient Physician Communication

Patients with diarrhea more than 5–7 days duration and negative evaluations for bacteria and parasites should be evaluated for inflammatory bowel disease.

Key Points

- Community-acquired diarrhea is defined as diarrhea presenting at the time of admission or within 3 days of admission to the hospital; nosocomial diarrhea occurs after 3 days of hospitalization.

- Hospital-acquired diarrhea in an otherwise healthy patient, in the absence of an obvious outbreak, necessitates scrutiny of the medication list and evaluation for *C. difficile*. The majority of patients with hospital-acquired diarrhea should have only a cytotoxin assay for *C. difficile* on diarrheal stool sent to the laboratory. Stool cultures in patients hospitalized more than 3 days are rarely positive. Clinical criteria will dictate whether additional testing is necessary.

- Stool testing in patients with community-acquired diarrhea should be guided by the clinical presentation, risk factors, and past medical history. Routine testing for ova and parasites is not cost effective. Patients with particular clinical risk factors and those with persistent community-acquired or hospital-acquired diarrhea will need stool cultures. Inflammatory markers may add additional supporting evidence for an invasive enteric pathogen.

- Additives to medications in liquid form (sorbitol, mannitol, or lactose) can lead to an osmotic diarrhea. Tube feeds can also be associated with an osmotic diarrhea; however, tube-fed patients also frequently receive liquid medications that may contribute to loose stool.

- Bowel rest is typically unnecessary during a diarrheal illness; early feeding has not been shown to prolong the course of diarrheal illnesses.

- Patients with a noninflammatory, community-acquired, watery diarrhea, without additional risk factors, may safely receive antimotility agents. Most patients with traveler's diarrhea can safely receive bismuth or loperamide, combined with antibacterials. Patients with suspected *C. difficile* infection, dysentery, or comorbidities should have additional testing before antidiarrheals are initiated

SUGGESTED READING

Aranda-Michel J, Giannella RA. Acute diarrhea: a practical review. Am J Med 1999; 106:670–676.

Bauer TM, Lalvani A, Fehrenbach J, et al. Derivation and validation of guidelines for stool cultures for enteropathogenic bacteria other than Clostridium difficile in hospitalized adults. JAMA 2001; 285:313–319.

Bartlett JG. Antibiotic associated diarrhea. N Engl J Med 2002; 346:334–339.

Gore JI, Surawicz C. Severe acute diarrhea. Gastroenterol Clin North Am 2003; 32:1249–1267.

Guerrant RL, Van Gilder T, Steiner TS, et al. Practice guidelines for the management of infectious diarrhea (IDSA guidelines). Clin Infect Dis 2001; 32:331–351.

Manatsathit S, Dupont HL, Farthing M, et al. Working party report: guideline for the management of acute diarrhea in adults. J Gastroenterol Hepatol 2002; 17(Suppl.):S54–S71.

Thielman NM, Guerrant RL. Acute infectious diarrhea. N Engl J Med 2004; 350:38–47.

CHAPTER ELEVEN

Hospital Discharge

Sunil Kripalani, MD, MSc, Amy K. Trobaugh, PharmD, and Eric A. Coleman, MD, MPH

INTRODUCTION

Along with admission to a hospital, discharge is a core process experienced by every living patient. For the majority of patients, it is a time of transition from hospital to home, but as many as 20% go to a continuing care venue, most commonly a skilled nursing facility (SNF). During this time, a shift in responsibility occurs from the inpatient provider or hospitalist to the outpatient primary care physician, or perhaps a SNF-based practitioner. Medication regimens are revised, with patients being asked to stop some medications, while starting or changing the doses of others. Patients must also prepare to assume greater self-care responsibilities as they return home. Negotiating these changes is often challenging for patients and their families.

When executed poorly, care coordination can adversely affect patient satisfaction, increase adverse events, and result in higher rates of hospital readmissions.[1,2] One study showed that 49% of patients experienced at least one medical error in the period following hospital discharge, including errors in medication continuity, diagnostic work-up, and test follow-up.[1] In another investigation, 19% of patients suffered an adverse event, most commonly an adverse drug event (ADE).[3] Half of these adverse events were judged preventable or ameliorable. Most were the result of poor communication between hospital caregivers and the patient or primary care physician.[3]

This chapter will review the key challenges to providing effective care around the time of hospital discharge, and review recent evidence behind solutions to improve communication and ease the care transition.

CHALLENGES

Inpatient-Outpatient Physician Discontinuity

Under the traditional model, primary care physicians (PCPs) usually admitted their own patients, coordinated their care in the hospital (while seeing patients in the office all day), and continued to treat them after discharge. This model promoted continuity of care, but struggled in the face of increasing inpatient and outpatient severity of illness, rapidly advancing technology, and a push to reduce hospital costs and length of stay.[4] The rapid growth of hospital medicine was largely fueled by increased efficiency and quality of hospital care, while permitting PCPs to remain devoted to their outpatient duties.[4] With about 15,000 hospitalists currently practicing in the United States and a projected workforce of approximately 30,000 by the year 2010, it is now increasingly common for patients' care to be transferred from a hospital-based physician to the PCP at the time of discharge.[5]

The patient discharge summary is the most common vehicle for communication between the inpatient and outpatient physician. However, a number of studies have shown that discharge summaries often lack important administrative and medical information, may arrive too late to be helpful, and sometimes never reach the PCP.[6]

Audits of discharge communications have revealed that they frequently do not identify[6]:

- Dates of admission and discharge (20–42%)
- The responsible hospital physician (2–27%)
- Primary diagnosis (2–39%)
- Results of abnormal diagnostic testing (20–75%)
- Hospital course (22–45%)
- Pending test results (65–88%)
- Follow-up plans (2–48%)
- Patient or family counseling (90–97%)

The lack of communication about pending test results is concerning, since approximately 40% of patients have test results that return after discharge, and many of these require action.[7]

Delays in the preparation and delivery of discharge summaries mean that most patients follow up with their PCP before the summary has arrived.[8,9] PCPs estimate that such delays limit their ability to provide adequate follow-up in approximately 15% of cases.[6]

Changes in the Medication Regimen

The period following hospital discharge is a vulnerable time for adverse drug events to occur, due in part to changes in the medication regimen, as well as poor patient comprehension of discharge diagnoses and medication instructions.[10] The medication regimen prescribed at discharge frequently differs from the pre-hospital regimen for several reasons.

First, physicians may not obtain a complete and accurate medication history at the time of admission. Omitting a medication taken at home is the most common error in the admission medication history.[11] Additionally, a nurse and even a pharmacist may obtain a medication history on the same patient. Discrepancies among the histories obtained by these different health care providers are rarely recognized or rectified. Approximately 50% of patients in a recent study had at least one unintended medication discrepancy on hospital admission orders, and 39% of these discrepancies were deemed potentially serious.[11] The quality of the information obtained from a patient at the time of admission can be affected by health literacy, language barriers, current health status, medication history interview skills, and time constraints.[12]

Second, significant changes in a patient's medication regimen can occur multiple times during hospitalization. Acute illness may prompt certain medications to be held, discontinued, or dosed differently during hospitalization. Few hospitals with advanced electronic health information systems are capable of prompting physicians at the time of discharge to consider restarting routine medications held upon admission to the hospital. The more complex a patient's hospitalization, the more likely it is errors may occur at crucial points of care. Critical transition points include transferring the patient from one service or level of care to another and resumption of medications after surgery.

Third, closed drug formularies at most hospitals require the therapeutic interchange of one medication for another drug in the same class during the patient's hospital stay. This practice increases the risk of ADEs due to duplication if the medications are not reconciled at the time of discharge.

Self-Care Responsibilities and Social Support

Patients now leave the hospital "quicker and sicker" than before, due to the economic pressures on our health care system. Upon returning home, patients also experience a "voltage drop" in the intensity of services provided. They no longer have multidisciplinary providers continually reviewing their health status and needs, but rather must follow up with their outpatient provider over a period of days to weeks. Unfortunately, hospital personnel may inaccurately estimate patients' functional status and self-care needs at discharge,[13] leaving them to fend for themselves. In the interim, patients must assume self-care responsibilities, such as monitoring for worsening symptoms, performing self-directed physical therapy exercise, or even administering subcutaneous medications. Additionally, patients may lack the level of social and family support needed to perform these activities effectively.

Ineffective Physician–Patient Communication

Although physician–patient communication is a cornerstone of medical practice, a large gap exists between physicians' provision of information and patients' comprehension.[14] Some of the problems noted in physician communication include[13,14]:

- Use of medical jargon
- Communication of a large amount of information in a short time
- Failure to distinguish the major points from the minor points
- Presentation of instructions verbally, without use of audiovisual materials or patient education handouts
- Inadequate opportunity for questions, clarification, or demonstration of the skills being taught
- No confirmation of patient comprehension

Adding to the challenges of effective physician–patient communication is the fact that approximately half of adult Americans have limited functional literacy skills. They commonly have difficulty reading and interpreting medical instructions, medication labels, and appointment slips.[15] Not surprisingly, patients with limited literacy skills are less knowledgeable about chronic diseases and their management. Low literacy is also associated with greater use of emergency department services, increased risk of hospitalization, and increased health care costs.[16] Patients with limited English proficiency face similar or even greater challenges, and they have increased hospital length of stay.[17]

Limited Guidelines

Evidence-based guidelines for improving the discharge process are lacking, except for special populations such as the elderly and patients with certain high-volume illnesses (e.g., congestive heart failure and community-acquired pneumonia).[18] The Society of Hospital Medicine has convened task forces to review the available evidence and make recommendations applicable to hospitalists and other inpatient physicians. The Continuity of Care Task Force has developed recommendations on information transfer from inpatient to outpatient physician at hospital discharge (see below). The Ideal Hospital Discharge Workgroup developed a checklist of steps to enhance patient safety when discharging the elderly or other patients.

Regulations to enforce evidence-based practice at the point of discharge are becoming more common. As a National Patient Safety Goal, the Joint Commission on Accreditation of Healthcare Organizations (JCAHO) now requires accredited health care organizations to "accurately and completely reconcile medications across the continuum of care."[19] JCAHO also supports the development of standardized hand-off procedures, acknowledging that poor communication is the most common root cause of sentinel and adverse events.[19]

SOLUTIONS

Improving Physician Information Transfer and Continuity

Improving information transfer from inpatient to outpatient physician requires attention to the content, format, and timely delivery of discharge communications. Based on a systematic review of the literature, the Society of Hospital Medicine/Society of General Internal Medicine Continuity of Care Task Force provided the recommendations outlined in Box 11-1.[6]

The discharge summary content areas specified in the box are based on the items most likely to contribute to adverse events (medications and pending test results),[3,7] as well as surveys of what PCPs find most helpful in discharge summaries.[8,20] In a study of hospitalist communication at discharge, PCPs rated the following items as most important: discharge medications, diagnoses, results of procedures, scheduled follow-up, and pending test results.[8] Because patients may follow up with their PCP within a few days of discharge, it is important to provide the PCP with at least this information on the day of discharge itself. A quick telephone call, facsimile, or email update to the PCP serves this function. A hand-written note, which the patient delivers to

Box 11-1 Recommendations to Improve the Transfer of Information from Inpatient to Outpatient Physician at Discharge

1. Confirm the name, address, phone number, fax number, and/or email address of primary care physician (PCP) upon admission, and convey this information to the transcription service at the time of dictation.

2. Have a system in place to ensure the timely preparation and delivery of patient information at discharge. Consider automatic, computer-generated summaries or reminders.

3. Using email, fax, or telephone, provide the PCP with a brief summary of the hospitalization on the day of discharge. At minimum, include the discharge medications, diagnoses, results of procedures, follow-up needs, and pending test results.

4. Send a detailed discharge summary to the PCP within 7 days.

5. Ensure summaries include:

   - Brief description of problem(s) that precipitated the hospitalization

   - Primary and secondary diagnoses

   - Dates of hospitalization, treatment provided, brief hospital course

   - Results of procedures and abnormal labs

   - Reconciled discharge medication regimen, with reasons for any changes and indications for newly prescribed medications

   - Appointments scheduled or needed

   - Follow-up needs and pending tests

   - Recommendations of any subspecialty consultants

   - Name of the responsible hospital physician

   - Documentation of patient education and confirmation of patient understanding through teach-back[38]

6. Use structured discharge summaries with subheadings to organize information

7. Consider computer-generated templates for common diagnoses

From Kripalani S, Phillips CO, Basaviah P, Williams MV, Saint SK, Baker DW. Deficits in information transfer from inpatient to outpatient physician at hospital discharge: a systematic review. J Gen Intern Med 2004; 19 (S1):135.

the outpatient physician at the first follow-up visit, can also be effective.

A detailed discharge summary should be delivered within 1 week. Computer-generated summaries are able to capture quickly and completely the most salient elements of the hospitalization, and they are available for delivery sooner than traditional dictated summaries.[21] Whether using computer-generated, handwritten, or dictated summaries, structuring the information with required subheadings leads to more complete and organized documents, which are preferred over unstructured narrative summaries.[22]

Medication Reconciliation and Education

Medication reconciliation is an active process that should occur throughout the hospital stay.[19] The most important times for reconciliation are transition points, such as patient transfer or discharge, when changes in the medication regimen are more likely. Reconciliation also provides an opportunity to review the safety and appropriateness of the regimen, and to discontinue undesirable or unnecessary medications.[23] The process of medication reconciliation includes the following steps:

1. Obtain an accurate history of medications prior to admission.

2. Compare the list of medications prior to admission to medications ordered at admission, throughout the hospital stay, and at discharge.

3. Rectify unintentional discrepancies; document the rationale for intentional discrepancies.[24]

4. Communicate a complete reconciled list of medications to the patient at discharge.

Medication reconciliation begins with actively involving the patient or caregiver in the medication history process and documenting the most accurate list possible, including the dose, route, and frequency (Box 11-2). It is important to adopt a standardized, highly visible location in the patient chart for the list of medications prior to admission. The responsibility and process of obtaining the list of medications prior to admission should be well delineated and based on the resources available at each institution. Ultimately, it is the physician's responsibility to ensure accurate and complete patient information. Partnering with clinical pharmacists, a tremendous resource when available, offers many advantages. Pharmacists have had formal education and experience in taking medication histories and may be ideal interviewers for all patients entering the inpatient setting. Unfortunately, pharmacists conduct the medication history interview in only 5% of US hospitals, and they are involved in drug counseling in only 48% of hospitals.[25]

The evidence for medication reconciliation is expanding and compelling.

- When nurses obtained and recorded the home medications on an order form that allowed prescribers to indicate whether the home medication should be continued or stopped, the accuracy of admission medication orders increased from 40% to 95%.[26]

- When pharmacists led admission medication reconciliation, they identified discrepancies in 27% of patients' admission orders, and physicians accepted 71% of their suggested interventions. Researchers estimated that, without these interventions, 22% of the underlying discrepancies may have resulted in patient harm during hospitalization, and 59% of the discrepancies could have resulted in patient harm if the error continued after discharge.[27]

- At the time of ICU transfer to the floor, nurse-led reconciliation of medications prior to admission, medication orders in the ICU, and medication orders at ICU transfer resulted in some change in patients' order in 94% of cases.[28]

Additional strategies to improve medication safety at transitions of care include the following:

- Avoid blanket orders such as "continue home medications" and "resume all medications."

- Provide patients with a complete list of their medication regimen with indications and administration instructions, in lay language.
- Indicate clearly to the patient and next provider any changes to the patient's previous regimen, such as medications that should be discontinued after discharge.
- Provide the PCP with the indication for new medications.
- Use inpatient pharmacist counseling when available, particularly for patients who are elderly, have limited literacy skills, take more than five medications daily, or take high-risk medications such as insulin, warfarin, cardiovascular drugs (including antiarrhythmics), inhalers, antiseizure medications, eye medications, analgesics, oral hypoglycemics, and oral methotrexate or other immunosuppressants.[29]

Providing Adequate Medical and Social Support

A multidisciplinary discharge planning team can help ensure meeting the social needs of patients and their families. Members of this team may include a nurse case manager and social worker, but also a physical therapist, occupational therapist, pharmacist, and other health care providers. After discussion with the patient and family and consideration of existing rules governing eligibility, the team may recommend home health services to provide additional medical support during the transition home.[30]

It is also important to make follow-up arrangements prior to discharge. Some tips for making such arrangements are:
- Give the patient a specific appointment, as this increases the likelihood of attending follow-up appointments compared to simply asking patients to call and schedule their own visit.
- Coach patients to clearly state that they were just discharged from the hospital when they speak to the scheduling person if they must schedule their own appointment.
- Typically, outpatient follow-up within two weeks of hospital discharge is appropriate. However, this may need to occur sooner, depending on the patient's status, tests pending at discharge, and the need for medication monitoring or follow-up testing.
- Following up with the same physician who provided hospital care can result in a lower combined rate of readmission and 30-day mortality.[31] A hospitalist-staffed follow-up clinic should be considered, particularly for patients who lack an established PCP.

Contacting patients by telephone a few days after discharge is also an excellent way to bridge the inpatient–outpatient transition. It provides an opportunity to address any patient questions, new or worrisome symptoms, and medication-related problems (e.g., not filling the discharge prescriptions, or difficulty understanding the new medication regimen).[10] Such telephone follow-up may be performed by a physician, physician assistant, advanced practice nurse, registered nurse, pharmacist, or care manager. Irrespective of who performs the telephone call, this individual should be familiar with the patient's recent course of events and plan of care made at discharge. Telephone follow-up not only promotes patient satisfaction, but also reduces rates of subsequent emergency room visits and hospital readmission.[32]

For certain patient populations, such as the frail elderly, home visits may be appropriate. A home visit provides the opportunity to assess the patient's daily needs and safety (e.g., fall risk). It can also be an enlightening way to assess medication use, reviewing old prescription bottles that may still be in the medicine cabinet, for example.[33] Close follow-up of at-risk or elderly patients after discharge can reduce hospital readmission and total health care costs.[34–37]

More Effective Physician–Patient Communication

Physicians may overcome many of the challenges above through more effective communication during hospitalization and at discharge. Recognizing that most patients struggle to understand medical information,[10,14] such communication should occur in

Box 11-3 Enhancing Physician–Patient Communication at Hospital Discharge

- Focus counseling on the few key points of greatest interest to patients (e.g., major diagnoses, medication changes, dates of follow-up appointments, self-care instructions).
- Ask hospital staff (i.e., nurses and pharmacists) to reinforce these key messages.
- Consider using patient education videos to provide standard instructions for common conditions (e.g., cardiac catheterization).
- When a language gap exists, use a trained interpreter rather than relying on rudimentary language skills or family members.[41]
- Provide illustrated take-home materials written in lay language.
- Effectively encourage patient questions.
- Confirm patient comprehension of key instructions through a teach-back.[38]
- Ask patients to demonstrate self-care behaviors.

lay terms, focus on the points of greatest concern to patients, and include confirmation of patient understanding (Box 11-3).

A new JCAHO National Patent Safety Goal is to "encourage the active involvement of patients and their families in the patient's own care."[19] This requires providing ample opportunity for questions. Unfortunately, physicians tend to either not invite patient questions, or when they do so, they use yes/no statements like, "Any questions?" or "Do you have any questions?" Knowing that the physician (who may have already stood up or have his/her hand on the doorknob) is busy, it is easy for patients to simply reply, "No." A far more effective way to invite patient and family questions is to ask in a more open-ended manner, "What questions do you have?" (while seated, making eye contact, and not darting for the door!).

Perhaps the most important step in the effective communication of discharge instructions is to confirm patient comprehension by asking the patient to "teach-back" the key points.[38] This is accomplished by asking the patient to repeat back his or her understanding of the discharge instructions. Use of this simple technique is advocated as one of the top methods to improve patient safety.[39] Patients should also be asked to demonstrate any new self-care behaviors that they will be required to perform at home, such as using an inhaler.

CONCLUSION

The period following hospital discharge is a vulnerable time of discontinuity and potential adverse events. Hospitalists should not see their commitment to the patient as ending with the discharge orders; rather, they should take steps to promote a safe and smooth transition of care. Through appropriate discharge planning and effective communication with patients, their family members, and outpatient physicians, hospitalists can play an important role in bridging the "voltage drop" between inpatient and outpatient care.

Key Points

- Medical errors and adverse events are common in the period immediately after hospital discharge.
- Hospitalists should strive to promote an effective transition of care back to the outpatient provider.
- Major challenges include:
  - Discharge summaries, the primary means of communication between inpatient and outpatient physician, are commonly incomplete, inaccurate, or delayed.
  - Medication regimen changes are common during hospitalization.
  - Patients are discharged rapidly from acute-care hospitals and have significant self-care responsibilities upon returning home, often without adequate family support.
  - Physician–patient communication is often too complex for patients to fully understand and remember.
  - Evidence-based guidelines about the discharge process are needed.
- Recommendations in this chapter provide guidance regarding:
  - More effective communication between inpatient and outpatient physician (Box 11-1).
  - Taking an accurate medication history as part of medication reconciliation (Box 11-2).
  - Bridging the care transition through effective follow-up appointments, telephone contact, and home visits.
  - More effective physician–patient communication, including confirmation of patient understanding (Box 11-3).

SUGGESTED READING

Coleman EA. Falling through the cracks: challenges and opportunities for improving transitional care for persons with continuous complex care needs. J Am Geriatr Soc 2003; 51(4):549–555.

Coleman EA, Smith JD, Frank JC, et al. Preparing patients and caregivers to participate in care delivered across settings: the care transitions intervention. J Am Geriatr Soc 2004; 52(11):1817–1825.

Dudas V, Bookwalter T, Kerr KM, et al. The impact of follow-up telephone calls to patients after hospitalization. Am J Med 2001; 111(9B):26S–30S.

Forster AJ, Murff HJ, Peterson JF, et al. The incidence and severity of adverse events affecting patients after discharge from the hospital. Ann Intern Med 2003; 138:161–167.

Moore C, Wisnivesky J, Williams S, et al. Medical errors related to discontinuity of care from an inpatient to an outpatient setting. J Gen Intern Med 2003; 18:646–651.

Roy CL, Poon EG, Karson AS, et al. Patient safety concerns arising from test results that return after hospital discharge. Ann Intern Med 2005; 143(2):121–128.

Sullivan C, Gleason KM, Rooney D, et al. Medication reconciliation in the acute care setting: opportunity and challenge for nursing. J Nurs Care Qual 2005; 20(2):95–98.

van Walraven C, Mamdani M, Fang J, et al. Continuity of care and patient outcomes after hospital discharge. J Gen Intern Med 2004; 19(6):624–631.

van Walraven C, Seth R, Laupacis A. Dissemination of discharge summaries: not reaching follow-up physicians. Can Fam Physician 2002; 48:737–742.

Williams MV, Davis TC, Parker RM, et al. The role of health literacy in patient-physician communication. Fam Med 2002; 34(5):383–389.

Section

Two

Preventive Services in the
Hospitalized Patient

12 Vaccination
Vaishali Singh

13 Smoking Cessation in Hospitalized Patients
Ursula Whalen, Sunil Kripalani

14 Prophylaxis for Venous Thromboembolism (VTE)
in the Hospitalized Medical Patient
Greg Maynard, Jason Stein

15 Osteoporosis
Laura J. Martin

16 Substance Abuse and Dependence
in the Hospitalized Patient
Jeffrey L. Greenwald, Jeffrey Samet

17 Preventing Nosocomial Infections
Armando Paez, James C. Pile

CHAPTER TWELVE

Vaccination

Vaishali Singh, MD, MPH, MBA

INTRODUCTION

The decline of vaccine-preventable diseases is one of the most remarkable global successes of the twentieth century. Vaccination has enabled the eradication of small pox and eliminated cases of indigenous poliomyelitis[1] Despite dramatic declines in infectious diseases, mortality and morbidity from vaccine-preventable disease still remain substantial. Between 50,000 and 70,000 adults die from pneumococcal disease, influenza, and hepatitis infections in the United States annually.[1] In fact, pneumonia and influenza still remain in the top 10 leading causes of annual death (ranked 7th in 2001).

In 1994, The National Vaccine Advisory Committee (NVAC) reviewed the status of adult immunization in the United States and reported that although vaccines were proven to be life saving and cost effective, they remain highly underutilized.[1] Hospitalized patients are particularly at risk for subsequent influenza and pneumococcal disease; however, immunization is often not considered and/or administered at that time. Studies indicate that up to 46% of patients hospitalized for influenza and approximately 66% of influenza deaths occurred in elderly patients who were discharged previously during the same flu season.[2] Similar data are shown for up to 66% of hospitalized patients with serious pneumoccoal infections who have been previously hospitalized within 5 years.[2] Reasons for vaccine underutilization include inadequate awareness by health care providers and the public of the importance of vaccination, missed opportunities by health care providers in both outpatient and inpatient settings, and inadequate reimbursement or funding for adult immunization by public and private health insurers.[1]

In an attempt to promote consistent vaccination practices, many national organizations and health care groups have provided detailed vaccination schedules for adults and other specific high-risk groups such as the elderly, immunocompromised persons, health care workers, and travelers. Immunization is also a prominent feature of "Healthy People 2010," a comprehensive nationwide health program agenda from the US Department of Health and Human Services.[3] Notably, this program has targeted 90% coverage in the elderly for pneumococcal and annual influenza immunization among adults 65 and older, and 62% for tetanus toxoid. In support of this goal, the American College of Physicians, in collaboration with the Infectious Diseases Society of America, has recommended age 50 to be a time for review of preventive health measures, with special emphasis on evaluating risk factors that would indicate a need for immunization.[3] Furthermore, several studies have already indicated the benefits of interventions such as standing orders at hospital discharge and in long-term care facilities or provider reminders to increase vaccination rates.[5] As noted below, the Joint Commission on Accreditation for Healthcare Organizations (JCAHO) now includes vaccination as a quality measure. The Centers for Disease Control and Prevention (CDC)'s Advisory Committee on Immunization Practices (ACIP) also endorsed these practices to promote hospital-based vaccination of adults, particularly for prevention of influenza and pneumococcal disease.[5] In 1993, federal legislation was passed that established reimbursement for the cost of influenza vaccination and administration.[6]

Below is a basic review of vaccine-preventable diseases and associated adult vaccination schedule (Tables 12-1 and 12-2). For further detailed information, please refer to the Centers for Disease Control and Prevention (CDC) web portal (www.cdc.gov).

REVIEW OF VACCINE-PREVENTABLE DISEASES AND SPECIFIC VACCINES

Pneumococcal Vaccine

Streptococcus pneumoniae is a bacterial organism that colonizes the upper respiratory tract and can cause bacteremia, meningitis, and pneumonia, as well as other upper and lower respiratory tract infections such as otitis media and sinusitis. Pneumococcal infection causes an estimated 40,000 deaths annually in the United States, accounting for more deaths than any other vaccine-preventable bacterial disease.[6] Case-fatality rates are highest for meningitis and bacteremia, and the highest mortality occurs among the elderly and patients who have underlying medical conditions.[7]

The pneumococcal vaccine contains 23 purified capsular polysaccharide antigens of *S. pneumoniae*, which represent at least 85%–90% of the serotypes that cause invasive pneumococcal infections in the United States.[7] The vaccine is administered intramuscularly or subcutaneously as one 0.5-mL dose and may be given with other vaccines, such as influenza or tetanus, without change in antibody response. Adverse reactions include

Table 12-1 Recommended Adult Immunization Schedule, by Vaccine and Age Group
United States, October 2005–September 2006

Vaccine ▼ / Age Group ▶	19–49 Years	50–64 Years	≥65 Years
Tetanus, diphtheria (Td)[1]*	1-dose booster every 10 yrs		
Measles, mumps, rubella (MMR)[2]*	1 or 2 dose	1 dose	
Varicella[3]*	2 doses (0, 4–8 wks)	2 doses (0, 4–8 wks)	
Vaccines below broken line are for selected populations			
Influenza[4]*	1 dose annually	1 dose annually	
Pneumococcal (polysaccharide)[5,6]	1–2 doses		1 dose
Hepatitis A[7]*	2 doses (0, 6–12 mos, or 0, 6–18 mos)		
Hepatitis B[8]*	3 doses (0, 1–2, 4–6 mos)		
Meningococcal[9]	1 or more doses		

NOTE: These recommendations must be read along with the footnotes.
*Covered by the Vaccine Injury Compensation Program.

▮ For all persons in this category who meet the age requirements and who lack evidence of immunity (e.g., lack documentation of vaccination or have no evidence of prior infection)

▮ Recommended if some other risk factor is present (e.g., based on medical, occupational, lifestyle, or other indications)

This schedule indicates the recommended age groups and medical indications for routine administration of currently licensed vaccines for persons aged ≥19 years. Licensed combination vaccines may be used whenever any components of the combination are indicated and when the vaccine's other components are not contraindicated. For detailed recommendations, consult the manufacturers' package inserts and the complete statements from the ACIP (www.cdc.gov/nip/publications/acip-list.htm).

Report all clinically significant postvaccination reactions to the Vaccine Adverse Event Reporting System (VAERS). Reporting forms and instructions on filing a VAERS report are available by telephone, 800-822-7967 or from the VAERS website at www.vaers.hhs.gov.

Information on how to file a Vaccine Injury Compensation Program claim is available at www.hrsa.gov/osp/vicp or by telephone, 800-338-2382. To file a claim for vaccine injury, contact the U.S. Court of Federal Claims, 717 Madison Place, N.W., Washington D.C. 20005, telephone 202-357-6400.

Additional information about the vaccines listed above and contraindications for vaccination is also available at www.cdc.gov/nip or from the CDC-INFO Contact Center at 800-CDC-INFO (232–4636) in English and Spanish, 24 hours a day, 7 days a week.

mild erythema and swelling at site of injection, and systemic symptoms of fever, or myalgia are rare. Severe anaphylactic reaction to the vaccine is rare. Contraindications include moderate illness and severe allergic reaction from a prior dose. The safety of the vaccine during pregnancy has not been adequately studied; however, there have been no reported adverse consequences for mothers who were inadvertently vaccinated. Females at high risk should be vaccinated before pregnancy if possible.[16] There have been no reported deaths caused by the vaccine.

Several clinical studies have demonstrated the cost effectiveness of this vaccine since its licensure in 1983, and its efficacy ranges from 55–80%, varying between different risk groups.[7] The vaccine is recommended for people aged 65 or over, aged 2 to 64 with chronic illness (e.g., diabetes, emphysema, congestive heart failure, cirrhosis), those with functional or anatomic asplenia, and/or people in living environments that increase the risk for invasive pneumococcal disease (e.g., nursing homes and long-term care facilities). Persons who are immunocompromised (e.g., leukemia, lymphoma, patients receiving chemotherapy, HIV infection, long-term corticosteroids), have chronic renal failure, or had the first dose before age 65 are considered to be at high risk for more rapid decline of antibody levels and may need revaccination after 5 years.

Influenza

Influenza virus causes a myriad of constitutional and respiratory symptoms (fever, myalgia, nonproductive cough, rhinitis,

headache) and can exacerbate underlying chronic cardiopulmonary disease and lead to secondary bacterial infection. It causes 36,000 deaths annually in the United States.[6] Influenza epidemics usually occur in the winter months, and the risk of severe illness, hospitalization, and death is higher among those aged ≥65 and among persons with underlying chronic disease.

The primary way of reducing the risk of influenza and its complications in the United States is by use of inactivated trivalent vaccine. Due to viral antigenic change, antibodies produced against one influenza virus type confer limited or no protection against another. Therefore, incorporation of one or more new strains is needed annually for revaccination. Efficacy of the vaccine depends on the degree of antigenic similarity between the vaccine and the actual circulating virus, as well as the immunocompetence of the recipient. If well matched, prevention of influenza occurs in 70–90% of healthy adults and results in decreased absence from work and use of health care resources.[8]

The vaccine also is beneficial in reducing secondary complications, and it is cost effective in reducing risk of influenza-related hospitalization and deaths among adults aged ≥65 with or without chronic underlying illness.[8] However, recent CDC recommendations have decreased the target age to ≥50 years, as recent studies have elucidated the potential of capturing this age group, as well as the indication that age-based strategies (as opposed to patient-risk strategies) are superior in producing higher immunization rates.[4,8] See recommendations for annual influenza vaccination in Box 12-1. Adverse effects of the vaccine

> **Box 12-1 CDC Advisory Committee on Immunization Practices (ACIP) Recommendations for Annual Influenza Vaccination**[8,9]
>
> Persons aged ≥50 years
>
> Residents of nursing homes or long-term care facilities who have chronic illness, adults with chronic cardiopulmonary illness
>
> Adults requiring regular medical follow-up or hospitalization in the ensuing year because of chronic illness (diabetes, renal dysfunction, immunosuppression caused by medications, or illness such as HIV)
>
> Women who will be pregnant (after 14 weeks' gestation during influenza season)
>
> Health care workers or caregivers (can transmit influenza virus to persons at high risk for complications from influenza)

include local erythema and induration at injection site, systemic reactions mimicking a mild "flu-like" illness, and allergy/hypersensitivity reaction (often related to residual egg protein in the vaccine). Of particular interest, the 1976 swine flu vaccine was linked with risk of a paralytic illness later named Guillain-Barré syndrome (GBS). While a causal relationship has remained unclear, investigations to date indicate no substantial increase in GBS associated with influenza vaccines.[8,9] Data also indicate that the rate of these symptoms is approximatly the same after placebo vaccination. Contraindication to use of the vaccine includes egg allergy and previous hypersensitivity reaction.

Measles, Mumps, Rubella

Measles, mumps, and rubella (MMR) are viral illnesses that are highly contagious and have potential for severe secondary complications. Measles produces a syndrome of fever, cough, coryza, rash, conjunctivitis, and the classic Koplik's spots (bluish-white spots on the buccal mucosa).[10] Pneumonia and subacute sclerosing panencephalitis are severe secondary complications with high mortality rates.[11] The clinical characteristics of mumps include unilateral or bilateral parotitis, fever, headache, myalgia, and anorexia. Complications of mumps are more common in adults than children, and they include orchitis (up to 38%), sterility in postpubertal men, aseptic meningitis, and deafness.[11] Rubella (German measles) illness is characterized by fever, postauricular lymphadenopathy, arthralgia, and pruritic rash. The most important complications of rubella are miscarriage and fetal anomalies.[11]

MMR are generally diseases of childhood, and their incidence has dramatically declined worldwide with the implementation of vaccination. However, in 1989–1991, a measles epidemic occurred in the United States, thus reemphasizing the importance of maintaining immunization levels in the general public.[11–13]

MMR vaccines are available separately, or in combination, as it is commonly used in recommended immunization schedules. The MMR vaccine is a live attenuated form of the virus and is generally given in 2 intramuscular doses, one at about 12 months and then repeated at age 4–6 or 11–12 years. Adults born before 1957 are considered immune to these diseases. Adults should receive ≥1 dose to confer immunity in the following cases: 1) born after 1957, 2) recent exposure to measles outbreak, 3) vaccinated with killed form of vaccine, 4) health care workers, 5) international travel, and 6) students in postsecondary educational institutions.[11] For women of childbearing years, regardless of age, MMR immunity should be determined and ensured, but vaccination is contraindicated in pregnant patients or those planning to become pregnant within the month.[9,11] Severe adverse reactions to the vaccine are rare; more commonly symptoms may include pain at injection site, fever (5%), rash, and temporary thrombocytopenia. Cases of thrombocytopenia have been reported to occur approximately 2 months after vaccination, with an incidence of approximately 1 per 30,000. Higher rates may be seen with those who previously have had idiopathic thrombocytopenic purpura, particularly for those who had thrombocytopenic purpura after an earlier dose of MMR vaccine.[14] MMR vaccination is associated with false negative purified protein derivative (PPD) results.[9] It is recommended to give the PPD either before MMR, or 4–6 weeks after MMR vaccination.

Diphtheria, Tetanus

Diptheria is an acute toxin-mediated disease caused by *Corynebacterium diptheriae*. The illness is typified by fever, anorexia, and exudative pharyngitis with membrane formation. The most severe complications are myocarditis and neuritis. While diphtheria was a major cause of death in the 1920s (~200,000 cases and ~15,000 deaths in 1921), the number of cases has fallen dramatically since implementation of the toxoid vaccine (formalin inactivated *Diptheriae* toxin) in the late 1940s.[15,16] Only 54 cases have been reported since 1980, with 58% of those in persons 20 years and older.[15]

Tetanus is primarily a disease of adults in the United States and is caused by the exotoxin produced by *Clostridium tetani*. Symptoms include fever, elevated blood pressure, generalized muscle rigidity and spasm, and lock jaw.[15] Complications include laryngospasm with respiratory distress, spine and long bone fracture due to sustained contracture, and autonomic nervous system hypersensitivity. The most common method of transmission is by contaminated injury or wound—specifically puncture wounds. Consequently, heroin users have been found to be at higher risk for tetanus. Tetanus toxoid (formaldehyde-treated toxin) was introduced to the routine vaccination schedule in the 1940s, causing reported incidence rates of tetanus to fall from ~500 cases at that time to ~50 cases in the 1970s. From 1980–2000, 70% of reported cases were in persons 40 and older.[16]

Diptheriae toxoid (formalin inactivated *Diptheriae* toxin) combined with tetanus toxoid is recommended for adults, including pregnant women, who have an uncertain history of a complete primary vaccination series in youth (three doses). Revaccination

Table 12-2 Recommended Adult Immunization Schedule, by Vaccine and Medical and Other Indications United States, October 2005–September 2006

Vaccine ▼ / Indication ▶	Pregnancy	Congenital immunodeficiency; leukemia[10]; lymphoma; generalized malignancy; cerebrospinal fluid leaks; therapy with alkylating agents, antimetabolites, radiation, or high-dose, long-term corticosteroids	Diabetes; heart disease; chronic pulmonary disease; chronic liver disease, including chronic alcoholism	Asplenia[10] (including elective splenectomy and terminal complement component deficiencies)	Kidney failure, end-stage renal disease, recipients of hemodialysis or clotting factor concentrates	Human immunodeficiency virus (HIV) infection[2,10]	Health care workers
Tetanus, diphtheria (Td)[1]*	1-dose booster every 10 yrs						
Measles, mumps, rubella (MMR)[2]*						1 or 2 doses	2 dose
Varicella[3]*				2 doses (0, 4–8 wks)			
Influenza[4]*	1 dose annually			1 dose annually			
Pneumococcal (polysaccharide)[5,6]	1–2 doses			1–2 doses			1–2 doses
Hepatitis A[7]*				2 doses (0, 6–12 mos, or 0, 6–18 mos)			
Hepatitis B[8]*	3 doses (0, 1–2, 4–6 mos)					3 doses (0, 1–2, 4–6 mos)	
Meningococcal[9]	1 doses					1 doses	

NOTE: These recommendations must be read along with the footnotes.
*Covered by the Vaccine Injury Compensation Program.

█ For all persons in this category who meet the age requirements and who lack evidence of immunity (e.g., lack documentation of vaccination or have no evidence of prior infection)

█ Recommended if some other risk factor is present (e.g., based on medical, occupational, lifestyle, or other indications)

█ Contraindicated

Recommended Adult Immunization Schedule, United States, October 2005–September 2006

1. **Tetanus and Diphtheria (Td) vaccination.** Adults with uncertain histories of a complete primary vaccination series with diphtheria and tetanus toxoid-containing vaccines should receive a primary series using combined Td toxoid. A primary series for adults is 3 doses; administer the first 2 doses at least 4 weeks apart and the third dose 6–12 months after the second. Administer 1 dose if the person received the primary series and if the last vaccination was received ≥10 years previously. Consult ACIP statement for recommendations for administering Td as prophylaxis in wound management (www.cdc.gov/mmwr/preview/mmwrhtml/00041645.htm). The American College of Physicians Task Force on Adult Immunization supports a second option for Td use in adults: a single Td booster at age 50 years for persons who have completed the full pediatric series, including the teenage/young adult booster. A newly licensed tetanus-diphtheria-acellular pertussis vaccine is available for adults. ACIP recommendations for its use will be published.

2. **Measles, Mumps, Rubella (MMR) vaccination.** *Measles component:* adults born before 1957 can be considered immune to measles. Adults born during or after 1957 should receive ≥1 dose of MMR unless they have a medical contraindication, documentation of ≥1 dose, history of measles based on health care provider diagnosis, or laboratory evidence of immunity. A second dose of MMR is recommended for adults who 1) were recently exposed to measles or in an outbreak setting, 2) were previously vaccinated with killed measles vaccine, 3) were vaccinated with an unknown type of measles vaccine during 1963–1967, 4) are students in postsecondary educational institutions, 5) work in a health care facility, or 6) plan to travel internationally. Withhold MMR or other measles-containing vaccines from HIV-infected persons with severe immunosuppression. *Mumps component:* 1 dose of MMR vaccine should be adequate for protection for those born during or after 1957 who lack a history of mumps based on health care provider diagnosis or who lack laboratory evidence of immunity. *Rubella component:* administer 1 dose of MMR vaccine to women whose rubella vaccination history is unreliable or who lack laboratory evidence of immunity. For women of childbearing age, regardless of birth year, routinely determine rubella immunity and counsel women regarding congenital rubella syndrome. Do not vaccinate women who are pregnant or might become pregnant within 4 weeks of receiving the vaccine. Women who do not have evidence of immunity should receive MMR vaccine upon completion or termination of pregnancy and before discharge from the health care facility.

3. **Varicella vaccination.** Varicella vaccination is recommended for all adults without evidence of immunity to varicella. Special consideration should be given to those who 1) have close contact with persons at high risk for severe disease (health care workers and family contacts of immunocompromised persons) or 2) are at high risk for exposure or transmission (e.g., teachers of young children; child care employees; residents and staff members of institutional settings, including correctional institutions; college students; military personnel; adolescents and adults living in households with children; nonpregnant women of childbearing age; and international travelers). Evidence of immunity to varicella in adults includes any of the following: 1) documented age-appropriate varicella vaccination (i.e., receipt of 1 dose before age 13 years or receipt of 2 doses [administered at least 4 weeks apart] after age 13 years); 2) born in the United States before 1966; 3) history of varicella disease based on health care provider diagnosis or self- or parental report of typical varicella disease for non-U.S.-born persons born before 1966 and all persons born during 1966–1997 (for a patient reporting a history of an atypical, mild case, health care providers should seek either an epidemiologic link with a typical varicella case or evidence of laboratory confirmation, if it was performed at the time of acute disease); 4) history of herpes zoster based on health care provider diagnosis; or 5) laboratory evidence of immunity. Do not vaccinate women who are pregnant or might become pregnant within 4 weeks of receiving the vaccine. Assess pregnant women for evidence of varicella immunity. Women who do not have evidence of immunity should receive dose 1 of varicella vaccine upon completion or termination of pregnancy and before discharge from the health care facility. Dose 2 should be given 4–3 weeks after dose 1.

4. **Influenza vaccination.** *Medical indications:* chronic disorders of the cardiovascular or pulmonary systems, including asthma; chronic metabolic diseases, including diabetes mellitus, renal dysfunction, hemoglobinopathies, or immunosuppression (including immunosuppression caused by medications or by HIV); any condition (e.g., cognitive dysfunction, spinal cord injury, seizure disorder or other neuromuscular disorder) that compromises respiratory function or the handling of respiratory secretions or that can increase the risk of aspiration; and pregnancy during the influenza season. No data exist on the risk for severe or complicated influenza disease among persons with asplenia; however, influenza is a risk factor for secondary bacterial infections that can cause severe disease among persons with asplenia. *Occupational indications:* health care workers and employees of long-term care and assisted living facilities. *Other indications:* residents of nursing homes and other long-term care and assisted living facilities; persons likely to transmit influenza to persons at high risk (i.e., in-home household contacts and caregivers of children birth through 23 months of age, or persons of all ages with high-risk conditions); and anyone who wishes to be vaccinated. For healthy nonpregnant persons aged 5–49 years without high-risk conditions who are not contacts of severely immunocompromised persons in special care units, intranasally administered influenza vaccine (FluMist®) may be administered in lieu of inactivated vaccine.

5. **Pneumococcal polysaccharide vaccination.** *Medical indications:* chronic disorders of the pulmonary system (excluding asthma); cardiovascular diseases; diabetes mellitus; chronic liver diseases, including liver disease as a result of alcohol abuse (e.g.,cirrhosis); chronic renal failure or nephrotic syndrome; functional or anatomic asplenia (e.g., sickle cell disease or splenectomy [if elective splenectomy is planned, vaccinate at least 2 weeks before surgery]); immunosuppressive conditions (e.g., congenital immunodeficiency, HIV infection [vaccinate as close to diagnosis as possible when CD4 cell counts are highest], leukemia, lymphoma, multiple myeloma, Hodgkin disease, generalized malignancy, organ or bone marrow transplantation); chemotherapy with alkylating agents, antimetabolites, or high-dose, long-term corticosteroids; and cochlear implants. *Other indications:* Alaska Natives and certain American Indian populations; residents of nursing homes and other long-term care facilities.

6. **Revaccination with pneumococcal polysaccharide vaccine.** One-time revaccination after 5 years for persons with chronic renal failure or nephrotic syndrome; functional or anatomic asplenia (e.g., sickle cell disease or splenectomy); immunosuppressive conditions (e.g., congenital immunodeficiency, HIV infection, leukemia, lymphoma, multiple myeloma, Hodgkin disease, generalized malignancy, organ or bone marrow transplantation); or chemotherapy with alkylating agents, antimetabolites, or high-dose, long-term corticosteroids. For persons aged ≥65 years, one-time revaccination if they were vaccinated ≥5 years previously and were aged <65 years at the time of primary vaccination.

7. **Hepatitis A vaccination.** *Medical indications:* persons with clotting factor disorders or chronic liver disease. *Behavioral indications:* men who have sex with men or users of illegal drugs. *Occupational indications:* persons working with hepatitis A virus (HAV)-infected primates or with HAV in a research laboratory setting. *Other indications:* persons traveling to or working in countries that have high or intermediate endemicity of hepatitis A (for list of countries, visit www.cdc.gov/travel/diseases.htm#hepa) as well as any person wishing to obtain immunity. Current vaccines should be given in a 2-dose series at either 0 and 6–12 months, or 0 and 6–18 months. If the combined hepatitis A and hepatitis B vaccine is used, administer 3 doses at C, 1, and 6 months.

8. **Hepatitis B vaccination.** *Medical indications:* hemodialysis patients (use special formulation [40 μg/mL] or two 20-μg/mL doses) or patients who receive clotting factor concentrates. *Occupational indications:* health care workers and public-safety workers who have exposure to blood in the workplace; and persons in training in schools of medicine, dentistry, nursing, laboratory technology, and other allied health professions. *Behavioral indications:* injection-drug users; persons with more than one sex partner in the previous 6 months; persons with a recently acquired sexually transmitted disease (STD); and men who have sex with men. *Other indications:* household contacts and sex partners of persons with chronic hepatitis B virus (HBV) infection; clients and staff of institutions for the developmentally disabled; all clients of STD clinics; inmates of correctional facilities; or international travelers who will be in countries with high or intermediate prevalence of chronic HBV infection for >6 months (for list of countries, visit www.cdc.gov/travel/diseases.htm#hepa).

9. **Meningococcal vaccination.** *Medical indications:* adults with anatomic or functional asplenia, or terminal complement component deficiencies. *Other indications:* first-year college students living in dormitories; microbiologists who are routinely exposed to isolates of *Neisseria meningitidis*; military recruits; and persons who travel to or reside in countries in which meningococcal disease is hyperendemic or epidemic (e.g., the "meningitis belt" of sub-Saharan Africa during the dry season [Dec–June]), particularly if contact with the local populations will be prolonged. Vaccination is required by the government of Saudi Arabia for all travelers to Mecca during the annual Hajj. Meningococcal conjugate vaccine is preferred for adults meeting any of the above indications who are aged ≤55 years, although meningococcal polysaccharide vaccine (MPSV4) is an acceptable alternative. Revaccination after 5 years may be indicated for adults previously vaccinated with MPSV4 who remain at high risk for infection (e.g., persons residing in areas in which disease is epidemic).

10. **Selected conditions for which *Haemophilus influenzae* type b (Hib) vaccine may be used.** *Haemophilus influenzae* type b conjugate vaccines are licensed for children aged 6 weeks–71 months. No efficacy data are available on which to base a recommendation concerning use of Hib vaccine for older children and adults with the chronic conditions associated with an increased risk for Hib disease. However, studies suggest good immunogenicity in patients who have sickle cell disease, leukemia, or HIV infection, or have had splenectomies; administering vaccine to these patients is not contraindicated.

Approved by the Advisory Committee on Immunization Practices (ACIP), the American College of Obstetricians and Gynecologists (ACOG), and the American Academy of Family Physicians (AAFP)

should be administered every 10 years. Adverse reactions include local erythema at site of injection, "arthus-type" reaction with exaggerated pain and swelling from shoulder to elbow, and severe systemic reactions including anaphylaxis and neurologic complications such as GBS and brachial neuritis.[16] The vaccine is contraindicated in persons with moderate illness, or severe prior dose-related allergic reaction or respiratory collapse.

Hepatitis A

Hepatitis A (HA) is caused by the hepatitis A virus (HAV) and is one of the most frequently reported diseases in the United States. From 1987–1997, the annual incidence of HA infection in the United States was 10 cases per 100,000.[16] Viral transmission occurs by fecal-oral route, and clinical illness is characterized by fever, malaise, anorexia, abdominal pain, and jaundice. Hospitalization rate for acute HA infection is 11–22%, with adults losing 27 days of work on average.[17] Severe liver failure or fulminant HA is responsible for 100 deaths annually in the U.S.[16] The HA vaccine (containing inactivated virus) is currently available in two formulations (adult and pediatric) and is recommended for groups at high risk for HA infection or severe complications, such as homosexual males, users of injectable and noninjectable illegal drugs, persons traveling in countries endemic with HA, occupational contact with primates, and chronic liver disease.[16,17] Adults ≥19 should receive one intramuscular dose of the adult formulation, with a booster 6–12 months later. Adverse reactions include local erythema at injection site, headache, anorexia, and fatigue; severe allergic reaction is rare.

Hepatitis B

The hepatitis B virus (HBV), which is transmitted by blood and sexual activity, causes hepatitis B (HB). HB causes acute and chronic liver inflammation and cirrhosis, and it is responsible for up to 80% of hepatocellular carcinomas.[16] Fulminant hepatitis progresses from acute hepatitis in 1–2% and has mortality rates between 63–93%. The CDC estimates 1.25 million people in the U.S. have HBV infection and that annually 80,000 people, mostly adults, get infected with HBV.[18]

Hepatitis B vaccine, available in the United States since 1981, is composed of recombinant HBV surface antigen made from yeast cells.[16,18] The adult immunization schedule consists of two intramuscular doses separated by 4 weeks, and a third dose 4–6 months after the second dose. The series confers adequate antibody response in >95% of children and >90% of healthy adults.[16,18] Furthermore, while antibody levels do decline from peak levels after the first year and slowly thereafter, numerous studies have indicated that individuals who appropriately respond to the primary vaccination series remain protected from HBV.[16] The vaccine is recommended for all adults who have not been previously immunized in childhood. Groups considered to be high risk for transmission of HBV include: health care workers, homosexual/bisexual men, heterosexuals with multiple partners or those who have been treated for sexually transmitted disease, injection drug users, household contacts of HBV carriers, hemodialysis patients, individuals in correctional or medical/long-term care facilities, international travelers to areas with endemic HBV infection, and victims of sexual assault.[16,18] Adverse reactions to the vaccine are local soreness at injection site and mild fever (1%); severe allergic reaction is rare. Since the vaccine contains noninfectious HBsAg particles, the CDC has stated that **neither pregnancy nor lactation should be considered a contraindication to vaccination of women.**[16] Of note, the FDA in 2001 approved a combination HAV and HBV vaccine for those individuals at risk for both infections.

Meningococcal Vaccine

Neisseria meningitides is a bacterial pathogen with several serotypes (A,C,Y,W-135) capable of causing meningitis and fulminant sepsis. Attack rates are generally higher in young children and steadily decline with older age groups. For persons aged 18–34, 41%, 25%, and 14% of cases were due to serotype B, C, and Y, respectively.[16] Groups considered at high risk for contracting meningococcal disease are those with asplenia, deficiencies in the terminal common complement pathway (C3, C5-C9), or immunosuppression and international travelers. Military recruits and college freshman have had high rates of meningococcal disease (serotype C), with outbreaks possibly related to common living situations (diverse background, crowded conditions).

The meningococcal polysaccharide vaccine contains the four most prominent serotypes and is administered in a single 0.5-mL subcutaneous injection. The serogroups A and C vaccines have demonstrated estimated clinical efficacies of 85–100% in adults, with a duration of protection of ~3 years. Routine vaccination is recommended only for high-risk groups as mentioned above, as well as in control of outbreaks. Adverse reactions to the vaccine are mild, most commonly due to local injection irritation (5–10%) or headache and transient fever (2–5%). Contraindications to the vaccine include hypersensitivity to the previous dose. Pregnancy, immunosuppression, and breastfeeding are not contraindications to meningococcal vaccine.[16]

Varicella

The varicella zoster virus is a herpes virus responsible for such contagious diseases as chickenpox and herpes zoster. Severe complications of varicella, including secondary bacterial infections of skin lesions, pneumonia, dehydration, encephalitis, hepatitis, and premature labor and delivery, often require hospitalization.[20] Varicella infection affects approximately 4 million people and results in 100 deaths per year.[21] Most adults are seropositive from prior infection in childhood and adolescence, but certain groups such as seronegative adults, health care workers, immunocompromised patients, and pregnant females are at high risk for severe infection, hospitalization, and mortality.[20] Although varicella infection is thought to be a childhood disease, review of its mortality data indicated a prominent increase in the proportion of adult deaths in the 1990–1994 period (54%). From 1970–1994 in the United States, adult deaths due to varicella increased three-fold, with similar increase seen in Great Britain.[21] This increased mortality has been thought to reflect increased immigration from countries where adults have more risk of contracting varicella, namely Mexico, the Philippines, China, Vietnam, and India. The sharp rise in infected adults has again highlighted the necessity of general public immunization.

The varicella vaccine was developed in 1995 and is estimated to provide 70–90% protection against infection and 95% protection against severe disease for 7–10 years after vaccination[20]. The vaccine is a live attenuated form of varicella zoster, and it is recommended (2 doses 4–8 weeks apart) for adult persons at high risk of complications, such as immunocompetent adults, family contacts of immunocompromised persons, health care workers, nonpregnant women of childbearing age (to reduce possible transmission to the fetus), and international travelers. Vaccination has been successful, as a review of data after the initiation of the vaccine has demonstrated sharp declines in mortality in all age groups under 50.[22] The vaccine is generally well tolerated, but adverse reactions include erythema and pain at the injection site, and less commonly a mild viral illness or rash. The vaccine contains live virus, and contraindications to its use are pregnancy and breastfeeding, anaphylaxis to prior dose, history of anaphylactic reaction to neomycin, cellular immunodeficiency, and immunosuppression.

VACCINATION IS A PERFORMANCE MEASURE FOR HOSPITAL QUALITY

The Joint Commission began development of performance measures with the inception of the Agenda for Change in 1987. Eventually, these activities were subsumed into what is now called the ORYX initiative. Since 1999, the Joint Commission has solicited input from a variety of stakeholders in health care, including clinical professionals, hospitals, consumers, state hospital associations, and medical societies about potential focus areas for a set of hospital core performance measures. Community acquired pneumonia (CAP) was one of the initial priority areas for hospital core measure development. Five pneumonia (PN) measures were implemented in July 2002, one of which was pneumococcal screening and/or vaccination (PN-2). In July 2004, additional PN measures were added, including influenza vaccination (PN-7). These measures are consistent with the Centers for Medicare and Medicaid Services 7th Scope of Work Project to improve health care quality.

PN-2 requires that hospitals identify inpatients 65 years of age and older with ICD-9-CM codes consistent with pneumonia, and screen for pneumococcal vaccine status with vaccination prior to discharge, if indicated. PN-7 requires hospitals to identify inpatients ≥50 years with pneumonia who were discharged during October, November, December, January, or February, and to screen them for influenza vaccine status with vaccination prior to discharge, if indicated.

CONCLUSION

As national implementation of hospital core measures continues to mature, the ability to compare health care organization data across systems and between measures will improve, and financial incentives based on measured performance of vaccination can be expected in the future. Hospitalists will likely play a leading role in improving vaccination performance measure rates.

Key Points

- Between 50,000 and 70,000 adults die from pneumococcal disease, influenza, and hepatitis infections in the United States annually,[1] with pneumonia and influenza among the top 10 leading causes of annual death.

- Pneumococcal vaccination is recommended prior to discharge for pneumonia patients age 65 and older following proper screening.

- Influenza vaccination is recommended prior to discharge for pneumonia patients age 50 years and older, who are hospitalized during October, November, December, January, or February.

- Tetanus is primarily a disease of adults in the United States.

- Hepatitis A is one of the most frequently reported diseases in the United States and has a hospitalization rate of 11–22%.

- Although varicella infection is commonly thought to be a childhood disease, recent increases in the proportion of adult deaths from it in the United States are believed to be due to increased immigration.

- Vaccination rates are hospital quality core measures assessed by JCAHO.

SUGGESTED READING

Atkinson W, Hamborsky J, McIntyre L, et al. Epidemiology and prevention of vaccine-preventable diseases. Centers for Disease Control and Prevention. Washington, DC: Public Health Foundation, 2006.

Bratzler DW, Houck PM, Jiang H, et al. Failure to vaccinate medicare patients. Acrh Intern Med 2002; 162:2349–2356.

Centers for Disease Control and Prevention. Vaccine-preventable diseases: improving vaccination coverage in children, adolescents, and adults. MMWR 1999; 48(RR-8):1–15.

Herzog NS, Bratzler DW, Houck PM. Effects of previous influenza vaccination on subsequent readmission and mortality in elderly patients hospitalized with pneumonia. Am J Med 2003; 115:454–461.

Prevention and control of influenza: recommendations of the Advisory Committee on Immunization Practices (ACIP). MMWR 2004; 53(RR-06):1–40.

Perry RT, Halsey, NA. The clinical significance of measles: A review. J Infect Dis 2004; 189(Suppl 1):S4–S16.

Diphtheria, tetanus, and pertussis: recommendations for vaccine use and other preventive measures recommendations of the Immunization Practices Advisory Committee (ACIP). MMWR 1991; 40(RR-10):1–28.

Prevention of hepatitis: a through active or passive immunization: recommendations of the Advisory Committee on Immunization Practices (ACIP). MMWR 1999; 48(RR-12):1–37.

Hepatitis B virus: A comprehensive strategy for eliminating transmission in the United States through universal childhood vaccination: recommendations of the Immunization Practices Advisory Committee (ACIP). Jan 2005 Update.

Prevention and control of meningococcal disease: Recommendations of the Advisory Committee on Immunization Practices (ACIP). MMWR 2000; 49(RR-7): 1–10.

Nguyen HQ, Jumaan AO, Seward JF. Decline in mortality due to implementation of varicella vaccination in the United States. N Engl J Med 2005; (352)5:450–458.

CHAPTER THIRTEEN

Smoking Cessation in Hospitalized Patients

Ursula Whalen, MD, and Sunil Kripalani, MD, MSc

BACKGROUND

Hospitalization presents a unique opportunity for smoking cessation. Because smoking in hospitals was banned in 1992 by the Joint Commission on Accreditation of Healthcare Organizations (now called The Joint Commission), inpatients are forced to live in a smoke-free environment.[1] While smoking cessation in hospitals may be involuntary for some tobacco users, a study performed prior to smoking bans revealed that up to 50% of adult smokers voluntarily quit smoking during their hospitalization.[2] Thus, hospitalization itself appears to motivate some smokers to quit smoking.

Many studies evaluating smoking cessation interventions in hospitalized patients have demonstrated increased long-term tobacco abstinence.[3–7] In fact, well-devised inpatient nicotine dependence programs not only attain higher long-term abstinence rates, but also are more cost effective than outpatient smoking cessation programs.[8,9] Moreover, inpatient smoking cessation programs help those who may not have access to outpatient services.[10] The US Department of Health and Human Services recommends that health care providers document smoking status on every hospitalized patient and provide appropriate counseling and pharmacotherapy for tobacco users.[11] Because health care provider interventions are effective in smoking cessation, the National Quality Forum has included smoking cessation advice or counseling as a measure of hospital care performance among smokers admitted with acute myocardial infarction, heart failure, or pneumonia.[12] Though smoking cessation programs for hospitalized patients have been proven effective and are recommended by the US Department of Health and Human Services as well as the National Quality Forum, a 2003 survey conducted by the American Hospital Association found that only 37% of hospitals in the United States offer a tobacco/nicotine dependence program for inpatients.[2] Several barriers to inpatient smoking cessation programs exist, such as a perceived lack of reimbursement for counseling or pharmacotherapy by some health insurance plans as well as a lack of skills and resources.[13]

ASSESSMENT

Epidemiology

Tobacco use claims 440,000 lives yearly and is the most common preventable cause of morbidity and mortality in the United States.[14] Furthermore, it costs an estimated $157 billion in annual health-related economic losses. Approximately 24% of Americans smoke.[15] Among patients hospitalized on a medical service, the prevalence of smoking may actually be lower due to over-representation of the elderly and patients with smoking-related comorbidities, who are more likely to have already quit.[16]

Screening

Given the high prevalence of smoking in the United States and its tremendous impact on morbidity and mortality, physicians must address tobacco use as an active medical problem.[17] Addressing tobacco use on every hospitalized patient is best accomplished by asking all patients about tobacco use and charting tobacco use as a fifth vital sign.[18]

Diagnosis

The Public Health Service–sponsored clinical practice guideline for treating tobacco use recommends an overall approach referred to as the 5-A's (Table 13-1).[11,19] The 5 A's strategy is designed to be brief, requiring no more than 3 minutes of direct clinician time.[11] The key elements of this approach pertaining to diagnosis are asking every patient about tobacco use and assessing the patient's readiness to quit and level of nicotine dependence. These diagnostic steps will help tailor the plan for smoking cessation counseling and pharmacologic management.

By understanding a useful model of behavior change, clinicians will be better prepared to counsel patients about lifestyle modifications. The model most frequently applied to smoking cessation is the "Stages of Change" model by Prochaska and DiClemente (Fig. 13-1).[20] This behavioral framework helps to determine the smoker's readiness to quit. Cessation counseling that is tailored to the patient's "stage" is more effective than generic counseling.[21]

The Fagerstrom test for level of nicotine dependence is helpful for assessing the patient's level of nicotine addiction and appropriate dose of nicotine replacement therapy (see Table 13-2).[22]

PROGNOSIS: Predictors of Successful Smoking Cessation

Predictors of Short-Term Cessation

Lando, et al.[23] conducted a study of 1,477 hospitalized smokers and determined several major predictors for short-term (7 days post-hospital discharge), self-reported smoking cessation. The key characteristics of the 467 patients (32.3%) who reported successful short-term smoking cessation included (1) age (smokers 45 and older were most successful with a 76% quit rate) (2)

admission for a smoking-related illness (49% quit rate) and (3) smokers in the action stage of change (77% quit rate).[23]

Predictors of Long-Term Cessation (12-Month Post–Hospital Discharge)

In the same study, long-term smoking cessation rates were collected and biochemically confirmed. Two hundred and forty-eight smokers (17%) had successfully quit at 1-month follow-up. The predictors of sustained smoking cessation were similar to the short-term predictors: age, stage of change, and admission for a smoking-related illness. Hospitalized smokers age 45 and older had high long-term quit rates (44%, vs. 18% for younger smokers). Those in the action stage of change on hospital admission were more likely to quit smoking successfully at 12 months (35%, vs. 16.6% for preparation stage, 16.6% for contemplation stage, and 6.1% for precontemplation stage). Twenty-nine percent of smokers admitted for a smoking-related illness quit at 12 months, versus 13.7% of those admitted for a problem not related to smoking.[24] Similarly, Goodman, et al.[24] found that smokers with coronary artery disease as their primary discharge diagnosis, which included admissions for myocardial infarction, unstable angina and chronic ischemic heart disease, had the highest rates of 6-month smoking abstinence. The authors attributed the increased abstinence in this population to two factors: (1) smokers admitted with coronary artery disease were more likely to believe that their coronary artery disease was linked to smoking, and (2) smokers with coronary artery disease were in more advanced stages of change compared to their counterparts without coronary artery disease.[24]

Another study of 154 hospitalized smokers found that patients' confidence in their ability to quit was the best predictor of long-term cessation. The authors' confidence scale is shown in Box 13-1. Subjects scoring 6 or higher on the scale were 10 times more likely to quit than those with a score below 6.[10] Administering such a tool prior to discharge could help hospitalists allocate limited resources toward patients most likely to quit.

MANAGEMENT

Only 7% of smokers successfully quit on their own, compared to success rates of 15–30% among smokers who receive intensive counseling and pharmacotherapy. While intensive counseling coupled with pharmacotherapy and outpatient follow-up

Table 13-1 The 5 A's	
Ask	Ask about tobacco use during every hospital admission.
Advise	Advise each patient to quit, using a firm, personalized message. Simply doing this doubles the quit rate. Use the reason for hospitalization or comorbid illness as a motivational tool.
Assess	Assess readiness to quit and nicotine dependence. For readiness, ask if patients are thinking about quitting in general and after they leave the hospital (see Fig. 13-1). For nicotine dependence, assess number of cigarettes per day and the time between waking and the first cigarette (see Table 13-2).
Assist	Assist in setting a quit date; consider pharmacologic therapy; provide advice or referral, and manage withdrawal symptoms.
Arrange	Arrange for follow-up (1–2 weeks post quit date) to congratulate success and help prevent relapse.

Table 13-2 The Fagerstrom Test for Level of Nicotine Dependence (Abbreviated Version)

How soon after waking do you smoke first cigarette?

<5 minutes = 3 points	5–30 minutes = 2 points	31–60 minutes = 1 point

How many cigarettes do you smoke per day?

>30 per day = 3 points	21–30 per day = 2 points	11–20 per day = 1 point

Interpretation

Total points	Level of dependence	Nicotine replacement therapy
5–6 points	**heavy nicotine dependence**	**consider 21-mg nicotine patch**
3–4 points	**moderate nicotine dependence**	**consider 14-mg nicotine patch**
0–2 points	**light nicotine dependence**	**consider 7-mg nicotine patch**

From Heatherton TF, Kozlowski LT, Frecker RC, et al. The Fagerstrom Test for Nicotine Dependence: a revision of the Fagerstrom Tolerance Questionnaire. Brit J Addict 1991; 86:1119–1127.

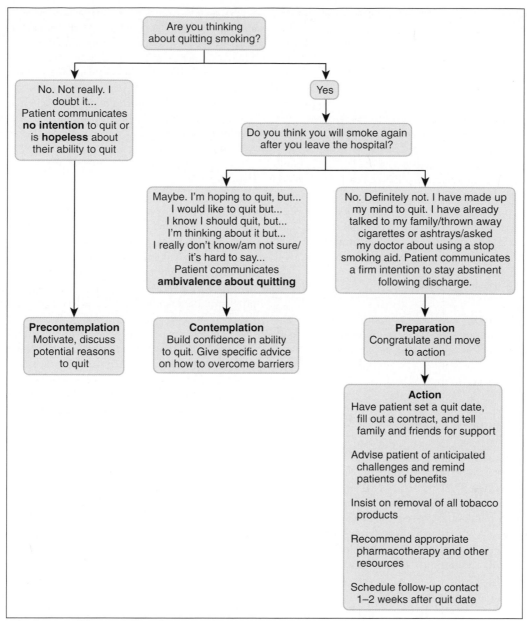

Figure 13-1 • Application of "Stages of Change" model in the hospital. Adapted from Dornelas EA, Sampson RA, Gray JF, et al. A randomized controlled trial of smoking cessation counseling after myocardial infarction. Prevent Med 2000; 30:261–268.

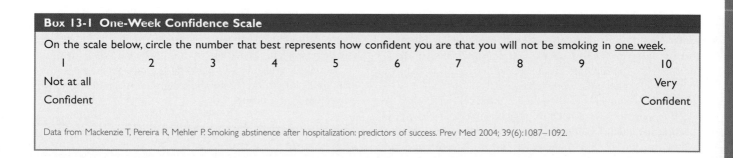

Box 13-1 One-Week Confidence Scale

On the scale below, circle the number that best represents how confident you are that you will not be smoking in <u>one week</u>.

1	2	3	4	5	6	7	8	9	10

Not at all
Confident

Very
Confident

Data from Mackenzie T, Pereira R, Mehler P. Smoking abstinence after hospitalization: predictors of success. Prev Med 2004; 39(6):1087–1092.

achieves the highest success rate, brief physician advice also increases cessation rates.[25,26]

Counseling

Ideally, well-trained smoking cessation counselors would be integrated into smoking cessation programs for hospitalized patients. Multiple studies have demonstrated high success rates with such an approach.[16,25,27] Physicians who are trained to counsel hospitalized smokers with brief, personalized messages, however, could make a significant impact on smoking cessation in this vulnerable group. However, interventions adding smoking cessation counseling to the job description of existing health care workers have had disappointing results. Training respiratory therapists to perform smoking cessation counseling in addition to their other duties yielded no significant difference between usual care and intervention at 1 year follow-up.[27]

Pharmacologic Management

While intensive smoking cessation counseling is an important component of smoking cessation interventions, pharmacologic therapy is just as critical and should be considered in every patient who is trying to quit.[11,26] Available first-line options include nicotine replacement therapy (NRT) or bupropion. Clonidine and nortriptyline are effective second-line agents.

Nicotine Replacement Therapy

Nicotine replacement may be given through a patch, gum, inhaler, or nasal spray. When combined with a behavior modification program, multiple clinical trials of NRT in the outpatient setting have demonstrated approximately double the quit rate, compared to placebo. Although inpatient evidence is limited, 12-week treatment with a nicotine patch was more effective than placebo (21% vs. 14%) when initiated in hospitalized smokers who expressed interest in quitting.[5] Other inpatient studies have shown similar results.[15]

Although the four major forms of NRT have approximately equal efficacy, the patch is easier to use and is often preferred by experts.[11] Nicotine patches are available over the counter (OTC) or by prescription. They vary in nicotine delivery from approximately 7 to 22 mg/hour. Nicotine gum is sold OTC in 2-mg or 4-mg pieces. The inhaler and nasal spray are available by prescription only. Individuals who smoke less than one pack per day should avoid the higher dose patches (21 mg) and gum (4 mg), as they would deliver more nicotine than the patient is currently obtaining through cigarettes. Recommended duration of therapy varies from 6 to 12 weeks with the patch and gum to 3–6 months with the nicotine nasal spray or inhaler. It is important that patients not smoke while taking NRT.

Potential side effects of the patch are a local, self-limited skin reaction in up to 50% of patients, which can usually be helped by rotating the patch location daily or by topical application of 5% hydrocortisone or 0.5% triamcinolone cream. Nicotine gum commonly causes mouth soreness, hiccups, dyspepsia, and jaw ache. The nasal spray irritates nasal passages in virtually all patients and should not be used in those with severe reactive airway disease. Finally, the nicotine inhaler can cause mild mouth and throat irritation, as well as coughing and rhinitis.

NRT is considered safe in patients with known cardiovascular disease when used in patients who, in the prior 2 weeks, are free from "unstable angina, myocardial infarction, coronary-artery bypass surgery or angioplasty, congestive heart failure, cor pulmonale, arrhythmia, peripheral vascular disease, cerebrovascular disease, stenosis of at least 50 percent in at least one major coronary artery as seen with coronary angiography, or a clinical history of angina."[28] There are little data available, however, concerning the safety of nicotine replacement therapy in individuals with unstable coronary disease.

Bupropion

Sustained-release bupropion (Zyban or Wellbutrin XL) is an antidepressant approved for smoking cessation; it can be used alone or in combination with NRT. Although data from inpatient studies are limited, bupropion has been successful in outpatient smoking cessation programs. The recommended duration of therapy is 7–12 weeks, starting 1 week before the quit date to provide a therapeutic level. It must be used with caution in patients who have a seizure or eating disorder.

In summary, patients admitted to the hospital who suffer from tobacco abuse should be counseled to quit by their hospitalist. The hospitalist should advise each patient to quit with a personalized message; determine whether the patient is thinking about quitting, and, if so, assist in setting a quit date as well as assess the level of nicotine dependence to facilitate discussion about pharmacologic therapy; and, finally, arrange for follow-up.

DISCHARGE AND FOLLOW-UP

Patient Education

Patient counseling about smoking cessation should be documented, particularly among patients with a smoking-related illness, such as myocardial infarction, chronic obstructive pulmonary disease, pneumonia, congestive heart failure, or cancer. As detailed above, tailoring such counseling to the patient's stage of change increases its relevance and likelihood of success (Fig. 13-1).

Physician Education

In the outpatient setting, even brief physician advice is associated with a higher likelihood of patient smoking cessation. However, this effect seems most prominent in unmotivated smokers and may not be generalizable to inpatient settings, where the acuity of illness itself can motivate many patients to quit. Because inpatient smoking cessation is most effective when delivered by a skilled professional, hospitalists may wish to acquire additional skills in this area. The resources in the following sections offer such training.

The Foundation for Innovations in Nicotine Dependence

www.findhelp.com

A nonprofit corporation established to research, educate, advocate, and assist in the treatment of nicotine dependence their web site is provided as a free resource to physicians, smokers, and anyone interested in current smoking cessation methods and medications.

Center for Tobacco Research and Intervention

www.cme.uwisc.org

Based at the University of Wisconsin School of Medicine. This site offers five web-based modules for continuing medical education to help clinicians implement the clinical practice guidelines for treating tobacco use and dependence.

Online Continuing Education

www.MedEdCME.com

Internet-based educational program offers ongoing continuing medical education, including a course for health care professionals on tobacco cessation treatment.

Outpatient Physician Communication

Similar to other chronic conditions, effective management of tobacco abuse in the hospital requires effective follow-up after discharge. Post-discharge telephone contact augments the impact of smoking cessation programs for hospitalized patients, and multiple phone calls were more successful than a single call in one study.[4] Other important strategies include enlisting the primary care physician's assistance in reinforcing the smoking cessation message, referring patients to established outpatient smoking cessation programs, and helping patients avoid relapse once they have quit.

Key Points

- Smoking is the most common preventable cause of morbidity and mortality in the United States.[14]

- Smoking cessation programs for hospitalized patients have been proven effective and are recommended by the US Department of Health and Human Services as well as the National Quality Forum.

- Treating tobacco use can be accomplished by using an overall approach referred to as the 5-A's (see Table 13-1), which

---

involves asking patients about tobacco use, and assessing the patient's readiness to quit and level of nicotine dependence.

- The "Stages of Change" model (see Fig. 13-1) is a useful tool to determine a smoker's readiness to quit. Cessation counseling that is tailored to the patient's "stage" is more effective than generic counseling.[22]

- Predictors of sustained smoking cessation are similar to short-term predictors and include: age, stage of change, and admission for a smoking-related illness.

- While intensive counseling coupled with pharmacotherapy and outpatient follow-up achieve the highest success rates, brief physician advice also increases cessation rates.[26,27]

- Nicotine replacement may be given through a patch, gum, inhaler, or nasal spray. When combined with a behavior modification program, multiple clinical trials of NRT in the outpatient setting have demonstrated approximately double the quit rate, compared to placebo.

- While data from inpatient studies are limited, bupropion has been successful in outpatient smoking cessation programs.

- Twelve-week treatment with a nicotine patch was more effective than placebo (21% vs. 14%) when initiated in hospitalized smokers who expressed interest in quitting.[5]

SUGGESTED READING

Fiore M, Bailer W, Cohen S. Treating tobacco use and dependence: clinical practice guideline. Rockville, MD: US Department of Health and Human Services, Public Health Service, 2000.

Lando H, Hennrikus D, McCarty M, et al. Predictors of quitting in hospitalized smokers. Nicotine Tob Res 2003; 5(2):215–222.

Mackenzie T, Pereira R, Mehler P. Smoking abstinence after hospitalization: predictors of success. Prev Med 2004; 39(6):1087–1092.

Rigotti N. Smoking cessation in the hospital setting: a new opportunity for managed care. Tob Control 2000; 9(Suppl 1):i55–i56.

Rigotti NA, Munafo MR, Murphy MF, et al. Interventions for smoking cessation in hospitalized patients. Cochrane Database Systemat Rev 2001; 2:CD001837. Review. Update in: Cochrane Database Systemat Rev 2003; 1:CD001837.

CHAPTER FOURTEEN

Prophylaxis for Venous Thromboembolism (VTE) in the Hospitalized Medical Patient

Greg Maynard, MD, MSc, and Jason Stein, MD

BACKGROUND

Over 2 million Americans suffer from deep venous thrombosis (DVT) each year, and 1 in 10 goes on to die from pulmonary embolism (PE). These 200,000 patients represent more annual deaths than those from breast cancer, AIDS, and traffic accidents combined.[1] Because of the silent nature of PE and declining rate of autopsies, this estimate in fact may be conservative.

The hospital is the most common place to acquire Venous Thromboembolism (VTE). Approximately half of all patients who develop VTE do so in the hospital. In a large registry trial capturing over 5,451 patients at 183 sites over a 6-month period, 50% (2,726) developed their VTE during hospitalization.[2]

Venous thromboembolism contributes significantly to hospital mortality. Pulmonary embolism is the most common preventable cause of death in the hospital. An estimated 10% of inpatient deaths are secondary to PE.[1] Patients who survive the initial diagnosis of PE face a mortality rate of 17.5% at 90 days.[3,4] Not only do patients with VTE suffer a 30% cumulative risk for recurrence, they are also at risk for the potentially disabling post-thrombotic syndrome.[5] These startling statistics emphasize the need for prevention.

While postoperative patients are traditionally recognized as being at highest risk for hospital-acquired VTE (see Chapter 100), the medical patient is also at high risk. Without prophylaxis, ranges of DVT risk are 10–26% in general medical patients,[6,7] 17–34% in patients with myocardial infarction,[8] 20–40% in patients with congestive heart failure,[9] 11–75% in patients with stroke,[8] and 25–42% in general medical intensive care patients.[10] Medical patients probably account for more than half of all hospital-acquired VTE events. In the DVT Free registry study, half the inpatients who suffered from VTE were nonsurgical and had no surgical procedures in the preceding 3 months.[2]

Underpinning the high prevalence of hospital-acquired VTE in medical patients is the underutilization of simple, cost-effective prophylactic measures. Of the 2,726 patients in the DVT Free registry who had their DVT diagnosed while hospitalized, only 1,147 (42%) received prophylaxis within the 30 days before diagnosis. Medical patients were much less likely to receive prophylaxis compared with surgical patients.[2]

The current reality in American hospitals is thus arrestingly substandard, especially considering what could be accomplished with simple, safe, and effective prophylaxis for the at-risk inpatient. Acknowledging the magnitude of this "implementation gap," the AHRQ report, *Making Healthcare Safer,* cited the provision of appropriate VTE prophylaxis as the paramount effective strategy to improve patient safety.[11]

Educational and awareness efforts alone have not proven adequate at increasing appropriate use of VTE prophylaxis. Similarly, order sets and critical pathways not supported by a healthy quality improvement framework are unlikely to succeed. Process redesign and continuous attention must include two essential elements:

1) Performance of a VTE risk assessment for every patient on admission and regularly throughout hospitalization
2) Selection of appropriate prophylaxis by linking the VTE risk to a corresponding menu of proven options

Following this rationale, we review optimal care for the individual patient and offer a practical section on implementing a protocol to optimize the prevention of VTE for the medical inpatient.

ASSESSMENT

Assessment of VTE Risk and Risk of Bleeding

Assessments of VTE risk should occur for each patient at the time of admission, transfers, and otherwise at regular intervals throughout the hospital stay. The risk assessment is derived from the history and physical examination. Simultaneously, an assessment of contraindications for pharmacologic prophylaxis should be performed.

Clinical Risk Factors

Specific medical conditions alone are not accurate predictors of VTE risk. For the same condition, moderate- and high-risk overlap, depending on severity of disease. Patient-related risk factors are at least as important as the admitting diagnosis. Advanced age, immobility, malignancy, pregnancy, estrogens, past medical history of VTE, inherited and acquired molecular risk factors, and metabolic abnormalities all increase risk. Medical interventions such as chemotherapy, invasive medical technologies, central venous catheters, and immobilization further increase a patient's VTE risk.

Table 14-1 Risk Factors for VTE in the Medical Patient

Clinical	Inherited or Acquired Thrombophilic Disorders
Increasing age >65	Activated Protein C Resistance (factor V Leiden)
Prolonged immobility, stroke, or paralysis	
Previous VTE	Prothrombin variant 20210A
Cancer or myeloproliferative disorders and their treatments	Antiphospholipid antibodies (lupus anticoagulant and anticardiolipin antibody)
Sickle cell crisis	Deficiency or dysfunction of antithrombin, protein C, protein S, or heparin cofactor II
Obesity	
Varicose veins	Dysfibrinogenemia
Cardiac dysfunction especially decompensated CHF	Decreased levels of plasminogen and plasminogen activators
Acute myocardial infarction	Heparin induced thrombocytopenia
Active lung disease, especially respiratory failure	Hyperhomocysteinemia
Indwelling central venous catheters	Myeloproliferative disorders such as polycythemia vera and primary thrombocytosis*
Inflammatory bowel disease	
Sepsis	
Dehydration or hyperviscosity	
Smoking	
Nephrotic syndrome	
Pregnancy or estrogen use	

*Geerts WH, Pineo GF, Heit JA, et al. Prevention of venous thromboembolism: the Seventh ACCP Conference on Antithrombotic and Thrombolytic Therapy. Chest 2004; 126 (3 Suppl):338S–400S.

Multiple risk factors have a cumulative effect. This reality should be taken into account when assigning VTE risk and deciding on a prophylactic strategy. Risk factors for VTE are summarized above in Table 14-1. Medical patients at the highest risk for VTE have decompensated heart failure or severe respiratory disease or are confined to bed with multiple risk factors as outlined in Table 14-1.

A checklist of VTE risk factors, posted in useful places in the hospital, may be helpful to serve as a memory aid for clinicians and to assist in formal assignment and documentation of VTE risk.

Highest and lowest risk patients are the easiest to classify. Patients with the very high-risk conditions of acute spinal cord injury and multiple major traumas are at very high risk for VTE—equivalent to the risk of major orthopedic surgery. In the absence of contraindications, these patients warrant low-molecular-weight heparin (LMWH) prophylaxis and consideration for supplementary intermittent pneumatic compression devices (IPC) or graduated compression stockings (GCS).

Low-risk patients are those who are ambulatory, have no risk factors, or are projected to have a short length of stay. These patients need no specific measures apart from being encouraged to ambulate.

Classifying patients who are not clearly in the highest or lowest risk categories can be challenging and at times may even seem arbitrary. Some generalizations can be useful. Sicker medical patients (e.g., ICU patient with severe respiratory disease or decompensated CHF) are generally considered high risk and have been studied in recent controlled trials.

Less clearly classified are medical patients with "classic" risk factors that have not been well studied in recent clinical trials. Such patients reasonably are considered to be at moderate risk for VTE. Individual physicians and institutions must define which prophylactic options are acceptable for these patients.

MANAGEMENT/PROPHYLAXIS FOR EACH LEVEL OF VTE RISK

Prophylaxis Options

Options for VTE prophylaxis are outlined in Table 14-2. An appreciation of the level of evidence supporting these agents for preventing VTE in the medical patient is valuable.

Aspirin has only a small benefit in preventing VTE and should not be used as a sole agent.

The Seventh American College of Chest Physicians (ACCP) Conference on Antithrombotic and Thrombolytic Therapy made this recommendation in 2004[12]:

In acutely ill medical patients who are admitted to the hospital with congestive heart failure or severe respiratory disease or who are confined to bed and have one or more additional risk factors including active cancer, previous VTE, sepsis, acute neurological disease, or inflammatory bowel disease, we recommended prophylaxis with LDUH (Grade 1A) or LMWH (Grade 1A).

This carefully phrased recommendation was framed to reflect the evidence available for the prevention of VTE, which is limited to the high-risk, acutely ill patient, and those with congestive heart failure or severe respiratory disease.

Older studies investigating prophylaxis with low-dose unfractionated heparin (LDUH) 5,000 units subcutaneously BID to TID in medical patients have important limitations. The limitations on these studies, predominantly from Europe, include: small populations, variations in endpoint measurements, and open label, nonrandomized design. What is clear is that evidence for the use of LDUH 5,000 units TID is more convincing than the evidence for LDUH 5,000 units BID.[7,13]

Table 14-2 VTE Prophylaxis Agents

Agent and Mechanism	Considerations
ES (aka GCS) Reduce venous stasis in legs	No risk for bleeding, as effective as LDUH in moderate-risk general surgery patients, can be combined with pharmacologic agent
IPC Enhance blood flow in deep veins of legs and reduces levels of PAI-1, thereby enhancing endogenous fibrinolytic activity	No risk for bleeding, as effective as LDUH in high-risk general surgery patients, can be combined with pharmacologic agent
	Comfort can affect compliance, contraindicated if patient immobilized >72 hours without any form of prophylaxis
LDUH Binds to antithrombin, potentiating its inhibition of thrombin and activated factor X	Well studied, no monitoring needed, no difference in major hemorrhage*
	Inadequate for high and highest risk, risk of HIT (1–5%) with overt vascular thrombosis in those with HIT (~50%)[†‡]
LMWH Same mechanism as LDUH	No monitoring needed, rates of major hemorrhage comparable to LDUH, can be dosed once daily, less likely than LDUH to produce HIT and thrombosis
	More expensive than LDUH, risk exists for HIT and thrombosis
Coumadin Inhibits vitamin K–dependent activation of cofactors II, VII, IX, and X with dose adjusted to target INR 2–3	Effective with dosing beginning day of surgery—or day after, conveniently continued into the outpatient setting
	Requires at least 3 days before therapeutic and required frequent monitoring until dose stable
Newer Agents —Fondaparinux SQ—catalyzes factor Xa inactivation by AIII without inhibiting thrombin	More study required. Promising characteristics: Fondaparinux—SQ route with no risk for HIT or thrombosis but most expensive option
—Hirudin IV—direct inhibitor of thrombin	Hirudin—approved in US only for HIT/thrombosis

ES = elastic stockings; GCS = graduated compression stockings; IPC = intermittent pneumatic compression PAI-1 = plasminogen activator inhibitor-1; LDUH = low-dose unfractionated heparin; LMWH = low-molecular-weight heparin; HIT = heparin-induced thrombocytopenia.

Additional Risk Factors: see Table "Additional Risk Factors for VTE".

*Compared with no prophylaxis

[†]Hirsh J, Warkentin TE, Raschke R, et al. Heparin and low-molecular-weight heparin: mechanisms of action, pharmacokinetics, dosing considerations, monitoring, efficacy, and safety. Chest 1998; 114(suppl):489S–510S.

[‡]Warkentin TE, Levine MN, Hirsh J, et al. Heparin-induced thrombocytopenia in patients treated with low-molecular-weight heparin or unfractionated heparin. N Engl J Med 1995; 332:1330–1335.

MORE RECENT STUDIES

LMWH versus Placebo

The landmark MEDENOX[14] study established again that acutely ill medical patients are at significant risk of VTE (15% total VTE, 5% proximal DVT). Enoxaparin 40 mg once daily given subcutaneously for 6–14 days was effective in reducing the risk of VTE by 63% compared to placebo, and benefit was maintained at 3-month follow-up. This result was achieved with no increase in adverse events, hemorrhage, or decreased platelets.

The PREVENT study[15] showed that the LMWH dalteparin 5,000 units daily for 14 days was more effective than placebo in the prevention of VTE in acutely ill patients hospitalized for at least 4 days with CHF (NYHA III, IV), acute respiratory failure, or with acute severe systemic disease plus one risk factor (RR = 0.55).

LMWH versus LDUH 5,000 Units TID

The PRINCE[16] and PRIME[17] studies both pitted enoxaparin 40 mg per day against LDUH 5,000 units TID in preventing VTE in high-risk medical patients. LMWH proved to be at least as efficacious and safe as LDUH in these trials.

SUMMARY OF HEPARIN PROPHYLAXIS IN MEDICAL PATIENTS: PREFERRED PROPHYLAXIS

Prophylactic doses of heparins will reduce the incidence of DVT and PE by 50–65%. The appropriate dose and frequency of LDUH for high-risk medical patients is 5,000 units TID. Little evidence exists to support lesser doses or frequency. For LMWH, enoxaparin 40 mg or dalteparin 5,000 units per day are the preferred regimens for high-risk patients. Choosing between LMWH and LDUH options should be an individual and institutional choice. LMWH is much more expensive per day, but is less likely to cause heparin-induced thrombocytopenia (HIT) and can be given once a day, which may improve patient acceptance and reduce nursing workload and overall cost.

For the moderate-risk medical patient, the current literature does not provide much guidance. Individuals and institutions need to make their own judgments.

ALTERNATIVE OPTIONS, NON-PHARMACOLOGIC OPTIONS, AND CONTRAINDICATIONS TO PHARMACOLOGIC PROPHYLAXIS

Low-dose unfractionated heparin at 7,500 units BID is empirically attractive. Given the half-life of LDUH, this dose and frequency might be as effective as LDUH 5,000 TID, and it would still retain a very significant cost advantage over LMWH. However, this regimen has not been well studied in randomized controlled trials in any patient population. Additionally, many pharmacies cannot obtain LDUH prepackaged in this dose, making it an impractical and fiscally unattractive choice.

Fondaparinux is a pentasaccharide that has been shown to reduce VTE in medical patients with an effect size similar to that of the LMWH trials.[18] It is very expensive compared to the other options, not as well studied, and should be considered primarily as an option in patients with HIT.

Should mechanical prophylaxis be used as frontline therapy? The 2004 ACCP consensus conference addresses this question as follows[12]:

We recommend that mechanical methods of prophylaxis be used primarily in patients who are at high risk of bleeding (Grade 1C+), or as an adjunct to anticoagulant-based prophylaxis (Grade 2A).

Although mechanical methods of prophylaxis have been studied and shown to be an effective prophylaxis option in surgical patients (though less studied than pharmacologic methods), there is an absence of meaningful data in the medical patient. Those using this method as a primary form of prophylaxis in the moderate-risk medical patient should do so with the appreciation that there is even less evidence for this approach than for pharmacologic options.

The 2004 ACCP consensus conference offered this niche role for lone mechanical prophylaxis in medical patients[12]:

In medical patients with risk factors for VTE, and in whom there is a contraindication for anticoagulant prophylaxis, we recommend the use of mechanical prophylaxis with GCSs or IPC (Grade 1C+).

A checklist of contraindications to pharmacologic prophylaxis is presented in Box 14-1. As with the timing of VTE risk assessment, patients should be screened for these contraindications on admission and periodically throughout their stay since status can change frequently. Whenever IPC or GCS is ordered, compliance should be noted and addressed. Educating the patient on the rationale for therapy may enhance compliance.

SPECIAL SITUATIONS AND DOSING ADJUSTMENTS

Malnourished, low weight, and elderly patients may need lower LDUH doses than 5,000 units TID to prevent excessive bleeding complications.

Patients with renal dysfunction (serum creatinine >2 or creatinine clearance <30) do not metabolize LMWH or fondaparinux well. Low-dose unfractionated heparins should be considered, or a reduction in dose of the LMWH prophylaxis.

Dosing in markedly obese patients is not well established.

SUBSEQUENT MONITORING AND THERAPY

All patients should periodically be assessed for changes in their VTE risk, contraindications to pharmacologic prophylaxis, and compliance with prophylactic measures.

Box 14-1 Contraindications to Pharmacologic DVT Prophylaxis

Absolute (check if applicable)

Active hemorrhage

Heparin/LMWH in patients with immune-mediated HIT.

Epidural/indwelling spinal catheter placement or removal

Severe trauma to head or spinal cord with hemorrhage in the last 4 weeks

Relative (check if applicable)

History of cerebral hemorrhage

Craniotomy within 2 weeks

Intraocular surgery within 2 weeks

GI, GU hemorrhage within the last 6 months

Thrombocytopenia (<50K) or coagulopathy (PT >18 seconds)

Active intracranial lesions/neoplasms

Neurosurgery

Uncontrolled hypertension

Platelet counts should be assessed at the initiation of any heparin prophylaxis and every third day thereafter. Even when the platelet count still falls in the normal range, a drop by 50% should spur further evaluation for HIT while alternative modes of prophylaxis are started.

Prophylaxis should be maintained until the VTE risk factors mandating prophylaxis are eliminated, or until the patient is discharged from the hospital. The benefit of continuing prophylaxis in medical patients after discharge is unknown, but may be reasonable practice in patients with ongoing high VTE risk. Studies evaluating the efficacy of continuing prophylaxis into the post-discharge period are underway.

Even when appropriate prophylaxis is used, medical inpatients can develop VTE. The risk reduction in clinical trials is approximately 50–65%. Thus, an index of suspicion for new VTE should be maintained.

INTEGRATING VTE PROPHYLAXIS INTO A HOSPITAL SYSTEM: LEADING AN IMPLEMENTATION TEAM

Without a supporting framework to prompt both regular VTE risk assessments and risk-appropriate prophylaxis, individual physicians and nurses have little hope of providing optimal VTE prevention for the medical patient. Hospitalists are ideally situated to lead efforts to systematize these steps.

Assembling a multidisciplinary team with front-line expertise is essential. The team should include nurses, pharmacists, hospitalists, and other physicians. An evaluation of your institution's current process should answer these questions:

- Do patients receive regular VTE risk assessments? If so, how often, who does them, and is the methodology standardized?
- Are VTE risk assessments and VTE prophylaxis orders incorporated into other order sets and protocols?

- Are the appropriate prophylaxis options readily available for each level of VTE risk?
- How many cases of hospital-acquired VTE were diagnosed in your institution last year? (Approximately half of all VTE diagnosed are hospital acquired.)
- How often is appropriate prophylaxis used in your institution? (Sampling methodology can give you a pretty good estimate with minimum effort, once the group defines what "appropriate" is for each level of risk.)

Setting a time-specific, measurable aim for the team is essential to gauge the team's success in reducing hospital acquired VTE. The websites of the Society of Hospital Medicine (www.hospitalmedicine.org) and the Institute for Healthcare Improvement (www.ihi.org) provide in-depth guidance for implementing an effective protocol to prevent hospital-acquired VTE in medical (and surgical) patients.

DISCHARGE/FOLLOW-UP PLANS

Patient Education

Patients should be encouraged to ambulate early. They should be advised of their VTE risk and of any measures that might mitigate that risk (e.g., stopping estrogen therapy). If pharmacologic prophylaxis is continued after hospital discharge, the risks and benefits should be discussed with the patient. Instructions to report signs or symptoms of bleeding, a new DVT, or PE should be clear.

Outpatient Physician Communication

Unless there is a complication of therapy or a high ongoing risk of VTE requiring outpatient prophylaxis, no specific communication is needed regarding routine prophylaxis limited to the hospital setting.

Key Points

- Fatal PE is the most common cause of preventable hospital deaths.
- Hospitalized medical patients are often at high risk for acquiring DVT or PE.

- Prophylaxis for VTE in medical patients is safe and effective—but significantly underutilized.
- Hospital processes should be designed to ensure that all eligible inpatients receive appropriate VTE prophylaxis. This can be accomplished through:

a. Performance of a VTE risk assessment for every patient on admission and regularly throughout hospitalization

b. Selection of appropriate prophylaxis by linking the VTE risk to a corresponding menu of proven options

- Platelet counts should be assessed at the initiation of any heparin prophylaxis and every third day thereafter. Even when the platelet count still falls in the normal range, a drop by 50% should spur further evaluation for HIT while alternative modes of prophylaxis are started.

SUGGESTED READING

Goldhaber SZ, Tapson VF. DVT Free Steering Committee: a prospective registry of 5,451 patients with ultrasound-confirmed deep vein thrombosis. Am J Cardiol 2004; 93(2):259–262.

Geerts WH, Pineo GF, Heit JA, et al. Prevention of venous thromboembolism: the seventh ACCP conference on antithrombotic and thrombolytic therapy. Chest 2004; 126(3 Suppl):338S–400S.

Samama MM, Cohen AT, Darmon JY, et al. The MEDENOX study: a comparison of enoxaparin with placebo for the prevention of venous thromboembolism in acutely ill medical patients. N Engl J Med 1999; 341:793–800.

Leizorovicz A, Cohen AT, Turpie AGG, et al. A randomized placebo controlled trial of dalteparin for the prevention of venous thromboembolism in 3706 acutely ill medical patients: the PREVENT medical thromboprophylaxis study. Circulation 2004; 110(7):874–879.

Lechler E, Schramm W, Flosbach CW, et al. The venous thrombotic risk in non-surgical patients: epidemiological data and efficacy/safety profile of a low-molecular-weight heparin (enoxaparin). The PRIME Study Group. Haemostasis 1996; 26(Suppl):49–56.

CHAPTER FIFTEEN

Osteoporosis

Laura J. Martin, MD

BACKGROUND

Fractures, a common consequence of osteoporosis, result in multiple hospitalizations, and hospitalists may be responsible for initiating therapy for osteoporosis in the hospital. Associated with increased risk of fracture, osteoporosis is a common bone disorder characterized by low bone mass and microarchitectural disruption of bone. Osteoporosis and osteopenia are defined by the World Health Organization based on bone mineral density T scores and presence or absence of fragility fractures[1] (Table 15-1). Major risk factors for primary osteoporosis include age >65, female sex, Caucasian ethnicity, current smoking, low body weight, personal history of fracture as an adult, and history of fragility fracture in a first-degree relative. These and additional risk factors are listed in Box 15-1. There are numerous medical conditions and medications that are associated with secondary osteoporosis (Box 15-2).

ASSESSMENT

Clinical Presentation

Prevalence

Although most prevalent in white postmenopausal females, osteoporosis occurs in all populations and in all age groups. In 1995, an estimated $13.8 billion was spent in the United States for treatment of osteoporosis-related fractures.[2] These osteoporotic fractures accounted for about 432,000 hospital admissions, with 57% of these admissions for hip fracture, 6.8% for vertebral spine fracture, 3.1% for forearm fractures, and 33% for fractures of other sites. Overall, vertebral spine compression fractures are the most frequently diagnosed osteoporosis-related fractures in the United States, with an incidence of 700,000 per year.[3]

The National Osteoporosis Foundation (NOF) estimated in 2002 that 7.8 million individuals in the United States have osteoporosis while 21.8 million have low bone density at the hip.[4] An estimated 20% of white women in the United States have osteoporosis at the hip while 52% have low bone density at the hip. It is estimated by the NOF that one of every two white women will have an osteoporotic fracture in her lifetime.

Differential Diagnosis

Osteoporosis can exist as a silent disease and commonly presents clinically with fractures. The three most prevalent types of osteoporotic fractures are vertebral, hip, and forearm fractures. Vertebral compression fractures are the most common, usually occurring in the thoracolumbar area; most are asymptomatic and diagnosed by x-ray. About one third of patients with osteoporotic vertebral fractures will present with acute back pain that usually subsides within 6 weeks. Hip fractures commonly occur in elderly patients with osteoporosis, the majority of these fractures occurring after a fall. The most common types of hip fracture are intertrochanteric, femoral neck, and subcapital. Distal radius fractures (Colles' fractures) usually occur after a fall onto outstretched hands.

Osteomalacia and hyperparathyroidism are other metabolic bone diseases besides osteoporosis/osteopenia that can lead to a decrease in bone density. In osteomalacia, there is disordered mineralization of newly formed organic matrix. Osteomalacia is seen in patients with vitamin D deficiency or small bowel disease and can be diagnosed definitively with a bone marrow biopsy. Hyperparathyroidism causes marrow fibrosis, changes in osteoid, and collections of osteoclasts. Laboratory tests including serum calcium and parathyroid hormone (PTH) are useful in the evaluation of suspected hyperparathyroidism.

Diagnosis

Preferred Studies

According to the NOF, routine bone mineral density testing is recommended in[4]:

1. All women aged 65 and older
2. Younger postmenopausal women who have one or more risk factors (other than being white, postmenopausal, and female)
3. Postmenopausal women who have suffered a fragility fracture to confirm the diagnosis and determine disease severity

The US Preventive services Task Force (USPSTF) recommends routine bone mineral density (BMD) testing in[5]:

1. Women aged 65 and older
2. Women aged 60 and over with increased risk for osteoporotic fractures

Table 15-1 Definitions of Osteoporosis and Osteopenia Based on World Health Organization Criteria

Classification	Bone Mineral Density T-score*	Previous Fragility Fracture
Normal	≥ −1 SD	None
Osteopenia	−1 to −2.5 SD	None
Osteoporosis	≤ −2.5 SD	None
Severe osteoporosis	≤ −2.5 SD	One

*T-score is expressed in standard deviations (SD), comparing the subject's BMD with the predicted mean peak BMD in a 30-year-old of the same sex. Adapted from: Assessment of fracture risk and its application to screening for postmenopausal osteoporosis: report of a WHO study group. World Health Organization Technical Report Series 843, 1994.

Box 15-1 Risk Factors for Osteoporosis

Age ≥ 65

Female sex

Caucasian race

Personal history of low-impact fragility fracture

History of fragility fracture in first-degree relative

Low body weight (<127 lbs)

Current smoking

Inadequate exercise

Excessive alcohol intake (>2 drinks/day)

Prolonged low calcium intake

Estrogen deficiency

Box 15-2 Medical Conditions and Medications Associated with Secondary Osteoporosis

Medical Conditions

    Hyperthyroidism

    Hyperparathyroidism

    Vitamin D deficiency

    Malabsorption syndromes

    Hypogonadism

    Chronic hepatic or renal disease

    Cushing's disease

    Multiple myeloma

    Prolonged immobilization

    Sarcoidosis

    Hyperprolactinemia

Medications

    Chronic use of glucocorticoids >3 months

    Antiseizure medications

    Excess thyroxine replacement

    Medroxyprogesterone

    Heparin

Methods of Measurement:

Dual x-ray absorptiometry (DXA) is the standard test to evaluate for osteoporosis. DXA produces a reliable result and is an accurate predictor for fracture risk. It measures BMD at clinically important sites such as the spine and hip. Results are reported in standard deviations as a T-score or Z-score. A T-score is based on standard deviation from mean peak bone density in a reference young adult population. A decrease of 1 standard deviation represents a 10–12% change in bone mineral density, and an increase in the risk of fracture by a factor of about 1.5. A Z-score is based on standard deviation from an age, sex, and ethnicity–matched reference population. A Z-score of −2.0 or less suggests a secondary cause of osteoporosis.

Evaluation for Secondary Causes of Osteoporosis

Although most postmenopausal women have the primary form of osteoporosis, secondary causes should be considered in postmenopausal women with abnormal Z-scores on DXA scan and/or medical conditions associated with the secondary form of osteoporosis. In premenopausal women and men diagnosed with osteoporosis, secondary causes are prevalent. Medical conditions and medications that contribute to secondary osteoporosis are listed in Box 15-2. Appropriate tests in the work-up of secondary osteoporosis should be based primarily on findings from the patient's medical history. Helpful tests sometimes include a serum calcium, thyroid stimulating hormone (TSH), and 25-hydroxy vitamin D level if deficiency is suspected.

Glucocorticoid-induced osteoporosis is the most prevalent medication-related cause of secondary osteoporosis. It should be suspected in patients treated with the equivalent of prednisone ≥5 mg/day for a 3 month or longer period of time. The American College of Rheumatology recommends routine BMD testing annually or biannually in patients receiving long-term glucocorticoids (prednisone equivalent of ≥5 mg/day).[6]

PREDICTION RULE

Common risk factors for osteoporosis are listed in Box 15-1. One well-validated instrument to aid in assessing patients at risk for low BMD is the Osteoporosis Risk Assessment Instrument (ORAI).[7] This instrument uses three variables (age, weight, and current use of hormone therapy) to predict risk of osteoporosis in postmenopausal women (Table 15-2). A score greater than 9 indicates that bone mineral testing is warranted. This tool has a sensitivity of 93.3% (95% confidence interval [CI] 86.3–97.0%) and specificity of 46.4% (95% CI 41.0–51.8%) in selecting women with low BMD. The sensitivity of the ORAI in identifying women with osteoporosis is 94.4% (95% CI 83.7–98.6%).

PROGNOSIS

During Hospitalization

Osteoporosis infrequently is a direct cause of mortality during hospitalization. It is a contributing factor in many patients hospitalized with fractures. Hip fracture is among the most serious diagnoses associated with osteoporosis. The estimated 30 day

Table 15-2 Scoring System for Osteoporosis Risk Assessment Instrument (ORAI)

Variable	Score
Age, yr	
≥75	15
65–74	9
55–64	5
45–54	0
Weight, kg	
<60	9
60–69	3
≥70	0
Current Estrogen Use	
No	2
Yes	0

Women with a total score of 9 or greater would be selected for bone densitometry.

Source: Cadarette SM, Jaglal SB, Kreiger N, et al. Development and validation of the osteoporosis risk assessment instrument to facilitate selection of women for bone densitometry. CMAJ 2000; 162(9):1289–1294. By permission of the publisher. © 2000 CMA Media Inc.

mortality in Medicare-insured patients hospitalized with a hip fracture is 11% for men and 6% for women.[8]

Postdischarge

The mortality rate from hip fracture is close to 25% at 1 year.[8]

MANAGEMENT

Preferred Treatment

The NOF recommends initiating therapy to reduce fracture risk in postmenopausal women with vertebral or hip fractures. In the outpatient setting, therapy is recommended for postmenopausal women with BMD DXA T score of below −2 in the absence of risk factors and in women with T-scores below −1.5 if one or more risk factors are present.[4]

Lifestyle Modification

Calcium and vitamin D are important components of the diet to maintain bone health. The NOF recommends advising all patients to consume at least 1,200 mg of calcium per day and 400–800 IU of vitamin D per day, including supplements if necessary. Regular weight-bearing exercise and balance-training exercises have been shown to reduce the risk of falls and fractures. Counseling on tobacco cessation and avoidance of excessive alcohol intake is recommended. All these lifestyle modification recommendations can be made both during hospitalization and at discharge.

Pharmacologic Therapy

There are two major types of drug therapy approved by the Food and Drug Administration (FDA) for the treatment of osteoporosis. Antiresorptive medications reduce bone loss by decreasing the activity of osteoclasts and increasing BMD. Approved antiresorptive agents include bisphosphonates, estrogen, selective estrogen receptor modulators (SERMs), and calcitonin. Human recombinant PTH (1–34), teriparatide is an anabolic therapy approved by the FDA.

Bisphosphonates

Alendronate, risedronate, and ibandronate are bisphosphonates approved by the FDA for treatment of osteoporosis. Bisphosphonates are synthetic analogs of pyrophosphate that bind to hydroxyapatite in bone, inhibit osteoclast activity, and reduce bone resorption.

Alendronate can increase BMD by about 8% at the spine and 6–7% at the hip in postmenopausal women over a 3-year period.[9] Alendronate has been shown to reduce fracture rates in the spine by 59%, hip by 63%, and wrist by about 34%.[10] Dosing for postmenopausal osteoporosis or osteoporosis in males is a 10-mg daily dose or 70-mg weekly dose.

Risedronate increases BMD of the spine by 5% and BMD of the hip by 2–3% over 3 years.[11] It has been shown to reduce spine fractures by 41% and nonspine fractures by 39%.[11] In elderly postmenopausal females with osteoporosis, it has been shown to reduce hip fractures by 30%.[12] Dosing for osteoporosis is 5 mg daily or 35 mg weekly.

Daily ibandronate increases BMD of the spine by 6.4% and hip by 3.1% over 3 years.[13] Ibandronate appears to reduce spine fractures by 52% at 3 years, but has not been shown to reduce nonvertebral fractures compared to placebo. A 1-year study comparing once-monthly ibandronate to the daily dosage showed similar efficacy and tolerability.[14] Dosing for postmenopausal osteoporosis is 2.5 mg daily or a once-monthly dose of 100 or 150 mg.

Because bisphosphonates are poorly absorbed, they should be taken first thing in the morning on an empty stomach with a full glass of water. Patients should avoid food for 30 minutes after dosing. To prevent the side effect of esophagitis, patients should be advised not to lie supine for 30 minutes after taking the medication. Bisphosphonates should be used with caution in patients with a history of esophageal stricture, gastric ulcers, or gastric reflux. Bisphosphonates should not be prescribed in pregnant women or in patients with significant renal dysfunction with creatinine clearance less than 30 mg/min.

Estrogen/Hormone Therapy

Estrogen is no longer considered to be a first-line therapy in many patients as a result of the Women's Health Initiative (WHI) trial.[15] This study found an increased risk of stroke and thrombotic problems in women taking hormone therapy and an increased risk of breast cancer in women taking the combination of estrogen and progesterone. The WHI did confirm the efficacy of estrogen in reducing fractures. Both hip and spine fractures were reduced by greater than 30% among those taking hormone therapy. The FDA now recommends that in women with postmenopausal osteoporosis estrogen/hormone therapy should only be considered for women at significant risk who cannot take nonestrogen medications.

Selective Estrogen Receptor Modulators

SERMs bind to estrogen receptors and have tissue-selective agonist and antagonist properties. Raloxifene is the only FDA-

Figure 15-1 • Vertebroplasty injection.

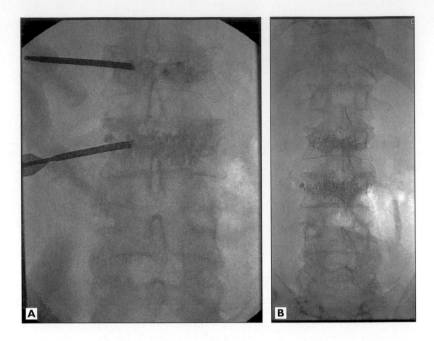

approved SERM; it increases spine BMD by about 2.6% and hip BMD by about 2.1–2.4% after 3 years.[16] It has been shown to reduce spine fractures by approximately 30–50%. No reduction in hip or nonspine fractures has been shown. Potential side effects include an increased risk of DVT and pulmonary embolism. Dosing for prevention and treatment of postmenopausal osteoporosis is 60 mg daily.

Calcitonin

Calcitonin is secreted by the parafollicular cells of the thyroid gland and inhibits bone resorption by osteoclasts. The Prevent Recurrence of Osteoporotic Fractures (Proof) trial showed a decrease in spine fractures by 33% with a calcitonin dose of 200 IU daily, but no reduction in fractures with a dose of 400 IU daily.[17] Based on these results, the efficacy of calcitonin in reducing fractures is in question. For this reason, calcitonin is considered a second-line therapy for osteoporosis. Calcitonin nasal spray is currently FDA-approved at 200 IU daily for treatment of osteoporosis in women who are at least 5 years postmenopause.

Parathyroid Hormone

Intermittent parathyroid hormone administration has been shown to have anabolic bone-building effects. Human recombinant PTH (1–34), also called teriparatide, has been shown to increase spine BMD by 9–13% and hip BMD by 3–6% after 21 months.[18] A reduction in spine fractures by about 65% and nonspine fractures by about 53% has been shown.[18] Teriparatide is FDA-approved for treatment of osteoporosis in postmenopausal women and in men. It is contraindicated in patients with hypercalcemia, renal dysfunction, bone cancer, or cancer with metastasis to bone. Recommended dosing is 20 microgram daily by subcutaneous injection.

Surgical Management—Vertebroplasty and Kyphoplasty (Fig. 15-1)

Vertebroplasty and kyphoplasty are two minimally invasive surgical procedures shown to provide rapid pain relief in patients who do not respond adequately to pain medications in the treatment of back pain from vertebral compression fractures. In a vertebroplasty procedure, polymethylmethacrylate cement is injected into the fractured vertebral body percutaneously under fluoroscopy. Kyphoplasty involves inserting a balloon-like catheter into the vertebral body, lifting the collapsed vertebra, and then injecting the cement. Kyphoplasty provides direct reduction of the vertebral fracture and frequently provides partial restoration of height and sagittal realignment of the spine. Nonrandomized studies show that 53–100% of patients achieve a rapid reduction of back pain 24 hours post-procedure.[19–25] To date, there are no randomized controlled trials evaluating these two treatment modalities. Possible complications include cement extravasation into the epidural or paravertebral areas, occasionally causing neurologic findings such as nerve root compression.[26] Additionally, there have been some case reports of extravasation into perivertebral veins, leading to pulmonary embolism.[27,28]

PREVENTION

There are several lifestyle modifications as described above—adequate calcium and vitamin D intake, regular weight-bearing exercise, and avoidance of tobacco and excessive alcohol intake—that are helpful in both the prevention and treatment of osteoporosis. Measures to help prevent falls in older patients include balance-training exercises, regular vision checks, and eliminating medications where possible that may lead to dizziness or confusion.

Helpful environmental measures include removing or taping down throw rugs and installing night-lights.

Osteopenia

Osteopenia is defined by the World Health Organization as a bone densiometry T-score of −1 to −2.5. Pharmacologic therapy is a consideration for prevention of the progression of osteopenia to osteoporosis. Bisphosphonates are FDA approved for prevention of osteoporosis. The recommended dose for osteoporosis prevention is similar for alendronate and risedronate, with dosing of 5 mg daily or 35 mg weekly. Estrogen/hormone therapy and raloxifene are also FDA approved for prevention of osteoporosis.

DISCHARGE/FOLLOW-UP PLANS

Patient Education

Patients should receive extensive counseling concerning lifestyle modifications helpful in both the prevention and treatment of osteoporosis as described previously.

Outpatient Physician Communication

Monitoring Osteoporosis

After initiation of pharmacologic treatment for osteoporosis, follow-up bone densiometry is recommended in an interval of 1–2 years.

Key Points

- Major risk factors for primary osteoporosis include age >65, female sex, Caucasian ethnicity, current smoking, low body weight, personal history of fracture as an adult, and history of fragility fracture in first-degree relative. One of every two white women will have an osteoporotic fracture in her lifetime.

- The three most prevalent types of osteoporotic fractures are vertebral, hip, and forearm fractures. Vertebral compression fractures are the most common, usually occurring in the thoracolumbar area; most are asymptomatic.

- Hip fracture is the most common cause of hospitalization secondary to osteoporosis; estimated 30 day mortality in Medicare-insured patients is 11% for men and 6% for women.

- Glucocorticoid-induced osteoporosis is the most prevalent medication-related cause of secondary osteoporosis.

- Physicians should initiate therapy to reduce fracture risk in postmenopausal women hospitalized with vertebral or hip fractures. This includes vitamin D and calcium supplements, lifestyle modification with increased weight-bearing exercise if possible, and tobacco cessation counseling for smokers.

- Vertebroplasty and kyphoplasty appear to provide rapid pain relief in patients who do not respond adequately to pain medications in the treatment of back pain from vertebral compression fractures. However, there are no RCTs evaluating their efficacy.

SUGGESTED READING

Assessment of fracture risk and its application to screening for postmenopausal osteoporosis: report of a WHO study group. World Health Organization Technical Report Series 843, 1994.

Cadarette SM, Jaglal SB, Kreiger N, et al. Development and validation of the osteoporosis risk assessment instrument to facilitate selection of women for bone densitometry. CMAJ May 2000; 162(9):1289–1294.

National Osteoporosis Foundation. Physician's guide to prevention and treatment of osteoporosis. Washington,DC: National Osteoporosis Foundation, 2003.

U.S. Department of Health & Human Services. Bone health and osteoporosis: a report of the surgeon general. Rockville, MD: Oct 2004. Available at http://www.surgeongeneral.gov/library/bonehealth/content.html. Accessed February 2006.

U.S. Preventive Services Task Force. Screening for osteoporosis in postmenopausal women: recommendations and rationale. Rockville, MD: Agency for Healthcare Research and Quality, 2002.

Diamond TH, Champion B, Clark WA. Management of acute osteoporotic vertebral fractures: a nonrandomized trial comparing percutaneous vertebroplasty with conservative therapy. Am J Med 2003; 114(4):257–265.

CHAPTER SIXTEEN

Substance Abuse and Dependence in the Hospitalized Patient

Jeffrey L. Greenwald, MD, and Jeffrey Samet, MD, MA, MPH

BACKGROUND

Unhealthy use of alcohol and other drugs is common in the United States. Almost a quarter of surveyed individuals in the United States over the age of 11 participated in binge drinking (≥5 units of alcohol in one sitting) at least once in the prior month; 7.6% met criteria for alcohol abuse or dependence in the prior year. The National Surveys on Drug Use & Health estimated that 11 million Americans had ever used oxycodone without a prescription and 1.9 million Americans had ever used heroin.[1]

It is unusual to admit a patient to an acute-care hospital solely because of substance abuse. However, a significant proportion of the patients admitted do have concurrent substance abuse issues either causing their presenting problems (e.g., decompensated cirrhosis, infective endocarditis, or pneumonia) or complicating their care (e.g., alcohol withdrawal syndrome or behavioral issues). Almost a quarter of a million hospital discharges in the United States in 2002 noted alcohol or drug abuse or dependence as a principal discharge diagnosis at a cost of over 1.75 billion dollars; 4 million hospitalizations in 2002 had secondary diagnoses for these problems.[2] Identification of these patients is critical to enable providers to anticipate complications of substance use and facilitate appropriate postdischarge services.

This chapter will focus on the most commonly used substances (i.e., opioids, alcohol, and cocaine), as the basic principles presented here will inform the approach to users of other substances. Issues related specifically to tobacco abuse and alcohol withdrawal are discussed in Chapter 13 and 89, respectively.

ASSESSMENT

The lexicon of addiction medicine includes the following common terms[3]:

Abuse: A destructive pattern of use, leading to significant social, occupational, or medical impairment.

Dependence: A condition involving three or more of the following:

- Tolerance: Either need for markedly increased amounts of the substance to achieve intoxication or markedly diminished effect with continued use of the same amount

- Withdrawal symptoms and/or the use of the substance to prevent the onset of these symptoms
- The substance often taken in larger amounts or over a longer period than was intended
- Persistent desire or unsuccessful efforts to cut down or control use
- Great deal of time spent in using or recovering from the substance
- Important social, occupational, or recreational activities given up or reduced because of use
- Use continued despite knowledge of having a persistent or recurrent physical or psychological problem that is likely to have been worsened by the substance

Unhealthy alcohol use: Alcohol use that includes abuse, dependence, and risky use (National Institute of Alcohol Abuse and Alcoholism [NIAAA] category of >14 drinks/week for men [>7 for women] and >4 per occasion for men [>3 for women]; for ages >65 the threshold for women apply to all).

Clinical Presentation

Patients who abuse or who are dependent upon drugs or alcohol may appear asymptomatic upon presentation. It is important to obtain a history of substance use by asking the questions listed in Box 16-1.

These factors will help the clinician to understand the severity of the patient's substance use and anticipate the possibility that a patient may have withdrawal symptoms. The questions in Table 16-1 should be asked, depending on which substances the patient uses.

In the following section, the clinical presentations and diagnostic considerations of opioid and cocaine intoxication and withdrawal are presented. Alcohol intoxication and withdrawal are reviewed in Chapter 89. Additional resources for clinicians are available on the NIAAA website: www.niaaa.nih.gov.

Opioid Intoxication

The clinical presentation of opioid-using patients can vary. For approximately 25% of heroin users, occasional use escalates to

Box 16-1 General Background Questions for Substance Using Patients

- Which substances—and often more than one[29,30,31]—are used?
- What route of administration?
- When was the substance last consumed?
- Does the patient exchange sex for drugs or alcohol?
- Have there been past periods of abstinence?
- What are the patient's current thoughts about his or her substance use?

Table 16-1 Important Historical Information Specific to Type or Route of Substance Used

Injection Drug Users

Where are needles obtained? (e.g., the street, a needle exchange, or a diabetic family member)

Are the needles reused or licked? (Dulling of the needle increases skin trauma and may increase skin infections, and licking may introduce oral flora.)

How are the "works" cleaned (the tools used to cook and administer the drugs)?

Are the needles shared with others?

Alcohol Users

What was the most number of drinks consumed in 1 day in the past month? What is the average number on a drinking day? How many days a week is alcohol consumed on a typical day?

What does the patient drink? ("Moonshine" consumption may increase the risk of lead poisoning.)

Is there a history of delirium tremens?

Cocaine Users

What form of cocaine is used (powder cocaine or crack)?
By what route is it taken (intranasal, smoked, injected)?

Table 16-2 Clinical Manifestations of Opioid Withdrawal

Opioid Withdrawal	
Grade 1	Lacrimation, rhinorrhea, diaphoresis, yawning, restlessness, and insomnia
Grade 2	Pupillary dilation, piloerction (so-called "gooseflesh"), muscle twitching, myalgias, arthralgias, and abdominal pain
Grade 3	Tachycardia, hypotension, tachypnea, fevers (typically low grade), anorexia, nausea, and restlessness
Grade 4	Diarrhea, vomiting, dehydration, hyperglycemia, hypotension, and fetal positioning

Modified from Fultz Jr, JM, Senay, EC. Guidelines for the management of hospitalized narcotic addicts. Ann Int Med 1975; 82:815–858.

physical dependence.[4] In those individuals, the initial euphoric feelings can wane completely and opioid use occurs mainly to avoid the dysphoric elements of the withdrawal reaction.

Physical manifestations of opioid use include miosis, constipation, and respiratory depression. Other central nervous system effects are sedation, obtundation, coma, and death, occurring in the setting of overdose.[5] Similar to the tolerance with euphoric effects, many physical effects of opioids decrease with ongoing use. However, less tolerance occurs with regard to respiratory and cognitive effects.

Opioid Withdrawal

Although exceedingly uncomfortable to the individual, opioid withdrawal alone is not fatal. Nonetheless, it is critical to recognize this syndrome, because patients experiencing it may be less willing or able to participate in their inpatient care. The onset of withdrawal symptoms depends on the opioid being taken. Heroin withdrawal may begin 4 to 6 hours after last use, with symptoms peaking in 24 to 48 hours and persisting for up to 2 weeks. Methadone withdrawal typically takes 36 to 48 hours to begin, due to its longer half-life, and it may last weeks.[6] Table 16-2 reviews the common clinical manifestations of the stages. Left untreated, patients may progress from stage 1 to 4, though not all patients will have all findings.

Cocaine Intoxication

Cocaine intoxication is associated with increased alertness, sexual arousal, increased energy, and euphoria. Over time, however, chronic users develop tolerance to these effects. Complications of cocaine use include tachyarrhythmias, marked hypertension, myocardial infarction, seizures, and strokes.[7] Polysubstance use may confuse the clinical presentation of cocaine intoxication.[6]

Cocaine Withdrawal

Unlike the more characterized withdrawal syndromes associated with opioids and alcohol, the withdrawal syndrome associated with cocaine is more variable. Although three phases have been described ("crash," lasting days characterized by depression, decreased appetite, and prolonged sleep; "withdrawal," lasting up to 10 weeks characterized by irregular sleep patterns, anhedonia, lethargy, anxiety, and high cocaine craving; and "extinction," characterized by improved mood with occasional cravings triggered by specific stimuli),[8] many have found that patients do not often experience all phases so distinctly. Minimal literature exists on cocaine withdrawal symptomatology in patients hospitalized for other medical or surgical reasons.

Diagnosis

Intoxication and withdrawal are clinical diagnoses based on a combination of patient history, physical examination, and selected laboratory tests. No specific diagnostic laboratory or radiographic test exists for these diagnoses.

History

When taking a substance use history (see Box 16-1), the clinician needs to communicate with a nonjudgmental attitude and demeanor; this approach will help to engender trust.[9] Drug and

Table 16-3 Differential Diagnosis of Cocaine and Opioid Intoxication and Withdrawal

	Cocaine	Opioid
Intoxication	Other intoxicants (e.g., amphetamines and caffeine) Mania Anxiety disorder Alcohol withdrawal Thyrotoxicosis	Other intoxicants (e.g., phencyclidine and benzodiazepines) Head trauma/intracranial hemorrhage Sepsis Meningoencephalitis Hypoglycemia Hypoxia Hypothermia[12]
Withdrawal	Other intoxicants (e.g., benzodiazepines and alcohol) Depression Head injury (e.g., postconcussion) Sepsis Meningoencephalitis Amphetamine withdrawal	Other intoxicants (e.g., cocaine or amphetamines) Anxiety disorder Gastroenteritis Viral illness Electrolyte abnormalities Acidosis

alcohol-related questions may sound punitive or accusative if the patient is not given respect and the complaint is not addressed with concern. Questions should explore the known consequences of the substance used. Histories of endocarditis, hepatitis C, pancreatitis, or human immunodeficiency virus (HIV) should alert the clinician to a possible history of substance abuse or dependence and withdrawal symptoms.

Physical Examination

In addition to the physical signs related to acute intoxication or withdrawal previously noted, certain physical examination findings may suggest substance abuse or dependence. These findings include: evidence of recent or prior physical trauma; scarring over veins on the arms, legs, feet, neck (i.e., "track marks"); nasal septal perforation (due to cocaine insufflation); jaundice, hepatomegaly, ascites, edema, neuropathy (due to alcohol abuse or alcoholic hepatitis); or cachexia (due to chronic stimulant or alcohol use or HIV infection).

Laboratory Tests

Routine laboratory tests provide limited additional clues to the presence of alcohol use, though none is specific for abuse or dependence. Helpful, though insensitive findings include: elevated alanine aminotransferase (AST) and aspartate aminotransferase (ALT) with AST/ALT ratios of 2 or more consistent with alcoholic hepatitis[10]; elevated gamma glutamyl transferase, an early marker of chronic alcohol ingestion; and macrocytosis as a result of three different potential mechanisms (a cell membrane effect, an associated folate deficiency, or an alcohol-related liver problem).[11]

Toxicology screens may also be useful. However, three caveats must be recognized:

1. Not all drugs will produce a positive toxicology screen on first-line (Level 1) screening tests.[12] For opioids, standard assays detect naturally occurring opiates or their derivatives (e.g., morphine, codeine, and heroin) but do not detect synthetic opioids (e.g., methadone, meperidine, propoxyphene, fentanyl, and tramadol). The identification of oxycodone is variable. Separate assays for many of these are available if needed in specific situations.

2. Toxicology screens will remain positive for variable amounts of time after last use. Cocaine is typically detectable for 2 days after an acute ingestion and up to 1 week for chronic users. Depending on the assay thresholds, opioids may be detected up to 4 days after an acute use and up to a week with chronic users.[12]

3. The presence of a positive toxicology screen for opioids, cocaine, or alcohol suggests that the patient may currently be intoxicated (if symptomatic). It may also suggest the possibility of a current or impending withdrawal syndrome. One cannot, however, definitively diagnose intoxication or withdrawal based solely on a toxicology screen.

A broad differential diagnosis should be considered before diagnosing a patient with intoxication or withdrawal (Table 16-3).

Non-Laboratory–Based Screening

Many patients with substance dependence problems will be asymptomatic at the time of admission. It is important to be able to identify these patients, due to implications for their comorbid diagnoses and for monitoring for withdrawal. Physicians frequently do not successfully identify inpatients with substance abuse or dependence,[13] so screening tools have been developed to help identify them.

Alcohol Abuse or Dependence Screening Tools

There are numerous alcohol screening tools in the literature, though only a few have been widely validated and used. The CAGE questions (Box 16-2) have been validated in inpatient settings.[14] A single positive response has diagnostic sensitivity for identifying an inpatient with alcohol abuse or dependence of 98% but a specificity of only 58%.[15] Two positive responses change the sensitivity and specificity to 87% and 77%, respectively. Thus, no positive responses would lower concern for an alcohol problem and two or more positive responses would heighten concern for a lifetime history of alcohol abuse or dependence.[16] Supplementary questions about the quantity of alcohol consumed and the frequency of consumption will improve the clinician's ability to identify unhealthy alcohol use that does not meet abuse or dependence criteria.

The Alcohol Use Disorders Identification Test (AUDIT)[17] is a 10-question screen (Box 16-3) that detects the spectrum of

Box 16-2 The CAGE Questions

Have you ever felt you should **c**ut down on your drinking?

Have people **a**nnoyed you by criticizing your drinking?

Have you ever felt **g**uilty about your drinking?

Have you ever had a drink first thing in the morning to steady your nerves or get rid of a hangover ("**e**ye-opener")?

unhealthy alcohol use (risky alcohol consumption, abuse and dependence). One study found that AUDIT identified more inpatients at risk than did the CAGE questions.[18] Identification of risky drinkers not meeting criteria for abuse or dependence still warrants addressing the alcohol use with the patient during hospitalization.

Opioid and Cocaine Abuse or Dependence Screening Tools

Few screening tests for opioid and cocaine abuse or dependence have been validated, and none has been broadly adopted.

Box 16-3 The Alcohol Use Disorders Identification Test (AUDIT): Interview Version

1. How often do you have a drink containing alcohol?

   (0) Never [Skip to Qs 9–10]

   (1) Monthly or less

   (2) 2 to 4 times a month

   (3) 2 to 3 times a week

   (4) 4 or more times a week

2. How many drinks containing alcohol do you have on a typical day when you are drinking?

   (0) 1 or 2

   (1) 3 or 4

   (2) 5 or 6

   (3) 7, 8, or 9

   (4) 10 or more

3. How often do you have six or more drinks on one occasion?

   (0) Never

   (1) Less than monthly

   (2) Monthly

   (3) Weekly

   (4) Daily or almost daily

   Skip to Questions 9 and 10 if total score for Questions 2 and 3 = 0

4. How often during the last year have you found that you were not able to stop drinking once you had started?

   (0) Never

   (1) Less than monthly

   (2) Monthly

   (3) Weekly

   (4) Daily or almost daily

5. How often during the last year have you failed to do what was normally expected from you because of drinking?

   (0) Never

   (1) Less than monthly

   (2) Monthly

   (3) Weekly

   (4) Daily or almost daily

6. How often during the last year have you needed a first drink in the morning to get yourself going after a heavy drinking session?

   (0) Never

   (1) Less than monthly

   (2) Monthly

   (3) Weekly

   (4) Daily or almost daily

7. How often during the last year have you had a feeling of guilt or remorse after drinking?

   (0) Never

   (1) Less than monthly

   (2) Monthly

   (3) Weekly

   (4) Daily or almost daily

8. How often during the last year have you been unable to remember what happened the night before because you had been drinking?

   (0) Never

   (1) Less than monthly

   (2) Monthly

   (3) Weekly

   (4) Daily or almost daily

9. Have you or has someone else been injured as a result of your drinking?

   (0) No

   (2) Yes, but not in the last year

   (4) Yes, during the last year

10. Has a relative or friend or a doctor or another health worker been concerned about your drinking or suggested you cut down?

    (0) No

    (2) Yes, but not in the last year

    (4) Yes, during the last year

From Lohr RH. Treatment of alcohol withdrawal in hospitalized patients. Mayo Clin Proc 1995; 70(8):777–782.

Clinicians should ask questions that allow an assessment of the DSM-IV criteria[3] for drug abuse and dependence. In addition, any nonprescription use of these substances may be considered "risky use" for subsequent problems, although no formal such definition exists comparable to the risky alcohol use definition.

PROGNOSIS: CLINICAL CONSEQUENCES

Withdrawal syndromes can complicate a patient's hospital course. A discussion of alcohol withdrawal and its predictors is presented in Chapter 89. Any hospitalized patient with a recent history of opioid or cocaine use is at risk for withdrawal symptoms. Patients with daily opioid use typically experience withdrawal if the opioids are stopped abruptly. It is important to identify these patients and treat them appropriately, as withdrawal symptoms may cloud their comorbid condition and make them less willing and able to participate in their care.

MANAGEMENT

Treatment

Pharmacotherapies for Withdrawal

Alcohol withdrawal is discussed in detail in Chapter 89. No specific medications have been shown to be efficacious for cocaine withdrawal.

Opioid Withdrawal

Several factors influence the treatment and course of opioid withdrawal: duration and quantity of use, time since last use, duration of action of the specific drug, and comorbid illnesses. It is helpful to divide opioid users into those who are receiving opioid maintenance treatment (e.g., methadone or buprenorphine) and those who are not. For those receiving opioid maintenance, it is critical to communicate with their program representative or physician to confirm their maintenance dose. Patients should continue their confirmed outpatient dose of medication while hospitalized without tapering.[19] If the clinician is unable to verify the maintenance dose and the patient begins to demonstrate withdrawal, the administration of 20 mg of methadone initially followed by 10 mg as needed should reduce physical symptoms sufficiently until the dose can be verified.[9] Until the maintenance dose is verified, no more than 40 mg of methadone should be given in the first 24 hours. Because of its very long half-life, methadone-maintained patients rarely suffer significant withdrawal symptoms within 36 hours of their last dose.

For patients not known to be on medication for opioid dependence, physicians should begin by evaluating the degree of withdrawal present. It is appropriate to consider treating all patients, even with mild withdrawal, with methadone. An initial dose in such situations is 20–30 mg.[20] This dose will not reduce craving but should reduce physical symptoms of withdrawal significantly in the majority of patients with some requiring 5–20 mg more (maximum: 40 mg/day initially). Attempting to dose methadone based on the amount of opioid used prior to admission is inexact at best and is not recommended. The key is to reevaluate the patient in 2 hours after an initial dose of methadone to assess for symptom control, as it takes 2 hours for the methadone effects to peak. An alternative, but less preferable approach, and only for patients with mild symptoms and who are medically stable, is the

use of clonidine therapy (0.1–0.2 mg orally every 4–6 hours as needed for withdrawal symptoms) with adjunctive therapy (Table 16-4).

On subsequent days, the cumulative methadone dose of the last 24 hours should be administered. Unless the patient requests it or the patient has established follow-up with a detoxification program, tapering the dose while in the hospital should not take place.

The inpatient clinician should not send a patient home with a prescription for methadone for opioid dependence, even as a taper. Outpatient prescriptions for methadone, except for pain management, may only be written legally by methadone treatment programs.

If a patient is unable to take oral medications, methadone may be given intramuscularly or subcutaneously. The daily dose is one half to two thirds of the oral dose divided over 3 doses.[20] For example, a patient receiving 100 mg of methadone orally could be converted to 20 mg IM every 8 hours.

A number of substances interact with methadone. Ritonavir, nevirapine, efavirenz, rifampin, barbiturates, carbamazepine, isoniazid, phenytoin, and alcohol may lower methadone levels, precipitate withdrawal, and require methadone dose adjustments. Cimetidine, erythromycin, ketoconazole, and fluvoxamine may raise the methadone level. Methadone may increase the level of other medications, including desipramine and zidovudine.[6,21]

The inpatient use of buprenorphine has not been extensively examined. One study of 30 patients evaluated the use of intravenous buprenorphine in medically ill patients and found it safe and effective.[22] However, no recommendations exist currently to guide its inpatient use. As buprenorphine is a partial opioid agonist, its use in an inpatient with pain may prove complicated, as it may block the effect of other opioids administered for analgesia. Until further studies exist, one should consider using methadone for opioid withdrawal in hospitalized patients who receive buprenorphine maintenance therapy as outpatients.

Pain Management in Patients with Opioid Abuse

Although pain is common among hospitalized patients, clinicians may feel uncomfortable prescribing opioids to opioid-dependent persons. Such logic results in poor pain control and an erosion of trust between clinician and patient. Additionally, chronic opioid users may require higher doses and less time between doses as a result of pharmacologic tolerance to the medications. Finally, evidence suggests that opioid-dependent persons may have lower thresholds for pain, making them appear needy or drug seeking.[9]

Assessment of pain is a clinical judgment. No proven method of measuring pain using physiologic or biochemical parameters exists. Patients in pain may not always develop tachycardia, for example. The clinician should attempt to develop trust surrounding pain complaints and gather input from other clinicians who know the patient's prior pain medication requirements and behaviors.

Daily methadone maintenance therapy does not provide significant analgesic effect. When used for pain, methadone is given 3 or 4 times daily. It is prudent to consider the methadone maintenance dose only as a treatment for the opioid dependence and not as an analgesic. Pain complaints should be addressed separately with medications in addition to the methadone. Long-acting oral medications are preferred. Scheduled medications reduce the need for patients to feel they always have to beg for pain medications. Patient-controlled analgesia (PCA) therapy is one approach to address this situation.[9] As with all patients, intravenous bolus

Table 16-4 Opioid Withdrawal Pharmacotherapies

Clinical Situation	Medication	Dosing Recommendations
Mild withdrawal—patient not in methadone maintenance program	methadone (oral)	Begin with 20 mg. Re-evaluate the patient 2 hours after the dose and add 5–10 mg more depending on severity of remaining physical symptoms. Give total dose of first 24 hours on subsequent days. Do not exceed 40 mg/day.
Moderate to severe withdrawal—patient not in a methadone maintenance program	methadone (oral)	Begin with 30 mg. Re-evaluate as above. Do not exceed 40 mg/day.
Patient established in methadone maintenance program	methadone (oral)	Confirm the patient's dose by communicating directly with the methadone program before giving first dose. Once confirmed, give dose as prescribed by methadone program and do not attempt a taper during hospitalization. If unable to reach the program, refer to recommendations above for patients not in a program until the dose is confirmed.
Patient is unable to take medications orally	methadone (intramuscular)	To convert to intramuscular dosing, lower the dose to one half to two thirds the oral dose, and divide *this* total dose into thirds for every 8 hour dosing.
Adjunctive medications to be considered in patient's withdrawing	clonidine	0.1–0.2 mg orally every 4–6 hours prn to control general withdrawal symptoms. Monitor blood pressure.
	ibuprofen	400–800 mg orally every 6–8 hours prn for body aches.
	dicyclomine	10–20 mg orally every 6 hours prn for abdominal cramping.
	lorazepam	0.5–2 mg at bedtime prn for sleep.
	promethazine	12.5–25 mg every 4–6 hours prn for nausea.

of pain medications and recurrent intramuscular injections are less desirable and should be reserved for patients for whom other methods are not available.

Addressing Other Medical Issues on the Inpatient Service

Since patients with substance abuse are less likely to have regular medical care,[23] and are at high risk for HIV, hepatitis B and C, tuberculosis, and sexually transmitted diseases, the inpatient clinician should consider screening for appropriate conditions. Additionally, a hospitalization may be an opportunity to update patients' vaccinations (e.g., influenza, tetanus, or pneumococcal vaccine).[9]

Nonpharmacologic Therapies for Substance-Abusing or Dependent Patients

Patients with substance abuse or dependence problems can benefit from psychological and spiritual support in addition to the pharmacologic treatment. The use of open-ended questions may provide the clinician with important insights into the lives of these patients.[9]

Brief, structured interventions may help patients address their alcohol use. In the review by Emmen et al.,[24] brief inpatient interventions yielded inconclusive benefits; however, those studies that utilized a psychologist or physician to offer the intervention had more promising effects.[24] Though the impact on cessation may be limited, the intervention should be guided toward engaging the patient in substance abuse aftercare. In addition, it is important to educate the patient about reducing the risk associated with illicit drug use, including the need to use clean needles, a behavior that is facilitated by utilizing needle exchange programs, not sharing needles, and cleaning drug paraphernalia. A brief intervention tool from the American Society of Addiction Medicine is available at www.asam.org/publ/12.pdf.

For clinicians caring for substance-abusing patients, it is helpful to be familiar with Prochaska and DiClimente's stages of change model.[26] This theory discusses the path that patients take from precontemplation (denial of the presence of the problem), to contemplation (considering the possible need for change), preparation (planning to change), action (a change is undertaken), and maintenance (ongoing behavioral change). A relapse phase is also part of the theory. Each phase requires a different approach tailored to the readiness of the patient, which may initially be assessed by a nonjudgmental question like "Do you think that your alcohol use is a problem?"[25] Success may be achieved with a clinician assisting a patient's movement from an early phase to a later one, not just when the patient enters a treatment program.

Discharge Planning

Substance abusers are at increased risk of leaving the hospital against medical advice (AMA).[9] Discussing patients' fears about possible withdrawal and the plan to address it may help mitigate their concerns and enable them to complete their hospital care. The clinician should also consider four aspects of aftercare: detoxification, sobriety maintenance, follow-up primary care, and the patient's living environment.

Significant detoxification may or may not have occurred during hospitalization. Ideally, patients who have not completed the withdrawal process, if willing, should enter a short-term detoxification program. The patient's hospitalizations, even for 2 or 3 days, may have permitted him or her to undergo the most challenging of the detoxification process while an inpatient. Outpatient programs are available in some areas. The use of other medications to assist in the detoxification process after discharge should be approached cautiously.

To achieve long-term abstinence, detoxification should transition to substance-abuse programs. It is important for clinicians to be aware of the substance-abuse services at their institutions and in their communities. Encouragement by physicians to join a program like Alcoholics or Narcotics Anonymous is worthwhile.[9,27] Primary care follow-up postdischarge can constructively address substance-abuse issues.[28] Adverse housing and social support factors may contribute to a patient's substance use, because easy access to substances may facilitate relapse. The clinician should be cognizant of this situation and should openly, frankly, and nonjudgmentally discuss it with the patient, examining alternatives.

- During the hospitalization, patients with substance-abuse issues should be assessed for potentially related medical illnesses (e.g., HIV, hepatitis B and C, tuberculosis, syphilis), and appropriate vaccinations should be administered (e.g., influenza, tetanus, or pneumococcal vaccines).

- Linkage to care postdischarge is important to ensure that the medical and substance-related issues are followed up. Primary care and substance-abuse counseling options should be sought for all patients after discharge.

Key Points

- Substance abuse and dependence are common on general inpatient services with a reported prevalence ranging between 8–29%.

- Recognition of these disorders requires proactive screening, because they are not always volunteered by patients or elicited during standard patient interviews.

- Assessment of patients identified by screening should lead to a brief intervention appropriate to the stage of readiness to address the substance use.

- Opioid withdrawal can be very distressing and requires treatment but is rarely life threatening unless it exacerbates an underlying condition.

- Many hospitalized patients with alcohol and opioid dependency will require medications to ameliorate withdrawal symptoms and improve their ability to engage in care.

- Patients in methadone treatment programs should continue this medication while hospitalized at the same dose after verification of the dose with the methadone program. Those patients not in a program should receive 20–30 mg daily with additional doses of 5–10 mg based strictly on the presence of withdrawal symptoms (maximum dose 40 mg/day if not enrolled in a methadone program after discharge). If a patient is unable to take oral medications, methadone may be given intramuscularly or subcutaneously. The daily dose is one half to two thirds of the oral dose divided over three doses. A number of substances interact with methadone, requiring adjustments in dose. Outpatient prescriptions for methadone, except for pain management, may only be legally written by methadone treatment programs.

ACKNOWLEDGMENTS

We would like to thank Drs. Richard Saitz and Daniel Alford, as well as Ms. Carly Bridden for their editorial contributions to this chapter.

SUGGESTED READING

Brown RL, Leonard T, Saunders LA, et al. The prevalence and detection of substance use disorders among inpatients ages 18 to 49: an opportunity for prevention. Prev Med 1998; 27:101–110.

Pennings EJ, Leccese AP, Wolff FA. Effects of concurrent use of alcohol and cocaine. Addiction 2002; 97(7):773–783.

Leri F, Bruneau J, Stewart, J. Understanding polydrug use: review of heroin and cocaine co-use. Addiction 2003; 98(1):7–22.

O'Connor PG, Fiellin DA. Pharmacologic treatment of heroin-dependant patients. Ann Int Med 2000; 133:L40–54.

Warner EA, Thomas TR, O'Connor PG. Pharmacotherapy for opioid and cocaine abuse. Med Clin N Am 1997; 81(4):909–925.

Hopper JA, Shafi T. Management of the hospitalized injection drug user. Inf Dis Clin N Am 2002; 16:571–587.

O'Connor PG, Samet JH, Stein MD. Management of hospitalized intravenous drug users: role of the internist. Am J Med 1994; 96:551–558.

Emmens MJ, Schippers GM, Bleijenberg G, et al. Effectiveness of opportunistic brief interventions for problem drinking in a general hospital setting: a systematic review. BMJ 2004; 328:318–320.

Prochask JO, DiClemente CC. Transtheoretical therapy toward a more integrative model of change. Psychother: Theory Res Pract 1982; 19(3):276–287.

Samet JH, Rollnick S, Barnes H. Beyond CAGE. Arch Intern Med 1996; 156:2287–2293.

Brown RL, Leonard T, Saunders LA, et al. The prevalence and detection of substance use disorders among inpatients ages 18 to 49: an opportunity for prevention. Prev Med 1998; 27:101–110.

Pennings EJ, Leccese AP, Wolff FA. Effects of concurrent use of alcohol and cocaine. Addiction 2002; 97(7):773–783.

Leri F, Bruneau J, Stewart J. Understanding polydrug use: review of heroin and cocaine co-use. Addiction 2003; 98(1):7–22.

CHAPTER SEVENTEEN

Preventing Nosocomial Infections

Armando Paez, MD, and James C. Pile, MD, FACP

Nosocomial infections are infections transmitted within hospitals. The implications of acquiring infections in a setting where sick individuals come to improve their health are important. Not only is it counterintuitive that one can become more ill in a place where cure of a disease is sought, but nosocomial infections are often difficult to treat because of a higher incidence of multidrug-resistant organisms. Prevention of nosocomial infections, therefore, is of critical importance to practicing hospitalists.

In the United States, it is estimated that about 2 million patients develop nosocomial infections annually.[1] The economic cost is significant because these infections increase patient morbidity and mortality, as well as prolong hospital stay.

INFECTION CONTROL

The key to prevention of hospital-acquired infections lies in the practice of infection control, part of the wider discipline of hospital epidemiology, which includes the analysis of infectious and noninfectious adverse outcomes. The main objective of an infection-control program is to prevent and reduce the rates of nosocomial infections through the application of scientific and statistical principles. The following functions contribute to the eventual success or failure of the program: infection surveillance, outbreak investigation, education regarding prevention of infections, hospital employee health programs, antimicrobial utilization and stewardship, policy development, environmental hygiene, new product evaluation, and quality assessment.[2]

Surveillance

The Study on the Efficacy of Nosocomial Infection Control (SENIC) of the Centers for Disease Control and Prevention (CDC) showed that surveillance for nosocomial infections could decrease the rates of infection by 32%.[3] This became the basis for development of hospital infection control programs across the United States. Since 1970, the Joint Commission on Accreditation of Healthcare Organizations (JCAHO) has mandated establishment of hospital infection committees as a requirement for hospital accreditation. This body, composed of representatives from different hospital departments, oversees the infection-control program. Since 1986, the CDC has recommended targeted hospital surveillance. Hospital-wide surveillance is no longer advocated, because it has proven to be too labor intensive and impractical. On a larger scale, a national surveillance system called the National Nosocomial Infection Surveillance System (NNIS) monitors nosocomial infections on a voluntary basis. More than 300 hospitals of 100 or more beds participate in this program.[4] Nosocomial infection rates of participating hospitals are benchmarked on a yearly basis.

Isolation Guidelines

In 1996, the CDC, through the Hospital Infection Control Practices Advisory Committee (HICPAC), published revised guidelines regarding isolation precautions.[5] The guidelines comprise standard as well as specific category precautions. The Standard Precautions consider all body fluids except sweat as potentially infectious. This requires an individual to wear gloves if contact with body fluids is likely and to wash his or her hands after glove removal. Full barrier protection may be necessary, depending on the situation. If this is required, a gown should be worn when splashes of body fluids are anticipated in addition to gloves and a mask, with or without eye protection, depending on whether fluids may potentially reach the eyes. The three specific isolation categories outline distinct measures based on the mode of infection transmission:

Contact Precaution

A private room for the patient is preferred, but cohorting of patients is allowed if necessary. Gloves are required to be worn and should be changed after contact with contaminated secretions. Gowns should be worn if clothing is anticipated to come in contact with contaminated surfaces. Hands should be washed before leaving the room. To the extent possible, environmental contamination should be minimized during patient transport, and noncritical items should be dedicated to a single patient. Examples of organisms spread by direct contact include *Clostridium difficile*, herpes simplex virus, and multidrug-resistant organisms such as methicillin-resistant *Staphylococcus aureus* (MRSA) and vancomycin-resistant *Enterococcus* (VRE).

Droplet Precaution

A private room for the patient is also preferred, but cohorting of patients is allowed if necessary. Masks should be worn by individuals who will be within 3 feet of the patient. Masks are likewise worn by patients during transport. Examples of organisms spread by respiratory droplets (>5 um) formed during coughing, sneezing, or talking that travel a short distance include influenza virus, rubella virus, *Haemophilus influenzae b*, *Neisseria meningitides,* and *Bordetella pertussis.*

Airborne Precaution

The patient is placed in a monitored negative-pressure room with at least 6–12 air exchanges per hour. A certified respirator mask or equivalent should be worn by individuals entering the patient's room. The patient, on the other hand, should wear a mask during transport. Examples of organisms that are spread by aerosolization of small particles (<5 um) that travel a long distance include but are not limited to *Mycobacterium tuberculosis,* varicella-zoster virus, and measles.

Hand Hygiene

Hand hygiene refers to any of the following: hand washing, hand antisepsis, hand disinfection, antiseptic handwash, or antiseptic handrub. Despite good evidence that appropriate hand hygiene reduces rates of nosocomial infections, overall compliance rates are only in the range of 40%.[6–8] Barriers to appropriate hand hygiene have been identified.[9,10] These include factors related to health care workers' lack of experience, knowledge, and education about the hand hygiene guidelines. Factors that relate to work environment, such as heavy workload and poor feedback, contribute to noncompliance. In many facilities, institutional policies and traditions that do not address and promote hand hygiene contribute to this problem. The factors mentioned previously need to be addressed by the infection-control program of each hospital if compliance in hand hygiene practice is to be achieved. Recently, guidelines in hand hygiene have been reviewed and updated.[11]

There is good evidence that alcohol-based hand disinfection is equal or superior to handwashing with standard soap and water. Alcohol-based products have effective antimicrobial effect against gram-positive and gram-negative organisms. Compared to both handwashing with soap and water and disinfecting with chlorhexidine gluconate, alcohol-based disinfectants require less time to achieve a comparable reduction in bacterial counts.[12,13] The equivalent efficacy of alcohol-based rubs with traditional handwashing in preventing nosocomial infection rates has been demonstrated.[14] However, the technique of handrub is important in its success.[15]

Occupational Exposure to Blood-Borne Pathogens

The Occupational Safety and Health Administration (OSHA) standardized the surveillance of occupational blood exposures in 1991. The CDC also established its own surveillance system in 1995. Introduction of safety-engineered devices has reduced the rates of needlestick injuries. The three blood-borne pathogens that pose the greatest risk to health care workers are the human immunodeficiency virus (HIV), hepatitis B virus (HBV), and hepatitis C virus (HCV). Hospitals are required to have policies and protocols regarding the management of needlestick injuries.

Occupational risk of HIV infection from a single HIV-contaminated needle stick is estimated to be approximately 0.3%.[16] There is evidence that risk of transmission is decreased with the use of antiretroviral postexposure prophylaxis (PEP).

Combination PEP (i.e., a two- or three-drug combination taken for 4 weeks) is more effective than monotherapy. The CDC recommends differing PEP regimens depending on the level of risk of transmission.[17] Currently recommended two-drug regimens include zidovudine/lamivudine and stavudine/lamivudine. Possible roles for tenofovir and lopinavir/ritonavir in PEP are being evaluated. Options for the third drug in three-drug regimen include indinavir, nelfinavir, abacavir, and efavirenz. Recommendations may be expected to change in the future as data on the use of new antiretrovirals in PEP are gathered. Information on PEP can be viewed at http://www.cdc.gov/ncidod/dhqp/bp.html and www.ucsf.edu/hivcntr/PEPline/. A 24-hr PEP hotline can be reached at 1-888-HIV-4911.

Unlike HIV, hepatitis B virus is very contagious. Susceptible health care workers who sustain needlestick injuries from HBsAg-positive patients in the absence of PEP have an approximate 30% risk of HBV infection, and a 5% risk of developing acute hepatitis B. The risk is even higher if the source patient is HBeAg-positive. Therefore, hepatitis B vaccination of health care workers is mandated in every hospital. However, this does not ensure adequate protection, as about 5–10% of the adult population will not respond to standard hepatitis B vaccination. Guidelines therefore recommend testing for adequate development of anti-HBs IgG in vaccinated health care workers. Hepatitis B revaccination should be performed if the level is not protective (<10 mIU/mL). Postexposure management of susceptible workers includes both active HBV immunization and passive prophylaxis consisting of HBV immunoglobulin (HBIG) (800 IU or 0.06 mL/kg), ideally given within 24 hours, but of some utility if given up to 7 days after exposure.[17]

The average transmission rate for HCV infection following occupational exposure is somewhere between HIV and HBV rates, ranging from 0–10%. However, transmission risk factors in occupationally acquired hepatitis C infection have not been fully defined. At this time, there is no recommended prophylaxis for hepatitis C exposure.[17] When suspected hepatitis C exposure occurs, the exposed health care worker should be tested for development of anti-HCV antibodies at baseline and 4–6 months after the exposure. Positive results should be confirmed by immunoblot testing. An HCV RNA test may be done 4–6 weeks after exposure if earlier diagnosis is needed.

PREVENTING SPECIFIC NOSOCOMIAL INFECTIONS

Urinary Tract Infections

Urinary tract infection (UTI) is the most common nosocomial infection, comprising more than 40% of all hospital-acquired infections.[18] About a quarter of patients with indwelling urinary catheters develop bacteriuria and hence increased risk for symptomatic infection. The need for urinary catheterization should always be reevaluated periodically, because the catheter is oftentimes unnecessarily left in place. Maintenance of a closed drainage system is central to the prevention of infection. An open system invariably leads to urinary tract infection. Alternatives to indwelling catheterization (including intermittent, condom, and suprapubic catheterization) should be considered in certain situations. However, whether these measures definitively decrease the rate of UTI is still not entirely clear. Other measures useful in preventing nosocomial UTI include use of sterile catheters and avoidance of unnecessary catheter manipulation. The use of antimicrobial-coated catheters has reduced the rates of urinary tract infections.[19] However, neither the periodic use of an antiseptic in meatal care nor the use of systemic antibiotic prophylaxis has been proven to be effective in decreasing UTI rates in catheterized patients.

Short-Term Catheter-Related Line Infection

Approximately 250,000 cases of central line-related blood stream infections occur annually in the United States. The associated mortality is somewhat uncertain, but it is estimated to be approximately 29%.[20]

There are several factors related to the development of line-related infections. Firstly, the skill of the operator in inserting and caring for a central line is inversely related to the risk of line-related complications and infections. Use of staff in a team approach in caring for the central line has been shown to decrease rates of line-related infection.[21] Secondly, the site of line placement is also associated with the risk of infection. Placement of short-term venous catheters in the femoral vein conveys a greater risk of infection compared to placement into the subclavian and internal jugular veins.[22] Thirdly, the type of line material influences infection rate. Polyurethane catheters are associated with lower rates of infection than those of polyvinyl chloride or polyethylene composition. Use of antibiotic/antiseptic-impregnated catheters such as chlorhexidine/silver and minocycline/rifampin has been shown to decrease the rate of infection. However, the use of prophylactic systemic antibiotics does not. Careful observance of antiseptic technique, including the use of maximal barrier protection during central line insertion, reduces the risk of line-related infection.[23] The use of 2% percent chlorhexidine gluconate in skin preparation is associated with a lower risk of infection than use of 10% povidone iodine or 70% alcohol.[24] On the other hand, the risk of infection with different types of dressings (i.e., transparent or gauze) does not appear to influence infection risk.[25] Guidelines for the prevention of intravascular catheter-related infections have been published by the CDC.[26]

Nosocomial Pneumonia

Hospital-associated or nosocomial pneumonia accounts for approximately 15% of all nosocomial infections. The main risk factor for the development of nosocomial pneumonia is mechanical ventilation. Nosocomial pneumonia is generally defined as a lung infection that is neither present nor incubating at the time of hospital admission. On the other hand, ventilator-associated pneumonia is defined to occur after 48 hours of endotracheal intubation. The lack of a gold standard in the diagnosis of this entity leads to considerable confusion in the literature.

Nosocomial pneumonias are most commonly caused by bacteria. However, the importance of viral infections may be underestimated, because viral testing is not commonly done in many institutions, apart from testing for influenza. The most common bacteria responsible for nosocomial pneumonia are gram-negative bacilli and *S. aureus*. Anaerobes, on the other hand, appear to be an unusual cause.

There are several risk factors associated with the development of hospital-acquired pneumonia. These include oropharyngeal, tracheal, and gastric colonization; aspiration of sinus, oropharyngeal, and gastric bacterial flora; endotracheal intubation and mechanical ventilation; contamination of respiratory devices and the patient's underlying immune status. Guidelines in the management of health care–associated pneumonia are published and updated periodically.[27,28] The use of orotracheal rather than nasotracheal intubation using an endotracheal tube with a dorsal lumen to allow drainage of respiratory secretions has been recommended. A trial of noninvasive ventilation rather than proceeding directly to invasive mechanical ventilation is likewise advised where feasible. Other category IA recommendations for the prevention of hospital-acquired pneumonia that are promoted by experts and supported by experimental and epidemiologic studies include: (a) staff education and involvement in infection prevention, (b) effective equipment cleaning and high level disinfection of semicritical equipment, (c) changing of soiled breathing circuits and decontaminating the hands if in contact with the fluids (d) pneumococcal and influenza vaccination of high-risk individuals and influenza vaccination of hospital personnel, (e) maintenance of an appropriate degree of suspicion for Legionnaire's disease and health care–associated pulmonary aspergillosis in high-risk patients, (f) use of sterile water in nebulization, (g) prevention of exposure to *Aspergillus* during construction or renovation of building structures, (h) use of rapid diagnostic tests for influenza in patients who are at high risk for serious complications, and (i) administration of prophylactic treatment in known exposures with discontinuation of the drug when the laboratory does not confirm the infection.

Combination versus monotherapy for nosocomial pneumonia remains controversial. No single empiric regimen has been demonstrated to be more effective than others. The duration of therapy is likewise controversial, but recently 8 days of antibiotic treatment was reported to be adequate for the treatment of most hospital-acquired pneumonia.[29] The key to success in treating nosocomial pneumonia lies in the use of appropriate therapy at the right time for an adequate duration. This entails making an effort to gather more clinical data, such as performing a bronchoscopy if necessary, with the goal of tailoring antibiotics to the specific pathogen(s) infecting the patient. This will help prevent the development of multidrug-resistant isolates, while at the same time ensuring the pneumonia is treated optimally.

Surgical Site Infection

Surgical site infections (SSI) are the third most common nosocomial infection. As is the case with nosocomial pneumonia, the definition of surgical site infections is not well standardized in the literature. A consensus from the Association of Professionals in Infection Control and Epidemiology (APIC), the Society for Healthcare Epidemiology of America (SHEA), and the Surgical Infection Society (SIS) produced a common definition of surgical site infection.[30] The consensus divides infections into incisional and organ/space categories, with the former accounting for approximately two thirds of all surgical site infections. The definition of superficial incisional SSI requires any of the following, occurring within 30 days of the surgery: (a) purulent discharge from the wound, (b) isolation of organisms that are aseptically obtained, (c) any symptom or sign of infection, and (d) a

Table 17-1 Preventive Strategies in Nosocomial Infections

Nosocomial Infection	Preventive Measures
1. Catheter-related urinary tract infection	a. Establish and periodically reevaluate the need for indwelling catheterization. b. Care properly for the indwelling catheter with attention to maintaining a closed system. c. Consider alternatives to indwelling catheterization. d. Consider use of antimicrobial-coated catheters.
2. Central line–related infection	a. Establish and periodically reevaluate the need for central access. b. Use aseptic and proper technique of line placement with use of full barrier protection. c. Choose the most appropriate site of placement. Consider subclavian or internal jugular rather than femoral approaches when possible. d. Use 2% chlorhexidine as preferred antiseptic. e. Consider use of antibiotic/antiseptic-impregnated catheters.
3. Hospital-associated pneumonia	a. Use noninvasive mechanical intubation if this is appropriate. b. Ensure effective equipment cleaning at all times. c. Gather clinical and microbiologic data with use of bronchoscopy, if appropriate, prior to use of empiric therapy. d. A targeted antibiotic approach in the treatment of nosocomial pneumonia should be used based on available data. Consider 7–8 days of therapy and reevaluate the need to continue therapy. e. Vaccinate high-risk individuals, including health care workers if appropriate with influenza and pneumococcal vaccine.
4. Surgical site infection	a. Infuse appropriate prophylactic antibiotics within 60 minutes of incision time. b. Consider β-lactam antibiotics first. Use vancomycin in the setting of high rates of MRSA infection. Other antibiotics should be considered depending on the individual risk of intraoperative infection. c. Maintain intraoperative normothermia, adequate supplemental oxygenation, fluid resuscitation, and tight glucose control.
5. *Clostridium difficile* colitis	a. Always use appropriate antibiotics to treat infection. b. Observe handwashing, appropriate barrier protection, and environmental cleaning.

diagnosis of infection made by a physician. In addition, an infection involving implants occurring within 1 year of the surgical procedure is also considered an SSI.

Recently, the national Surgical Infection Prevention (SIP) project of the Centers for Medicare and Medicaid Services and the CDC was launched. The goal of this project is to decrease the morbidity and mortality associated with SSIs. Recommendations to prevent SSIs include infusion of the first dose of preferred antibiotic within 60 minutes before the incision, with the goal of achieving adequate serum and tissue drug levels. These should exceed the MICs of organisms likely to be encountered during the surgery. Antibiotic prophylaxis should not exceed 24 hours in duration, with the possible exception of cardiothoracic surgery procedures.[31] Antimicrobial prophylaxis after wound closure is unnecessary. β-lactam antimicrobials are the prophylactic agents of choice. When there is a history of penicillin allergy, vancomycin and clindamycin are alternative options. In institutions where MRSA rates are high, vancomycin should be considered. The use of additional agents depends on the possibility of exposure to other organisms likely to be encountered during the surgery. Nasal mupirocin decreases the rates of nasal carriage of *S. aureus* but has not been shown to lead to a reduction in SSI rates.[32,33] Dosing of prophylactic antimicrobials in such a manner that adequate antimicrobial levels are achieved until time of wound closure depends in part on the drug half-life. In general,

the antibiotic should be redosed if the operation is still in progress two half-lives after the first dose. Adjunctive measures to prevent SSIs are maintenance of intraoperative normothermia, adequate supplemental oxygen, appropriate fluid resuscitation, and tight glucose control.[34]

There are many options for antimicrobial prophylaxis. Factors to consider in the choice of the antibiotic include the cost of the agent, safety, drug half-life, and the risk of promoting antimicrobial resistance. First- or second-generation cephalosporins such as cefazolin, cefuroxime, cefotetan, or cefoxitin are recommended in several guidelines for orthopedic and cardiovascular surgeries. In the case of a documented or uncertain penicillin allergy, vancomycin or clindamycin can be used. For gynecologic or obstetric surgeries, cefotetan may be the drug of choice. In the patient with a β-lactam allergy, an aminoglycoside, aztreonam, or quinolone may be added to gram-positive coverage in this situation. For colorectal surgery, an orally administered antimicrobial bowel preparation in conjunction with parenteral antimicrobials is used. The recommended oral prophylaxis is a combination of neomycin with erythromycin, or neomycin with metronidazole given 18–24 hours before the operation along with mechanical bowel preparation. Parenteral prophylaxis includes cefotetan or cefoxitin, or a combination of cefazolin with metronidazole. Clindamycin with gentamicin, aztreonam, or a quinolone can be used in penicillin-allergic patients.[35]

Clostridium difficile Colitis

C. difficile–associated diarrhea remains an important nosocomial infection. The major risk factor for this type of infection is the administration of antibiotics. Appropriate use of antibiotics, therefore, helps to prevent this infection. *C. difficile* may be acquired directly or indirectly from another individual. Distortion of the normal fecal flora in an individual whose gut is colonized by *C. difficile* facilitates development of the disease. Transmission may occur via hands of health care professionals or via fomites. Handwashing, barrier protection, and environmental cleaning with hypochlorite solutions help prevent spread of the infection.[36] Importantly, alcohol-based antiseptic handrub may not kill *C. difficile* spores, and therefore handwashing with soap and water is advised in this setting. This topic is discussed in detail in Chapter 61.

Key Points

- A good infection control program is key to prevention of nosocomial infections.

- Standard and specific isolation precautions (contact, droplet, and airborne) are utilized depending on the nature of the risk of disease transmission.

- Good hand hygiene practice that is effective and promotes compliance, such as the use of alcohol-based products, is important in preventing nosocomial infection. Alcohol-based hand cleansers are *not* effective against *C. difficile* spores, however.

- Guidelines to the prevention of infection of health care workers with blood-borne pathogens exist and are updated regularly.

- Relatively simple strategies exist that can decrease the rates of certain nosocomial infections. These include urinary tract infection, catheter-related bloodstream infection, nosocomial pneumonia, surgical site infection, and *C. difficile*–associated diarrhea.

SUGGESTED READING

National Nosocomial Infections Surveillance (NNIS) System Report, data summary from January 1992 to June 2004. Am J Infect Control 2004; 32:470–485.

Garner JS. Guideline for isolation precautions in hospitals. The Hospital Infection Control Practices Advisory Committee. Infect Control Hosp Epidemiol 1996; 17:53–80.

Pittet D, Boyce JM. Revolutionising hand hygiene in health care settings: guidelines revisited. Lancet Infect Dis 2003; 3(5):269–270.

Kampf G, Kramer A. Epidemiologic background of hand hygiene and evaluation of the most important agents for scrubs and rubs. Clin Microbiol Rev 2004; 17:863–893.

Updated US Public Health Service Guidelines for the Management of Occupational Exposures to HBV, HCV and HIV and Recommendations for Postexposure Prophylaxis. MMWR 2001; 50:1–52.

Rupp ME, Fitzgerald T, Marion N, et al. Effect of silver-coated urinary catheters: efficacy, cost-effectiveness, and antimicrobial resistance. Am J Infect Control 2004; 32:445–450.

O'Grady NP, Alexander M, Dellinger EP, et al. Guidelines for the prevention of intravascular catheter-related infections. Center for Disease Control and Prevention. MMWR 2002; 51:1–29.

Tablan OC, Anderson LJ, Besser R, et al. Guidelines for preventing health care-associated pneumonia, 2003. Recommendations of the CDC and the Healthcare Infection Control Practices Advisory Committee. MMWR 2004; 53:1–36.

Guidelines for the management of adults with hospital-acquired, ventilator-associated and health care-associated pneumonia. Am J Respir Crit Care Med 2005; 171:388–416.

American Society of Health-System Pharmacists. ASHP therapeutic guidelines on antimicrobial prophylaxis in surgery. Am J Health Syst Pharm 1999; 56:1839–1888.

Laupland KB, Conly JM. Treatment of *Staphylococcus aureus* colonization and prophylaxis for infection with topical intranasal mupirocin: an evidence-based review. Clin Infect Dis 2003; 37:933–938.

Bratzler D, Houck PM. Surgical infection prevention guidelines writers workgroup. Antimicrobial prophylaxis for surgery: an advisory statement from the National Surgical Infection Prevention Project. Clin Infect Dis 2004; 38:1706–1715.

Section
3hree

Cardiovascular

18 Chest Pain
Ashish Aneja, Vesselin Dimov, Paul Grant

19 Acute Coronary Syndromes: Acute MI
Jennifer Kleinbart, Douglas C. Morris

20 Acute Coronary Syndromes: Unstable Angina and Non-ST
Segment Elevation Acute Myocardial Infarction
Jennifer Kleinbart

21 Heart Failure
Wassim H. Fares, Franklin A. Michota

22 Bradyarrhythmias
Arthur C. Kendig, Mina K. Chung

23 Tachyarrhythmias
Arthur C. Kendig, Mina K. Chung

24 Cardiac Arrest
David V. Gugliotti

25 Syncope
Anitha Rajamanickam, Saira Noor, Franklin A. Michota

26 Deep Vein Thrombosis
Amir K. Jaffer

27 Pulmonary Embolism
Steven B. Deitelzweig

28 Acute Aortic Dissection
Eric M. Siegal

29 Valvular Heart Disease
Leonardo Rodriguez, Brian P. Griffin

30 Acute Pericarditis
Lorenzo Di Francesco

31 Peripheral Arterial Disease (PAD)
Henna Kalsi, John R. Bartholomew

32 Hypertensive Crises
Erica Brownfield

CHAPTER EIGHTEEN

Chest Pain

Ashish Aneja, MD, Vesselin Dimov, MD, and Paul Grant, MD

BACKGROUND

Chest pain accounts for nearly 6 million visits to emergency departments each year in the United States, representing the most common reason for evaluation after abdominal pain.[1] This number does not include the countless episodes of chest pain that occur on hospital floors after admission, many of which are unrelated to the patient's admitting diagnosis. Among patients presenting to the emergency department (ED), more than 1.4 million individuals are hospitalized for unstable angina (UA) and non-ST-segment elevation myocardial infarction (NSTEMI). The National Registry for Myocardial Infarction-4 (NRMI-4) data suggest that of the 1.68 million discharges for acute coronary syndrome (ACS) in the year 2001, approximately 0.5 million were diagnosed as ST-elevation myocardial infarctions (MI).[2,3] Since several noncardiac conditions can masquerade as chest discomfort indistinguishable from cardiac causes by historical data alone, extensive and costly laboratory and radiographic evaluations often become inevitable. Despite advances that help differentiate more efficiently between cardiac and noncardiac causes of chest pain, approximately 2–8% of patients with myocardial infarction are discharged from the emergency department.[4–7] Almost a fifth of all money disbursed as the result of litigation against emergency room physicians is related to either overlooking or incorrectly managing acute coronary syndromes. Intuitively, these statistics invoke a cautious, expensive, and often defensive decision-making approach in the ED, leading to excessive hospital admissions. In addition to the potential patient harm caused by unnecessary and often invasive investigations, it is estimated that the additional health care costs incurred are approximately $5 billion annually in the United States.

CLINICAL PRESENTATION

General Approach

Chest pain is the cardinal manifestation of ACS. It may originate not only in the heart but also in a variety of intrathoracic structures, such as the aorta, pulmonary artery, bronchopulmonary tree, pleura, esophagus, and diaphragm. Alternatively, the cause may lie in the tissues of the thoracic wall, including the thoracic muscles, cervicodorsal spine, sensory nerves, and abdominal structures, such as the stomach. When managing a patient with chest pain, the primary emphasis is to rule out the most ominous diagnoses first. The main focus of the initial assessment should be on rapidly diagnosing patients with ACS, pulmonary embolism (PE), aortic dissection, and tension pneumothorax. When collecting the history of a patient with chest pain, it is important to have a mental checklist. The clinician must collect all relevant information regarding pain location, onset, character, radiation, alleviating and exacerbating factors, time course, history of prior similar episodes, severity on a numerical scale, and associated symptoms such as diaphoresis, shortness of breath, dizziness, palpitations, and nausea.

Location

If the chest pain is localized to a small area of the chest wall and can be reproduced with local pressure, the probability of a cardiac origin is diminished but not eliminated. Pain due to myocardial ischemia is usually more diffuse and often radiates to the arm, neck, or jaw. Sometimes, the patient cannot qualify the nature of the chest discomfort and places his or her clenched fist over their sternum ("Levine sign"), suggestive of pain arising from cardiac ischemia. Epigastric pain is more likely to be secondary to gastroesophageal or upper abdominal causes, but does not exclude pain of cardiac etiology.

Onset and Duration

Chest pain due to stable angina pectoris often occurs in brief episodes lasting from 2 to 10 minutes during physical exertion and is relieved by rest. If the episode is very brief, lasting only seconds, the cause is unlikely to be cardiac. Chest pain that lasts longer than 10 minutes can be due to myocardial infarction, unstable angina, aortic dissection, or PE, among other important causes. Pain associated with a pneumothorax, aortic dissection, or acute PE usually has an abrupt onset and is worse at the beginning of the episode. By contrast, the onset of ischemic chest pain is often gradual with a crescendo pattern. Nontraumatic musculo-skeletal pain usually has a vague onset, and patients do not often recall the circumstances of how the pain started.

Alleviating and Exacerbating Factors

Angina pectoris typically occurs on exertion, but may also be provoked by a heavy meal or strong emotion. Chest pain from cardiac ischemia may be relieved by rest or sublingual nitroglycerin. However, the diagnostic value of pain relief with sublingual nitroglycerin has been questioned in a recent study. The authors suggested that relief of pain after nitroglycerin administration does not predict active coronary artery disease and should not be used to guide diagnosis.[8] Chest discomfort that is precipitated by a meal suggests gastroesophageal causes but may also occur with severe multivessel coronary artery disease. Pleuritic chest pain is characteristically worsened by respiration, especially with a deep breath or cough, and also decreases the likelihood of ACS.

Associated Symptoms

The combination of severe chest discomfort and profuse sweating is strongly suggestive of myocardial infarction. Other important considerations include acute PE and aortic dissection, because they are also associated with a high mortality. Additional symptoms in this setting may include shortness of breath, nausea, and vomiting. Dyspnea is more likely to originate in pulmonary structures (e.g., pneumothorax, PE, pleurisy). A recent study has questioned this and suggested that dyspnea, independent of its origin, carries a poor prognosis in the setting of suspicion for coronary artery disease.[9] Palpitations may be the presenting symptom of cardiac arrhythmias in the setting of an acute myocardial infarction or PE. Hemoptysis can sometimes be seen in patients with PE but can also be secondary to bronchitis or pneumonia. Fever and chills are more characteristic of an inflammatory process such as pneumonia, pleurisy, or pericarditis.

DIFFERENTIAL DIAGNOSIS

Coronary Artery Disease

The characteristics of ischemic chest pain have been described in further detail in the Acute Coronary Syndrome section of this text. Apart from the classical symptoms, a significant number of patients may present without chest pain but rather "anginal equivalents." These symptoms include jaw, neck, ear, or arm discomfort, new-onset dyspnea, nausea, vomiting, diaphoresis, and unexplained fatigue. Elderly patients, women, and diabetics are at particular risk of experiencing atypical angina. Features that *suggest* noncardiac cause are pleuritic chest pain (sharp or knife-like pain exacerbated by cough or breathing), middle or lower abdominal pain, reproducible pain with movement or palpation of the chest wall, constant pain lasting several hours, brief episodes of pain lasting a few seconds or less, and pain that radiates to the lower extremities. However, pain that is sharp, stabbing, or reproducible *does not exclude* ACS. The Multicenter Chest Pain Study of patients presenting to ED found that 22% with sharp or stabbing pain, 13% with pleuritic pain, and 7% with pain reproduced on palpation were subsequently diagnosed with ACS.[10]

Pulmonary Embolism

Acute PE is a relatively uncommon cause of chest pain in the primary-care setting but must be considered in hospitalized patients with risk factors for deep vein thrombosis. Chest pain due to embolism is usually pleuritic in nature and associated with dyspnea. The most common symptoms of PE are dyspnea (73%), pleuritic chest pain (66%), and cough (37%). Hemoptysis is noted in 13% of patients. Fifty percent of patients diagnosed with PE have nonspecific electrocardiographic abnormalities, and 84% have an abnormal chest x-ray film.[11] (*See* Chapter 27 for more detail.)

Aortic Dissection

Chest pain due to aortic dissection is usually of sudden onset and is often described as "ripping" or "tearing." The pain may substernal, or it may be felt in the back. Aortic dissection is most commonly seen in men in their sixties with uncontrolled hypertension or other risk factors, including Marfan's syndrome, congenital bicuspid aortic valve, and coarctation of the aorta. Due to the high mortality associated with this condition, physicians should have a high index of suspicion for aortic dissection. Findings that should prompt a rapid investigation and treatment include sudden-onset chest pain, widened mediastinum on chest x-ray, congestive heart failure, neurologic deficits, change in mental status, syncope, hypotension, difference in pulse pressure of the upper extremities, and lower extremity ischemia. The diagnosis of aortic dissection is most commonly made with computed tomography (CT) scan of the chest. However, other modalities may include transesophageal echocardiogram, magnetic resonance imaging (MRI), and aortogram. (*See* Chapter 28 for more detail.)

Pericarditis

Chest pain in pericarditis is usually of acute onset and more localized than ischemic pain. Patients often report that the pain is sharp and exacerbated by a deep breath. It classically worsens in the supine position and improves when the patient sits up or leans forward. Other features that aid in diagnosing pericarditis include auscultation of a pericardial friction rub, widespread ST-segment elevation on the electrocardiogram, and the presence of a pericardial effusion seen on chest x-ray or echocardiogram. Minor elevations of cardiac injury biomarkers are not uncommon in these patients because of mild coexisting myocardial damage. (*See* Chapter 30 for more detail.)

Pleuritis

Pleuritic chest pain is often of stabbing quality and worsens with inspiration. Pleuritic symptoms can be associated with pneumonia due to bacterial, viral, or immunologic causes. Pleural effusions typically present with shortness of breath rather than chest pain, and are usually located laterally as opposed to precordially.

Pneumothorax

Pain from a pneumothorax is typically sudden in onset and accompanied by marked dyspnea. These symptoms develop more rapidly and can be life threatening in a tension pneumothorax. In this condition, a one-way valve mechanism leads to progressive air trapping in the intrapleural space, causing compression of vascular structures in the thorax. Emergent treatment consists of decompression by inserting a large-bore needle into the second intercostal space in the midclavicular line on the affected side.

Esophageal Causes

Chest pain due to gastroesophageal reflux disease (GERD) or esophageal spasm can mimic angina pectoris and is often described by patients as a squeezing or burning sensation. This pain may last from minutes to hours; it is variably relieved by antacids in the case of GERD and calcium channel antagonists and nitrates in the case of esophageal spasm. GERD is the most common cause of noncardiac chest pain. Esophageal spasm, described as a cause of chest pain by William Osler in 1892, occurs considerably less often.

Musculoskeletal Chest Pain

Musculoskeletal chest pain, characterized by its long duration of hours to days, tends to be localized to a specific area of the chest wall. Approximately 10–15% of chest pain cases in the emergency room are due to musculoskeletal causes, and this percentage is even greater in primary care settings. Musculoskeletal chest pain occurs more frequently among women than men. Its association with exertion, fever, cough, numbness, and atypical locations such as the axilla or midthoracic spine often characterizes this type of pain.

Psychogenic Chest Pain

Patients with anxiety or panic disorders, depression, or hypochondriasis may present with chest pain without an obvious cause. According to one study, approximately 20% of patients seen in the emergency department for chest pain were diagnosed as having panic disorder.[12] Physicians should be cautious when diagnosing chest pain due to psychogenic causes because 20–30% of patients with ischemic chest pain also have a coexisting psychiatric disorder.[12] It is very important to rule out organic causes before ascribing chest pain to a psychogenic etiology.

Other Causes

Chest pain can also be caused by valvular heart disease, specifically aortic and mitral valve stenosis. Mitral valve prolapse has been described in association with nonischemic chest pain as well as panic episodes. Rheumatic diseases such as rheumatoid arthritis, ankylosing spondylitis, psoriatic arthritis, and fibromyalgia may cause musculoskeletal chest pain. Pre-eruptive herpes zoster can cause chest pain in the absence of the initial characteristic vesiculated skin lesions. Table 18-1 summarizes the differential diagnosis of chest pain.

INITIAL ASSESSMENT

History and Physical Examination

Apart from the differential diagnosis of chest pain as previously discussed, every ED should have a policy that enables rapid evaluation of patients with suspected ACS. The initial decision-making process may have significant economic and clinical ramifications.[13] As per the American College of Cardiology/American Heart Association (ACC/AHA) guidelines, telephone calls from patients with chest pain syndromes suggestive of ACS should not be evaluated on the phone. These patients should be referred to a facility that allows for physician evaluation and the performance and interpretation of a 12-lead electrocardiogram (ECG). Patients with previously diagnosed coronary artery disease (CAD) who complain of chest pain require referral to an ED that can offer immediate reperfusion therapy. Evidence suggests that patients with acute chest pain should be referred to a facility that is adequately staffed and equipped to manage chest pain, even if the initial transport time to such a facility may be longer.[14] The probability of a patient suffering with an STEMI (ST-elevation myocardial infarction) increases with unremitting chest pain lasting greater than 20 minutes. The National Heart Attack Alert Program notes that patients with chest pain, pressure, tightness or heaviness; pain that radiates to neck, jaw, shoulders, back, or one of the arms; indigestion or "heartburn"; nausea and/or vomiting associated with chest discomfort; persistent shortness of breath; or weakness, dizziness, lightheadedness, and loss of consciousness are at high likelihood of having a myocardial infarction.[15]

Depending upon the initial history and physical examination, patients are often classified into several "rule-in" diagnostic categories with the "worst-possible" diagnosis receiving the highest priority. The physician then determines the initial investigations, which are usually the most sensitive tests available for detection of the diagnosis in question.

When ACS is the prime suspicion, initial assessment should address two vital questions. First, what is the likelihood that the signs and symptoms represent ACS secondary to obstructive CAD? Table 18-2 classifies patients into risk categories according to this question. The second question the physician must attempt to answer is the likelihood of adverse clinical outcomes including death, MI, stroke, heart failure, recurrent symptomatic ischemia, and serious arrhythmia in a patient with chest pain suspected to be the result of ACS. Table 18-3 answers this question according to risk as determined from the initial assessment.

In order to classify patients into these event risk groups, a focused history and physical examination are essential. The five most important factors derived from the initial history that relate to the likelihood of ischemia due to CAD, ranked in the order of importance, are 1) the nature of the anginal symptoms, 2) prior history of CAD, 3) sex, 4) age, and 5) the number of traditional risk factors present.[16–18] Traditional risk factors for CAD (e.g., hypertension, diabetes, dyslipidemia, cigarette smoking) predict acute ischemia only weakly in isolation and should not be the sole criteria for admission.[19,20] The presence of all these factors, except smoking, is predictive of poorer outcomes in patients who have been diagnosed with ACS by standard ECG and cardiac markers.

Table 18-1 Differential Diagnosis of Chest Pain with Associated Characteristics

Diagnosis	Location	Character	Duration	Alleviating or Exacerbating Factors	Associated Symptoms or Signs
Angina	Substernal, radiates to arm, neck or jaw	Pressure, squeezing, heaviness, tightness	2–10 min	May be relieved with rest or sublingual nitroglycerin* Precipitated by exercise, extremes of weather, or emotional stress	Dyspnea
Myocardial infarction	Same as angina	Same as angina, but may be more severe	Sudden onset, 20 min or longer	Unrelieved by rest or nitroglycerin*	Dyspnea, diaphoresis, nausea, vomiting, S_4 gallop
Pulmonary embolism	Substernal or over region of pulmonary infarction	Pleuritic	Sudden onset; minutes to 1 hour	Aggravated by deep breathing	Dyspnea, tachypnea, tachycardia; hypotension if large emboli; syncope; pleural rub, hemoptysis with pulmonary infarction
Aortic dissection	Substernal or back	Tearing, knife-like, often the worst pain of lifetime	Sudden onset, unrelenting	Predisposed by uncontrolled hypertension	Pulse or blood pressure difference between arms, aortic insufficiency murmur
Pericarditis	Substernal, more localized than angina	Sharp, pleuritic	Lasts hours to days; may wax and wane	Aggravated by deep breathing, or supine position; relieved by sitting up	Pericardial friction rub; elevated JVP and distant heart sounds if pericardial effusion present
Pneumothorax	Over region of pneumothorax	Pleuritic, sharp	Sudden onset	Aggravated by deep breathing, relieved by needle decompression in tension pneumothorax	Dyspnea, decreased or absent breath sounds and hyperresonance to percussion on the affected side Mediastinal shift and hypotension in tension pneumothorax
Pleuritis	Over the region of effusion	Pleuritic, sharp	Lasts hours to days	Aggravated by deep breathing	Pleural rub, dullness, egophony and high-pitched breathing if significant effusion
Esophageal causes	Substernal, no radiation	Deep, burning	Minutes to hours	Exacerbated by food and lying down; relieved by antacids in GERD Relieved with calcium channel antagonists in esophageal spasm	Heartburn, regurgitation, dysphagia
Musculoskeletal	Chest wall	Insidious and persistent, may be sharp	Hours to weeks	Exacerbated by deep breathing or movement	May be associated with dysesthesia
Psychogenic	Nonspecific	Nonspecific	Minutes to hours	Aggravated by a panic attack	Hyperventilation, diaphoresis

JVP—Jugular Venous Pressure; GERD—gastroesophageal reflux disease
*Caveat in text

In younger patients, especially those less than 40 years (though cocaine is used by patients in their 50s and 60s), cocaine use should be considered and a urine drug screen obtained. The seven-point TIMI risk score developed by Antman et al. from the TIMI 11B trial is currently among the most widely utilized scales in the ED to predict adverse outcomes[21] (*see* Table 18-4). This risk score for chest pain (age >65 years, more than three coronary risk factors, prior angiographic coronary obstruction, ST-segment deviation, more than two angina events within 24 hours, use of aspirin within 7 days, and elevated cardiac markers) has been validated in several large clinical trials for predicting optimal therapy. Similar risk-stratification models have been developed in other parts of the world to predict patient outcomes but need further validation before attaining widespread acceptance.[22]

Table 18-2 Likelihood That Signs and Symptoms Represent an Acute Coronary Syndrome

Feature	High likelihood (any of the following)	Intermediate likelihood (absence of high-likelihood features and presence of any of the following)	Low likelihood (absence of high- or intermediate-likelihood features but may have any of the following)
History	– Chest or left arm pain or discomfort as chief symptom similar to prior documented angina – Known history of CAD, including MI	– Chest or left arm pain or discomfort as chief symptom – Age >70 years – Male sex – Diabetes mellitus	– Probable ischemic symptoms in absence of any of the intermediate likelihood characteristics – Recent cocaine use
Examination	– Transient MR, hypotension, diaphoresis, pulmonary edema, or rales	– Extracardiac vascular disease	– Chest discomfort reproduced by palpation
ECG	– New transient ST segment deviation (≥0.05 mV) or T-wave inversion (≥0.2 mV) with symptoms	– Fixed Q waves – Abnormal ST-segments or T-waves not documented to be new	– T-wave flattening or inversion in leads with dominant R-waves – Normal ECG
Cardiac markers	Elevated TnI, TnT, or CK-MB	Normal	Normal

CAD = coronary artery disease
MI = myocardial infarction
MR = mitral regurgitation
ECG = electrocardiogram
TnI = Troponin I
TnT = Troponin T
CK-MB = Creatine Kinase MB isoenzyme

From Braunwald E, Mark DB, Jones RH, et al. Unstable angina: diagnosis and management. Rockville, MD; Agency for Health Care Policy and Research and the National Heart, Lung, and Blood Institute, US Public Health Service, US Department of Health and Human Services. APHCR Publication No. 94–0602. Copyright ACC/AHA 2002.

Electrocardiogram

The 12-lead ECG remains the single most important test in chest pain evaluation. It requires cautious and diligent interpretation, even in the busiest emergency department setting. An ECG should be obtained in every patient with ongoing chest pain within 10 minutes of presentation. A recording made during an episode of the presenting symptom is ideal, but every effort must be made to get a recording expeditiously, even if symptoms have subsided. The accidental omission of the ECG in the initial work-up for chest pain or incorrect interpretation if performed are the most important factors in ED medical malpractice cases.

The presence of new ST-segment changes (≥0.05 mV) and T-wave abnormalities (≥0.2 mV) that appear consistent with ischemia requires risk stratification to a higher level. ST elevations of ≥0.1 mV in at least two contiguous leads is indicative of myocardial infarction in >90% cases. Marked symmetrical T-wave inversion (≥0.2 mV) strongly suggests ischemia in the left anterior descending artery.[23] Nonspecific ST-segment changes (<0.05 mV) or T-wave changes (<0.2 mV) are less helpful. Of all patients with acute chest pain but a normal ECG, 1–6% are eventually diagnosed with MI, and approximately 4% with unstable angina.[24] Common causes of ST-elevation other than MI include left ventricular aneurysm, pericarditis, Prinzmetal's angina, early repolarization, and Wolff-Parkinson-White syndrome.

In addition to being a pivotal diagnostic tool for chest pain, the 12-lead ECG has prognostic value. Patients with ACS and bundle-branch block, paced rhythm, or left ventricular hypertrophy are at higher risk for death, followed by patients with ST-segment deviation. Patients with an isolated T-wave inversion or a normal ECG are considered lower risk.

Myocardial Injury Markers

Markers of myocardial injury have important diagnostic and prognostic value. Until recently, creatine kinase MB isoenzyme (CK-MB) had been most frequently utilized, despite several short-comings. It is normally detected in small quantities in serum and is released with skeletal muscle injury, including ubiquitous causes such as ethanol overuse or trauma. CK-MB isoforms exist in only one form in myocardial tissue (CK-MB2) but in different isoforms in plasma (CK-MB1). The use of an absolute level of CK-MB2 of greater than 1 units/L and a ratio of CK-MB2 to CK-MB1 of greater than 1.5 has improved sensitivity for the diagnosis of MI within the first 6 hours compared with conventional assays for CK-MB, but are not widely available. A "CK-MB mass index" (ratio of total CK to CK-MB) greater than 2.5% is suggestive of myocardial damage but may be inaccurate when the skeletal muscle injury produces large amounts of total CK. This ratio is also considered unreliable in chronic skeletal muscle injuries, which tend to release greater amounts of CK-MB. Despite these limitations, CK-MB remains heavily utilized in conjunction with troponins because of early detection, widespread availability, and low cost.

The cardiac troponins (troponin I [cTnI] and troponin T [cTnT]) have a sensitivity of 84–89% for the detection of an acute MI. Troponins have been described as having a lower specificity

Table 18-3 Short-Term Risk of Death or Nonfatal Myocardial Ischemia in Patients with Unstable Angina

Feature	High risk (at least one of the following features must be present)	Intermediate risk (no high-risk features but must have one of the following)	Low risk (no high- or intermediate-risk features but may have any of the following)
History	Accelerating tempo of ischemic symptoms in preceding 48 h	– Prior MI, peripheral vascular disease, cerebrovascular disease, or CABG – Prior aspirin use	
Character of pain	Prolonged ongoing rest pain (>20 min)	– Prolonged (>20 min) rest angina, now resolved, with moderate or high likelihood of CAD – Rest angina (<20 min) or relieved with rest or sublingual NTG	New-onset or progressive CCS Class III or IV angina in the past 2 weeks without prolonged (>20 min) rest pain but with Moderate or high likelihood of CAD (see Table 18-2)
Clinical findings	– Pulmonary edema, most likely due to ischemia – New or worsening MR murmur – S_3 or new/worsening rales – Hypotension, bradycardia, tachycardia – Age >75 years	Age >70 years	
ECG	– Angina at rest with transient ST-segment changes >0.05 mV – Bundle-branch block, new or presumed new – Sustained ventricular tachycardia	– T-wave inversions >0.2 mV – Pathologic Q waves	Normal or unchanged ECG during an episode of chest discomfort
Cardiac markers	Elevated (e.g., TnT or TnI >0.1 ng/mL)	Slightly elevated (e.g., TnT >0.01 but <0.1 ng/mL)	Normal

MI—myocardial infarction; CABG—coronary artery bypass grafting; CAD—coronary artery disease; NTG—nitroglycerin; CCS Class—Canadian Cardiovascular System Class; MR—mitral regurgitation; ECG—electrocardiogram; TnI—troponin I; TnT—troponin T

From Braunwald E, Mark DB, Jones RH, et al. Unstable angina: diagnosis and management. Rockville, MD; Agency for Health Care Policy and Research and the National Heart, Lung, and Blood Institute, US Public Health Service, US Department of Health and Human Services. APHCR Publication No. 94–0602. Copyright ACC/AHA 2002.

for MI than traditional CK-MB assays, but this may be related to their greater sensitivity for smaller degrees of myocardial damage. "False-positive" troponin elevations represent myocardial damage from causes other than coronary disease. Such damage may be the result of myocarditis, acute decompensated heart failure, sepsis, and PE. Elevated levels are also commonly reported in patients with chronic renal disease and collagen-vascular diseases. In these patients, the temporal variability in troponin values may provide vital clues to the presence of myocardial injury. Changes in troponin levels are important from a therapeutic and prognostic standpoint in the perioperative high-risk surgery setting because patients are often obtunded from narcotic and anxiolytic use. Troponins T and I have almost the same diagnostic performance when compared head to head. Rapid bedside assays for cTnT and cTnI are becoming more available and have demonstrated comparable efficacy to standard enzyme assays.

Myoglobin is a low-molecular-weight heme protein found in both skeletal and cardiac muscle. It is considered most valuable for its early detection of MI in appropriate clinical circumstances.

It may be detected as early as 2 hours after the onset of myocardial necrosis but its efficacy is limited due to its rapid decline to normal (usually within 24 hours) and lack of specificity to myocardial tissue.

Risk Stratification and Initial Management

Once the patient has been classified into a risk category based upon the above algorithms and the physician's clinical suspicion, several different courses of action can be taken. Patients requiring immediate reperfusion therapy usually receive either thrombolysis or percutaneous coronary intervention (PCI) based on clinical and logistic factors. Patients deemed to be "high-risk" but not necessitating immediate reperfusion are admitted to intensively monitored units (e.g., coronary care units). Several hospitals have short stay units (e.g., Clinical Decision Units or Chest Pain Units) where patients at "intermediate risk" are monitored electrocardiographically while awaiting biochemical tests

Table 18-4 TIMI Score Stratification For Patients with Unstable Angina or NSTEMI

Risk Factors—1 Point for Each	Yes	No
Age ≥65		
≥3 risk factors for CAD*		
Known coronary stenosis >50%		
ASA use in last 7 days		
≥2 episodes of angina in last 24 hours		
ST deviation ≥0.5 mm		
Elevated cardiac markers		
TOTAL Points		

*Cardiac risk factors
– Diabetes
– Cigarette smoking
– Positive family history
– Hypertension
– Hypercholesterolemia

Risk	TIMI Score	Rate of Events%*
High (≥5)	6 or 7	41
	5	26
Intermediate (3 or 4)	4	20
	3	13
Low (≤2)	2	8
	0 or 1	5

TIMI risk score correlated with increasing number of events (all cause mortality, new or recurrent MI, or severe ischemia requiring revasucularization) within 14 days of assessment. Adapted from Antman et al. National hospital medical care survey; 2002 emergency department summary. JAMA 2000; 284:835–42.

and diagnostic imaging. "Low-risk" patients often need further evaluation with exercise testing or radionuclide imaging techniques, but this can sometimes be performed in the outpatient setting. Acute MI or unstable angina is eventually confirmed in no more than 30% of patients who are admitted with suspected ACS.

Treadmill exercise stress ECG testing can be performed safely with minimal complications in low-risk patients, provided no contraindications exist. Patients who are not candidates include those with a noninterpretable baseline ECG, ECG changes consistent with ischemia, ongoing chest pain, and evidence of heart failure. Two sets of cardiac enzymes should be negative before exercise stress testing is performed. Patients with a normal exercise ECG test have a 6-month cardiac event rate of approximately 2% in contrast to 15% among patients with a positive or equivocal test.[25] Pharmacologic stress echocardiography or radionuclide imaging is preferred in patients who are physically unable to perform treadmill stress testing. Rest perfusions scans that are read as high risk predict an increased subsequent event rate in contrast to low-risk scans that portend a much lower subsequent event rate at 30 days of <2%.[26] The presence of wall motion abnormalities on echocardiography at rest or with stress is predictive of a worse prognosis.

CONSIDERATIONS IN THE HOSPITALIZED PATIENT WITH CHEST PAIN

Although the approach to chest pain is fairly standard regardless of the clinical setting, there are several points to consider in the hospitalized patient. Postoperatively, for example, patients are at increased risk for cardiac ischemia, given the perioperative stress response, increase in myocardial oxygen consumption, fluid shifts, hypercoagulation, changes in endothelial function, and variability in blood pressure (see Chapter 110).

Hospitalized patients are also at risk for many noncardiac causes of chest pain. By virtue of immobilization, patients may experience atelectasis, gastroesophageal reflux, aspiration pneumonia or pneumonitis, and PE via deep venous thrombosis. Of note, oncology patients are at particular risk for PE secondary to their thrombophilic state. Hospital-acquired infections, particularly pneumonia, can cause chest pain that is usually pleuritic in nature. Pneumothorax is oftentimes iatrogenic from procedures such as central venous line placement or thoracentesis. Many hospitalized patients experience anxiety or even panic attacks that may include chest pain or discomfort as part of their presentation.

NOVEL APPROACHES TO CHEST PAIN DIAGNOSIS

Several novel approaches have recently emerged as potential diagnostic tools to distinguish cardiac from noncardiac etiologies of chest pain in the urgent setting. Although new laboratory biochemical markers and diagnostic imaging techniques show promise, further research is needed before they can be routinely utilized in clinical practice.

Myeloperoxidase is a leukocyte enzyme that appears to be a powerful measure of vascular wall inflammation. In a study of 604 patients presenting to the ED with chest pain, elevated levels of plasma myeloperoxidase independently predicted the risk of acute MI, even in patients with negative cTnT values.[27] Although further studies are needed, it appears myeloperoxidase may have the potential to prognosticate patients presenting with chest pain.

Damaged endothelium from a variety of disorders elevates blood levels of circulating endothelial cells. Studies are now assessing the relationship of circulating endothelial cells and CAD. One study measured circulating endothelial cells in patients admitted with non–ST-elevation ACS and found their levels to be a specific and independent diagnostic marker of future adverse cardiovascular events.[28] These elevations in circulating endothelial cells occurred earlier than cTnT levels.

A third biochemical marker showing potential to identify high-risk patients with ACS is soluble CD40 ligand, a marker of inflammatory thrombotic activity that is released after platelet stimulation. Not only did soluble CD40 ligand predict an increased risk of cardiovascular events in patients with unstable CAD in a recent randomized clinical trial, it also showed that these patients benefit from treatment with a glycoprotein IIb/IIIa inhibitor.[29]

In addition to laboratory testing, advances in diagnostic imaging can also improve the clinical assessment of acute chest pain. The most promising imaging modality is that of multi-detector computed tomography (MDCT), also known as 64 slice CT, to directly assess coronary artery stenosis. In the assessment of chest pain in the emergency department, one prospective study using MDCT in addition to standard evaluation reported a sensitivity and specificity of 83% and 96%, respectively for the diagnosis of a cardiac cause of chest pain.[30] It seems undeniable that diagnostic accuracy will only improve with the advancement of imaging technology.

Key Points

- The main focus in the initial assessment of a patient complaining of chest pain should be on rapidly diagnosing the potentially life-threatening conditions of ACS, PE, aortic dissection, and tension pneumothorax.

- Pain that is sharp, stabbing, or reproducible *does not exclude* ACS. Among patients presenting to the ED, up to 22% with sharp or stabbing pain, 13% with pleuritic pain, and 7% with pain reproduced on palpation were subsequently diagnosed with ACS.

- Dyspnea, independent of its origin, carries a poor prognosis in the setting of chest pain.

- GERD is the most common cause of noncardiac chest pain.

- The seven-point TIMI risk score is currently among the most widely utilized scales in the ED to predict adverse outcomes. The 12-lead ECG remains the single most important data tool in chest pain evaluation.

- Acute MI or unstable angina is eventually confirmed in no more than 30% of patients who are admitted with suspected ACS.

SUGGESTED READING

Heart Disease and Stroke Statistics—2004 Update. Dallas, TX: American Heart Association, 2003.

ACC/AHA 2002 Guideline update for the management of patients with unstable angina and non-ST-segment elevation myocardial infarction.

McCarthy BD, Beshansky JR, D'Agostino RB, et al. Missed diagnosis of acute myocardial infarction in the emergency department: results from a multicenter study. Ann Emerg Med 1993; 22:579–582.

Lee TH, Cook EF, Weisberg M, et al. Acute chest pain in the emergency room: identification and examination of low-risk patients. Arch Intern Med 1985; 145:65–69.

Selker HP, Beshansky JR, Griffith JL, et al. Use of the acute cardiac ischemia time-insensitive predictive instrument (ACI-TIPI) to assist with triage of patients with chest pain or other symptoms suggestive of acute cardiac ischemia: a multicenter, controlled clinical trial. Ann Intern Med 1998; 129:845–855.

National Heart Attack Alert Program: Emergency Department: Rapid identification and treatment of patients with acute myocardial infarction. US Department of Health and Human Services, US Public Health Service, National Institute of Health, National Heart, Lung, and Blood Institute. September 1993; NIH Publication No. 93-3278.

Antman EM, Cohen M, Bernink PJ, et al. The TIMI risk score for unstable angina/non-ST elevation MI: a method for prognostication and therapeutic decision making. JAMA 2000; 284:835–842.

Abidov A, Rozanski A, Hachamovitch R, et al. Prognostic significance of dyspnea in patients referred for cardiac stress testing. N Engl J Med 2005; 353:1889–1898.

CHAPTER NINETEEN

Acute Coronary Syndromes: Acute MI

Jennifer Kleinbart, MD, and Douglas C. Morris, MD

BACKGROUND

Over 1.4 million Americans die of heart disease yearly, making it the leading cause of death in the United States among all races and ethnic groups.[1] Acute coronary syndromes (ACS) represent a spectrum of disease resulting from acute coronary obstruction that impedes myocardial blood flow. Complete arterial occlusion may result in transmural infarction, which acutely manifests with ST segment elevation on the electrocardiogram, thus distinguishing ST elevation myocardial infarction (STEMI) from non-ST segment elevation myocardial infarction (NSTEMI). In 2001, there were over 1.6 million hospital discharges for acute coronary syndrome, of which an estimated 500,000 were due to STEMI.[1]

Acute coronary obstruction typically results from rupture or erosion of a preexisting atherosclerotic plaque, which leads to platelet activation and thrombus formation that may occlude the arterial lumen. Prompt recognition of STEMI is critical, as the management of acute STEMI centers on emergent reperfusion of the infarct-related artery, with the goal of limiting infarct size and consequently preventing or reducing infarct expansion and ventricular remodeling. Preventing transmural progression of the infarct can reduce the potential for life-threatening arrhythmias.

ASSESSMENT

Clinical Presentation

Prompt recognition of symptoms by patients and clinicians is critical to reduce treatment delays. The GRACE National Registry of myocardial infarction found that the median time from symptom onset to seeking medical attention for acute myocardial infarction (AMI) was 2.3 hours (mean delay, 4.7 hours).[2]

When considering the likelihood that a patient has ACS, it is important to consider the patient's risks for coronary disease as well as the presenting symptoms. Close to 90% of patients with AMI are likely to have traditional risk factors for coronary disease.[3] Among patients with STEMI, approximately 50–60% have hypertension; 40–50% have hyperlipidemia; 15–25% are diabetic; 65% are overweight; and 70% of men and 46% of women smoke cigarettes.[3–5] The median age of patients with STEMI is 65 years (median age for men and women is 61 years and 69 years, respectively). Of patients with ACS, the likelihood of STEMI (versus NSTEMI) is greater among men, diabetics, Caucasians, and current smokers.[3] Patients who present with STEMI are less likely to have a history of coronary disease, or to be on aspirin, a β-blocker, or a statin.[3]

While chest pain is a frequent reason for emergency care visits, only 10% of men and 6% of women presenting to the emergency department (ED) with symptoms suspicious for myocardial ischemia are diagnosed with myocardial infarction.[6] Yet, in the more than 90% of patients with AMI who present with chest pain, there is considerable overlap in characteristics of cardiac and noncardiac pain (see Chapter 18).[3,7,8] Typical pain of infarction is described as a tightness or pressure located in the retrosternal area and commonly radiating to the left or both arms, neck, or jaw. Associated dyspnea, diaphoresis, nausea, and vomiting are frequent. One study found that pain of the left chest and arm was described in 55% of patients with cardiac chest pain and in 46% of those with noncardiac pain, and retrosternal pain was present in 34% of those with cardiac and in 66% of those with noncardiac pain.[8] Pain of infarction may occur with exertion, stress, or at rest and, in contrast to anginal pain, is generally prolonged more than 20 minutes.

Approximately 9% of patients with ACS present without chest pain.[9] Such atypical presentation leads to an incorrect diagnosis in almost 25% of cases. These patients most commonly present with dyspnea (49%), diaphoresis (26%), nausea and vomiting (24%), or syncope (19%).[9] While elderly patients, women, and those with diabetes are generally regarded as groups most likely to present with symptoms other than chest pain, it is important to recognize that many patients with such presentations actually may not fit these categories. In a series of 20,881 patients with ACS, of the 1,763 patients presenting without chest pain, two thirds were under age 75, over 50% were male, and two thirds were nondiabetic.[9] Compared to patients who present with chest pain, STEMI patients who present with other manifestations of ischemia are less likely to receive fibrinolytics or primary Percutaneous intervention (PCI) (36% vs 66%), and have higher in-hospital mortality (19% vs. 6.3%, P < 0.001).[9]

Prevalence and Presenting Signs and Symptoms

Partly due to the relatively low prevalence of MI among patients presenting with chest pain, individual historical features have not been found to have adequate specificity to markedly increase the

Table 19-1 Prevalence and Presenting Signs and Symptoms of Patients with Acute MI

Symptom	Frequency (%)
Chest pain	91
Arm and shoulder pain	22–55
Diaphoresis	50
Dyspnea	48
Nausea/vomiting	38
Indigestion, epigastric pain	11
Syncope	3

Presenting complaints of 4.497 patients with AMI. From: Meischke H, Larsen P, Eisenberg M. Gender differences in reported symptoms for acute myocardial infarction: impact on prehospital delay time interval. Am J Emerg Med 1998; 16(4):363–366.

Table 19-2 Differential Diagnosis of Chest Pain and Distinguishing Features

Disorder	Distinguishing Features
Aortic dissection	Pain radiating to back Unequal pulses and blood pressures Hematuria/acute renal failure
Pericarditis	Pleuritic pain Positional Pericardial rub ECG: diffuse ST elevation and PR depression
Pulmonary embolism	Pleuritic chest pain Hypoxia Prominent dyspnea ECG: SI-QIII-TIII pattern (RV strain)
Pulmonary edema	Prominent dyspnea Rales Elevated JVP, S3
Peptic ulcer disease and esophageal disorders	Postprandial or nocturnal symptoms (reflux disease) Nonexertional Pain radiating to back (posterior gastric ulcer)
Musculoskeletal disorders (chest wall pain)	Reproducible tenderness Pain with movement of shoulders or arms

ECG—electrocardiogram; RV—right ventricle; JVP—jugular venous pressure.

likelihood of MI (Table 19-1). The following clinical features were found to have likelihood ratios in the range of 2–3 (leading to small increases in disease likelihood):

- Pain in chest or left arm
- Pain radiating to left arm or right shoulder
- Chest pain most important symptom
- Nausea or vomiting
- Diaphoresis
- Past history of MI

Characteristics that moderately decrease the likelihood of infarction (likelihood ratios 0.2–0.3) are pain that is sharp or stabbing, pleuritic, positional, or reproduced with palpation.[10]

Physical examination: Physical examination should focus on evaluating the patient's hemodynamic stability and identifying complications of MI. Hypotension may indicate cardiogenic shock or tamponade. Patients should be evaluated for signs of heart failure (rales, elevated jugular venous pressure [JVP], S₃); heart murmurs should be characterized, and peripheral pulses should be assessed.

Differential Diagnosis

Acute chest pain may be caused by a variety of cardiac, pulmonary, gastrointestinal, and musculoskeletal disorders as delineated in Table 19-2 and described in detail in Chapter 18.

Diagnostic Studies

Diagnostic Criteria

In 2000, the European Society of Cardiology and American College of Cardiology proposed the following definition of acute myocardial infarction, including troponins as a diagnostic criteria.[11]

Typical rise and gradual fall (troponin) or more rapid rise and fall (creatinine kinase-MB [CK-MB]) of biochemical markers of myocardial necrosis with at least one of the following:

a. Ischemic symptoms
b. Development of pathologic Q waves on the electrocardiogram (ECG)
c. ECG changes indicative of ischemia (ST segment elevation or depression)
d. Coronary artery intervention (e.g., angioplasty)
OR
e. Pathologic findings of an acute MI

STEMI is diagnosed in the presence of characteristic ST segment elevation or left bundle branch block (LBBB) on electrocardiogram. Cardiac enzymes are used to confirm diagnosis, assess the effect of reperfusion therapy, and provide prognostic information. Importantly, initial management, including reperfusion, should not be delayed while waiting for the results of cardiac enzyme testing.

Preferred

Preferred Diagnostic Approach

- 12-lead ECG immediately on presentation. If suspicion of acute myocardial infarction (AMI) is high, repeat several serial ECGs every 10–15 minutes to evaluate for ST segment changes.
- Measure CK-MB, total CK, and troponin (T or I) at presentation and 6 hours later. Undetectable troponin and normal CK-MB/CK ratio at these times rule out MI. If even a slight increase in troponin level occurs, continued enzyme monitoring is indicated.
- If suspicious ischemic symptoms recur, enzymes should be repeated until at least 6 hours after onset of recurrent symptoms.
- If enzyme levels are elevated, continue to monitor enzymes until they have begun to decline.

Alternative

- In addition to above recommendations, myoglobin levels may be measured at 0 and 2 hours for earlier identification of infarction (high sensitivity, but low specificity).

Evidence and Rationale

I. Electrocardiogram

Acute transmural infarction causes a current of injury directed toward the affected myocardium that manifests on ECG as ST segment elevation. STEMI is diagnosed by ST segment elevation of at least 1 mm in at least two contiguous leads or new LBBB. Specificity for AMI is increased if a cutoff of 2 mm ST elevation in anteroseptal precordial leads is used (sensitivity 56%, specificity 94%).[12] As ST segment elevation occurs in healthy individuals and as a result of nonischemic disorders, it is critical to recognize the typical "tombstone" or convex morphology of ST elevation due to infarction. Reciprocal ST-segment depression in leads opposite from those with ST elevation may be seen with STEMI.

The diagnosis of STEMI based on LBBB can be challenging, especially if an old ECG is not available for comparison. The validated scoring system below has been shown to markedly improve diagnostic accuracy. Findings that independently predict AMI in the presence of LBBB are:

1. ST elevation > 1 mm in leads with a positive QRS   5 points
2. ST depression > 1 mm in leads V_1, V_2, or V_3 3 points
3. ST elevation > 5 mm in leads with a negative QRS   2 points

The presence of any of these findings has a sensitivity of 44–79%. A total score of three or more points (i.e., criteria 1 or 2) is considered diagnostic of AMI (90% specificity), and a score of two points is suggestive of AMI (80% specificity).[13,14]

Other causes of ST elevation

Over 90% of healthy young males have ST elevation on ECG, which has led this to be considered a normal male pattern. The ST segment elevation is usually in the anterior precordial leads, and ranges from 1–3 mm with a concave upward appearance.[15,16] This finding is seen in only 20–30% of women and men over age 75. Early repolarization, commonly seen in young black males, results in ST elevation from 1–4 mm in mid-precordial leads. This pattern is characterized by concave upward ST segments, tall upright T waves, and notching of the J point (Fig. 19-1).

Other causes of ST segment elevation that can be confused with STEMI, and their distinguishing features, are listed below (Fig. 19-2):

- **Pericarditis:** Diffuse ST elevation and PR segment depression except in lead avR which shows ST **depression** and PR **elevation**
- **Myocarditis**
- **Left ventricular hypertrophy (LVH):** ST elevation is concave upward in right precordial leads.
- **LV aneurysm:** Persistent ST-elevation in anterior leads following MI
- **Hypothermia:** Prominent convex ST elevation at the J-point (Osborne waves) that occur with body temperature below 30°C (86° F).
- **Hyperkalemia:** Downsloping ST elevation; other findings may include tall peaked T waves and low amplitude P waves
- **Brugada syndrome:** ST-segment elevation is primarily limited to leads V_1 and V_2. Typically, a downsloping ST segment begins from the top of the R′ wave and ends with an inverted T wave.

The area of infarcted myocardium should be identified on ECG based on the leads with ST segment elevation. This is important in anticipating complications that vary with infarct location and directing treatment (Table 19-3).

2. Cardiac biomarkers

Elevation of cardiac enzymes, with a characteristic time course of their rise and fall, confirms the diagnosis of acute myocardial infarction. Currently available markers include CK, CK-MB, tro-

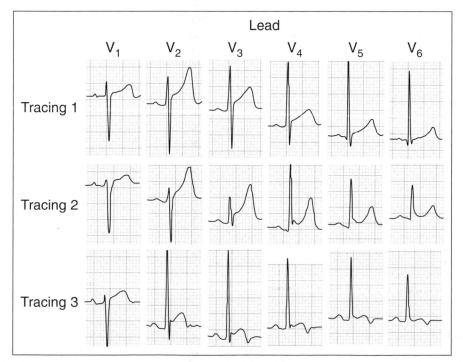

Figure 19-1 ● From Wang, Asinger, Marriott. ST-Segment Elevation in Conditions Other than Acute Myocardial Infarction. N Engl J Med. November 27, 2003; 349:2128–2135.

Figure 19-2 • Examples of ST segment elevation not due to acute infarction. From: Sgarbossa EB, Pinski SL, Barbagelata A, et al. Electrocardiographic diagnosis of evolving acute myocardial infarction in the presence of left bundle-branch block. N Engl J Med 1996; 334(8):481–487.

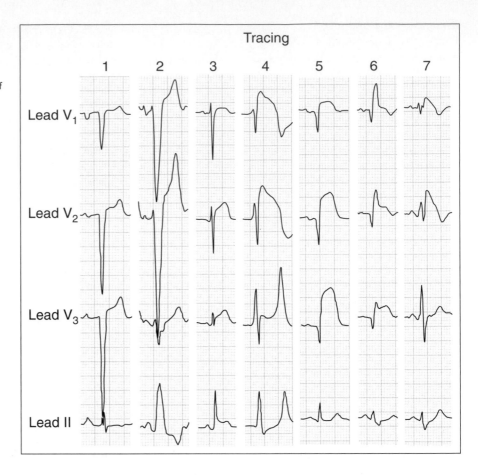

Table 19-3 ECG Findings Based on Site of Infarct

Territory	Leads with ST elevation	Vessel
Anteroseptal	V_{1-3}	LAD
Lateral	V_{4-6}, I, avL	LCX
Inferior	II, III, avF	RCA, less commonly LCX
	Elevation in lead III > II	Proximal or mid RCA
	Elevation in lead II ≥ III (especially if ST depression in I, avL or ST elevation in V_1, V_2)	Distal occlusion of dominant RCA or LCX
Posterior	V_{1-3} or V_4: **ST depression**, tall R waves, upright T waves	LCX
Right ventricle	ST elevation in V_3 or V_4 on right sided ECG	Proximal RCA
	MI with ST elevation in V_1	

LAD—left anterior descending; LCX—left circumflex; RCA—right coronary artery; MI—myocardial infarction; ECG—electrocardiogram.

ponin T and I, and myoglobin. Because STEMI is diagnosed by ECG changes, cardiac markers are useful for diagnostic confirmation, monitoring effectiveness of reperfusion after fibrinolytic therapy, and as a prognostic tool.

CK-MB and myoglobin are released from both cardiac and skeletal muscle, and they are therefore normally detectable in healthy individuals. Levels of both markers increase with skeletal muscle disease or injury (including heavy exercise and rhabdomyolysis) and with renal disease. Using the ratio of CK-MB to total CK increases accuracy, especially when total CK is elevated due to skeletal muscle release.

Unlike CK-MB, cardiac troponins T and I are found only in cardiac smooth muscle and therefore are not detectable in healthy individuals. However, minor troponin T elevation (0.05–0.10 ng/dL) has been documented among trauma patients without suspected myocardial injury.[17] In addition to myocardial ischemia, troponins may be elevated in decompensated heart failure, severely elevated hypertension, pulmonary embolism, myositis, and renal disease.[17,18]

Approximately 5% of troponin is free in the cytoplasm and may be released rapidly after cell injury, while the majority of troponin is bound in the myofibrillar apparatus and released over the next several hours. One third of patients with STEMI have elevated troponin levels at presentation (>0.1 ng/dL) using the standard third-generation assays; however, rapid bedside assays detect baseline elevations in fewer than 10%.[19,20] By 8 hours, the

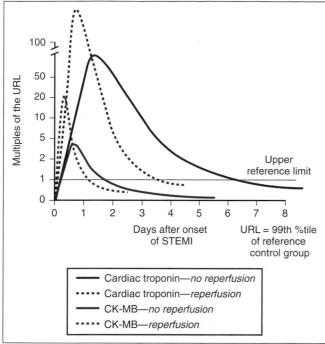

Figure 19-3 • Typical rise and fall of troponins and CK-MB in patients who receive immediate reperfusion and those who do not. From: Alpert, et al. J Am Col Cardiol 2000; 36(233):959; and Wu, et al. Clin Chem 1999; 451104 (234).

Table 19-4 Killup Classification of Heart Failure and Associated Mortality

Killip Class	Description	In Hospital Mortality, 2004(%)[24,31]	30 Day Mortality(%)[26,30]
I	No rales or S3	3	5
II	Rales < 50%	10	14
III	Pulmonary edema	20	32
IV	Cardiogenic shock	45–60	47–58

median troponin level of STEMI patients is 7.1 ng/dL, compared to levels of <0.5 ng/dL in NSTEMI patients with ST segment depression or T wave inversion.[19] Patients with anterior infarction, signs of heart failure, and longer duration of symptoms are more likely to have elevated baseline troponin.[20] Serial measurement of troponin and CK-MB at presentation with repeat levels 6 hours later is highly sensitive, with negative results effectively ruling out infarction.[21,22]

In patients with STEMI, time to peak levels of troponin and CK-MB depends on the timing and effectiveness of reperfusion. Troponin levels peak at 24–48 hours and may be detectable for 7–10 days. CK-MB typically peaks by 12–24 hours, returning to normal by 24–48 hours. Early peaking CK-MB (by 12–18 hours) indicates effective reperfusion. A subsequent rise in CK-MB levels signifies recurrent infarction (Fig. 19-3).

Myoglobin is released from injured cardiac and skeletal muscle, and it therefore is a sensitive but very nonspecific marker for AMI. Levels increase rapidly after myocardial injury, making myoglobin appealing for early exclusion of AMI, particularly in Emergency Department Chest Pain Units. Despite this, myoglobin levels have not been found to provide significant additional information to troponins and CK-MB, and therefore their use remains limited.[17,21] In addition, as both the rise and fall of myoglobin occur rapidly after myocardial damage, levels may be declining in patients who present several hours after symptom onset.

Prognosis

Data from the international GRACE registry of acute coronary syndromes show overall in-hospital mortality of close to 8% following STEMI.[5] In addition, stroke complicates approximately 0.5–2% of STEMIs.[5,23] Of patients who survive hospi-

talization, mortality is 5% over the next 6 months.[5] In addition, 18% of patients will be readmitted, and 14% will require revascularization.[5]

However, rates of death and complications following STEMI vary considerably, depending on the patient's risk factors (i.e., age, gender), the site and extent of the infarct, and the treatment provided. Identifying a patient's risk of adverse events is important to guide therapy and provide counseling to patients. Factors that independently increase mortality in patients with STEMI include increasing age,[5,24,25] heart failure and cardiogenic shock,[24] and anterior location of infarction.[26] Additional predictors of mortality include female sex, in-hospital stroke,[5] atrial fibrillation that develops more than 24 hours after presentation (OR 2.48 for mortality at 7 years),[27] depression (OR 2.01 at 14 months),[28] elevated B-type natriuretic peptide (BNP) levels, troponin levels, and ECG findings.

Cardiogenic shock and heart failure: The severity of heart failure is one of the strongest predictors of in-hospital and 30-day mortality for patients with STEMI patients (Table 19-4). Up to one third of STEMI patients have signs of heart failure at presentation or developing during hospitalization, with a higher incidence among those with anterior wall MI, women, hypertension, and diabetes[29] (Fig. 19-4). These patients have a four-fold increase in

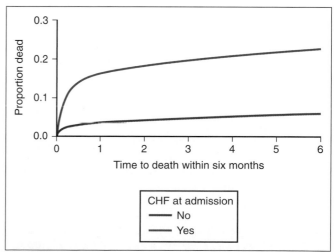

Figure 19-4 • Six-month mortality of STEMI patients who presented with heart failure compared to those who did not. From: Steg PG, Dabbous UH, Feldman LJ, et al. Determinants and prognostic impact of heart failure complicating acute coronary syndromes: observations from the Global Registry of Acute Coronary Events (GRACE). Circulation 2004; 109(4):494–499.

30-day and 6-month mortality.[24,29] Cardiogenic shock carries the highest in-hospital mortality, with rates of approximately 50–60%, and 80–85% for elderly or renal failure patients.[30,31] Even with successful reperfusion, in-hospital mortality for STEMI with cardiogenic shock is 50%. However, mortality of over 80% has been reported among patients with failed PCI.[31] For the patients with cardiogenic shock who survive hospitalization, few additional deaths occur over the next 6 months.[30]

Age: In-hospital mortality increases with age and is almost doubled in patients over age 75, compared with those age 65–75 years (10.7% vs. 5.6%, P < 0.0001) (Fig. 19-5).[25] For patients who survive hospitalization, 6-month mortality is nine times higher among those over age 74 compared to younger patients, and three times higher among those age 65–74 years old.[5]

Gender: Among patients younger than age 75, mortality is higher for women. Women with AMI who are <50 years old have a two-times increased mortality compared to men of this age group[25] (*see* Fig. 19-5).

Troponins: Troponin levels provide important prognostic information for STEMI patients: mortality increases with increasing baseline and peak levels.[19,20] Among STEMI patients from the GUSTO III study, mortality at 24 hours was three times higher among patients with elevated troponin (6.7% vs. 2.2%), and remained significantly higher at 30 days (6.2% vs. 15.7%).[20]

ECG: ECG findings of ST segment elevation and depression are associated with higher mortality compared to ST elevation alone.[69] Resolution of ST segment elevation is a marker of restored tissue perfusion that correlates with improved outcomes. In the TIMI 14 trial, resolution of ST segment elevation by at least 70% corresponded with significantly lower 30-day mortality, compared to patients with less than 30% resolution of ST segment elevation (1.0% vs. 5.9%).

Risk Stratification tools

Several validated scoring systems are useful for estimating mortality following STEMI.

TIMI Score

The TIMI Risk Score is a validated scoring system to predict short-term risk of mortality following STEMI.[32,33] Mortality increases with higher TIMI Score[33] (Fig. 19-6).

GRACE score

The GRACE Prediction Score is a validated tool to predict 6-month postdischarge mortality following ACS. Points are assigned for medical history (age, history of CHF and MI); findings at initial presentation (heart rate, systolic blood pressure, and presence of ST-segment depression); and findings during hospitalization (initial serum creatinine, elevated cardiac enzymes, and absence of in-hospital PCI).[34] The same GRACE scoring system was derived and validated among both STEMI and NSTEMI patients, allowing one prediction tool for both groups of patients (Fig. 19-7).

MANAGEMENT

Treatment

Preferred

Initial

The primary goals in management of STEMI are hemodynamic stabilization, management of life-threatening complications, and reperfusion therapy to restore flow to the infarct-related artery. Patients with STEMI should be admitted to a CCU for continuous cardiac monitoring. After 12–24 hours of clinical stability, patients may be transferred to a step-down unit. Low-risk patients who have undergone successful PCI may be admitted directly to intermediate care. Patients with heart failure or a hemodynamically tolerated arrhythmia (i.e., rate-controlled atrial fibrillation) may be monitored in a step-down unit if appropriate monitoring and skilled nursing care are available.[35]

For patients with STEMI, the foundation of acute therapy is reperfusion of the infarct-related artery. Additional treatment includes antiplatelet and antithrombotic therapy and anti-ischemic therapy.

Figure 19-5 • Relationship of in-hospital mortality with age and gender in patients with STEMI. From: Vaccarino V, Parsons L, Every NR, et al. The National Registry of Myocardial Infarction: Sex-based differences in early mortality after myocardial infarction. N Engl J Med 1999; 341(4):217–225.

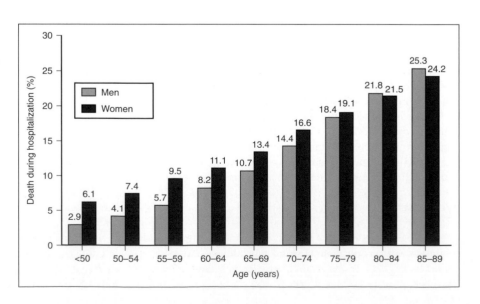

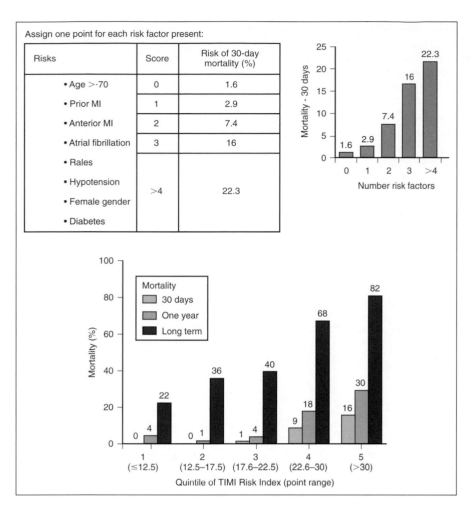

Assign one point for each risk factor present:

Risks	Score	Risk of 30-day mortality (%)
• Age >·70	0	1.6
• Prior MI	1	2.9
• Anterior MI	2	7.4
• Atrial fibrillation	3	16
• Rales		
• Hypotension		
• Female gender	>4	22.3
• Diabetes		

Figure 19-6 • The TIMI Risk Score for predicting 30-day mortality in patients with STEMI. From: Morrow DA, Antman EM, Charlesworth A, et al. TIMI risk score for ST-elevation myocardial infarction: a convenient, bedside, clinical score for risk assessment at presentation. Circulation 2000; 102(17):2031–2037.

Antiplatelet and antithrombotic therapy

1. **Aspirin** irreversibly inhibits platelet function and reduces short-term mortality in patients with STEMI. In the ISIS-II trial, STEMI patients randomized to aspirin had a 23% reduction in 35-day mortality, with a number needed to treat of 42.[36]

Recommendations: All patients suspected of acute MI should immediately receive ASA 162–325 mg chewed, unless they have a true aspirin allergy (anaphylaxis) or have active major bleeding.

2. **Heparins**
• **Unfractionated heparin:** UFH is routinely used in patients with ACS, despite limited data to support its benefit.[37,38] When used with fibrinolytics, lower dosing should be used to reduce risk of intracranial hemorrhage (ICH) (Table 9).
• **Low Molecular Weight Heparin (LMWH):** Among STEMI patients who receive fibrinolytic therapy, LMWH is more effective than UFH in reducing mortality.[39,42,77] In the ENTIRE-TIMI 23 Trial, 483 patients received either full dose tenecteplase or half dose tenecteplase plus abciximab, a glycoprotein IIb/IIIa inhibitor, and were randomized to enoxaparin or UFH. Enoxaparin led to a significant reduction in the combined outcome of 30-day death/reinfarction compared to UFH (4.9 vs. 11.3%). There was no significant difference in risk of major hemorrhage or of ICH, however, the study excluded patients >75 years old, who may be at higher bleeding risk.[42]

The largest trial comparing LMWH to UFH randomized 20,506 patients with STEMI receiving fibrinolytic therapy to enoxaparin given for up to 8 days or weight based unfractionated heparin for 48 hours. At 30 days there were fewer deaths and nonfatal MIs in the enoxaparin group (9.9% vs. 12%; P < .001; number needed to treat [NNT] = 48), at the expense of a small increase in major bleeding (2.1% vs. 1.4%; P < .001; number needed to harm = 142). Intracranial bleeding was not increased. Enoxaparin was dose adjusted for patients >75 years old and those with renal disease.

Intracranial bleeding is a major concern for patients >75 years old receiving in conjunction with thrombolytics.[39] Based on the EXTRACT-TIMI 25 results, it appears safe among these patients if the lower dose is used.[77]

3. **Fondaparinux:** The OASIS-6 trial showed that compared to UFH or placebo, fondaparinux given for 8 days reduced mortality and severe bleeding in STEMI patients who received fibrinolytic therapy or were not reperfused. Benefit was not seen among patients who underwent primary PCI.[43]

4. **Clopidogrel:** Clopidogrel is an oral antiplatelet agent that improves outcomes when given as initial treatment to STEMI patients receiving thrombolytic therapy.[75,76] A large randomized trial of clopidogrel versus placebo for patients with STEMI receiving fibrinolytics showed a significant mortality reduction among clopidogrel treated patients. Major bleeding and ICH were not increased, even in the subset of patients >75 years old.[75]

Risk calculator for 6-month postdischarge mortality after hospitalization for Acute Coronary Syndrome

Record the points for each variable at the bottom left and sum the points to calculate the total risk score. Find the total score on the x-axis of the nomogram plot. The corresponding probability on the y-axis is the estimated probability of all-cause mortality from hospital discharge to 6 months.

Medical History		**Findings at Initial Hospital Presentation**		**Findings During Hospitalization**	
① Age in years	Points	④ Resting heart rate, beats/min	Points	⑦ Initial serum creatinine, mg/dL	Points
≤29	0	≤49.9	0	0–0.39	1
30–39	0	50–69.9	3	0.4–0.79	3
40–49	18	70–89.9	9	0.8–1.19	5
50–59	36	90–109.9	14	1.2–1.59	7
60–69	55	110–149.9	23	1.6–1.99	9
70–79	73	150–199.9	35	2–3.99	15
80–89	91	≥200	43	≥4	20
≥90	100				
② History of congestive heart failure	24	⑤ Systolic blood pressure, mm Hg		⑧ Elevated cardiac enzymes	15
		≤79.9	24	⑨ No in-hospital Percutaneous Coronary invervention	14
③ History of myocardial infarction	12	80–99.9	22		
		100–119.9	18		
		120–139.9	14		
		140–159.9	10		
		160–199.9	4		
		≥200	0		
			1		
		⑥ ST-segment depression	11		

Points

① _____
② _____
③ _____
④ _____
⑤ _____
⑥ _____
⑦ _____
⑧ _____
⑨ _____

Total risk score _____ (sum of points)

Mortality risk _____ (from plot)

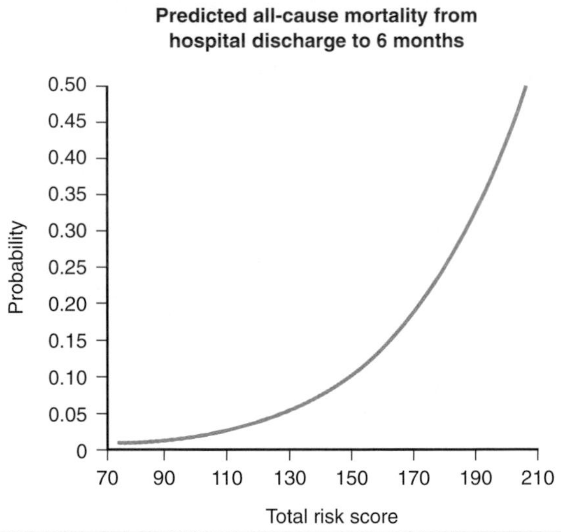

Predicted all-cause mortality from hospital discharge to 6 months

Figure 19-7 • The GRACE Prediction Score

5. Glycoprotein IIb/IIIa Inhibitors:

- For patients undergoing primary PCI, IIb/IIIa inhibitors should be initiated as early as possible.[35] Five randomized trials have compared abciximab to placebo in a total of 3,666 patients undergoing primary PCI for STEMI. The primary benefits appear to be in recurrent ischemia, manifested by reductions in urgent target vessel revascularization and reinfarction.[44–48] Other IIb/IIIa agents have been less well studied in STEMI.

- Combination therapy with the IIb/IIIa inhibitor abciximab and half-dose fibrinolytic therapy (reteplase or tenecteplase) may be considered for prevention of reinfarction in patients with anterior MI, age <75 years, and no risk factors for bleed-

ing. Bleeding was increased in older patients. For patients managed with fibrinolytic therapy, IIb/IIIa Inhibitors in combination with half-dose thrombolytics do not reduce mortality.[49,50]

6. **β-blockers:** As a result of negative inotropic and chronotropic activity, β-blockers reduce heart rate and myocardial contractility, decreasing myocardial oxygen demand. Both atenolol and metoprolol have been studied in patients. Trials conducted before fibrinolytic therapy was available showed that early β-blocker administration reduced mortality as soon as day 1, a benefit that was sustained at 2 weeks (ISIS-I, MIAMI). More recent with AMI[71,72] studies of early intravenous versus delayed β-blocker use in patients receiving fibrinolytics have not shown mortality

reductions. The TIMI IIB trial showed reductions in reinfarction and recurrent ischemia, but not mortality, at 42 days with early versus delayed (starting at day 6) administration of metoprolol, with the greatest benefit when given within 2 hours of symptom onset.[73] The larger COMMIT trial found that early IV β-blocker use was associated with a reduction in reinfarction and ventricular fibrillation, however, this benefit was offset by an increase in cardiogenic shock in the first 24 hours. There was no difference in mortality rates. Given these findings, routine use of early IV β-blockers is not recommended. As most of the adverse effects occurred in the first day, use of oral β-blockers after hemodynamic stabilization is a safer approach.[74]

Contraindications to β-blockers include bradycardia (HR < 60), hypotension, moderate-to-severe decompensated heart failure, and active bronchospasm. Recommendations to avoid use of β-blockers in patients with cocaine-induced infarction are based on theoretical concerns of exacerbating coronary spasm; however, adverse effects from β-blockers have not been clearly substantiated.

7. **Reperfusion therapy:** Reperfusion therapy restores flow through the infarct-related artery to the jeopardized myocardium. All patients with STEMI should be immediately evaluated for emergent reperfusion in attempts to limit infarct size. Reperfusion may be achieved with primary percutaneous coronary intervention (PCI: balloon angioplasty and/or stenting) or fibrinolytic therapy. With either method of reperfusion, the primary aim is to minimize delays in restoration of blood flow. The goal for primary PCI is "door to balloon" time of <90 minutes, and for thrombolytic therapy, a "door-to-needle" time of <30 minutes. When available, PCI is generally the favored approach. However, in many institutions where rapid access to PCI is not feasible, thrombolytic therapy should be administered immediately if no contraindications exist.

As PCI is generally considered advantageous over thrombolytic therapy, centers without PCI capability may consider transfer to another institution for emergent PCI rather than use of fibrinolytic therapy. In making the decision as to whether to administer fibrinolytics or transfer for PCI, the following factors should be considered:

- Time from onset of symptoms: The earlier in the course, the greater the imperative to initiate thrombolytic therapy
- Patient age: The older patient is at greater risk with thrombolytic treatment.

Table 19-5 Absolute Benefit of Thrombolytic Therapy Based on Presenting Characteristics

	Lives saved per 1,000	NNT
Symptoms < 6 hours	30	33
Symptoms 7–12 hours	20	50
Anterior infarction	37	27
Inferior infarction	8	125

From: Fibrinolytic Therapy Trialists'[FTT] Collaborative Group. Indications for fibrinolytic therapy in suspected acute myocardial infarction: collaborative overview of early mortality and major morbidity results from all randomised trials of more than 1000 patients. Lancet 1994; 343:311–322.

- Infarct location: Anterior infarction places the patient at greater risk of complications, and PCI may be favored.
- **Fibrinolytic therapy: Fibrinolytics (thrombolytics)** activate plasminogen by enzymatically exposing the active center of plasmin. When administered to STEMI patients within the first 12 hours following symptom onset, thrombolytic therapy significantly reduces short- and long-term mortality (Table 19-5). Meta-analysis of large randomized trials comparing fibrinolytic therapy to placebo confirmed a significant overall 21% mortality reduction at 35 days in patients treated with thrombolytics. The greatest benefit was found among patients presenting within 12 hours of symptom onset and those with anterior infarction.[51]

The most feared complication of fibrinolytic therapy is ICH, which occurs in approximately 1% of treated patients.[52,53] Most ICH that complicates thrombolytic use occurs within the first 24–48 hours. Thrombolytics result in approximately four extra strokes per 1,000 patients treated in the first 24 hours (NNH 250). In-hospital mortality for STEMI patients who develop ICH is approximately 50–80%, and residual neurologic deficits are present in 25% of survivors.[23,41] To reduce the rate of this complication, patients considered for thrombolytics should be carefully screened for risks of intracerebral bleed (Tables 19-6 and 19-7). Advancing age and prior history of stroke are the two strongest risk factors for ICH due to thrombolytics. The incidence of ICH among patients under age 65 is 0.4%, compared to 2.1% among patients over age 75.[23] Using lower-dose unfractionated

Table 19-6 Contraindications to Thrombolytic Therapy

Absolute	Relative
Prior intracranial hemorrhage	BP >180/110 mmHg
Intracranial neoplasm or cerebrovascular lesion	Ischemic stroke >3 months prior
Ischemic stroke within 3 months (except within 3 hours)	Dementia
Suspected aortic dissection	Traumatic or prolonged CPR (>10 minutes) within 3 weeks
Active bleeding or bleeding diathesis (excluding menses)	Major surgery or internal bleeding within 3 weeks
Significant closed-head or facial trauma within 3 months	Pregnancy Active peptic ulcer Current use of anticoagulants

BP—blood pressure; CPR—cardiopulmonary resuscitation.
From: Antman E, Anbe D, Armstrong P, et al. ACC/AHA guidelines for management of patients with ST elevation myocardial infarction. J Am Coll Cardiol 2004; 44:671–719.

Table 19-7 Risk of Intracerebral Hemorrhage in STEMI Patients receiving specific Fibrinolytic Therapy

CCP: alteplase (rtPA)	Number of risks	Risk of ICH
Age >75	0–1	0.7
Weight: women <65 kg men <80 kg	2	1.0
Female	3	1.6
Black race	4	2.5
SBP >159 on admission	5+	4.1
Prior stroke		
Thrombolytic use		
Excessive anticoagulation		
IN-TIME: lanoteplase (ntPA)		
Age >75	0	0.25
Weight: <67 kg	1	0.7
Black race	2	1.0
SBP >159 on admission	3	2.0
Prior stroke	4	2.4
Thrombolytic use		
Prior nifedipine use		

From: InTIME-II. Intravenous NPA for the Treatment of Infarcting Myocardium Early; InTIME-II, a double-blind comparison of single-bolus lanoteplase vs accelerated alteplase for the treatment of patients with acute myocardial infarction. Eur Heart J 2000; 21:2005–2013.

Table 19-8 PCI versus Fibrinolytic Therapy

Invasive favored (Primary PCI)	Fibrinolysis favored
Skilled PCI laboratory with surgical backup available*	Skilled PCI laboratory is not available or will be delayed (door-to-balloon time >90 min)
Door-to-balloon time <90 min	
Cardiogenic shock or Killup class 3	
Increased risk of intracranial bleeding	
Diagnosis of MI in question	

*Skilled PCI laboratory: operator performs >75 primary PCI cases/year, team experience >36 primary PCI cases/year.

heparin reduces the risk of ICH without affecting overall mortality.[53] If an acute change in mental status occurs, particularly in the first 24 hours after thrombolytic treatment, the patient should undergo immediate evaluation for ICH with noncontrast head computed tomography (CT), and all antiplatelet, anticoagulant, and fibrinolytic therapy should be discontinued pending results.

Choice of Fibrinolytic Agent: Currently available fibrinolytic agents include streptokinase, alteplase (tPA), reteplase, lanoteplase (nTPA), and tenecteplase (TNK-tPA). Streptokinase is antigenic, can lead to allergic reactions and hypotension, and causes marked systemic fibrinolysis, while the other agents are considered fibrin specific. In addition, as tPA results in a small but significant 35-day mortality show benefit over streptokinase, fibrin-specific agents are preferred for treatment of STEMI.[55]

Each of the fibrin-specific thrombolytics has been compared to alteplase in large randomized trials, with each showing equivalent mortality at 30-days.[56-60] Whereas tPA is administered as a bolus followed by IV infusion, the other fibrinolytics are given as a single weight-based bolus, which may facilitate administration. More important than the particular agent chosen is the need to eliminate delay to administration, as increased time-to-treatment results in higher mortality.[59]

Recommendations: In the absence of contraindications, the ACC recommends thrombolytic therapy in the following settings:

• **ACC Class I:** Patients with STEMI with symptom onset within the prior 12 hours and ST elevation >0.1 mV in at least two consecutive leads or new or presumably new LBBB

• **ACC Class IIa:** Symptoms within 12 hours and ECG findings of posterior MI or symptoms 12–24 hours with ongoing symptoms of ischemia and ST elevation

8. **Percutaneous Coronary Intervention (PCI) versus Thrombolytic Therapy:**

The invasive approach to management of STEMI involves immediate angiography with revascularization of the culprit lesion by PCI or coronary artery bypass grafting (CABG) (Fig. 19-8). Compared to fibrinolytic therapy, primary PCI significantly reduces short- and long-term rates of death, nonfatal reinfarction, and stroke (Table 19-8). Among 14 randomized trials comparing primary PCI to fibrin-specific thrombolytics, 30-day mortality was reduced by 20% with PCI (5.3% vs. 6.6%, p = 0.0004; NNT = 77).[61] Combined data from five randomized trials that compared emergent transfer for PCI with on-site thrombolysis showed significant reductions in nonfatal reinfarction and total stroke and a nonsignificant mortality reduction from PCI, despite a delay of approximately 40 minutes due to hospital transfer.[61] For patients with cardiogenic shock, who have the highest mortality, PCI provides a significant reduction in short- and long-term mortality: 30-day mortality 47% vs. 56% and 1-year mortality 53% vs. 66%, for PCI compared to fibirnolytics.[30]

A summary of treatment modalities and recommendations for STEMI is outlined in Table 19-9.

Adverse events associated with PCI include the need for vascular repair (0.4–2%) and development of acute renal failure (0.5%).[61] In patients with cardiogenic shock, PCI was shown to reduce acute renal failure by approximately 50% (13% vs. 24% with PCI vs. fibrinolytic therapy)[30] (Table 19-10).

Additional Medications That Should be Added During Hospitalization

1. Clopidogrel: For all patients following coronary intervention
2. Angiotensin converting enzyme inhibitors (ACE-inhibitors): Shown to reduce mortality in patients with coronary artery disease (CAD) (HOPE trial) and in patients with systolic heart failure
3. Lipid lowering: The goal for patients with established CAD is to lower LDL below 70. Unless contraindicated, all patients should be discharged with a statin. If patients on a high-dose statin have not reached goal low density lipoprotein (LDL), ezetimibe or niacin may be added.
4. Aldosterone antagonists: For patients with EF <0.40 and symptomatic heart failure or diabetes mellitus

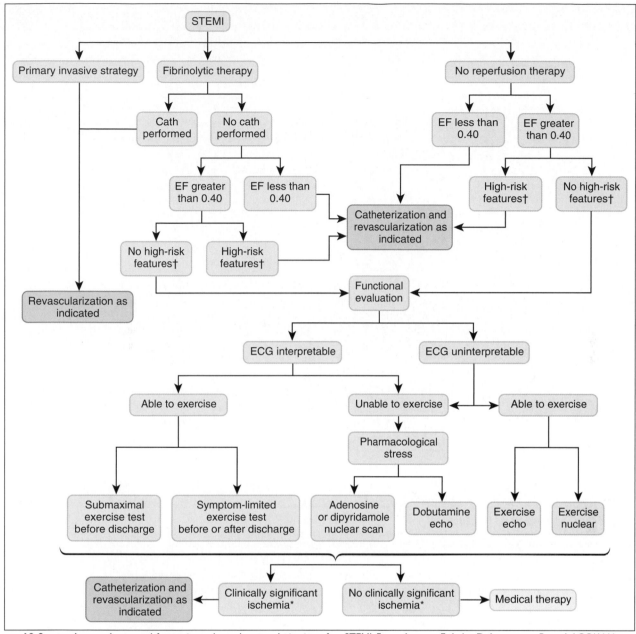

Figure 19-8 • Approach to need for angiography and revascularization after STEMI. From: Antman E, Anbe D, Armstrong P, et al. ACC/AHA guidelines for management of patients with ST elevation myocardial infarction. J Am Coll Cardiol 2004; 44:671–719.

Alternative Options

- Angiotensin receptor blockers may be used in patients intolerant of ACE inhibitors due to cough.
- Long-acting calcium channel blockers are acceptable anti-anginals for patients who are unable to tolerate β-blockers or who need additional blood pressure lowering.

Indications for AICD

Patients with ventricular fibrillation or ventricular tachycardia that is sustained or hemodynamically significant >48 hours after AMI should have an AICD placed prior to discharge.[35] In the absence of sustained ventricular tachycardia or fibrillation, automatic implantable cardiac defibrillator (AICD) placement should be considered for patients with an ejection fraction <30% 1

month following MI and those with EF 31–40% who have non-sustained ventricular tachycardia.[65]

PREVENTION

Risk factor modification should be stressed to patients hospitalized with ACS. Patients should receive counseling as part of patient instruction at discharge on the following that apply:

1. Smoking cessation with outpatient referral
2. Diet: low cholesterol, low saturated fat
3. Exercise and cardiac rehabilitation referral
4. Weight loss
5. Substance abuse
6. Medication compliance

Table 19-9 Recommended Initial Treatment for STEMI and Dosing

Antiplatelet	Aspirin	162–325 mg (nonenteric) chewed followed by 75–325 mg PO daily
Antithrombotic	Unfractionated heparin	Bolus 60 units/kg (up to 4,000 units), then infusion 12 units/kg/h (up to 1,000 units) with goal PTT 1.5–2.0 times control
		Reduce to 50 units/kg if using glycoprotein IIb/IIIa inhibitor
	Enoxaparin	30 mg IV bolus, then 1 mg/kg SQ q 12 hours
	Clopidogrel	75 mg q day
		For patients >75 years old; omit bolus, and reduce dose to 0.75 mg/kg q 12 hours; for Cr clearance <30 mL/min, reduce dose to 1 mg/kg q 24 hours
Antianginal	Nitroglycerin	Sublingual: 0.4 mg SL q 5 minutes for pain relief
		IV: start at 10–30 mcg/min, titrate to relief of pain, keeping SBP >90 mm Hg
		Topical: 1–1½ inches paste applied q 8 hours
	β-blockers[†]	Initial IV dose, then maintenance oral dose
	Metoprolol	Maintenance: begin at 6.25–12.5 mg q 8–12 hours, increase as tolerated
	Atenolol	Maintenance: begin at 25 mg daily, increase as tolerated
Fibrinolytic therapy	Alteplase (tPA)	15 mg IV bolus followed by 0.75 mg/kg over 30 minutes (up to 50 mg), then 0.5 mg/kg over the next 60 minutes (up to 100 mg total)
	Tenecteplase	One weight-based IV bolus over 10–15 seconds

Weight (kg)	Dose
<60	30 mg
60–69	35 mg
70–79	40 mg
0–89	45 mg
90	50 mg

ACE inhibitors Angiotensin Receptor Blockers	In first 24 hours, start short-acting oral ACE inhibitor in all patients with anterior infarction, pulmonary edema, EF <40%, and absence of hypotension or contraindications (i.e., captopril 6.25 12 mg q 8 hours). Use ARB if ACE intolerant due to cough.

[†]β-blockers without intrinsic sympathomimetic activity (ISA) are recommended: metoprolol, atenolol, esmolol, propranolol.

Table 19-10 Complications

Mechanical Complication	Incidence	Manifestations	Infarct Location
Papillary muscle rupture (usually posterior papillary muscle)	1%	Sudden-onset dyspnea and hypotension MR murmur (may be soft), pulmonary edema, cardiogenic shock	Inferior
Septal rupture	No reperfusion: 1–3% Fibrinolytics: 0.2–0.3%[63]	Chest pain, dyspnea, hypotension Harsh systolic murmur, pulmonary edema, S₃, biventricular failure, cardiogenic shock Persistent ST elevation In-hospital mortality with complex vs. simple rupture 78% vs. 38%; RV vs. no RV extension 71% vs. 29%[62]	Anterior, inferior, septal
LV free wall rupture	Risk reduced with primary angioplasty vs. fibrinolytics: 3.7% vs. 8.1% (anterior MI)[64] 1.8% vs. 3.3% (all MI)[65]	Chest pain, nausea, syncope, arrhythmia, sudden death Hemodynamic collapse, tamponade with pulsus paradoxus, PEA	Anterior

MR—mitral regurgitation; PEA—pulseless electrical acivity; RV—right ventricle

Each complication has a bimodal occurrence, with most occurring within the first 24 hours, and between days 3–5, but may occur up to 14 days post-MI.

DISCHARGE/FOLLOW-UP PLANS

Patient Instruction

1. Activity: Recommendations from ACC/AHA Guidelines[35]
   - **All patients should be given a referral for Cardiac Rehabilitation at the time of discharge.** Cardiac rehabilitation is a comprehensive long-term program that involves medical evaluation, prescribed exercise, cardiac risk factor modification, education, and counseling.
   - Based on risk assessment or exercise testing, daily walking should be initiated immediately, with a goal of at least 30 minutes of aerobic activity daily, but at a minimum of 3 or 4 times a week.

Table 19-11 Discharge Medications

All patients without contraindications should receive
1. ASA 75–162 mg daily
1. Clopidogrel 75 mg daily
3. β-blocker
4. ACE inhibitor (ARB if intolerant)
5. Statin with additional lipid lowering as needed to achieve LDL <70 mg/dL

Additional or Alternative Medications for Special Conditions:

EF <0.40 with symptomatic heart failure or DM	• Aldosterone blockade (eplerenone): patients should be tolerating an ACE-inhibitor or ARB
	*contraindications:
	  • Cr >2.5 mg/dL (men) or >2.0 mg/dL (women)
	  • K⁺ >5.0 mEq/L

Hypertriglyceridemia (TG >500 mg/dL):	• Fibrate

Indication for anticoagulation	• **Stent placed:**
	  • Aspirin plus warfarin with target INR 2.0–3.0
	• **No stent placed: do NOT use clopidogrel**
	  • Aspirin plus warfarin (target INR 2.0–3.0)
	  OR
	  • Warfarin alone (target INR 2.5–3.5)

ARB—angiotensin receptor blocker; EF—ejection fraction; TG—triglycerides; DM—diabetes mellitus

• In stable patients without complications, sexual activity can be resumed within 7 to 10 days.
• Timing of return to work must be individualized, based on physical and emotional stress involved, whether successful reperfusion was achieved, severity of heart failure symptoms, and complications during hospitalization. Patients with successful reperfusion who return to work in the first month following STEMI do not have an increase risk of adverse events.[63] In the PAMI-II trial, low-risk patients (i.e., age <70 years, ejection fraction >0.45, 1- or 2-vessel disease, and good PTCA result) encouraged to return to work at 2 weeks experienced no adverse events.[64]
• Driving can begin 1 week after discharge, with restrictions per individual state laws. Patients who experienced serious arrhythmias or cardiogenic shock or required CPR should delay driving 2–3 weeks after symptoms have stabilized.
• Air travel is safe within 2 weeks in stable patients, but should be avoided in those with rest angina or dyspnea and with fear of flying, as the reduced oxygen tension in aircrafts may lead to hypoxia.
2. Diet
• Low saturated fat: <7% of total calories as saturated fats, <200 mg of cholesterol per day, and increased consumption of omega-3 fatty acids
• Low sodium: for patients with heart failure or hypertension
• Weight management: desirable BMI between 18.5 and 25 kg/m²

Outpatient Physician Communication

Patients should be given a follow-up appointment with their primary care provider within 2–4 weeks of discharge. A hospital discharge summary should be provided to the primary care provider (PCP) along with list of discharge medications in a timely manner, prior to the first follow-up visit (Table 19-11).

Key Points

• Close to 90% of patients with AMI are likely to have traditional risk factors for coronary disease.

• Compared to patients who present with chest pain, patients with STEMI who present with other complaints (9%) are less likely to receive fibrinolytics or primary PCI (36% vs. 66%), and they have higher in-hospital mortality (19% vs. 6.3%, p < 0.001).

• Minor troponin elevation can occur in trauma patients without suspected myocardial injury, decompensated heart failure, severely elevated hypertension, pulmonary embolism, myositis, and renal disease.

• Factors that independently increase mortality in patients with STEMI include increasing age, heart failure and cardiogenic shock (one of the strongest predictors), and anterior location of infarction.

• The TIMI Risk Score is a validated scoring system to predict short-term risk of mortality following STEMI.

• For patients with STEMI, the foundation of acute therapy is reperfusion of the infarct-related artery.

• All patients should be given a referral for cardiac rehabilitation at the time of discharge.

SUGGESTED READING

Eagle K, Lim M, Dabbous O, et al. A validated prediction model for all forms of acute coronary syndrome. Estimating the risk of 6-month postdischarge death in an international registry. JAMA 2004; 291:2727–2733.

Antman E, Anbe D, Armstrong P, et al. ACC/AHA guidelines for management of patients with ST elevation myocardial infarction. J Am Coll Cardiol 2004; 44:671–719.

CREATE TGI. Effects of reviparin, a low-molecular-weight heparin, on mortality, reinfarction, and strokes in patients with acute myocardial infarction presenting with ST-segment elevation. JAMA 2005; 293(4):427–435.

Topol E. (The GUSTO V Investigators). Reperfusion therapy for acute myocardial infarction with fibrinolytic therapy or combination reduce fibrinolytic therapy and platelet glycoprotein IIb/IIIa inhibition. The GUSTO V randomised trial. Lancet 2001; 357:1905–1914.

Keeley EC, Boura JA, Grines CL. Primary angioplasty versus intravenous thrombolytic therapy for acute myocardial infarction: a quantitative review of 23 randomised trials. Lancet 2003; 361:13–20.

CHAPTER TWENTY

Acute Coronary Syndromes: Unstable Angina and Non-ST Segment Elevation Acute Myocardial Infarction

Jennifer Kleinbart, MD

BACKGROUND

Acute coronary syndrome (ACS) is the term encompassing clinical symptoms of acute myocardial ischemia, and it represents a spectrum of disease resulting from acute coronary obstruction that impedes myocardial blood flow. Non–ST elevation ACS (NSTE-ACS) includes both non ST-elevation myocardial infarction (NSTEMI) and unstable angina (USA), which both result from incomplete or transient coronary occlusion with decreased myocardial perfusion. NSTEMI and USA may be indistinguishable on presentation, and their initial management is the same. NSTEMI is differentiated from USA by elevated levels of cardiac biomarkers.

NSTE-ACS develops when myocardial oxygen demand exceeds supply, most commonly as a result of disruption of a previously nonocclusive atherosclerotic plaque.[1] Unstable coronary disease may result from dynamic obstruction, including Prinzmetal's angina, nonfocal vasoconstriction (as with cocaine or cold immersion), and microcirculatory angina. Prinzmetal's angina refers to focal spasm of an epicardial artery that impedes blood flow either in a nondiseased segment of an epicardial vessel or adjacent to a nonobstructive plaque.[2]

ASSESSMENT

Clinical Presentation

Prompt recognition of symptoms by patients and clinicians is critical to reduce treatment delays. Initial assessment of the patient with chest pain should focus on (1) the likelihood, or pretest probability, that a patient's symptoms are due to cardiac ischemia and (2) the risk of adverse cardiac events.

When considering the likelihood that a patient has ACS, consider both the patient's risk factors for coronary disease as well as the presenting symptoms. Risk factors include male sex, increasing age, family history of coronary disease, diabetes mellitus, cigarette smoking, peripheral arterial disease, hypertension, dyslipidemia, and renal disease. Close to 90% of patients with AMI are likely to have traditional risk factors for coronary disease.[3] Forty percent of NSTEMI patients are female; one third have diabetes, and one third have had a prior myocardial infarction (MI).[4]

ACS patients may present with atypical chest pain histories, especially in description of the quality of chest pain. The following features are associated with pain caused by cardiac ischemia:
1. Pain is retrosternal.
2. Pain radiates to the arm, neck, or jaw.
3. Pain is precipitated by stress or exertion and relieved within 10 minutes by rest or nitroglycerin.

Patients with all three features are considered to have "typical" angina; two out of three features, "atypical angina"; and those with one out of three features are classified as having nonanginal chest pain. Significant angiographic coronary disease was found in 89% of patients with typical pain, 50% of patients with atypical pain, and 16% with nonanginal pain.[5] Adding age and gender to this model even more accurately predicts ischemia as the cause of chest pain (Table 20-1). For example, a 35-year-old female with typical angina has a 26% risk of coronary disease, while the risk in a 55-year-old male with typical angina is 92%.[5]

In addition to history, age, and gender, clinical risk factors, physical examination findings, electrocardiogram (ECG) changes, and elevation of cardiac markers are useful for predicting the probability of coronary disease (Table 20-2).[6]

Among patients who present with ischemic pain, the symptom severity should be assessed, as well as a determination as to whether symptoms are stable or unstable. The Canadian Cardiovascular Society Classification (CCSC) provides a standard classification for angina severity (Table 20-3). Unstable angina includes ischemic pain that is accelerating (increasing in severity, duration, or with less exertion), particularly to CCSC Class III or IV within the last 2 weeks, new angina, and rest angina. As opposed to ischemic pain, pain of infarction may occur at rest and be prolonged (*see* Chapter 19).

Prevalence and Presenting Signs and Symptoms

A study comparing pain characteristics among patients with significant coronary disease compared to those with normal angiograms found that two out of the three features below were present in 85% of patients with significant disease while in only 26% of those with normal angiograms[7]:
1. Pain duration <5 minutes
2. Rest pain in <2/10 episodes
3. 10/10 episodes being reproduced by a similar level of exertion.

Table 20-1 Likelihood of Coronary Disease (%) Based on History, Age, and Gender

Age, (yrs)	NONANGINAL PAIN		ATYPICAL PAIN		TYPICAL PAIN	
	Men	Women	Men	Women	Men	Women
30–39	5	0.8	22	4	70	26
40–49	14	3	46	13	87	55
50–59	22	8	59	32	92	79
60–69	28	19	67	54	94	91

From: Diamond G, Forrester J. Analysis of probability as an aid in the clinical diagnosis of coronary-artery disease. N Engl J Med 1979; 300:1350–1358.

Table 20-2 Likelihood That Signs and Symptoms Represent an ACS

Feature	High Likelihood Any of the Following:	Intermediate Likelihood Absence of High-Likelihood Features and Presence of Any of the Following:	Low Likelihood Absence of High- or Intermediate-Likelihood Features But May Have:
History	Chest or left arm pain or discomfort as chief symptom reproducing prior documented angina	Chest or left arm pain or discomfort as chief symptom Age >70 years	Probable ischemic symptoms in absence of any of the intermediate likelihood characteristics
	Known history of CAD, including MI	Male sex Diabetes mellitus	Recent cocaine use
Examination	Transient MR, hypotension, diaphoresis, pulmonary edema, or rales	Extracardiac vascular disease	Chest discomfort reproduced by palpation
ECG	New, or presumably new, transient ST-segment deviation (≥0.05 mV) or T-wave inversion (≥0.2 mV) with symptoms	Fixed Q waves Abnormal ST segments or T waves not documented to be new	T-wave flattening or inversion in leads with dominant R waves Normal ECG
Cardiac markers	Elevated cardiac TnI, TnT, or CK-MB	Normal	Normal

CAD—coronary artery disease; MI—myocardial infarction; MR—mitral regurgitation; TnI—troporin I; TnT—troponin T; ECG—electrocardiogram
Braunwald E, Mark DB, Jones RH, et al. Unstable angina: diagnosis and management. Rockville, MD: Agency for Health Care Policy and Research and the National Heart, Lung, and Blood Institute, US Public Health Service, US Department of Health and Human Services; 1994; AHCPR Publication No. 94-0602.

Table 20-3 Canadian Cardiovascular Society Classification of Angina

Class	Angina occurs with:
I	Prolonged exertion
II	Moderate activity: can walk >2 blocks
III	Mild activity: symptoms occur walking <2 blocks
IV	Minimal activity or at rest

Physical examination: Physical examination should focus on evaluating the patient's hemodynamic stability and identifying complications of MI, such as heart failure. Among patients with NSTEMI, tachycardia and congestive heart failure (CHF) are each presenting signs in approximately 25% of patients, with hypotension or cardiogenic shock in approximately 4% of patients.[4]

Differential Diagnosis

Acute chest pain may be caused by a variety of cardiac, pulmonary, gastrointestinal, and musculoskeletal disorders, as described in Chapter 18 and Chapter 19.

Diagnosis

Diagnostic Criteria

Unstable angina is a clinical diagnosis based on characteristic chest pain or anginal equivalents (i.e., dyspnea, arm pain, nausea) that are typically associated with activity and relieved by rest. ECG changes support the diagnosis, especially when dynamic (i.e., occurring with symptoms and normalizing following symptom resolution); however, they are not necessary for the diagnosis.

Preferred

Preferred Diagnostic Approach

Among patients presenting with chest pain or symptoms suspicious for acute ischemia or infarction, the diagnosis of STEMI or NSTEMI should be pursued. This includes a 12-lead ECG and cardiac enzymes (CK-MB and troponin T or I) at presentation and again 6–8 hours later. The diagnosis of NSTEMI is made when characteristic ischemic symptoms are accompanied by a rise and fall of cardiac biomarkers in the absence of ST segment elevation. If troponins are still undetectable at 6–8 hours after presentation,

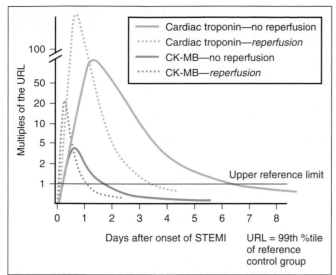

Figure 20-1 • Typical rise and fall of troponins and CK-MB in patients who receive immediate reperfusion and those who do not. Modified with permission from: Antman E, Bassand J, Klein W, et al. Myocardial infarction redefined—a consensus document of The Joint European Society of Cardiology. J Am Coll Cardiol 2000; 36(233):959; *and* Wu A, Apple F, Gibler WB, et al. National Academy of Clinical Biochemistry standards of laboratory practice: recommendations for the use of cardiac markers in coronary artery diseases. Clin Chem 1999; 45(234):1104.

MI is ruled out; however, significant coronary stenosis with ischemia has not been excluded, and should be pursued if symptoms or ECG suggests this.

Acute ischemia may cause ST-segment depression, transient ST-segment elevation, or T-wave inversions. ST-segment depression is the most common ECG abnormality among NSTEMI patients, and it is highly predictive of coronary thrombosis, especially when changes occur with symptoms.[8] T-wave inversions that are symmetric and >2 mV deep are suggestive of ischemia. Up to 6% of chest pain patients with normal ECGs will have a NSTEMI.

Evidence and Rationale

Cardiac Biomarkers

Elevation of cardiac enzymes, with a characteristic time course of their rise and fall, confirms the diagnosis of acute myocardial infarction. Currently available markers include creatinine kinase (CK), CK-MB, troponin T and I, and myoglobin (Fig. 20-1).

CK-MB and myoglobin are released from both cardiac and skeletal muscle and are therefore normally detectable in healthy individuals. Levels of both markers increase with skeletal muscle disease or injury (including heavy exercise and rhabdomyolysis) and with renal disease. Using the ratio of CK-MB to total CK is more accurate for diagnosing infarction than total CK alone, especially when total CK is elevated due to skeletal muscle damage.

Unlike CK and CK-MB, cardiac troponins are found only in cardiac muscle. Therefore, troponins should not be detectable in healthy individuals, and even minor elevations should raise suspicion for an acute cardiac process. However, elevations may occur in diseases other than acute ischemia, including decompensated heart failure, severely elevated hypertension, pulmonary embolism, and myositis. Minor troponin elevations have been documented among trauma patients without suspected myocardial injury, and in renal failure patients without overt coronary disease.[9,10] In one study, half of patients with heart disease who presented with chest pain not considered to be ischemic had troponin I levels greater than 0.07 mcg/L, and one fourth had levels over 0.1 mcg/L.[11]

Approximately 5% of troponin is free in the cytoplasm and may be released rapidly after cell injury, while the majority of troponin is bound in the myofibrillar apparatus and released over the next several hours. Serial measurement of troponin T and I and CK-MB/CK at presentation with repeated 6 to 8 hours later is highly sensitive, with negative results effectively ruling out infarction.[13,14]

Myoglobin is released from injured cardiac and skeletal muscle, and it therefore is a sensitive but very nonspecific marker for AMI. Levels increase rapidly after myocardial injury, making myoglobin appealing for early exclusion of AMI, particularly in emergency department chest pain units. Despite this, myoglobin levels have not been found to provide significant additional information to troponins and CK-MB, and therefore their use remains limited.[9,13] In addition, as both the rise and fall of myoglobin occur rapidly after myocardial damage, levels may be declining in patients who present several hours after symptom onset.

Prognosis

While trial data show 7-day mortality rates of 1.5–2.0%, data from nontrial NSTE-ACS registries show inhospital mortality rates of 3.8–7.3%.[4,15,16] Following NSTE-ACS, mortality at 1 year and 4 years is approximately 9% and 22%, respectively.[16] Other inhospital complications following NSTEMI/USA include reinfarction (2%), heart failure (7%), shock (2%), stroke (0.6%), and RBC transfusion (10%).[4]

Assessing a patient's risk for short-term adverse events is a critical step in determination of appropriate management, including intensity of monitoring, and treatments such as glycoprotein IIb/IIIa inhibitors, and early revascularization. Risk of death or recurrent MI is higher in patients with particular historical, clinical, and electrocardiographic findings, as well as among those with elevated levels of troponin[6] (Table 20-4). Mortality is significantly higher among patients with diabetes mellitus and those with renal disease.[17,18] Key clinical features on admission that are associated with increased risk of death or MI include age over 75, elevated cardiac enzymes on admission, more severe anginal symptoms prior to admission (CCSC Class III or IV), pulmonary rales, and ST-segment depression.[19] Tachycardia, bradycardia, and hypotension also predict higher adverse outcomes.[20]

Age—Age greater than 60 years increases mortality among NSTE-ACS patients, with a mortality risk almost five times greater in patients over age 70.[16]

ECG—Among patients with isolated T-wave inversion, 30-day mortality was 1.7%, compared with mortality of 5.1% among patients with either ST depression or ST-elevation AMI.[8] Mortality differences persisted at 6 months (3.4% for T-wave inversion, 8.9% for ST-depression, and 6.8% for ST-elevation).[8]

Troponins—Mortality increases with increasing baseline and peak levels. The GUSTO-IIa study showed that 1-year mortality was significantly higher in patients with elevated troponin-T levels compared to those without troponin elevations (14% vs. 5%).

Table 20-4 Short-Term Risk of Death or Nonfatal MI in Patients with Unstable Angina

Feature	High Risk At Least One of the Following Features Must Be Present:	Intermediate Risk No High-Risk Feature But Must Have One of the Following	Low Risk No High- or Intermediate-Risk Feature But May Have Any of the Following Features:
History	Accelerating tempo of ischemic symptoms in preceding 48 hr	Prior MI, peripheral or cerebrovascular disease, or CABG, prior aspirin use	
Character of pain	Prolonged ongoing (>20 minutes) rest pain	Prolonged (>20 min) rest angina, now resolved, with moderate or high likelihood of CAD Rest angina (<20 min) or relieved with rest or sublingual NTG	New-onset or progressive CCS Class III or IV angina in the past 2 weeks without prolonged (>20 min) rest pain but with moderate or high likelihood of CAD (see Table 20-5)
Clinical findings	Pulmonary edema, most likely due to ischemia New or worsening MR murmur S_3 or new/worsening rales Hypotension, bradycardia, tachycardia Age >75 years	Age >70 years	
ECG	Angina at rest with transient ST-segment changes >0.05 mV Bundle-branch block, new or presumed new Sustained ventricular tachycardia	T-wave inversions >0.2 mV Pathologic Q waves	Normal or unchanged ECG during an episode of chest discomfort
Cardiac markers	Elevated (e.g., TnT or TnI >0.1 ng/mL)	Slightly elevated (e.g., TnT >0.01 but <0.1 ng/mL)	Normal

*Estimation of the short-term risks of death and nonfatal cardiac ischemic events in UA is a complex multivariable problem that cannot be fully specified in a table such as this; therefore, this table is meant to offer general guidance and illustration rather than rigid algorithms.

Adapted from AHCPR Clinical Practice Guideline No. 10, Unstable Angina: Diagnosis and Management, May 1994. Braunwald E, Mark DB, Jones RH, et al. Unstable angina: diagnosis and management. Rockville, MD: Agency for Health Care Policy and Research and the National Heart, Lung, and Blood Institute, US Public Health Service, US Department of Health and Human Services; 1994; AHCPR Publication No. 94-0602.

Risk Stratification Tools

In the early assessment of the patient with suspected ACS, risk stratification is critical to guide initial management. Early risk stratification takes into consideration patient demographics, coronary disease risk factors, and results of initial testing. A number of risk assessment guides and scoring systems can aid with this.

Thrombolysis in Myocardial Infarction Trials (TIMI) Score

The TIMI Risk Score is a validated scoring system to predict short-term risk of mortality in patients with NSTEMI/USA. Mortality increases with higher TIMI Score[21] (Fig. 20-2).

Rates of combined all-cause mortality, MI, and severe recurrent ischemia prompting urgent revascularization through 14 days after randomization are associated with number of TIMI risk factors. Event rates increase significantly as the TIMI risk score increases (P < 0.001 for trend).[21] Patients with a score of ≤2 are considered low risk; 3-4, intermediate risk; and ≥5, high risk. Cardiology consultation in the hospital is reasonable for all patients with intermediate and high risk.

GRACE Score

The GRACE Prediction Score (Fig. 20-3) is a validated tool to predict 6-month postdischarge mortality following ACS

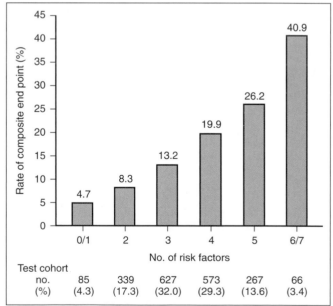

Test cohort						
no.	85	339	627	573	267	66
(%)	(4.3)	(17.3)	(32.0)	(29.3)	(13.6)	(3.4)

Figure 20-2 • The TIMI Risk Score for predicting 14-day risk of mortality/MI/urgent revascularization in patients with NSTEMI/USA. From: Antman E, Cohen M, Bernink P, et al. The TIMI Risk Score for unstable angina/non-ST elevation MI: a method for prognostication and therapeutic decision making. JAMA 2000; 284:835–842.

RISK CALCULATOR FOR 6-MONTH POSTDISCHARGE MORTALITY
AFTER HOSPITALIZATION FOR ACUTE CORONARY SYNDROME

Record the points for each variable at the bottom left and sum the points to calculate the total risk score.
Find the total score on the x-axis of the nomogram plot. The corresponding probability on the y-axis is
the estimated probability of all-cause mortality from hospital discharge to 6 months.

Medical history	Findings at initial hospital presentation	Findings during hospitalization
1 Age in years Points	**4 Resting heart rate, beats/min** Points	**7 Initial serum creatinine, mg/dL** Points
≤29 — 0	≤49.9 — 0	0–0.39 — 1
30–39 — 0	50–69.9 — 3	0.4–0.79 — 3
40–49 — 18	70–89.9 — 9	0.8–1.19 — 5
50–59 — 36	90–109.9 — 14	1.2–1.59 — 7
60–69 — 55	110–149.9 — 23	1.6–1.99 — 9
70–79 — 73	150–199.9 — 35	2–3.99 — 15
80–89 — 91	≥200 — 43	≥4 — 20
≥90 — 100		
2 History of congestive heart failure — 24	**5 Systolic blood pressure, mm Hg**	**8 Elevated cardiac enzymes** — 15
3 History of myocardial infarction — 12	≤79.9 — 24	**9 No in-hospital percutaneous coronary intervention** — 14
	80–99.9 — 22	
	100–119.9 — 18	
	120–139.9 — 14	
	140–159.9 — 10	
	160–199.9 — 4	
	≥200 — 0	
	6 ST-segment depression — 11	

Points

1 ____
2 ____
3 ____
4 ____
5 ____
6 ____
7 ____
8 ____
9 ____

Total risk score ____ (Sum of points)

Mortality risk ____ (From plot)

PREDICTED ALL-CAUSE MORTALITY
FROM HOSPITAL DISCHARGE TO 6 MONTHS

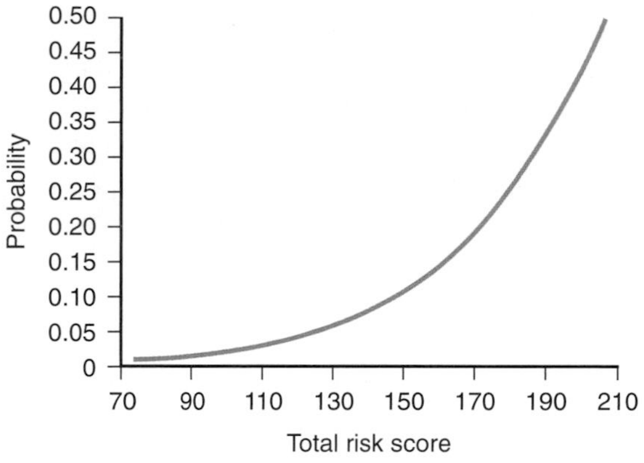

Figure 20-3 • GRACE Score.

MANAGEMENT

(see Chapter 19). Points are assigned for medical history (age, history of CHF and MI), findings at initial presentation (heart rate, systolic blood pressure, and presence of ST-segment depression), and findings during hospitalization (initial serum creatinine, elevated cardiac enzymes, and absence of inhospital PCI).[22] The same GRACE scoring system was derived and validated among both STEMI and NSTEMI patients, allowing one prediction tool for both groups of patients.

Treatment

Preferred

Initial

The primary goals in management of NSTEMI are relief of ischemia and prevention of life-threatening complications, with

Table 20-5 Recommended Initial Treatment for NSTEMI/USA and Dosing

Antiplatelet	Aspirin	162–325 mg (nonenteric) chewed followed by 75–325 mg PO daily
	Clopidogrel	300 mg PO × 1, then 75 mg PO daily
Antithrombotic	Unfractionated heparin	Bolus 60 units/kg (up to 4,000 units), then infusion 12 units/kg/h (up to 1,000 units) with goal PTT 1.5–2.0 times control Reduce to 50 units/kg if using glycoprotein IIb/IIIa inhibitor
	Enoxaparin	30 mg IV bolus, then 1 mg/kg SQ q 12 hr
Glycoprotein	Eptifibatide (Integrilin)	135 mcg/kg bolus, then
IIb/IIIa		0.5 mcg/kg/min × 20–24 hr
Inhibitor	Tirofiban (Aggrastat)	0.4 mcg/kg/min × 30 min, then 0.1 mcg/kg/ming × 48 + hr
	Abciximab (ReoPro)	0.25 mcg/kg bolus, then 0.125 mcg/kg/min × 12 hr
Antianginal	Nitroglycerin	Sublingual: 0.4 mg q 5 minutes for pain relief IV: start at 10–30 mcg/min, titrate to relief of pain, keeping SBP >90 mm Hg Topical: 1–1½ inches paste applied q 8 hr
	β-blockers* Metoprolol Atenolol	Initial IV dose, then maintenance oral dose Begin at 6.25–25 mg q 8–12 hr, increase as tolerated Begin at 25 mg daily, increase as tolerated
ACE inhibitors		In first 24 hours, start oral ACE inhibitor in all patients with anterior infarction, pulmonary edema, EF <40%, and absence of hypotension or contraindications.
Angiotensin receptor blockers		Use ARB if ACE intolerant due to cough.

*β-blockers without intrinsic sympathomimetic activity (ISA) are recommended: metoprolol, atenolol, esmolol, propranolol.

anti-ischemic, antiplatelet, and antithrombotic therapy. Treatment recommendations are summarized in Table 20-5.

Antiplatelet and Antithrombotic Therapy

Aspirin

Aspirin irreversibly inhibits platelet function, and has been found to significantly reduce short-term mortality in patients with acute MI and USA. Pooled data from four randomized trials comparing aspirin to placebo found a 25–30% reduction in the risk of death or MI.[6]

Recommendations: All patients suspected of acute MI should immediately receive ASA 160–325 mg chewed, unless they have a true aspirin allergy (anaphylaxis) or have active major bleeding.

Thienopyridines: Clopidogrel and Ticlopidine

Clopidogrel is a thienopyridine, which acts by irreversibly antagonizing platelet adenosine diphosphate (ADP) receptors. Patients with NSTE-ACS who are allergic to aspirin and those who are not expected to undergo early revascularization should be treated with clopidogrel on presentation. For patients planned for early intervention, clopidogrel is initiated following percutaneous coronary intervention (PCI). As clopidogrel significantly increases surgical bleeding and need for transfusion, it should be withheld for 5–7 days if coronary artery bypass grafting (CABG) is indicated.[23]

The recommendations for clopidogrel are largely based on the CURE trial, which evaluated clopidogrel in more than 12,000 patients with NSTE-ACS. The risk of cardiovascular death, MI, or stroke was significantly reduced in clopidogrel-treated patients (11.4% vs. 9.3%, P < 0.001, NNT 45). Approximately 75% of patients did not undergo early intervention, and fewer than 10%

received glycoprotein IIb/IIIa inhibitors. Major bleeding was significantly increased (NNH 100).[24] The PCI-CURE trial compared clopidogrel to placebo in 2,658 patients with NSTE-ACS undergoing PCI. The composite endpoint of cardiovascular death, MI, or urgent target-vessel revascularization with in 30 days of PCI was reduced by 30% (number needed to treat [NNT] 53).[25]

Heparins

- **Unfractionated heparin (UFH):** UFH is routinely used in patients with ACS. A 1996 meta-analysis that included six randomized trials comparing unfractionated heparin plus aspirin with aspirin alone in a total of 1,353 patients with USA and non–Q wave MI found a reduced risk of MI or death during treatment that approached statistical significance (RR 0.67, 95% CI, 0.44–1.02; P = 0.06) in the heparin-treated group; however, this benefit did not persist at 2–12 weeks following treatment. There was no significant increase in major bleeding.[26]
- **Low-molecula-weight-heparin (LMWH):** Enoxaparin is at least as safe and effective as UFH for reducing 30-day mortality and reinfarction, and two meta-analyses suggest that enoxaparin may be more effective than UFH for reducing death or MI.[27,28] Other LMWHs, particularly nadroparin and dalteparin, have not shown the same benefit as enoxaparin.[29,30]

Meta-analysis of six randomized trials comparing enoxaparin with UFH, including 21,946 patients, found no difference in 30-day mortality, but did find a small although significant reduction in the combined outcome of death or MI at 30 days in patients treated with enoxaparin (OR 0.91, 95% CI 0.83–0.99, NNT 107). When patients who received prerandomization antithrombin therapy were excluded, the benefit with enoxaparin was larger (OR 0.81, 95% CI 0.70–0.89, NNT 72). There was no significant difference in blood transfusion or major bleeding at 7 days.[28] The INTERACT trial showed that in high-risk patients receiving the glycoprotein (GP) IIb/IIIa inhibitor eptifibatide, enoxaparin was more effective than UFH for improving early outcomes.[31] Follow-up at 2.5 years showed a sustained benefit in the enoxaparin group, with a 39% reduction in the risk of death or MI (NNT 17).[32]

Recommendations: Patients with NSTE-ACS should receive either UFH or enoxaparin, unless contraindicated based on high bleeding risk or history of HITT. Enoxaparin offers the convenience of easier administration, and it avoids the need for monitoring serum levels and drip adjustments. Despite higher drug acquisition costs, overall costs may be lower with enoxaparin than with UFH.[33]

Glycoprotein (GP) IIb/IIIa Inhibitors

The GP IIb/IIIa inhibitors act by occupying the platelet GP IIb/IIIa receptors, preventing fibrinogen binding, and thereby preventing platelet aggregation. A GP IIb/IIIa inhibitor is indicated for patients with NSTE-ACS who are planned to undergo early revascularization and for high-risk patients (ST depression, elevated troponin, or ongoing ischemia) who are managed medically. Due to results of the GUSTO-IV trial, which showed that high-risk NSTE-ACS patients treated with abciximab had a small but significant increase in mortality at 48 hours (NNH 100), abciximab is not indicated for patients not planned for revascularization.[34] For these patients, either tirofiban or eptifibatide should be administered.

GP IIb/IIIa inhibitors have the clearest benefit among patients who undergo revascularization.[35–38] For example, in the PURSUIT trial of eptifibatide, the risk of death/nonfatal MI at 30 days was reduced by 31% among patients who underwent revascularization compared to a nonsignificant 7% reduction among patients who were not revascularized.[37] Meta-analysis of randomized trials including more than 31,000 patients not planned to undergo early revascularization who were randomized to a IIb/IIIa inhibitor versus placebo showed a significant reduction in death and non-fatal MI at 5 days and at 30 days (OR 0.91, 95% CI 0.85–0.98, NNT 100).[39] GP IIb/IIIa inhibitors were associated with a 1% absolute risk increase of major bleeding but did not increase intracranial bleeding.[39] Of note, when the patients who did undergo revascularization were excluded from the analysis, the benefit of IIb/IIIa inhibitors did not reach statistical significance.

β-Blockers

As a result of negative inotrope and chronotropic activity, β-blockers reduce heart rate and myocardial contractility, decreasing myocardial oxygen demand. While not specifically studied among US patients, β-blockers have been shown to reduce morbidity or mortality in patients with acute MI, recent MI, and stable angina. The TIMI IIB trial showed reductions in reinfarction and recurrent ischemia, but not mortality, at 42 days with early versus delayed (starting at day 6) administration of metoprolol, with the greatest benefit when given within 2 hours of symptom onset.

Contraindications to β-blockers include bradycardia (HR <60), hypotension, moderate to severely decompensated heart failure, and active bronchospasm. Recommendations to avoid use of β-blockers in patients with cocaine-induced infarction are based on theoretical concerns of exacerbating coronary spasm; however, adverse effects from β-blockers have not been clearly substantiated in this setting.

Early Invasive versus Noninvasive Strategy

An early invasive strategy refers to the practice of routine cardiac catheterization for NSTEMI/USA patients with revascularization as indicated, while a noninvasive strategy (also called conservative or ischemia-guided) manages patients medically unless indicators of ongoing or recurrent ischemia are present. The 2002 ACC/AHA Guidelines recommend an early invasive strategy for patients who have the following characteristics: recurrent ischemia, elevated troponin, new ST segment depression, new heart failure, high-risk stress test, EF <40%, hemodynamic instability, sustained ventricular tachycardia, PCI within 6 months, or prior CABG.[6]

These recommendations are based on the results of three randomized trials (FRISC-II, TACTICS-TIMI 18, and RITA-3) comparing early invasive versus noninvasive strategies for patients with NSTE-ACS.[40–43] Patients in each trial were treated with ASA and heparin or LMWH, with a IIb/IIIa inhibitor. Each trial found that patients in the early invasive group had improved outcomes (recurrent angina or revascularization), although mortality was only reduced in the FRISC-II trial. Meta-analysis of early invasive versus conservative strategies showed reduction in MI, severe angina, and rehospitaliztion. A subgroup analysis that included these three trials (but excluded three earlier trials before use of GP IIb/IIIa inhibitors which showed benefit to conservative treatment) found reductions in mortality and MI in troponin-positive patients who were managed with the early invasive approach.[44]

However, the more recent ICTUS trial that compared early invasive management (within 48 hours) to selectively invasive management in high-risk NSTE-ACS patients did not find a reduction in the primary endpoint of death, nonfatal MI, or rehospitalization for anginal symptoms within 1 year after randomization. Mortality in both arms was 2.5%. In contrast to findings from earlier trials, the early invasive group had a higher rate of MI, although there were fewer rehospitalizations.[45] While results of this trial are in contrast to earlier randomized trials, it is possible that improvements in medical treatment may have narrowed the gap between the two strategies.

Risk Stratification: Noninvasive Testing

Selection of Patients

Noninvasive stress testing is recommended for patients with confirmed NSTEMI/USA who did not undergo early invasive testing or for confirmation of the diagnosis of ischemia (among patients in whom MI has been excluded). Patients with NSTEMI/USA who are being managed medically should have evaluation of left ventricular (LV) function prior to discharge and should be referred for catheterization if systolic dysfunction is present. If LV function is normal, patients should undergo predischarge stress testing to evaluate for recurrent ischemia. Low-risk patients (TIMI score ≤2) should be symptom free for at least 12 hours, and intermediate patients (TIMI score of 3 or 4) should be free of symptom for at least 48 hours prior to testing.[6]

Selection of Test

A number of tests are available to evaluate cardiac ischemia. The choice of tests should be based on local availability and experience, the patient's ability to exercise, gender, and baseline ECG abnormalities.

1. The exercise treadmill test is appropriate for patients able to exercise in whom the ECG is free of baseline ST-segment abnormalities, bundle branch block, LV hypertrophy, intraventricular conduction defect, paced rhythm, preexcitation, and digoxin effect. Adding an imaging modality provides greater accuracy for women.[6,46] If above ECG abnormalities are present, a nuclear imaging (i.e., exercise thallium) should be used to add sensitivity to low-level exercise testing.

2. For patients unable to exercise, pharmacologic stress testing with imaging, such as dipyridamole thallium or dobutamine stress echocardiography (sensitivity 78%, specificity 88%) are tests with similar accuracy. Newer tests for diagnosing ischemia include positron emission tomography (PET) scanning, coronary magnetic resonance angiogram (MRA), 64-slice CT, and computed tomography (CT)-angiography.

Diagnostic accuracy of noninvasive tests has generally been evaluated in patients who do not have acute ischemia. Meta-analysis of pharmacologic stress testing that included studies with varying prevalences of CAD (33%–100%) found the sensitivity and specificity of both dipyridamole and dobutamine echocardiography to be 76–79% and 86–89%, respectively, with no gender differences noted.[47] PET scanning appears be diagnostically superior to sestamibi SPECT, with sensitivity of 87% versus 82% and specificity of 93% versus 73%, using a definition of 70% angiographic stenosis as significant ischemia.[48]

In terms of risk stratification for conservatively treated patients, the presence of recurrent ischemia or high-risk findings on stress testing predicts higher mortality. In the VANQWISH trial of invasive versus conservative management for NSTE-ACS, mortality at 1 month and 1 year among conservatively treated patients with high-risk stress tests was 3% and 13%, compared to rates of 1% and 6% among patients without these findings.[49]

Additional Medications That Should Be Added During Hospitalization

1. Clopidogrel: For all patients following coronary intervention
2. ACE-inhibitors: Shown to reduce mortality in patients with CAD (HOPE trial) and in patients with systolic heart failure
3. Lipid lowering: The goal for patients with established CAD is to lower low-density lipoprotein (LDL) <70. Unless contraindicated, all patients should be discharged on a statin. If patients on a high-dose statin have not reached goal LDL, ezetimibe or niacin may be added.

Alternative Options

- Angiotensin receptor blockers may be used in patients intolerant of ACE inhibitors due to cough.
- Long-acting calcium channel blockers are acceptable anti-anginals for patients who are unable to tolerate β-blockers or who need additional blood pressure lowering.

PREVENTION

Risk-factor modification should be stressed to patients hospitalized with ACS. Patients should receive counseling on the following that apply (*see* "Patient Instruction"):
1. Smoking cessation with outpatient referral
2. Diet: low cholesterol, low saturated fat
3. Exercise and cardiac rehabilitation referral
4. Weight loss
5. Substance abuse
6. Medication compliance

DISCHARGE/FOLLOW-UP PLANS

Patients diagnosed with acute coronary syndrome and believed to have coronary artery disease should be prescribed five medications at discharge if there are no contraindications: aspirin, β-blocker, statin, ACE inibitor (or ARB), and clopidogrel. Recommended discharge medications are summarized in Table 20-6.

Patient Instruction

1. Activity: Recommendations from ACC/AHA Guidelines[50]
   - **All patients should be given a referral for cardiac rehabilitation at the time of discharge.** Cardiac rehabilitation is a comprehensive long-term program that involves medical evaluation, prescribed exercise, cardiac risk-factor modification, education, and counseling.

Table 20-6 Discharge Medications

All patients without contraindications should receive
1. Aspirin 75–162 mg daily
2. Clopidogrel 75 mg daily
3. β-blocker
4. ACE inhibitor (ARB if intolerant)
5. Statin with additional lipid lowering as needed to acheive LDL <70 mg/dL

Additional or Alternative Medications for Special Conditions:

Hypertriglyceridemia (TG >500 mg/dL):	• Fibrate
Indication for anticoagulation	• **Stent placed:**
	• Aspirin plus warfarin with target INR 2.0–3.0
	• **No stent placed: do NOT use clopidogrel**
	• Aspirin plus warfarin (target INR 2.0–3.0)
	OR
	• Warfarin alone (target INR 2.5–3.5)

ACE—angiotensin converting enzyme; ARB—angiotensin receptor blocker; LDL—low density lipoprotein; TG—triglycerides; IINR—international normalized enzyme

- Based on risk assessment or exercise testing, daily walking should be initiated immediately, with a goal of at least 30 minutes of aerobic activity daily, but at a minimum of three or four times a week.
- In stable patients without complications, sexual activity can be resumed within 7–10 days.
- Timing of return to work must be individualized, based on physical and emotional stress involved, whether successful reperfusion was achieved, severity of heart failure symptoms, and complications during hospitalization. Patients with successful reperfusion who return to work in the first month following STEMI do not have an increase risk of adverse events.[51] In the PAMI-II trial, low-risk patients (i.e., age <70 years, ejection fraction greater than 0.45, 1- or 2-vessel disease, and good PTCA result) encouraged to return to work at 2 weeks experienced no adverse events.[52]
- Driving can begin 1 week after discharge, with restrictions per individual state laws. Patients who experienced serious arrhythmias, cardiogenic shock, or required cardiopulmonary resuscitation (CPR) should delay driving 2–3 weeks after symptoms have stabilized.
- Air travel is safe within 2 weeks in stable patients, but should be avoided in those with rest angina or dyspnea and with fear of flying, as the reduced oxygen tension in aircrafts may lead to hypoxia.

2. Diet
- Low saturated fat: <7% of total calories as saturated fats, <200 mg of cholesterol per day, and increased consumption of omega-3 fatty acids.
- Low sodium: for patients with heart failure or hypertension
- Weight management: desirable body mass index (BMI) between 18.5 and 25 kg/m^2

Outpatient Physician Communication

Patients should be given a follow-up appointment with their primary care provider within 2–4 weeks of discharge (See Chapter 19).

Key Points

- USA is a clinical diagnosis based on characteristic chest pain or anginal equivalents (i.e., dyspnea, arm pain, nausea) that is typically associated with activity and relieved by rest. ECG changes support the diagnosis; however, they are not necessary for the diagnosis.
- About 90% of patients with AMI are likely to have traditional risk factors for coronary disease.
- All patients suspected of acute MI should immediately receive ASA 160–325 mg chewed, unless they have a true aspirin allergy (anaphylaxis) or have active major bleeding.

- Recent research comparing early invasive management (within 48 hours) to selectively invasive management in high-risk NSTE-ACS patients did not find a reduction in the primary endpoint of death, nonfatal MI, or rehospitalization for anginal symptoms within 1 year after randomization.
- Patients diagnosed with ACS due to CAD should be prescribed five medications at discharge if there are no contraindications: aspirin, β-blocker, statin, ACE inibitor (or ARB), and clopidogrel.
- All patients diagnosed with ACS and CAD should be given a referral for cardiac rehabilitation at the time of discharge.

SUGGESTED READING

CRUSADE. www.crusade.com. 2006.

James S, Lindahl B, Timmer J, et al. Usefulness of biomarkers for predicting long-term mortality in patients with diabetes mellitus and non-ST-elevation acute coronary syndromes (a GUSTO IV substudy). Am J Cardiol 2006; 97:167–172.

Eagle K, Lim M, Dabbous O, et al. A validated prediction model for all forms of acute coronary syndrome: Estimating the risk of 6-month postdischarge death in an international registry. JAMA 2004; 291:2727–2733.

Yusuf S, Zhao F, Mehta S, et al. Effects of clopidogrel in addition to aspirin in patients with acute coronary syndromes without ST-segment elevation. N Engl J Med 2001; 345:494–502.

Mehta S, Yusuf S, Peters R. Effects of pretreatment with clopidogrel and aspirin followed by long-term therapy in patients undergoing percutaneous coronary intervention: the PCI-CURE study. Lancet 2001; 358:527–533.

Petersen J, Mahaffey K, Hasselblad V, et al. Efficacy and bleeding complications among patients randomized to enoxaparin or unfractionated heparin for antithrombin therapy in non-ST-segment elevation acute coronary syndromes: A systematic overview. JAMA 2004; 292:89–96.

Fitchett D, Langer A, Armstrong P, et al. Randomized evaluation of the efficacy of enoxaparin versus unfractionated heparin in high-risk patients with non-ST-segment elevation acute coronary syndromes receiving the glycoprotein IIb/IIIa inhibitor eptifibatide. Long-term results of the Integrilin and Enoxaparin Randomized Assessment of Acute Coronary Syndrome Treatment (INTERACT) trial. Am Heart J 2006; 151:373–379.

Mehta S, Cannon C. Routine vs selective invasive strategies in patients with acute coronary syndromes: a collaborative meta-analysis of randomized trials. JAMA 2005; 293:2908–2917.

deWinter R, Windhausen F, Cornel J, et al. Invasive versus conservative treatment in Unstable Coronary Syndromes (ICTUS) Investigators: Early invasive versus selectively invasive management for acute coronary syndromes. N Engl J Med 2005; 353:1095–1104.

Kim C, Kwok Y, Heagerty P, et al. Pharmacologic stress testing for coronary disease diagnosis: a met-analysis. Am Heart J 2001; 142:934–944.

Antman E, Anbe D, Armstrong P, et al. ACC/AHA guidelines for management of patients with ST elevation myocardial infarction. J Am Coll Cardiol 2004; 44:671–719.

CHAPTER TWENTY-ONE

Heart Failure

Wassim H. Fares, MD, and Franklin A. Michota, MD

BACKGROUND

Congestive heart failure, now referred to as heart failure (HF), is a clinical syndrome characterized by a decreased ability of the heart to effectively pump blood out of the lungs and/or the venous system into the arterial system. Approximately five million Americans suffer from HF, with 300,000 deaths and 550,000 new cases annually. It accounts for approximately one million hospital admissions in the United States, costing an estimated $38 billion or 5.4% of the total US health care budget.[1] Six to ten percent of people older than 65 years of age carry this diagnosis, and the elderly population continues to grow. HF is the most common discharge diagnosis for US hospitals today and currently represents the single largest expense for the Medicare program.

CLINICAL PRESENTATION

Presenting Signs and Symptoms

HF is a chronic, remitting, and relapsing illness. Most patients spend most of their time in a compensated phase, yet the natural history of HF is a progressive course that ultimately ends in repeated decompensated episodes and death. The most common reasons for decompensation include: nonadherence to medications and/or diet, inadequate dose of medications, progression of disease, acute coronary syndrome (ACS), uncontrolled hypertension, arrhythmia, thyroid disease, valvular decompensation, and viral myocarditis. Certain medications, through various mechanisms, may increase the body's retention of fluids and electrolytes (e.g., nonsteroidal anti inflammatory drugs [NSAIDs], steroids, insulin sensitizers [e.g., rosiglitazone]), or directly compromise the heart's ability to adequately shift blood from the venous to the arterial system (e.g., calcium channel blockers [CCB], certain antiarrhythmics, chemotherapeutic agents [e.g., adriamycin] and cardiotoxic drugs), and thus induce acute decompensated heart failure (ADHF) (Table 21-1).

The clinical presentation of ADHF is variable. Patients may have symptoms ranging from generalized daily fatigue or mild shortness of breath at rest, to full cardiogenic shock, or even sudden death. HF is often categorized in terms of the type (systolic or diastolic) or ventricle involved (left or right). In systolic HF, there is a decreased ventricular ejection fraction (EF) while in diastolic HF there is decreased ventricular compliance. Left HF symptoms are mainly related to pulmonary congestion, with or without decreased cardiac output. Right HF leads to systemic venous congestion, manifesting as jugular venous distention (JVD), ascites, and lower extremity edema. The most common cause of right HF is left HF, and the separation of the symptoms between right and left HF is often artificial.

Congested patients often present with pulmonary complaints such as shortness of breath (dyspnea) on exertion or at rest, difficulty breathing while lying flat (orthopnea), paroxysmal nocturnal dyspnea (PND) or awakening from sleep with shortness of breath, and cough that is typically nonproductive or productive of pinkish-colored sputum. Additional congestive symptoms include lower extremity edema, abdominal distention (if ascites is present), abdominal pain, anorexia, and early satiety. Perfusion abnormalities do not tend to result in physical complaints and are more often detected on blood chemistries and/or physical examination. Change in mental status and impaired kidney function may signify decreased perfusion. Patients with abnormal perfusion but no congestion are known as "cold and dry." Those with normal perfusion but evidence of congestion are referred to as "warm and wet." "Cold and wet" patients tend to be the sickest, as they have poor perfusion and congestion (Table 21-2).[2]

Since HF is a disease of the elderly,[15] the influence of comorbidities will alter the presentation of ADHF. Patients with dysrhythmias, such as new-onset or uncontrolled atrial fibrillation, may have signs and symptoms of HF along with palpitations. Cerebrovascular accidents or transient ischemic attacks may also present with HF in the setting of intracardiac thrombi and peripheral emboli. Any uncompensated chronic disease may precipitate HF and will be associated with a varied symptom complex. Common comorbid examples include coronary ischemia with chest pain; chronic obstructive pulmonary disease (COPD) with wheezing and purulent cough; pneumonia with shortness of breath and fever; thyroid disease with weight loss, tremors, diaphoresis, or ophthalmologic signs; and diabetes mellitus with polyuria or polydipsia.

Physical examination findings in ADHF depend upon the type of HF and the severity of the decompensated state. Patients are generally noted to be in distress with abnormal vital signs. Tachycardia and tachypnea with Cheyne-Stokes respirations are often present. Blood pressure may be elevated or low. Confusion or mental status change is suggestive of poor perfusion. Findings in right HF include JVD with or without a hepatojugular reflex,

Table 21-1 Medication "Usual Suspects" for Inducing Heart Failure Exacerbation

Mechanism	Direct Cardiac Effect	Fluid retention	Miscellaneous
Medication	CCB Beta-blockers Antiarrhythmics	NSAIDS Alpha-blockers Corticosteroids Insulin sensitizers	Chemotherapeutic agents Cardiotoxic drugs

CCB—calcium channel blocker; NSAIDS—nonsteroidal anti-inflammatory drugs.

Table 21-2 Low Perfusion vs. Congestion at Rest in Heart Failure

	CONGESTION AT REST	
Low Perfusion at Rest	**No**	**Yes**
No	Warm and dry PCWP and CI normal	Warm and wet PCWP elevated and CI normal
Yes	Cold and Dry PCWP low/normal and CI decreased	Cold and wet PCWP elevated and CI decreased

PCWP—Pulmonary capillary wedge pressure; CI—cardiac index.

lower extremity edema, ascites, and right upper quadrant pain with palpation (due to congestion of the liver). Left HF is associated with a cardiac gallop (i.e., S_3 or S_4), displaced point of maximal impulse (PMI), and congestion of the lungs with crackles, wheezing, tachypnea, and hypoxia. Other signs include a narrow pulse pressure, a parasternal heave (seen with right ventricular hypertrophy and right HF), cardiac murmurs (with associated valvular pathology), a friction rub, diminished heart sounds, and decreased extremities temperature.

DIFFERENTIAL DIAGNOSIS

Many HF symptoms are nonspecific (dypsnea), and HF may coexist or be precipitated by other diagnoses. Life-threatening conditions that can present with shortness of breath with or without hypotension should be investigated expeditiously and include ACS with anginal equivalent, pulmonary emboli, tension pneumothorax, and cardiac tamponade. Pulmonary diseases, including but not limited to COPD exacerbation, asthma exacerbation, or pneumonia, are also high on the differential diagnosis list. The possibility of anxiety or panic attacks or other psychiatric pathologies also exists. Finally, any condition that can cause noncardiogenic pulmonary edema may mimic or coexist with ADHF.

Diagnostic Studies

Preferred

Patients presenting with suspected ADHF should have a chest radiograph (CXR) and an electrocardiogram (ECG). Blood should be drawn for basic electrolytes, magnesium, kidney function, liver enzymes, albumin, a complete blood count (CBC), cardiac enzymes, and a plasma B-type natriuretic peptide (BNP) level. New ADHF patients should also have a transthoracic echocardiogram performed to characterize the HF as systolic, diastolic, or both.

CXR findings should support acute pulmonary edema and can range from mild pulmonary vascular redistribution to marked

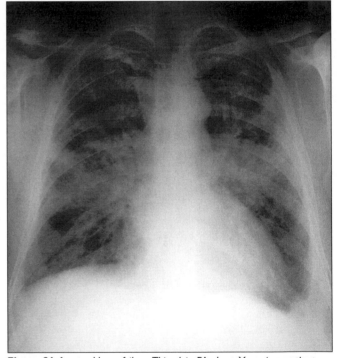

Figure 21-1 • Heart failure. This plain PA chest X-ray in a patient with heart failure shows cardiomegaly, upper lobe diversion, and hilar congestion. Kerley B septal lines were present in the original film but are not visible in this reproduced image. From Burkitt HG, Quick CRG. Essential surgery: problems, diagnosis and management, 3rd Edition. Edinburgh: Churchill Livingstone, 2001.

cardiomegaly and extensive bilateral interstitial markings with Kerley B lines (Figure 21-1). The presence of bilateral perihilar alveolar edema may give the typical "butterfly" appearance. Pleural effusions are often absent, given the acute nature of the accumulation of pulmonary edema. Other significant CXR findings include noncardiac pathology that might explain the patient's symptoms, such as infiltrates, pneumothorax, chest masses, or adenopathy. A normal CXR does not rule out ADHF. Twenty percent of echocardiogram-confirmed cardiomegaly is missed on CXR, and radiograph sensitivity for increased pulmonary capillary wedge pressure (PCWP) is only 65%.

The value of an ECG is not so much to diagnose ADHF as it is to eliminate ACS or arrhythmia as a precipitating cause. The ECG may also provide clues for pericardial disease, or a constrictive (low QRS, electric alternans) or restrictive (such as amyloidosis or other infiltrating diseases) cardiac condition. All patients with ADHF should be evaluated for the presence of ischemic heart disease, and in the absence of a confirmed precipitant for ADHF, should generally have a "rule-out myocardial injury" protocol with cardiac biomarkers and ECGs every 8 hours for the first 24 hours.

Plasma BNP has proven to be of great value in distinguishing between HF and noncardiac diseases, such as COPD, pneumonia, and noncardiac pulmonary edema. BNP is a peptide that is secreted by the cardiac ventricles, and it is responsible for natriuresis, diuresis, and vasodilation in response to increased ventricular pressure. BNP levels have been directly associated with the PCWP and thus the diagnosis of ADHF.[7] In patients with dyspnea, a low BNP level (<100 pg/mL) practically rules out ADHF. Moderate levels of BNP (100–480 pg/mL) indicate that ADHF is likely contributing (alone or in concert with other illnesses) to the patient's symptoms. A very high BNP level (>480 pg/mL) almost always implicates HF as a contributing factor to the patient's symptoms, indicating the need for ADHF treatment (Table 21-3).[9] However, there are factors that can influence the BNP level, and the BNP level should not be used to diagnose or exclude ADHF alone. Any process causing stretch or increased pressure of the ventricles, whether it is systolic or diastolic HF, valvular heart disease, or any pulmonary process that causes increased pressure in the right ventricle (e.g., pulmonary embolism, pulmonary hypertension, emphysema) can elevate the BNP. In addition, advanced age and impaired renal function can elevate the BNP, while morbid obesity is associated with low BNP levels. Table 21-4 outlines other factors that can influence the BNP level.

Transthoracic echocardiography is essential in evaluating the function of the left ventricle (systolic and diastolic) and in identifying the presence of wall motion abnormalities and/or significant valvular heart disease. ADHF therapy is directed toward the type of HF (systolic versus diastolic), and new HF patients should have an echocardiogram to optimize their treatment regimen. Obtaining an echocardiogram in the setting of new ADHF is a Joint Commission Quality-of-Care measure for HF (Table 21-5).

Alternative Options

Additional studies are obtained as directed by the history and physical examination. Patients with tachyarrhythmias and suspected thyroid disease should have a thyroid-stimulating

Table 21-3 BNP Diagnostic Characteristics for HF with A 100 pg/mL Cut-Point

Sensitivity	90%
Specificity	76%
Predictive accuracy	83%
Odds ratio	29.60

Table 21-4 Conditions That Can Influence BNP Levels Other than HF

Increase	Decrease
Advanced age	Flash pulmonary edema
Renal failure	Acute mitral regurgitation
Hypoalbuminemia	Cause of pulmonary edema: upstream of left ventricle (e.g., mitral stenosis)
Lung disease with right-sided failure	
Acute, large pulmonary embolism	
Acute coronary syndrome	
Myocardial infarction	
Cause of pulmonary edema: left ventricle or downstream	

Table 21-5 Joint Commission Quality-of-Care Indicators for HF

	Quality Indicator	Specifications
HF-1	Discharge instructions	Activity level, diet, discharge medications, follow up appointment, weight monitoring, and what to do if symptoms worsen
HF-2	Left ventricular function assessment	Documentation in the hospital record that left ventricular function was assessed before admission, during hospitalization, or is planned for after discharge
HF-3	ACEI or ARB for left ventricular systolic dysfunction	Prescription of ACEI or ARB for heart failure patients with left ventricular systolic dysfunction and without ACEI and ARB contraindications
HF-4	Adult smoking cessation advice/counseling	Documentation in the hospital record of smoking cessation counseling or advice for heart failure patients that are cigarette smokers

HF—heart failure; ACEI—angiotensin converting enzyme inhibitor; ARB—angiotensin receptor blocker

hormone checked. Patients with asymmetric or profound peripheral edema may benefit from a duplex of lower extremities or a D-dimer level. If other etiologies for hypoxia or chest pain remain on the differential, then computed tomography pulmonary angiography should be entertained. Other studies may include electrophysiologic testing (usually limited to those with a history of sustained or symptomatic ventricular tachycardia, unexplained syncope, or cardiac arrest), endomyocardial biopsy (suspected primary cardiac amyloidosis, giant cell myocarditis, active cardiac sarcoidosis, or eosinophilic myocarditis), iron studies for hemochromatosis, HIV load, alcohol level, urine toxicology, antinuclear antibodies, viral serologies, antimyosin antibodies, or genetic testing.

Algorithms

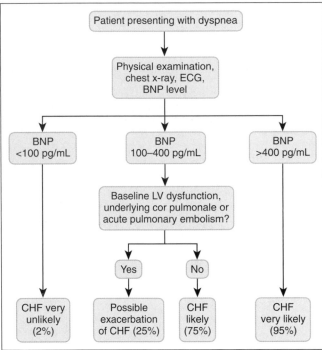

Figure 21-2 • Diagnostic algorithm for HF using BNP.

PROGNOSIS

During Hospitalization

Inhospital mortality rate may vary between 2% and 22%, depending on the patient's risk factors (the average is 4–5%). Kidney function and vital signs upon presentation are the most important prognostic factors of in-hospital mortality (Table 21-6).

Postdischarge

After an index hospitalization for ADHF, the overall prognosis is guarded. You can expect up to 50% of patients to be readmitted to the hospital within 6 months, and the 5-year survival is only 50%. Advanced age, presence of comorbidities, low ejection fraction, advanced New York Heart Association (NYHA) class (Table 21-7), presence of hyponatremia, low exercise capacity, and continued presence (despite aggressive treatment) of an audible S_3 sound or jugular venous distension (JVD) are all poor prognostic factors.[16–19]

Some parameters that have prognostic implications may vary with time, such as NYHA classification or ejection fraction. Moreover, if the etiology of the HF is a reversible one, such as viral infection, the prognosis (depending on the variable being followed) may improve. Arrhythmias, elevated activity of the renin-angiotensin-aldosterone system, elevated blood pressure, decreased renal perfusion, fluid retention, and increased sympathetic activity (manifested by tachycardia, HTN, anxiety, or agitation) are poor prognostic features. Concomitant cardiac

Table 21-6 Mortality in HF Patients Stratified by Blood Pressure and Renal Function				
	BUN	SBP	Cr	Inhospital Mortality (%)
Low risk	<43	<115	N/A	2.14
Intermediate 3	<43	<115	N/A	5.49
Intermediate 2	<43	>115	N/A	6.41
Intermediate 1	<43	<115	<2.75	12.42
High risk	<43	<115	>2.75	21.94

Table 21-7 Classifications of HF	
ACC/AHA Stages of HF	**NYHA Classification**
A: At high risk for developing HF. No symptoms. No structural or functional abnormalities	N/A
B: Developed structural heart disease, but no symptoms	N/A
C: Current or prior symptoms of HF	**I:** No symptoms from ordinary activities **II:** Mild limitation with ordinary activity **III:** Marked limitation with ordinary activity **IV:** Symptomatic even at rest
D: End-stage HF	

Source: Adapted from ACC/AHA 2005 Guideline Update for the Diagnosis and Management of Chronic Heart Failure in the Adult.

diseases generally portend a poorer prognosis for HF patients. Specifically, concomitant diastolic dysfunction, coronary artery disease, right ventricular failure, ventricular tachycardia, and hypotension have significant impact on the overall prognosis. Comorbidities such as diabetes mellitus, systemic or pulmonary hypertension, thyroid disease, obesity, renal insufficiency, or liver disease can negatively affect the HF patient's prognosis. Serum sodium is a very sensitive indicator of the patient's overall state of compensation. Hyponatremia, a sodium of ≤134 mEq/L, is a presumed sign of increased fluid retention and thus is an indication of HF progression (Table 21-8).

TREATMENT

The treatment of patients with ADHF depends on the presence or absence of congestion and poor perfusion.[22] Those who are congested are treated with oral or intravenous (IV) diuretics and vasodilators for afterload reduction. Patients with perfusion abnormalities often require vasoactive therapies such as vasodilators with or without positive inotropic agents. The immediate goals of treatment are to reverse acute hemodynamic abnormalities and to relieve symptoms. Other hospitalization goals include identifying the reason for decompensation; and initiating treatments that will slow disease progression, reduce the risk for rehospitalization, and improve long-term survival.

Table 21-8 Poor Prognostic Variables in HF Patients

1. Laboratory work:
   a. Hyponatremia (Na ≤134 mEq/L)
   b. Renal failure (serum creatinine ≥2.0 mg/dL, increased blood urea nitrogen (BUN))
   c. Elevated BNP
   d. Low EF

2. Functional status:
   a. Six minute walk distance less than 300 meters
   b. Dependency with activities of daily living
   c. Peak oxygen consumption during exercise testing of less than 14 mL/kg/min (4 METS)
   d. NYHA class III or IV for 3 months

3. Symptoms:
   Persistent orthopnea

4. Medical history:
   COPD, dementia, hepatic cirrhosis, cancer, cerebrovascular disease

5. Demographics:
   Age >70 years

6. Vital signs:
   Tachycardia, tachypnea, abnormal blood pressure

METS—metabolic equivalents; COPD—chronic obstructive pulmonary disease; NYHA—New York Hear Association

Preferred

Initial

General Measures

Until there is some relief of symptoms, ADHF patients will generally require bed rest along with a modest fluid restriction. Patients with hypoxia should receive supplemental oxygen to achieve normal oxygen saturations. All comorbidities should be optimized as appropriate.

Medications

Although loop diuretics have not been shown to improve survival, they are the most commonly used medication for HF patients, as they readily improve symptoms in congested patients. Intermittent metolazone, which is a thiazide-like diuretic that inhibits sodium reabsorption in the distal tubule, may be used in conjunction with loop diuretics to enhance diuresis. Thiazide drugs are weak diuretics and are not recommended as a sole diuretic in the setting of HF. The use of an aldosterone antagonist, spironolactone or eplerenone, in patients with NYHA class III and IV HF is associated with a survival benefit in addition to symptomatic relief in the outpatient setting.[3] Despite a suggestion that there is decreased gut absorption of oral diuretics due to gut edema in HF requiring IV diuretic use, no convincing evidence for this phenomenon exists. The oral dose of furosemide is equivalent to half the IV dose (e.g., 40 mg of oral furosemide is equivalent to 20 mg of IV furosemide).

ADHF patients are in a neurohormonally vasoconstricted state. Diuretics do not block the neurohormonal cascade, and following the initial administration of diuretics is documented to potentiate renin secretion, increase PCWP, increase mean arterial pressure, and increase circulating norepinephrine levels. Theoretically, vasodilators should return the ADHF patient to a homeostatic balance in a way that diuretics cannot; thus, there is a renewed emphasis on initial vasodilator therapy in ADHF. The three most commonly used vasodilators are nitroglycerine, sodium nitroprusside, and nesiritide (Table 21-9). They all share the side effect of hypotension. Nitroglycerine exerts its vasodilatory effect by dilating both the arterial and, more significantly, the venous system, thus reducing the preload. It is relatively cheap, but tolerance develops within 24 hours. The most common adverse effect is severe headache, which can be seen in up to 20% of patients. Sodium nitroprusside causes vasodilation by directly relaxing the venous and arteriolar smooth muscles. There is the potential for cyanide toxicity, especially when its use is prolonged, high doses are used, or the patient has renal insufficiency; however, the greatest limitation with nitroprusside therapy is that it requires careful IV titration, generally requiring invasive arterial blood pressure monitoring in an intensive care unit (ICU)

Table 21-9 Vasodilators in HF

Vasodilator agent	t½	Key Point
Nitroglycerine	3–5 minutes	Causes tachyphylaxis, leads to severe headache in 20% of patients
Nesiritide	20 minutes	Neurohormonal blocker, no titration needed, some questions as to safety
Nitroprusside	4 hours	Toxic metabolites, requires ICU care

setting. Routinely placing ADHF patients in an ICU for initial vasodilator therapy would be cost prohibitive.

Nesiritide is recombinant human B-type natriuretic peptide. It causes an increase in intracellular cyclic guanylate monophosphate (cGMP), and thus causes relaxation of vascular smooth muscle and endothelial cells. As expected, nesiritide is believed to promote diuresis, natriuresis, and ventricular relaxation in the same fashion as endogenous BNP; and unlike the aforementioned vasodilators, nesiritide is an intravenous neurohormonal blocker.[8] Nesiritide causes significantly fewer headaches than nitroglycerine, and it does not lead to tachyphylaxis. Nesiritide does not require titration and can be administered on a regular telemetry floor, thus reducing the cost of HF therapy. When compared to IV nitroglycerine or placebo, nesiritide showed improved outcomes of dyspnea, global clinical scores, and reduction in PCWP. Two meta-analyses have raised concerns about adverse renal effects and a potential increase in short-term mortality with nesiritide infusion.[5] However, a review of all the available clinical studies involving nesiritide neither confirms nor refutes these concerns. There is a known dose-dependent effect on creatinine with nesiritide infusion, likely related to excessive hypotension. A review of the phase III FDA labeling study for nesiritide (VMAC trial) demonstrated no difference in hypotension compared to nitroglycerine. Patients who did have a >0.5-mg/dL increase in serum creatinine with nesiritide infusion did not demonstrate an increased risk for death. Furthermore, analysis of the ADHERE registry does not support an increased risk of death with nesiritide infusion compared to nitroglycerin, dobutamine, or milrinone. Presently, nesiritide is FDA labeled for the inpatient treatment of ADHF in patients with dyspnea at rest, but no studies demonstrate significant advantage compared to optimal standard therapy with diuretics and other vasodilators. Hospitalists would benefit patients by using an order set or guidelines to manage patients with ADHF.[6]

For the vast majority of ADHF patients, vasodilators and diuretics will be sufficient as initial therapy. However, patients with poor perfusion and cardiogenic shock will need inotropic support, despite potentially adverse consequences. Positive inotropic agents have been shown to independently increase mortality, exacerbate underlying ischemia, and induce ventricular arrhythmias, especially with prolonged use (more than 72 hours). It is important to carefully select those ADHF patients for which the risk/benefit ratio favors inotropic therapy. Two commonly used inotropic agents are dobutamine and milrinone. Dobutamine is an adrenergic agonist, given intravenously for short periods of time for acute resuscitation for cardiac decompensation. As a beta-agonist, dobutamine usually increases heart rate, blood pressure, and ventricular response (e.g., ectopy or ventricular tachycardia), which in turn increases myocardial oxygen demand, which may be detrimental to cardiac compensatory mechanisms. Milrinone is a phosphodiesterase enzyme inhibitor that is also given intravenously for short periods of time in ADHF. It increases the levels of cyclic adenosine monophosphate (cAMP) and thus increases calcium influx into myocardial cells increasing contractility. It may also cause systemic arterial and venous dilation via inhibition of peripheral phosphodiesterase, and thus should be avoided in severe obstructive aortic and pulmonic valvular disease. Like dobutamine, arrhythmias and increased mortality are the main risks of milrinone infusion.

Subsequent

General Measures

New HF patients will need education about their disease and the monitoring of their volume status at home by weighing themselves daily. This process should begin in the hospital if possible. Inpatient dietitian counseling will introduce the patient to the services that are offered by the nutritionist as well as creating a point of contact for outpatient follow up. Similarly, although an exercise program is not appropriate during ADHF, education and referral to outpatient services should be initiated in the hospital. It is also important that the HF patient understand his or her medications, and an inpatient visit by a clinical pharmacist will help reinforce any discharge day education provided by the clinician or nurse.

Medications

Studies have consistently shown that the neurohormonal effects of aldosterone can advance the progression of HF. Angiotensin-converting enzyme inhibitors (ACEI) block the formation of aldosterone by inhibiting conversion of angiotensin I to angiotensin II. Therefore, unless contraindicated, all patients with left ventricular dysfunction, a history of myocardial infarction, or those at high risk for cardiovascular disease (e.g., diabetes mellitus, atherosclerotic vascular disease, or multiple cardiovascular risk factors) should be on an ACEI.[12] ACEIs, as a class, decrease mortality in HF patients. Cough is a common side effect, with renal failure, hypotension, and angioedema being the most serious potential side effects. An angiotensin receptor blocker (ARB) may replace an ACEI, if a patient is intolerant to the ACEI because of angioedema, cough, or rash, as these side effects are due to elevated levels of bradykinin that occur from blockade of the conversion of kinins (by ACEI) to its inactive metabolites. Patients who develop renal failure, hyperkalemia, and hypotension with an ACEI are likely to develop the same with an ARB, as these effects are secondary to decreased stimulation of the angiotensin II receptors, directly by the ARBs, and indirectly through decreased conversion of angiotensin I to angiotensin II by ACEIs. Hydralazine and isosorbide dinitrate are an alternative combination substitute for ACEI, or if the HF is not well managed using the other medical regimens, including an ACEI. Amlodipine or felodipine is an alternative for ACEI and hydralazine/isosorbide dinitrate. These might be very helpful if other medications do not control the blood pressure.

The initiation of beta-blockers (BB) in ADHF patients is associated with poor outcomes due to their negative hemodynamic effects. However, in stable HF patients, multiple randomized controlled studies have shown that BBs reduce total mortality, cardiovascular mortality, cardiovascular or HF hospitalizations, HF symptoms, need for cardiac transplantation, and myocardial infarction in patients with NYHA class II–IV HF. Therefore, BBs should be initiated when the patient is euvolemic, excluding patients with bradycardia, severe bronchoconstrictive disease, and hypotension. Initial doses should be low and titrated up slowly, especially in the elderly. Sustained release metoprolol and carvedilol are both FDA-approved BBs for HF management.

Spironolactone has been shown to reduce morbidity and mortality in HF patients with an EF <35%,[3] and it should be added to a regimen that already includes an ACEI, BB, and loop diuretic. Special attention should be given to the creatinine and potassium levels; potassium supplementation should be withheld or reduced when initiating spironolactone. Gynecomastia occurs in 10% of patients on spironolactone.

Digoxin decreases morbidity by improving HF symptoms and decreasing hospitalizations, especially in those with advanced HF (low EF and NYHA class III or IV), but it has no survival benefit.[4] Digoxin is inexpensive, which is an important advantage, yet this must be balanced against the lack of survival benefit and a narrow therapeutic window.

Anticoagulation

It is not uncommon to see HF patients on systemic anticoagulation with vitamin K antagonists (warfarin). HF patients have a higher incidence of thromboembolism than other patients with a preserved ventricular function, with recent studies showing a thromboembolic incidence in the range of 1.8–2.5% per year.[11,10] Low cardiac output, decreased activity, and peripheral edema predispose to thrombosis. In addition, HF patients are in a relative hypercoagulable state, as manifested by increased blood viscosity, platelet activation, and other markers. Yet despite all of this, HF alone is not an indication for systemic anticoagulation. HF patients need a history of embolic phenomenon or documented intracardiac thrombus prior to meeting the treatment threshold. However, HF is a contributing risk factor for thromboembolism in patients with atrial fibrillation, and thus anticoagulation is indicated in this setting.

Medications to Avoid

Research has shown some medications to be of no benefit in HF, and in some cases they might cause harm. These include, but are not limited to, calcium channel blockers (except amlodipine) for treatment of HF, starting an ARB instead of an ACEI in the absence of contraindications, long-term intermittent use of a positive inotrope infusion, antioxidants, coenzyme-Q, taurine, carnitine, growth hormone, or thyroid hormone. Additional drugs to avoid due to their deleterious effects in HF patients include antiarrhythmics (except amiodarone), nonsteroidal anti-inflammatory drugs (NSAIDS), tricyclic antidepressants, corticosteroids, and lithium.

Alternative Options

Patients with refractory symptoms should be carefully reevaluated to ensure that reversible etiologies and aggravating factors are not missed. Patients with diuretic resistance may benefit from ultrafiltration to maintain euvolemia. If symptoms persist despite such an evaluation, the patient likely has end-stage HF (5% of all HF patients). Treatment options for patients with end-stage HF include heart transplantation, automated implantable cardiac defibrillator (AICD), cardiac resynchronization therapy (CRT), intra-aortic balloon counterpulsation pump (IABP), left ventricular assist device (LVAD), palliative care, and hospice. Patients with a peak oxygen consumption at maximal exercise of <10–14 mL/kg/min usually benefit from heart transplantation. Other indications for heart transplantation included inotrope dependence, recurrent HF hospitalizations despite maximal therapy, severe ischemic symptoms, and refractory cardiogenic shock. Defibrillators were shown to improve survival in patients with history of surviving a sustained ventricular tachycardia or fibril-

lation event, or EF <35% with history of myocardial infarction or HF symptoms. CRT, also called biventricular pacing, is used for HF patients with interventricular conduction delay, low ejection fraction, and moderate-to-severe symptoms despite optimal medical therapy. The rationale for the use of CRT is primarily to avoid dyssynchrony of the ventricles and thus optimize cardiac pump function.[13,14] IABP and LVAD are mechanical devices that support the cardiopulmonary system until a more definitive therapy becomes available, such as heart transplantation or reversal of hemodynamic collapse. If the HF is advanced enough that it is deemed that extra intervention might have greater risks than potential benefits, referral to hospice care is appropriate.

END-OF-LIFE CARE

Discussions concerning end-of-life care are an important part of managing the HF patient. Not having these discussions in a timely manner may subsequently have detrimental effects. Ongoing patient and family education regarding prognosis for function and survival is a class I recommendation by the American College of Cardiology and the American Heart Association (ACC/AHA). Education should cover at least the anticipated course of illness, different management options including their respective side effects and success potential, and overall prognosis. Other ACC/AHA class I recommendations include: patient and family education about options for formulating and implementing advance directives, and making use of components of hospice care that are appropriate to the relief of suffering. A focus on symptom control, and other comfort measures, such as inactivation of implantable defibrillators, may be appropriate in end-stage HF. These discussions ideally should be done at the early stages of the disease (if not even earlier), rather than during hospitalization for ADHF. Yet, inpatient end-of-life discussions may be warranted, particularly if the available HF management options are not relieving symptoms and the overall prognosis for functional recovery is poor.

DISCHARGE/FOLLOW-UP PLANS

Patient Instruction

Documentation of discharge instructions is a Joint Commission quality indicator for HF (see Table 21-5). HF patients should be instructed to monitor their weight frequently and report significant changes to their heath care provider. They should be counseled on the importance of a salt- and fluid-restricted diet, alcohol and smoking cessation, exercise, and routine health maintenance. Patients should fully understand what to do if symptoms should worsen and be provided with a full list of medications. Elevating the legs and the use of compression stockings can cosmetically improve lower extremity edema. A follow-up appointment with a primary care provider should be arranged prior to discharge. All instructions should be given both orally and in a written form.

Outpatient–Physician Communication

HF is a chronic disease that is best cared for within a formal disease-management program and a multidisciplinary team.[20,21] The primary care provider needs a detailed discharge summary

Table 21-10 Reduction in Readmission with a Structured Discharge Program in HF

	Reduction in Readmission (%)	95% CI
Home visit	24	7, 37
Clinic visit	36	−28, 68
Home visit with Phone contact	21	9, 31
Extended home care	18	0, 34

of the hospitalization, the etiology of the decompensated episode, and a full medication list. Multiple discharge programs have been studied, and many have been shown to be very successful. A well-structured discharge program can be as effective as many of the HF medications in reducing mortality and avoiding rehospitalizations (Table 21-10).

Key Points

• The four JCAHO quality indicators for ADHF patients are: checking left ventricular function if not recently checked, starting/continuing an ACEI/ARB for patients with ventricular dysfunction unless contraindicated, discharge instructions, and smoking cessation counseling for smokers.

• Therapy for HF patients should aim at reversing the neurohormonal changes that are the core of the pathophysiology of HF.

• Investigating the cause of the decompensation of HF and trying to correct it may prevent another admission and might be life saving.

• Signing out the patient to the physician who is going to follow up on the patient is crucial for the continuity of care.

• If the prognosis is still poor even with the potential use of evidence-based management that might include high-tech options such as CRT, AICD, or heart transplantation, then consider hospice.

SUGGESTED READING

Hunt SA, Abraham WT, Chin MH, et al. ACC/AHA 2005 guideline update for the diagnosis and management of chronic heart failure in the adult: summary article a report of the American College of Cardiology/American Heart Association Task Force on Practice Guidelines (writing Committee to Update the 2001 Guidelines for the Evaluation and Managment of Heart failure). K Am Coll Cardiol 2005; 46:1116–1143.

Ware LB, Matthay MA. Acute pulmonary edema. N Engl J Med 2005; 353:2788–2796.

Nohria A, Lewis E, Stevenson LW. Medical management of advanced heart failure. JAMA 2002; 287(5):628–640.

Doust JA, Pietrzak E, Dobson A, et al. How well does B-type natriuretic peptide predict death and cardiac events in patients with heart failure: systematic review. BMJ 2005; 330:625–633.

Harrison A, Morrison LK, Krishnaswamy P, et al. B-type natriuretic peptide predicts future cardiac events in patients presenting to the emergency department with dyspnea. Ann Emerg Med 2002; 39(2):131–138.

Bettencourt P, Feneira A, Dias P, et al. Predictors of prognosis in patients with stable mild to moderate heart failure. J Cardiac Failure 2000; 6(4):306–313.

Fonarow GC, Adams KF Jr, Abraham WT, et al. (for the ADHERE Scientific Advisory Committee, Study Group, and Investigators). Risk stratification for in-hospital mortality in acutely decompensated heart failure: classification and regression tree analysis. JAMA 2005; 293:572–580.

Fonarow GC. ADHERE Scientific Advisory Committee. The Acute Decompensated Heart Failure National Registry (ADHERE): opportunities to improve care of patients hospitalized with acute decompensated heart failure. Rev Cardiovasc Med 2003; 7(4 supp):S21–30.

Publication committee for the VMAC investigators. Intravenous nesiritide versus nitroglycerine for treatment of decompensated congestive heart failure: the VMAC trial. JAMA 2002; 287:1531–1540.

Sackner-Bernstein JD, Kowalski M, Fox M, et al. Short-term risk of death after treatment with nesiritide for decompensated heart failure: a pooled analysis of randomized controlled trials. JAMA 2005; 293(15):1900–1905.

Phillips CO, Wright SM, Kern DE, et al. Comprehensive discharge planning with postdischarge support for older patients with congestive heart failure: a meta-analysis. JAMA 2004;291(11): 1358–1367.

Peacock WF 4th, Remer EE, Aponte J, et al.. Effective observation unit treatment of decompensated heart failure. Congest Heart Fail 2002; 8(2):68–73.

Peacock WF, Aponte JH, Craig MT, et al. Inpatient versus emergency department observation unit management of heart failure. Ann Emerg Med 1998; 32:S46.

CHAPTER TWENTY-TWO

Bradyarrhythmias

Arthur C. Kendig, MD, and Mina K. Chung, MD

BACKGROUND

Significant bradycardias consist of arrhythmias with rates of <60 beats/min. The appropriate diagnosis and assessment of the risk associated with arrhythmias are important to their treatment.

SPECIFIC BRADYARRHYTHMIAS: PRESENTATION, PHYSICAL EXAMINATION, DIAGNOSIS, AND TREATMENT

Sinus Node Dysfunction

Sinus node dysfunction ("sick sinus syndrome") includes a range of abnormalities, including sinus bradyarrhythmias (e.g., sinus pauses, sinus bradycardias, chronotropic incompetence, sinus pauses/arrest, sinoatrial exit block) and tachycardia-bradycardia syndrome (e.g., paroxysmal or persistent atrial tachyarrhythmias with periods of bradyarrhythmia). Other forms of sinus node dysfunction that cause tachycardias (e.g., sinus tachycardia, inappropriate sinus tachycardia, sinus node reentry) are discussed in Chapter 23. Treatment depends on the basic rhythm disturbance and etiology. Drug therapy for rapid atrial arrhythmias may aggravate the bradyarrhythmias, and permanent pacing may be required if patients are symptomatic.[2]

Sinus Bradycardia

Sinus bradycardia, which is defined as sinus rates of <60 beats/min, is common in young, healthy adults (especially in athletes), with normal rates during sleep falling to as low as 35–50 beats/min. Though usually benign, it can be associated with diseases such as hypothyroidism, vagal stimulation, increased intracranial pressure, myocardial infarction (MI); and drugs, such as β-blockers (including those used for glaucoma), calcium channel blockers, amiodarone, clonidine, lithium, and parasympathomimetic drugs. Usually, treatment is unnecessary if the patient is asymptomatic. Patients with chronic bradycardia or chronotropic incompetence and symptoms of congestive heart failure or low cardiac output, however, may benefit from permanent pacing.[2]

Sinus Pauses or Sinus Arrest

Sinus pauses or arrest may result from degenerative changes of the sinus node, acute MI, excessive vagal tone or stimuli, digitalis toxicity, sleep apnea, or stroke. Symptomatic or very long pauses may require permanent pacing.

Hypersensitive Carotid Sinus Syndrome

Carotid sinus hypersensitivity can produce sinus arrest or atrioventricular block leading to syncope, and it may be demonstrable with carotid sinus massage. With carotid sinus massage, two types of responses are noted: (1) a cardioinhibitory component with pauses of longer than 3 seconds or (2) a vasodepressor component with a decrease in systolic blood pressure. Symptomatic patients may require pacemaker implantation to treat the cardioinhibitory component. Continued symptoms caused by vasodepressor reactions, even after pacemaker implantation, may require further treatment, including support stockings, high-sodium diets, or sodium-retaining drugs.

Atrioventricular Dissociation

Atrioventricular dissociation refers to independent depolarization of the atria and ventricles. It may be caused by physiologic interference resulting from slowing of the dominant pacemaker (e.g., sinus node) and escape of a subsidiary or latent pacemaker (e.g., junctional or ventricular escape), physiologic interference resulting from acceleration of a latent pacemaker that usurps control of the ventricle (e.g., accelerated junctional tachycardia or ventricular tachycardia [VT]), or atrioventricular block preventing propagation of the atrial impulse from reaching the ventricles, thus allowing a subsidiary pacemaker (e.g., junctional or ventricular escape) to control the ventricles.[2]

Note that patients with complete atrioventricular block have atrioventricular dissociation and, generally, a ventricular rate that is slower than the atrial rate. Patients with atrioventricular dissociation, however, may have complete atrioventricular block or dissociation, resulting from physiologic interference, with the latter typically having an atrial rate that is slower than the ventricular rate.

Figure 22-1 • ECGs showing second-degree AVB, Mobitz type I.

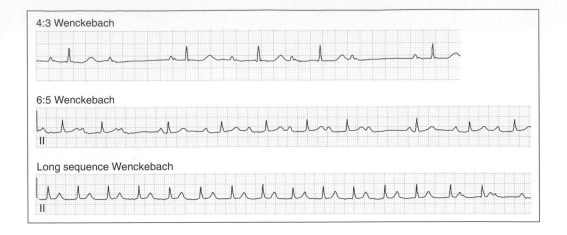

4:3 Wenckebach

6:5 Wenckebach

II

Long sequence Wenckebach

II

Figure 22-2 • ECGs showing second-degree AVB, Mobitz type II.

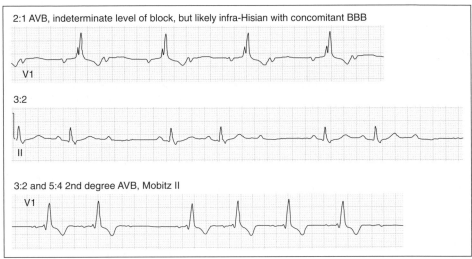

2:1 AVB, indeterminate level of block, but likely infra-Hisian with concomitant BBB

V1

3:2

II

3:2 and 5:4 2nd degree AVB, Mobitz II

V1

BBB—bundle branch block; AVB—artrioventricular block

Atrioventricular Block

Atrioventricular block occurs when the atrial impulse either is not conducted to the ventricle or is conducted with delay at a time when the atrioventricular junction is not refractory. It is classified on the basis of severity into three types.

In first-degree atrioventricular block, conduction is prolonged (PR interval >200 ms), but all impulses are conducted. The conduction delay may occur in the atrioventricular node, the His-Purkinje system, or both. If the QRS complex is narrow and normal, the atrioventricular delay usually occurs in the atrioventricular node.

In second-degree atrioventricular block, an intermittent block in conduction occurs. In Mobitz type I (i.e., Wenckebach) second-degree atrioventricular block, progressive prolongation of the PR interval occurs before the block in conduction. In the usual Wenckebach periodicity (Fig. 22-1), the PR interval gradually increases, but with a decreasing increment, thus leading to a gradual shortening of the RR intervals. The longest PR interval usually precedes the block, and the shortest PR interval usually occurs after the block, thereby resulting in the long RR interval of the blocked impulse being shorter than twice the basic PP interval. Variants of this pattern are not uncommon. In Mobitz type II second-degree atrioventricular block (Fig. 22-2), PR intervals before the block are constant, and there are sudden blocks in

P-wave conduction. Advanced or high-degree atrioventricular block refers to a block of two or more consecutive impulses. In Mobitz type I block, the level of the block is almost always at the atrioventricular node. Rarely, type I Wenckebach periodicity in the His-Purkinje system may be seen in patients with bundle branch block (BBB). In contrast, Mobitz type II block is almost always at the level of the His-Purkinje system and has a higher risk of progressing to complete atrioventricular block.

In third-degree (i.e., complete) atrioventricular block (Fig. 22-3), no impulses are conducted from the atria to the ventricles. The level of the block can occur at the atrioventricular node (usually congenital), His bundle, or in the His-Purkinje system (usually acquired). Escape beats that are junctional at rates of 40–60 beats/min generally occur with congenital complete atrioventricular block. Escape beats that are ventricular in origin often are slow, ranging from 30–40 beats/min.[2,4]

TREATMENT: INDICATIONS FOR PACING

Indications for Permanent Pacing

Conditions for which permanent pacing is or is not indicated are outlined in Table 22-1 and are based on a three-part classification of indications as follows:

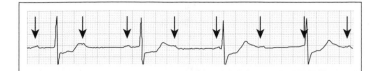

Figure 22-3 • ECG showing third-degree AVB (with escape beats).

Table 22-1 Indications for Permanent Pacemakers

Disorder	Class of Indication	Indication	Optimal Pacing Mode
Sinus node dysfunction	I	Sinus node dysfunction with documented symptomatic bradycardia, possibly a consequence of necessary long-term drug therapy; symptomatic chronotropic incompetence	AAI if no AV node or other conduction tissue disease; DDD if concomitant AV node or conduction disease present; DDDR if chronotropic incompetence; DDIR or automatic mode switching if episodes of supraventricular arrhythmias present
	IIa	Sinus node dysfunction with heart rates <40 beats/min, no clear associations between symptoms and bradycardia; in minimally symptomatic patients, chronic heart rate <30 beats/min while awake. Also, syncope without known origin or sinus node dysfunction diagnosed during an EP study.	
	IIb	Chronic HR <40 bpm while awake	
	III	No symptoms; symptoms clearly documented as not associated with slow heart rate; symptomatic bradycardia due to nonessential drug therapy	
AV block	I	Advanced second- or third-degree AV block with symptomatic bradycardia, arrhythmias requiring drugs causing bradycardia, asystole ≥3 seconds or escape rhythm <40 bpm, after AV junction ablation, postoperative AV block not expected to resolve, or neuromuscular diseases with AV block. Second degree AV block with symptomatic bradycardia	DDD if chronotropically competent; VVI(R) if no organized atrial activity; DDDR or VVIR if chronotropically incompetent
	IIa	Asymptomatic second-degree type II or third-degree AV block with heart rates >40 beats/min (Class I indication if wide QRS); asymptomatic second-degree type I at intra-His or infra-His levels; first-degree with symptoms similar to pacemaker syndrome.	—
	IIb	Marked first-degree block (>0.30 s) with left ventricular dysfunction and congestive heart failure in which shorter AV interval results in hemodynamic improvement; neuromuscular disease with any AV block.	
	III	Asymptomatic first-degree AV block or asymptomatic second-degree AV block type I at the AV node level; AV block expected to resolve and unlikely to recur (e.g., drug toxicity, Lyme disease, OSA)	—
AV block associated with myocardial infarction	I	Persistent advanced second-degree AV block or third-degree AV block with block in the His-Purkinje system (bilateral BBB); transient advanced AV block and associated BBB; persistent and symptomatic second- or third-degree AV block	DDD if chronotropically competent; VVI(R) if no organized atrial activity; DDDR or VVIR if chronotropically incompetent
	IIb	Persistent advanced AV block at the AV node	—
	III	Transient AV block in the absence of intraventricular conduction defects or in the presence of isolated left anterior fascicular block; acquired left anterior fascicular block without AV block; persistent first-degree AV block with BBR not demonstrated previously	—

AV—atrioventricular; OSA—obstructive sleep apnea

Table 22-1 Indications for Permanent Pacemakers—cont'd

Disorder	Class of Indication	Indication	Optimal Pacing Mode
Bifascicular or trifascicular block	I	Fascicular block with intermittent third-degree AV block, second-degree type II AV block, with or without symptoms, or alternating BBB	DDD if chronotropically competent; VVI(R) if no organized atrial activity; DDDR or VVIR if chronotropically incompetent
	IIa	His to ventricular electrogram interval >100 ms or fascicular block associated with syncope that cannot be ascribed to other causes; pacing-induced infra-His block	
	IIb	Neuromuscular disease with fascicular block.	
	III	Asymptomatic fascicular block or fascicular block with associated first-degree AV node block	—
Neurocardiogenic syncope or carotid sinus hypersensitivity	I	Recurrent syncope provoked by carotid sinus stimulation; pauses of >3 s induced by minimal carotid sinus pressure	DDD or DDI
	IIa	Syncope associated with bradycardia reproduced by head upright tilt; recurrent syncope without clear provocative events and with a hypersensitive cardioinhibitory response; syncope of unexplained origin when major abnormalities of sinus node or AV conduction function are discovered or provoked in electrophysiology studies; syncope with bradycardia	—
	IIb	Reproducible neurally mediated syncope	
	III	Recurrent syncope in the absence of a cardioinhibitory response; asymptomatic or minimally/vaguely symptomatic hyperactive cardioinhibitory response to carotid sinus stimulation; recurrent syncope in the absence of a hyperactive cardioinhibitory response; situational vasovagal syncope in which avoidance behavior is effective	—
Cardiomyopathy	I	None	DDD if chronotropically competent; DDDR if chronotropically incompetent
	IIb	Severely symptomatic patients with hypertrophic obstructive cardiomyopathy refractory to drug therapy and significant resting or provoked left ventricular outflow tract obstruction; symptomatic drug-refractory dilated cardiomyopathy with prolonged PR interval when acute hemodynamic studies have demonstrated hemodynamic benefit of pacing	
	III	Asymptomatic or medically controlled patients with hypertrophic obstructive cardiomyopathy or dilated cardiomyopathy; symptomatic patients without left ventricular outflow tract obstruction; symptomatic ischemic cardiomyopathy	—

AV—atrioventricular; BBB—bundle branch block.; OSA—obstructive sleep apnea

Adapted from: Kusumoto FM, Goldschlager N. Cardiac pacing. N Engl J Med 1996; 334:8998; *and* Gregoratos G, Abrams J, Epstein AE, et al. ACC/AHA/NASPE 2002 Guideline update for implantation of cardiac pacemakers and antiarrhythmia devices: summary article: a report of the American College of Cardiology/American Heart Association Task Force on Practice Guidelines (ACC/AHA/NASPE committee to update the 1998 guidelines). Circulation 2002; 106:2145–2161.

Class I: Conditions for which there is general agreement that permanent pacemakers should be implanted

Class II: Conditions for which pacemakers frequently are used but for which there is disagreement regarding their necessity

Class III: Conditions for which there is general agreement that pacemakers are unnecessary

Indications for Temporary Pacing

In general, temporary pacing is indicated for patients with medically refractory, symptomatic bradyarrhythmias without contraindications to pacing. In the absence of acute MI, particularly while awaiting implantation of a permanent pacemaker (if indicated), temporary pacing can be warranted for patients with medically refractory, symptomatic or hemodynamically compromising sinus node bradyarrhythmias, second- or third-degree atrioventricular block, or third-degree atrioventricular block with a wide QRS complex escape rhythm or a ventricular rate of <50 beats/min.

In the presence of acute MI, temporary pacing is indicated for the following:

Third-degree atrioventricular block

Second-degree atrioventricular block

Mobitz II with anterior MI

Mobitz II with inferior MI and wide QRS complex or recurrent block with narrow QRS complex

Mobitz I with marked bradycardia and symptoms

Atrioventricular block associated with marked bradycardia and symptoms (e.g., hypotension, heart failure, low cardiac output)

BBB

New bifascicular block

Alternating BBB

New BBB with anterior MI

    Bilateral BBB of indeterminate age with anterior or indeterminate MI

    Bilateral BBB with first-degree atrioventricular block[3]

Key Points

- Though usually benign, sinus bradycardia can be associated with diseases, such as hypothyroidism, vagal stimulation, increased intracranial pressure, MI, and medications (the most common cause).

- Patients with atrioventricular dissociation may have complete atrioventricular block or dissociation resulting from physiologic interference, with the latter typically having an atrial rate that is slower than the ventricular rate.

- In general, temporary pacing is indicated for patients with medically refractory, symptomatic bradyarrhythmias without contraindications to pacing.

SUGGESTED READING

Gregoratos G, Abrams J, Epstein AE, et al. ACC/AHA/NASPE 2002 Guideline update for implantation of cardiac pacemakers and antiarrhythmia devices: summary article: a report of the American College of Cardiology/American Heart Association Task Force on Practice Guidelines (ACC/AHA/NASPE committee to update the 1998 guidelines). Circulation 2002; 106:2145–2161.

Mangrum JM, DiMarco JP. The evaluation and management of bradycardia. N Engl J Med 2000; 342:703–709.

Kaushik V, Leon AR, Forrester JS Jr, et al. Bradyarrhythmias, temporary and permanent pacing. Crit Care Med 2000; 28(10 Suppl):N121–N128.

Kusumoto FM, Goldschlager N. Cardiac pacing. N Engl J Med 1996; 334:89–98.

Task Force of the Working Group on Arrhythmias of the European Society of Cardiology. The Sicilian Gambit. Circulation 1991; 84:1831–1851.

CHAPTER TWENTY-THREE

Tachyarrhythmias

Arthur C. Kendig, MD, and Mina K. Chung, MD

BACKGROUND

Cardiac arrhythmias can be categorized on the basis of mechanisms, rates, and associated risk. Tachyarrhythmias have rates of more than 100 beats/min. The mechanisms underlying cardiac arrhythmias usually are categorized into disorders of impulse formation, impulse conduction, or a combination of both. The appropriate diagnosis and assessment of the risk associated with arrhythmias influence their treatment.

PATIENT HISTORY AND PHYSICAL EXAMINATION

A key to diagnosing and appropriately treating patients with tachyarrhythmias is determination of the underlying, predisposing cardiac substrate. Known structural heart disease can greatly influence both treatment and diagnosis. The concomitant occurrence of syncope with rapid palpitations or pulse should prompt concerted efforts to document the nature of the arrhythmia associated with symptoms. Triggering agents or events may be important to longer term treatment and subsequent prevention of arrhythmias. In addition to hemodynamic status and evidence of underlying valvular or ventricular dysfunction, helpful physical findings include evidence of atrioventricular dissociation (i.e., cannon A waves in the jugular venous pulse) and termination or slowing with vagal maneuvers or adenosine.

Differential Diagnosis and Diagnostic Studies

Tachyarrhythmias can be classified into wide versus narrow QRS complex and regular versus irregular tachycardia (Table 23-1). Electrocardiographic (ECG) evaluation of tachycardias should begin by assessing the rate, regularity, and QRS complex width. Narrow QRS complex tachycardias, which are defined as having a QRS complex less than 120 ms, imply ventricular activation over the rapidly conducting His-Purkinje system, which suggests a supraventricular tachycardia (SVT). Irregularity of the ventricular rate during an SVT suggests atrial fibrillation, atrial flutter with variable block, or multifocal atrial tachycardia. A wide QRS complex tachycardia may result from ventricular tachycardia (VT) or SVT and is discussed later.

TACHYARRHYTHMIAS: NARROW QRS COMPLEX

Diagnostic Studies: ECG

ECG evaluation of narrow QRS complex tachycardias should include assessment of the following:
Rate
Regularity
QRS complex width
Atrial activation pattern and relationship to the QRS complex (RP/PR relationship, morphology of the P wave)
QRS complex morphology
Effect of bundle branch block (BBB) aberration (if present)
Mode of initiation
Effect of vagal maneuvers and drugs

In narrow QRS complex tachycardias, the relationship of the QRS complex and P waves can be important in establishing the diagnosis. The QRS complex and P-wave relationships and configurations commonly seen in patients with various SVTs are shown in Figures 23-1 and 23-2, and they are discussed further in later sections on specific arrhythmias.

Specific Supraventricular Narrow QRS Complex Arrhythmias: Presentation, Physical Examination, Diagnosis, and Treatment

Atrial Premature Depolarizations

Atrial premature depolarizations can be frequent and occasionally symptomatic. Although not associated with significant risk, they can be associated with underlying cardiovascular or pulmonary disease. Treatment includes reassurance, avoidance of precipitating factors (e.g., caffeine, sympathomimetic agents), and occasionally beta-blockers or calcium channel blockers.

Sinus Tachycardia

Sinus tachycardia is defined in an adult as a sinus rate of greater than 100 beats/min. The sinus node is located in the high right atrium and is sensitive to catecholamines and autonomic tone. Therefore, sinus tachycardia may be secondary to many physiologic and pathologic states. It is a normal response to exertion, anxiety, and a variety of stresses, including fever, hypotension, hypovolemia, congestive heart failure, pulmonary embolism,

Table 23-1 Differential Diagnosis of Tachycardias

Regular Rhythm	Irregular Rhythm
Narrow QRS Complex	
Sinus node tachycardias	
Inappropriate sinus tachycardia	
Sinus node reentry	
Atrial tachycardias	Multifocal atrial tachycardia
Reentrant	Atrial fibrillation
Atrial flutter, fixed AV block	Atrial flutter, variable AV block
Junctional tachycardias	
Atrioventricular nodal reentry	
Typical	
Atypical	
Atrioventricular reciprocating tachycardia and other	
SVTs associated with accessory pathways	
Wide QRS Complex	
Ventricular tachycardia	Ventricular tachycardia
Supraventricular tachycardia with:	Atrial fibrillation with:
Preexisting BBB	Preexisting BBB
Functional BBB	Functional BBB
Preexcitation	Preexcitation
Antidromic AV reentry	Torsades de pointes
Bystander accessory pathway	
AV,BBB	

AV—atrioventricular; SVT—supraventricular tachycardia; BBB—bundle branch block
From: Chung MK. Arrhythmias. In: Stoller JK, Michota FA, Mandell BF, eds. The Cleveland Clinic Intensive Review of Internal Medicine. 4th ed. Philadelphia: Lippincott, Williams & Wilkins, 2005.

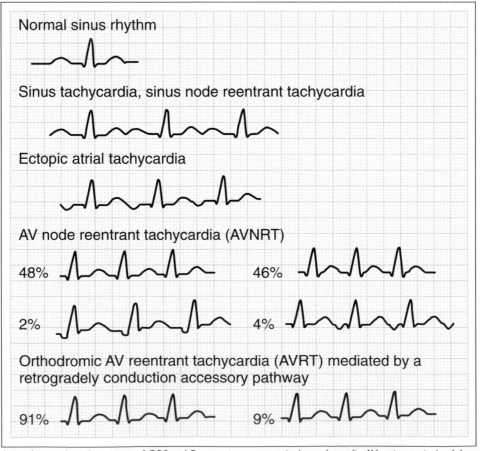

Figure 23-1 • Relationships and configurations of QRS and P waves in supraventricular tachycardia. AV, atrioventricular. Adapted from: Josephson ME. Clinical Cardiac Electrophysiology: Techniques and Interpretation, 2nd ed. Malvern, PA: Lea & Febiger, 1993. 269.

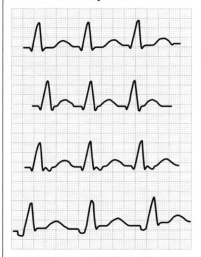

Normal sinus rhythm

Short R-P tachycardias

AVNRT
Other junctional tachycardias
Orthodromic AVRT mediated by a
retrogradely conducting AP

AVNRT
Other junctional tachycardias
Orthodromic AVRT mediated by a
retrogradely conducting AP

Orthodromic AVRT mediated by a
retrogradely conducting AP
AVNRT

AVNRT

Long R-P tachycardias

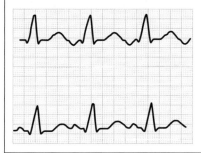

Atypical AVNRT (anterograde
fast, retrograde slow conduction
pathway)
Orthodromic AVRT mediated by a
slow, decrementally conducting
retrograde AP
Atrial tachycardia

Atrial tachycardia
Sinus node reentrant tachycardia
Sinus tachycardia

Figure 23-2 • Differential diagnosis of supraventricular tachycardias by RP/PR relationships and P-wave configurations. *, most common; AP, accessory pathway; AVNRT, atrioventricular nodal reentrant tachycardia; AVRT, atrioventricular reentrant tachycardia. Adapted from: Josephson ME. Clinical Cardiac Electrophysiology: Techniques and Interpretation, 2nd ed. Malvern, PA: Lea & Febiger, 1993; 270.

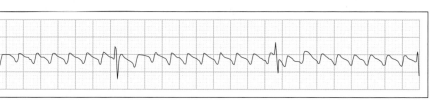

Figure 23-3 • ECG demonstrating atrial flutter.

myocardial ischemia or infarction, inflammation, and drugs. Physiologic sinus tachycardia has normal P-wave morphology and exhibits gradual rate acceleration and deceleration that vary with changes in the autonomic tone and volume. Treatment should focus on the cause of sinus tachycardia, avoidance of stimulants, fluid replacement in patients with hypovolemia, fever reduction, and, possibly, beta-blockers or calcium channel blockers.[5]

Multifocal Atrial Tachycardia

Multifocal atrial tachycardia is characterized by a heart rate of greater than 100 beats/min; multiple (three or more) P-wave morphologies; and variable PP, PR, and RR intervals. The multiple P-wave morphologies result from multiple depolarizing foci in the atria. The irregularly irregular ventricular rate can mimic atrial fibrillation, and differentiation from "coarse" atrial fibrilla-

tion can be made by isoelectric periods between P waves. Multifocal atrial tachycardia predominantly occurs in patients who are elderly or critically ill with advanced chronic pulmonary disease. In critically ill patients, it is associated with high hospital mortality.

Treatment is directed toward the underlying disease. Antiarrhythmic agents often are ineffective, and beta-blockers can be effective but often are contraindicated in patients with severe bronchospastic disease. Verapamil, amiodarone, and potassium as well as magnesium replacement have been helpful. The mechanism underlying multifocal atrial tachycardia may be enhanced automaticity or triggered activity.[5]

Atrial Flutter (Fig. 23-3)

Atrial flutter can occur in patients without structural heart disease, but chronic, persistent atrial flutter most often occurs in

Figure 23-4 • ECG demonstrating atrial fibrillation.

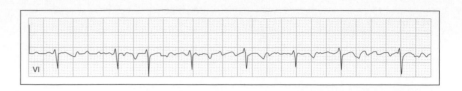

patients with underlying heart disease. The incidence of atrial flutter is lower than that of atrial fibrillation, and two general categories of atrial flutter have been described.

The typical (type I) form is caused by macroreentry in the right atrium with conduction utilizing the right atrial isthmus between the tricuspid annulus and inferior vena cava. This inscribes the typical saw-tooth flutter waves on the surface ECG. In untreated patients with type I atrial flutter, the atrial rate usually is 300 beats/min, with 2 : 1 atrioventricular conduction and a ventricular rate of 150 beats/min. Occasionally, 1 : 1 atrioventricular conduction can be seen in patients with preexcitation syndromes, or atrial flutters slowed by antiarrhythmic medications. Vagal maneuvers or adenosine can help to establish the diagnosis by blocking the ventricular response and enhancing appreciation of the flutter waves. Esophageal or intracardiac atrial electrogram recordings can help in patients for whom the diagnosis remains unclear.

Atypical (type II) atrial flutter has an atrial rate that usually is 250–400 beats/min and may not be influenced or terminated by atrial pacing. In type II atrial flutter, the right atrial isthmus, involved in type I atrial flutter, is generally not a critical component of the reentrant circuit with other right or left atrial pathways of conduction participating in the arrhythmia.

Treatment of atrial flutter commonly involves controlling the ventricular response with agents such as verapamil, diltiazem, beta-blockers, or digoxin. Long-term prevention of atrial flutter has been difficult with medical treatment. Synchronized, direct current (DC) cardioversion is effective and may require only low energies (i.e., 25–100 J). Rapid atrial overdrive pacing may also terminate type I atrial flutter.

Type I atrial flutter can be cured, with a success rate of 75–90%, by radiofrequency ablation. Atypical atrial flutter may also be approached with catheter ablation methods and advanced mapping techniques, although success rates are lower than for those of type I atrial flutter. Radiofrequency ablation also has been used successfully as adjunctive therapy in patients on antiarrhythmic agents to cure the atrial flutter that can be facilitated by these agents.

Atrial Fibrillation (Fig. 23-4)

Atrial fibrillation is the most common sustained tachyarrhythmia. During atrial fibrillation, electrical activation of the atria occurs in rapid, multiple waves of depolarization, with continuously changing pathways, and the atrial activation rate may exceed 300–400 beats/min. This pattern of rapid, disordered atrial activation results in loss of coordinated atrial contraction and irregular electrical inputs to the atrioventricular node, leading to irregular ventricular rates. Focal or micro-reentrant pulmonary vein triggers initiating atrial fibrillation have been recognized as a more common cause of atrial fibrillation than previously appreciated. These most frequently arise from the ostia

Table 23-2 American College of Chest Physicians Guidelines for Antithrombotic Therapy for Atrial Fibrillation		
Risk Factors	**Number**	**Recommendation**
High[a]	1	Warfarin[b]
Moderate[c]	>1	Warfarin[b]
	1	Warfarin[b] or aspirin[d]
None	0	Aspirin[d]

[a]Prior transient ischemic attack, stroke or systemic embolus, hypertension, poor left ventricular function, congestive heart failure, rheumatic mitral valve disease or prosthetic heart valve, diabetes mellitus, or age >75 years.

[b]Warfarin target international normalized ratio: 2.5 (range, 2.0–3.0).

[c]Age 65–75 years, diabetes mellitus, coronary artery disease with preserved left ventricular systolic function.

[d]Aspirin, 325 mg/day.

From: Singer DE, Albers GW, Dalen JE, et al. Antithrombotic therapy in atrial fibrillation. Chest 2004; 126:(Suppl)429S-456S.

of the pulmonary veins and can potentially be catheter ablated with long-term cure.[4]

The incidence of atrial fibrillation increases with age. The most common underlying cardiovascular diseases associated with atrial fibrillation are hypertension and ischemic heart disease, but atrial fibrillation may also occur in the absence of structural heart disease ("lone" atrial fibrillation).

On the surface ECG, atrial fibrillation is characterized by absence of discrete P waves, presence of irregular fibrillatory waves, or both, and an irregularly irregular ventricular response. Complete BBB or aberrancy (e.g., Ashman's phenomenon) can mimic VT. At physical examination, the pulse is irregularly irregular; variable stroke volumes may produce pulse deficits, and the jugular venous waveform lacks A waves.

One of the most important clinical consequences of atrial fibrillation is its association with thromboembolic events and stroke. Recommended guidelines for antithrombotic therapy are listed in Table 23-2 and Box 23-1.

Acute treatment of atrial fibrillation that is symptomatic with an increased heart rate should include urgent cardioversion if the patient is hemodynamically unstable or has evidence of ischemia or pulmonary edema. For moderate to severe symptoms, acute control of the ventricular rate usually can be achieved with intravenous beta-blockers, verapamil, diltiazem, or digoxin (Table 23-3). Digoxin can be used safely in patients with heart failure, but it has a delayed peak onset of heart rate-lowering effect and a narrow therapeutic window. Pharmacologic or electrical cardioversion, use of antiarrhythmic agents, and anticoagulation should be considered. Pharmacologic conversion can be

Box 23-1 Guidelines for Electrical Cardioversion

Anticoagulation (e.g., warfarin, INR 2.0–3.0) should be given for 3 weeks before elective cardioversion of patients who have been in atrial fibrillation for >48 hours and continued until normal sinus rhythm has been maintained for 4 weeks. In some circumstances, a transesophageal protocol may be substituted for conventional therapy but adjusted-dose warfarin should be continued until sinus rhythm has been maintained at least 4 weeks.

Consideration should be given to treating patients in atrial flutter in the same manner as patients in atrial fibrillation.

Long-term anticoagulation beyond the fourth week after cardioversion should be considered if the patient has had previous episodes of AF and if there is a history of cardiomyopathy, previous embolism, mitral valve disease, or other indications for long-term anticoagulation, as listed previously.

Heparin anticoagulation followed by oral anticoagulation may be indicated for patients requiring emergency cardioversion for hemodynamic instability. For atrial fibrillation <48 hours, risk of embolism after cardioversion appears low, but pericardioversion anticoagulation is recommended.

Note: Many of these patients were excluded from the multicenter trials on atrial fibrillation. There is an increased risk of bleeding that correlates with the level of anticoagulation (i.e., INR >4). A marked decrease in efficacy is noted at international normalized ratio <2. Contraindications to anticoagulation include hemorrhagic tendencies, recent intracranial hemorrhage or neurosurgery, recent major hemorrhage or trauma, and uncontrolled diastolic hypertension with blood pressure >105 mm Hg. Other critical considerations include patients at risk of falling, alcohol abuse, drug interactions, poor compliance or follow-up, and concomitant use of nonsteroidal antiinflammatory drugs.

AF—atrial fibrillation; INR—international normalized ratio

Adapted from: Singer DE, Albers GW, Dalen JE, et al. Antithrombotic therapy in atrial fibrillation. Chest 2004; 126:(Suppl)429S-456S.

attempted intravenously, using procainamide, ibutilide, or amiodarone, or orally, using class I or III antiarrhythmic agents (Table 23-4). If the duration of atrial fibrillation is more than 48 hours, anticoagulation with warfarin for 3 weeks versus transesophageal echocardiographically guided cardioversion with anticoagulation should be considered (*see* Box 23-1). For shorter durations of atrial fibrillation (i.e., <48 hours), anticoagulation should be considered if the patient has underlying heart disease or risk factors for thromboembolism, and pericardioversion anticoagulation is recommended.[2,4]

Long-term treatment of atrial fibrillation should include evaluation for underlying structural heart disease, risk factors, and, potentially, other precipitating arrhythmias. Anticoagulation with warfarin or aspirin should be considered (*see* Table 23-2). Control of the ventricular rate with beta-blockers, calcium channel blockers, or digoxin also may be required (*see* Table 23-3). In addition, restoring and maintaining sinus rhythm with cardioversion, maintenance antiarrhythmic therapy, or both can be considered. Antiarrhythmic agents that may effectively maintain sinus rhythm include class IA, class IC, class IA/B/C, and class III antiarrhythmic drugs (*see* Table 23-4). Nonpharmacologic approaches for symptomatic patients include catheter-based atrial fibrillation ablation with pulmonary vein ostial isolation or surgical pulmonary vein isolation or the maze procedure. Complete atrioventricular junction ablation with implantation of a rate-responsive, permanent pacemaker could be considered for refractory atrial fibrillation and poorly controlled ventricular rates, although this procedure causes permanent AV block and renders the patient pacemaker dependent.[8]

Atrioventricular Nodal Reentrant Tachycardia

The most common form of paroxysmal reentrant SVT is atrioventricular nodal reentrant tachycardia (AVNRT), which accounts for 60–70% of patients with paroxysmal SVT. The rate of AVNRT usually is 150–200 beats/min. In typical AVNRT, anterograde conduction occurs via a slow-conducting pathway and retrograde conduction via a fast-conducting pathway. Rapid retrograde activation of the atrium via the fast pathway occurs nearly simultaneously with the ventricular activation, and it usually causes the P wave to be simultaneous with, or buried within, the QRS complex, and it either is not visible or is detected at the end of the QRS complex (within 80 ms) in 94% of cases. A small r′ (second positive deflection on EKG) in the QRS of lead V_1 has been strongly associated with AVNRT (Fig. 23-5).[5]

In 5–10% of patients with AVNRT, atypical or uncommon AVNRT occurs, in which anterograde conduction takes place via the fast pathway and retrograde conduction via the slow pathway. This causes retrograde P waves that usually are negative in the inferior and are separated from the QRS complex, with an RP interval that is longer than the PR interval.

Clinically, AVNRT commonly occurs in patients with no structural heart disease, and 70% of patients are women. It may occur at any age, but most patients present during the fourth or fifth decade of life. Symptoms may include palpitations, lightheadedness, near syncope, weakness, dyspnea, chest pain, rarely syncope, and frequently neck pounding with prominent A waves that can be seen on the jugular pulse, representing atrial contraction against a closed tricuspid valve.

Vagal maneuvers may slow or terminate the tachycardia. Adenosine is the initial drug of choice. Termination of a narrow-complex tachycardia by vagal maneuvers or adenosine can be helpful diagnostically by suggesting that the atrioventricular node may be a component of the conduction pathway.

Beta-blockers, verapamil, or diltiazem also can be successful. Long-term use of these agents or of class IA, IC, or III antiarrhythmic drugs can be successful; but radiofrequency catheter ablation has become the standard therapy for cure of AVNRT, with success rates that can exceed 95% and less than a 1% risk of inducing complete atrioventricular block or need for a permanent pacemaker.[5]

Atrioventricular Reentrant Tachycardia

During AVRT, the accessory pathway, the atria, and ventricles are essential parts of the circuit (Fig. 23-6). Orthodromic AVRT (Fig. 23-7) is the most common SVT in patients with accessory pathways, occurring in 90% of those who are symptomatic. Anterograde conduction occurs via the atrioventricular node and retrograde via the accessory pathway inscribing a narrow QRS complex (with no preexcitation) on the surface ECG unless BBB aberrancy occurs. Spontaneous or induced BBB during orthodromic AVRT that slows the tachycardia rate indicates participation of an accessory pathway ipsilateral to the side of the BBB. The heart rate of the tachycardia usually is 150–250 beats/min, and is usually initiated by an atrial or ventricular premature depolarization.[5]

Table 23-3 Medical Treatment for Ventricular Rate Control in Supraventricular Arrhythmias, Including Atrial Fibrillation

Agent	Loading Dose	Maintenance Dose	Side Effects/Toxicity	Comments
Class II (beta-blockers)				
Propranolol	1 mg IV every 2–5 min to 0.1–0.2 mg/kg	10–80 mg PO TID to QID	Bronchospasm, congestive heart failure, decreased blood pressure	Effective in heart rate control even with exercise, rapid onsets of action
Metoprolol	5 mg IV every 5 min to 15 mg	25–100 mg PO BID		
Esmolol	500 mcg/kg IV over 1 min	50 mcg/kg IV for 4 hr, repeat load as needed and ↑ maintenance to 20–50 µg/kg/min every 5–10 min as needed		Esmolol short-acting
Class IV (calcium channel blockers)				
Verapamil	2.5–10 mg IV over 2 min	5–10 mg IV every 30–60 min or 40–160 mg PO TID	Decreased blood pressure, congestive heart failure	Rapid onset, can be used safely in chronic obstructive pulmonary disease and diabetes mellitus
Diltiazem	0.25 mg/kg over 2 hr, repeat as needed every 15 min at 0.35 mg/kg	5–15 mg/h IV or 30–90 mg PO QID	Increased digoxin level	—
Class III				
Sotalol	—	80–240 mg PO BID	Bradycardia, congestive heart failure, bronchospasm, decreased blood pressure, increased QT, torsades de pointes, proarrhythmia	—
Amiodarone	600–1,600 mg/day, divided	100–400 mg PO daily	Bradycardia, pulmonary, thyroid, liver, skin, gastrointestinal, ophthalmologic	Drug interactions
Digoxin	0.25–0.50 mg IV, then 0.25 mg IV every 4–6 hr to 1 mg in the first 24 hr	0.125–0.250 mg PO or IV daily	Anorexia, nausea, AV block, ventricular arrhythmias; accumulates in renal failure	Used in congestive heart failure, vagotonic effects on the AV node, delayed onset of action, narrow therapeutic window, less effective in paroxysmal atrial fibrillation or high adrenergic states
Adenosine	6–18 mg IV rapid bolus	—	Transient sinus bradycardia, sinus arrest, AV block, flushing, chest discomfort, bronchospasm; may precipitate atrial fibrillation by shortening of atrial refractoriness	Not effective in controlling ventricular rate in atrial fibrillation flutter, but may be useful diagnostically; can terminate reentrant paroxysmal supraventricular tachycardias using the AV node

AV 3|—atrioventricular.

Modified from: Chung MK. Arrhythmias. In: Stoller JK, Michota FA, Mandell BF, eds. The Cleveland Clinic Intensive Review of Internal Medicine. Fourth Edition. Philadelphia: Lippincott, Williams & Wilkins, 2005.

Table 23-4 Class I and III Antiarrhythmic Agents

Antiarrhythmic Drug	Dose	Side Effects/Comments
Class IA		Increased QT, proarrhythmia/TdP, potential increased AV node conduction can be seen with all three
Quinidine	200–400 mg PO TID to BID	Diarrhea, nausea, increased digoxin levels
Procainamide	10–15 mg/kg IV at 50 mg/min or 500–1,000 mg PO every 6 h (sustained release)	Decreased blood pressure, congestive heart failure, drug-induced lupus; metabolite N-acetylprocainamide (class III) can accumulate in renal failure
Disopyramide	100–300 mg PO TID	Anticholinergic effects (e.g., urinary retention, dry eyes/mouth), congestive heart failure
Class IB		
Lidocaine	50–100 mg IV (0.5–1.5 mg/kg) bolus, infusion of 1–4 mg/min, and rebolus in 5–15 min	Reduce dosage in congestive heart failure, elderly, hepatic dysfunction, bradycardia, hypotension, CNS side effects (tremors, seizures, altered mental status)
Mexiletine	150–300 mg PO every 8 hr	Gastrointestinal side effects (nausea, vomiting) common, may be minimized by dosing with meals; CNS effects (tremor, dizziness, nervousness)
Tocainide	400–600 mg PO every 8 hr	Gastrointestinal side effects (nausea, vomiting), CNS less common (dizziness, vertigo, nervousness); rare but potentially life-threatening agranulocytosis and pulmonary fibrosis
Class IC		Proarrhythmia
Flecainide	50–200 mg PO BID	Visual disturbance, dizziness, congestive heart failure, avoid in coronary artery disease or left ventricular dysfunction
Propafenone	150–300 mg PO TID	Congestive heart failure, avoid in coronary artery disease/left ventricular dysfunction
Class IA/B/C		
Moricizine	200–300 mg PO TID	Proarrhythmia, dizziness, gastrointestinal/nausea, headache, caution in coronary artery disease/left ventricular dysfunction
Class III		
Sotalol	80–240 mg PO BID	Congestive heart failure, bronchospasm, bradycardia, increased QT, proarrhythmia/TdP; renally excreted
Bretylium	5–10 mg/kg IV bolus; 1–2 mg/min IV infusion	Hypotension; transient increased arrhythmias possible due to initial norepinephrine release; reduce dose in renal failure
Amiodarone	600–1,600 mg/day loading in divided doses PO, 100–400 mg PO daily maintenance; IV available	Pulmonary toxicity, bradycardia, hyperthyroidism or hypothyroidism, hepatic toxicity, gastrointestinal (nausea, constipation), neurologic, dermatologic, and ophthalmologic side effects, drug interactions
Ibutilide	1.0 mg IV over 10 min, may repeat in 10 min	Monitor for QT prolongation, TdP
Dofetilide	125–500 mcg PO every 12 hr; initial dose: CrCl (mL/min) >60: 500 mcg BID; 40–60: 250 mcg BID; 20–40: 125 mcg BID	In-hospital initiation mandated; exclude if CrCl <20 mL/min; monitor for QT prolongation, proarrhythmia/TdP; headache, muscle cramps

AV—atrioventricular; CNS—central nervous system; TdP—torsades de pointes; CrCl—creatinine clearance

Modified from: Chung MK. Arrhythmias. In: Stoller JK, Michota FA, Mandell BF, eds. The Cleveland Clinic Intensive Review of Internal Medicine. Fourth Edition. Philadelphia: Lippincott, Williams & Wilkins, 2005.

Antidromic AVRT is uncommon, occurring in <5–10% of patients with Wolff-Parkinson-White syndrome. In antidromic AVRT, anterograde conduction occurs via an accessory pathway and retrograde conduction via the atrioventricular node or a second accessory pathway. Because ventricular activation occurs via an accessory pathway, the QRS complex is wide, bizarre, and preexcited. Other accessory pathway-associated tachycardias include atrial fibrillation, atrial flutter, atrial tachycardia, or AVNRT with conduction via a bystander accessory pathway, in which the accessory pathway is not integral to the tachycardia but conducts to the ventricle. Slowly conducting, concealed accessory pathways, which usually are located in the posteroseptum, can mediate near-incessant orthodromic SVT with retrograde, slow conduction via the accessory pathway (i.e., permanent form of junctional reciprocating tachycardia); these can present as a tachycardia-mediated cardiomyopathy. The most common tachycardias associated with accessory pathways are discussed in the following sections; their treatment is summarized in Box 23-2.

Short-term treatments of the two common, regular, narrow complex tachycardias (i.e., orthodromic AVRT and AVNRT) are similar because the atrioventricular node is an integral part of the

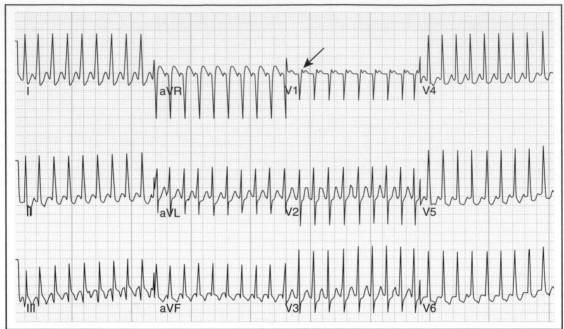

Figure 23-5 • Atrioventricular nodal reentrant tachycardia (AVNRT). Note small r′ in V₁, representing retrograde atrial activation occurring nearly simultaneously with ventricular activation.

Figure 23-6 • Tachycardias associated with accessory pathways (APs). AVRT, atrioventricular reentrant tachycardia.

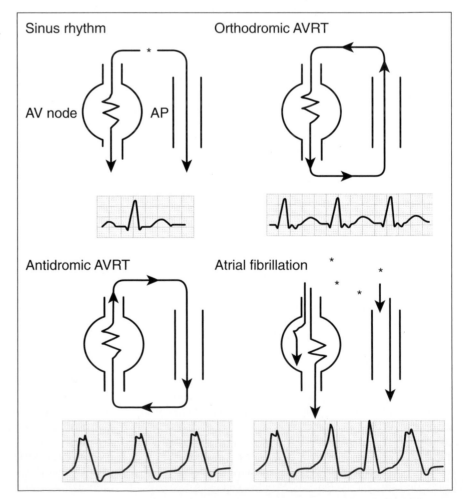

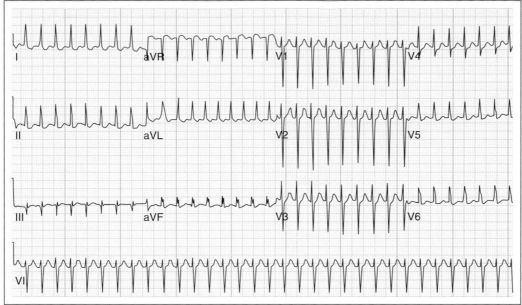

Figure 23-7 • Orthodromic atrioventricular reentrant tachycardia (AVRT). In orthodromic AVRT, a narrow QRS complex occurs (in the absence of aberration). This confirms anterograde conduction occurring through the AV node. Thus, this acute SVT can usually be treated successfully with AV nodal blocking maneuvers or drugs (e.g., vagal maneuvers, adenosine, beta-blockers).

circuit in the anterograde direction. To terminate the tachycardia, vagal maneuvers or adenosine are the first options of choice, followed by intravenous beta-blockers, verapamil, or diltiazem. Adenosine can shorten atrial refractory periods but occasionally may precipitate atrial fibrillation with a rapid ventricular response. In patients with very rapid SVT and hemodynamic impairment, DC cardioversion is the initial treatment of choice. Longer-term treatment may include beta-blockers, verapamil, diltiazem, digoxin, or class IA, IC, or III antiarrhythmic drugs. Radiofrequency catheter ablation, however, can be curative with high success rates; in many patients, it can be considered as a first-line or early therapeutic option. However, in antidromic AVRT, if the atrioventricular node makes up the retrograde limb, then vagal maneuvers or adenosine may terminate the tachycardia, but these measures will not be effective if both limbs are accessory pathways. In the short term, treatment may require DC cardioversion or procainamide.[5]

Atrial Fibrillation and Wolff-Parkinson-White Syndrome

In patients with manifest accessory pathways having a short refractory period, rapid conduction to the ventricles during atrial fibrillation via the accessory pathway can provoke ventricular fibrillation. The shortest preexcited RR interval during atrial fibrillation gives an indication as to the refractory period of the accessory pathway. Short refractory periods (<250 ms) are associated with increased risk of sudden death. Diagnostically, atrial fibrillation with ventricular preexcitation should be suspected for rapid, irregularly irregular rhythms with varying QRS morphology and widths due to variable degrees of ventricular fusion (Fig. 23-8). Verapamil can increase the ventricular rate during atrial fibrillation; intravenous verapamil may precipitate ventricular fibrillation and should not be given. The treatment of choice is procainamide or DC cardioversion.[4]

TACHYARRHYTHMIAS: WIDE QRS COMPLEX

Clinical Presentation

Wide complex tachycardia (WCT) has a QRS duration of 120 ms or longer, with a ventricular rate of 100 beats/min or more. In multiple studies, VT was the correct diagnosis in more than 80% of patients presenting with WCT. VT is more likely to occur in older patients, but age alone is not a useful marker. In very young patients (<20 years), SVT is a more frequent cause of WCT. Hemodynamic instability is a poor discriminating factor because hemodynamic stability depends on rate, ventricular function, cardiac disease, and concomitant pharmacologic therapy. A history of structural heart disease, particularly of coronary artery disease with previous myocardial infarction (MI), is important. In patients with a history of MI, 98% of WCTs result from VT; a history of MI and symptoms of tachycardia starting only after the MI strongly favor VT.[1]

Physical Examination

Rate and blood pressure are not useful in determining the cause of WCTs. The finding of atrioventricular dissociation, however, strongly favors VT because approximately two thirds of patients with VT have atrioventricular dissociation at electrophysiology study, and atrioventricular dissociation is rare in SVT. Asynchronous contraction of the atria and ventricles can cause cannon A waves in the jugular venous pulsation, wide split heart sounds, variable S_1, and variability in blood pressure resulting from changes in stroke volume with atrioventricular dissociation.

Box 23-2 Management of Preexcitation Syndromes

Initial evaluation

    Determine presence or absence of symptoms

    Characterize symptoms, including frequency and severity

    Determine previous treatment regimens and effectiveness

    Document specific arrhythmias present during symptoms

    Determine presence of concomitant heart disease

Acute treatment of arrhythmias associated with preexcitation syndromes

    Orthodromic SVT

        Vagal maneuvers (e.g., Valsalva's, carotid sinus massage)

        Adenosine IV (6–12 mg rapid bolus)

        Verapamil IV (5–10 mg), beta blocker, or diltiazem

        Procainamide IV (1 g over 20–30 min)

        Cardioversion

    Antidromic SVT (retrograde conduction may occur via a second AP or the AV node)

        Procainamide IV

        Cardioversion

    Atrial fibrillation (digoxin and verapamil may accelerate ventricular rate and should not be used)

        Procainamide IV

        Cardioversion

Long-term treatment of patients with preexcitation syndromes

    Pharmacologic management

        Concealed AP

            Digoxin/verapamil/beta-blocker

            Class IC: flecainide/propafenone

            Class IA: disopyramide/quinidine/procainamide

            Class III: sotalol/amiodarone

        Manifest AP

            Class IC: flecainide/propafenone

            Class IA: disopyramide/quinidine/procainamide

            Class III: sotalol/amiodarone

Indications for nonpharmacologic management

    Life-threatening ventricular rate during atrial fibrillation/flutter

    SVT refractory to medical therapy

    Intolerance to medical therapy

    Alternate first-line therapy in patients with symptomatic arrhythmias, high-risk occupations, or preference for nonpharmacologic treatment

Nonpharmacologic approaches

    Radiofrequency catheter ablation

    Surgical ablation (rarely required)

    Indications for electrophysiology studies

    Delineation of the mechanism of arrhythmias

    Localization/mapping of pathways for ablation

    Assess efficacy of antiarrhythmic agents

    Assessment of the refractory periods of the AP as an indicator of the risk of sudden death

AP = accessory pathway; AV = atrioventricular; SVT = supraventricular tachycardia.

From: Chung MK. Arrhythmias. In: Stoller JK, Michota FA, Mandell BF, eds. The Cleveland Clinic Intensive Review of Internal Medicine. Fourth Edition. Philadelphia: Lippincott, Williams & Wilkins, 2005.

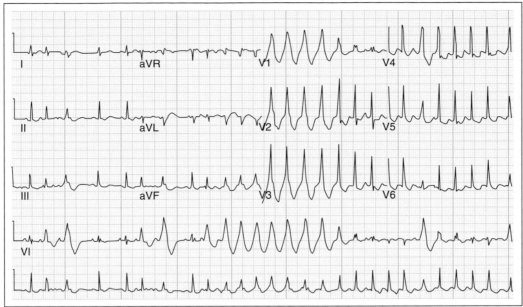

Figure 23-8 • Atrial fibrillation with Wolff-Parkinson-White syndrome (ventricular preexcitation). The rhythm is irregular and often quite rapid. The QRS is variable in morphology and duration due to variable degrees of fusion between conduction through the AV node vs. an anterogradely conducting accessory pathway.

Differential Diagnosis of Wide QRS Complex Tachycardias

Considerations include:

SVT

SVT with preexisting BBB or intraventricular conduction defect

SVT with aberrant His-Purkinje system conduction (i.e., functional BBB)

Ashman's phenomenon after long-short RR interval

Rate-related, acceleration-dependent BBB

Maintenance of functional BBB by transseptal concealed conduction (i.e., linking)

SVT with antegrade conduction via an accessory pathway

Antidromic SVT with antegrade conduction via an accessory pathway

Atrial fibrillation/flutter/tachycardia with antegrade conduction via an accessory pathway

AVNRT with antegrade conduction down a bystander accessory pathway

SVT with slowed conduction because of electrolyte or metabolic imbalance or an antiarrhythmic drug

The diagnosis of WCT often can be established on the basis of clinical presentation, physical examination, ECG findings, and provocative maneuvers. As a general rule, however, treat it as a VT when in doubt, particularly in patients with structural heart disease.

Diagnostic Studies: ECG

The ECG should be analyzed with specific attention to the atrioventricular relationship, presence of capture or fusion beats (Fig. 23-9). QRS morphology may also be helpful (Figs. 23-10, 23-11). In patients with preexisting complete BBB, the QRS complex is wide, and comparison with previous ECGs can be helpful. The QRS complex may be wide in any supraventricular

rhythm, however, if functional aberrancy occurs. Most SVTs with aberrancy have QRS complex durations of 140 ms or less, but wide QRS complex durations can be seen with preexcitation and marked baseline intraventricular conduction defects. In addition, 15–35% of patients with VT also may have QRS complex durations of 140 ms or less. A QRS complex duration of longer than 140 ms with WCT of right BBB morphology or of longer than 160 ms with left BBB morphology favors the diagnosis of VT. Patients receiving antiarrhythmic drugs may particularly develop rate-related aberrancy. Preexcitation via an anterograde-conducting accessory pathway also causes a wide QRS complex.[7,10]

Atrioventricular dissociation strongly favors the diagnosis of VT (see Figure 23-9), but this feature is not always identifiable on surface ECGs. One third of VTs may have 1:1 ventriculoatrial (VA) conduction. Even so, variable retrograde VA conduction, or VA Wenckebach conduction, strongly suggests VT. Rare SVTs may exhibit VA dissociation. Recording of an atrial electrogram by a right atrial or an esophageal electrode may facilitate assessment.

A commonly used four-level algorithm for distinguishing VT from SVT (Brugada criteria) is shown in Figure 23-12. This algorithm was prospectively validated for more than 500 WCTs with electrophysiologic diagnoses. It had a high sensitivity (0.987) and specificity (0.965).[3]

Treatment

For hemodynamically unstable WCT, including pulmonary edema or severe angina, cardioversion should be performed. Sedation should be given before cardioversion if the patient is awake. For hemodynamically stable WCT, a clinical history should be elicited and physical examination performed (including inspection for cannon A waves). A 12-lead ECG and laboratory studies to exclude electrolyte and metabolic abnormalities,

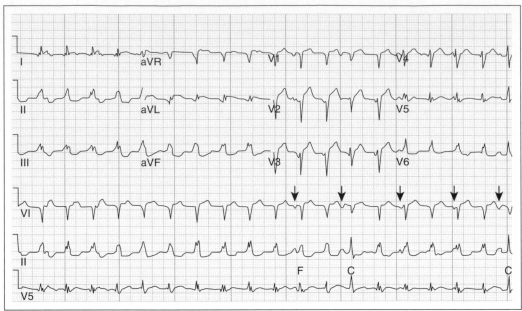

Figure 23-9 • Wide complex tachycardia due to slow ventricular tachycardia. Demonstrated are AV dissociation with P waves indicated by arrowheads, as well as fusion (F) and capture (C) beats. Ventricular fusion beats occur with a narrower QRS when the ventricle is activated from two different sites (e.g., supraventricular conduction to the ventricles during ventricular tachycardia; or premature ventricular complex during supraventricular tachycardia with aberrancy). Sinus capture beats during ventricular tachycardia are form of fusion, but the narrow complex occurring with a shorter coupling interval (than the ventricular tachycardia interval) denotes a sinus beat has captured the ventricle during ventricular tachycardia. This indicates the rhythm is ventricular tachycardia, as a shorter coupling interval during supraventricular tachycardia with aberrancy would result in no change in or a wider QRS duration.

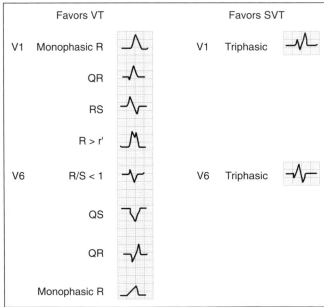

Figure 23-10 • Right bundle branch block morphologic criteria for distinguishing ventricular tachycardia (VT) from supraventricular tachycardia (SVT). Adapted from: Wellens HJJ, Bar FWHM, Lie KI. The value of the electrocardiogram in the differential diagnosis of a tachycardia with a widened QRS complex. Am J Med 1978; 64:27–33.

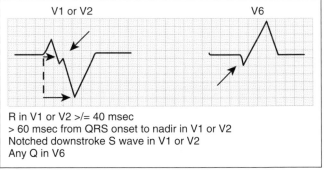

R in V1 or V2 >/= 40 msec
> 60 msec from QRS onset to nadir in V1 or V2
Notched downstroke S wave in V1 or V2
Any Q in V6

Figure 23-11 • Left bundle branch block morphologic criteria for ventricular tachycardia in leads V1 and V6. Adapted from: Kindwall KE, Brown J, Josephson ME. Electrocardiographic criteria for ventricular tachycardia in wide complex left bundle branch block morphology tachycardias. Am J Cardiol 1988; 61:1279–1283.

ischemia, hypoxia, or drug toxicity should be obtained. If the diagnosis is in doubt, placement of an esophageal lead can be considered. If supraventricular tachycardia or atrial flutter is suspected, adenosine, 6–12 mg delivered intravenously as a rapid bolus, can be given. Lidocaine or procainamide can be attempted as well, and if the WCT persists, bretylium or intravenous amiodarone can be considered. Intravenous verapamil should not be used to treat WCT because hemodynamic collapse and death have

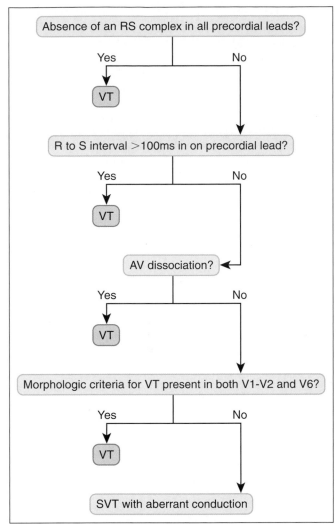

Figure 23-12 • Brugada criteria for distinguishing ventricular tachycardia (VT) from supraventricular tachycardia (SVT) in tachycardia with widened QRS complexes. From: Brugada P, Brugada J, Mont L, et al. A new approach to the differential diagnosis of a regular tachycardia with a wide QRS complex. Circulation 1991; 83:1649–1659.

been reported, regardless of the cause of the WCT. Cardioversion under anesthesia or overdrive pace termination can be attempted for persistent WCT. If WCT is incessant, consider the possibility of electrolyte abnormalities, digitalis toxicity, acute severe ischemia, reperfusion arrhythmias, proarrhythmia, or TdP. Consideration also should be given to empiric magnesium sulfate (MgSO₄), treatment for acute ischemia or MI, and intravenous amiodarone.

Evaluation after termination of WCT should include consideration of electrophysiologic testing to determine the WCT etiology. Subsequent therapy depends on the diagnosis but can include pharmacologic, ablation, or device therapies.

SPECIFIC VENTRICULAR ARRHYTHMIAS: PRESENTATION, PHYSICAL EXAMINATION, DIAGNOSIS, AND TREATMENT

VT is defined as three or more consecutive ventricular beats at a rate of 100 beats/min or more. Nonsustained VT is defined as VT lasting three or more beats under 30 seconds in duration and that does not require intervention for termination. Sustained VT is VT lasting 30 seconds or more or requiring intervention for termination. QRS complex morphology may be either monomorphic (i.e., uniform) or polymorphic (i.e., variable). The usual heart rate of VT ranges from 100–280 beats/min. VT is wide because of the slower rate of conduction through ventricular tissue compared with that through Purkinje's fibers. Hemodynamic stability depends on the rate, underlying cardiac disease, ventricular function, and concomitant pharmacologic treatment.

Premature Ventricular Depolarizations

Isolated premature ventricular depolarizations are not associated with significant risk in patients without structural heart disease, but frequent premature ventricular complexes can be markers for potential increased risk in those with structural heart disease. Treatment of isolated, symptomatic premature complexes generally includes assessment of risk if there is structural heart disease or risk factors, avoidance of precipitating factors (e.g., caffeine, sympathomimetic agents), and reassurance with occasional beta-blockers or rarely other antiarrhythmic agents for persistently symptomatic patients. Electrophysiology study with mapping and catheter ablation of focally originating premature ventricular complexes or tachycardias also has been performed for frequent and refractory symptoms.

Sustained Ventricular Tachycardia or Fibrillation: Aborted Sudden Cardiac Death

The patient who survives hemodynamically compromising sustained ventricular arrhythmias or aborted sudden cardiac death in the absence of reversible causes or acute MI faces a high recurrence rate. Implantation of an implantable cardioverter-defibrillator (ICD) is usually indicated. Randomized studies (e.g., the Antiarrhythmics versus Implantable Defibrillator Trial) have demonstrated superiority of ICDs over medical therapies with antiarrhythmic drugs in these high-risk patients.[11]

Ventricular Tachyarrhythmias after Myocardial Infarction

Premature ventricular complexes, nonsustained or sustained VT, ventricular fibrillation, and polymorphic VT can occur during the acute phases of ischemia and infarction. Coronary reperfusion has been associated with accelerated idioventricular rhythms and ventricular tachyarrhythmias. Nonsustained or sustained VT, which often results from reentry, can occur late after MI.

Use of lidocaine as prophylaxis for ventricular fibrillation in patients with suspected acute MI has been controversial. Current data suggest that routine use of prophylactic lidocaine in patients with suspected acute MI should be avoided when facilities and personnel for prompt resuscitation are available, but when defibrillation is unavailable, it might be beneficial.

Short-term treatment of ventricular arrhythmias after MI depends on the hemodynamic status of the patient and presence of ongoing or recurrent ischemia. The long-term prognosis depends on the timing of these arrhythmias in relation to the acute infarction as well as to the degree of ventricular dysfunction. Early VT and fibrillation that is sustained are associated with an increased inhospital mortality. Among hospital survivors, however, it may not signify a worsened long-term prognosis. Short-term therapy may require DC countershock, antiarrhythmic therapy, correction of electrolyte and metabolic imbalances, or assessment and treatment of associated recurrent or ongoing ischemia.

Long-term treatment requires assessment of prognostic significance. Frequent or complex ventricular arrhythmias occurring after the acute phase of MI (i.e., the first 48–72 hours) are more frequent in patients with significant myocardial dysfunction. They also are an independent prognostic factor. Empiric suppression of PVCs or nonsustained VT using antiarrhythmic agents, however, with the possible exception of amiodarone, is associated with the potential for an increased mortality. Patients greater than 1 month after MI with left ventricular ejection fraction (LVEF) ≤30% should undergo ICD implantation based on superior survival seen in the Multicenter Automatic Defibrillator Implantation Trial II (MADIT II).[12] Results of the Sudden Cardiac Death in Heart Failure Trial (SCDHeFT) support ICD implantation in patients with LVEF of 35% or less and NYHA functional class II greater congestive heart failure.[13] For patients with nonsustained VT and a left ventricular ejection fraction of <40% after MI, consideration should be given for electrophysiology study with implantation of an ICD if the study induces sustained VT or reproducible ventricular fibrillation. Sustained ventricular arrhythmias after the acute phase of MI are associated with a high rate of recurrence, and ICD implantation is usually indicated. Beta-blockers and angiotensin-converting enzyme inhibitors also have been associated with improved survival rates in many studies and should be routinely advocated in the absence of contraindications.

Ventricular Arrhythmias Associated with Nonischemic Cardiomyopathy

The presence of nonsustained VT in patients with nonischemic cardiomyopathy has been associated with increased risk of mortality. Based on results of the SCD-HeFT trial, ICD implantation is justified for patients with ischemic cardiomyopathy, LVEF ≤35%, and NYHA FC II or greater heart failure symptoms. Sustained ventricular arrhythmias, including those in sudden cardiac death survivors, are associated with a high rate of recurrence, and ICD implantation is usually indicated.

Torsades de Pointes

A form of polymorphic VT, Torsades de Pointes (TdP) is a potentially life-threatening condition that can occur as a complication of several medications or in association with congenital long QT syndromes. The heart rate ranges from 150 to 250 beats/min with twisting of the QRS complexes around the baseline. QT prolongation and QTU abnormalities are characteristic but may be present only in beats preceding TdP. TdP typically is rate dependent; and sinus bradycardia, bradycardia resulting from atrioventricular block, or abrupt prolongation of the RR interval (e.g., with a pause after a premature complex) can trigger its onset. It usually initiates with "long-short" coupled intervals, which may occur because of a PVC on the previous, long QT-associated T wave. A pause followed by a subsequent sinus or supraventricular beat and another PVC with a short coupling interval then may initiate TdP.

Acquired and congenital forms of long QT syndromes also can predispose an individual to TdP. Acquired conditions and drugs associated with TdP are listed in Box 23-3.

Treatment includes avoidance of offending agents and may require acceleration of the heart rate, which can be accomplished with either pharmacologic agents (e.g., isoproterenol) or pacing,

---

Box 23-3 Conditions and Medications That Prolong the QT Interval

Antiarrhythmic drugs that prolong QT interval:

- Quinidine
- Procainamide (including its metabolite N-acetylprocainamide)
- Disopyramide
- Sotalol
- Amiodarone
- Bepridil
- Dofetilide

Tricyclic antidepressants

- Phenothiazines

Antibiotics:

- Erythromycin
- Pentamidine
- Trimethoprim-sulfamethoxazole
- Ampicillin
- Ketoconazole
- Itraconazole
- Spiramycin

Antihistamines:

- Terfenadine
- Astemizole
- Diphenhydramine

Other QT-prolonging drugs:

- Probucol
- Ketanserin
- Cisapride
- Organophosphates

Electrolyte abnormalities:

- Hypokalemia
- Hypomagnesemia
- Hypocalcemia (uncommon)

Bradyarrhythmias

Hypothyroidism

Liquid protein and other diets, anorexia

Central nervous system abnormalities, particularly affecting sympathetic outflow

Subarachnoid hemorrhage

Brainstem, cervical cord lesions

From: Chung MK. Arrhythmias. In: Stoller JK, Michota FA, Mandell BF, eds. The Cleveland Clinic Intensive Review of Internal Medicine. Fourth Edition. Philadelphia: Lippincott, Williams & Wilkins, 2005.

and intravenous magnesium. Lidocaine, mexiletine, or phenytoin can be tried as well. Long-term treatment of high-risk patients with long QT syndrome, including survivors of cardiac arrest, may include ICD implantation or beta-blockers. Electrolyte balance should be maintained. Genetic testing for long QT mutations is also clinically available.

GENERAL PHARMACOLOGIC THERAPY FOR TACHYARRHYTHMIAS

The most commonly accepted classification of antiarrhythmic drugs is the modified Vaughan-Williams classification. Class I antiarrhythmic drugs block Na^+ channels, thereby decreasing action potential upstroke velocity (i.e., phase 0) and slowing conduction. Class I drugs are further divided into three subdivisions. Class IA agents, which prolong repolarization or action–potential duration, have a moderate effect on conduction slowing and depression of phase 0. Class IB drugs have little effect on conduction and phase 0 in normal tissue, but they exhibit moderate effects in abnormal tissue. In addition, they show either no effect or a shortening of repolarization/action potential duration. Class IC agents have a marked effect on conduction slowing and phase 0, with mild or no effects on repolarization or action potential duration. Class II contains the β-adrenergic blocking agents, and in class III the potassium channel–blocking agents prolong repolarization/action potential duration. Class IV contains calcium channel blockers. Tables 23-3 and 23-4 list commonly used antiarrhythmic agents and their suggested dosages.[9]

Key Points

- Treatment should focus on the cause of sinus tachycardia, not just on slowing the rate.

- Multifocal atrial tachycardia in critically ill patients is associated with high hospital mortality.

- Atrial fibrillation is the most common sustained tachyarrhythmia, and its incidence increases with age. One of the most important clinical consequences is its association with thromboembolic events and stroke.

- If the duration of atrial fibrillation is more than 48 hours, anticoagulation with warfarin for 3 weeks versus transesophageal echocardiographically guided cardioversion with anticoagulation should be considered.

- AV nodal reentrant tachycardia commonly occurs in patients with no structural heart disease, and 70% of patients are women. Most patients present during the fourth or fifth decade of life, and adenosine is the initial drug of choice.

- Among patients with Wolff--Parkinson-White Syndrome, verapamil can increase the ventricular rate during atrial fibrillation; intravenous verapamil may precipitate ventricular fibrillation in this setting should not be given.

- In patients with very rapid SVT and hemodynamic impairment, DC cardioversion is the initial treatment of choice.

- Among patients with wide complex tachycardia, VT is the correct diagnosis in more than 80% of patients. In patients with a history of MI, 98% of WCTs result from VT.

SUGGESTED READING

Akhtar M, Shenasa M, Jazayeri M, et al. Wide QRS complex tachycardia: reappraisal of a common clinical problem. Ann Intern Med 1988; 109:905–912.

Singer DE, Albers GW, Dalen JE, et al. Antithrombotic therapy in atrial fibrillation. Chest 2004; 126 (Suppl): 429S–456S.

Brugada P, Brugada J, Mont L, et al. A new approach to the differential diagnosis of a regular tachycardia with a wide QRS complex. Circulation 1991; 83:1649–1659.

Fuster V, Ryden LE, Asinger RW, et al. ACC/AHA/ESC guidelines for the management of patients with atrial fibrillation: executive summary. A Report of the American College of Cardiology/American Heart Association Task Force on Practice Guidelines and the European Society of Cardiology Committee for Practice Guidelines and Policy Conferences (Committee to Develop Guidelines for the Management of Patients With Atrial Fibrillation) Developed in Collaboration with the North American Society of Pacing and Electrophysiology. Circulation 2001; 104:2118–2150.

Ganz LI, Friedman PL. Supraventricular tachycardia. N Engl J Med 1995; 332:162–173.

Gregoratos G, Abrams J, Epstein AE, et al. ACC/AHA/NASPE 2002 guideline update for implantation of cardiac pacemakers and antiarrhythmia devices: summary article: a report of the American College of Cardiology/American Heart Association Task Force on Practice Guidelines (ACC/AHA/NASPE committee to update the 1998 guidelines). Circulation 2002; 106:2145–2161.

Kindwall KE, Brown J, Josephson ME. Electrocardiographic criteria for ventricular tachycardia in wide complex left bundle branch block morphology tachycardias. Am J Cardiol 1988; 61:1279–1283.

Kusumoto FM, Goldschlager N. Cardiac pacing. N Engl J Med 1996; 334:89–98.

Task Force of the Working Group on Arrhythmias of the European Society of Cardiology. The Sicilian gambit. Circulation 1991; 84:1831–1851.

Wellens HJJ, Bar FWHM, Lie KI. The value of the electrocardiogram in the differential diagnosis of a tachycardia with a widened QRS complex. Am J Med 1978; 64:27–33.

CHAPTER TWENTY-FOUR

Cardiac Arrest

David V. Gugliotti, MD

BACKGROUND

Sudden cardiac arrest is defined by the International Liaison Committee on Resuscitation (ILCOR) as the cessation of cardiac mechanical activity as confirmed by the absence of signs of circulation.[1] This definition was established to improve standardization of cardiopulmonary resuscitation evaluation and reporting. ILCOR was formed to systematically review resuscitation science and develop evidence-based consensus guidelines for resuscitation worldwide. The term sudden cardiac death (SCD) has been used interchangeably with sudden cardiac arrest; however, in cases when resuscitation is successful, the event may be referred to as aborted SCD.

Resuscitation guidelines were updated in 2005, based on evidence evaluation from the 2005 International Consensus Conference on Cardiopulmonary Resuscitation (CPR) and Emergency Cardiovascular Care (ECC) Science With Treatment Recommendations.

These guidelines were incorporated into individual resuscitation council guidelines. The American Heart Association guidelines for CPR and ECC were published as a supplement to *Circulation* in December 2005, and they represent a comprehensive review of available resuscitation literature. One major emphasis of the new AHA guidelines is to improve survival from cardiac arrest by increasing the number of cardiac arrest victims who receive early, high-quality CPR.

Sudden cardiac death is a leading cause of death in the United States, accounting for more than 400,000 deaths per year. An estimated 250,000–400,000 are victims of out-of-hospital cardiac arrest. In addition, an estimated 370,000–750,000 patients will have cardiac arrest and receive attempted resuscitation in the hospital each year.[2,3] Survival from cardiac arrest remains poor, despite efforts for improved response times for out-of-hospital arrest and standardized practices for cardiac arrest resuscitation.

Most victims of cardiac arrest have some form of underlying heart disease, though arrest can occur in apparently healthy individuals. Sudden cardiac arrest accounts for a high proportion of cardiac disease-related deaths in persons aged 35–44 years.

Cardiac resuscitation in or out of the hospital depends on a standard sequence of events known as the Chain of Survival. The chain of survival concept has evolved through several decades of research into sudden cardiac arrest. Effective execution of steps in the chain of survival increases the chance that a person can survive cardiac arrest in or out of the hospital.

The major chain of survival links of resuscitation include:

1. Rapid access—activate Emergency Medical Services (EMS) system in the community or code team in the hospital; also recognition of early warning signs
2. Rapid cardiopulmonary resuscitation—CPR as a bridge until advanced help arrives
3. Rapid defibrillation—quick and accurate assessment of heart rhythm and defibrillation of the heart if indicated
4. Rapid advanced care—administration of medications and adequate ventilation, including intubation

ASSESSMENT

Clinical Presentation

Cardiopulmonary arrest is diagnosed by the triad of pulselessness, unconsciousness, and apnea. Most patients have sudden onset of symptoms related to rapid collapse of cerebral and cardiac circulation. Sudden loss of circulation generally results in loss of consciousness within 15 seconds, though agonal respirations may persist for 60 seconds. Primary respiratory arrest (acute airway obstruction, decreased respiratory drive, or respiratory muscle weakness) results in transient hemodynamic instability that progresses to loss of consciousness, bradycardia, and pulselessness usually within 5 minutes.[4] The differential diagnosis of cardiac arrest is broad (Table 24-1), and understanding possible causes helps to guide diagnostic testing and therapy.

Prodromal symptoms of cardiac arrest may include chest pain, shortness of breath, weakness or fatigue, syncope, palpitations, or a variety of nonspecific complaints. Information from bystanders or medical personnel is critical. Circumstances surrounding the event, including whether the arrest was witnessed, time of arrest, condition prior to arrest, and recent medications or ingestions, should be noted. Of particular note, in hospitalized patients suffering cardiac arrest, physicians should identify preceding evidence of a significant change in vital signs (BP <90 mmHg despite treatment or pulse rate >130 per min), unexplained decrease in consciousness, increased or decreased respiratory rate (>30 or <6 breaths per min), and unexplained ventricular ectopy.

Table 24-1 Common Causes of Nontraumatic Cardiac Arrest

General	Specific	Disease/Agent
Cardiac		Coronary artery disease
		Cardiomyopathy
		Structural abnormalities
		Valve dysfunction
Respiratory	Hypoventilation	CNS dysfunction
		Neuromuscular disease
		Toxic and metabolic
	Upper airway obstruction	CNS dysfunction
		Foreign body infection
		Trauma
		Neoplasm
	Pulmonary dysfunction	Pneumonia
		Asthma, COPD
		Pulmonary edema
		Pulmonary embolus
Circulatory	Mechanical obstruction	Tension pneumothorax
		Pericardial tamponade
		Pulmonary embolus
	Hypovolemia	Hemorrhage
	Vascular tone	Neurogenic
		Sepsis
Metabolic	Electrolyte abnormalities	Hypocalcemia
		Hypokalemia or hyperkalemia
		Hypomagnesemia
		Hypocalcemia
Toxic	Prescription medications	β-blockers
		Calcium channel blockers
		Digitalis
		Antidysrhythmics
		Tricyclic antidepressants
	Drugs of abuse	Heroin
		Cocaine
	Toxins	Cyanide
		Carbon monoxide
Environmental		Lightning
		Drowning/near-drowning
		Hypothermia/ hyperthermia
		Electrocution

Adapted from: Adult resuscitation. In: Marx. Rosen's Emergency Medicine: Concepts and Clinical Practice, 5th ed. St. Louis, 2002. 64–83.

Cardiac arrest and resuscitation in the hospitalized patient are much more complex than in out-of-hospital arrest. Hospital patients have varying degrees of cardiac and pulmonary dysfunction that cannot be characterized as cardiac arrest, such as hypotension or shock. Respiratory patterns may be abnormal and range from normal to gasping or agonal breaths. In addition, some patients suffering cardiac arrest are already mechanically ventilated in an intensive care unit (ICU) setting.[5]

Physical examination focuses mainly on evaluation and maintenance of adequate airway; palpation of the pulse in a large artery (to confirm cardiac arrest—though people actually do not accurately detect the presence or absence of pulses in this stressful setting); and detecting any physical examination findings that may indicate a cause for the arrest—these include evidence of gastrointestinal hemorrhage, other signs of blood loss, tense or distended abdomen, engorged jugular veins, upper airway obstruction, and asymmetric breath sounds with initial ventilation. The physical examination reveals little information about the duration of arrest, except for the first few minutes after the event.[4]

Diagnosis

The diagnosis of cardiac arrest is confirmed with the findings of a pulseless, unconscious, apneic patient. A rapid sequence of events must follow to activate the medical emergency response system in the hospital (code team).

Prognosis

The chance of survival from cardiac arrest is highest when an arrest is witnessed, prompt CPR is initiated, the initial rhythm is ventricular tachycardia or ventricular fibrillation, and defibrillation is administered quickly. These findings are particularly true when applied to out-of-hospital cardiac arrest.

The prognosis after in-hospital cardiac arrest has been difficult to evaluate. Diverse hospital settings make standardized data collection difficult, and cardiac arrest event reporting is inconsistent. During an actual inpatient arrest, estimation of an individual patient outcome is even more complicated. Cardiac arrest is a complex pathway for a diverse collection of diseases and varied conditions present before or arising during the hospitalization.[6] Comorbid conditions may or may not directly contribute to the development of cardiac arrest. Detailed discussion of the severity of comorbid conditions is often lacking in research studies, and this makes interpretation of morbidity and mortality from outcome studies difficult.

In one study of pre-arrest morbidity and associated outcomes from resuscitation, 553 CPR events were recorded and 120 (21.7%) patients survived to discharge.[7] Factors independently associated with low survival include age of 70 years and older, stroke, or renal failure before hospital admission (OR = 0.6, 0.3, 0.3), and congestive heart failure during admission (OR = 0.4). Angina pectoris and ventricular arrhythmia as the main hospital admission diagnosis were associated with higher survival (30.1% and 70%; OR 2.1 and 11, respectively).

A Canadian study of general medical inpatients revealed a similar survival to discharge of 13.4% among 247 patients experiencing cardiac arrest.[8] In this study, 143 events were witnessed with a survival to discharge of 22.4%. In contrast, 104 unwitnessed events resulted in a survival to discharge rate of only 1%.

The National Registry of Cardiopulmonary Resuscitation (NRCPR) evolved from American Heart Association models for in-hospital CPR recording. The NRCPR registry is the largest, standardized reporting of in-hospital resuscitation in the United States. NRCPR data from January 2000 through June 2002 include 14,720 cardiac arrests that met inclusion criteria occurring in adults at 207 participating hospitals.[9] The three most common reasons for cardiac arrest were (1) cardiac arrhythmia (49%), (2) acute respiratory insufficiency (37%), and (3) hypotension (32%). About half of in-hospital cardiac arrests occurred in an ICU. Overall, 44% of adult in-hospital cardiac arrest victims had a return of spontaneous circulation (ROSC); 17% survived to hospital discharge.

Ventricular fibrillation (VF) or pulseless VT was the initial pulseless rhythm in only 25% of in-hospital cardiac arrest victims. ROSC occurred in 58% of VF cases, yielding a survival-to-hospital-discharge rate of 34% in this group of patients. Survival to discharge for patients with a presenting rhythm of PEA or asystole was only 10%. Of particular note in the NRCPR data was that 86% of patients had witnessed events and/or were monitored at the time of the event.

Van Walraven et al. developed a clinical decision rule to address discontinuation of in-hospital cardiac arrest resuscitation.[10] Outcome data, information about the arrest, and patient statistics from 1,077 in-hospital cardiac resuscitation events were analyzed. Death in the hospital was significantly more likely in patients older than 75 years, when the arrest was not witnessed, if resuscitation lasted longer than 10 minutes, and if the initial rhythm was not VT or VF. The decision rule identified all 103 study patients who survived to hospital discharge. In this study, all patients with no pulse after 10 minutes of resuscitation, an initial rhythm not VT or VF, and having an unwitnessed arrest died. The initial cardiac rhythm was VT or VF in 31.4%.

This clinical decision aid was validated in a secondary analysis of a resuscitation registry at the Medical Center of Central Georgia.[6] Some patients in the study who were predicted to have no chance of recovery (and did not survive to discharge) did have short-term recovery of consciousness, which may have been considered significant. However, overall this validation study had 99.1% sensitivity to predict some chance of survival to hospital discharge.

MANAGEMENT

Treatment

Initiation of BLS (Basic Life Support)

The key components of the BLS algorithm are initiated as rapidly as possible by the first responder to an arrest (usually hospital nursing staff who are BLS certified). The goal of BLS is to restore circulation of oxygenated blood to vital organs until further workup and definitive therapy can be given. Victims of cardiac arrest need immediate CPR. CPR prolongs the time that VF is present and increases the likelihood that a shock will terminate VF to an effective cardiac rhythm. The following steps comprise the international BLS algorithm and represent the primary ABCD survey of the cardiac arrest victim (Fig. 24-1)[11]:

1. Check responsiveness.
2. Activate the emergency response system.
3. Open the **airway,** and check **breathing.**
4. Give two effective breaths.
5. Assess **circulation (pulse check for health care providers only—limit to 10 seconds).**
6. Compress chest (no signs of circulation detected).
7. Employ **defibrillation.**

Components of BLS

Assess Responsiveness

Shake or tap the patient and ask, "Are you alright?" or "Can you hear me?"

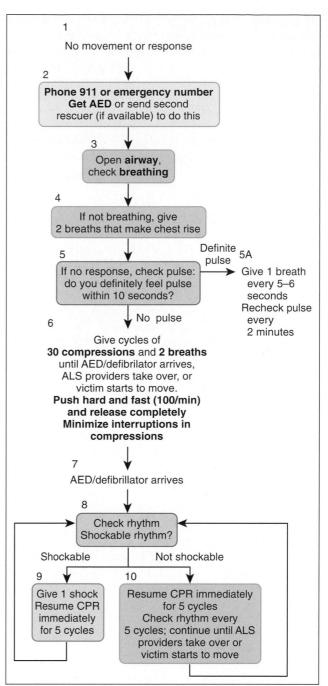

Figure 24-1 • Adult BLS Healthcare Provider Algorithm. General guideline for BLS. From: 2005 American Heart Association Guidelines for Cardiopulmonary Resuscitation and Emergency Cardiovascular Care, Part 4: Adult Basic Life Support. Circulation 2005; 112(suppl IV):IV22.

Airway and Breathing

The victim should be placed on a hard surface in the supine (face-up) position. Signs of airway obstruction should be assessed and relieved with manual maneuvers or suction if indicated. Use the head tilt–chin lift maneuver to open the airway. The head tilt–chin lift maneuver involves placing one hand on the forehead of a supine patient and applying firm pressure with the palm of hand, tilting the head back. With the other hand, the fingers are placed under the bony part of lower jaw, and the jaw is lifted upward to bring the chin forward.

The absence of spontaneous breaths should be confirmed by observation, and two rescue breaths at 1 second per breath are given with bag-valve mask, mouth-to-mask, or mouth-to-mouth ventilation. Effective breaths should result in a visible chest rise and avoid rapid or forceful breaths. Chest compressions should then be started. Breaths should be continued between chest compressions at compression-to-breath ratio of 30:2 until the patient has a stable airway (endotracheal intubation). Once a stable airway is present, breaths should be delivered at a rate of 8–10 breaths per minute, and compressions should not stop for delivery of ventilations.

Chest Compressions

"Push Hard, Push Fast" Serial, rhythmic chest compressions should be applied to the lower half of the sternum at a rate of 100 compressions per minute. The depth of each compression should be approximately 4–5 cm. The chest should be allowed to recoil completely after each compression, with approximately equal compression and relaxation times. Research data indicate that a rate of at least 80 compressions per minute is needed to achieve optimal blood flow during CPR—the goal of 100 compressions per minute was established to ensure that an adequate amount of compressions are applied in a 1-minute period.[10] Chest compressions create blood flow by increasing intrathoracic pressure or directly compressing the heart. Some evidence suggests that victims are more likely to survive if a higher number of chest compressions are delivered with CPR, even if fewer ventilations are given. Coronary perfusion pressure increases with each sequential chest compression, leading to the recommended 30:2 compression to breath ratio (compared to 15:2).

Defibrillation

Defibrillation is the most vital intervention for BLS in out-of-hospital arrest. For a patient in VF, the probability of successful resuscitation and subsequent survival to hospital discharge is directly related to the shortest time interval between onset of VF and delivery of the first shock. Many out-of-hospital interventions have focused on decreasing the time to recognize shockable heart rhythms and delivery of the first shock. Automatic external defibrillators (AEDs) have been successful in improving survival from out-of-hospital cardiac arrest. Prompt BLS and early defibrillation should be available throughout all hospital and outpatient medical facilities, and in-hospital resuscitation goals should focus on decreasing the time to defibrillation. The use of defibrillation transcends both ACLS and BLS care and is further discussed below as applied to in-hospital arrest.[12]

Initiation of ACLS (Advanced Cardiopulmonary Life Support)

The foundation of ACLS care is good BLS care. Prompt CPR and early defibrillation can significantly increase the chance for survival to hospital discharge.[13] Advanced cardiopulmonary life support includes BLS and initiation of the secondary ABCD survey. The secondary ABCD survey includes:

1. **Airway** management with endotracheal intubation
2. **Breathing** assessment by checking tube placement and ventilation
3. **Circulation** management with IV placement and ECG assessment

4. **Differential diagnosis** for evaluating reversible causes of arrest

Team aspects of resuscitation efforts should always be stressed. An effective resuscitation team exhibits defined roles, including leadership and organization skills for the team leader and specific performance skills for individual team members. ACLS treatment algorithms are initiated based on the presenting cardiac rhythm. See Figure 24-2 for ACLS algorithm based on presenting cardiac rhythm.

Components of ACLS

Defibrillation

Defibrillation techniques provide current flow through the heart to achieve defibrillation while minimizing electrical current injury to the heart. Monophasic defibrillators deliver current in one direction, varying the speed and amount of waveform decline and the speed of return to zero voltage. When a monophasic defibrillator is used, a dose of 360 Joules (J) should be used for all shocks. If ventricular fibrillation recurs during an arrest, the previous energy needed for defibrillation should be chosen for ensuing shocks.

Biphasic defibrillation delivers electrical current in two directions. Current flows in a positive direction for a specified time, then reverses and flows in a negative direction for the duration of the electrical discharge. The optimal energy for first-shock biphasic waveform defibrillation has not been completely determined and is dependent on the specific device. Successful defibrillation has been demonstrated with first-shock energy of 150–200 J. Familiarity with each device used for clinical care is essential. If the provider is not aware of the optimal effective biphasic energy for that device to terminate VF, then 200 J should be selected for the first shock and equal or higher dose for subsequent shocks.[12] Increasingly, biphasic defibrillators are replacing monophasic versions.

Medications for Cardiovascular Support[13,14]

Epinephrine Dosage: 1 mg IV every 3–5 minutes (endotracheal administration 2–2.5 mg)

Increases coronary and cerebral blood flow by alpha-adrenergic stimulation and increased peripheral vasoconstriction. No proven role for high-dose epinephrine—high-dose epinephrine may increase return of spontaneous circulation (ROSC), but does not improve survival to discharge.

Vasopressin Dosage: 40 units IV once
Nonadrenergic peripheral vasoconstriction.

Vasopressin may be used as an alternative agent to epinephrine for cardiac arrest with any presenting heart rhythm.

One dose of vasopressin 40 units IV may replace either the first or second dose of epinephrine in the management of pulseless arrest.

Agents for Arrhythmias:

Amiodarone Dosage: 300 mg IV push, 150 mg repeat dose if needed, and initial infusion 1 mg/min.

Complex drug with effects on sodium, potassium, and calcium channels; as well as alpha- and beta-adrenergic blocking properties.

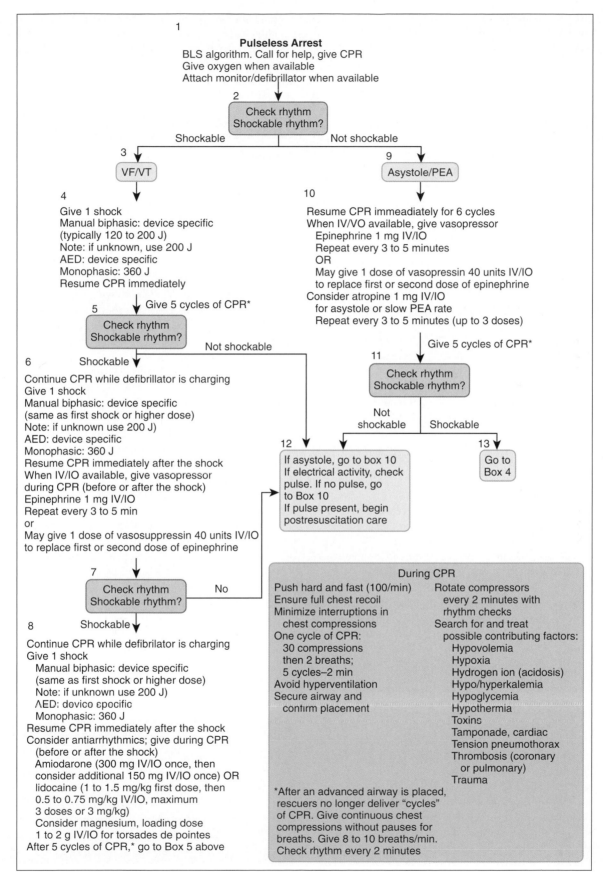

Figure 24-2 • AGLS Pulseless Arrest Algorithm. Algorithm for AGLS care. From: 2005 American Heart Association Guidelines for Cardiopulmonary Resuscitation and Emergency Cardiovascular Care, Part 7.2: Management of Cardiac Arrest. Circulation 2005; 112(Suppl 4):IV59.

Amiodarone is the preferred antiarrhythmic with impaired cardiac function.

Recommended after defibrillation and epinephrine/vasopressin in cardiac arrest with persistent VF or VT.

Lidocaine Dosage: 1–1.5 mg/kg IV initial bolus, additional bolus 0.5–0.75 mg/kg if necessary (total dose should not exceed 3 mg/kg or 200–300 mg total during a 1-hour period.)

Continuous infusion after rhythm restoration is controversial (1–4 mg/min infusion).

Exerts blocking effects on sodium channels.

Lidocaine can effectively suppress ventricular arrhythmias, especially associated with myocardial ischemia or infarction, and may be used for refractory VF.

Magnesium Dosage: 1–2 g IV push.
Recommended in arrest if torsades de pointes or hypomagnesemia is present.

Atropine Dosage: 0.5 mg IV push, with repeat doses every 3–5 minutes (total dose 3 mg.)

Anticholinergic agent.

Recommended for asystole or slow PEA.

Other Agents and Interventions:

Sodium Bicarbonate Dosage: 1 mEq/kg IV bolus.
May be beneficial in certain circumstances, including preexisting acidosis, hyperkalemia, or tricyclic or phenobarbital overdose.
Use should generally be guided by measured bicarbonate concentrations.

End-Tidal CO_2 Monitoring Devices measure the concentration of CO_2 from the lungs, and the presence of exhaled CO_2 is usually a reliable indicator of correct endotracheal tube placement.

End-tidal CO_2 may be employed as a noninvasive indicator of cardiac output and is a prognostic indicator for ROSC.

Arterial Blood Gases (ABGs) ABG monitoring is not a reliable indicator of tissue hypoxemia, hypercarbia, or tissue acidosis during cardiac arrest. ABGs are not indicated in cardiac arrest management.

PREVENTION

A significant number of men and women with serious coronary atherosclerotic heart disease (CAD) may present in a dramatic fashion with sudden cardiac arrest. Risk factors for sudden cardiac death are considered the same as those for CAD. Prevention of cardiac arrest involves aggressive CAD risk factor recognition and modification.

In the inpatient setting, prevention of cardiac arrest involves prompt recognition of signs of clinical deterioration. Changes in vital signs, neurologic condition, and symptoms of shortness of breath or chest pain should prompt aggressive investigation and intervention. So-called "pre-arrest" conditions may signal impending full cardiopulmonary arrest. Many hospitals have introduced Rapid Response Teams (RRT) or Medical Emergency Teams (MET) to respond to patients with acute physiologic deterioration, and these interventions have had success in decreasing the number of cardiac arrests in some situations.

An additional aspect of cardiac arrest prevention is appropriate and comprehensive assessment of do not resuscitate (DNR) status in the hospital. Each patient or designated family member should be asked about the patient's wishes regarding resuscitation (i.e., advance directive). This is reviewed in more detail in Chapter 95, Palliative Care.

DISCHARGE/FOLLOW-UP PLANS

Postresuscitation care of the cardiac arrest victim is complex and incurs high risk of short- and long-term complications. Components of postresuscitation care include: (1) optimizing hemodynamic, respiratory, and neurologic support; (2) identifying and treating reversible causes of arrest; and (3) monitoring and treating temperature and metabolic derangements. Some evidence points to improved outcomes with permissive hypothermia or active induction of hypothermia. Hemodynamically stable patients with mild hypothermia (>33°C) should not be actively rewarmed because this degree of hypothermia may be beneficial to neurologic outcome. Glucose should be monitored closely to avoid hypoglycemia, while also avoiding elevated sugars which are detrimental to critically ill patients (particularly in regards to infectious complications).[15]

ECG monitoring, supplemental oxygen, and IV saline infusion are common interventions after arrest. Antiarrhythmic therapy may be considered, especially if the arrest was VF or VT, or if there is suspicion of acute myocardial infarction. Evaluation of the cause of arrest should be undertaken, focusing on myocardial infarction, electrolyte abnormalities, or primary arrhythmia as the etiology. Hemodynamic instability is common after resuscitation, and it requires close cardiac monitoring and further evaluation, along with hemodynamic support. Finally, the patient should be transferred to an intensive care unit for continued laboratory and other evaluations to assess organ dysfunction and complications that arise related to arrest. A recent meta-analysis of 11 studies involving 1914 patients documented five clinical signs that strongly predict death or poor neurologic outcome.[16]

- Absent corneal reflex at 24 hours
- Absent pupillary response at 24 hours
- Absent withdrawal response to pain at 24 hours
- No motor response at 24 hours
- No motor response at 72 hours

Assistance from a palliative care consult service may be highly useful in communicating the dire prognosis in these situations.

Key Points

- Factors independently associated with low survival rates from cardiac arrest include age ≥70 years, stroke, or renal failure before hospital admission, and congestive heart failure during admission. Angina pectoris and ventricular arrhythmia as the main hospital admission diagnosis are associated with higher survival.

- Applying a clinical decision rule can identify patients for whom in-hospital resuscitation probably can be stopped, as all will not survive to discharge; criteria include: patients with no pulse after 10 minutes of resuscitation, an initial rhythm not VT or VF, and those having an unwitnessed arrest.

SUGGESTED READING

Eisenberg MS, Mengert TJ. Cardiac resuscitation. N Engl J Med 2001; 344(17):1304–1313.

van Walraven C, Forster AJ, Parish DC, et al. Validation of a clinical decision aid to discontinue in-hospital cardiac arrest resuscitations. JAMA 2001; 285(12):1602–1606.

Brindley PG, Markland DM, Mayers I, et al. Predictors of survival following in-hospital adult cardiopulmonary resuscitation. CMAJ 2002; 167(4):343–348.

Peberdy MA, Kaye W, ORnata JP, et al. Cardiopulmonary resuscitation of adults in the hospital: a report of 14720 cardiac arrest from the National Registry of Cardiopulmonary Resuscitation. Resuscitation 2003; 58:297–308.

Booth CM, Boone RH, Tomlinson G, et al. Is this patient dead, vegetative, or severely neurologically impaired? Assessing outcome for comatose survivors of cardiac arrest. JAMA 2004; 291:870–879.

CHAPTER TWENTY-FIVE

Syncope

Anitha Rajamanickam, MD, Saira Noor, MD, and Franklin A. Michota, MD

BACKGROUND

Syncope is a sudden, temporary, and partial or complete loss of consciousness associated with a loss of postural tone and with spontaneous, rapid, and complete recovery not requiring electrical or chemical cardioversion, drugs, or a pacemaker to restore normal mental status and cardiac rhythm. Syncope, derived from the Greek word *synkope*, or "pause," is caused by transient hypoperfusion to the areas of the brain necessary for consciousness (the brainstem reticular activating system and the bilateral cerebral cortices). A 35% reduction in cerebral blood flow or complete disruption of cerebral perfusion for 5–10 seconds results in syncope. This needs to be differentiated from other causes of altered consciousness, such as seizures, hysteria, anxiety attacks, drop attacks, head trauma, narcolepsy, metabolic or drug-induced encephalopathy, and sudden cardiac death (Box 25-1). Near syncope is a sense of impending loss of consciousness or weakness. Near syncope occurs more frequently than syncope and often provides important diagnostic clues, as the patient has a better recollection of the event.

Syncope may be the first manifestation of a potentially life-threatening disorder. Syncope-associated morbidity includes lacerations, extremity fractures, head injuries, and motor vehicle accidents. Observational studies confirm that cardiac causes of syncope have a much higher mortality rate than syncope from noncardiac causes. Physicians must distinguish high-risk syncope patients with potentially fatal conditions who require admission to the hospital from low-risk syncope patients who may be safely discharged home with outpatient follow-up. For those patients who are hospitalized, the mean length of stay ranges from an average of 3–5 days, with an average cost of $5,500. Cost-benefit analysis suggests that hospitalization for syncope without comorbidity leads to an economical loss for most hospitals.

ASSESSMENT

Clinical Presentation

Prevalence

Syncope is common, representing the cause of 1–3% of emergency room visits and about 1% of hospitalizations. One third of individuals are expected to have at least one episode of syncope during their lifetime. In addition, recurrent syncope occurs in 20% of patients within 1 year of the initial episode. Syncope occurs in all age groups, although the incidence increases with advancing age especially after age 70. In the Framingham Hearts study, the prevalence of syncope was about 11% each for men and women during an average of 17 years of follow-up.

Presenting Signs and Symptoms

History should be meticulously recorded and should focus on the circumstances immediately prior to the syncopal episode, its onset, and how the episode resolved. A detailed medication history, including illicit drugs, is necessary, as many drugs can precipitate syncope through a variety of mechanisms such as orthostasis (antihypertensives, antidepressants), decreased cardiac output (beta-blockers, antiarrhythmics), sinoatrial node depression (antiarrhythmics, digoxin), or prolongation of the Q-T interval (antidepressants, phenothiazines, antiarrhythmics).

The physical examination should focus on vital signs, including bilateral blood pressure and orthostatic measurements, and a comprehensive cardiovascular assessment. This should include auscultation for valvular heart disease, palpation of pulses and auscultation of carotid and femoral arteries, assessment of volume status and occult blood loss (guaiac stool), and checking for the presence of a rhythm disturbance. Neurologic examination should look for focal neurologic deficits and include cranial nerve and fundoscopic assessments.

Differential Diagnosis

There are many etiologies for syncope (Box 25-2), but they can be categorized into cardiovascular (arrhythmias and blood flow obstruction), reflex-mediated (vasovagal and carotid hypersensitivity), orthostatic, neurologic, psychiatric, and unknown (about 20%). The following reviews historical and physical findings specific to an etiology.

Cardiovascular Syncope

It is imperative that physicians recognize syncope secondary to a cardiac etiology causing inadequate cardiac output and cerebral hypoperfusion, as it is associated with increased risk of premature death or subsequent cardiovascular events. Factors predictive of

Box 25-1 Disorders That Mimic Syncope

1. Seizures
2. Psychiatric causes
   a. Panic disorder, anxiety disorder, major depression, somatization, conversion, breath holding
3. Drop attacks
4. Narcolepsy
5. Hypoxia
6. Hypoglycemia
7. Hyperventilation
8. Carbon monoxide and other chemical and natural gas poisoning
9. Cataplexy
10. Transient ischemic attack
11. Vertigo
12. Pregnancy (changes in vascular autoregulation and anatomy lead to maternal fainting in about 8% of women during **early** pregnancy)

cardiac syncope include presence of heart disease, history of ventricular arrhythmias, supine position at the onset of the episode (arrhythmias, heart block), or syncope during exertion (aortic outflow obstruction, aortic stenosis, long Q-T syndrome, catecholamine-sensitive ventricular tachycardia). Blurred vision; convulsion during syncope but without a postictal phase; palpitations prior to syncope; pain in the chest, neck, shoulder, or epigastric area; dyspnea; and quick post event recovery of mentation all strongly suggest cardiac syncope. A family history of sudden death may suggest hypertrophic cardiomyopathy (HOCM), anomalous origin of left coronary artery from the sinus of Valsalva, long Q-T syndrome, or catecholamine-sensitive ventricular tachycardia. Syncope that occurs multiple times in a day and without warning suggests arrhythmia. Patients with mechanical heart valves warrant especially close evaluation and will likely require hospitalization in the setting of syncope.

Syncope is associated with pulmonary embolism (PE) in up to 14% of cases of PE. This diagnosis must be considered any time a patient complains of dyspnea and chest pain with an episode of syncope. Signs and symptoms for deep vein thrombosis and pulmonary embolism should be sought. Aortic dissection may also present with syncope, emphasizing the importance of a thorough evaluation of all pulses.

Reflex-Mediated Syncope

Reflex-mediated syncope is due to activation of cardiopulmonary baroreceptors and/or mechanoreceptors causing inappropriate bradycardia and/or peripheral vasodilatation. Reflex-mediated syncope has many variations, but includes vasovagal (neurocardiogenic), carotid sinus, situational syncope, and syncope from glossopharyngeal or trigeminal neuralgia. There is no increased risk for cardiovascular morbidity or mortality associated with reflex-mediated syncope, but the syncope can result in death if it occurs at an inopportune time such as while driving a car.

Vasovagal syncope is the most common type of syncope in young adults and is colloquially referred to as a "fainting spell." It usually occurs in a standing position and is precipitated by fear, apprehension, emotional stress, pain, fatigue, sleep or food deprivation, warm ambient environment, alcohol consumption, instrumentation, or pregnancy. It is brief in duration (3 seconds versus up to 3 minutes as seen with cardiac syncope). Autonomic symptoms predominate; and nausea, diaphoresis, blurred or faded vision, epigastric discomfort, and light-headedness usually precede syncope by a few minutes. Patients are usually pale and diaphoretic with dilated pupils.

Patients with the carotid sinus hypersensitivity have an exaggerated baroreceptor response resulting in periods of inappropriately high vagal tone and sympathetic suppression. Carotid sinus massage (gentle) is the diagnostic maneuver of choice, but the technique has not been standardized. Contraindications to carotid sinus massage include carotid bruits, history of stroke or transient ischemia attack, ventricular tachycardia, or recent myocardial infarction. Symptoms of syncope or presyncope should be reproducible by gentle carotid sinus massage. Association with precipitating factors such as neck twisting, shaving, head turning or wearing tight-fitting collars, neck tumors, extensive neck scarring secondary to radical surgery dissection or radiation fibrosis, or neck trauma reinforces the diagnosis.

Certain situations (micturition, defecation, coughing, or gastrointestinal stimulation) may be associated with syncope. The history is diagnostic. Cough-induced syncope occurs after prolonged bouts of coughing, usually due to chronic obstructive pulmonary disease or emphysema. Postprandial syncope, common in elderly patients, has no clear mechanism, although it is thought to be caused by inadequate sympathetic compensation to pooling of blood in the splanchnic circulation and/or a peripheral vasodilatation induced by insulin.

Orthostatic Syncope

Orthostatic hypotension is defined as a drop in blood pressure of at least 20 mm Hg systolic or 10 mm Hg diastolic within 3 minutes of standing. Tachycardia during testing indicates volume depletion. A blunted heart rate response suggests baroreceptor impairment that may occur normally in older patients. Syncope due to orthostasis leads to pallor that is usually striking and is not accompanied by cyanosis or respiratory disturbances. Medications are often associated with orthostatic syncope and include most antihypertensives (including diuretics) and antidepressants. Orthostasis secondary to occult blood loss will usually be associated with anemia or evidence of blood in the stool.

Neurologic Syncope

Patients with syncope from neurologic cause are at greater risk for both fatal and nonfatal stroke. Following neurologic syncope, the patient's face is florid, and the breathing is usually slow and stertorous. Only two central nervous system lesions can cause syncope: bilateral cortical dysfunction or reticular activating system injury (vertebrobasilar insufficiency). Syncope from vertebrobasilar insufficiency (VBI) generally has other associated symptoms of posterior circulation insufficiency, such as vertigo, diplopia, ataxia, and dysarthria. Severe bilateral carotid artery stenosis or unilateral stenosis with contralateral carotid occlusion may rarely cause syncope in a patient with upright posture. Historical clues include focal weakness; abdominal discomfort

Box 25-2 Etiology of Syncope

1. Cardiovascular syncope (20%)
   a. Arrhythmia
      i. Tachyarrhythmias (VT, torsades de pointes, long Q-T, SVT)
      ii. Bradyarrhythmias (SSS, AVB, drug induced, pacer malfunction)
   b. Structural heart disease
      i. Valvular
         • AS, prosthetic valve thrombus, MS
      ii. Obstructive
         • HOCM, myxoma
      iii. Pump failure
         • Acute MI, tamponade
         • Low flow states, such as those associated with advanced cardiomyopathy, severe heart failure, and valvular insufficiency
      iv. Vascular (rare)
         • PE, PPH, aortic dissection, SC steal, air embolism
2. Reflex-mediated syncope (40%)
   a. Vasovagal (neurocardiogenic)
   b. Situational (micturition, posttussive, postprandial, defecation, deglutition, weightlifters)
   c. Carotid sinus hypersensitivity
3. Orthostatic syncope (15%)
   a. Volume depletion, severe hemorrhage, venous pooling
   b. Medication-induced
   c. Dysautonomic
      i. Primary disorders
      ii. Secondary disorders (DM, renal failure, HIV, collagen-vascular disease)
4. Neurologic syncope (1%)
   a. Cerebrovascular disease (vertebrobasilar insufficiency)
   b. Subarachnoid hemorrhage, increased intracranial pressure (tumor, trauma, ventricular obstruction), migraine
5. Psychiatric (5%)
6. Metabolic derangements (<1%)
   a. Hypokalemia, hypomagnesemia, hypocalcemia (prolonged Q-T)
7. Unknown (20%)

VT—ventricular tachycardia; SVT—supraventricular tachycardia; SSS—sick sinus syndrome; AVB—atrioventricular block; AS—aortic stenosis; MS—mitral stenosis; HOCM—hypertrophic obstructive cardiomyopathy; MI—myocardial infarction; PE—pulmonary embolism; PPH—primary pulmonary hypertension; SC steal—subclavian steal; COI—chronic orthostatic intolerance; POTS—postural orthostatic tachycardia syndrome; DM—diabetes mellitus; HIV—human immunodeficiency virus.

prior to event; nausea and diaphoresis during recovery; and changes in speech, sensation, coordination, or balance. Sudden severe headache with accelerated hypertension, nausea, vomiting, focal neurological and meningeal signs may indicate subarachnoid hemorrhage.

Mimics of Syncope

Syncope should be differentiated from other causes of altered consciousness such as seizure, hysteria, anxiety attacks, drop attack, head trauma, narcolepsy, metabolic or drug-induced encephalopathy, and sudden cardiac death (see Box 25-1). History of spontaneous, rapid, and complete recovery is specific for syncope and not common with other etiologies of altered consciousness. Psychiatric disorders (especially anxiety and depression) may be associated with hyperventilation-induced syncope and should be considered if the initial evaluation is unrevealing. In the setting of an unwitnessed episode of loss of consciousness, the physician should consider hypoglycemia or other metabolic disorders which can provoke loss of consciousness.

Syncope versus Seizures

The differentiation between syncope and seizures is important, and it is not always obvious. Tongue biting or oral trauma, incontinence (especially fecal), lack of pallor or cyanosis, persistent tonic-clonic movements, slow return to consciousness, post event headache or confusion, or myalgias indicate seizures. Symptoms of nausea or diaphoresis prior to the event suggest syncope, whereas an aura (an auditory phenomenon, an upset stomach, complex visual experiences, or unpleasant olfactory sensations) is associated with seizures. Patients with syncope do not remember actually hitting the ground. Post event confusion has been described with syncope, but the confusion should not last more than 30 seconds. Seizure-like activity can occur with syncope (convulsive syncope) if the patient is held in an upright posture. However, convulsive syncope is not sustained and also rarely lasts longer than 30 seconds. Seizures generally last for at least 1–2 minutes. Seizures are associated with stertorous breathing and tachycardia, whereas syncope is usually associated with pallor and a slow, thready pulse.

Diagnosis

There are four pathophysiologic etiologies for syncope: cardiovascular, reflex-mediated, orthostatic, and neurologic. However, the underlying cause of syncope remains unidentified in as many as 20% of patients, even after a thorough evaluation. A comprehensive history and a thorough physical examination are the most sensitive and specific diagnostic tools at our disposal, with a diagnostic yield of 50% (Table 25-1). Subsequent testing provides an additional diagnosis in only 8–15% of cases. Consultation with a cardiologist may be worthwhile.

Preferred Studies

Initial evaluation consists of a comprehensive history, thorough physical examination including orthostatic blood pressures, and 12-lead electrocardiogram (ECG) (Fig. 25-1). This initial evaluation provides a working cause of syncope in approximately 45–55% of the patients. Abnormal ECG findings are common, occurring in over 80% of patients with cardiovascular syncope, but in only 5% of patients with neurologic or reflex-mediated syncope. ECG findings of ischemia indicate risk for acute coronary syndromes, including myocardial infarction, even in the absence of chest pain, and these patients should be hospitalized for further evaluation (Box 25-3). Patients with other ECG abnormalities, such as arrhythmia or bundle branch block, should also be strongly considered for hospitalization.

Additional Studies

Neurologic syncope is uncommon; and tests to detect cerebrovascular disease, such as head computed tomography (CT), magnetic resonance imaging (MRI), electroencephalography (EEG), and carotid ultrasonography are often overused. These tests should only be obtained when the history and physical examination point to a neurologic etiology or after testing for cardiovascular or reflex-mediated causes of syncope have been nondiagnostic.

Twenty-four hour (Holter) ECG monitoring is indicated in patients with a family history of sudden cardiac death, syncope with palpitations, known or suspected cardiac disease, exertional syncope, or abnormal findings on ECG. Typically, patients will warrant hospitalization in this instance and will be on a 24-hour telemetry monitor during their hospital stay. Syncope episodes without arrhythmia on monitoring, or arrhythmia in the absence of symptoms, may help exclude a cardiovascular cause of syncope. Occasionally, asymptomatic arrhythmias (ventricular tachycardia, prolonged sinus pause, heart block) will require additional investigation. If no arrhythmias or syncope events occur during the Holter monitoring, then prolonged ECG monitoring via an ambulatory loop monitor can be undertaken if suspicion of arrhythmia is still high.

Echocardiography is helpful in the setting of known cardiac disease, a history suggestive of cardiac disease, or an abnormal ECG. In the absence of these findings, echocardiography is not indicated. Similarly, cardiac enzymes are of little value if drawn routinely on elderly patients with syncope, unless other signs or symptoms suggestive of myocardial ischemia are present.

Exercise testing can help diagnose ischemia or exercise-induced tachyarrhythmias. These tests are only helpful for the investigation of exertional syncope and should be used with caution in patients already suspected to have syncope secondary to myocardial ischemia. In this instance, direct coronary vessel visualization may be preferred.

Signal-averaged ECG may be helpful in excluding a cardiac cause of syncope. This special ECG identifies signals at the end of the QRS complex that represent delayed conduction through diseased myocardium. They are indicated in patients with a history of ventricular tachycardia (VT), but otherwise are known to have structurally normal hearts. Most patients where VT is suspected, however, will need further electrophysiologic testing.

Intracardiac **electrophysiologic studies (EPS)** use electric stimulation and monitoring to discover conduction abnormalities that predispose to arrhythmias. The diagnostic yield of EPS is greater in patients with heart disease and is not indicated in the setting of a normal heart and ECG findings. EPS is frequently performed in patients with structural heart disease after noninvasive attempts have failed to provide an explanation for syncope. Several studies in this group of patients have shown that 45–80% with syncope originally determined to be of unknown cause actually have a cardiovascular etiology by EPS and that the risk of death is higher in these patients than in the general population.

Head-up tilt-table (HUTT) testing is used in patients with unexplained syncope, particularly those patients with structurally normal hearts. A positive HUTT is defined as provocation of a hypotensive episode associated with clinical symptoms. Once arrhythmias have been excluded, a positive HUTT is considered diagnostic for reflex-mediated vasovagal syncope. However, with the sensitivity of this test being about 80%, specificity suffers, and false positives occur. Psychiatric disorders should be considered for patients who lose consciousness during HUTT, but without blood pressure or heart rate changes.

Laboratory testing should include basic chemistries, glucose, and pregnancy test in women of childbearing age. Testing for illicit drug use may also be warranted, depending on the history.

Some patients will continue to have intermittent syncope despite a negative workup outlined above. In these cases, an implantable loop recorder (ILR) may be helpful. ILR should only be used in patients with syncope and a negative cardiovascular evaluation including EPS studies, HUTT, and a psychiatric evaluation.

Algorithms

Figure 25-1 represents an approach to the patient presenting with syncope.

Table 25-1 Diagnostic Modalities for Syncope

Test	What	Approximate Cost	Diagnostic Yield	Indications
History and physical examination	Family history, orthostatics blood pressures, cardiovascular and neurologic examinations	$150	45–55%	All patients
ECG		$100	Identifies etiology in 2–11% (but abnormal in 50%)	All patients
Laboratory testing	Not required except based on history and physical	Can get expensive	Very low (abnormalities in 2–3%, but not necessarily etiology of syncope)	Consider blood glucose, CBC, BMP or β-hCG if indicated
Neurologic testing	EEG CT/MRI head Carotid Doppler	$400 $900 $450	All-comers: 1.5% neurologic signs and symptoms: >30%	Focal neurologic signs and symptoms to suggest seizure, CVA, or CVD
Carotid massage	1. Cardiac monitor 2. Head rotated contralateral 3. Firm massage 5–10 sec 4. Vital sign measures before and after 5. Contraindicated: bruits, recent MI, CVA, or VT		Unknown estimated yield of 25–30% in men >50 years old with syncope	Carotid sinus Hypersensitivity: Sinus pause >3 sec or SBP drop of >50 mm Hg or >30 mm Hg with symptoms
Echocardiogram	Evaluation of cardiac anatomy and function	$450–$800	No studies have assessed diagnostic yield (estimated 5–10%)	Known or suspected structural cardiovascular disease
Stress-testing		$450–$700+		Exertional ischemia or arrhythmia
Holter monitor (only useful if symptoms present)	Continuous recording of 2–3 leads while patient keeps symptoms diary	$500 per 24 hour	Overall: 19% (includes positive and negative yield) 24 hr → 15% 48 hr → 25%	Organic heart disease, abnormal ECG, or high suspicion for arrhythmia
Ambulatory loop monitor	Records 1–4 min before and 30–60 sec after activation	$300 per 30 days	25–35% (positive and negative yield in selected population)	Frequent syncope, suspicion for arrhythmia
Implantable loop monitor (invasive)	Records 20 min before and 1–4 min after activation	$10,000	59% (positive and negative yield in very selected patient populations)	Infrequent syncope, negative cardiac evaluation, negative tilt table, negative psychiatric evaluation
Signal-averaged ECG	Identifies signals at end of QRS complex that represent delayed conduction through diseased myocardium	$150+	Negative predictive value: 90% (selected population)	Patients without known cardiac disease with VT, but relatively suspected low risk
EPS testing (invasive)	Assesses inducible VT or severe AVB through cardiac conduction intervals	$5000 (excludes ablation)	30–60% in very selected patient populations (organic heart disease and/or ECG changes and appropriate history)	Organic heart disease and high suspicion for arrhythmia or normal heart with high suspicion for bradyarrhythmia
Tilt-table testing	Evaluates predisposition to vasovagal syncope by exaggerating reduction in venous return with upright posture	$650	49% without isoproterenol use in very selected patient population (BUT note results not reproducible in 15–35% of patients)	Recurrent unexplained syncope without organic heart disease or with negative CV workup (suspected reflex-mediated, dysautonomic, or psychogenic syncope)
Psychiatric testing	Evaluate for panic, anxiety, depression, alcohol dependence	$150+	21% (selected patients)	Young patients with multiple symptoms who faint frequently without injury

Diagnostic modalities for syncope. ECG = electrocardiogram, B-hCG = beta human chorionic gonadotropin, EEG = electroencephalogram, CT = computed tomography, MRI = magnetic resonance imaging, CVA = cerebrovascular accident, CVD = cerebrovascular disease, VT = ventricular tachycardia, EPS = electrophysiologic studies, AVB = atriaventricular block, CV = cardiovascular.

Adapted from: Schnipper JL, Kapoor WN. Diagnostic evaluation and management of patients with syncope. Med Clin North Am 2001; 85(2):423–456, xi.

Figure 25-1 • Algorithm for evaluation of patients with syncope. The European society of Cardiology's Guidelines on management (Diagnosis and Treatment) of syncope provides recommendation on the evaluation of syncope. From: Brignole M, Alboni P, Benditt D, et al. Guidelines on management (diagnosis and treatment) of syncope. Eur Heart J 2001; 22(15):1256–1306.

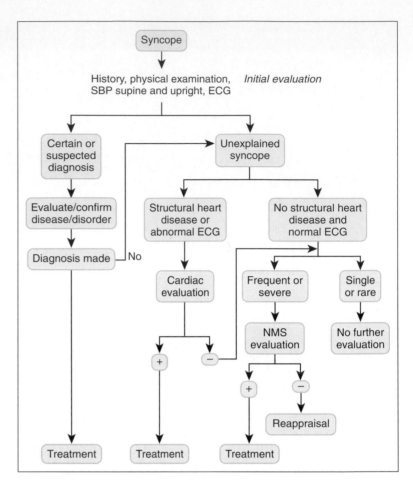

Prognosis

During Hospitalization

Cardiac syncope is associated with increased risks of premature death and cardiovascular events. Patients with neurologic syncope are at greater risk for both fatal and nonfatal stroke. The San Francisco Syncope Rule, derived from a cohort of 684 ER visits for syncope, identifies patients who are at immediate risk for serious outcomes within 7 days of syncope, based on the presence of dyspnea, hypotension, history of CHF, hematocrit <30, and abnormal ECG findings.[33] This rule, if properly applied, has 96% sensitivity and 62% specificity at identifying patients at risk for short-term serious outcomes. This tool was further validated in a prospective cohort study of 791 consecutive visits to the emergency room (ER) for syncope. There is no increased risk for cardiovascular morbidity or mortality associated with reflex-mediated syncope.[34]

Postdischarge

Martin and colleagues described a syncope risk stratification system that predicts a 10-fold increase in the incidence of serious arrhythmia and or death at 1 year, based on the presence of three out of four of the following—abnormal ECG, age >45, history of congestive heart failure, or history of ventricular arrhythmia. Patients that have cardiac and neurologic syncope excluded have a benign prognosis, regardless of whether the etiology is specifically determined or not.

MANAGEMENT

Patients with syncope should be placed on a cardiac monitor with an intravenous line started. A rapid assessment for airway, breathing, circulation, and injuries should be performed. ECG, pulse oximetry, and rapid blood glucose evaluation should be performed promptly, and intravenous dextrose and low-flow oxygen administered as needed. After the initial assessment, the syncope patient may need to be admitted to the hospital for observation, 24-hour telemetry monitoring, and further investigation for any potential life-threatening etiologies. There is significant variation across the United States in regard to hospitalization for syncope. There are no controlled clinical trials comparing the advantages and disadvantages of managing patients with syncope on an outpatient basis as compared with an inpatient basis. General guidelines on hospitalization for syncope are shown in Box 25-3.

Treatment

The treatment of syncope depends on the underlying etiology. Thus, full treatment of the various causes of syncope is beyond the scope of this chapter. This section will briefly review common treatment strategies for the four etiologic groups of syncope.

Orthostatic Syncope

Patients orthostatic from volume depletion will need rehydration.[23] Medications that can decrease blood pressure or cause

Box 25-3 Guideline Criteria for Hospitalization in Syncope

Hospitalization for syncope is indicated:

- Complaints of chest pain
- Focal neurologic deficits
- History or examination findings suggesting coronary artery disease, congestive heart failure, ventricular arrhythmia or valvular disease
- Electrocardiographic findings of ischemia, infarction, arrhythmia, or bundle branch block
- Signs and symptoms suggesting pulmonary embolism, cardiac tamponade, aortic dissection, or subarachnoid hemorrhage

Hospitalization for syncope should be strongly considered:

- A history of exertional syncope (in the absence of physical examination evidence of aortic stenosis or other left ventricular outflow obstruction), frequent syncope
- Age >70 yr
- Physical examination findings of tachycardia, orthostatic changes, or injury
- Suspected cardiac disease
- Syncope causing severe injury
- Family history of sudden death
- Patients without heart disease but with sudden onset of palpitations shortly before syncope
- Syncope in supine position
- Frequent recurrent episodes
- High suspicion of cardiac syncope

Adapted from: Linzer M, Yang EH, Estes NA, et al. Diagnosing syncope. Part 2: Unexplained syncope. Clinical Efficacy Assessment Project of the American College of Physicians. Ann Intern Med 1997; 127(1):76–86.

---

negative chronotropic effects should be reviewed in the context of orthostasis and whether the benefits of the medication outweigh harmful side effects. Drug-related hypotension was the most frequent cause of orthostatic syncope in a large (n = 650) prospective, observational study of emergency room patients.[18] Adjusting dosages or discontinuation of certain medications may be warranted in severe cases.

Autonomic dysfunction may also cause orthostatic syncope. Increasing salt intake increases orthostatic tolerance and improves cerebrovascular and peripheral vascular control.[19] Wearing waist-high compression stockings and abdominal binders may be beneficial. Moderate exercise training improves symptoms and increases orthostatic tolerance without increasing resting blood pressure.[20] Tilt-training is also an effective treatment option for recurrent reflex-mediated syncope and severe orthostatic intolerance.[21] The medication of choice in autonomic dysfunction is fludrocortisone (mineralocorticoid for volume expansion), starting at 0.1 mg/day and increasing doses according to the response. Midodrine is an α_1-agonist with vasopressor activity that increases peripheral resistance. A 10-mg dose of midodrine prescribed two to three times daily is effective in increasing orthostatic blood pressure and may ameliorate symptoms.[22]

Vasovagal Syncope

Vasovagal (neurocardiogenic) syncope is the most commonly diagnosed cause of syncope and has a relatively benign prognosis. Treatment begins with reassurance of the benign course and counseling regarding recognition of prodromal symptoms. Avoidance of precipitating factors such as excess alcohol, prolonged standing, and exercising in hot weather is recommended. Patients with susceptibility to reflex-mediated syncope should increase dietary salt intake. Maintenance of hydration, tilt-training exercises, lower extremity muscle strengthening and toning, lower extremity pressure stockings, and biofeedback may also be beneficial. An uncontrolled retrospective report found that oral fluid therapy significantly reduced the number of syncope episodes in a cohort of adolescent subjects.[8]

Several medications have been investigated to reduce recurrent vasovagal syncope. β-blockers have been the most frequently studied and most widely prescribed. Other drugs that have been investigated include paroxetine, clonidine, and midodrine. One short-term randomized trial and a large number of uncontrolled studies claim effectiveness of β-blockers in reducing syncope events, but several controlled trials have not confirmed these findings. A randomized, placebo-controlled, double-blind trial of 208 patients with two or more syncope episodes and a positive tilt-test found no difference between metoprolol and placebo in preventing vasovagal syncope over a 1-year treatment period. However, in another randomized, double blind, crossover trial of 20 patients with vasovagal syncope, metoprolol was found more effective than clonidine in preventing recurrent syncope.[9–11] A small, randomized trial of paroxetine showed a reduced rate of recurrence after 2 years of treatment.[12] Midodrine has been shown in a number of small trials and one randomized control study (n = 61) to be more beneficial in reducing syncope than hydration with oral fluids, salt tablets, and counseling in patients with reflex-mediated syncope.[13] Uncontrolled studies using ephedrine, pseudoephedrine, dextroamphetamine, and methylphenidate have also shown some benefit, but the only randomized controlled study in this group (etilefrine) found no benefits over placebo.

Pacemakers may be considered in patients with severe recurrent syncope resistant to pharmacologic therapy, particularly those patients with significant bradycardia. A randomized trial (n = 54) using permanent pacemakers, which provided pacing at a high rate if a predetermined drop in the heart rate occurred, in patients with severe symptoms (six or more episodes in their lives) and bradycardia on tilt-testing, showed an 85% relative risk reduction for recurrent syncope. Six open-label studies of permanent pacing have also demonstrated that pacemaker therapy is associated with considerable improvement over medical therapy alone. Nonetheless, a large double-blind, randomized trial of 100 patients at 15 centers from September 1998 to April 2002 found pacing therapy did not reduce the risk of recurrent reflex-mediated syncope. More randomized trials are needed to determine appropriate drug therapy and to define the role of pacemakers in reflex-mediated syncope.[14–17]

Cardiovascular Syncope

Arrhythmias

Transient ventricular tachycardia (VT) and bradyarrhythmias are the most common cardiac causes of syncope. Tachyarrhythmias include VT, long Q-T syndrome, and supraventricular tachycardia (SVT). In patients with structural heart disease, the risk of ventricular arrhythmias and sudden death increases with the severity of ventricular dysfunction. Patients surviving an episode of witnessed VT-associated syncope will ultimately probably require the insertion of an automatic implantable cardioverter-defibrillator (AICD), unless some other definitive treatment is possible (e.g., CABG or PCI for CAD). SVT is generally managed initially by vagal maneuvers such as carotid massage. If the SVT does not terminate by vagal maneuvers, then intravenous adenosine is indicated. Approximately 90% or more of SVTs caused by AV nodal reentry are terminated by adenosine. Long-term therapy of SVT includes β-blockers or calcium channel blockers. Recurrent tachycardias may require catheter ablation of accessory pathways.

Bradyarrhythmias include sinus node dysfunction and AV nodal conduction delays. They are initially managed with vagolytic drugs such as atropine, followed by permanent pacemaker. Iatrogenic causes of bradycardia (such as drug therapy) must be excluded prior to pacemaker insertion. Sinoatrial and AV nodes are relatively resistant to permanent injury by infarction or infection, and normal function returns over time; thus, permanent pacing is rarely required. However, even transient but complete AV block of the HIS–Purkinje system justifies the insertion of a pacemaker.

Structural Heart Disease

Structural heart disease includes valvular disorders, pump failure, and obstructive diseases. Treatment will depend on the specific condition. Critical aortic stenosis needs to be treated surgically. Cardiac outflow obstruction may be treated with β-blockers to decrease outflow obstruction and myocardial workload. Brugada syndrome presents with right bundle branch block,

J point elevation, and concave elevation of ST segments in the presence of normal coronaries. It has a fairly grim prognosis if left untreated and usually warrants an implantable defibrillator. Myocardial infarction (Chapter 19), pulmonary embolism (Chapter 27), cardiac tamponade, and aortic dissection (Chapter 28) are all medical emergencies and are discussed elsewhere in this reference.

Neurologic Syncope

Neurologic causes of syncope are rare. If a stroke is confirmed by imaging, then blood pressure and glucose control and avoidance of increased intracranial pressure are the primary treatment goals. Seizure activity is controlled with intravenous phenytoin and then by oral antiseizure medications as warranted. Vertebrobasilar insufficiency requires ICU management with assistance from a neurologist. If bilateral carotid artery stenosis is deemed the cause of the syncope, then carotid endarterectomy may be advisable.

DISCHARGE/FOLLOW-UP PLANS

Discharge instructions will vary, depending on whether the etiology of syncope has been determined. Patients without a determined etiology for syncope should be referred for further outpatient follow-up and testing. This may include an event recorder, HUTT, consultation for further electrophysiology study (EPS) studies, or psychiatric evaluation. Patients with documented cardiovascular or neurologic syncope will generally receive definitive treatment in the hospital. Patients will need instructions regarding their ability to drive.

Obviously, syncope during driving can be hazardous to self and others. State laws vary with respect to the physician and patient responsibilities for reporting medical conditions that affect the ability to drive. Physicians should be aware of the pertinent laws in their own state. Syncope patients with ventricular tachycardia or SVT treated with medical therapy or by an automatic implantable cardiac defibrillator may resume driving after being free of arrhythmia for 6 months. Patients with bradycardia and syncope may resume driving 1 week after successful pacemaker insertion.

Patients determined in the hospital to have reflex-mediated syncope generally do very well; however, recurrent syncope can be debilitating. Situational syncope requires patient education with respect to syncope triggers. Patients with carotid sinus hypersensitivity should be instructed not to wear tight collars and to maintain good hydration. Patients with orthostatic syncope need to be taught about avoiding postprandial drops in blood pressure, elevating the head of their beds, and the importance of assuming an upright posture slowly. Patients may need instruction on how to apply compression stockings.

Patients with reflex-mediated syncope should also be informed of the possibility of pacemaker placement in the future. With respect to driving, patients with reflex-mediated syncope with presyncopal symptoms, clear warning, and a clear precipitant may resume driving immediately. Patients with frequent syncope of unknown cause, no warning, or known precipitating factors should not resume driving until the cause is clarified and appropriate therapy has been initiated and proven to be successful.

Key Points

- The basics of evaluating a patient with syncope include a meticulous history that includes all medications (OTC, prescribed, and illicit), physical examination targeted to the cardiovascular and neurologic system, and ECG. Laboratory testing should be focused based on findings from this evaluation.

- It is imperative that physicians recognize syncope secondary to a cardiac etiology, as it is associated with increased risk of premature death or subsequent cardiovascular events.

- Patients presenting with syncope and complaints of dyspnea should be evaluated for pulmonary embolism.

- Syncope secondary to a neurologic etiology is uncommon, and tests such as head CT, MRI, EEG, and carotid ultrasonography are not indicated in the evaluation, unless there are concerning neurologic symptoms or findings on examination.

- Patients discharged from the hospital after an episode of syncope should be warned about driving based on state laws and etiology if determined.

SUGGESTED READING

Pavri BB, Ho RT. Syncope: identifying cardiac causes in older patients. Geriatrics 2003; 58(5):26–32.

Georgeson S, Linzer M, Griffith JL, et al. Acute cardiac ischemia in patients with syncope: importance of the initial electrocardiogram. J Gerontol Series A: Bio Sci Med Sci 2003; 58(11):1055–1058.

Kapoor WN. Syncope. N Engl J Med 2000; 343:1856–1862.

Sheldon R, Connolly S, Rose S, et al. Prevention of syncope trial (POST): a randomized, placebo-controlled study of metoprolol in the prevention of vasovagal syncope. Circulation 2006; 113(9):1164–1170.

Connolly SJ, Sheldon R, Thorpe KE, et al. Second vasovagal pacemaker study (VPS II): rationale, design, results, and implications for practice and future clinical trials. JAMA 2003; 289(17):2224–2229.

Linzer M, Yang E, Estes NA, et al. Clinical guideline: diagnosing syncope. II. Unexplained syncope. Ann of Int Med 1997; 127:76–86.

Soteriades ES, Evans JC, Larson MG. Incidence and prognosis of syncope. N Engl J Med 2002; 347:878–885.

Linzer M, Yang EH, Estes M, et al. Diagnosing syncope. I. Value of history, physical examination, and electrocardiography. Ann Intern Med 126:989–996.

Quinn J, McDermott D, Stiell I, et al. Prospective validation of the San Francisco Syncope Rule to predict patients with serious outcomes. Ann Emerg Med 2006; 47(5):448–454.

Schnipper JL, Kapoor WN. Diagnostic evaluation and management of patients with syncope. Med Clin North Am 2001; 85(2):423–456, xi.

Grubb BP. Clinical practice: Neurocardiogenic syncope. N Engl J Med 2005; 352(10):1004–1010.

Brignole M, Alboni P, Benditt D, et al. Guidelines on management (diagnosis and treatment) of syncope. Eur Heart J 2001; 22(15):1256–1306.

CHAPTER TWENTY-SIX

Deep Vein Thrombosis

Amir K. Jaffer, MD

BACKGROUND

Deep vein thrombosis (DVT) and pulmonary embolism (PE) are a continuum of the same disease process termed venous thromboembolism (VTE). VTE is the third-leading cause of cardiovascular death in the United States after myocardial infarction and stroke.[1] A common disease requiring hospitalization with an average annual incidence of approximately 117 cases per 100,000, over two thirds are attributable to DVT with or without PE.[2] Autopsy studies demonstrate large numbers of silent events leading to widely reported estimates of 2 million DVT cases and up to 200,000 deaths annually related to PE.[3] Studies utilizing ventilation perfusion scanning suggest that approximately half the patients with DVT have silent PE as well.[4,5] The focus of this chapter is on DVT; PE is reviewed separately in Chapter 27.

ASSESSMENT

Clinical Presentation

Prevalence and VTE Risk Factors

The prevalence of DVT is influenced by the presence of VTE risk factors and three underlying etiologic factors for thrombosis: venous stasis, endothelial injury, and hypercoagulability. These factors have been referred to as "Virchow's triad," named for the nineteenth-century pathologist, Rudolf Virchow, who showed that pulmonary thrombi generally originate in the deep veins of the systemic circulation and are carried to the pulmonary circulation by venous blood flow.[6,7] Increasing age, major surgery, and other established DVT risk factors (Box 26-1) reflect these underlying pathophysiologic processes. Both thrombophilia (hereditary factors such as factor V Leiden; G20210A prothrombin gene mutation; deficiencies of protein C, S, or antithrombin; listed in Table 26-1) and acquired risk factors (estrogen replacement, cancer, cardiovascular disease, surgery, trauma, immobility, use of central venous catheters, autoimmune disease such as antiphospholipid syndrome) contribute to the risk of DVT. Many times, the cause of thrombophilia may not be evident unless patients are tested.[8] However, the magnitude of risk conferred by thrombophilia and other risk factors varies, as outlined in Box 26-1. It is not currently known how the various factors interact to determine a single patient's individual VTE risk, yet there is

evidence that overall VTE risk increases in proportion to the number of predisposing factors present.[6] There is a clear relationship between age and overall health and the prevalence of VTE. The annual incidence of DVT increases from approximately 5 per 100,000 people in those <20 years of age to approximately 500 cases per 100,000 in those >80 years.[9] In a recent population-based study, over 60% of patients with first-time DVT either were nursing home residents or had been recently discharged from the hospital. These data support the importance of trying to prevent DVT in hospitalized patients.

Presenting Signs and Symptoms

Patients with DVT can present with symptoms of lower extremity swelling, calf pain, redness, dilated superficial veins, and warmth.[10] Physical examination signs include unilateral edema, palpable cords, erythema, tenderness along the deep venous distribution, calf pain on dorsiflexion of the foot (positive Homan's sign), and fever. Unfortunately, neither the signs nor symptoms of DVT are sensitive or specific.[11] For a positive Homans' sign, the sensitivity varies from 13% to 48%, and the specificity from 39–84%,[12] essentially no better than flipping a coin.

Differential Diagnosis

Given the low specificity of DVT symptoms, the majority of patients presenting with clinical signs and symptoms of DVT will not have the disease (i.e., ~80% will instead have one of the following: leg trauma, internal derangement of the knee, cellulitis, obstructive lymphadenopathy, lymphedema, drug-induced edema, calf muscle pull or tear, superficial thrombophlebitis, postphlebitic syndrome or a Baker cyst).[11] Quantifying the patient's VTE risk factors will help create a clinical pretest probability for the presence of DVT. Thus, a detailed history should include questions about a prior history of thrombosis and a family history of thrombosis.[13] In addition, patients should be questioned regarding the presence of certain significant disorders, such as collagen-vascular disease, myeloproliferative disease, atherosclerotic disease, or nephrotic syndrome. The use of medications such as oral contraceptive pills, hormone replacement therapy, and antipsychotic drugs that have been associated with the development of VTE should also be recorded.[14–16] Cancer

Box 26-1 Risk Factors for VTE

Strong risk factors (odds ratio >10)

Fracture (hip or leg)

Hip or knee replacement

Major general surgery

Major trauma

Spinal cord injury

Moderate risk factors (odds ratio 2–9)

Arthroscopic knee surgery

Central venous lines

Chemotherapy

Congestive heart or respiratory failure

Hormone replacement therapy

Malignancy

Oral contraceptive therapy

Paralytic stroke

Pregnancy/postpartum

Previous venous thromboembolism

Thrombophilia

Weak risk factors (odds ratio <2)

Bed rest >3 days

Immobility due to sitting (e.g., prolonged car or air travel)

Increasing age

Laparoscopic surgery (e.g., cholecystectomy)

Obesity

Pregnancy/antepartum

Varicose veins

Reproduced from: Anderson FA Jr, Spencer FA. Risk factors for venous thromboembolism. Circulation 2003; 107(23 Suppl 1):I9–16.

Table 26-1 Approximate Prevalence of Genetic Thrombophilias by Population

Genetic Abnormality	Caucasian	African	Asian
Factor V Leiden	5%	<0.1%	<0.1%
Prothrombin G20210A	3%	<0.1%	<0.1%
Protein S	0.003–0.2%	?	?
Protein C	0.2–0.4%	?	?
Antithrombin	0.02–0.2%	?	?

Reproduced from Feero, WG. Genetic thrombophilia. Primary Care 2004; 31:685–709.

is a risk factor for DVT; the patient should also be questioned about a past history of cancer or a recent cancer diagnosis. Review of system questions should include constitutional symptoms such as loss of appetite, weight loss, fatigue, pain, hematochezia, hemoptysis, or hematuria, which may be seen as a result of various malignancies. The physical examination should be focused on the chest, heart, and lower extremities. Even

Table 26-2 Diagnostic Approach to Acute DVT*

Testing Modality	Sensitivity (%)	Specificity (%)
Compression ultrasound	97	94
Impedance plethysmography (IPG)	65–97	83–94
Contrast venography MRI	100	100
Pelvic/thigh	90–100	95–100
Calf	80–87	97–100
D-Dimer (ELISA)	97	47

*Lower values for calf DVT

though the examination is often unrevealing, signs on examination can further strengthen pretest probability.

Diagnosis

Accurate diagnosis of DVT remains challenging, due to the nonspecificity of the clinical examination, and it has undergone a change over the last 20 years, with a greater reliance on diagnostic testing. Tests clinically available to assist in DVT diagnosis include: D-dimer testing, compression duplex ultrasound, contrast venography, and magnetic resonance imaging (MRI) (Table 26-2). In clinical practice today, the two most commonly used tests are the D-dimer and the compression ultrasound. Despite the availability of objective tests for DVT, the cornerstone of DVT diagnosis is the development of a pretest clinical probability. The importance of estimating pretest clinical probability of disease became readily apparent upon publication of the Prospective Investigation of the Pulmonary Embolism Diagnosis (PIOPED) study.[17] Formal clinical prediction rules have since been created and validated that can help even the novice clinician determine the pretest probability for DVT. An example of one commonly used clinical prediction rule is presented in Table 26-3.

Preferred Studies

Compression ultrasonography is the preferred diagnostic test because it is noninvasive, relatively inexpensive, and readily available. The test, however, relies heavily on the operator. It assesses compressibility of the external iliac, deep and superficial femoral, popliteal, and calf veins. It is very sensitive and specific for detecting proximal DVT (noncompressibility is diagnostic of DVT, whereas compressibility excludes DVT). The sensitivity and specificity of compression ultrasound for proximal vein DVT are >90%. The sensitivity and specificity decline dramatically when compression ultrasonography is used to evaluate asymptomatic patients (22% and 58%, respectively) versus symptomatic patients (96% and 96%, respectively). Ultrasound is also relatively insensitive to DVT isolated to the calf. Several diagnostic algorithms using serial compression ultrasonography have been validated and published. Serial testing with compression ultrasound may be necessary in patients with high clinical pretest probability of DVT but a negative initial compression ultrasound. Conversely, a low or intermediate pretest probability of disease

Table 26-3 Clinical Model for Predicting Pretest Probability for Deep Vein Thrombosis Finding Points*

Active cancer (treatment ongoing or within previous 6 months or palliative)	+1
Paralysis, paresis, or recent plaster immobilization of the lower extremities	+1
Recently bedridden for more than 3 days or major surgery within 4 weeks	+1
Localized tenderness along the distribution of the deep venous system	+1
Entire leg swollen†	+1
Calf swelling by more than 3 cm when compared with the asymptomatic leg (measured 10 cm below the tibial tuberosity)†	+1
Pitting edema (greater in the symptomatic leg)	+1
Collateral superficial veins (nonvaricose)	+1
Alternative diagnosis as likely or greater than that of deep vein thrombosis	−2

*Score	Clinical Probability of DVT
≤0	Low
1 or 2	Moderate
≥3	High

†Among patients with symptoms in both legs, the more symptomatic leg is used.
Reproduced from: Wells PS, et al. Value of assessment of pretest probability of deep-vein thrombosis in clinical management. Lancet 1997; 350(9094):1795–98.

combined with a negative compression ultrasound may help rule out DVT.

D-dimer (a fibrin split product) assays are useful adjuncts to noninvasive testing for suspected DVT because they have high sensitivity and, therefore, high negative predictive values. A D-dimer is formed when crossed-linked fibrin contained within a thrombus undergoes proteolysis by plasmin. Various D-dimer assays are available, including enzyme-linked immunosorbent assays (ELISA), latex agglutination assays, and a whole blood agglutination test. Based on a recent rigorous systematic review of all the available D-dimer tests, the ELISA appears to have the highest sensitivity and specificity.[18] Recent studies show that DVT can be reliably excluded in emergency department patients with suspected DVT who have a normal ELISA D-dimer assay and low pretest probability of disease.[19,20]

Alternative Options

Today, contrast venography is a second-line test for the diagnosis of DVT, even though it is still considered the diagnostic gold standard. It is very accurate for both proximal and calf DVT, with a sensitivity and specificity of close to a 100%. However, venography is invasive and expensive and can be technically difficult. Approximately 10% of patients experience inadequate contrast visualization or difficulty in cannulating the appropriate vein. Sometimes, this test may also induce thrombophlebitis, a complication in about 3% of patients. The contrast dye itself may be

associated with contrast-induced renal failure and idiosyncratic reactions that may include urticaria, angioedema, bronchospasm, or cardiovascular collapse.

MRI appears to have a sensitivity and specificity in the 90% range, compared to contrast venography for detecting proximal DVT. MRI is not as good as compression ultrasound for calf vein DVT, but better for noniliac pelvic vein thrombosis. One of the disadvantages of MRI is being able to distinguish acute from chronic DVT. Other potential problems include contraindications such as patients with metallic devices and significant claustrophobia. Finally, it is more expensive than compression ultrasound.[21]

Prediction Rule

Although several clinical prediction rules have been studied, the one that has been validated as part of sequential testing algorithms and is most commonly used in practice is shown in Table 26-3. It is essential to incorporate a tool such as this to help in developing a pretest probability that can then be incorporated into the diagnostic algorithm, and ultimately to guide appropriate management.

Algorithms

Algorithms that combine pretest probability of disease, D-dimer testing, and ultrasonography, have both been developed and validated in practice. In a randomized controlled trial involving 1,096 outpatients presenting with suspected lower-extremity DVT, a clinical prediction rule was used to categorize them as likely or unlikely to have DVT. Five-hundred thirty patients were then randomly assigned to undergo ultrasound imaging alone (control group), and 566 underwent D-dimer testing (D-dimer group) followed by ultrasound imaging unless the D-dimer test was negative in combination with low clinical suspicion (as determined by the clinical prediction rule). The overall prevalence of DVT or PE was 15.7%. Among patients for whom DVT had been ruled out by the initial diagnostic strategy, there were two confirmed VTE events in the D-dimer group (0.4%; 95% confidence interval, 0.05–1.5%) and six events in the control group (1.4%; 95% confidence interval, 0.5–2.9%; P = 0.16) during 3 months of follow-up. The use of D-dimer testing resulted in a significant reduction in the use of ultrasonography, from a mean of 1.34 tests per patient in the control group to 0.78 in the D-dimer group (P = 0.008). Two hundred eighteen patients (39%) in the D-dimer group did not require ultrasound imaging. This study concluded that DVT could be ruled out in patients who are judged clinically unlikely to have DVT and a negative D-dimer test—thus obviating the need for ultrasound testing.

The algorithms use Bayes' theorem as their basis. This theorem dictates that the posttest odds of disease are equal to the pretest odds of disease multiplied by the likelihood ratio of the diagnostic test used.[22,23] Positive and negative likelihood ratios of the D-dimer and ultrasound tests used most commonly in the evaluation of DVT are shown in Table 26-4. A full discussion of the application of Bayesian analysis to the diagnosis of DVT is beyond the scope of this chapter, but a key concept is that a diagnosis of DVT can generally be secured or excluded when the pretest clinical probability is concordant with an appropriate diagnostic test.[22] For example, a low pretest clinical suspicion of DVT in conjunction with a negative D-dimer test can exclude the diagnosis. Likewise, a high pretest clinical suspicion of DVT

Table 26-4 Approximate Likelihood Ratios of Commonly Used Diagnostic Tests for The Evaluation of DVT*

Diagnostic Test	Likelihood Ratio*	Clinical Setting	Comments
D-dimer[18] – Quantitative ELISA 　Negative test 　Positive test – Other assay types 　Negative test 　Positive test	 0.07–0.12 1.5–3.0 0.11–0.36 1.6–5.0	Evaluation of suspected acute DVT or PE in symptomatic, non-anticoagulated outpatients	Questionable reliability in patients on anticoagulant medications, those with nonacute symptom onset, and in hospitalized patients.[55]
Duplex ultrasound[56] 　Negative 　Positive	 0.05 24	Suspected symptomatic proximal lower-extremity DVT	Accuracy may be lower for distal DVT, for asymptomatic DVT (e.g., postoperative surveillance), and for upper-extremity thrombosis. Since most PEs arise from thrombi in the legs, duplex ultrasound can also be used in the evaluation of suspected PE.

*When likelihood ratios were not specifically reported, they were calculated using standard formulas.[22] Likelihood ratios are interpreted as follows using Bayes' theorem:
(Pretest odds of disease) × (Likelihood ratio for given finding) = (Posttest odds of disease)

Odds and probabilities can be interconverted using the formulas:
Odds = probability/(1-probability) or
Probability = odds/(1+ odds)

For example: In a patient with an estimated pretest probability of 80% for DVT (very high pretest suspicion), the probability of DVT after a negative compression ultrasound can be calculated as follows:

Pretest probability of 80% is converted to pretest odds of 80/20 (= 4)
Likelihood ratio of disease with a negative duplex ultrasound is approximately 0.05

Posttest odds of DVT = 4 × 0.05 = 0.20
Posttest probability of DVT = 0.20 /(1 + 0.20) = 16.7%
Further testing may be indicated, since this patient still has an ~16% chance of having a DVT despite the negative compression ultrasound.

Modified from: Jaffer AK, Brotman DJ, Michota F. Current and emerging options in the management of venous thromboembolism. Cleve Clin J Med 2005; 72 (Suppl 1): S14–S23. Reprinted with permission. Copyright (c) 2005. Cleveland Clinic Foundation. All rights reserved.

with a discordant (i.e., negative) test result mandates additional testing. An algorithm in Figure 26-1 outlines this approach.

PROGNOSIS

During Hospitalization

Some of the problems patients may develop include recurrent DVT, PE, or bleeding on anticoagulation. The rates of recurrent VTE range from 5–8%, despite acute phase treatment with low-molecular-weight heparin (LMWH) or unfractionated heparin (UFH). The rate of major bleeding can range from 0.5–7% with anticoagulation. The numbers are higher with UFH compared to LMWH, and mortality ranges from about 4–8%. Heparin-induced thrombocytopenia (HIT) can also occur, and this number is <1% with LMWH while closer to 3% with UFH.[24]

Postdischarge

HIT can occur postdischarge.[25] If patients develop recurrent VTE shortly after discharge and return to the hospital with a new arterial or venous event, HIT should be suspected. A platelet count that was falling toward the last few days of a patient's hospitalization may be a clue. However, diagnosis requires a strong suspicion based on the clinical presentation and laboratory findings.

Confirmation of this diagnosis requires a typical clinical picture along with positive heparin-induced platelet activation testing using functional assays in addition to antigen assays that measure antibodies against platelet factor 4 (PF4). High suspicion requires cessation of UFH or LMWH and use of direct thrombin inhibitor anticoagulant therapy, even prior to the confirmation of this diagnosis.[26]

Some patients who develop bleeding on warfarin require readmission to the hospital. The risk of recurrent thrombosis is higher in patients without a reversible VTE risk factor. This includes patients with idiopathic DVT and in those with certain biochemical abnormalities, including antiphospholipid antibodies, hyperhomocysteinemia, and homozygous factor V Leiden. Among patients with cancer, DVT frequently is associated with serious clinical outcomes. Its treatment is resource intensive and costly.[27]

Postthrombotic syndrome (PTS) after an acute symptomatic DVT affects approximately 37% of patients; PTS typically develops within 2 years. A frequent and burdensome complication of proximal DVT, even among patients maintained on long-term oral anticoagulation,[28] PTS is more likely in the setting of proximal, recurrent DVT with significant thrombus burden. A study of 180 patients with proximal DVT showed that the use of compression stockings (30–40 mm Hg at the ankle) could reduce the rate of postthrombotic sequelae by 50% (p = 0.011).[29]

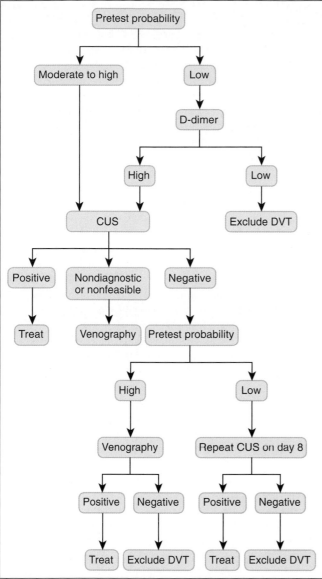

Figure 26-1 • Approach to the Diagnosis of DVT.
CUS—compression ultrasound
Reproduced from: Kyrle PA, Eichinger S. Deep-vein thrombosis. Lancet 2005; 365:1163–1174.

Table 26-5 FDA-Approved Initial Therapy for DVT

UFH
Use normogram—80 U/kg bolus followed by continuous IV drip 18 U/kg/hr
Goal aPTT* = 60–80

LMWH
Enoxaparin 1 mg/kg SC q12h or Enoxaparin 1.5 mg SC q24h or dalteparin 200 IU/kg SC q24h or tinzapain 175 IU/kg SC q24h

Factor Xa-inhibitor
Fondaparinux   5 mg SC qd if Wt < 50 kg
                 7.5 mg SC qd if wt 50–100 kg
                 10 mg SC qd if wt > 100 kg

*May vary from institution to institution. Maintain activated partial thromboplastin time (aPTT) in therapeutic range which must correspond to heparin levels of 0.3–0.7 U/ml.

MANAGEMENT

Treatment

Initial Therapy

Preferred

Prompt initiation of anticoagulant therapy is essential in the acute management of DVT, except in patients who are actively bleeding or in whom the risk of bleeding clearly outweighs benefits. Currently, several groups of drugs are available to treat DVT, including: UFH, LMWH, and factor Xa inhibitors (pentasaccharides). Parenteral direct thrombin inhibitors (DTI) are approved for use in patients with acute VTE and concomitant HIT. Based on clinical trial data regarding the various classes of anticoagulants, the recommendations for initial anticoagulant therapy for DVT are shown in Table 26-5.

The preferred initial agent is LMWH. In December of 1996, the FDA approved enoxaparin for outpatient treatment of DVT. Prior to this approval, patients with DVT were traditionally treated in the hospital with UFH. Registry data confirm that this approach still continues today, despite studies showing that LMWH dosed subcutaneously is just as effective as inpatient UFH with shorter lengths of stay and significant cost savings.[30] With coordinated protocols in place, patients can be safely treated as outpatients directly from the emergency department or doctor's office. Exceptions may include homeless patients and those with inadequate social support at home. An algorithm for the treatment of DVT is outlined in Figure 26-2.

LMWH has several advantages over UFH. LMWH can be dosed subcutaneously once or twice daily with more predictable pharmacokinetics, good bioavailability, and less HIT potential (~1%); in most clinical situations, it does not require special monitoring.[31] The safety and efficacy of LMWH for the outpatient therapy of DVT have been directly studied.[32,33] A recent meta-analysis of 11 clinical trials with a total of 3,566 patients compared LMWH to UFH for treatment of acute DVT. The three outcomes evaluated included prevention of recurrent thromboembolism, major bleeding, and mortality. The analysis included studies using different LMWH preparations (dalteparin, enoxaparin, ardeparin, reviparin, and tinzaparin) and showed that LMWH therapy was superior to UFH by decreasing mortality by approximately 30% (absolute risk reduction = 1.65%, number needed to treat (NNT) = 61, P = 0.02%). Of note, the rates of recurrent thromboembolism and major bleeding were similar for both LMWH and UFH groups.

Alternative Options

If UFH is used, a weight-based dosing normogram (80 U/kg bolus followed by 18 U/kg/h IV infusion) helps achieve a therapeutic, activated, partial thromboplastin time (aPTT) faster within the first 24 hours and decreases the rate of recurrent thromboembolism in patients with underlying VTE, compared to traditional empiric dosing (5,000 U bolus followed by 1,000 U/h IV infusion.[34] The American College of Chest Physicians (ACCP) recommends that each institution determine its own therapeutic aPTT range to correspond to a heparin level of 0.3–0.7 IU/ml of anti-Xa activity. This aPTT range validation is important if clinicians are to provide optimal anticoagulation with UFH. Some problems associated with UFH use include: a higher rate of HIT (about 3% compared to LMWH), low bioavailability and the need for a

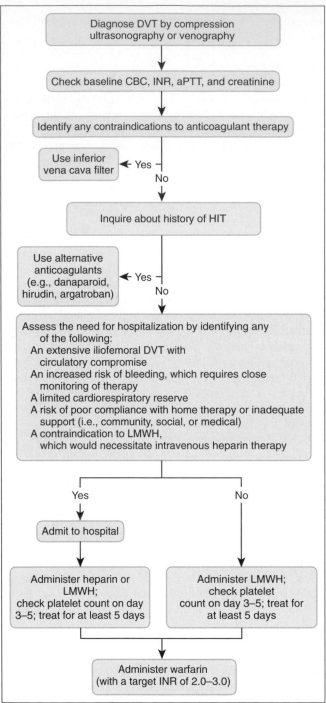

Figure 26-2 • Management of DVT.
Reproduced from: Bates SM Ginsberg JS. Clinical practice: Treatment of deep-vein thrombosis. N Engl J Med 2004; 351:268–277.

ment of DVT and PE, based on two double blind, non-inferior, randomized clinical trials.[35] It inhibits both free and platelet-bound factor Xa. It binds antithrombin with high affinity, has close to 100% bioavailability, and a plasma half-life of 17–21 hours that permits once daily administration. The drug is excreted unchanged in urine and is contraindicated in patients with severe renal impairment (creatinine clearance <30 ml/min). It does not bind PF4 and therefore should not cause HIT. One important limitation is the lack of an antidote if uncontrolled bleeding does occur. A procoagulant, such as factor VIIa, might be effective, but is not available commercially.[36]

Another group of drugs that can be used to treat DVT includes the DTIs. Currently, there are four FDA-approved parenteral DTIs (argatroban, lepirudin, bivalirudin, and hirudin). Three of these four agents are indicated to treat thrombosis in HIT. Presently, no DTI is FDA approved for VTE treatment alone. The only oral DTI that has also been evaluated in phase III clinical trials is Ximelagatran. Ximelagatran is a prodrug that is rapidly hydrolyzed to form melagatran—the active drug that binds thrombin. It has a plasma half-life of 4–5 hours and is given twice daily in fixed doses. It does not have drug and food interactions like warfarin, and it is renally cleared. The drug has been shown in phase III trials to be effective for VTE prevention after major orthopedic surgery, stroke prevention in atrial fibrillation, and both acute treatment of VTE and for the secondary prevention of VTE after an acute episode.[37] However, it was rejected by the FDA in 2004, due to concerns about increased liver enzymes and the potential for adverse cardiac events. Ximelagatran was approved for use in several European countries for VTE prevention after major orthopedic surgery, but recently pulled off the market worldwide due to concerns of safety.

Catheter-directed thrombolytic therapy for VTE, although performed routinely in tertiary centers, should generally be reserved for patients with severe iliofemoral DVT where there is risk of limb ischemia and/or a high-risk for subsequent PTS.[31] Other options used to restore patency of thrombosed veins include open surgical thrombectomy and percutaneous mechanical thrombectomy. Surgical thrombectomy had previously been abandoned secondary to poor long-term results. However, recently with improved techniques and better selection of patients, surgical thrombectomy has started to regain some therapeutic role in treating acute DVT in young patients with short segment occlusions. Percutaneous techniques have allowed thrombolysis, percutaneous mechanical thrombectomy, and stenting to be used in conjunction with each other—allowing for better resolution of venous clot burden. Practitioners who treat patients with DVT should be familiar with all the options available to restore venous patency, preserve valvular function, and thereby minimize the risk of late postthrombotic complications.[38]

The use of inferior vena cava (IVC) filters has increased markedly during the last two decades in patients with PE, patients with DVT alone, and patients at risk for VTE without documented acute disease.[39] IVC filters should generally be reserved for patients with an acute DVT or PE and an immediate contraindication to anticoagulation or patients with an acute recurrent DVT or PE, despite adequate anticoagulant therapy.[40] The FDA recently approved three different types of retrievable IVC filters. Although long-term safety data for these devices are not yet available, these removable IVC filters may be an attractive option for

continuous IV infusion, the need for titration of anticoagulant effect with frequent monitoring of aPTT, time needed to validate the aPTT range, osteopenia, and osteoporosis.[31]

Fondaparinux is a synthetic analog of a unique pentasaccharide sequence that mediates the interaction of heparin with antithrombin. Fondaparinux is approved by the FDA for the treat-

Table 26-6 Coumadin Dosing Nomogram: Original 10 mg[41]

Day	INR	Dose (mg)
1	<1.5	10
2	<1.8	10
	1.8–2.0	5
	2.1–3.0	2.5
	>3.0	0
3	<1.6	15
	1.6–2.0	10
	2.1–3.0	5
	3.1–3.5	2.5
	>3.5	0
4	<1.6	15
	1.6–2.0	10
	2.1–2.5	7.5
	2.6–3.0	5
	3.1–3.5	2.5
	>3.5	0

INR = international normalized ratio.

Reproduced from: Kovacs MJ, et al. Comparison of 10-mg and 5-mg warfarin initiation nomograms together with low-molecular-weight heparin for outpatient treatment of acute venous thromboembolism: a randomized, double-blind, controlled trial. Ann Intern Med 2003; 138:714–19.

patients with transient contraindications to anticoagulation therapy.

SUBSEQUENT THERAPY

Acute VTE treatment begins with antithrombin therapy as discussed previously. Subsequent therapy involves chronic oral anticoagulation (OAC) with vitamin K antagonists (VKA) such as warfarin to reduce the likelihood of VTE recurrence. OAC should be started as soon as the patient has received the initial dose of antithrombin therapy and he or she is considered adequately anticoagulated. Warfarin exerts its effect by inhibiting the vitamin K–dependent gamma-carboxylation of coagulation factors II, VII, IX, and X in the intrinsic clotting pathway. Since it affects *production* of these factors, its effect is delayed 36–72 hours or until the body clears coagulation factors in circulation. Of note, initial prolongation of the prothrombin time (INR) with warfarin treatment is due to reduction in factor VII (half-life of 5–7 hours). However, clotting is still somewhat functional until about 5 days of adequate warfarin dosing sufficiently reduces factors II, IX, and X. For this reason, heparin and warfarin treatment should overlap by 4–5 days to minimize DVT recurrence.

The debate over the starting dose of warfarin and the duration of therapy continues. Recent evidence suggests initiation of warfarin therapy with 10 mg daily may result in a therapeutic INR much faster than 5 mg without increasing the risk of bleeding or thrombembolic complications.[40] Randomized trials have previously shown that patients are more likely to have a therapeutic INR 3–5 days after initiating warfarin with a 5-mg dose rather than a 10-mg dose. Also, the 10-mg dose more frequently resulted in supratherapeutic INR values.[42,43] Experts now recommend that clinicians consider patient-specific factors such as age,

weight, concomitant medications, and comorbid diseases when deciding on the starting warfarin dose. Some commonly encountered medications that require warfarin initiation with a lower starting dose include: amiodarone, trimethoprim-sulfamethoxazole, and metronidazole. Some commonly encountered comorbidities that also require a lower warfarin starting dose include liver disease and congestive heart failure. If the 10-mg dose is chosen as the starting dose, it is important to use a detailed titration scheme as outlined in Table 26-6.

Choosing the duration of warfarin therapy requires balancing the risks of recurrent and fatal VTE of warfarin therapy against the risks of major and fatal bleeding on warfarin therapy. Making this decision requires a tailored approach specific to the individual patient while using the available evidence from clinical studies.

The rate of recurrent VTE at 1 year following 3 months of OAC in the setting of a reversible VTE risk factor (such as surgery) is approximately 3–5%. The rate of recurrent VTE at 1 year following 6 months of OAC in the setting of long-haul air travel, trauma, or hormone replacement therapy is also approximately 5%. However, in the setting of unprovoked or idiopathic VTE, the 1-year recurrence rate jumps to approximately 10%; and in the setting of cancer, it is 20%. Five to ten percent of recurrent VTE events are fatal. The rate of major bleeding with OAC is not insignificant and varies from 1–4% per year in clinical trials with case fatality rates for major bleeding ranging from 9–13%. The rate of intracranial bleeding varies from 0.65–1% per year on OAC.[44,45] Prospective studies have also shown that the rate of bleeding in clinical practice is much higher than that demonstrated in clinical trials.[44]

Two recent studies on OAC intensity and duration for patients with idiopathic VTE have been published, with some conflicting results. The PREVENT study randomized 508 patients with idiopathic VTE to either conventional therapy with warfarin (target INR 2–3) or to a low-intensity warfarin group (target INR 1.5–1.9). The study concluded that long-term, low-intensity warfarin therapy (target INR 1.5–1.9) was a highly effective method of preventing recurrent VTE while minimizing the bleeding risk. Subsequently, the ELATE trial investigators concluded that conventional-intensity warfarin therapy (INR 2–3) is more effective than low-intensity warfarin therapy (INR 1.5–1.9) for the long-term prevention of recurrent VTE, as the low-intensity warfarin regimen did not appear to reduce the risk of clinically important bleeding. Ultimately, the take-home message from both studies is that patients with idiopathic VTE benefit from lifelong OAC; however, the intensity of OAC therapy that best balances efficacy and safety remains unclear.[46] Evidence-based recommendations are summarized in Table 26-7.

Patients with cancer have higher rates of warfarin-resistant thrombosis and warfarin-associated bleeding compared to VTE patients without cancer.[47] The CLOT investigators[48] recently examined the safety and efficacy of dalteparin (200 IU/kg/day for the first month, followed by 150 IU/Kg/day for 5 months) compared to traditional therapy with dalteparin for 5–7 days followed by OAC with warfarin for the treatment of VTE in cancer patients. Eight percent of patients (27 of 336) in the LMWH group suffered recurrence, compared to 16% (53 of 336) in the OAC group (hazard ratio 0.48; p = 0.002). Most recurrences occurred while on therapeutic anticoagulation. The frequencies of major and

TABLE 26-7 Guidelines for Duration of Anticoagulant Therapy for VTE*

Risk Factor for VTE	Duration of Treatment (Target INR 2.5, Range 2.0–3.0)
Major transient risk factor*	3 mo
Minor risk factor†	6 mo†
Unprovoked	Indefinite‡
If unprovoked and also:	
Isolated calf DVT; anticoagulant therapy a burden; or moderate to high risk of bleeding§	6 mo
Uncontrolled malignancy	Indefinite (preferably with LMWH)‡
If uncontrolled malignancy and also:	
A very high risk of bleeding§; or an additional reversible provoking risk factor	Consider 6 mo rather than indefinite therapy

*Major transient risk factors include within 3 months of surgery with general anesthesia; plaster cast immobilization of a leg; hospitalization.

†Minor transient risk factors include within 6 weeks of estrogen therapy; prolonged air travel (i.e., >10 hours); pregnancy; less marked leg injuries; or immobilization. Six months of treatment reflects the author's preference but 3 months is also reasonable.

‡Decision should be reviewed annually to consider new developments in antithrombotic therapy or change in the patient's risk of bleeding. Additional factors favoring indefinite therapy include PE versus proximal DVT at presentation; >1 episode of unprovoked VTE; antiphospholipid antibodies; protein C, protein S, or antithrombin deficiency; homozygous factor V Leiden or G20210A prothrombin mutation; combined thrombophilic abnormalities; inferior vena caval filter; and patient preference.

§Risk factors for bleeding include age 65 years or older; previous stroke; previous bleeding (e.g., gastrointestinal); active peptic ulcer disease; renal impairment; anemia; thrombocytopenia; liver disease; diabetes mellitus; use of antiplatelet therapy; poor patient compliance; poor control of anticoagulation; and structural lesion (including tumor) expected to be associated with bleeding. One or two risk factors suggests moderate risk and three or more risk factors suggest high risk of bleeding.

Reproduced from: Kearon C. Long-term management of patients after venous thromboembolism. Circulation 2004; 110(9 Suppl 1):110–18.

minor bleeding were similar. Although this trial did not specifically enroll patients with postoperative VTE, the relatively high recurrence rates illustrates that cancer patients with VTE are at high risk for recurrence, even in the face of ongoing warfarin therapy. A smaller study using enoxaparin 1.5 mg/kg daily demonstrated a similar risk reduction that failed to reach statistical significance.[47] The major limitation of chronic outpatient subcutaneous therapy with LMWH in the treatment of cancer-associated VTE is the cost of the drug,[49] and the willingness of the patient or family members to administer daily injections over several months. Nonetheless, the ACCP currently recommends 3–6 months of LWWH for DVT in the setting of cancer.[31]

PREVENTION

Approximately two thirds of all DVT in the community develops in patients who have been recently hospitalized. Traditionally, surgical patients have been the focus of inpatient DVT prevention, and this topic is specifically reviewed in Chapter 100. However, medical patients are also at significant risk for VTE and its complications. The problem of inadequate and omitted prophylaxis for DVT in medical patients was clearly demonstrated in the U.S. DVT-Free Registry. This registry was conducted at 183 US hospitals and included 5,451 patients, both inpatients and outpatients, with ultrasound-confirmed DVT. Approximately 50% developed symptomatic VTE in the hospital after being admitted with another diagnosis. Of these, only 42% (1,147 of 2,726) had received any prophylaxis prior to their VTE diagnosis. The number of medical inpatients overall who received prophylaxis in the 30 days prior to diagnosis was only 28%. This was lower than the 48% of the surgical patients who received prophylaxis in the 30 days prior to diagnosis. This study suggests that the utilization of VTE prophylaxis is far from optimal in hospitalized medical patients at risk for VTE.[50] Chapter 14 reviews the approach to DVT prevention among medical patients in the hospital.

DISCHARGE/FOLLOW-UP PLANS

Patients hospitalized on anticoagulant therapy require a complete blood count (CBC) at least every other day for monitoring the platelet count; a decrease by 50% may represent HIT. UFH therapy requires a PTT monitoring every 6 hours for the duration of therapy. For those patients being discharged home on outpatient LMWH therapy, a CBC should be checked on Day 3 and Day 7 of therapy. In addition, patients need their INR checked at least every other day until the INR is consistently >2.0. At that time, the frequency of the INRs can be decreased.

Patients discharged on outpatient LMWH will need patient education (see below) and prescriptions for both the LMWH and warfarin. Enoxaparin is the only LMWH currently FDA approved for outpatient use at the dose of 1 mg/kg subcutaneously every 12 hours.

Patient Education

The pharmacist or nurse and the supervising physician need to coordinate the clinical, nonclinical, and educational aspects of the outpatient treatment of DVT. A case manager or coordinator can help verify that the patient's prescription provider covers the cost of LMWH.

The nurse or pharmacist must educate the patient and/or caregiver about the following:
1. How to perform LMWH injections, including technique, sites for injection sites, and proper disposal of syringes
2. Understanding the condition of acute DVT and the associated risks and complications
3. Understanding the treatment regimen of LMWH and warfarin (what the drugs do, dosing schedule, potential side effects and drug and food interactions)
4. Education about the signs of bleeding and other adverse events and how to respond to them
5. An explanation of laboratory tests and subsequent dose changes
6. How to access emergency assistance
7. Period and time of next follow-up appointment

Table 26-8 Testing Recommendations for Thrombophilia

Patients to Consider for Testing	Tests to Consider
Any patient with DVT <50 years old	Prothrombin G20210A gene testing
Idiopathic DVT any age	Activated protein C resistance/factor V Leiden gene testing
Strong family history of thrombosis	Protein S level
Venous thrombosis in unusual site	Protein C level
Recurrent venous thrombosis	Antithrombin level
Life-threatening thrombotic event	Thrombin time
Relatives of patients with thrombophilia	Activated partial thromboplastin time*
Recurrent adverse pregnancy outcome	Lupus anticoagulant*
Stillbirth	Anticardiolipin antibodies* Homocysteine level†

DVT: deep venous thrombosis.

Factor VIII, IX, and XI levels†

Reproduced from: Feero WG. Genetic Thrombophilia. Primary Care 2004; 31:685–709.

Outpatient Physician Communication

Communication with the patient's primary care physician (PCP) is an important step in successful DVT treatment. Anticoagulation therapy initiated in the hospital must be transferred to the PCP for further management and follow-up in the outpatient setting. A follow-up appointment with the PCP is necessary to ensure that the INR is being followed, and that the dose of warfarin is adjusted to a target INR of 2.0 to 3.0. In addition, the PCP should be encouraged to perform age-appropriate cancer screening.

The hospital is generally not the most appropriate setting for evaluation of hypercoaguability, and thus related tests should not be routinely ordered by the hospitalist. It has long been known that some patients have a tendency to develop thrombosis. However, a laboratory diagnosis of a hypercoagulable state such as factor V Leiden mutation, hyperhomocysteinemia, protein S deficiency, or prothrombin gene mutation 20210A often does not change patient care, may not be cost effective, and may lead to unnecessary anxiety among patients who test positive. Therefore, testing for hypercoagulability should only be performed when it will directly affect the plan of care. PCPs should recognize that testing is costly and that no large prospective studies have really examined the efficacy of testing. The use of hypercoabulability panels (though common) should be discouraged, and testing should be individualized as outlined in Table 26-8.[13] Even in patients with laboratory-diagnosed thrombophilia, thrombotic events are often triggered by a situational risk factor,[51,52] and once the situational factor has resolved and the thrombosis has been treated, there is little reason for indefinite anticoagulation. Most such patients do not suffer recurrent events.[53,54]

Key Points

- Signs and symptoms of DVT are neither sensitive nor specific; therefore, it helps to generate a pretest probability of disease using a clinical prediction rule.

- A D-dimer ELISA has a high negative predictive value and therefore is good at ruling out disease when the pretest probability of disease is low.

- Ultrasounds of the lower extremities have a very high sensitivity and specificity for above the knee DVT.

- Prompt initiation and maintenance of parenteral anticoagulant therapy for at least 5 days and until the INR is >2 is the mainstay for the acute management of DVT.

- IVC filters should be reserved for patients who either have a contraindication to anticoagulation or who develop a new DVT in the presence of therapeutic anticoagulation.

- Subcutaneous anticoagulant therapy such as LMWHs and pentasaccharides can facilitate early discharge of inpatients with DVT.

- Catheter-directed thrombolytic therapy should be reserved for patients with severe ileofemoral DVT and concern for limb ischemia.

- Patients suffering from idiopathic VTE may benefit from life-long oral anticoagulation.

SUGGESTED READING

Meignan M, et al. Systematic lung scans reveal a high frequency of silent pulmonary embolism in patients with proximal deep venous thrombosis. Arch Intern Med 2000; 160(2):159–164.

Anderson FA, Jr, Spencer FA. Risk factors for venous thromboembolism. Circulation 2003; 107(23 Suppl 1):I9–16.

Anand SS, et al. Does this patient have deep vein thrombosis? JAMA 1998; 279(14):1094–1099.

Stein PD, et al. D-dimer for the exclusion of acute venous thrombosis and pulmonary embolism: a systematic review. Ann Intern Med 2004; 140(8):589–602.

Tick LW, et al. Practical diagnostic management of patients with clinically suspected deep vein thrombosis by clinical probability test, compression ultrasonography, and D-dimer test. Am J Med 2002; 113(8):630–635.

Wells PS, et al. Evaluation of D-dimer in the diagnosis of suspected deep-vein thrombosis. N Engl J Med 2003; 349(13):1227–1235.

Bates SM, Ginsberg JS. Clinical practice: treatment of deep-vein thrombosis. N Engl J Med 2004; 351(3):268–277.

Bartholomew R, Begelman SM, Almahameed A. Heparin-induced thrombocytopenia: principles for early recognition and management. Cleve Clin J Med 2005; 72(Suppl 1):S31–36.

Elting LS, et al. Outcomes and cost of deep venous thrombosis among patients with cancer. Arch Intern Med 2004; 164(15):1653–1661.

Kahn SR, et al. Predictors of the post-thrombotic syndrome during long-term treatment of proximal deep vein thrombosis. J Thromb Haemost 2005; 3(4):718–723.

Buller HR, et al. Antithrombotic therapy for venous thromboembolic disease: The Seventh ACCP Conference on Antithrombotic and Thrombolytic Therapy. Chest 2004; 126(3 Suppl):401S–428S.

Buller HR, et al. Fondaparinux or enoxaparin for the initial treatment of symptomatic deep venous thrombosis: a randomized trial. Ann Intern Med 2004; 140(11):867–873.

Stein PD, Kayali F, Olson RE. Twenty-one-year trends in the use of inferior vena cava filters. Arch Intern Med 2004; 164(14):1541–1545.

Kovacs MJ, et al. Comparison of 10-mg and 5-mg warfarin initiation nomograms together with low-molecular-weight heparin for outpatient treatment of acute venous thromboembolism: a randomized, double-blind, controlled trial. Ann Intern Med 2003; 138(9):714–749.

Kearon C. Long-term management of patients after venous thromboembolism. Circulation 2004; 110(9 Suppl 1):I10–18.

Lee AY, et al. Low-molecular-weight heparin versus a coumarin for the prevention of recurrent venous thromboembolism in patients with cancer. N Engl J Med 2003; 349(2):146–153.

Goldhaber SZ, Tapson VF. A prospective registry of 5,451 patients with ultrasound-confirmed deep vein thrombosis. Am J Cardiol 2004; 93(2):259–262.

CHAPTER TWENTY-SEVEN

Pulmonary Embolism

Steven B. Deitelzweig, MD, RVT, CMD, FACP, FSVMB

BACKGROUND

Syndromes characterized by embolization of material into the pulmonary venous circulation causing cardiopulmonary dysfunction represent life-threatening situations for patients and require rapid diagnosis and treatment by hospital medicine practitioners. This chapter will focus on venous thromboembolism (VTE) causing pulmonary embolism (PE). PE of nonthrombotic material (e.g., fat, amniotic fluid, air, septic, and tumor) will also be briefly discussed in the context of the thrombotic paradigm. Deep Vein Thormbosis is reviewed in Chapter 26.

Venous thrombi typically form (due to platelet aggregation as well as altered venous flow dynamics) along the valve cusps within the soleal sinuses of the calf. These thrombi can overwhelm the endogenous fibrinolytic system within minutes. The propensity of a thrombus to propagate and/or embolize to the lungs is greatest during the first 7 days. Ventilation perfusion ($\dot{V}/\dot{Q}$) mismatch is the principal physiologic effect of PE, and it leads to hypoxemia in 85% of patients.

The hemodynamic response to PE is variable, depending on the degree of occlusion of the pulmonary arterial bed, neurohumoral activation, and underlying cardiovascular disease. The resultant decrease in the cross-sectional area of the pulmonary arterial bed causes an increase in the pulmonary vascular resistance (PVR). The increase in PVR impedes right ventricular outflow, and thus cardiac output (CO) is diminished. Increasing levels of vascular obstruction produce worsening hypoxemia, which stimulates vasoconstriction and a further rise in pulmonary artery pressure (PAP). The right ventricle eventually fails when it cannot generate sufficient systolic pressure to overcome the increasing PAP and preserve pulmonary perfusion. In patients without underlying cardiopulmonary disease, a greater than 50% obstruction of the pulmonary circulation is generally required for a significant increase in the mean PAP. When the extent of obstruction of the pulmonary circulation approaches 75%, the right ventricle must generate a systolic pressure in excess of 50 mm Hg and a mean pulmonary artery pressure of >40 mm Hg to preserve pulmonary perfusion.[7] Patients with underlying cardiopulmonary disease experience more substantial deterioration in cardiac output from PE.

PE can be the primary reason for admission to the inpatient medical units, or it can arise as a complication of critical illness. Most frequently, PE results from proximal deep venous thrombosis (DVT) from the legs, but upper extremity thrombi (particularly common in patients with central venous catheters) may also embolize. Accurate diagnosis followed by effective therapy unequivocally reduces the morbidity and mortality of PE. Use of decision rules aids the diagnostic process.

ASSESSMENT

Clinical Presentation

Prevalence

PE afflicts over 500,000 American annually, causing 10% of all inhospital deaths, and it remains the single most important cause of maternal deaths associated with live births in the United States. Given that only one third of proximal DVTs are clinically recognized, the actual rate of DVT may be as high as two million per year. It is also estimated that 600,000 patients develop PE each year and that 60,000 die of this complication. Regrettably, the rate of diagnosis of PE has not improved much since 1970. Although advanced age increases the risk of VTE, any member of the population can be afflicted with a 10.7% probability by the age of 80 years. Unfortunately, autopsy studies continue to show that most cases of fatal PE are unrecognized and undiagnosed.[1–7]

Presenting Signs and Symptoms

The history and physical examination are insensitive and nonspecific for the clinical diagnosis of both DVT and PE. It should be emphasized that *clinical suspicion may imply the need for further evaluation but cannot, by itself, be relied upon to confirm or exclude the diagnosis of PE.*

Pulmonary embolism should always be considered whenever unexplained dyspnea is present. Dyspnea, pleuritic chest pain, and hemoptysis are common in PE, but are nonspecific. Anxiety, lightheadedness, sudden hypotension, and syncope are all symptoms that may be caused by PE but may also result from a number of other disorders. Tachypnea and tachycardia are the most common signs of PE but are also nonspecific. The cardiac and pulmonary physical examinations are both nonspecific. The index of clinical suspicion becomes a more useful parameter when considered in conjunction with $\dot{V}/\dot{Q}$ scanning.[8] Diagnostic efforts for suspected PE may be appropriate, even in the setting of alternative explanations if risk factors and the clinical setting are suggestive. Dyspnea and tachypnea with clear lung fields and

Table 27-1 Acute Pulmonary Embolism: Symptoms

	All Patients (N = 383) (%)	No Previous Cardiopulmonary Disease (N = 117) (%)
Dyspnea	78%	73%
Pleuritic chest pain	59%	66%
Cough	43%	37%
Leg pain	27%	26%
Hemoptysis	16%	13%
Palpitations	13%	10%
Wheezing	14%	9%
Angina-like pain	6%	4%

From: The PIOPED study—The PIOPED Investigators. Value of the ventilation/perfusion scan in acute pulmonary embolism: Results of the prospective investigation of pulmonary embolism diagnosis. JAMA 1990; 263:2753–2759; and Stein PD, ed. Pulmonary Embolism. Baltimore: Williams and Wilkins, 1996.

Table 27-2 Predicting the Pre-test Probability of Pulmonary Embolism

Clinical Characteristics	Score
Active cancer (treatment with 6 month or palliative)	1
Surgery or bedridden for ≥3 days for past 4 weeks	1.5
History of deep venous thrombosis or pulmonary embolism	1.5
Hemoptysis	1
Heart rate >100 beats/min	1.5
Pulmonary embolism judged to be the most likely diagnosis	3
Clinical signs and symptoms compatible with deep venous thrombosis	3

Probability of PE	Total Score
Low	≤4
Moderate	4.5–6
High	>6

Adapted from: Wells PS, Anderson DR, Rodger M, et al. Derivation of a simple clinical model to categorize patients, probability of pulmonary embolism: increasing the model's utility with the SimpliRED D-dimer. Thromb Haemost. 2000; 83:416–420.

hypoxemia may mistakenly be attributed to a flare of chronic obstructive lung disease or asthma when underlying PE may be present.[9] Symptoms of acute PE and their frequency based upon the PIOPED study are presented in Table 27-1.

As no single finding predicts the presence or absence of PE, a clinical prediction rule should be used to formulate the probability of pulmonary embolism prior to diagnostic testing (i.e., determine pretest probability of PE). Wells and his colleagues developed a clinical model to determine the pretest probability of PE based on certain simple clinical parameters (Table 27-2). The validity of this prediction rule has been demonstrated in diagnostic studies when paired with D-dimer testing (see below).

Diagnosis

The key to the diagnosis of PE begins with a high clinical suspicion for this diagnosis. The diagnostic technology for acute PE has evolved considerably. While $\dot{V}/\dot{Q}$ scanning followed by pulmonary arteriography has been the gold-standard approach for decades, spiral (helical) computed tomography (CT) angiograms, especially using multidetector scanners, and magnetic resonance angiogram (MRA) scanning have been increasingly utilized. In most hospitals, CT angiogram is the procedure of choice for evaluating patients with suspected PE.

Diagnostic algorithms for acute PE are presented in Figures 27-1 and 27-2.

Chest Radiography

Most patients with PE have an abnormal but nonspecific chest radiograph. In PIOPED,[8] the chest radiograph was abnormal in 98 of 117 (84%) patients, with the most common abnormalities being atelectasis and/or parenchymal abnormalities occurring in 79 of 117 (68%) individuals. Common radiographic findings include atelectasis, pleural effusion, pulmonary infiltrates, and elevation of a hemidiaphragm. Classic findings of pulmonary infarction, such as a juxtapleural wedge-shaped opacity at the costophrenic angle indicating pulmonary infarction (Hampton's hump) or decreased vascularity (Westermark's sign), may suggest the diagnosis, but they are infrequent. A normal chest radiograph in the setting of severe dyspnea and hypoxemia without evidence of bronchospasm or anatomical cardiac shunt is strongly suggestive of PE. The chest radiograph cannot be used to conclusively diagnose or exclude PE. Other processes such as pneumonia, congestive heart failure, pneumothorax, or rib fracture may cause symptoms similar to acute PE and should be considered.

Electrocardiography

The electrocardiogram also cannot be relied upon for the diagnosis of acute PE, but is usually abnormal. Findings in acute PE are generally nonspecific and include T-wave changes, ST-segment abnormalities, and left or right axis deviation. In the Urokinase Pulmonary Embolism Trial (UPET), electrocardiographic abnormalities were demonstrated in 87% of patients with proven PE without underlying cardiac or pulmonary disease.[10] Even with massive or submassive PE, manifestations such as the S1Q3T3 pattern, right bundle branch block, P-wave pulmonale, or right axis deviation occurred in only 26% of patients. The low frequency of specific ECG changes associated with PE was confirmed in the PIOPED study.[8] Nonspecific ST-segment or T-wave changes were the most common electrocardiographic abnormalities and were noted in 44 of 89 (49%) patients. The presence of T-wave inversion in the precordial leads may correlate with more severe right ventricular dysfunction.

Arterial Blood Gas Analysis

Hypoxemia is common in acute PE. Certain individuals, particularly young patients without underlying lung disease, may have a normal PaO_2. In PIOPED, the A-a difference was increased by more than 20 mm Hg in 76 of 88 (86%) patients with PE. The

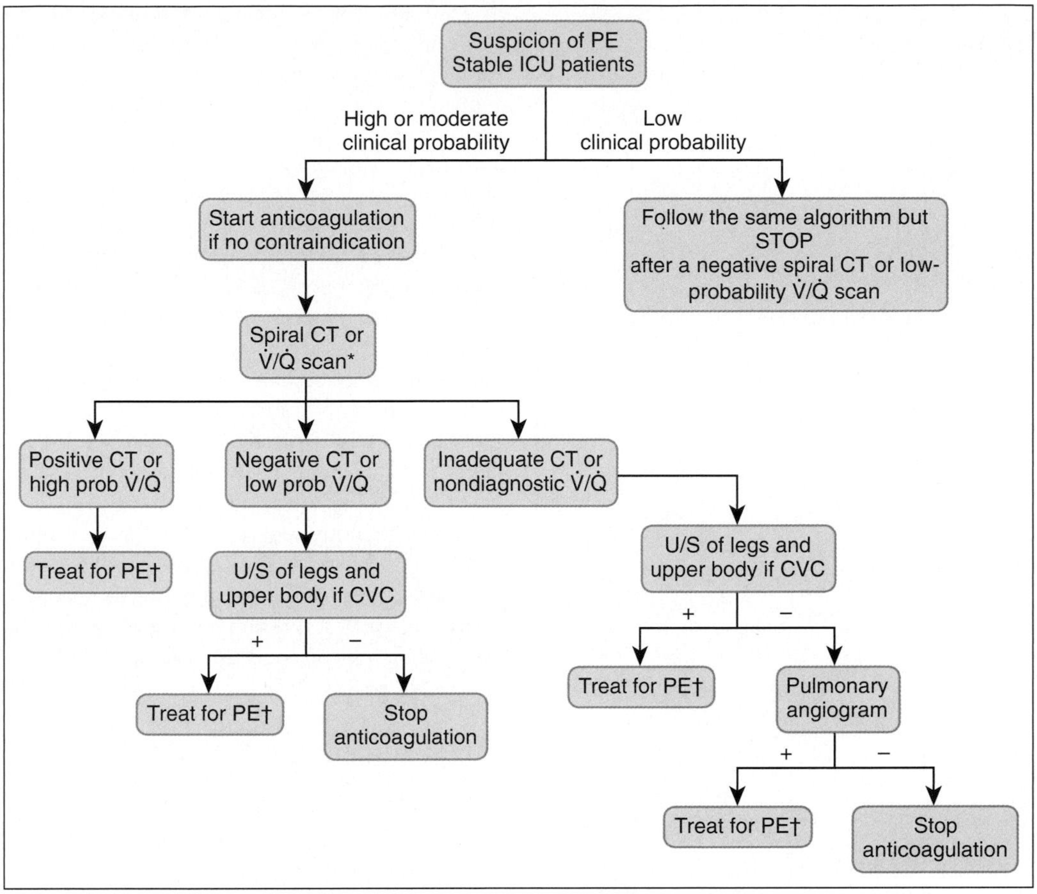

Figure 27-1 • Diagnostic algorithm for suspected pulmonary embolism in stable intensive care unit patients.

*V/Q scan is most useful when the chest radiograph is normal or near normal.

†Treatment may include consideration of thrombolytics even in stable patients, depending on clot burden; consider echocardiography to help stratify patients.

Abbreviations: PE = pulmonary embolus; ICU = intensive care unit; CT = computed tomography; V/Q = ventilation-perfusion; U/S = ultrasound; CVC = central venous catheter.

alveolar-arterial (A-a) difference was elevated in all patients, with the pCO_2 usually low. The diagnosis of acute PE cannot be excluded based upon a normal PaO_2. Although the A-a difference is usually elevated in PE, it may rarely be normal in patients without preexisting cardiopulmonary disease. It is important to realize that an elevated pCO_2 (caused, for example, by preexisting lung disease or metabolic alkalosis), does not rule out the possibility of acute PE.

D-Dimer Testing

D-dimer represents a specific derivative of cross-linked fibrin and has been extensively evaluated in the setting of suspected acute PE. A normal enzyme-linked immunosorbent assay (ELISA) appears quite sensitive in excluding PE. When a positive D-dimer level is considered to be 500 mcg/L or greater, the sensitivity and specificity for PE have been shown to be 98% and 39%, respectively.[11] Of note, a systematic review in 2004 documented that the ELISA form of D-dimer is more sensitive than latex agglutination.[14] However, many clinical conditions in addition to acute thromboembolism are associated with an elevated D-dimer level (i.e., low specificity). Thus, the D-dimer test is useful when negative, not positive.

A negative D-dimer assay together with a respiratory rate <20 breaths/min, and a pO2 >80 mm Hg, has proven to be very sen-

sitive in ruling out acute PE.[12] Neither symptoms, signs, radiographic findings, electrocardiography, nor the plasma D-dimer measurement can be considered diagnostic of PE or DVT; and when these entities are suspected, further evaluation with noninvasive or invasive testing is necessary.

Clinical probability scores (*see* Table 27-2) have been used together with a negative D-dimer test to *help to exclude PE.* A prospective clinical trial confirmed the utility of combining a D-dimer assay with a simplified scoring system utilizing readily available clinical parameters.[13] This was validated in a 2006 study of more than 1,000 patients. If patients have a "low" probability of PE and negative D-dimer results, additional diagnostic testing can be withheld without increasing the frequency of VTE during follow-up. Fortunately, the combination of low clinical probability and negative D-dimer results occurs in 50% of outpatients and in 20% of inpatients with suspected PE.[13a] Several prospective, well-designed studies offer reliable evidence that prediction scores, sometimes utilizing D-dimer testing, may lessen the need for additional diagnostic testing.[14] While such scoring systems appear useful in characterizing patients with suspected PE, they have not yet been as widely adopted into clinical practice as they probably should.[14a]

Another clinical outcome study of more than 3,000 patients in the Netherlands with clinically suspected PE evaluated them using a diagnostic algorithm with a dichotomized clinical deci-

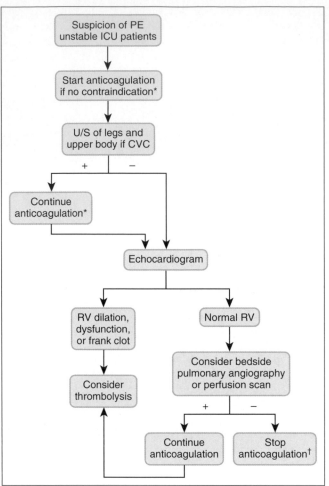

Figure 27-2 • Diagnostic algorithm for suspected pulmonary embolism in unstable intensive care unit patients.

*Consider inferior vena cava filter if DVT present and anticoagulation is contraindicated, or also in the setting of massive pulmonary embolism with DVT when it is believed that any further emboli might be lethal and thrombolytic use is prohibited.

†Stop anticoagulation after a negative pulmonary angiography or a normal or low-probability perfusion scan.

PE = pulmonary embolus; ICU = intensive care unit; U/S = ultrasound; CVC = central venous catheter; RV = right ventricle; DVT = Deep Vein Thrombosis

sion rule (unlikely or likely PE), D-dimer testing, and CT.[14b] Based on Wells' decision rule, moderate and high clinical probability of PE were combined into likely, while low probability was described as unlikely. Again, the situation of unlikely clinical probability and a negative D-dimer result appeared safe to withhold anticoagulant therapy. This was a common finding, occurring in one third of patients presenting with suspected PE.

For patients with high clinical suspicion of VTE, D-dimer results should not affect clinical decisions (i.e. patients need additioinal diagnostic studies). These conclusions are supported by the findings of a recent systematic review examining D-dimer for the exclusion of acute venous thrombosis and PE.[14]

Cardiac Biomarkers

Patients with PE sometimes have elevated troponin levels. Elevated troponin is specific for cardiac myocyte damage, and the right ventricle appears to be the source of the enzyme elevation in acute PE. Not surprisingly, both cardiac troponin T and troponin I levels have been found to be elevated in acute PE, especially in massive PE in which myocyte injury due to right ventricular strain might be expected. Several studies have suggested that troponin levels may be elevated in acute PE,[15–19] and a recent investigation suggested that an elevated level might be of prognostic value.[18] In this study of 38 patients with acute PE, 18 (47%) had elevated cardiac troponin I levels. Of the 18 patients, 12 of 18 (67%) had right ventricular dilation/hypokinesis compared with only 3 of 20 (15%) without elevation of cTnI (P = 004). Furthermore, cTnI-positive patients had significantly higher right ventricular systolic pressures, as well as having a higher chance of developing cardiogenic shock (33% vs. 5%, P = 01). The most important application of elevated cardiac troponin levels is that in a clinically compatible setting, an elevated value might serve as a clue to the diagnosis of PE and lead to further investigation. Plasma brain natriuretic peptide (BNP) levels may be a supplementary tool for evaluating right ventricular function in patients with acute PE. The exact utility is yet unclear and is currently under evaluation. Importantly, somewhat elevated BNP levels (e.g., 300–700) should not mislead the physician to make the misdiagnosis of heart failure as the etiology of dyspnea in a patient with PE.

Ventilation-Perfusion Scanning and Pulmonary Arteriography

Spiral CT and $\dot{V}/\dot{Q}$ scanning are the most common diagnostic tests utilized specifically for suspected PE. Based upon well-designed, prospective clinical trials, when the $\dot{V}/\dot{Q}$ scan is nondiagnostic, it should be interpreted together with the index of clinical suspicion.[8] In the PIOPED study, the utility of $\dot{V}/\dot{Q}$ scanning combined with clinical assessment of patients with suspected PE was prospectively evaluated.[8] Thirty-three percent of patients with intermediate probability scans and 12% of patients with low-probability scans were definitively diagnosed with PE by pulmonary arteriography. When the clinical suspicion of PE was considered very high, PE was found to be present in 96% of patients with high probability scans, 66% of patients with intermediate scans, and 40% of patients with low-probability scans. If the clinical scenario suggests PE, the diagnosis of PE should be rigorously pursued, even when the lung scan reveals low or intermediate probability. Based upon reliable evidence (well-designed clinical trials) together with expert opinion and experience, when there is high clinical suspicion for PE, a high-probability $\dot{V}/\dot{Q}$ scan is diagnostic. When the $\dot{V}/\dot{Q}$ scan is normal, PE is effectively excluded. A nondiagnostic scan requires further evaluation.

Several potential diagnostic pathways may be appropriate after a nondiagnostic $\dot{V}/\dot{Q}$ scan. Pulmonary arteriography (the gold standard) should be considered, and a nondiagnostic $\dot{V}/\dot{Q}$ scan may help guide the vessels selected for arteriogram, thus limiting the amount of contrast required. Arteriography is considered safe in experienced hands. Another option is to do lower extremity studies. If, in the setting of a nondiagnostic $\dot{V}/\dot{Q}$ scan, a leg ultrasound is performed and is positive for DVT, treatment can be instituted, and no additional studies are needed. While a negative D-dimer suggests the absence of VTE, additional imaging should be performed when the clinical setting suggests that PE is likely. Another diagnostic option is to perform a multidetector CT angiogram.

Spiral (Helical) CT Scan Angiography—A Preferred Study Option

The use of CT angiography is replacing V̇/Q̇ scanning for suspected PE. A contrast bolus is required for vascular imaging of the pulmonary vessels, and thus patients at risk of renal failure may not be able to undergo this test. Spiral CT may reveal emboli in the main, lobar, or segmental pulmonary arteries with >90% sensitivity and specificity. Three-dimensional reconstruction techniques (multiplanar reformation) can be applied to the opacified pulmonary vasculature to better define vessels located within the plane that has been sectioned. Studies evaluating spiral CT to determine sensitivity and specificity for acute PE have revealed a range of 53–100% and 81–97%, respectively, for these parameters.[20–27] Different study designs, patient exclusion criteria, levels of experience, and reading protocols have accounted for some of the differences.

The results of PIOPED II were published in 2006, documenting that multidetector (mainly four-slice) CT angiography is preferred to V̇/Q̇ scan in the diagnosis of PE.[27a] With a specificity of 96% and sensitivity of 83%, there was still a 17% false negative rate. However, these were predominantly subsegmental clots of uncertain clinical significance. The combination of low probability by Wells' clinical prediction rule (*see* Table 27-2) and a negative CT angiogram had a 96% negative predictive value, while intermediate probability resulted in an 89% probability of no PE. However, if a patient had a high probability of PE before the test, then the negative predictive value was only 60%. The positive predictive value of multi-detector CT angiography was 92–96% among patients with intermediate to high clinical probability, but just 58% among those with low likelihood of PE. Of note, this study was conducted on outpatients, and CT venography of the leg veins did not seem to add much to the diagnostic process.[27b]

The sensitivity for PE in smaller (subsegmental) vessels remains suboptimal, and the importance of such small emboli also is controversial. A potential concern would be a patient with small, undiscovered subsegmental emboli in whom silent DVT might be present. Not treating such a patient could result in recurrent PE, or possibly contribute to the development of postphlebitic syndrome. Thus, considering leg studies in a patient with high clinical suspicion for acute PE and a negative CT would appear prudent. In a prospective study, patients with suspected PE, a negative chest CT, and negative ultrasound of the legs had good outcomes without a significant number of recurrences.[28] Perhaps a better measure of the usefulness of a diagnostic technique is whether or not it misses *clinically important* events. Evidence of moderate quality (from controlled clinical trials and expert opinion) suggests that if spiral CT is used, the addition of negative leg studies or D-dimer testing improves the negative predictive value for clinically significant PE.

An important advantage of spiral CT over V̇/Q̇ scanning is direct visualization of the thrombus and the ability to define alternative nonvascular pathology. In a recent clinical study, the use of CT scanning for suspected PE resulted in 31 new diagnoses other than PE.[29] These included diagnoses such as aspiration pneumonia, pulmonary edema, lung cancer, esophageal cancer, and invasive aspergillosis—all entities that could not be diagnosed by V̇/Q̇ scan. The most common relative contraindications to performing contrast-enhanced spiral CT scanning are renal insufficiency and contrast allergy. The cost-effectiveness of utilizing spiral CT scanning for suspected PE has been studied, and it would appear that because of the frequency of nondiagnostic V̇/Q̇ scans, spiral CT scanning may prove to reduce cost in the evaluation of patients with suspected PE.

Although the evidence supporting the use of spiral CT for suspected emboli at the segmental level or greater is of only moderate quality (based upon multiple controlled trials and expert opinion), this technique is the most common initial diagnostic test at many hospitals and has multiple advantages over V̇/Q̇ scanning.[30] The advantages and limitations of spiral CT scanning for suspected acute PE are listed in Table 27-3.

Magnetic Resonance Imaging

Magnetic resonance imaging (MRI) has been utilized to evaluate clinically suspected PE.[24,31,32] This technique has several potential advantages, including no use of ionizing radiation, safer contrast agents, and excellent sensitivity and specificity for the diagnosis

Table 27-3 Advantages and Limitations of Spiral Computed Tomography (CT) Scanning for the Diagnosis of Acute Pulmonary Embolism

Advantages	Limitations
Availability	Intravenous contrast required
Sensitivity for central emboli*	Reader expertise required
Specificity*	Not portable
Relative rapidity of procedure	Morbid obesity may prevent scanning
Diagnosis of other disease entities	
Multiplanar reformation (3 dimensions)	**Relative contraindications**
Safety	Renal insufficiency‡
Advancing technology	Contrast allergy
Nondiagnostic readings unusual†	
Potential for CT venography	

*In clinical trials to date, high sensitivity and specificity have been limited to emboli in the main, lobar, and segmental vessels. Sensitivity is inadequate for subsegmental vessels.

†CT scans are read as nondiagnostic in approximately 10% of cases (much lower than for ventilation-perfusion scans).

‡Mild renal insufficiency is not a contraindication.

of VTE.[33] Unfortunately, MRI is often time-consuming and too difficult for critically ill patients with respiratory distress to tolerate this technique. In addition, CO_2 angiography would be a viable option in the setting of chronic kidney disease when an interventionist with expertise for this procedure is available.

Echocardiography

Echocardiography, which can often be obtained more rapidly than either lung scanning or pulmonary arteriography, may reveal findings that strongly suggest hemodynamically significant PE.[34] Patients with PE often have underlying cardiopulmonary disease such as chronic obstructive lung disease; therefore, neither right ventricular dilation nor hypokinesis can be reliably used even as indirect evidence of PE. Direct visualization of massive PE may occasionally be possible, particularly if transesophageal echocardiography is performed. Echocardiography is sometimes used to gauge the extent of right ventricular dysfunction in the setting of proven acute PE (see treatment).[35] Intravascular ultrasound (IVUS) has been used to directly visualize acute PE at the bedside. Although this technique appears sensitive for more proximal emboli, it has not achieved widespread use.

Massive Pulmonary Embolism

The presence of suspected massive PE presents both difficulties as well as potential diagnostic advantages.[36] When patients present as severely ill with extreme hypoxemia and/or hypotension, the diagnostic evaluation must be performed as quickly as possible. Critically ill patients may be difficult to transport to the radiology department. Portable perfusion scanning may be useful in such individuals since the chances for a high-probability diagnostic scan are likely to be higher with a massive PE. It would be exceedingly unlikely also for CT scanning to be negative in the setting of massive PE with larger, more proximal emboli likely. Echocardiography would be even more likely to reveal dramatic right ventricular dilation and dysfunction, which in the absence of other potential causes would suggest the possibility of acute PE. Potential therapeutic implications of such findings will be reviewed later in the management segment.

Management

Treatment

Several pharmacologic and nonpharmacologic options have been studied for the treatment of VTE with different efficacy and safety results. Unfractionated heparin (UFH), low-molecular-weight heparins (LMWHs), warfarin, thrombolytics, inferior vena cava filters, surgical thrombectomy, and several new agents are available as treatment options. An early question that was answered by Barritt and Jordan in the first prospective randomized anticoagulation trial in patients with acute venous thromboembolism in 1960 was the need for anticoagulation in patients with acute PE. In a trial stopped prematurely after only 35 patients enrolled, the mortality rate from PE in the untreated group was >25%, compared to no deaths from PE in the anticoagulation group.[37] Standard of care dictates aggressive anticoagulation in patients with acute PE.

There are two phases in the treatment of patients with symptomatic venous thromboembolism: acute or initial treatment,

and chronic or secondary prophylaxis. Acute-phase treatment options include continuous IV UFH infusion, subcutaneous (SC) low molecular weight heparin (LMWH), the use of an inferior vena caval filter, and thrombolytic therapy.

Acute VTE Management

Unfractionated Heparin (UH)

All heparins are heterogeneous mixtures of glycosaminoglycans derived from animal products that catalyze the blood enzyme antithrombin (AT). UFH has a narrow therapeutic window and has been cited as a common cause of drug-related deaths in hospitalized patients. Significant bleeding occurs in 7–30% of patients on IV UFH, and complication rates of 1–2% per day have been reported. However, a weight-based dosing protocol was shown to result in a 97% likelihood of therapeutic heparin effect with an intravenous bolus of 80 units/kg followed by continuous IV infusion of 18 units/kg/hr.[38a]

Using the activated partial thromboplastin time (APTT), the dosage of heparin should be adjusted to maintain an anticoagulant intensity above the lower limit of a defined therapeutic range.[39] Most physicians are familiar with an APTT of 1.5–2.5 times the control as a therapeutic range for heparin. There are alternatives to this standard of monitoring, such as heparin levels via either thrombin/protamine titration with a target of 0.2–0.4 units/mL, or an anti-Xa level of 0.5–1.1 units/mL.

Warfarin may be started within the first 24–48 hours at a dose of 5.0–7.5 mg a day.[44] The disadvantages of "loading doses" of warfarin of 10 mg per day have been well described, including a high incidence of overanticoagulation. However, heavier patients may require a larger 10 mg initial dose.

Both heparin and warfarin must be used concomitantly for at least 4 days until the international normalized ratio (INR) is within therapeutic range (INR at 2.0–3.0), preferably for 2 consecutive days, at which time heparin administration can be discontinued to avoid early prothrombotic conditions.[40]

The most common and serious adverse effect of anticoagulation is bleeding. The risk of major hemorrhage with UFH is higher with intermittent compared with continuous IV infusion. No difference in major bleeding was detected between continuous IV and subcutaneous heparin.[41]

LMWH is less often associated with major hemorrhage, most probably due to the complexities of UFH administration, which involves pump infusion, varying techniques and laboratory reagents, dosing manipulation, and intrinsic pharmacologic properties. Patient characteristics associated with increased major bleeding include age >70 years and the presence of comorbid conditions. Those who are healthy have a 2% incidence, while debilitated, severely ill patients have a 25% risk of bleeding. Aspirin is known to increase the hemorrhagic risk when combined with heparin but has been administered commonly without serious bleeding.[42,43] Wound and soft tissue hemorrhage comprise 31% of bleeding sites. Combined gastrointestinal and genitourinary hemorrhage accounts for 46%. Although infrequent at 1%, the clinical presentation of bleeding into the retroperitoneum, adrenal glands, and central nervous system can be devastating.

Bleeding with UFH can be managed by discontinuation and observation, as the half-life is only 90 minutes on reversal with 1 mg per 100 units of UFH of protamine sulfate. Side effects of protamine sulfate administration are anaphylaxis, hypotension, and possible bleeding. Equimolar concentrations of protamine sulfate neutralize anti-IIa activity but only partial anti-Xa activity of LMWHs, probably because protamine sulfate does not bind to very low molecular weight components. It remains unknown whether protamine affects clinically important bleeding.

A serious adverse effect with all forms of heparin is heparin-induced thrombocytopenia (HIT). HIT occurs at an incidence of 3.5% with UH and 0.6% with LMWH.[44] Typically, after at least 5 days of heparin administration, a 50% reduction in the platelet count when compared to pretreatment platelet counts, or an absolute reduction to 100,000 per mm³, suggests the development of HIT. This is an antigen–antibody reaction between heparin and platelet factor 4.[45] If this complication occurs or is suspected, a direct thrombin inhibitor such as hirudin or argatroban needs to be administered because of the potential for cross-reactivity with other heparins and LMWHs. (This is covered in more detail in Chapter 78.)

Due to an increase in osteoclast activating factor, heparin-induced osteoporosis can be a serious complication, especially with long-term administration (i.e., the pregnant patient with pregnancy-induced venous thrombosis in the first trimester). The risk of osteoporosis occurs less frequently with prolonged administration of LMWH than with UFH.[47]

The absolute contraindications to anticoagulant therapy include intracranial hemorrhage, active internal bleeding, peptic ulcer disease with hemorrhage, malignant hypertension, intracranial neoplasm, recent and significant trauma or surgery, and history of heparin-induced thrombocytopenia.

Low-Molecular-Weight Heparin Preferred Option

LMWHs possess a number of significant advantages over UFH. LMWH has favorable pharmacokinetics with 90% bioavailability at both low (prophylaxis) and high (treatment) doses. A prolonged half-life independent of dose allows for subcutaneous injection once or twice daily with a predictable dose response, most often without monitoring (anti-Xa level). In fact, the response is so predictable that, with the exception of certain high-risk situations, no dose monitoring is necessary. LMWHs have fewer pentasaccharide units, the high-affinity binding sites for antithrombin III; and the anti-factor Xa to IIa ratio is 2:1 to 4:1 for LMWHs, as opposed to 1:1 for UFH. Several major randomized, prospective multicenter trials and meta-analyses in the mid-1990s demonstrated no statistical advantage of LMWH over UFH in the treatment of VTE when comparing VTE recurrence, hemorrhage, and death.

For acute PE, several randomized trials have demonstrated that LMWHs are at least as safe and effective as UFHs in preventing recurrent emboli.[48–50] Currently, enoxaparin (Lovenox) is approved by the United States Food and Drug Administration (FDA) at a dosage of 1 mg/kg given subcutaneously twice daily or 1.5 mg/kg once daily to inpatients with DVT, with or without PE. The outpatient regimen is a dosage of 1 mg/kg twice daily for DVT without PE. Dalteparin (Fragmin) is not yet approved for the treatment of VTE but has been used in dosages of 100 anti-factor Xa units/kg given subcutaneously twice daily and 200 anti-Xa units/kg given once daily for the management of DVT. Tinzaparin is FDA-labeled at a dosage of 175 international units/kg for DVT with or without PE, but data have been established only for use in hospitalized patients.

Thrombolytic Therapy

Thrombolytic agents cause the direct acceleration of clot lysis and a reduction in clot burden. These agents activate plasminogen to form plasmin, which then results in fibrinolysis as well as fibrinogenolysis. Defining those patients in whom the benefit of a rapid reduction in clot burden outweighs the increased hemorrhagic risk of thrombolytic therapy may be difficult. Catheter-directed and systemic thrombolytic therapy have both been investigated. There are three FDA-approved thrombolytic agent regimens for PE utilizing weight-based monograms (Box 27-1).

The case for thrombolytic use is strongest in patients with massive PE complicated by shock, which occurs in about 10% of PE patients and for which the mortality rate may be 25%. Thrombolysis in these patients results in a more rapid resolution of abnormal right ventricular function. There are emerging data to suggest that patients with acute submassive embolism (extensive clot burden without shock or severe hypoxemia) may also benefit from thrombolysis. A recent prospective, randomized, clinical trial demonstrated that patients with acute PE without hypotension but with right ventricular dysfunction on echocardiogram had an improved clinical course when given thrombolytic therapy plus heparin versus heparin alone. Thrombolysis seemed to prevent clinical deterioration and the need for escalation of care.

No clear data have shown one thrombolytic agent as superior to the others, though shorter infusion regimens and even bolus dosing may be favored in the case of massive PE. Each of the approved regimens is administered at a fixed dose, making measurements of coagulation unnecessary during infusion. The APTT should be measured after the thrombolytic infusion is completed and repeated at 4-hour intervals until the aPTT is less than twice the upper limit of normal. At this point, continuous intravenous UFH should be administered without a bolus loading dose when thrombolytic therapy is given.

Thrombolytic therapy is contraindicated in patients at high risk for hemorrhage, as both the lysis of hemostatic fibrin plugs and fibrinogenolysis can lead to severe bleeding. Intracranial

---

Box 27-1 FDA-Approved Thrombolytic Regimens for Pulmonary Embolism

Streptokinase

250,000 IU loading dose over 30 min followed by 100,000 IU/24 hr IV

Urokinase

4400 IU/kg loading dose over 10 min followed by 4,440 IU/kg/hr for 12–24 hr IV

Urokinase: (2,000 U/lb IV (loading dose over 10 minutes); then 2,000 U/lb/hr for 12–24 hours

rt-PA

100 mg continuous IV infusion over 2 hr

FDA = Food and Drug Administration
IU = international unit
U = unit

hemorrhage is the most devastating complication of thrombolytic therapy and is generally stated to occur in about 2% of patients. Invasive procedures should be minimized, as bleeding commonly occurs at sites of pulmonary arteriography or arterial line placement. Retroperitoneal hemorrhage may result from a vascular puncture above the inguinal ligament and is often clinically silent but may be life threatening. The decision for thrombolysis should be made on a case-by-case basis. There should be a lower threshold to administer thrombolytic therapy in the setting of a relative contraindication if a patient is extremely unstable from life-threatening PE.

Mechanical thrombectomy devices have recently been evaluated for therapy of large occlusive acute venous thrombi either in the lower extremities or pulmonary vasculature. Interventional radiologists are gaining experiences with this treatment, and it avoids the potential complications of thrombolytic therapy.

Vena Cava Interruption

Inferior Vena Cava (IVC) filter placement can be performed to minimize the risk of PE from lower extremity thrombi. The primary indications for IVC filter placement include contraindications to anticoagulation, recurrent embolism while on adequate therapy, and significant bleeding during anticoagulation. Filters can also be placed in the setting of massive PE when it is believed that any further emboli might be lethal. A number of filter designs exist and can be inserted via the jugular or femoral veins. The vena cava recovery filter is a novel, IVC filter that is one of a new class referred to as "optional" filters. An optional IVC filter can be left indwelling as a permanent device, or it may be retrieved when the clinical need for mechanical IVC interruption no longer exists. The device does not have a time limit for removal, but gives clinicians the flexibility to assess a patient's risk and determine the appropriate time of removal. Rare complications include insertion-related complications, filter migration, direct thrombus extension through the filter, and IVC thrombosis. Recently, temporary filters have been utilized in patients in whom the risk of bleeding appears to be short term.

Surgical Embolectomy

Although surgical embolectomy is most commonly performed for chronic thromboembolic pulmonary hypertension, rare circumstances warrant its consideration in acute PE. A candidate for acute embolectomy should have a documented massive PE with refractory shock, failure of or contraindication to thrombolytic therapy, and the availability of an experienced surgical team. Interventional radiologists are able to remove clots via mechanical thrombectomy, which is replacing the use of surgery.

Special Treatment Considerations: Massive PE

Once massive PE with hypotension and/or severe hypoxemia is suspected, aggressive supportive treatment should be initiated immediately. Cautious infusion of intravenous saline may augment preload and improve impaired right ventricular function. Dopamine and norepinephrine are the favored vasopressors if hypotension persists. Although dobutamine may boost right ventricular output, it may worsen hypotension. Supplemental oxygen, intubation, and mechanical ventilation are instituted as needed to support respiratory failure. Anticoagulation and thrombolytic therapy should be considered as previously described above. Pulmonary embolectomy may be appropriate in patients with massive embolism in whom thrombolytic therapy is contraindicated.

Nonthrombotic Pulmonary Emboli

Although the differential diagnosis of acute PE predominantly includes other cardiopulmonary diseases, other nonthrombotic sources of emboli may rarely occur in certain clinical settings. Through venous blood return to the lungs, the pulmonary vascular bed is exposed to a variety of potentially obstructing substances. These substances may be exogenous or endogenous in origin, and they may result in various clinical consequences, including dyspnea, chest pain, hypoxemia, and sometimes death. Nonthrombotic sources of emboli include fat embolism, amniotic fluid embolism, air embolism, schistosomiasis, septic embolism, and tumor embolism.[51–55]

Fat Embolism

Fat embolism most commonly occurs in the setting of the traumatic fracture of long bones.[52] This disorder is usually a more impressive clinical syndrome when multiple fractures of larger bones are involved. However, orthopedic procedures and trauma to other fat-replete tissues such as the liver or subcutaneous tissue can sometimes result in similar consequences. After the inciting event, there is generally a delay of 24–48 hours before symptoms develop. Neutral fat enters the vascular system, and a characteristic syndrome of dyspnea, petechiae, and mental confusion often develops. It is unclear why the syndrome develops in some patients and not in others.

The obstruction of numerous vessels by neutral fat particles as well as the deleterious effects of free fatty acids released from neutral fat by lipases account for the pathophysiologic consequences of fat embolism.[51] These free fatty acids cause a diffuse vasculitis with capillary leakage from cerebral, pulmonary, and other vascular beds. The diagnosis is made from the clinical and radiographic findings in the setting of risk factors such as surgery or trauma. Fat droplets by oil red O stain in bronchoalveolar lavage fluid may be suggestive of fat embolism, but clinical studies to date suggest that this finding is neither sensitive nor specific. Treatment is generally supportive, including oxygen and mechanical ventilation, and the prognosis is generally good. Therapy with corticosteroids remains controversial. Steroid prophylaxis has been suggested in high risk patients.

Amniotic Fluid Embolism

Amniotic fluid embolism is uncommon, but it represents one of the leading causes of maternal death in the United States. This disorder occurs during or after delivery when amniotic fluid gains access to uterine venous channels and then to the maternal pulmonary and general circulations. The delivery may be either spontaneous or by cesarean section and usually has been without complication. There are no identifiable risk factors in either the patient or the fetus.

The syndrome manifests as a sudden onset of severe respiratory distress and hypotension, and death frequently results. The primary mechanism of injury appears to involve the thromboplastic activity of amniotic fluid. Extensive fibrin deposition then develops in the pulmonary vasculature and sometimes in other organs. A consumptive coagulopathy ensues, with marked hypofibrinogenemia. An enhanced fibrinolytic state frequently develops after the acute event. Left ventricular dysfunction may result from the potential role of a myocardial depressant effect of amniotic fluid. The resulting pulmonary edema may be both hydrostatic and noncardiogenic.

The differential diagnosis includes PE, septic and hemorrhagic shock, venous air embolism, aspiration pneumonia, congestive heart failure (from acute myocardial infarction or other causes), placentae abruptio, and ruptured uterus. The diagnosis should be suspected based upon the clinical picture. Examination of the pulmonary arterial blood may or may not reveal the amorphous fragments of vernix caseosa, squamous cells, or mucin.

The administration of heparin, antifibrinolytic agents such as α-aminocaproic acid, and cryoprecipitate has been suggested for treatment. However, the primary treatment is supportive, with oxygen and mechanical ventilation. Even with aggressive support, maternal mortality may be as high as 80%.

Air Embolism

The increased frequency of air embolism reflects the variety of invasive surgical and medical procedures now available, the frequent use of indwelling venous and arterial catheters, and the frequency of thoracic and other forms of trauma.[53,54] The consequences of air embolism range from minimal to life threatening. With venous embolism in the setting of a patent foramen ovale, embolization to the coronary or cerebral circulation is a great concern. In the absence of a patent foramen ovale, the lungs can filter modest amounts of air, but large single or continuous episodes of air embolism can still gain access to the systemic arterial circulation.

Symptoms and signs are dependent upon the severity of the episode. Air in the systemic circulation may be difficult to recognize because even small quantities may cause significant symptoms, and intravascular air clears quickly from the circulation. Dyspnea, wheezing, chest pain, cough, agitation, confusion, tachycardia, and hypotension may be evident. A "mill wheel murmur" (air in the right ventricle) may sometimes be auscultated. Hypoxemia and hypercapnia are present in more severe cases, and the chest radiograph may reveal pulmonary edema or air-fluid levels.

Treatment includes immediate placement of the patient in the Trendelenburg/left lateral decubitus position and administration of 100% oxygen. If a central venous catheter is in place near the right atrium, air aspiration should be attempted. Occasionally, hyperbaric oxygen is indicated. Anticonvulsants are administered in the presence of seizures. Prevention of air embolism, as well as a high index of suspicion when it occurs, is crucial.

Schistosomiasis

This parasitic disorder causes severe pulmonary vascular obstruction and pulmonary hypertension via both anatomical obstruction by the organism itself and an inflammatory vasculitic response to the organism. In endemic areas (e.g., Egypt), schistosomal disease is a common cause of cor pulmonale.

Septic Embolism

Intravenous drug abuse is by far the most common cause of septic embolism. Prior to the drug era, this entity was nearly always a complication of septic pelvic thrombophlebitis due to both septic abortion and postpartum uterine infection. Infections secondary to indwelling intravenous catheters are increasingly common as well. Subcutaneous injections can cause local infections that subsequently invade peripheral veins.

Other Emboli

Pulmonary embolic phenomena may develop from a variety of other substances.[55] Cancer cells may enter and adhere to pulmonary vessels, mimicking pulmonary embolism. Brain tissue has been discovered in the lungs after head trauma, as have liver cells after abdominal trauma. Bone marrow has been reported in lung tissue after cardiopulmonary resuscitation.

Noninfectious vasculitic-thrombotic complications also occur in intravenous drug users. Materials such as talc used to "cut" heroin or cocaine may occasionally themselves provoke vascular inflammation and secondary thrombosis. Perfusion scans can demonstrate segmental or smaller defects. Distinguishing these from emboli due to deep venous thrombosis can be difficult. Repetitive insults can lead to chronic pulmonary hypertension.

DISCHARGE/FOLLOW-UP PLANS

Patient education and discharge follow-up plans for patients suffering PE do not differ from those of patients diagnosed and treated for DVT. These are covered in detail in Chapter 26. The main focus is on appropriate education of the patient regarding use of warfarin and management of the anticoagulation, ideally with follow-up in a clinic specializing in this.

Key Points

- As no single finding predicts the presence or absence of PE, a clinical prediction rule should be used to formulate the probability of pulmonary embolism prior to diagnostic testing

- Patients with a low clinical probability of PE and negative D-dimer test results can be observed and followed without further testing.

- Both troponins and BNP may be elevated in patients with large PEs.

- Multidetector CT angiography has better test characteristics than V̇/Q̇ scanning to diagnose PE.

- LMWHs have a number of advantages compared to unfractionated heparin, including: ease of use, lack of need for PTT monitoring, and ability to be given as an outpatient.

- Thrombolytic therapy or mechanical thrombectomy by an interventional radiologist should be considered for patients with massive PE.

SUGGESTED READING

The PIOPED investigators. Value of the ventilation/perfusion scan in acute pulmonary embolism: Results of the prospective investigation of pulmonary embolism diagnosis. JAMA 1990; 263:2753–2759.

Kearon C, Ginsberg JS, Douketis J. An evaluation of D-dimer in the diagnosis of pulmonary embolism: a randomized trial. Ann Int Med 2006; 144:812–821.

Stein PD, Hull RD, Patel KC, et al. D-Dimer for the exclusion of acute venous thrombosis and pulmonary embolism: a systematic review. Ann Int Med 2004; 140:589–602.

Sox H. Better care for patients with suspected pulmonary embolism. Ann Int Med 2006; 144:210–212.

Writing Group for the Christopher Study Investigators. Effectiveness of managing suspected pulmonary embolism using an algorithm combining clinical probability,D-dimer testing, and computed tomography. JAMA 2005; 295:172–179.

Stein PD, Fowler SE, Goodman LR, et al. Multidetector computed tomography for acute pulmonary embolism. N Engl J Med 2006; 354:2317–2327.

Perrier A, Bounameaux H. Accuracy or outcome in suspected pulmonary embolism. N Engl J Med 2006; 54:2383–2385

Chunilal SD, Eikelboom JW, et al. Does this patient have pulmonary embolism? JAMA 2003; 290: 2849–2858.

Fedullo PF, Tapson VF. The evaluation of suspected pulmonary embolism. N Engl J Med 2003; 349:1247–1256.

Goldhaber SZ. Echocardiography in the management of pulmonary embolism. Ann Intern Med 2002; 136:691–700.

Goldhaber SZ. Pulmonary embolism. Lancet 2004; 363:1295–1305.

Hyers TM, Agnelli G, Hull RD, et al. Antithrombotic therapy for venous thromboembolic disease. Chest 2004.

Konstantinides S, Geibel A, Heusel G, et al. Heparin plus alteplase compared with heparin alone in patients with submassive pulmonary embolism. N Engl J Med 2002; 347:1143–1150.

Robinson G. Pulmonary embolism in hospital practice. BMJ 2006; 332:156–160.

Rocha AT, Tapson VF. Venous thromboembolism in intensive care patients. Clin Chest Med 2003; 24:103–122.

Tapson VF, Carroll BA, Davidson BL, et al. The diagnostic approach to acute venous thromboembolism: clinical practice guideline. Am J Resp Crit Care Med 1999; 160:1043–1066.

CHAPTER TWENTY-EIGHT

Acute Aortic Dissection

Eric M. Siegal, MD

BACKGROUND

Introduction

Fewer than 0.5% of all patients presenting with chest or back pain to an emergency department suffer from aortic dissection.[1] Although it is a rare disease, aortic dissection is frequently lethal and can easily be mistaken for less serious pathology. In one series, aortic dissection was missed in 38% of patients at presentation, with 28% of patients first diagnosed at autopsy.[2] Early recognition and management of aortic dissection are crucial. In the first 48 hours after presentation, the mortality rate for untreated acute aortic dissection may exceed 1% per hour.[3] Generally, cardiothoracic surgeons or cardiologists experienced with managing aortic dissection should direct evaluation and treatment. Hospitalists, however, are increasingly assuming responsibility for the initial triage and management of patients with acute chest pain syndromes and therefore must be able to rapidly identify aortic dissection, initiate supportive therapy, and refer patients to appropriate specialty care.

Pathophysiology

Aortic dissection is defined as separation of the layers of the aortic wall due to infiltration of high-pressure arterial blood. The proximate cause is elevated shear stress across the aortic lumen in the setting of a concomitant defect in the aortic media. Shear stress is caused by the rapid increase in luminal pressure per unit of time (dP/dt) that results from cardiac systole. As the aorta traverses away from the heart, an increasing proportion of the kinetic energy of left ventricular systole is stored in the aortic wall as potential energy, which facilitates anterograde propagation of cardiac output during diastole. This conversion of kinetic to potential energy also attenuates shear stress. As the proximal aorta is subject to the steepest fluctuations in pressure, it is at highest risk of dissection.

Once the aortic intima is compromised, blood dissects longitudinally through the aortic media with proximal or distal propagation, creating a false lumen that may communicate with the true lumen of the aorta. Blood may flow through the true lumen, false lumen, or both. Propagation of the dissection causes much of the morbidity associated with aortic dissection by disrupting blood flow across branch vessels or by directly compromising the pericardium or aortic valve. The dissection may traverse the entire aortic wall, causing aortic rupture and exsanguination (Figs. 28-1 and 28-2).

Types of Aortic Dissection

Acute aortic dissection is classified as any aortic dissection diagnosed within 2 weeks of the onset of symptoms, the period of highest risk for mortality. Patients who survive more than 2 weeks without treatment have chronic dissection. Aortic dissections are further classified according to their anatomic location. The fundamental distinction is whether the dissection is proximal (involving the aortic root and ascending aorta) or distal (below the left subclavian artery). Proximal aortic dissections are surgical emergencies, while distal dissections can often be managed medically. The Stanford and DeBakey classification systems are most commonly used.

Variants of aortic dissection exist. Aortic intramural hematomas are caused by intramural hemorrhage of the vasa vasorum without an identifiable intimal tear.[4] Penetrating atherosclerotic ulcers are focal defects in the aortic wall with surrounding hematoma but no longitudinal tissue plane dissection. They typically result from advanced atherosclerotic disease, and they may progress to aortic dissection, rupture, or aneurysm formation. The pathophysiologic distinctions between aortic intramural hematoma (IMH), penetrating atherosclerotic ulcer (PAU), and classic aortic dissection remain somewhat controversial. Both IMH and PAU may progress to aortic aneurysm formation, frank dissection or aortic rupture, suggesting that these entities represent a spectrum of disease with broad overlap[5-7] (Fig. 28-3, Table 28-1).

ASSESSMENT

Prevalence and Risk Factors

Aortic dissection is a rare disease, with an estimated incidence of approximately 5–30 cases per 1 million people per year.[8,9] Two thirds of patients are male, with an average age at presentation of approximately 65 years. A history of systemic hypertension, found in 72% of patients, is by far the most common risk factor.[2,9] Other major risk factors are atherosclerosis, history of prior cardiac surgery, and known aortic aneurysm.[9] Hypertension and

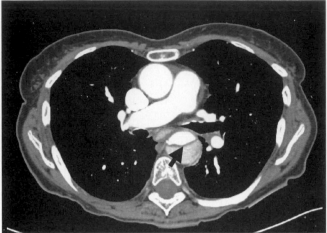

Figure 28-1 • Transverse CT angiogram of a Stanford Type I aortic dissection. An intimal flap (arrow) demarcates the true lumen (top) and the false lumen (bottom). Courtesy Dr K. Ed Adib, UW Health and Meriter Hospital, Madison, WI.

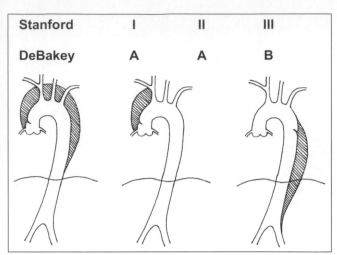

Figure 28-3 • Stanford and DeBakey classification systems of aortic dissection.

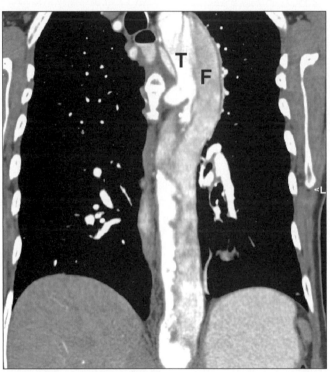

Figure 28-2 • Coronal CT Angiogram of an extensive Stanford Type I Aortic Dissection. T: True Lumen. F: False Lumen. Image Courtesy of Dr K. Ed Adib, UW Health and Meriter Hospital, Madison, WI.

Table 28-1 Composite Schema for Classification of Aortic Dissection

Acuity
- **Acute:** <2 weeks after onset
- **Chronic:** >2 weeks after onset

Anatomic location:
- **Ascending aorta:** Stanford type A, Debakey type II
- **Ascending and descending aorta:** Stanford type A, Debakey type I
- **Descending aorta:** Stanford type B, Debakey type III

Pathophysiology:
- **Class 1:** Classical aortic dissection with intimal flap between true and false lumen
- **Class 2:** Aortic intramural hematoma without identifiable intimal flap
- **Class 3:** Intimal tear without hematoma (limited dissection)
- **Class 4:** Atherosclerotic plaque rupture with aortic penetrating ulcer
- **Class 5:** Iatrogenic or traumatic aortic dissection (intra-aortic catheterization, high-speed deceleration injury, blunt chest trauma)

atherosclerosis are significantly less common in younger patients (<40 years of age), occurring respectively in 34% and 1% of cases.[10] Several other risk factors for acute aortic dissection, most of which are more prevalent in younger patients, have been identified (Box 28-1).

- Collagen diseases (e.g., Marfan syndrome and Ehlers-Danlos): In the International Registry of Acute Aortic Dissection (IRAD), 50% of young patients presenting with aortic dissection had Marfan syndrome.[9]
- Bicuspid aortic valve (BAV): Individuals with BAV are 5–18 times more likely to suffer aortic dissection than those with a trileaflet valve.[11,12] In one survey, 52% of asymptomatic young men with BAV were found to have aortic root dilatation, a frequent precursor of dissection.[12]
- Aortic coarctation
- Turner's syndrome: As many as 6.3% of patients with Turner syndrome may have aortic root dilatation with or without dissection.[13]
- Strenuous exercise: Multiple case reports have associated aortic dissection with high-intensity weightlifting. Most affected individuals were subsequently found to have at least one other risk factor, including hypertension and cocaine abuse.[14–16]
- Large vessel arteritis: Giant cell, Takayasu's, syphilis
- Cocaine and methamphetamine ingestion[17–18]

Box 28-1 Risk Factors for Aortic Dissection

Hypertension

Atherosclerotic disease

History of cardiac surgery

Aortic aneurysm

Collagen diseases (e.g., Marfan syndrome and Ehlers-Danlos)

Bicuspid aortic valve (BAV)

Aortic coarctation

Turner's syndrome

Strenuous exercise

Large vessel arteritis: Giant cell, Takayasu's, syphilis

Cocaine and methamphetamine ingestion

Third-trimester pregnancy

Blunt chest trauma or high-speed deceleration injury

Iatrogenic injury, typically from intra-aortic catheterization

Box 28-2 Findings in Acute Aortic Dissection

Hypotension or shock due to:

• Hemopericardium and pericardial tamponade

• Acute aortic insufficiency due to dilatation of the aortic annulus

• Aortic rupture

Acute myocardial ischemia/infarction due to coronary ostial occlusion

Pericardial friction rub due to hemopericardium

Syncope

Pleural effusion or frank hemothorax

Acute renal failure due to dissection across the renal arteries

Mesenteric ischemia due to dissection across intra-abdominal arteries

Neurologic deficits:

• Stroke due to occlusion of the arch vessels

• Limb weakness

• Spinal cord deficits due to cord ischemia

• Horner syndrome due to compression of the superior sympathetic ganglion.

• Hoarseness due to compression of the left recurrent laryngeal nerve

• Third-trimester pregnancy, especially in patients with diseases of collagen. Recent data from IRAD have called into question the significance of pregnancy as a risk factor. Of 346 enrolled women with aortic dissection, only 2 were pregnant, suggesting that the previously held association of pregnancy with aortic dissection may be an artifact of selective reporting.[19,20]

• Blunt chest trauma or high-speed deceleration injury

• Iatrogenic injury, typically from intra-aortic catheterization

Clinical Presentation

Acute aortic dissections are rarely asymptomatic; in fact, the absence of sudden-onset chest pain decreases the likelihood of dissection (negative LR 0.3).[21] In IRAD, approximately 95% of patients with aortic dissection complained of pain in the chest, back, or abdomen; 90% characterized their pain as either "severe" or "the worst ever"; and 64% described it as "sharp."[9] The pain of acute aortic dissection is classically described as "tearing" or "ripping" in nature. Although the presence of tearing or ripping chest or back pain is suggestive of aortic dissection (positive LR 1.2–10.8), its absence does not reliably exclude the diagnosis.[9] The clinical findings associated with aortic dissection depend largely upon the anatomic location of the dissection. This variability of presentation compounds the challenge of establishing a diagnosis. Women who develop aortic dissection are generally older and present later after the onset of symptoms than men. Their symptoms are less typical and are more likely to be confounded by altered mental status.[20] A diagnosis of aortic dissection should be strongly considered for patients presenting with acute chest or back pain and otherwise unexplained aortic insufficiency, focal neurologic deficits, pulse deficits, or end-organ injury (Box 28-2).

Differential Diagnosis

The differential diagnosis of acute aortic dissection is the same as for any presentation of acute, severe chest or back pain, and includes acute coronary syndrome, pulmonary embolus, pneu-

mothorax, pneumonia, musculoskeletal pain, acute cholecystitis, esophageal spasm or rupture, acute pancreatitis, and acute pericarditis.

Diagnosis

Electrocardiogram (ECG): Electrocardiographic abnormalities are commonly seen in aortic dissection and may include ST-segment or T-wave abnormalities or left ventricular hypertrophy. Proximal aortic dissections may compromise coronary artery perfusion, generating ECG findings compatible with acute myocardial infarction, which may lead the clinician to diagnose and treat myocardial infarction while missing the underlying diagnosis.[22] In a recent survey, 9 of 44 patients (21%) presenting with acute aortic dissection were initially diagnosed with acute coronary syndrome and anticoagulated, with two deaths.[23] ECGs must therefore be interpreted with extreme caution in aortic dissection.

Chest x-ray: Chest radiography is a mainstay in the evaluation of acute chest pain in the emergency department. Unfortunately, the diagnostic utility of plain-film radiography in aortic dissection is limited. Mediastinal widening (>8 cm) and abnormal aortic contour, the "classic" radiographic findings in aortic dissection, are present in only 50–60% of cases, and 12% of patients have a completely normal chest x-ray.[9] Nonspecific radiographic findings, most notably pleural effusion, may also be seen.[24] If the index of suspicion is elevated, a confirmatory study must be obtained (Fig. 28-4).

Transthoracic Echocardiography (TTE). While it is an excellent tool to evaluate many aspects of cardiac anatomy and function, surface echocardiography can reliably visualize only limited portions of the ascending and descending aorta. As a

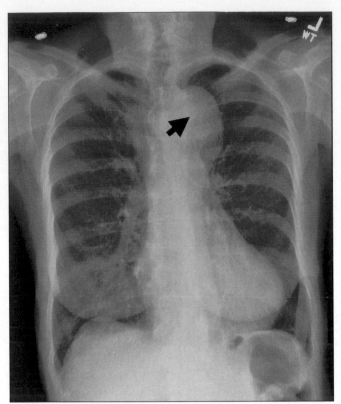

Figure 28-4 • Chest Radiograph of a proximal aortic dissection. The aortic knob is displaced superiorly and laterally (arrow). Courtesy Dr K. Ed Adib, UW Health and Meriter Hospital, Madison, WI.

consequence, it is neither sufficiently sensitive nor specific to diagnose aortic dissection.[25,26] TTE does, however, play a role in rapidly assessing patients at the bedside for aortic valve or pericardial compromise when these complications are suspected.

Preferred Imaging Studies

The ideal imaging modality should identify aortic dissection with high sensitivity and specificity. It should also identify the entry and exit points of the dissection, the extent of the aortic thrombus, and compromise of branch vessels, the aortic valve and the pericardium. Four imaging modalities meet most of these criteria.

Aortography: Previously the "gold standard" for diagnosing aortic dissection, aortography has been supplanted by newer, less-invasive imaging modalities. The sensitivity and specificity of aortography are at best equivalent and possibly inferior to less invasive imaging modalities.[27] False negatives may occur if both the true and false lumens opacify equally with contrast, or if the false lumen is sufficiently thrombosed to preclude any instillation of contrast. Aortography cannot identify aortic intramural hematomas, is invasive and highly operator-dependent, requires nephrotoxic contrast, and generally takes longer to obtain than other modalities. Aortography uniquely offers excellent visualization of the coronary arteries and branch vessels and is preferred when such information is necessary. Percutaneous aortic endovascular stent-grafting has been recently employed to repair distal aortic dissections.[28–30] As a result, aortography is gaining new life as a therapeutic modality.

CT angiography (CTA): Spiral CTA is probably the most commonly used modality for diagnosing aortic dissection. It is emergently available at most hospitals, and images can be obtained in minutes. Sensitivity and specificity approach 100%, and CTA may be more sensitive than MRA or TEE in evaluating arch vessel involvement.[31,32] Like conventional angiography, CTA requires administration of nephrotoxic contrast. It frequently cannot visualize the entry and exit sites (intimal flaps) of a dissection, and it provides no information about the coronary arteries or the competency of the aortic valve.[24,33] Thus, if aortic dissection is identified by CTA, a second study may be needed to provide further diagnostic information and guide surgical intervention.

Magnetic Resonance Angiography (MRA): MRA provides excellent noninvasive evaluation of the thoracic aorta. Sensitivity and specificity are similar to spiral CTA, but MRA effectively identifies the location of the intimal tear and provides some functional information about the aortic valve.[31,34] MRA is not emergently available at many hospitals. Scanning is time intensive, requiring the patient to remain motionless and relatively inaccessible for up to an hour. Furthermore, patient claustrophobia and the presence of pacemakers or ferromagnetic foreign bodies may preclude MRA.

Transesophageal echocardiography (TEE): The sensitivity and specificity of TEE are also excellent—on par with CTA and MRA.[35,36] TEE provides superb images of the pericardium and detailed assessment aortic valve function. It also is extremely effective at visualizing the aortic intimal flap. A significant advantage of TEE is its portability, allowing bedside diagnosis in a matter of minutes. For this reason, TEE is particularly useful for evaluation of hemodynamically unstable patients with suspected aortic dissection. TEE is somewhat invasive and usually requires patient sedation. It is also highly operator dependent, and its effective use requires the rapid availability of an experienced and technically skilled operator.

Recommendations

CTA, MRA, and TEE are all highly sensitive and specific modalities for diagnosing aortic dissection. Therefore, the patient's condition, the information needed, and the resources and expertise available should drive the choice of study. MRA is generally considered the gold standard and is the preferred modality for hemodynamically stable patients with suspected aortic dissection. Due to slow data acquisition and inaccessibility of patients in the scanner, it is generally unsuited for unstable patients, including those with ongoing chest or back pain. Bedside TEE is an excellent choice for patients who are too unstable for MRA. Arch aortography is generally reserved to confirm questionable diagnoses or to specifically image branch arteries.

Most trials comparing CTA, MRA, and TEE were performed in the early 1990s. Computed tomography has evolved significantly over the intervening decade, and many of the diagnostic limitations previously ascribed to CTA, such as the inability to generate 3-D reconstructed images, no longer exist. Furthermore, CT angiography is widely available and is gaining increasing acceptance as a first-line imaging modality for patients with noncardiac chest pain.[37] Medical centers that maintain round the clock CT capability may have limited or delayed access to TEE, MRA, or aortography. Given the potential for rapid and dramatic patient deterioration, it is imperative to quickly establish a diagnosis when aortic dissection is suspected. Thus, when the choice is

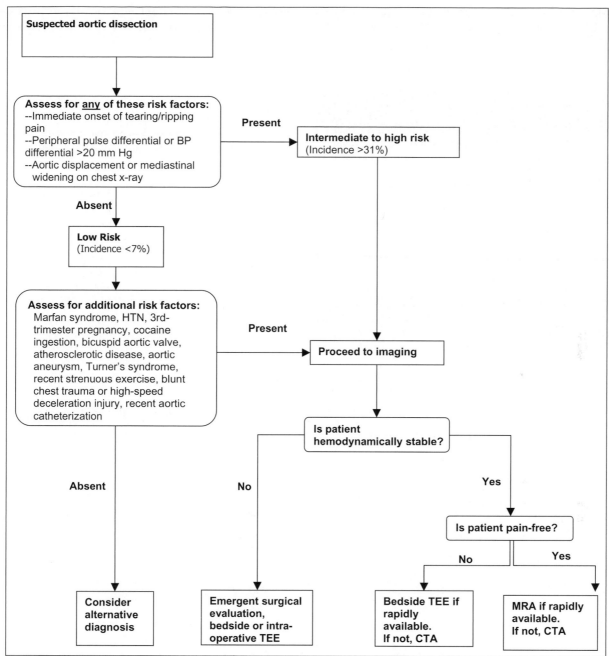

Figure 28-5 • Decision tree for the diagnosis of acute aortic dissection.

TEE—Transesophageal echocardiogram; CTA—computed tomographic angiogram; MRA—magnetic resonance angiogram

obtaining an immediate CTA or a delayed TEE or MRA, CTA is generally the better choice (Fig. 28-5, Table 28-2).

Clinical Prediction Tool

Three clinical features were demonstrated to be effective in identifying aortic dissections in patients presenting with acute chest or back pain: immediate onset of tearing or ripping chest pain, mediastinal widening (>8 cm) or aortic enlargement/displacement on chest x-ray, and blood pressure differential between arms exceeding 20 mm Hg. When all three findings were absent, dissection was unlikely (7%). If either chest pain or radiographic findings was present, the likelihood was intermediate (31%–39%). With any other combination of findings, dissection

was likely (>83%). This prediction tool effectively identified 96% of all patients who presented to an emergency department with acute aortic dissection.[1] However, 4% of the patients categorized as low risk were ultimately diagnosed with aortic dissection. Given the exceptionally high mortality of a missed diagnosis, a 4% false negative rate is unacceptably high. Thus, the absence of any of the aforementioned findings should not dissuade the clinician from obtaining a confirmatory imaging study if the pretest probability for acute aortic dissection is elevated.

Prognosis

Despite significant medical and surgical advances, aortic dissection remains exceptionally lethal. Patients with proximal dissections are more likely to die than those with distal dissections. Medical treatment of proximal dissection is generally reserved for patients too ill, unstable, or frail to undergo surgery; hence the extremely high mortality rate. In contrast, the

majority of patients with distal dissection are managed medically, with surgery generally reserved for acute complications (Table 28-3).

MANAGEMENT

Approximately half of all patients who present with acute aortic dissection are acutely hypertensive.[9] This is a true hypertensive emergency that mandates immediate decrease in blood pressure to the lowest level that maintains organ perfusion. As a rule, short-acting, parenteral, titratable antihypertensive agents should be used. Intravenous beta-adrenergic blockers are the mainstay of therapy. Their negative inotropic and chronotropic effects decrease shear stress (dP/dt) across the aortic lumen and decrease the likelihood of dissection propagation. Vasodilators (e.g., nitroprusside, nitroglycerin) should be initiated if beta-blockers prove insufficient to lower blood pressure. They should never be used alone, as they may cause reflex tachycardia and consequently increase intraluminal shear stress. Analgesia and anxiolysis further decrease blood pressure by controlling the severe pain and anxiety often associated with acute dissections (Table 28-4).

Hypotension or shock, which develops in 15%–30% of patients with acute aortic dissection, is an ominous finding that frequently

Table 28-2 Comparative Diagnostic Utility of Imaging Techniques in Aortic Dissection

	TEE	CTA	MRA	Aortography
Sensitivity	++	++	+++	++
Specificity	+++	++	+++	++
Classification	+++	++	++	+
Intimal flap	+++	–	++	+
Aortic regurgitation	+++	–	++	++
Pericardial effusion	+++	++	++	–
Branch vessel involvement	+	++	++	+++
Coronary artery involvement	++	+	+	+++

Adapted from: Recommendations of the task force on aortic dissection, European Society of Cardiology. In: Erbel R, Alfonso F, Boileau C, et al. Diagnosis and management of aortic dissection: task force report of the European Society of Cardiology. Eur Heart J 2001; 22:1642–1681.

Table 28-3 Mortality in Acute Aortic Dissection

	PROXIMAL (DEBAKEY I, II; STANFORD A)		DISTAL (DEBAKEY III; STANFORD B)	
	Surgical (%)	Medical (%)	Surgical (%)	Medical (%)
In-hospital mortality	26	58	31	11
Average	35		15	

From: Hagan PG, Nienaber CA, Isselbacher EM, et al. The international registry of acute aortic dissection (IRAD). JAMA 2000; 283:897–903.

Table 28-4 Drugs for Hypertensive Emergency/Acute Aortic Dissection

Name	Mechanism	Dose	Cautions/Contraindications
Esmolol	Cardioselective beta-1 blocker	Load: 500 mcg/kg IV Drip: 50 mcg/kg/min IV Increase by increments of 50 mcg/min	Asthma or bronchospasm/ Bradycardia 2nd or 3rd degree AV block/ Cocaine or methamphetamine abuse
Labetalol	Nonselective beta-1,2 blocker Selective alpha-1 blocker	Load: 20 mg IV Drip: 2 mg/min IV	Asthma or bronchospasm/ Bradycardia 2nd or 3rd degree AV block/ Cocaine or methamphetamine abuse
Enalaprilat	ACE inhibitor	0.625–1.25 mg IV q6h Max dose: 5 mg q6h	Angioedema/ Pregnancy Renal artery stenosis/ Severe renal insufficiency
Nitroprusside	Direct arterial vasodilator	Begin at 0.3 mcg/kg/min IV Max dose 10 mcg/kg/min	May cause reflex tachycardia/ Cyanide/thiocyanate toxicity—especially in renal insufficiency
Nitroglycerin	Vascular smooth muscle relaxation	5–200 mcg/min IV	Decreases preload—contraindicated in tamponade or other preload-dependent states/ Concomitant use of sildenafil or similar agents

portends hemodynamic collapse.[9,38] Patients who develop hypotension are at five-fold increased risk of death (55.0% vs. 10.3%) and have markedly increased risk of developing neurologic deficits as well as myocardial, mesenteric, and limb ischemia. Hypotension may result from pump failure, aortic rupture, systemic lactic acidosis, or spinal shock. Bedside transthoracic echocardiography may be particularly useful in evaluating hypotensive patients, as it can be used to quickly and noninvasively determine the integrity of the aortic valve and pericardium. Although hypotension may transiently respond to volume resuscitation, all hypotensive patients with aortic dissection, regardless of type, should be immediately referred for emergent surgical evaluation. Pericardiocentesis in the setting of pericardial tamponade remains controversial; a small study suggested that decompression of the pericardial sac may hasten hemodynamic collapse by accelerating blood loss.[39]

Facilities that do not have urgent cardiopulmonary bypass capability should emergently transport patients with aortic dissection to a tertiary care facility. Transfer should not be delayed to confirm a questionable diagnosis. Proximal (DeBakey I, II; Stanford A) aortic dissections frequently compromise the pericardium, aortic valve, or arch vessels and therefore should be managed surgically. Medically treated proximal dissections carry a dismal 60% in-hospital mortality rate.[9] Distal (DeBakey III; Stanford B) aortic dissections are generally treated medically, with surgical intervention limited to patients with expanding aortic aneurysm, risk of aortic rupture, refractory hypertension, intractable pain, or intraluminal hematoma expansion of sufficient magnitude to prevent perfusion of end organs. Individual branch vessel occlusion may be effectively ameliorated with conventional arterial stenting.

Endovascular stent grafting has been successfully utilized in patients with distal aortic dissections who would have otherwise required surgery.[28–30] The stent graft is deployed across the proximal intimal tear, obliterating the false lumen and allowing the aorta to heal. A recent meta-analysis showed medium-term outcomes for endovascular stent grafting that compared favorably with conventional surgery for distal (DeBakey B; Stanford III) dissections.[40]

FOLLOW-UP

Survivors of aortic dissection, especially those with diseases of collagen, should be viewed as having a systemic disease that predisposes them to further aortic and great vessel events. Almost one third of survivors of acute aortic dissection will develop dissection propagation, aortic rupture, or require aortic surgery within 5 years of presentation.[41] All patients should be maintained on life-long beta-blockade to reduce shear stress to the aortic lumen, with blood pressure maintained below 135/80. Progression to aortic aneurysm is common, and patients should undergo serial imaging of the aorta at 1, 3, 6, and 12 months after discharge and annually thereafter. Dilatation of the proximal aorta to >5.0 cm and of the distal aorta to >6.0 cm should prompt referral for surgical repair.

Despite little supporting data, it is generally accepted that patients should moderate their physical activity to avoid extremes of blood pressure elevation. Patients should also be warned to seek immediate medical attention if they develop recurrent chest or back pain or focal neurologic deficits.

Key Points

- Aortic dissection is most commonly a disease of hypertensive, elderly men.

- Look for three key findings when evaluating a patient for acute aortic dissection: immediate onset of tearing or ripping chest/back pain, mediastinal widening or abnormal aortic contour on chest radiograph, and variance of blood pressure (>20 mm Hg) between arms. If all three findings are absent, acute aortic dissection is unlikely. The presence of any of these findings should prompt further workup.

- Think aortic dissection in patients who present with acute chest, back, or abdominal pain with unexplained acute neurologic deficits or acute end-organ damage.

- A normal chest radiograph does *not* rule out aortic dissection. Only TEE, CT, and MR angiography are sufficiently sensitive to rule out dissection. Conventional angiography is rarely used as a first-line diagnostic tool, but it may be useful as a confirmatory test or to provide additional anatomic information.

- Patients with proximal aortic dissection, or any aortic dissection with concomitant hypotension are at exceptionally high risk for early mortality. They should be immediately referred for surgical evaluation.

- Parenteral beta-blockers are the mainstay of therapy for non-hypotensive aortic dissection.

SUGGESTED READING

Von Kodolitsch Y, Schwartz A, Nienaber CA. Clinical prediction of acute aortic dissection. Arch Int Med 2000; 160:2977–2982.

Hagan PG, Nienaber CA, Isselbacher EM, et al. The international registry of acute aortic dissection (IRAD). JAMA 2000; 283:897–903.

Klompas, M. Does this patient have an acute thoracic aortic dissection? JAMA 2002; 287(17):2262–2272.

Nienaber CA, Eagle KA. Aortic dissection: new frontiers in diagnosis and management. Part II: Therapeutic management and follow-up. Circulation 2003; 108:772–778.

Moore AG, Eagle KA, Bruckman D, et al. Choice of computed tomography, transesophageal echocardiography, magnetic resonance imaging, and aortography in acute aortic dissection: International Registry of Acute Aortic Dissection (IRAD). Am J Cardiol 2002; 89:1235–1238.

Erbel R, Alfonso F, Boileau C, et al. Diagnosis and management of aortic dissection: task force report of the European Society of Cardiology. Eur Heart J 2001; 22;1642–1681.

CHAPTER TWENTY-NINE

Valvular Heart Disease

Leonardo Rodriguez, MD, FACC, and Brian P. Griffin, MD, FACC

BACKGROUND

Valvular heart disease (VHD) commonly results in referral for cardiovascular evaluation, and patients with VHD represent the largest portion of patients undergoing cardiovascular surgery at our institution (Figure 29-1). VHD can give rise to stenosis, regurgitation, or a combination of lesions at one or more valves. With the increasing age of the US population, aortic stenosis is becoming more prevalent, and degenerative mitral valve disease has replaced rheumatic valve disease as the most common etiology for mitral regurgitation in the United States. Valvular lesions can occur as a result of pathologic changes in the valve leaflets or supporting structures (i.e., the chordae or papillary muscles). VHD tends to progress over time as degenerative changes are superimposed on the primary pathology. In many cases, the hemodynamic impact on the ventricle determines the prognosis.

ETIOLOGY

Congenital Disorders

Valvular abnormalities, common in many congenital syndromes, mainly affect the aortic and pulmonic valves among adults afflicted with them. For example, valve abnormalities can be seen in specific developmental syndromes, such as supravalvular aortic stenosis in Williams' syndrome.

Myxomatous Degeneration

Myxomatous degeneration most often involves the mitral or tricuspid valve. In this condition, leaflet and particularly chordal tissue is abnormally redundant and weak. This tissue abnormality leads to prolapse and mitral regurgitation. Chordal rupture is common and may precipitate a rapid clinical deterioration from sudden severe regurgitation. The precise abnormality in valve tissue is unknown but is thought to involve the structural proteins such as collagen.[1] A familial tendency to the disease is often noted.[2] Inherited connective tissue diseases such as Marfan syndrome produce valve abnormalities similar to those found in myxomatous degeneration.

Rheumatic Disease

Rheumatic heart disease remains the most common cause of mitral stenosis and a frequent cause of aortic regurgitation. It is the most common cause of multivalvular heart disease. Rheumatic heart disease remains a significant problem in immigrants, especially those from Latin America and Southeast Asia. Isolated outbreaks of rheumatic fever continue to be reported in the United States, even in affluent communities.[3] Rheumatic fever appears to cause valvular heart disease by an autoimmune phenomenon whereby antibodies against streptococcal antigens cross-react with valvular tissue. Valvular involvement can present acutely as a result of edema of valvular tissue. Progressive fibrosis, superimposed calcification, and scarring with retraction of leaflet tissue lead to valvular stenosis, incompetence, or both. The interval between the occurrence of rheumatic fever and clinical manifestations varies, as does the degree of involvement, and it may be related to the number of episodes of rheumatic fever.

Degenerative Disease

Degenerative calcification causes aortic stenosis in the elderly and in patients with renal dysfunction; it results from calcium deposition on the body of the valve leaflets rather than on the commissures. Factors found to promote degenerative valvular changes are increasing age, a low body mass index, hypertension, and hyperlipidemia. Histologic changes that simulate atheroma and involve lipid deposition and inflammatory cell infiltration of the leaflets have been described in patients with early degenerative changes in the aortic leaflets. Even mild degenerative changes in the aortic valve have been reported to have an adverse prognostic impact.[4,5] Calcification of the mitral annulus is common in the elderly; it is more common in women than men and can produce mitral regurgitation. Occasionally, mitral annular calcification extends onto the valve leaflets, causing stenosis. Restriction of the posterior leaflet by severe annular calcification may cause mitral regurgitation.

Endocarditis

Endocarditis usually occurs on previously abnormal valves, although overwhelming sepsis or IV drug abuse can lead to infec-

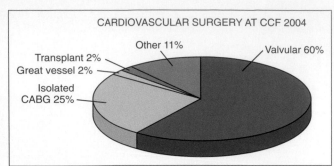

Figure 29-1 • Distribution of surgical cases at CCF in 2004. Valvular heart disease constitutes more than half of the surgical caseload. Source: Cardiothoracic Surgery Department Cleveland Clinic Foundation—CCF

CABG—coronary artery bypass graft

tion of normal valves. The predominant hemodynamic manifestation of endocarditis is valvular regurgitation caused by leaflet perforation or deformity of the free edges. Scarring and retraction of infected tissue also contributes to regurgitation in the chronic stages of healed endocarditis.

Coronary Artery Disease

Mitral regurgitation is common in coronary artery disease, and its presence carries an adverse prognosis. During acute infarction, the papillary head, or more rarely papillary muscle, may rupture, leading to catastrophic regurgitation that is often fatal. In chronic ischemic heart disease, elongation of an infarcted papillary muscle or regional wall motion abnormalities at the base of the papillary muscle can lead to malcoaptation of the leaflets and mitral regurgitation.

Connective Tissue Disease

Libman-Sacks endocarditis consists of noninfected warty vegetations involving predominantly the mitral valve; it is characteristic of systemic lupus erythematosus.[6] Significant regurgitation and stenosis rarely occur acutely but are seen with scarring from chronic disease. Valvular involvement in rheumatoid arthritis is common and leads to valve thickening but is usually not of hemodynamic significance. Aortitis in ankylosing spondylitis may produce significant aortic regurgitation. As mentioned above, patients with Marfan syndrome often have mitral prolapse and aortic regurgitation.

IATROGENIC CAUSES OF VALVULAR HEART DISEASE

Iatrogenic causes include radiation therapy, the use of serotonin agonists such as methysergide, and the use of anorexiants such as fenfluramine and phentermine in combination.[7] Radiation leads to scarring and calcification of valve leaflets many years after the initiating radiation. Although less common than initially anticipated, both methysergide and anorexiant agents' effects on valve tissue often simulate rheumatic disease, but regurgitation rather than stenosis predominates as the hemodynamically prominent lesion. Serotonin is also thought to play a role in the valvulopathy produced by anorexiants; the precise mechanism remains to be elucidated.

OTHER CAUSES OF VALVULAR HEART DISEASE

Amyloid disease causes valvular thickening but rarely causes significant stenosis. The carcinoid syndrome most often involves the valves on the right side of the heart and leads to stenosis or incompetence of the tricuspid or pulmonary valve.

Secondary Involvement

Left ventricular dilatation can cause dilatation of the mitral annulus and, thereby, mitral regurgitation. Common secondary causes of mitral regurgitation include coronary artery disease, aortic valve disease, and dilated cardiomyopathy. Similarly, tricuspid regurgitation results from right ventricular enlargement secondary to pulmonary hypertension or an atrial septal defect. Dilatation of the ascending aorta, especially involving the annulus of the aortic valve, can lead to aortic regurgitation. This is seen in hypertension and in aneurysms of the ascending aorta.

ASSESSMENT AND MANAGEMENT

Valvular heart disease often remains asymptomatic for many years, but once symptoms develop survival is reduced if the lesion is not corrected. Characterization of the lesions and assessment of hemodynamic severity are often possible on physical examination but are aided by additional testing such as Doppler echocardiography and cardiac catheterization. Doppler echocardiography measures the flow velocity across a narrowed valve. Echocardiography allows an integral evaluation of the anatomical lesion, ventricular size, and ejection fraction as well as hemodynamic evaluation using Doppler. In stenotic lesions, it is possible to estimate the pressure gradients using the modified Bernoulli equation, $P = 4v^2$; P is pressure in mm Hg, and v is the maximal velocity obtained with Doppler. Another advantage of echocardiography is the possibility of serial studies to assess the progression of disease. Cardiac catheterization is restricted to cases where echoDoppler is equivocal and for evaluation of the coronary anatomy. Use of multislice computed tomography (CT) may replace this last indication in patients with low probability of coronary disease. The decision to intervene in patients with VHD is generally based on symptoms, ventricular function, and presence of coronary artery disease. However, other factors are also taken into account, such as surgical risk, atrial arrhythmias, and pulmonary hypertension.

SPECIFIC VALVULAR LESIONS

Mitral Stenosis

The normal mitral valve is at least 4 cm² in cross-sectional area. Reduction in valve area from mitral stenosis is considered severe when the valve area is less than 1 cm². To maintain flow through the valve, left atrial pressure rises, leading to an increase in the pressure gradient across the valve and to increased pulmonary venous and capillary pressures with resultant dyspnea (Fig. 29-2). Flow through the stenotic mitral valve is dependent on the duration of diastole. Tachycardia shortens diastole disproportionately and causes a further elevation in left atrial pressure and can precipitate symptoms even in relatively mild stenosis. Left

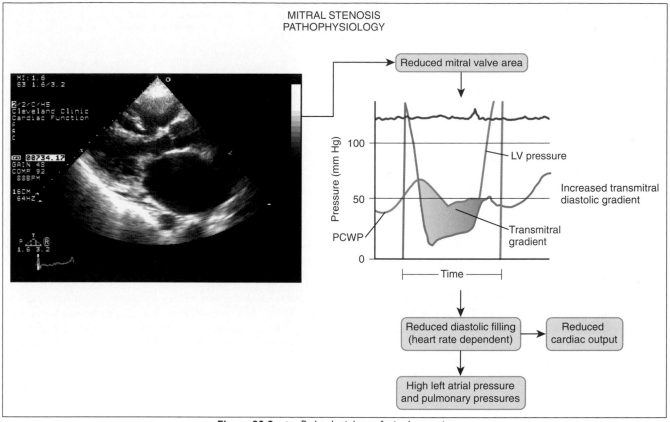

Figure 29-2 • Pathophysiology of mitral stenosis.

atrial enlargement develops, which in turn predisposes to atrial fibrillation, atrial thrombus formation, and thromboembolism. Severe mitral stenosis is often associated with an increase in pulmonary arterial pressure, leading to right-sided heart failure and secondary tricuspid and pulmonary incompetence. In severe pulmonary hypertension, cardiac output at rest is reduced, yielding a relatively low-pressure gradient across the mitral valve even in patients with severe stenosis.

Symptoms and Signs

Mitral stenosis is often asymptomatic at presentation and for many years thereafter. Symptomatic patients usually present with dyspnea, but can also present with angina, right-sided heart failure, atrial arrhythmia, or embolism. The physical findings in mitral stenosis depend on the severity of the stenosis, the mobility of the valve, and the rhythm (Fig. 29-3). The principal sign is a rumbling diastolic murmur that is best heard at the apex with the stethoscope bell. In sinus rhythm, the murmur increases in intensity with atrial contraction (presystolic accentuation). Increased severity of stenosis is associated with a longer murmur and a thrill. With a pliable valve, an opening sound—the opening snap—is heard, and the sudden closure of the stenotic valve at end-diastole gives rise to a loud first heart sound. When the valve calcifies and becomes less mobile, the opening snap and loud first heart sound disappear. A loud pulmonary component of the second heart sound is heard with pulmonary hypertension. The signs and symptoms of mitral stenosis are simulated by left atrial myxoma. In this condition, functional mitral stenosis results from prolapse of a mobile tumor arising from the mitral septum into the mitral valve opening.

Diagnostic Evaluation

Electrocardiography can reveal left atrial enlargement if the patient is in sinus rhythm. Left atrial enlargement, mitral valve calcification, and signs of pulmonary congestion can all be present on chest x-ray. Doppler echocardiography is the test of choice in confirming the diagnosis, establishing the severity of stenosis, detecting complications, and determining the most appropriate treatment. Echocardiography also allows accurate differentiation of mitral stenosis from a left atrial myxoma. The severity of stenosis is determined by measuring the pressure gradient across the valve with Doppler echocardiography and by calculating the valve area. Mitral stenosis should be suspected if the mean gradient exceeds 5 mm Hg; it typically exceeds 10 mm Hg in severe stenosis. Transesophageal echocardiography is more useful than transthoracic echocardiography in excluding atrial thrombus and assessing the severity of mitral regurgitation and is usually performed if balloon valvuloplasty is contemplated. Cardiac catheterization is rarely needed to establish the diagnosis but is used to confirm the severity of stenosis and to evaluate the coronary anatomy.

Management

Once symptoms develop in mitral stenosis, survival decreases without surgical or balloon dilatation or valve replacement. In the absence of symptoms, management is directed at preventing recurrence of rheumatic fever.[8] Patients in atrial fibrillation require heart rate control with a beta-blocker, digoxin, or both. Systemic anticoagulation with warfarin is definitely indicated to prevent thromboembolism when (1) atrial fibrillation is present,

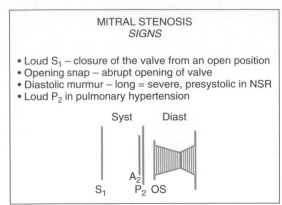

Figure 29-3 • Signs on physical examination of patients with pure mitral stenosis.

S1—first heart sound; A2—aortic component of second heart sound; P2—pulmonary component of second heart sound; OS—opening snap; NSR—normal sinus rhythm

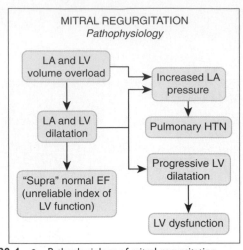

Figure 29-4 • Pathophysiology of mitral regurgitation.

EF—ejection fraction; HTN—hypertension; LA—left atrium; LV—left ventricle

(2) there is a history of embolism, or (3) a thrombus is detected in the atrium. Anticoagulation should be considered in patients with paroxysmal atrial fibrillation, dilated left atrium (>50 mm in diameter on echocardiography), or those with severe atrial stasis (as evidenced by swirling echoes or "smoke" in the left atrium on echocardiography).[12] In symptomatic patients in whom surgical intervention poses a relatively high risk, the judicious use of diuretics and drugs to control heart rate (i.e., digoxin, calcium channel blockers, or beta-blockers) may allow symptomatic relief. Interventions to increase valvular area are indicated before the onset of symptoms of dyspnea in the following patients: women with severe stenosis who wish to become pregnant and in whom the volume load of pregnancy is unlikely to be tolerated; patients with recurrent thromboembolic events; and patients with severe pulmonary hypertension.

A number of interventions are currently available in patients with mitral stenosis. These include percutaneous balloon valvuloplasty, performed in the cardiac catheterization laboratory; surgical commissurotomy; and replacement of the mitral valve with prosthesis. Balloon valvuloplasty is performed by inflating a specially designed balloon catheter in the mitral orifice to split the fused commissures. Excellent symptomatic relief is obtained in suitable patients.[13,14] This is currently the initial intervention of choice in mitral stenosis in suitable patients. Typically, the mitral valve area doubles in size from 1.0 cm^2 to 2.0 cm^2, with a concomitant reduction in the pressure gradient. Complications of balloon mitral valvuloplasty include mortality (<1%), severe mitral regurgitation (3%), thromboembolism (3%), and residual atrial septal defect with significant shunting (10–20%).[14,15] Contraindications to balloon mitral valvuloplasty include significant mitral regurgitation, as this will likely increase after balloon inflation; left atrial thrombus, which can be dislodged at the time of the procedure; and significant subvalvular involvement or leaflet calcification, which increase the risk of complications and limit the degree of dilatation produced.[13] In pregnant patients with symptomatically severe mitral stenosis that has not responded to conservative measures such as bed rest and rate control, balloon valvuloplasty is the technique of choice to increase the valve area.[16]

Surgical commissurotomy is now usually performed under direct vision after institution of cardiopulmonary bypass. Surgi-

cal commissurotomy may be feasible when balloon valvuloplasty is impossible, such as in patients with significant mitral regurgitation, subvalvular stenosis, or atrial thrombus. A number of studies comparing surgical commissurotomy with balloon commissurotomy have shown equivalent immediate and medium-term (3- to 4-year) results in terms of increase in valvular area, improvement in symptoms, and freedom from repeat intervention in appropriately selected patients.[13] However, commissurotomy, whether performed with a balloon or surgically, is a palliative procedure, and in most cases a further intervention is eventually required. Repeat commissurotomy is sometimes feasible, but most often, mitral valve replacement is then necessary.[17] A prosthetic replacement is also indicated if the valve is heavily scarred or calcified, or if severe mitral regurgitation is present. Prosthetic replacement has higher mortality and morbidity than either surgical or balloon commissurotomy.

Mitral Regurgitation

Mitral regurgitation leads to volume overload of the left ventricle, which must increase in size to achieve a normal stroke output to accommodate the leakage of blood back into the left atrium (Fig. 29-4). Progressive left ventricular dilatation eventually leads to an increase in afterload, contractile impairment, reduction of cardiac output, and heart failure. In acute mitral regurgitation (such as can occur with chordal rupture, ischemia, or endocarditis), left atrial and pulmonary venous and arterial pressures increase quickly, giving rise to dyspnea and, often, acute pulmonary edema. In more chronic forms of mitral regurgitation, an increase in left atrial pressure is often offset by a concomitant increase in atrial compliance. Consequently, symptoms appear late in the course of the disease. Left atrial enlargement predisposes to atrial fibrillation and atrial thromboembolism. In long-standing mitral regurgitation, pulmonary hypertension can develop, which in turn leads to tricuspid regurgitation and right heart failure.

Symptoms and Signs

In most patients, mitral regurgitation remains asymptomatic for many years. Dyspnea, fatigue from low cardiac output, and edema occur late in the course of the disease. Mitral regurgita-

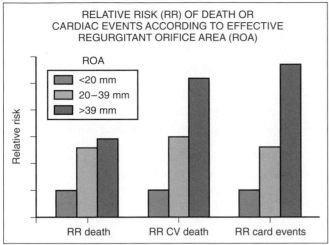

Figure 29-5 • Relative risk of death in asymptomatic patients with severe mitral regurgitation according to size of regurgitant orifice area (ROA). The severity of mitral regurgitation and RR of death increases with the size of ROA. From: Enriquez-Sarano M, Avierinos JF, Messika-Zeitoun D, et al. Quantitative determinants of the outcome of asymptomatic mitral regurgitaion. N Engl J Med 2005; 352:875–883.

tion is recognized clinically by a systolic murmur at the apex, radiating to the axilla and increasing on expiration. In patients with a posteriorly directed jet of mitral regurgitation, the murmur is heard well at the back. In more severe cases, the murmur lasts throughout systole. The intensity of the first sound varies according to the etiology; it can be normal or loud in rheumatic MR and faint in holosystolic prolapse/flail. Second heart sounds are soft or difficult to hear, and a third heart sound is present. A midsystolic click can be present in myxomatous disease; in less severe cases, this click can precede the murmur. The murmur can also be confined to late systole with papillary muscle dysfunction. Mitral regurgitant murmurs caused by ischemia can be variable in duration and intensity, depending on the degree of ischemia and the loading conditions. In general, the intensity of the murmur correlates with the severity of the mitral regurgitation.

Diagnostic Evaluation

Chest X-ray may show left atrial and ventricular enlargement. Doppler echocardiography is the noninvasive method of choice to confirm the presence of mitral regurgitation. Echocardiography is used to diagnose the mechanism of the regurgitation (e.g., prolapse or annular dilatation); color flow mapping is used to provide a semiquantitative assessment of severity on the basis of the size and penetration of the left atrium by the regurgitant jet. Additionally, echocardiography can be used to assess the effects of the regurgitation on left ventricular size and function. Quantitative measurements of regurgitation, such as the regurgitant volume, regurgitant fraction (regurgitant volume divided by [regurgitant volume plus stroke volume]), and regurgitant orifice area (the area through which the valve leaks) are now possible with newer Doppler techniques. These are useful in determining the true severity of the lesion and following it over time, and they have recently been associated with prognosis in asymptomatic patients.[18] The larger the regurgitant orifice area, the worse the prognosis, even in asymptomatic patients[18] (Fig. 29-5). Left ventricular size and volume, as well as contractile function, are used to determine the need for surgical intervention. Transesophageal

echocardiography is very sensitive in the detection of mitral regurgitation and is used mainly in those patients who are difficult to evaluate by the transthoracic approach.[19] Contrast ventriculography is used to determine the severity of mitral regurgitation in patients undergoing cardiac catheterization.

Management

Symptomatic severe mitral regurgitation is considered an indication for surgical intervention if the valve is primarily involved. Symptomatic patients with ischemic mitral regurgitation often require mitral valve surgery in addition to revascularization. Mitral regurgitation secondary to left ventricular dilatation often improves with afterload reduction, and surgical intervention is not usually indicated.

Asymptomatic mitral regurgitation is more difficult to assess and manage than other valvular lesions because in this condition, the true contractile function of the left ventricle is difficult to determine with conventional measures such as the ejection fraction. Such measurements of contractility are confounded by the increase in ventricular preload caused by the extra volume of blood in the left atrium and the variable effect on afterload. Afterload is increased by left ventricular dilatation, but this effect is offset as the ventricle ejects much of its blood into a relatively low-pressure system (the left atrium). Left ventricular ejection fraction can appear falsely elevated in mitral regurgitation and usually falls after surgical correction. *An ejection fraction of <60% should be considered abnormally low in mitral regurgitation.* Thus, in the management of mitral regurgitation, it should be borne in mind that left ventricular dysfunction is often latent and that, once present, the dysfunction cannot be corrected by operative intervention.[20] Therefore, it is important to refer patients for surgery before the onset of true left ventricular dysfunction, even in the absence of symptoms. Stress echocardiography is useful in detecting latent left ventricular dysfunction not evident on a resting study. Failure of the left ventricular ejection fraction to increase or the left ventricular end-systolic volume to decrease on exercise is predictive of incipient left ventricular dysfunction and should be considered an indication for early surgery.[21]

Recent studies indicate a better long-term survival rate in severe mitral regurgitation when surgery is performed early.[22,23] In primary asymptomatic mitral regurgitation with preserved left ventricular function, afterload reduction has not been shown to delay surgery or improve left ventricular function in the few small studies that have addressed this issue; afterload reduction is not currently recommended to treat such patients.[24]

Patients with moderately severe or severe left ventricular dysfunction (ejection fraction <35%) and significant mitral regurgitation were thought in the past to be poor surgical candidates due to high operative risk. More recently, experience shows these patients may be operated on with an acceptable risk. Symptomatic improvement usually results, but a survival benefit of operating in this group has not yet been shown.[25,26] Patients who are not considered suitable for surgery because of left ventricular dysfunction often benefit from afterload reduction and diuretics.[27] Afterload reduction is beneficial in stabilizing patients with hemodynamically significant acute mitral regurgitation in preparation for surgery.

Mitral valve repair is currently the technique of choice in the surgical management of mitral regurgitation because the operative mortality is lower, ventricular function is better preserved, and long-term complications such as thromboembolism and infection are lower with repair than with replacement.[28,29] Long-term failure of repair occurs at a rate of 1–2% a year but is higher with rheumatic disease. The surgical mortality for mitral valve repair for myxomatous degeneration is less than 1% in experienced centers. If mitral valve repair is not possible, a mitral prosthesis is implanted.[30] Chordal and papillary muscle preservation is increasingly being employed when a mitral prosthesis is inserted, as this has been shown to help conserve left ventricular function postoperatively.[31]

Mitral Valve Prolapse

Mitral valve prolapse is a common condition in which the mitral valve leaflets are displaced in systole into the left atrium.[32] It is usually caused by myxomatous degeneration of the valve and can occur in some form in up to 3% of the general population; it is more common in women than in men. In the majority of cases, mitral valve prolapse represents a benign abnormality; in a minority, mainly older men, significant mitral regurgitation results from rupture of a chord or from endocarditis and requires surgical intervention. Mitral valve prolapse is associated with low body weight, low blood pressure, and thoracic skeletal abnormalities such as pectus excavatum. Patients with mitral valve prolapse have a slightly increased risk of stroke, myocardial ischemia, and sudden death. Ventricular extrasystoles are common and can be symptomatically troublesome. Mitral valve prolapse has historically been associated with multiple nonspecific symptoms such as atypical chest pain, presyncope, anxiety, and panic attacks. A causal relation between these symptoms and mitral valve prolapse has not been established.[2]

Diagnosis

A midsystolic click at the mitral area during cardiac auscultation is often the finding that first brings mitral valve prolapse to the attention of the examiner. The click has been attributed to tensing of the redundant valve tissue with cardiac contraction. A late systolic murmur can follow the click. Maneuvers that reduce intracardiac volume, such as having the patient stand or perform the Valsalva maneuver, cause the click to occur earlier in systole and cause an increase in the duration of the murmur if it is present. The typical auscultatory findings and their response to these maneuvers are sufficient to make a diagnosis of mitral valve prolapse. Two-dimensional echocardiography is the method of choice to confirm the diagnosis. Doppler echocardiography is used to detect and quantify associated regurgitation.

Management

Asymptomatic mitral valve prolapse requires no specific treatment. Periodic examination is indicated to detect any progression in the severity of mitral regurgitation. Prophylaxis for endocarditis is indicated if both a click and a murmur are present but is not indicated in the absence of mitral regurgitation.[8] Symptomatic ventricular ectopy often responds to beta-blockade. Many patients with atypical chest pain and other nonspecific symptoms improve when reassured of the relatively benign nature of the condition. Empirical treatment with small doses of beta-blockers can also provide symptomatic relief. Mitral regurgitation should be treated as described earlier.

Aortic Stenosis

The normal aortic valve is 3–4 cm^2 in area when fully open. Aortic stenosis is considered severe when the valvular area is 1 cm^2 or less and considered critical when the area is <0.75 cm^2. Aortic stenosis causes concentric left ventricular hypertrophy as a compensatory mechanism that maintains cardiac output at rest despite the increased pressure gradient across the valve. If untreated, eventually this compensatory mechanism is overcome, causing the left ventricle to fail and dilate and the resting cardiac output to decline (Fig. 29-6).

It is now recognized that multiple risk factors can predispose to progression of aortic stenosis. Factors associated with aortic stenosis are elevated cholesterol and triglycerides, smoking, hypertension, diabetes, and renal failure.

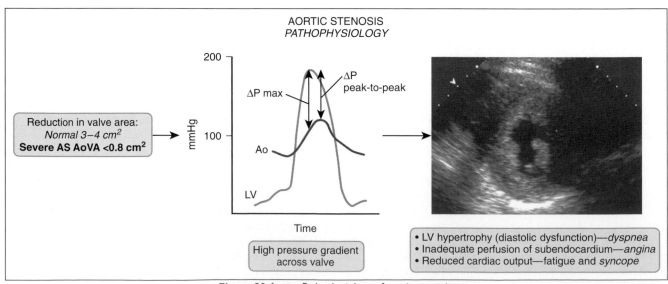

Figure 29-6 • Pathophysiology of aortic stenosis.

AS—aortic stenosis; AoVA—aortic valve area

Symptoms and Signs

There is a variable relation between the severity of stenosis and symptoms. Many patients with critical aortic stenosis are asymptomatic, whereas patients in states of volume overload, such as pregnancy, may have symptoms with stenosis of lesser severity. Dyspnea is often the presenting feature; it reflects increased left atrial pressure and pulmonary venous hypertension from the increased left ventricular pressure in systole and the diastolic ventricular dysfunction imposed by left ventricular hypertrophy. Angina is common even in the absence of significant obstruction in the epicardial coronary blood vessels because of impaired supply of blood to the subendocardium in the hypertrophied left ventricle. Exertional syncope also occurs with stenosis and can result from the inability to increase cardiac output sufficiently to supply both skeletal muscle and the cerebral vasculature, resulting in impaired cerebral blood supply or from abnormal baroreceptor reflexes. Serious arrhythmia can also cause syncope and even sudden death in severe aortic stenosis. Fatigue is common, owing to low cardiac output.

In severe aortic stenosis, the carotid pulse typically is reduced in intensity and has a slow delayed upstroke. This can be difficult to evaluate in the elderly patient with hardened carotid arteries. Aortic stenosis gives rise to a systolic murmur that is heard over the aortic area and that can radiate to the carotid arteries and to the apex. In severe stenosis, the murmur peaks later in systole and can be associated with a thrill. A fourth heart sound is usually present. Although the physical findings are important in alerting the clinician to the presence of aortic valve disease, the degree of hemodynamic severity is more reliably determined with Doppler echocardiography.

Diagnostic Evaluation

The presence of left ventricular hypertrophy on electrocardiography provides useful supporting evidence for significant aortic stenosis. Doppler echocardiography is used to determine the mechanism and the hemodynamic severity of the stenosis, as well as the effects on left ventricular size and function. Continuous wave Doppler echocardiography is used to measure the peak velocity across the valve and thus the aortic pressure gradient; the mean pressure gradient across the valve is often 50 mm Hg or more in severe aortic stenosis. However, the pressure gradient is determined not only by the degree of stenosis but also by flow through the valve and can be relatively low despite severe aortic stenosis if cardiac output is reduced. In most instances, therefore, the valve area should be calculated in addition to the pressure gradient. Because Doppler echocardiography and invasive measurements of aortic valve severity have been shown to agree when both are performed expertly, cardiac catheterization is now used less often as the primary diagnostic tool in assessing aortic stenosis. Cardiac catheterization is used to confirm the echocardiographic findings in patients being considered for surgery or when there is significant discrepancy between the clinical findings and echocardiographic findings but more often only to know the coronary anatomy.

Course and Management

Aortic stenosis is a progressive disease that can remain asymptomatic for many years. The rate of progression varies greatly but increases with age, associated coronary artery disease, and the severity of the stenosis. Preliminary evidence suggests that in the earlier stages of the disease treatment with statins may slow the progression of aortic stenosis.[34] This is a subject under active investigation.[34–36] Progression to symptoms or intervention is likely within 2 years in older patients with severe asymptomatic aortic stenosis.[37] Sudden death can occur with aortic stenosis; this is rare in the absence of symptoms. Once symptoms become manifest, survival without surgical treatment is reduced.[38] Thus, mean survival in patients with angina is 5 years; with syncope, 3 years; and with heart failure, 2 years or less.

Operative mortality increases with severe symptoms, advanced age, and the presence of left ventricular dysfunction. The onset of symptoms, therefore, is the major indication for surgical intervention. Left ventricular dysfunction attributable to aortic stenosis is another indication for intervention, because it demonstrates failure of compensatory mechanisms and incipient symptoms. Selected patients presenting with severe AS, severe LV dysfunction, and profound heart failure may benefit from IV sodium nitroprusside to improve cardiac output.[39] Surgical relief of aortic stenosis usually leads to symptomatic relief and improvement in left ventricular function when such function was abnormal preoperatively. Aortic valve surgery in the very elderly is associated with an increased mortality but provides excellent palliation of symptoms; surgery should be considered in such patients provided they are otherwise viable.[40] Patients with severe left ventricular dysfunction resulting from aortic stenosis should also be considered for surgery, because significant improvement in ventricular function and symptoms often results; without surgery, survival is poor.

Surgical intervention in aortic stenosis usually involves insertion of a prosthesis or human valve. In congenital aortic stenosis, valve repair or commissurotomy can be feasible, although significant aortic regurgitation can result. Balloon valvuloplasty has proved disappointing in the long-term treatment of adult calcific aortic stenosis.[41] However, stenosis recurs in as many as 50% of patients within 6 months, and fewer than 25% survive more than 3 years. Balloon valvuloplasty is now indicated in the palliative treatment of adult patients with aortic stenosis who are not surgical candidates because of significant comorbidity; it is also used to stabilize critically ill patients for whom surgery is planned at a later stage. Balloon dilatation is effective in young patients with congenital aortic stenosis and is an alternative to surgery in symptomatic aortic stenosis during pregnancy.

Aortic Regurgitation

Aortic regurgitation causes volume overload of the left ventricle. In chronic aortic regurgitation, the volume overload is well tolerated for years. The left ventricle dilates to accommodate the increased volume load and thereby maintains a normal resting cardiac output. Unlike in mitral regurgitation, the left ventricle in aortic regurgitation must expel all of the increased volume of blood into the systemic circulation; severe enlargement of the left ventricle is common. Because of a compensatory increase in ventricular compliance, left ventricular diastolic pressure often remains in the normal range, despite the increase in ventricular size. The ventricle hypertrophies to maintain normal wall stress. Eventually, compensatory mechanisms fail, and contractile impairment and increased diastolic pressure result in elevated left atrial and pulmonary venous pressures and symptoms

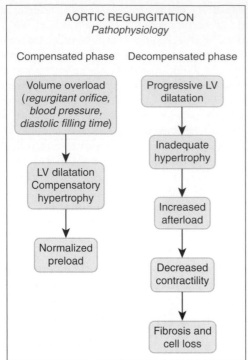

Figure 29-7 • Pathophysiology of aortic regurgitation.

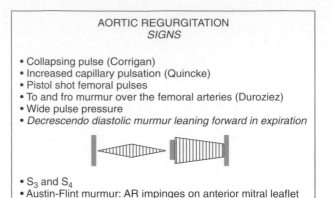

Figure 29-8 • Signs on physical examination of patients with aortic regurgitation. AR: aortic regurgitation.

(Fig. 29-7). Acute aortic regurgitation can develop as a result of sudden disruption of the valve apparatus with endocarditis or aortic dissection. This is poorly tolerated because the left ventricle is unable to dilate fast enough to compensate for the volume load. Left ventricular diastolic pressure rises rapidly and leads to pulmonary congestion and edema. Cardiac output falls, and shock and even death can follow.

Symptoms and Signs

In chronic aortic regurgitation, symptomatic presentation occurs late in the course of disease; dyspnea and fatigue are the usual findings. Angina can occur in the absence of coronary artery disease because of the increased demand for oxygen caused by severe left ventricular enlargement and hypertrophy together with the reduced supply of oxygen resulting from the underperfusion of the coronary arteries. Such underperfusion is caused by the low diastolic pressure characteristic of this condition.

The cardinal signs on physical examination of aortic regurgitation are summarized in Figure 29-8. A decrescendo diastolic murmur in the left sternal border and wide pulses are the typical findings in patients with significant aortic stenosis. Even in the absence of significant stenosis, an aortic systolic murmur is audible, reflecting the increased flow through the valve. A wide pulse pressure characterizes severe chronic aortic regurgitation and an elevated systolic pressure caused by the increased stroke output; also characteristic is a reduction in the diastolic pressure, which occurs as blood leaks back into the left ventricle throughout diastole. If the aortic regurgitant jet hits the mitral valve leaflet, it can cause partial closure of the valve, creating an apical diastolic murmur that simulates mitral stenosis (Austin-Flint murmur). The ejection of a large volume of blood into the systemic circulation and its rapid leak backward into the heart cause many peripheral circulatory manifestations that confirm rather

than establish the diagnosis. Acute aortic regurgitation can be more difficult to recognize because the murmur is often short and the reduced cardiac output leads to a reduction in the intensity of the murmur.

Diagnostic Evaluation

Marked cardiomegaly and prominence of the ascending aorta are often present on chest x-ray in chronic severe aortic regurgitation. Doppler echocardiography establishes the mechanism and severity of aortic regurgitation and its effect on left ventricular size and function. In severe aortic regurgitation, early closure of the mitral valve and diastolic mitral regurgitation can occur as a result of the increased pressure in the left ventricle in diastole. Confirmation of the severity of aortic regurgitation is obtained by aortography. Aortography for assessing the severity of aortic regurgitation should be performed if there is any discrepancy between the clinical findings and the findings on Doppler echocardiography. Stress ventriculography and echocardiography have both been used to determine the response of the left ventricle to the effects of exercise: a significant fall in left ventricular ejection fraction or an increase in end-systolic volume suggests incipient contractile dysfunction and can be an indication for early surgical intervention. Assessment of the ascending aorta should be part of the integral evaluation of patients with aortic regurgitation. Dilatation of the ascending aorta and aortic aneurysms may be associated with aortic regurgitation. The ascending aorta is often visualized with transthoracic echo, but if this is not possible, transesophageal echo, CT, MRI, or contrast angiography should be used.

Course and Management

Chronic aortic regurgitation is well tolerated for many years.[43] Operative mortality is increased and long-term survival reduced if the left ventricle is greatly enlarged or if left ventricular dysfunction has been present for more than 1 year. Left ventricular dysfunction that is present for a shorter period is likely to improve and even resolve after surgery. Several studies have shown that asymptomatic patients with normal left ventricular function can be safely followed for a long period (up to 11 years in one study) with serial physical examination and Doppler echocardiographic examination performed at least yearly and then more frequently as left ventricular dilatation progresses.[43] Surgery is indicated once symptoms develop. In asymptomatic patients, surgery is indicated once resting left ventricular function declines or if severe left ventricular dilatation (end-systolic dimension >5 cm, end-diastolic dimension >7 cm) occurs.[44] Recent evidence suggests that these dimensions should be normalized for body size and surgery considered at an earlier stage, especially in women. Afterload reduction with vasodilators such as hydralazine, captopril, and nifedipine has been shown to reduce regurgitant volume and ventricular size in aortic regurgitation.[24] Treatment with nifedipine, 20 mg twice a day, has been shown to delay the need for surgical intervention in chronic asymptomatic aortic regurgitation but has not been widely used for this indication.[45] Acute severe aortic regurgitation requires urgent surgery. Intravenous vasodilatation with sodium nitroprusside or other vasodilators can reduce the regurgitant volume and can help stabilize the patient awaiting surgery.

Surgical intervention in aortic regurgitation usually leads to improvement in symptoms and left ventricular size. Although the operative risk is increased when severe left ventricular dilatation or dysfunction is present, significant improvement in symptoms and ventricular function often occurs after surgery; the prognosis without surgery is very poor.[44] Aortic regurgitation usually requires insertion of a prosthesis or human valve. Occasionally, repair is feasible, especially in prolapsing bicuspid valves or when the aortic root is dilated.

Tricuspid and Pulmonary Disease

Tricuspid regurgitation is most often secondary to right ventricular dilatation and is the most common valvular problem of the right heart. Tricuspid regurgitation is recognized on physical examination by the characteristic large V waves in the jugular venous pulse and by a systolic murmur heard at the base of the sternum that increases on inspiration. In severe cases, pulsatile hepatomegaly is present. Doppler echocardiography allows rapid detection and assessment of the severity of the regurgitation. Presentation often includes fatigue from reduced forward output and peripheral edema. Severe tricuspid regurgitation is usually treated with surgical repair. If a repair is not possible, a bioprosthesis is usually implanted because of the increased risk of thrombosis of a mechanical prosthesis at this position. Secondary tricuspid regurgitation can improve if the primary condition leading to pulmonary hypertension is treated and leads to a decrease in right heart size.

Tricuspid stenosis occurs in approximately 5–10% of patients with severe mitral stenosis. The characteristic physical findings are a large A wave in the jugular venous pressures and a diastolic murmur over the tricuspid area. Doppler echocardiography and right heart catheterization are both used to assess severity. The mean gradient across the tricuspid valve is typically greater than 5 mm Hg. In cases with significant stenosis, either balloon dilatation or surgical repair or replacement is indicated.

Congenital pulmonary stenosis occurs in isolation or as part of various syndromes and is usually detected before adulthood. Significant pulmonary stenosis is treated with balloon dilatation or surgery. Significant pulmonary insufficiency is rare but can occur with a carcinoid tumor or endocarditis or secondary to pulmonary hypertension. Pulmonary allograft implantation is indicated for severe cases.

PROSTHETIC VALVES

In-depth discussion of prosthetic valves is beyond the scope of this chapter. However, some general concepts are important to be discussed. Prostheses can be classified into two groups, mechanical and biologic, each having different properties, problems, and indications.

Mechanical Prostheses

The major advantage of mechanical prostheses is durability. Mechanical prostheses can remain functional for decades and are used especially in young or middle-aged patients to reduce the need for reoperation. Their main disadvantage is the associated risk of thromboembolism, which necessitates long-term anticoagulation and carries a risk of hemorrhage. An increased incidence of subsequent infection, hemolysis, thrombosis of the valve, and mechanical failure is another problem associated with mechanical prostheses.

Bioprosthesis

Three classes of biologic valves are currently available: xenografts, allografts, and autografts. A xenograft is a prosthesis fashioned from animal tissue (porcine, bovine, or equine). Allografts (homografts) are human valves that have been harvested postmortem and either cryopreserved or treated with antibiotics. An autograft is a valve from the patient's own body that is moved to a different anatomical site. The most common autograft is the pulmonary valve inserted at the aortic position. Biologic valves have a lower risk of thromboembolism than mechanical prostheses and do not usually require chronic anticoagulation. They are indicated for patients in whom anticoagulation is inappropriate. Homografts are the valve of choice in patients with aortic endocarditis, particularly if a periaortic abscess is present.

In elderly patients, xenografts are a better option, given their increased risk for chronic anticoagulation. The duration of xenografts has improved considerably and has contributed to the increased use of this type of prosthesis.[46]

Problems and Complications of Valve Prostheses

The main complications related to prosthetic valves are valvular thrombosis, thromboembolic disease, prosthetic failure, and infection.[47]

When present, these complications are often severe, with inherent high morbidity and mortality. Some of these complications can be minimized with regular follow-up visits, adequate anticoagulation, and echocardiographic surveillance. Prosthetic valve endocarditis carries a high mortality and is often an indication for reoperation.

ANTICOAGULATION

Systemic anticoagulation with warfarin or dicumarol decreases but does not eliminate the incidence of thromboembolism with mechanical valves. The incidence of thromboembolic events is lowest in patients younger than 50 years, lower with aortic prostheses than with mitral or multiple prostheses, and lower with bileaflet disk valves than with single-leaflet valves.[48,49] Hemorrhagic events are more common in older patients. Recent studies have indicated that the level of anticoagulation required to prevent thromboembolism is less than was previously thought. A large study of anticoagulation in mechanical prostheses has suggested that an international normalized ratio (INR) of 2.5 to 4.0 is desirable in most instances and minimizes hemorrhagic and thromboembolic complications.[48,49] The appropriate INR for an individual patient will vary, depending on past history of embolic or bleeding events, age, and type, position, and number of prostheses. Antiplatelet agents such as aspirin or clopidogrel may be added to the anticoagulation regimen in patients who have sustained recurrent thromboembolic events despite adequate anticoagulation.

Thromboembolic risk with xenografts is greatest in the first 3 months after surgery.[50] During this period, oral anticoagulation medications are recommended in high-risk patients (e.g., patients with mitral prostheses or paroxysmal atrial fibrillation); for patients who are not at high risk, aspirin, 325 mg/day, is recommended.

PROBLEMS ASSOCIATED WITH PREGNANCY

Despite the increase in intravascular volume, pregnancy is usually well tolerated in previously asymptomatic patients with valvular heart disease.[9] During pregnancy, regurgitant lesions are better tolerated than stenosis. Prophylactic intervention to increase the valve area is recommended before pregnancy in patients with hemodynamically severe stenosis.

Pregnancy is contraindicated in women with mechanical prostheses because of the considerable risk to mother and fetus. The risk to the mother is associated with a difficulty in maintaining effective anticoagulation; the risk to the fetus is associated with potential teratogenic effects of warfarin.[51,52] If possible, valve repair or insertion of an allograft or an autograft should be attempted in a woman of childbearing age who wishes to become pregnant. The management of patients with mechanical prostheses who become pregnant or who desire pregnancy is controversial. Warfarin is associated with an embryopathy and increases the risk of fetal wastage. Optimal anticoagulation is also difficult with heparin, especially when given by the subcutaneous route, and it is associated with increased maternal risk for thromboembolism and hemorrhage. Different approaches have been advocated for the management of pregnant patients with mechanical prostheses, but none is ideal. Low-molecular-weight heparin has been associated with valve thrombosis and death in pregnant women.[51] Evaluation by a cardiologist and a high-risk obstetrician is essential for the successful management of this difficult group of patients.

ANOREXIANT-INDUCED VALVE DISORDER

Anorexiants, drugs that suppress appetite, have been reported to cause a valve disorder similar to that caused by ergot derivatives and carcinoid syndrome. This was first reported in 1997, and a number of large studies since confirmed an increased prevalence of valve disorders in populations treated with fenfluramine, dexfenfluramine, phentermine, or a combination of these drugs.[7,53-56] Over 18 million prescriptions were filled for these drugs in 1996 alone. The precise pathophysiology of the valve disorder is still unclear. All of these anorexiant agents affect central serotonergic receptors. A causal relationship of serotonin to this disorder is also suggested by its similarity to carcinoid disease in which serotonin is also implicated as a causative factor. Initial reports suggested a high prevalence of valve disease in patients treated with these anorexiant agents, and they were withdrawn from the market in September 1997. More recently, the prevalence of clinically symptomatic valve-related disease in patients receiving these drugs has been reported to be 1 in 1,000.[57]

Anorexiant drug valvulopathy affects mainly the aortic and mitral valve. Leaflet thickening, restricted leaflet motion, chordal thickening, and valve regurgitation without stenoses are the most common abnormalities seen. Although valve disease severe enough to warrant valve surgery has been reported, in many instances, the valve lesion appears to be mild or moderate in severity. Factors that are thought to increase the likelihood of more severe disease are longer duration of treatment with anorexiant therapy, use of drug combinations, and higher dose treatment. Those who received <3 months of treatment appear to have a relatively low likelihood of significant valve disease.[57] Patients exposed to anorexiant drugs should undergo a thorough cardiovascular examination for signs of mitral or aortic regurgitation.

Echocardiography is indicated if the physical findings suggest valve disease or if the duration of treatment was more than 3 months. Patients with evidence of valve disease on echocardiography should be followed serially and receive prophylactic antibiotics for dental and other procedures associated with significant bacteremia.

OUTPATIENT PHYSICIAN COMMUNICATION AND PATIENT EDUCATION

In all patients with structural valvular heart disease, endocarditis prophylaxis should be considered at the time of dental or other procedure that produce significant bacteremia. The prophylactic regimens recommended by the American Heart Association have been revised.[8]

Patients with hemodynamically significant valvular heart disease should generally avoid participation in competitive sports. Recommendations of the American College of Cardiology provide guidance regarding specific lesions.[10] Valvular heart disease is a chronic disease requiring periodic examination and follow-up, even in asymptomatic patients and in those who have had corrective surgical or other procedures. Among patients with mitral regurgitation, serial echocardiographic evaluation should be performed at least yearly and more frequently as ventricular dilatation progresses in severe asymptomatic mitral regurgitation. Patients with aortic stenosis should be instructed to report the onset of any symptoms and should undergo regular follow-up evaluation with physical examination and Doppler echocardiography. Doppler examination should be performed at least yearly and more frequently in patients with severe stenosis and in older patients. Patients with prosthetic valves should be seen at least yearly.

Key Points

- Rheumatic heart disease remains the most common cause of mitral stenosis and is the most common cause of multivalvular heart disease. Rheumatic heart disease remains a significant problem in immigrants, especially those from Latin America and Southeast Asia.

- The predominant hemodynamic manifestation of endocarditis is valvular regurgitation caused by leaflet perforation or deformity of the free edges.

- Mitral regurgitation is common in coronary artery disease, and its presence carries an adverse prognosis.

- Interventions to increase valvular area in mitral stenosis are indicated before the onset of symptoms of dyspnea in the following patients: women with severe stenosis who wish to become pregnant and in whom the volume load of pregnancy is unlikely to be tolerated; patients with recurrent thromboembolic events; and patients with severe pulmonary hypertension.

- An ejection fraction of <60% should be considered abnormally low in mitral regurgitation. Left ventricular dysfunction is often latent and, once present, the dysfunction cannot be corrected by operative intervention. Refer patients for surgical evaluation before the onset of true left ventricular dysfunction, even in the absence of symptoms.

- Acute severe aortic regurgitation requires urgent surgery. Intravenous vasodilatation with sodium nitroprusside or other vasodilators can reduce the regurgitant volume and can help stabilize the patient awaiting surgery.

SUGGESTED READING

Gardin JM, Schumacher D, Constantine G, et al. Valvular abnormalities and cardiovascular status following exposure to dexfenfluramine or phentermine/fenfluramine. JAMA 2000; 283:1703–1709.

Dajani AS, Taubert KA, Wilson W, et al. Prevention of bacterial endocarditis. Recommendations by the American Heart Association. JAMA 1997; 277:1794–1801.

Gohlke-Barwolf C, Acar J, Oakley C, et al. Guidelines for prevention of thromboembolic events in valvular heart disease. Study Group of the Working Group on Valvular Heart Disease of the European Society of Cardiology. Eur Heart J 1995; 16:1320–1330.

Enriquez-Sarano M, Avierinos JF, Messika-Zeitoun D, et al. Quantitative determinants of the outcome of asymptomatic mitral regurgitation. N Engl J Med 2005; 352:875–883.

Levine HJ, Gaasch WH. Vasoactive drugs in chronic regurgitant lesions of the mitral and aortic valves. J Am Coll Cardiol 1996; 28:1083–1091.

Otto CM. Aortic stenosis and hyperlipidemia: establishing a cause-effect relationship. Am Heart J 2004; 147:761–763.

Otto CM, Burwash IG, Legget ME, et al. Prospective study of asymptomatic valvular aortic stenosis. Clinical, echocardiographic, and exercise predictors of outcome. Circulation 1997; 95:2262–70.

Khot UN, Novaro GM, Popovic ZB, et al. Nitroprusside in critically ill patients with left ventricular dysfunction and aortic stenosis. N Engl J Med 2003; 348:1756–1763.

Vesey JM, Otto CM. Complications of prosthetic heart valves. Curr Cardiol Rep 2004; 6:106–111.

Cannegieter SC, Torn M, Rosendaal FR. Oral anticoagulant treatment in patients with mechanical heart valves: how to reduce the risk of thromboembolic and bleeding complications. J Intern Med 1999; 245:369–374.

Bonow BO, Carabello BA, Kanu C, et al. ACC/AHA 2006 guidelines for the management of patients with valvular heart disease: a report of the American College of Cardiology/American Heart Association Task Force on Practice Guidelines. Circ 2006; 114(5):e84–231.

CHAPTER THIRTY

Acute Pericarditis

Lorenzo Di Francesco, MD, FACP

BACKGROUND

The normal pericardium covers the heart within the middle mediastinum, protects the heart from adjacent organs, and provides constraint during the diastolic filling period. It is composed of both a visceral and parietal layer about 1–2 mm thick and is separated by a pericardial space that contains approximately 15–35 cc of a specialized pericardial fluid that acts as a lubricant during the cardiac cycle.

Pericarditis results from acute inflammation of the pericardium that can either occur as an isolated event or be part of a more generalized systemic disorder. While the exact incidence of acute pericarditis is not entirely clear, it accounts for at least 5% of patients seen in the emergency room setting with nonischemic chest pain.[1] The possible causes for a given case of acute pericarditis are numerous; categories include: idiopathic (unknown), infectious, autoimmune (vasculitis, connective tissue disease), neoplastic, metabolic, traumatic, secondary to diseases in surrounding organs (myocardial infarction [MI], pneumonia, pulmonary embolism, aortic dissection), and a large number of rarer miscellaneous causes. See Box 30-1 for a more extensive differential of causes. Given the clinical difficulty of determining a clear cause for a patient's pericarditis, the majority of causes by default fall into the idiopathic variety. In three large case series of unselected patients with acute pericarditis (631 patients total), the most common diagnoses were: idiopathic, specific etiology (i.e., post infarction, drug induced etc.), autoimmune, neoplastic, tuberculosis, and, rarely, purulent pericarditis.[2–4]

Pericarditis can be characterized as dry, fibrinous, or effusive, with its clinical course being highly dependent on the underlying cause. While most cases will be determined to be idiopathic (cause unknown), probably a postviral infection and self-limited, a number of cases of varying causes can progress and lead to more troubling sequelae that include recurrent pericarditis, pericardial effusion, cardiac tamponade, constrictive pericarditis, and, rarely, subacute effusive pericarditis with signs of constriction ("effusive-constrictive pericarditis"). A reasonable classification system for pericardial syndromes is listed in Box 30-2.

Certain secondary causes of pericarditis need special attention. Obviously, patients with a clinical picture of sepsis and underlying purulent pericarditis need aggressive antibiotic treatment and fast pericardial drainage. In addition, there are two types of post MI pericarditis. The early form, pericarditis epistenocardiaca, occurs secondary to direct extension of an acute transmural MI,

but is rarely discovered given the clinical presentation is usually overshadowed by the presentation of myocardial pain and a ST segment injury pattern of an acute MI on electrocardiogram (ECG) with the focal pericarditis often not heard. The second late form is called Dressler's syndrome, which is characterized by development of acute pericarditis with fever and elevated acute phase reactants (Erythrocyte sedimentation rate [ESR], white blood cell count [WBC], etc.). Classically, pericardial pain develops more than 1 week after an MI and is felt to represent an autoimmune response to previously released myocardial antigens. Again, the ECG changes of the acute pericarditis here may be obscured by evidence of a recent MI.[5] Pericarditis that occurs after cardiac surgery, postpericardiotomy syndrome, typically develops around 4 weeks after surgery in up to 20% of patients. Finally, acute pericarditis secondary to fulminant renal failure or during hemodialysis in a patient with end-stage renal failure is important to diagnose, given its known associated higher mortality, risk for progression to cardiac tamponade and need to escalate the patient's dialysis regimen.[6]

ASSESSMENT

Clinical Presentation

Symptoms

The most common symptom of acute pericarditis is chest discomfort, found in >90% of cases. Typically described as acute onset, left-sided retrosternal pain that is often pleuritic in quality, it is notably positional, found to be worse in the supine position, and improves when the patient sits upright and leans forward. Similar to myocardial ischemic pain, it can radiate to the patient's neck, arms, and left shoulder. Unlike myocardial ischemic pain that can radiate across to one or both shoulders or to the patient's back between the scapula, chest pain that radiates to one or both of the trapezius muscle ridges is more consistent with pericarditis, given that the phrenic nerve, which innervates those muscles, can be irritated as it traverses through the inflamed pericardial space. If patients have a large or rapidly accumulating pericardial effusion, they may complain of local compression symptoms such as dyspnea, dysphagia, hoarseness, or singultus. Those patients with rare progression to cardiac tamponade often complain of severe shortness of breath, dyspnea on exertion, palpitations, orthopnea, cough, and occasionally delirium secondary to cerebral hypoperfusion. Patients who develop constrictive pericarditis

Box 30-1 Causes of Acute Pericarditis

Idiopathic

Infections

Bacterial, tuberculous, viral (coxsackie, influenza, HIV, etc.), fungal, rickettsial, mycoplasma, leptospiral, listeria, parasitic, and others

Vasculitis and connective-tissue disease

Rheumatoid arthritis, rheumatic fever, systemic lupus erythematosus, scleroderma, Sjögren's syndrome, Reiter's syndrome, ankylosing spondylitis, Wegener's granulomatosis, giant-cell arteritis, polymyositis (dermatomyositis), Behçet's syndrome, familial Mediterranean fever, dermatomyositis, polyarteritis, Churg-Strauss syndrome, thrombotic thrombocytopenic purpura, leukocytoclastic vasculitis, and others

Diseases in adjacent structures

Myocardial infarction, aortic dissection, pneumonia, pulmonary embolism, empyema

Metabolic disorders

Uremia, dialysis-related, myxedema, gout, scurvy

Neoplastic disorders

Primary

Mesothelioma, sarcoma, fibroma, lipoma, and others

Secondary (metastatic or direct spread)

Carcinoma, lymphoma, carcinoid, and others

Trauma

Direct

Pericardial perforation (penetrating injury, esophageal or gastric perforation) and cardiac injury (cardiac surgery, percutaneous procedures)

Indirect

Radiation, nonpenetrating chest injury

Association with other syndromes

Postmyocardial and pericardial injury syndromes, inflammatory bowel disease, Lofflers' syndrome, Stevens-Johnson syndrome, giant-cell aortitis, hypereosinophilic syndromes, acute pancreatitis, others

Adapted from Troughton RW, Asher CR, Klein AL. Pericarditis. Lancet 2004; 363:717–27.

Box 30-2 Classification of Pericardial Syndromes

Acute pericarditis (<3 months)

– Idiopathic

– Secondary

Chronic pericarditis (>3 months)

Recurrent pericarditis

– Intermittent type

– Incessant type

Pericardial effusion

Cardiac tamponade

Constrictive pericarditis

Subacute effusive pericarditis with signs of constriction ("effusive-constrictive pericarditis")

---

pericardial rub is a three-component (atrial systole, ventricular systole, and early diastole), high-pitched, scratchy sound heard best at the left lower sternal border at end expiration with the patient leaning forward. Studies show the rub to be triphasic in a half, biphasic in a third, and monophasic in the rest.[7] Importantly, a pericardial rub should always be differentiated from a pleural friction rub (which only occurs during the respiratory cycle) by its lack of disappearance when a patient holds his or her breath. Those patients with significant pericardial effusion may have clinical evidence of compression of the base of the left lung, which results in dullness under the left scapula called the Bamberger-Pins-Ewart sign.[5] Progression to full-blown cardiac tamponade physiology is usually associated with Beck's triad, consisting of systemic hypotension, quiet heart sounds, and elevated central venous pressure (CVP). Evaluation of the normal inspiratory drop in the systolic blood pressure (<10 mm Hg) might reveal evidence of significant pulsus paradoxus (>10 mm Hg inspiratory drop in systolic blood pressure). Those rare patients who develop constrictive pericarditis with chronic fibrous thickening and/or calcification of the pericardial sac will manifest right > left heart failure signs. Signs include a decreased apical impulse, an early diastolic heart sound (pericardial knock), bilateral pleural effusions, and elevated CVP, which may also manifest elevation or a failure to fall with inspiration (Kussmaul's sign) in association with a prominent y descent (Friedreich's sign), a pulsatile liver, hepatomegaly, clinical ascites, and bilateral lower extremity edema.

Electrocardiogram

Classic ECG Changes

The ECG typically undergoes a series of changes, quite helpful in the diagnosis of this condition, that reflect the acute pericardial inflammatory process and its ultimate resolution. Daily ECGs usually elucidate all the stages. Classically, there are four serial electrocardiographic changes that have been well documented to occur in acute pericarditis; however, one or more of these stages may be absent if the pericardial process resolves quickly or evolves too fast.[8] The four classic electrocardiographic stages of acute pericarditis are summarized in Table 30-1.

---

either acutely (days) or subacutely (months to years) following their bout of pericarditis will present with symptoms of left and right heart failure due to abnormal diastolic filling with raised left- and right-sided filling pressures due to the reduced compliance of a rigid pericardium. Common symptoms in this setting include shortness of breath, dyspnea on exertion, cough, orthopnea, paroxysmal nocturnal dyspnea, abdominal swelling, and lower extremity edema.

Signs

A pericardial friction rub is considered the pathognomonic sign of pericarditis. It is deceptively intermittent, highly positional, and can vary in intensity even during the same day. Typically, a

Electrical Basis for ECG Changes in Acute Pericarditis

Given that the pericardium produces no detectable electrical phenomenon, the electrical basis of the ECG abnormalities in the PR segment, ST segment, and T waves that occur during acute pericarditis result primarily from the secondary myocardial inflammation restricted to the subepicardial "shell." Given that the entire subepicardial region is involved, all the ECG changes found during the course of pericarditis develop in phase with each other, and because the secondary myocarditis is mainly superficial, no Q waves form; R waves are not affected; QRS duration is not prolonged, and QT interval prolongation is unusual.

The Stage 1 ECG with its marked ST segment injury pattern (primarily in leads I, II, aVL, aVF, V3-V6) is felt to reflect the generalized pericardial inflammatory process and its associated myocarditis (Fig. 30-1). The Stage 2 ECG represents resolution of the superficial myocarditis as the ST segments return to normal but often accentuates the associated PR depression (seen in lead aVR), which is felt to represent the generalized epicardial atrial injury. The Stage 3 ECG and its generalized T wave inversion result from a delay in repolarization of the whole subepicardial healing myocardium (Fig. 30-2). The Stage 4 ECG reflects resolution of the pericarditis with return to the patient's baseline ECG. Given the right patient clinical picture, the evolution of the patient's ECG through the following stages over time is virtually diagnostic of acute pericarditis: Stage 1 to 2 to 3 to 4; Stage 1 to 2 or 4 (omitting 3); Stage 2 to 3 and/or 4.

Differential Diagnosis of the ECG Findings in Acute Pericarditis

ECG changes of early repolarization and MI may confuse the diagnosis of acute pericarditis. Differentiation between the ECG in pericarditis, early repolarization, and acute MI requires careful analysis of the ST segment configuration, presence of Q waves, presence of reciprocal ST segment changes, location of the ST elevation, measurement of the ST/T amplitude ratio in lead V6 or V5, loss of R wave voltage, and PR segment depression.[9] See Table 30-2 for comparison. In a study of patients with acute pericarditis versus those with early repolarization, an ST/T amplitude ratio in V6 > 0.25 separated all patients with pericarditis from those patients with early repolarization when a Stage 1 type ECG was analyzed.[10]

ECG Changes Associated with Pericardial Effusion and Cardiac Tamponade

Patients with significant pericardial effusion may manifest significant lowering of their overall ECG voltage, and a number of patients with pericardial effusion might manifest QRS electrical alternans (beat to beat variation in the amplitude of the QRS). One study of hospitalized patients with and without pericardial effusions and cardiac tamponade showed that the "low-voltage ECG" had a sensitivity of 2% and specificity 100%, while "QRS electrical alternans" had sensitivity of 6% and specificity of 89% for pericardial effusion. In addition, a "low-voltage ECG" had a sensitivity 25% and specificity of 99%, and "QRS electrical alternans" had a sensitivity of 8% and specificity of 93% for cardiac tamponade. Thus, these signs are helpful when present if your pretest probability is intermediate to high, but not helpful to rule out both concomitant pericardial effusion or cardiac tamponade when absent.[11]

Laboratory Tests

Routine Laboratory Tests

There are no pathognomonic laboratory findings in acute pericarditis, given that the cause in most cases is idiopathic. Inflammatory markers such as the white blood cell count (WBC), C reactive protein (CRP), and erythrocyte sedimentation rate (ESR) might be elevated to various degrees but are all nonspecific and do not necessarily point to a specific diagnosis. The presence of

Table 30-1 ECG Stages in Acute Pericarditis

Stage 1	Concave ST segment elevation particularly "epicardial" leads I, II, aVL, aVF, V3-V6. No true reciprocal ST segment depressions except in "cavity pattern" leads such as aVR, V1, and, rarely, in V2.
Stage 2	ST junctions return to baseline with little T wave changes, PR segment depression in "epicardial leads," which may give the false impression of continued ST segment elevation if the T-P interval used as the baseline.
Stage 3	Diffuse T wave inversion.
Stage 4	ECG resolution to normal.

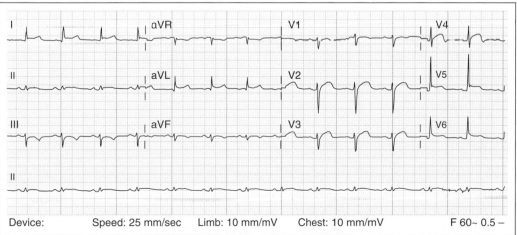

Figure 30-1 • ECG Acute Pericarditis Stage I.

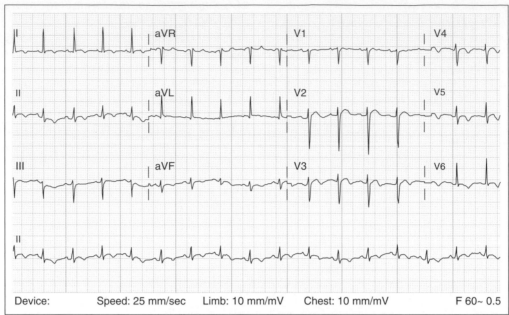

Figure 30-2 • ECG Acute Pericarditis Stage 3.

Table 30-2 Separating Acute Pericarditis, Early Repolarization, and Acute Myocardial Infarction (MI) by ECG Changes

ECG Changes	Pericarditis	Early Repolarization	Acute MI
ST-segment configuration	Concave	Concave	Convex
Q waves	None	None	Present
Reciprocal ST-segment changes	None	None	Present
Location of ST elevation	Limb/prec	Precordial > limb	Area of MI
ST/T ratio in lead V6 or V5	>0.25	<0.25	—
Loss of R wave voltage	Absent	Absent	Present
PR-segment depression	Present	Absent	Absent

Adapted from Marinella MA. Electrocardiographic manifestations and differential diagnosis of acute pericarditis. American Family Physician 1998; 57(4):699–704.

advanced renal failure might help support a diagnosis of uremic pericarditis. Rheumatologic tests such as antinuclear antibodies and rheumatoid factor should be obtained if the clinical history and examination suggest a particular connective tissue disease (i.e., systemic lupus erythematosus, rheumatoid arthritis, etc.) or vasculitis.

Cardiac Troponins

Importantly, because most cases of acute pericarditis are associated with a "superficial myocarditis," the presence of abnormal serum cardiac troponin I (cTnI) is not uncommon and may lead to confusion in the diagnosis. Three studies of acute pericarditis patients revealed that between 32–71% had elevations in cTnI, usually on the day of admission or by the second day.[12,14] Confusingly, troponin leak can be detectable for up to a week, with a rise and fall pattern that resembles that seen in acute MI and therefore not helpful in differentiating acute coronary syndrome from acute pericarditis. Factors found to be associated with troponin leak during acute pericarditis included younger patients (typically males) with a recent infection, diffuse ST elevation on presentation, and the presence of a pericardial effusion on echocardiogram (ECHO). While the troponin leak during acute pericarditis is related to the extent of superficial epicardial myocardial inflammation, it has not been found to be a negative prognostic factor (like in cases of acute coronary syndrome with associated troponin leak).

Chest Radiography

The role of chest radiography is primarily to raise the suspicion of an alternative diagnosis (i.e., pulmonary edema, pneumonia, pleural effusion, pulmonary mass, or mediastinal mass). Most cases of uncomplicated acute pericarditis will be associated with a normal cardiac silhouette. Occasionally, a patient with symptoms of pericarditis might have concomitant cardiomegaly and pulmonary edema, suggesting that the patient has a myopericarditis or constrictive pericarditis. Likewise, patients with pericarditis and slowly developing pericardial effusion will have a "water bottle" shaped enlargement of their cardiac silhouette indicating at least 250 cc of pericardial fluid (Fig. 30-3). Those rare patients with recurrent pericarditis who develop constrictive pericarditis may have pericardial calcification on their chest radiograph, but this finding is not sensitive.

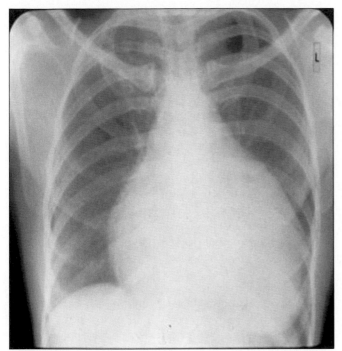

Figure 30-3 • Chest x-ray (CXR) Large pericardial effusion "water bottle heart." Photograph from late Dr. Harry Shawdon, permission granted by Ian Maddison, FRCR.

Echocardiography

While transthoracic echocardiography is recommended in all patients with known or suspected pericarditis by the American College of Cardiology (ACC), American Heart Association (AHA), and American Society of Echocardiography (ASE) guidelines, the presence of an associated significant pericardial effusion only confirms the clinical diagnosis and is not required for the definitive diagnosis. Transthoracic echocardiography can be extremely helpful to identify those rare patients with acute pericarditis and accompanying cardiac tamponade or constrictive pericarditis. There are a number of important Doppler echocardiographic features that suggest cardiac tamponade and include the following: abnormal respiratory changes in ventricular dimensions, right atrial compression, right ventricular diastolic collapse, abnormal respiratory flow velocities at the tricuspid and mitral valves, a dilated inferior vena cava (IVC) demonstrating no inspiratory collapse, left atrial compression, left ventricular diastolic compression, and the "swinging heart."[15]

DIAGNOSIS

The diagnosis of acute pericarditis is purely clinical. It requires that the patient exhibit at least two out of three criteria that include: a classic history of pericardial pain, physical examination revealing a pericardial friction rub, and/or an ECG revealing changes consistent with acute pericarditis (stage 1) or serial ECG changes consistent with resolving pericarditis (stage 1 to 2 to 3 to 4; stage 1 to 2 or 4; stage 2 to 3 and/or 4).

PROGNOSIS

The majority of patients with acute pericarditis have a good prognosis. A systematic review of the literature identified a number of clinical features among patients with acute pericarditis (called "poor prognostic predictors") that were found to be associated with either an increased short-term risk of complications or identified patients with a higher likelihood that an invasive evaluation (usually involving pericardiocentesis) might lead to a specific diagnosis.[16] A prospective study in Spain of over 300 patients with acute pericarditis stratified patients without any of the following "poor prognostic predictors": fever >38°C, subacute onset, immunosuppression, pericarditis associated with trauma, use of oral anticoagulants, myopericarditis, severe pericardial effusion by ECHO (defined by >20 mm anterior and posterior effusion), or cardiac tamponade to a "low-risk" outpatient management protocol versus direct hospital admission for evaluation and treatment.

They classified 254/300 patients as "low risk," and these were managed as outpatients with a regimen of high-dose aspirin 800 mg orally every 6 or 8 hours for 7–10 days. In follow-up only 33/254 patients required hospitalization for aspirin failure. Importantly, there was no mortality among the patients treated as outpatients over a mean follow-up period of 38 months, with only 43 relapses, four cases of constriction, and no cases of cardiac tamponade. Subgroup analysis of the data revealed a greater complication rate among low-risk patients who were aspirin nonresponders.

While exhaustive diagnostic studies were not routinely utilized, they diagnosed 90.3% of low-risk patients as having an idiopathic/viral cause and 9.4% with a specific identifiable cause. For the 46 patients found to have at least one "poor prognostic predictor," 21.7% were subsequently diagnosed as idiopathic/viral, while 78.3% were diagnosed with a specific cause after extensive invasive workups.

MANAGEMENT

Outpatient or Inpatient

Patients with acute pericarditis can be managed conservatively without hospitalization if they do not have any "poor prognostic predictors," have not had a precipitating acute MI-related pericarditis, or represent a case of either uremic pericarditis or suspected purulent pericarditis, since these conditions require emergent hospitalization for more specialized evaluation and treatment. An appropriate triage protocol is found in Figure 30-4.

Outpatient Treatment

Despite the lack of large, randomized, prospective treatment trials, nonsteroidal anti-inflammatory drugs (NSAIDs) continue to represent the main form of effective therapy in the majority of patients with acute pericarditis. Choice of specific NSAID is usually left to the treating physician, who should strongly consider their individual efficacy as well as the potential associated side effects. The most commonly used NSAIDS with their dose ranges include aspirin (650–1625 mg q4–5 hr), ibuprofen (200–1200 mg q6 hr), naproxen (200–500 mg q12 hr), and indomethacin (25–50 mg q8–12 hr; SR 75 mg q12 hr). All patients should receive additional gastrointestinal protection with an oral proton pump inhibitor. One large prospective trial of patients with acute pericarditis showed that "low-risk patients" stratified to a standardized outpatient regimen (aspirin 800 mg

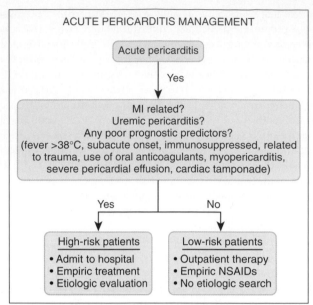

Figure 30-4 • Acute Pericarditis Management.

q6–8 hr in addition to gastrointestinal protection with either misoprostol or a proton pump inhibitor for 7–10 days with gradual aspirin tapering over 2–3 weeks) had a response rate of 87%.[16]

Recurrent pericarditis may occur in follow-up in between 15–32% of patients, presumably due to an immune-mediated antibody disease likely involving antimyocardial antibodies. A recent review of many small studies suggested that this entity is likely best treated with colchicine at doses of 1 mg/day for at least 1 year with a gradual tapering period thereafter. However, large randomized controlled trials are needed for a more definitive answer.[17]

Inpatient Treatment and Evaluation

Hospitalized patients should be started on empiric NSAID therapy with a focus on more intensive and invasive etiologic evaluation. Patients presenting with a clinical picture suspicious for purulent pericarditis should quickly be placed on empiric antibiotics and undergo diagnostic as well as therapeutic pericardiocentesis emergently. Obviously, patients with uremic pericarditis should begin hemodialysis if end-stage renal disease is newly diagnosed or undergo more aggressive hemodialysis if already on hemodialysis.[18] Patients with MI-related pericarditis, either the early form "pericarditis epistenocardiaca" or from direct extension of an acute transmural MI, should be aggressively managed as high-risk MI patients. Therapy for symptomatic MI-related pericarditis can be managed with aspirin 650 mg qid for 24 hours; if there is no significant response, the dose can be increased to 975 mg qid. An alternative is indomethacin 25 mg qid for 24 hours; if there is no significant response, the dose can be increased to 50 mg qid. If a patient fails to respond to aspirin, he or she can be switched to indomethacin and aspirin. If the patient's pericardial pain fails to respond to aspirin and indomethacin, prednisone 40 mg once a day can be given for 1 week and then tapered.[19] Clearly, all patients with cardiac tamponade by ECHO should undergo ther-

apeutic pericardiocentesis, and patients with evidence of constrictive pericarditis should be evaluated by cardiology and ultimately cardiothoracic surgery for consideration for pericardiotomy.

Invasive Testing and the Role of Pericardiocentesis and Pericardial Biopsy

Clearly, the benefits of pericardiocentesis and/or pericardial biopsy need to be weighed against the risks of the procedure. Diagnosis of neoplastic and tuberculous pericarditis can be particularly tricky. It is clear that the diagnostic yield of these procedures is highly dependent on patient selection. The most studied protocol for evaluating patients with acute pericarditis is the "Barcelona experience"[2] (Table 30-3). In the evaluation of 231 consecutive patients with primary pericardial disease (acute pericarditis or cardiac tamponade presenting without an apparent cause), the sensitivity and specificity of pericardiocentesis and pericardial biopsy were reasonably high (79%/98% and 78%/95%, respectively). However, their diagnostic value was dependent on whether the procedure was indicated for "diagnostic" versus "therapeutic" reasons. For pericardiocentesis, the diagnostic yield was 6% for "diagnostic" indications and 29% for "therapeutic" indications. Likewise, for pericardial biopsy, the diagnostic yield was 5% if done for "diagnostic" indications and 54% for "therapeutic" indications. Similarly, an etiologic evaluation led to a specific diagnosis in 78.3% of patients (n = 46) hospitalized for treatment and considered to have moderate- to high-risk features as defined by any of the "poor prognostic predictors."[16] So far, no study has prospectively evaluated the Barcelona protocol versus the use of "poor prognostic predictors" to determine the best strategy for definitively diagnosing the cause among patients with acute pericarditis. Currently accepted clinical indications for performing acute pericardiocentesis in acute pericarditis include patients with clinical tamponade, high suspicion for purulent pericarditis, suspicion for neoplastic pericarditis, and large and/or symptomatic pericardial effusion not responding to treatment after 1 week (Table 30-3).

Pericardial Fluid Analysis

There have been very few studies of normal pericardial fluid composition. One recent evaluation of 30 patients undergoing elec-

---

Box 30-3 Indications for Pericardiocentesis*

Clinical tamponade

High suspicion for purulent pericarditis

Suspect neoplastic pericarditis

Large or symptomatic pericardial effusion not responding to treatment after 1 week

*Contraindications: acute aortic dissection associated pericardial effusion, uncorrected coagulopathy, anticoagulant therapy, platelets <50 K, small, posterior or loculated effusions. Traumatic or purulent pericarditis ultimately requires cardiothoracic surgical intervention emergently.

tive open-heart surgery suggests that pericardial fluid contains the same concentration of small molecules (glucose, urea, uric acid, creatinine) as serum with fluid:serum ratios very close to 1 in accordance with the theory that pericardial fluid is an ultrafiltrate of plasma. Interestingly, the mean WBC was 1,430 (800–2,100) with a differential consisting of 53% (±14%) lymphocytes. Unlike pleural fluid, it was noted that the LDH and protein content of normal pericardial fluid was higher than expected with pericardial fluid LDH:serum LDH ratio of 2.4 (1.3–3.5) and pericardial fluid protein:serum protein ratio of 0.6 (0.5–0.7), thereby making it impossible to use traditional Light's criteria for pleural fluid analysis to separate pericardial effusions into "transudative or exudative" processes.[20]

It is well known that patients with tuberculous or malignant pericarditis can have negative pericardial fluid analyses (including cultures and cytology) as well as normal pericardial biopsy results. Definitive proof of either tuberculous pericarditis or pericardial malignancy in these cases thus ultimately requires examination of the entire pericardium at pericardiostomy. A number of biological markers, including adenosine deaminase (ADA) and interferon γ, have been studied in small numbers of patients with pericarditis and/or pericardial effusions and found to be reliable markers for the presence of pericardial tuberculosis. ADA catalyzes the deamination of adenosine to inosine and ammonium. Its activity is 10–20 fold higher in T lymphocytes than B lymphocytes, and its level in pleural fluid has been found to be significantly higher in tuberculous pleural effusions than in other types of pleural exudative disorders.

In one study of 110 consecutive patients presenting with large pericardial effusions, ADA levels >30 U/L were found to have a sensitivity of 94% and specificity of 68% for diagnosing pericardial tuberculosis. More importantly, interferon γ levels >200 pg/L appear to have a sensitivity and specificity of 100% for predicting those patients with tuberculous pericardial disease.[21] A study of 24 patients with moderate to larger pericardial effusions suspected of having tuberculosis (14 of which had definitive tuber-

culosis and 8 malignancy) showed that a pericardial fluid ADA >40 U/L had a sensitivity of 93% and a specificity of 97% for tuberculosis, and interestingly a pericardial fluid carcinoembryonic antigen level (CEA) >5 ng/mL had a sensitivity of 75% and a specificity of 100% for diagnosing malignant pericarditis.[22]

Discharge/Follow-up Plan

In general, hospitalized patients can be discharged once they are clinically stable with improvement in their symptoms and signs, have shown no progression to cardiac tamponade or constrictive pericarditis, and do not require any further invasive evaluations for more definitive diagnosis, particularly for tuberculosis or malignancy. Appropriate follow-up should be based on the final diagnosis and therapy employed for each individual case. All patients triaged to initial outpatient management should receive follow-up within 1 week to assess their response to conservative NSAID therapy. Patients clearly responding to NSAID therapy should undergo gradual tapering of their NSAID therapy over 2–3 weeks. Patients with clinical worsening of their symptoms or progression of their pericardial process to clinical cardiac tamponade or constrictive pericarditis should be referred for emergent hospitalization and further evaluation with appropriate therapeutic management. Standardized guidelines on the diagnosis and management of pericardial diseases are currently now available.[23]

Patient Educational Materials

Patients diagnosed with acute pericarditis and managed as outpatients or discharged from the hospital with stable disease should not only be given appropriate close follow-up but also should be given appropriate educational materials such as those created by the JAMA patient education series about pericarditis written for patients (Fig. 30-5).

Table 30-3 Barcelona Experience Evaluation Protocol in Acute Pericarditis	
Step	**Procedures**
I	General clinical and laboratory evaluation, including ECG, CXR, and ECHO. For persistent illness >1 week, a specific etiologic search recommended.
II	Pericardiocentesis performed for patients with tamponade, suspected purulent pericarditis, or clinical activity with pericardial effusion lasting >1 week after NSAID treatment. Appropriate pericardial fluid studies were performed according to laboratory availability.
III	Pericardial biopsy was performed if the illness lasted >3 weeks without an apparent etiologic diagnosis.
IV	Empiric antituberculous therapy was instituted if the diagnosis was not established by the above procedures.

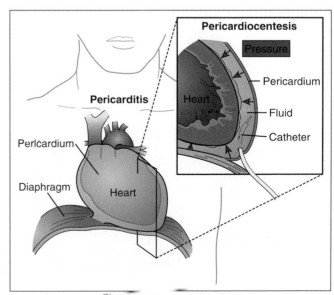

Figure 30-5 • Pericarditis.
From: Patient Education Page. JAMA 2003; 289(9):1194.

Key Points

- The diagnosis of acute pericarditis is purely clinical. It requires that the patient exhibit at least two out of three criteria that include: a classic history of pericardial pain, physical examination revealing a pericardial friction rub, and/or the classic ECG.

- Most cases of acute pericarditis are associated with a "superficial myocarditis," and the presence of abnormal serum cardiac troponins is not uncommon and may lead to confusion in the diagnosis.

- Patients with acute pericarditis can be managed conservatively without hospitalization if they do not have any poor prognostic predictors (fever >38°C, subacute onset, immunosuppressed, related to trauma, use of oral anticoagulants, myopericarditis, severe pericardial effusion, cardiac tamponade) or have not had a precipitating acute MI related pericarditis, or represent a case of either uremic or suspected purulent pericarditis since these conditions require emergent hospitalization for more specialized evaluation and treatment.

- Hospitalized patients should be started on empiric NSAID therapy with a focus on more intensive and invasive etiologic evaluation as needed.

- Currently accepted clinical indications for performing acute pericardiocentesis in acute pericarditis include patients with clinical tamponade, high suspicion for purulent pericarditis, suspicion for neoplastic pericarditis, and large and/or symptomatic pericardial effusion not responding to treatment after one week

SUGGESTED READING

Imazio M, Demichelis B, Parrini I, et al. Day-hospital treatment of acute pericarditis: a management program for outpatient therapy. J Am Coll Cardiol 2004; 43(6):1042–1046.

Troughton RW, Asher CR, Klein AL. Pericarditis. Lancet 2004; 363:717–727.

Imazio M, Demichelis B, Cecchi E, et al. Cardiac troponin I in acute pericarditis. J Am Coll Cardiol 2003; 42(12):2144–2148.

Maisch B. Pericardial diseases, with a focus on etiology, pathogenesis, pathophysiology, new diagnostic imaging methods, and treatment. Curr Opin Cardiol 1994; 9:379–388.

Imazio M, Trinchero R. Clinical management of acute pericardial disease: a review of results and outcomes. Ital Heart J 2004; 5:803–817.

Maisch B, Seferovic PM, Ristic AD, et al. Task Force on the Diagnosis and Management of Pricardial Diseases of the European Society of Cardiology: Guidelines on the diagnosis and management of pericardial diseases executive summary: The Task force on the diagnosis and management of pericardial diseases of the European Society of cardiology. Eur Heart J 2004; 25:587–610.

CHAPTER THIRTY-ONE

Peripheral Arterial Disease (PAD)

Henna Kalsi, MD, RVT, RPVI and John R. Bartholomew, MD

BACKGROUND

Peripheral arterial disease (PAD) refers to lower extremity arterial disease, causing substantial morbidity and mortality in our aging population. Atherosclerosis of the aorta, iliac, or femoral and tibial arteries is the most common cause of PAD. The main symptom of PAD, intermittent claudication, is defined as a cramping or tightness in the leg that occurs with fixed distances of walking. It is important to recognize, however, that the majority of patients with PAD have no symptoms of their disease.

Patients with PAD can also present with acute limb ischemia (ALI) or chronic limb ischemia (CLI). In ALI, there is a sudden decrease in limb perfusion often threatening limb viability, while in CLI patients may complain of rest pain, or present with tissue loss (ischemic ulcers, fissures or gangrene).[1]

Patients with PAD are at high risk for cardiovascular ischemic events including angina, myocardial infarction (MI), arrhythmias, stroke (CVA), and death. While loss of limb is uncommon, quality of life is profoundly affected. It is important for physicians to identify this high-risk population in order to pursue risk-factor modification and lifestyle interventions aggressively in an attempt to reduce adverse cardiovascular events and associated symptomatology.

ASSESSMENT

Clinical Presentation

Prevalence of Peripheral Arterial Disease

PAD affects 8–12 million individuals in the United States, and the prevalence of intermittent claudication (more common in individuals over 70 years of age) reportedly ranges from 1.8–7% of the population.[2–5] For every patient diagnosed with intermittent claudication, there are another three who do not complain of or recognize the symptoms.[1] Data from the PARTNERS program-PAD Awareness, Risk and Treatment: New Resources for Survival found higher rates than previously reported, with PAD found in 29% of high-risk patients (individuals age 70 or older or aged 50–64 years with a history of smoking or diabetes mellitus).[6] The ADI was calculated by the ratio of the systolic blood pressure measured at the ankle compared to the systolic pressure at the

brachial artery, and ABIs <0.9 (normal is ≥0.9) identified patients with PAD.

PAD is not a benign condition. In the Framingham Heart Study, the average annual mortality for men with intermittent claudication was 39 per 1,000 compared to 10 individuals per 1,000 without claudication.[7] Patients with severe and symptomatic large-vessel PAD have a 15-fold increase in rates of mortality due to cardiovascular disease and coronary heart disease. The presence of PAD is also associated with increased morbidity and mortality among older hypertensive adults and women with osteoporosis and PAD.[8–10]

Presenting Signs and Symptoms of Peripheral Arterial Disease

Patients with intermittent claudication complain of an aching or cramping pain, or fatigue or weakness in the leg while walking (Fig. 31-1). Their walking distance seldom varies from day to day, and simply stopping their walk (or slowing the pace) relieves the pain. Intermittent claudication is usually felt in the calves and results from arterial occlusive disease of the femoral, popliteal, or tibial arteries, but it may also be located in the buttocks, hips, or thighs due to aortoiliac disease. Many patients do not report their symptoms to their physician. They may assume their discomfort is part of growing old or related to their job or lifestyle.

Patients presenting with ALI mainly complain of sudden and severe pain. This is normally located in the forefoot, but may extend into the ankle or calf. The most common cause of ALI is an embolus, usually from a cardiac source in an individual with a recent MI or atrial fibrillation. Patients with acute embolic occlusion often have no prior symptoms of intermittent claudication. A less common cause for ALI is thrombosis *in situ*. This develops in patients with preexisting native arterial occlusive disease or in individuals with a history of a previous bypass surgical graft or an endovascular procedure. Symptoms resulting from thrombosis *in situ* are typically less dramatic because patients have already developed a collateral blood supply.

CLI in patients with significant underlying arterial disease results in breakdown of their skin or progresses to rest pain. This

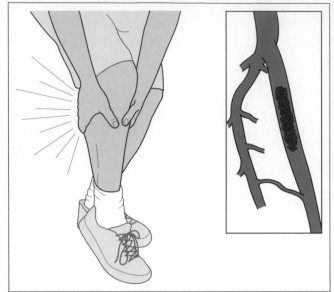

Figure 31-1 • Typical calf pain that is seen in an individual with intermittent claudication.

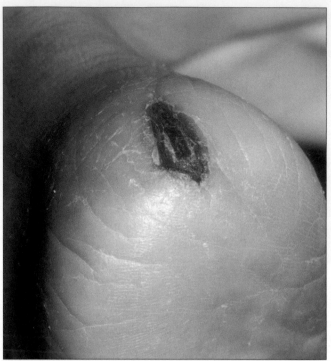

Figure 31-2 • A heel fissure, usually very painful and often seen in patients with PAD following minor trauma.

type of pain occurs in the foot and toes, and is aggravated by elevating the limb while relieved by placing the foot in a dependent position. Rest pain is usually worse at night, forcing the patient to sleep in a chair or bed with his or her leg hanging over the side.

Physical Examination in Peripheral Arterial Disease

The physical examination should include measurement of the blood pressure in both arms; auscultation for a heart murmur and for carotid, abdominal aorta, or ileofemoral artery bruits. Evaluation of the abdomen and legs looking for abdominal or popliteal artery aneurysms should also be performed as well as palpation of the femoral, popliteal, dorsalis pedis, and posterior tibial arteries. Of note, while vascular laboratory personnel have sufficient diagnostic precision in palpating peripheral pulses, generalist physicians have fair to poor agreement, and vascular surgeons appear to be better but also have variable agreement in studies. A handheld Doppler should be used if you cannot palpate the pulses, and it markedly increases diagnostic precision. Patients with intermittent claudication may have a normal physical examination, or diminished or absent pulses (Table 31-1). Approximately 10% of the normal population will not have palpable pedal pulses, and in those individuals, an anterior tibial pulse should be sought.

Poor skin condition, a lack of hair growth over the leg, thickened nails, and cold hands and feet are often considered signs of PAD. These are not reliable findings. However, other clues such as tendinous and tuberous xanthomas or xanthelasma of the eyelids are more predictive of PAD.

In ALI, pulses are generally absent; and the limb may be cold, mottled, and paralyzed. The contralateral extremity is often normal if the ALI is due to an embolism, while in patients with thrombosis *in situ*, pulses in both legs are generally diminished.

Table 31-1 The Pulse Examination in Patients with PAD

Palpable Pulse	Grade
Absent	0
Diminished	1
Normal	2

Management of peripheral arterial disease (PAD). (From: Trans Atlantic Inter-Society Consensus (TASC). J Vasc Surg 2000; 31: S54–S122.)

Box 31-1 The Six P's

Pain

Pulselessness

Pallor

Poikilothermia

Paresthesias

Paralysis

An important concept to remember in the examination of the patient with ALI is the six P's (Box 31-1).

Patients with CLI often have cyanosis of the toes or painful ischemic ulcers or fissures over areas exposed to pressure (Figs. 31-2 and 31-3), These are usually found on the distal portions of the toes, and around nail beds and bony prominences. Minor

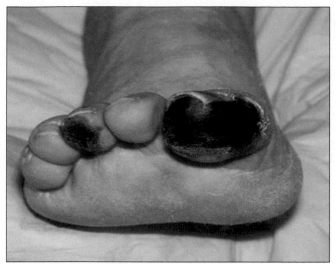

Figure 31-3 • Gangrenous changes of the toe in a patient with long-standing chronic limb ischemia.

episodes of trauma or ill-fitting shoes aggravate this condition. Ulcers are usually small and shallow with a gray, yellow, or black base. Granulation tissue is absent, and secondary infection may be present. A swollen leg is not an uncommon finding and results from placing the leg in a dependent position over an extended period of time to relieve rest pain.

Differential Diagnosis of Peripheral Arterial Disease

Several key principles help differentiate intermittent claudication from other causes of leg pain, in particular pseudoclaudication due to lumbar canal stenosis. Individuals with pseudoclau-

dication report that their walking distance to discomfort varies from day to day, and often complain of pain with sitting, standing, or lying in bed. They also must sit or lie down to get relief of their symptoms. With intermittent claudication from PAD, standing still for several minutes provides relief. A more detailed differential diagnosis of intermittent claudication is found in Table 31-2, and different causes for ALI and CLI are listed in Table 31-3.

DIAGNOSIS

Preferred Diagnostic Studies in Patients with Suspected Peripheral Arterial Disease

The ABI is one the most useful noninvasive tests to confirm the diagnosis of PAD. It objectively confirms or rules out the existence of hemodynamically significant occlusive arterial disease and provides a rough measure of the severity of PAD. It also aids in the differential diagnosis and can detect lesser disease in the contralateral leg, which may not be suspected.[1] Table 31-4 demonstrates the relationship of the resting ABI to the severity of PAD.

Pulse volume recordings (PVR) and segmental plethysmography are additional helpful physiologic tests. Doppler pressure measurements and plethysmographic waveforms are obtained at the arm, thigh, calf, ankle, transmetatarsal, and toes. Differences in the pressure at these levels are considered significant if a drop of >20 mm Hg is identified. Waveform analysis is particularly helpful in the diabetic patient with calcified arteries whose pressure readings may be falsely elevated. These methods accurately detect and localize hemodynamically significant large vessel occlusive disease. A treadmill exercise test can determine the

---

Table 31-2 Differential Diagnosis for Intermittent Claudication

Clinical Disorder	Location of Pain	Key Findings
Intermittent claudication	Calf, thigh, buttocks; depends on area involved	Cramping or tightness with walking, reproducible, relieved with rest
Pseudoclaudication	Radiation along the course of a nerve root, buttocks, hip, or thigh	Sharp, radiating discomfort occurs while standing, sitting, or walking. Associated with parasthesias. Discomfort varies from day to day, relieved with change in position, but usually requires the individual sit down. Common with back problems.
Venous claudication	Thigh or calf pain	
Baker's cyst	Behind the knee	Pain after exercise with slow relief, tight or bursting pain
Hip arthritis	Hip, thigh, buttocks	Pain at rest common; swelling and tenderness often present
Deep vein thrombosis	Groin, thigh, or calf	Aching pain worse with activity, usually relieved with sitting, but may occur at rest
Buerger's disease	Toes and feet	Diffuse pain, leg is swollen, pain at rest Distal extremity ischemia in hands or feet; smokers, ulcers, and foot claudication
Popliteal artery entrapment syndrome or cystic adventitial disease	Calf	Pain after severe exertion, usually younger male athletes, with nontraditional risk factors

Table 31-3 Etiologies for Limb Ischemia

Atherosclerotic Patient	Nonatherosclerotic Patient
Atheroembolism	Hypercoagulable state (antiphospholipid antibody syndrome, Heparin-induced thrombocytopenia)
Thrombosed or stenosed artery (superficial femoral artery)	Vasculitis: giant cell arteritis, Takayasu's arteritis, thromboangiitis obliterans
Thrombosed aneurysm (popliteal artery)	Trauma
Thrombosed bypass graft or previous endovascular procedure	Cystic adventitial disease Popliteal artery entrapment syndrome
Dissection	Drugs: ergotamines, cocaine
Embolism (heart, aneurysm, plaque)	Embolism: heart, paradoxical embolism Aneurysm

HIT—heparin induced thrombocytopenia
From: Management of peripheral arterial disease (PAD). Trans Atlantic Inter-Society Consensus (TASC). J Vasc Surg 2000; 31: S54–S122.

Table 31-4 Relationship of Resting Ankle-Brachial Index (ABI) to Severity of Disease

Highest Ankle Pressure (Dorsalis Pedis versus Posterior Tibialis Arteries) ABI = Highest Arm Pressure (Left versus Right Brachial Arteries)

ABI	Severity of Disease
0.9–1.0	Normal
0.7–0.89	Mild disease
0.4–0.69	Moderate disease
0.0–0.39	Severe disease

degree of intermittent claudication, and it can exclude other causes for limb pain when a strong clinical suspicion for PAD exists in a patient with a normal resting ABI.

Alternative Diagnostic Options for Patients with Suspected Peripheral Arterial Disease

Arteriography is still considered the gold standard for diagnosing PAD, but it should only be considered in the patient with life style-limiting intermittent claudication or in the individual with ALI or CLI where surgery or endovascular intervention is planned. Full arteriography using digital subtraction angiography remains the procedure of choice.

Arterial duplex ultrasonography, a noninvasive modality, can detect stenoses and occlusions, and alterations in the Doppler waveform and peak systolic velocities help determine the degree of stenosis, or if a complete arterial occlusion is present.

Magnetic resonance angiography (MRA) is gaining support for the assessment of PAD. It is especially useful in the patient at risk for contrast-induced renal failure who would normally require conventional arteriography. At the present time, it does not distinguish well between tight stenosis and occlusion, often overestimating the severity of disease. MRA is useful for aortoiliac disease, and several studies demonstrated its usefulness for identifying tibial vessels as potential sites for bypass surgery. MRA is limited by motion artifact and cannot be performed in patients with pacemakers, aneurysm clips, or metallic implants. Endovascular stents are MR compatible.

CT angiography is also being used for the noninvasive evaluation of aortoiliac disease. Similar to arteriography, patients are at risk for contrast-induced renal failure. Large-scale trials are needed to evaluate this technique further for this indication.

Supportive Tests in Patients with Peripheral Arterial Disease

About one third of patients with PAD have clinically significant coronary artery disease. Therefore, all patients should have a baseline ECG, and a stress test may be indicated in select individuals.[1,11] A carotid duplex should be performed if the patient has a carotid bruit or symptoms suggestive of a TIA or a history of stroke, and an ultrasound of the abdominal aorta or popliteal arteries should be performed if there is clinical suspicion for an aneurysm. Patients with ALI should also have a creatinine phosphokinase (CPK), their acid-base status assessed, and a two dimensional echocardiogram or transesophageal echocardiogram (TEE) to identify the source of their ischemic event. Heparin-induced thrombocytopenia (HIT) can also present as arterial thrombosis in patients receiving heparin or low-molecular-weight heparin (LMWH) and should be considered in the differential diagnosis of both ALI and CLI. Therefore, antigen testing for HIT may be indicated in select cases.

Other useful tests include a sedimentation rate, fibrinogen, lipoprotein (a), and a fasting plasma homocysteine level and, in select patients, a hypercoagulable profile that includes anticardiolipin antibodies and lupus anticoagulant. These later tests should be considered in evaluating younger patients with premature atherosclerosis who have a strong family history of thrombotic events or in individuals who lack traditional risk factors for atherosclerosis.

Algorithm

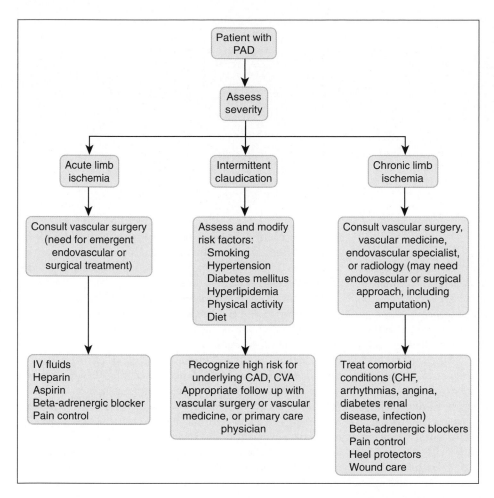

Figure 31-4 • Algorithm for evaluating the patient with PAD.

PAD—peripheral arterial disease; CAD—coronary artery disease; CVA—cerebrovascular accident; CHF—congestive heart failure

Patient with PAD

↓

Assess severity

Acute limb ischemia

Consult vascular surgery (need for emergent endovascular or surgical treatment)

↓

IV fluids
Heparin
Aspirin
Beta-adrenergic blocker
Pain control

Intermittent claudication

Assess and modify risk factors:
  Smoking
  Hypertension
  Diabetes mellitus
  Hyperlipidemia
  Physical activity
  Diet

↓

Recognize high risk for underlying CAD, CVA Appropriate follow up with vascular surgery or vascular medicine, or primary care physician

Chronic limb ischemia

Consult vascular surgery, vascular medicine, endovascular specialist, or radiology (may need endovascular or surgical approach, including amputation)

↓

Treat comorbid conditions (CHF, arrhythmias, angina, diabetes renal disease, infection)
  Beta-adrenergic blockers
  Pain control
  Heel protectors
  Wound care

PROGNOSIS

During Hospitalization

Patients with intermittent claudication should be properly identified, risk factor modification initiated, and appropriate follow-up arranged. Unless there are other related medical problems, they should require no special attention during their hospitalization other than recognition that these individuals have a high incidence of coronary artery and cerebrovascular disease.

If the patient is admitted for a nonvascular-related surgical procedure, a careful history with particular attention to the cardiovascular examination is important. Patients with unstable coronary symptoms, decompensated congestive heart failure (CHF), significant arrhythmias, or severe valvular heart disease require further evaluation and treatment. If the patient has had previous coronary revascularization (CABG or stent) within 5 years or a coronary evaluation within 2 years and has no new cardiac symptoms, he or she is at acceptable risk for surgery. See Chapter 102 for a more detailed description of preoperative assessment of cardiac risk.

The patient presenting with an acutely ischemic limb is at immediate risk for threat to life and limb and requires urgent attention. Clinical categories of ALI are listed in Table 31-5; these are helpful to determine treatment options. These individuals are particularly susceptible to arrhythmias and MI, two processes that contribute to most ALI deaths, and they are also at risk for developing renal failure (due to myoglobinuria or contrast-induced), infection, respiratory failure, and hemorrhagic and thrombotic (HIT) complications from anticoagulation. Reperfusion injury, sensory or motor impairment, and increased signs of ischemia may develop, necessitating fasciotomy and further complicating recovery. Recurrent limb ischemia or death may develop, and the 30-day operative mortality in several recent series ranged from 9.7% to 17%, but may be as high as 42% in the very elderly; almost half of these deaths are attributed to thromboembolic complications.[1,12] It is important to keep in mind the concept that not all limbs are salvageable, and life takes precedence over limb.

Patients with CLI are at risk from complications associated with diagnostic procedures and therapeutic interventions while hospitalized. Their comorbidities (especially diabetes) play an important role in their prognosis, and they are susceptible to many of the same complications listed for the patient with ALI. Amputation rates approach 10–40%, and perioperative mortality as high as 10% is reported for a below-the-knee amputation.[1]

Table 31-5 Clinical Categories of Acute Limb Ischemia (SVS/ISVS Classification)

Category	Prognosis	FINDINGS		DOPPLER SIGNALS	
		Sensory Loss	Motor Loss	Arterial	Venous
I Viable	Not immediately threatened	None	None	Audible	Audible
II Threatened					
A Marginally	Salvageable if or promptly treated.	Minimal (toes) none	None	Often inaudible	Audible
B Immediately	Salvageable with immediate revascularization.	More than toes, with rest pain	Mild, moderate associated	Usually inaudible	Audible
III Irreversible	Major tissue loss or nerve damage	Profound anesthetic	Profound paralysis	Inaudible	Inaudible

From: Management of peripheral arterial disease (PAD). Trans Atlantic Inter-Society Consensus (TASC). J Vasc Surg 2000; 31: S54–S122.

Postdischarge

Appropriate follow-up with a vascular specialist is important to improve outcome for patients with PAD. The majority of individuals (approximately 75%) with intermittent claudication followed over a 5-year period will not experience any change in their condition; however, as many as 25% will note a decline in their walking ability, and 5% will require intervention.[1] Earlier studies noted amputation rates of 5–6.8% over a 5-year period.[5,13] More current data suggest that only 1–2% will require an amputation over this same time frame.[1,14] Although the 5-year mortality rates in patients with intermittent claudication have decreased substantially over the last decade with more aggressive risk factor modification and newer treatments options, coronary artery disease causes most deaths.[8,15]

Long-term prognosis for patients with ALI depends on their immediate surgical outcome and underlying comorbidities. Loss of limb greatly affects lifestyle and longevity. Recurrence of ALI also affects the prognosis. In one study, long-term anticoagulation improved survival and decreased recurrence, largely due to the prevention of additional thromboembolic complications.[16]

The postdischarge prognosis for patients with CLI is usually poor, and approximately 50% of patients will be dead in 1 to 2 years.[1] Five years following a below-the-knee amputation, about 30% of patients will undergo a contralateral amputation, and only 20% will be alive with one intact leg.[1]

MANAGEMENT

Treatment

Preferred

Initial

Inpatient treatment depends on the severity of PAD found and the circumstances of the patient's hospitalization.

Patients with ALI need immediate restoration of blood flow. After initial therapy with intravenous fluids, heparin, aspirin, and pain control, definitive treatment should be undertaken with endovascular procedures such as catheter-directed thrombolysis or mechanical thrombectomy, or surgical embolectomy or revascularization. Definitive intervention should be performed with minimal delay and at least within 6 hours of the patient's initial symptoms. A surgical approach is usually best for embolic ALI, while endovascular therapy may be better for cases of thrombosis *in situ* of native or bypass grafts and when the cause is uncertain.

Individuals with CLI should be stabilized prior to any endovascular or surgical intervention, especially if unstable coronary syndromes, decompensated CHF, significant arrhythmias, or severe valvular heart disease coexist. Treatment of other comorbid conditions, including respiratory problems, associated infection, pain control, and renal function is also important.

The use of heel protectors and proper skin care is vital to prevent the development of, or worsening of, ulcers or fissures due to trauma or pressure. If the limb is potentially salvageable, appropriate imaging should be done to determine if the lesion is anatomically suitable for endovascular or surgical treatment. If an endovascular approach is not feasible, then surgical bypass should be done, depending on the type and location of the lesion. If neither percutaneous nor surgical treatment is possible, then primary amputation should be considered, especially in the patient who has overwhelming infection or pain that is poorly controlled or who is otherwise not a surgical candidate for a more extensive revascularization procedure.

For patients with intermittent claudication that is not lifestyle limiting, a walking exercise program is the primary modality used to improve symptoms, quality of life, and functional capacity. A supervised program (walking at least three to five time per week) is the cornerstone of treatment.[17,18] Patients are advised to walk until they develop moderate leg pain, rest until it subsides, and walk again.

Only two medications available in the United States may be useful for symptomatic relief of intermittent claudication, and both require 2 to 3 months before they are effective. Pentoxifylline (Trental) is a hemorrheologically active agent that reportedly increases red blood cell membrane flexibility and reduces blood viscosity, platelet aggregation, and fibrinogen concentration. Mixed results have been reported in randomized controlled trials, with some patients reporting improved walking distances, while others report little or no benefit.[19,20] Cilostazol (Pletal), a type III phosphodiesterase inhibitor, suppresses platelet aggregation and is a direct vasodilator. It improves maximal and pain-free walking distance as well as increases the quality of life in PAD patients and appears more effective than pentoxifylline at diminishing intermittent claudication.[21,22] Side effects include flatulence, diarrhea, headaches, and palpitations. Cilostazol is contraindicated in patients with CHF.

An indication for a more aggressive treatment approach to intermittent claudication is lifestyle-limiting claudication. Both endovascular and surgical techniques are optional, and patients with aorto-iliac lesions and select patients with femoropopliteal arterial disease appear to be the best candidates.

Alternative Treatment Options

Gene therapy for therapeutic angiogenesis is still mostly a research tool. Though recommended by some physicians, chelation therapy has no proven benefit. Pharmacotherapy including prostanoids (prostacyclin analogs—iloprost and beraprost), vasodilator drugs (papaverine), and L-arginine have met with various degrees of success, but most are not available (only L-arginine in nutritional supplements).[1]

Prevention

Risk Factor Management

Risk factors for PAD are identical to those for MI and cerebrovascular accident (CVA). Aggressive risk-factor modification to control weight and diet, diabetes, hypertension, hyperlipidemia, and smoking cessation is essential. Lifestyle modification is the most important intervention that physicians should prescribe and patients can take. All patients with newly diagnosed PAD should have a complete blood count (CBC), fasting blood sugar, hemoglobin A_1c level, serum creatinine and blood urea nitrogen (BUN), a fasting lipid profile, and a urinalysis. If present, impaired glucose tolerance, hyperhomocystinemia, hyperfibrinogenemia, low high-density lipoprotein (HDL), elevated C-reactive protein, and increased lipoprotein(a) need to be addressed in the discharge and follow-up plan.

Appropriate support for smoking cessation and constant encouragement are essential. Attempt behavioral modification counseling and prescribe pharmacotherapy using sustained-release bupropion hydrochloride and nicotine supplements available as gum, respiratory inhalers, nasal spray, or transdermal patches. Blood pressure should be vigorously controlled. The goal for nondiabetic patients is <140/90, and <130/80 is recommended for diabetic patients with PAD.[23] An ACE inhibitor should

be used as a first-line agent (if tolerated), and a beta-blocker should be considered in patients with underlying CAD.[23,24] Diabetic patients are more likely to present with CLI and should be given specific instructions to care for their feet to prevent ulcerations or gangrene. They should also strive to achieve a HbA_1c <6.5. The National Cholesterol Education Program guidelines (NCEP III) should be followed for dyslipidemia management (LDL <100 mg/dL), although recent evidence suggests that the target LDL should be even lower (<70 mg/dL).[25] A statin should be considered in all patients with PAD, regardless of their lipid values as confirmed by the British heart protection study.[26] Antiplatelet agents are recommended for all PAD patients, barring a contraindication to their use. Aspirin (81–325 mg daily) or clopidogrel (75 mg/day) could be used. In the Antithrombotic Trialists' Collaboration, antiplatelet therapy demonstrated a 23% reduction in vascular events in patients with intermittent claudication and lower extremity revascularization.[27] The CAPRIE trial (Clopidogrel Versus Aspirin in Patients at Risk of Ischemic Events study) demonstrated a significant relative risk reduction for combined cardiovascular outcomes in PAD patients taking clopidogrel versus those taking aspirin.[28] Whether clopidogrel should be the first-line therapy in all patients requires confirmation from additional studies.

DISCHARGE/FOLLOW-UP PLANS

Patient Education

The importance of patient education cannot be overemphasized. Patient compliance is essential. Guidelines listed in Table 31-6 should be given to all patients.

Outpatient Physician Communication

Aggressive risk factor modifications should be emphasized to the outpatient physician. Overall patient assessment including diagnostic test results and interventions performed during hospitalization should be communicated to assure appropriate follow-up.

For more in-depth information, we recommend Trans Atlantic Inter-Society Consensus (http://www.tasc-pad.org/html/index.html).[1]

Table 31-6 Patient Care Guidelines for PAD

Stop smoking	Behavior modification options Tobacco dependence pharmacotherapy: gum, nasal spray, transdermal patches, respiratory inhalers, or sustained-release bupropion hydrochloride
Diet control	Follow American Heart Association diet Weight maintenance (or loss)
Control high blood pressure	Take medications as prescribed ACE inhibitor, beta-blocker for CAD
Control diabetes mellitus	Maintain hemoglobin A_1c under 6.5, follow an appropriate diabetic diet
Know your cholesterol	LDL should be under 100 mg/dL, ideally 70 mg/dL Check liver function tests if on statin at baseline, then at 12 weeks and then annually
Care of your feet	Keep feet clean, trim toenails Break in new shoes slowly
Exercise therapy	30 minute at least three times per week

Key Points

- PAD increases with age and affects about 20% of individuals older than 55 years and up to 50% of elderly people with a history of smoking and diabetes mellitus. However, approximately half of all people with PAD are asymptomatic.

- Patients with PAD have an increased risk of mortality from cardiovascular disease, and those requiring surgery for non-vascular reasons are at increased risk for a cardiovascular event.

- Patients with PAD may have a normal physical examination or diminished or absent pulses. The findings of thickened nails, a lack of hair growth over the leg, or cold feet are not reliable signs of PAD. Use of a handheld Doppler has good diagnostic accuracy for detecting lower extremity peripheral arterial disease.

- Intermittent claudication must be differentiated from pseudo-claudication, due to lumbar canal stenosis. Individuals with intermittent claudication have symptoms only with walking, whereas the patient with pseudoclaudication often reports discomfort with standing, sitting, or lying in bed.

- The first test to perform in patients with suspected PAD is the ABI.

- A walking exercise program is the first line of treatment advised to patients with PAD who do not have lifestyle-limiting intermittent claudication, rest pain, or ischemic ulcers.

SUGGESTED READING

Khan NA, Rahim SA, Anand SS, et al. Does the clinical examination predict lower extremity peripheral arterial disease? JAMA 2006; 295:536–546.

Hankey GJ, Norman PE, Eikelboom. Medical treatment of peripheral arterial disease. JAMA 2006; 295:547–553.

Hiatt WR. Medical treatment of peripheral arterial disease and claudication. N Engl J Med 2001; 344:1608–1621.

Intermittent claudication in Transatlantic Inter-Society Consensus (TASC). Management of peripheral arterial disease. J Vasc Surg 2000; 31:S54–S122.

Ouriel K. Peripheral arterial disease. Lancet 2001; 358:1257–1264.

Pasternak RC, Criqui MH, Benjamin EJ, et al. Atherosclerotic Vascular Disease Conference. Circulation 2004; 109:2605–2612.

Antithrombotic Trialists Collaboration. Collaborative meta-analysis of randomized trials of antiplatelet therapy for prevention of death, myocardial infarction and stroke in high-risk patients. BMJ 2002; 324:71–86.

CHAPTER THIRTY-TWO

Hypertensive Crises

Erica Brownfield, MD, FACP

BACKGROUND

Definitions

Hypertensive crises refer to clinical situations in which the blood pressure is elevated and there is either acute (hypertensive emergencies) or impending end-organ damage (hypertensive urgencies). *Hypertensive emergencies* are severe elevations in blood pressure (no specific level criterion) that are complicated by acute end-organ damage and require immediate lowering of blood pressure to limit further damage.[1] Examples of end-organ damage include hypertensive encephalopathy, intracranial hemorrhage, cerebrovascular accident, acute myocardial infarction, unstable angina pectoris, dissecting aneurysm, acute left ventricular failure with pulmonary edema, acute renal failure, eclampsia, and microangiopathic hemolytic anemia. *Hypertensive urgencies* are less well defined as severe elevations in blood pressure with impending (but not acute) end-organ damage.[2] Examples include papilledema, shortness of breath, and pedal edema. Historically, hypertensive urgencies have been defined as diastolic blood pressures ≥120 mm Hg. It is important to remember, however, that the absolute blood pressure is not as critical as the degree and rate of increase from baseline blood pressure in determining what is or is not a hypertensive urgency. Someone with chronic severely elevated blood pressure (i.e., diastolic BP >120 mm Hg) who has chronic shortness of breath and pedal edema is less likely to be classified as having a hypertensive urgency, versus a patient with the acute onset of shortness of breath and pedal edema and with the same blood pressure but increased from a baseline in the normal range.

Epidemiology

Although approximately 60 million Americans have hypertension, only 1% develop hypertensive crises.[3] The typical patient who presents with a hypertensive crisis is 40–50 years of age, male, noncompliant with hypertensive therapy, lacks primary care, and uses illicit substances and/or alcohol.[4] Any disorder that causes hypertension can give rise to a hypertensive crisis, but the most common cause is poorly controlled essential hypertension. Other etiologies include medications and antihypertensive withdrawal syndromes, illicit drugs, renal and pregnancy-related diseases, vasculitis, postoperative hypertension, coarctation of the aorta, burns, and pheochromocytoma.

PATHOPHYSIOLOGY

The pathophysiology of hypertensive crises is not completely understood. With mild-to-moderate elevations in blood pressure, arterial and arteriolar vasoconstriction initially maintains tissue perfusion while preventing increased pressure from being transmitted to more distal vessels. With severe elevations in blood pressure (i.e., >180/110 mm Hg), this autoregulation fails, and increased pressure in capillaries leads to endothelial damage of the vascular wall, causing fibrinoid necrosis and perivascular edema. Fibrinoid necrosis obliterates the vascular lumen, resulting in organ damage.[5]

ASSESSMENT

Clinical Presentation

A hypertensive crisis should be considered in any and all patients who present with severely elevated blood pressure (usually >180/110 mm Hg), regardless of symptoms. Although patients who present with a hypertensive emergency may have more signs and symptoms than those with a hypertensive urgency (which is usually asymptomatic), a quick and focused, yet thorough evaluation is critical in establishing a diagnosis and initiating therapy.

History

A brief and focused history should address the presence of end-organ damage, the circumstances surrounding the hypertension, and any identifiable etiology (Box 32-1). One should address the duration as well as the severity of hypertension, all current medications including prescription and nonprescription drugs, the use of recreational drugs, and compliance with current antihypertensive therapy. A history of medical problems, specifically cardiovascular and renal disease, and date of last menstrual period in women is essential. Finally, the presence and duration of current symptoms, if any, are important. Although common symptoms of hypertensive crises include headache, blurry vision, and chest pain, the presence of any of these does not

Box 32-1 Targeted Historical Questions in Hypertensive Crises

Presence of neurologic or cardiovascular symptoms

Blurry vision

Sensory paresthesias, motor weakness

Confusion

Somnolence

Chest pain

Dyspnea

History of hypertension and antihypertensive therapies

History of illicit drug use

Any past medical history

History of noncompliance

Over-the-counter medication use

Last menstrual period in women

Box 32-2 Focused Physical Examination in Hypertensive Crises

CNS

  Focal neurologic findings

  Seizures

  Altered mental status

  Papilledema, hemorrhages, exudates

Cardiovascular

  Evidence of congestive heart failure

    Pulmonary edema

    Extra heart sounds

    Jugular venous distension

    Peripheral edema

  Equal and symmetric blood pressure and pulses bilaterally

  Abdominal masses and bruits

Box 32-3 Initial Laboratory and Other Tests in Hypertensive Crises

Chemistry panel with electrolytes and creatinine

Urinalysis with microscopy

Complete blood count with peripheral smear

Electrocardiogram

Chest radiography when indicated

Head imaging when indicated

Pregnancy test when indicated

Toxicology screen when indicated

Box 32-4 Examples of Hypertensive Emergencies

Ischemic stroke

Intracerebral hemorrhage

Hypertensive encephalopathy

Malignant hypertension

Aortic dissection

Acute coronary syndromes

Acute pulmonary edema

Acute renal failure

Scleroderma crises

Eclampsia

Microangiopathic hemolytic anemia

---

indicate a hypertensive crisis and can be seen with uncontrolled hypertension alone. In addition to asking about these common symptoms, one should ask about other symptoms such as dyspnea, back pain, and confusion.

Physical Examination

The physical examination should focus on the presence of end-organ damage and help with identifying secondary causes of hypertension (Box 32-2). It should begin with an assessment of blood pressure, with an appropriate-size cuff in both upper extremities and in a lower extremity. It is critical to measure blood pressure accurately, because it is common to see recordings of falsely elevated blood pressures from using the wrong technique (i.e., inappropriate small size cuff artificially elevating blood pressure, cuff over clothing, etc). It is helpful to use an organ system–based approach to identify signs of end-organ damage. The examination can aid in determining the degree of involvement of affected organs and provide clues to possible causes of secondary forms of hypertension. A careful cardiovascular, neurologic, and funduscopic examination, as well as checking for abdominal masses and bruits, should be conducted.

Laboratory and Other Studies

Initial studies should be limited and focused on assessing the presence of acute end-organ damage (Box 32-3). They should be performed in an expedited manner. Laboratory studies should include a chemistry panel consisting of electrolytes and creatinine, a urinalysis with microscopic examination of sediment, and a complete blood count with a peripheral smear. Additional laboratory studies including a toxicology screen and pregnancy test may be considered when appropriate. An electrocardiogram should be performed to assess for evidence of ischemia or infarction. Further studies, including chest and brain imaging (chest x-ray, head or chest CT), should be reserved for those in which the clinical examination suggests acute end-organ damage (i.e., asymmetric blood pressure and pulses, focal neurologic signs, coma).

DIAGNOSIS

Hypertensive Emergency

The diagnosis of *hypertensive emergency* is made when a patient presents with elevated blood pressure and acute end-organ damage (Box 32-4). Although commonly the diastolic blood pressure is >120 mm Hg, the degree of blood pressure elevation is *not* uniformly above a certain level, nor should it be defined by it. It is more important to establish the presence of *acute* end-organ damage in the setting of elevated blood pressure. In determining the acuity of organ damage, it becomes important to know historical data on patients before arriving at the diagnosis of hypertensive emergency. For example, if a patient presents with a diastolic blood pressure of 140 mm Hg and a creatinine of 3.0 mg/dL, but 6 months ago had a creatinine of 2.8 mg/dL, this finding alone is not a hypertensive emergency, but could rather be considered indicative of a hypertensive urgency or uncontrolled severe hypertension. Therefore, it is the responsibility of the treating physician to conduct the investigation necessary to obtain any relevant historical information on patients if possible. Arriving at the correct diagnosis is critical to treatment and prognosis and is also important in terms of cost. Admitting someone to the intensive care unit (ICU) for presumed, but incorrectly diagnosed, hypertensive emergency can lead to unnecessary increased costs.

Hypertensive Urgency

The diagnosis of *hypertensive urgency* is somewhat controversial. Although some use the diastolic blood pressure of ≥120 mm Hg,[2] it is important to make the diagnosis of hypertensive urgency on a case-by-case basis. Many patients with a diastolic blood pressure of 120 mm Hg or greater do not have an *urgent* need to lower blood pressure. A large number of patients with severe hypertension do not have impending target organ damage; rather, they have *chronic severe uncontrolled hypertension*, and they should be classified as such. Making the diagnosis of hypertensive urgency is not as critical as hypertensive emergency, because the management is not that different from chronic severe uncontrolled hypertension.

Prognosis

Patients with long-standing severe uncontrolled hypertension are at continued risk for coronary, cerebrovascular, and renal disease. For those who present with hypertensive emergencies, the approximate 1-, 5-, and 10-year survival rates are 75–85%, 60–70%, and 45–50%, respectively.[6,7] Patients who have renal insufficiency tend to do worse.[8]

MANAGEMENT

Treatment

The treatment of hypertensive crises must balance preventing further end-organ damage while maintaining tissue perfusion.

The initial goal for blood pressure reduction is *not* to obtain a normal blood pressure. Rapid and aggressive reductions in blood pressure can actually induce cerebral, myocardial, or renal ischemia or infarction if the blood pressure falls below the range at which tissue perfusion can be maintained by autoregulation.[9] The treatment of hypertensive crises is dictated by expert consensus rather than by the results of randomized controlled trials. Treating physicians should use effective regimens that are familiar to them and tailored to individual patients. Two questions that should be considered in all patients with hypertensive crises are at what rate and to what extent should the blood pressure be lowered. The answers depend on whether it is a hypertensive emergency or urgency.

HYPERTENSIVE EMERGENCIES

Hypertensive emergencies require immediate lowering of blood pressure. All patients should be admitted to an ICU where continuous arterial blood pressure monitoring can take place. Intravenous medications should be used so that predictable and controlled changes in blood pressure occur. The initial reduction in mean arterial pressure should not exceed 20–25% below the pretreatment blood pressure. A more gradual decrease in blood pressure should be sought over the next 24 hours. Excessively rapid reductions in blood pressure are dangerous and should be avoided. As the signs and symptoms of acute end-organ damage are controlled, parenteral therapy can be gradually weaned, while initiating oral medications. Typically, the initial doses of oral medications should be given before the parenteral therapy is stopped.

Patients who present with an ischemic stroke and marked hypertension represent a notable exception to immediate lowering of blood pressure in a hypertensive emergency. Reductions in blood pressure may adversely affect cerebral autoregulation, causing an expansion of an otherwise small ischemic area. There is no clear evidence to support the use of antihypertensive treatment during an acute stroke in the absence of other concurrent acute end-organ damage. Usually, hypertension associated with an acute stroke will spontaneously return to prestroke levels within several days. Thus, these patients should be allowed to remain hypertensive during the initial 48–72 hours after admission to optimize cerebral perfusion.

There are several parenteral antihypertensive drugs that can be used in hypertensive emergencies (Table 32-1). The choice of drugs varies with the clinical setting and also with the experience of the hospital and physician. Following is an overview of the most commonly used medications, as well as recommended therapies in specific hypertensive emergencies.

Antihypertensive Drugs

Nitroprusside

Nitroprusside is an arteriolar and venous dilator that has an immediate onset (seconds) and disappears within minutes. It is generally safe and very effective, working in a predictable manner. While nitroprusside has been the gold standard for many hypertensive emergencies, there are limitations to its use, including the need for constant monitoring, hypotension, and cyanide toxicity. This toxic risk is increased in patients with underlying renal

Table 32-1 Commonly Used Antihypertensive Drugs in Hypertensive Emergencies

Medication	Initial Dose	Maximum Dose
Nitroprusside	0.25–0.5 mcg/kg/min	8–10 mcg/kg/min
Nitroglycerin	5 mcg/min	100 mcg/min
Esmolol	Bolus: 500 mcg/kg, that can be repeated after 5 min	
	Infusion: 50–100 mcg/kg/min	300 mcg/kg/min
Labetalol	Bolus: 20 mg bolus, followed by 20–80 mg every 10 min	300 mg
	Infusion: 0.5–2mg/min	
Enalaprilat	1.25 mg every 6 hr	
Fenoldopam	0.1 mcg/kg/min titrated every 15 min	
Hydralazine	10 mg every 20–30 min	20 mg
Nicardipine	5 mg/hr	15 mg/hr
Phentolamine	5–10 mg every 5–15 min	

insufficiency and with use for more than 24–48 hours. There is a potential risk in cases of cardiac ischemia that nitroprusside causes "coronary steal," shunting blood away from ischemic areas.[10] Thus, nitroprusside should be avoided if possible in patients with cardiac ischemia. Nitroprusside should also be avoided in pregnant women, because it is teratogenic. The initial starting dose is 0.25–0.5 mcg/kg per minute; maximum dose is 8–10 mcg/kg per minute, but this high of a dose should be limited to a short period of time due to the increased risk of toxic metabolite (thiocyanate and cyanide) accumulation.

Nitroglycerin

Nitroglycerin is predominately a venodilator yielding arteriolar dilation with increased doses. It also has a quick onset, with effects lasting only minutes. Nitroglycerin is perhaps most effective in those patients with acute coronary syndromes and in those with hypertension following coronary bypass surgery. The initial dose is 5 mcg/min; maximum dose is 100 mcg/min. The main side effects of nitroglycerin include headache, tachycardia, and tachyphylaxis—increasing dosages will be necessary over time to sustain the same effect.

Esmolol

Esmolol is a cardioselective beta-blocker with a short half-life (9 minutes) and a relatively short duration of action (30 minutes). It has almost immediate onset of action, decreasing heart rate in addition to blood pressure. The main potential side effects are hypotension and bronchospasm. Esmolol can be administered as a 500 mcg/kg bolus injection, which may be repeated after 5 minutes. Alternatively, an infusion of 50–100 mcg/kg/min may also be initiated and increased to 300 mcg/kg/min as needed.

Labetalol

Labetalol is an alpha- and beta-adrenergic blocker with a rapid onset (5 minutes). It does not directly affect cerebral blood flow.

Labetalol can be given as a bolus (20 mg initially, followed by 20–80 mg every 10 minutes to a total dose of 300 mg) or as an infusion (0.5–2 mg/minute). The main side effects of labetalol include hypotension, heart block, and bronchospasm.

Enalaprilat

Enalaprilat is an intravenous form of enalapril. Although it has few side effects, the response to enalaprilat is unpredictable. Enalaprilat should be used with caution in patients who are hypovolemic and should be avoided in pregnant women. The initial dose is 1.25 mg, followed by up to 5 mg every 6 hours as necessary. The onset of action is usually 15 minutes, with the peak effect sometimes not observed for hours.

Fenoldopam

Fenoldopam is a peripheral dopamine-1 receptor agonist. It causes peripheral vasodilatation while maintaining or increasing renal perfusion. Fenoldopam is equivalent to nitroprusside in its ability to lower blood pressure. It is most effective during the first 48 hours of treatment. It can be used safely in all hypertensive emergencies and may be most beneficial in patients with renal insufficiency. The initial starting dose is 0.1 mcg/kg per minute; the dose can be titrated at 15-minute intervals. Many hospitals do not have fenoldopam on formulary because it is much more expensive than older medications such as nitroprusside. Fenoldopam is contraindicated in patients with glaucoma.

Hydralazine

Hydralazine is an arterial vasodilator that causes unpredictable hypotension and reflex tachycardia. It has prolonged effects and should be primarily limited to pregnant women, because it increases uterine blood flow. Hydralazine is given as a 10-mg bolus, with the maximum dose being 20 mg.

Nicardipine

Nicardipine is a dihydropyridine calcium channel blocker that is as effective as nitroprusside in lowering blood pressure. It is given as an intravenous infusion with an initial dose of 5 mg/hr and can be increased to a maximum of 15 mg/hr. It may potentially have favorable effects in patients with cardiac and cerebral ischemia by relaxing coronary smooth muscle and increasing vasodilatation, respectively. Nicardipine has a longer half-life than nitroprusside; therefore, rapid titration is not usually possible.

Phentolamine

Phentolamine is an alpha-adrenergic blocker that should be restricted to hypertensive emergencies induced by catecholamine excess (i.e., pheochromocytoma, tyramine ingestion in a patient on monoamine oxidase inhibitors). Phentolamine can cause angina and arrhythmias. When used, phentolamine is given as a 5- to 10-mg bolus every 5–15 minutes.

Treatment of Specific Hypertensive Emergencies

Aortic Dissection

Optimal drugs to treat a dissection are those that decrease not only mean arterial blood pressure, but also the rate at which blood pressure increases (dp/dt). This is usually achieved by the combination of nitroprusside and an intravenous beta-blocker such as esmolol or labetalol. Nitroprusside should not be given alone.

Acute Coronary Syndromes

Cardiac ischemia or infarction commonly increases the systemic blood pressure. Intravenous parenteral vasodilators, such as nitroglycerin, are effective. Beta-blockers are also beneficial in hypertensive patients with acute coronary syndromes. One should be careful in using nitroglycerin and beta-blockers in those patients with posterior wall or right ventricle ischemia (e.g., inferior myocardial infarction), as these patients are preload and volume dependent. Drugs that increase cardiac work (hydralazine) should be avoided.

Acute Pulmonary Edema

Patients with acute pulmonary edema and hypertension should be treated with vasodilators (nitroprusside or nitroglycerin) and loop diuretics. Enalaprilat is an alternative treatment. Beta-blockers should be used with caution, if at all.

Acute Renal Failure

In patients with hypertension and acute renal failure, choices of therapy include fenoldopam, nicardipine, and beta-blockers. The use of nitroprusside should be limited to a brief period (i.e., <24 hours), because its toxic metabolite, thiocyanate, can accumulate.

Ischemic Stroke

There is no proven benefit from rapid reduction of blood pressure in patients with an acute ischemic stroke. Antihypertensive treatment may adversely affect cerebral autoregulation in acute stroke. Most patients presenting with this scenario have increased blood pressure that gradually returns toward baseline after the event. Therapy should be individualized and generally initiated only if other acute end-organ damage is present.

Intracerebral Hemorrhage

Recent animal evidence suggests that modest control of blood pressure after intracerebral hemorrhage is probably safe.[11] Since hypertension after intracerebral hemorrhage may be self-limiting, delayed hypotension can occur with oral antihypertensive medications. Therefore, if parenteral medications are used to lower pressure initially, oral antihypertensives should be avoided until baseline blood pressure is determined posthemorrhage. Theoretically, beta-blockers, nicardipine, labetalol, and enalaprilat are ideal choices since they have little effect on intracranial pressure. Nitroprusside and nitroglycerin should be avoided, because they cause cerebral venodilation.[12]

Pregnancy

In pregnant women with severe hypertension (preeclampsia, eclampsia), intravenous hydralazine is the treatment of choice because it increases uterine blood flow. Beta-blockers and nicardipine can also be used if hydralazine is contraindicated or if the blood pressure response is not optimal.

HYPERTENSIVE URGENCIES

In the past, a relatively rapid reduction in blood pressure has been recommended.[13] There is no proven benefit, however, from such a rapid reduction in asymptomatic patients who have no evidence of acute target end-organ damage. In fact, a deleterious effect on cerebral, cardiac, and/or renal perfusion can occur with uncontrolled and unpredictable large blood pressure reductions.[14]

How quickly hypertensive urgencies need to be treated is debatable. Individualized decisions need to be made with each patient, taking into consideration the patient's history, degree of compliance, symptoms, and likelihood of target end-organ damage. It is imperative that an accurate blood pressure be recorded and problems of noncompliance and use of illicit drugs be documented. Whether the blood pressure is lowered over hours, days, or weeks is more a matter of preference and comfort among treating physicians and not as a result of outcome data. Since most patients who present with hypertensive urgencies are those who have long-standing uncontrolled severe hypertension, making adjustments to their antihypertensive regimen, or reinitiating therapy in a noncompliant patient, is usually all that is required.

If the decision has been made to acutely decrease blood pressure, the initial goal should be to reduce the blood pressure to a target of 160/110 mm Hg over several hours to days with conventional oral therapy.[15] Allowing the patient rest in a quiet room can also be beneficial. Most patients will require at least two antihypertensive medications. It is important to remember that the benefit seen with many oral medications will not be reflected in blood pressures measured hours to days after beginning a new agent; it will likely require 1 to 2 weeks.

In general, there is no need to hospitalize patients with hypertensive urgencies.[16] Ongoing outpatient management of blood pressure is necessary, however, to gradually return blood pressure to a normal and safe level and to decrease complications.

DISCHARGE/FOLLOW-UP PLANS

A normal blood pressure should *not* be the discharge goal of patients admitted with hypertensive emergencies. Aiming for a diastolic blood pressure of 100–110 at discharge may be reasonable. Patient education is critical in helping to prevent future hypertensive crises and in managing blood pressure in general. Stressing compliance with diet, weight reduction if necessary, avoidance of illicit drugs and other substances (i.e., sympathomimetics), and adherence to antihypertensive therapy is important. Consultation with a dietician prior to discharge may enhance compliance with a low-salt diet. Scheduling a 2-week follow up with a primary care physician should be coordinated at the time of discharge. Patients should be instructed to call their doctor or return to seek medical attention if any acute symptoms return or appear.

Key Points

- The absolute blood pressure is not as critical as the degree and rate of increase from baseline blood pressure in determining what is or is not a hypertensive urgency.

- Many patients with a diastolic blood pressure of 120 mm Hg or greater do not have an *urgent* need to lower blood pressure. A large number of patients with severe hypertension do not have impending target organ damage; rather, they have *chronic severe uncontrolled hypertension,* and they should be classified as such.

- The initial goal for blood pressure reduction is *not* to obtain a normal blood pressure; rapid and aggressive reductions in blood pressure can actually induce cerebral, myocardial, or renal ischemia or infarction.

- Patients with hypertensive emergencies require ICU admission and immediate and predictable lowering of blood pressure with IV medications, but the initial reduction in mean arterial pressure should not exceed 20–25% below the pretreatment blood pressure.

- The choice of parenteral antihypertensive drugs varies with the clinical setting and also with the experience of the hospital and physician.

- There is no proven benefit from rapid reduction of blood pressure in patients with an acute ischemic stroke, and this may worsen outcomes.

- A normal blood pressure should *not* be the discharge goal of patients admitted with hypertensive emergencies. Aiming for a diastolic blood pressure of 100–110 at discharge is reasonable.

SUGGESTED READING

Cherney D, Straus S. Management of patients with hypertensive urgencies and emergencies. A systematic review of the literature. *JGIM* 2002; 17:937–945.

Vaughan CJ, Delanty N. Hypertensive emergencies. Lancet 2000; 356:411–417.

Qureshi AI, Wilson DA, Hanley DF, et al. Pharmacologic reduction of mean arterial pressure does not adversely affect regional cerebral blood flow and intracranial pressure in experimental intracerebral hemorrhage. Crit Care Med 1999; 27:965–971.

Manno EM, Atkinson JLD, Fulgham JR, et al. Emerging medical and surgical management strategies in the evaluation and treatment of intracerebral hemorrhage. Mayo Clin Proc 2005; 80(3):420–433.

Chobanian AV, Bakris GL, Black HR, et al. The seventh report of the joint national committee on prevention, detection, evaluation, and treatment of high blood pressure: the JNC 7 report. *JAMA* 2003; 289:2560–2672.

Varon J, Marik PE. The diagnosis and management of hypertensive crises. Chest 2000; 118:214–227.

Section

4 Four

Infectious Diseases

33 Community-Acquired Pneumonia (CAP)
Bradley A. Sharpe, Scott A. Flanders

34 Nosocomial Pneumonia
Scott A. Flanders

35 Urinary Tract Infections
Carol E. Chenoweth, Sanjay Saint

36 Skin and Soft Tissue Infections
Lakshmi K. Halasyamani

37 Acute Bacterial Meningitis
Christopher Kim, James C. Pile

38 Infective Endocarditis
Suzanne F. Bradley

39 Vascular Catheter-Related Infections
Carol E. Chenoweth, Sanjay Saint

40 Septic Arthritis
Vikas I. Parekh, James Riddell IV

41 HIV and AIDS
Daniel R. Kaul, Powel Kazanjian

42 Bioterrorism
James C. Pile

43 Fever in the Hospitalized Patient
Daniel R. Kaul

CHAPTER THIRTY-THREE

Community-Acquired Pneumonia (CAP)

Bradley A. Sharpe, MD, and Scott A. Flanders, MD

BACKGROUND

"Pneumonia may well be called the friend of the aged. Taken off by it in an acute, short, not often painful illness, the old man escapes those 'cold gradations of decay' so distressing of himself and to his friends."

—William Osler, MD, 1898

Community-acquired pneumonia (CAP) continues to be a common and serious illness, causing substantial morbidity and mortality in the adult population. There are an estimated 5–6 million cases a year in the United States, with more than 1 million hospitalizations. Community-acquired pneumonia is one of the most common admitting diagnoses among adults, and with a 30-day mortality between 10 and 14% for patients admitted to the hospital, it is the leading cause of infectious death in the U.S.[1]

Community-acquired pneumonia is a model illness in hospital medicine—it is a common disease that allows for evidence-based and cost-effective management. In addition, many national organizations have proposed multiple quality indicators for community-acquired pneumonia, thus providing an opportunity for institutional quality improvement. This chapter outlines the assessment and management of patients admitted to the hospital with community-acquired pneumonia.

ASSESSMENT

Clinical Presentation

Presenting Signs and Symptoms

Patients admitted to the hospital with CAP typically present with a brief history of respiratory complaints, including cough (>90%), dyspnea (66%), sputum production (66%), and pleuritic chest pain (50%).[2,3] In 10–30% of patients, nonrespiratory complaints can predominate, including headache, myalgias, fatigue, and gastrointestinal symptoms.[4] Elderly patients, an increasing percentage of hospitalized patients, are less likely to present with typical CAP symptoms (such as cough) and more likely to have altered mental status as a presenting symptom.[4]

On physical examination, patients with CAP usually have signs of fever (80%), tachypnea (70%), and tachycardia (50%). Most will have a focal lung examination (>90%) with findings ranging from crackles to bronchial breath sounds.[6] No examination finding is specific for the diagnosis of pneumonia, but the absence of fever, tachycardia, *and* tachypnea significantly reduces the probability of CAP in patients with suspected pneumonia.[6] Furthermore, similar to the clinical history, the physical examination of elderly patients with community-acquired pneumonia is not specific or sensitive for the diagnosis of CAP, as up to 40% of patients will not have fever.[7]

Leukocytosis is common in patients with CAP; however, its absence does not rule out disease.[8] A number of guidelines recommend laboratory evaluation of electrolytes, urea nitrogen, creatinine, liver enzymes, and bilirubin, although these are used primarily for prognostication and are not specifically useful in the diagnosis of CAP.

Differential Diagnosis

Given the nonspecific nature of the symptoms and signs associated with CAP, there is no single clinical feature or combination of clinical features that adequately rules in or out the diagnosis of CAP. Consequently, the differential diagnosis to be considered in patients with suspected CAP is broad. Noninfectious diseases can often present with similar clinical syndromes; these include congestive heart failure, chronic obstructive pulmonary disease (COPD), exacerbation, asthma, pulmonary embolism, and hypersensitivity pneumonitis. These diseases can often be distinguished with a thorough history and physical examination.

Additionally, there are other upper and lower airway infectious diseases that can result in similar nonspecific signs and syndromes. In particular, pneumonia must often be differentiated from acute bronchitis, which as a diagnosis accounts for up to 40% of patients evaluated for cough (vs. 5% for pneumonia). Patients with acute bronchitis frequently do not present with high fevers or hypoxia and in general will not benefit from antibiotic therapy. Patients felt to have CAP might also be suffering from other "pneumonia syndromes," including aspiration pneumonia, postobstructive pneumonia, and pneumonia in immunocompromised patients (e.g., those with HIV, on steroids, chemotherapy, etc.). Determining the correct diagnosis can have implications for therapy and prognosis.

DIAGNOSIS

Preferred Studies

The diagnosis of CAP requires both: (1) the signs and symptoms consistent with pulmonary infection *and* (2) evidence of a new radiographic infiltrate. Therefore, most guidelines recommend that *all* patients with the possible diagnosis of CAP should be evaluated with chest radiography.[9–11]

The specific radiographic findings in CAP range from lobar consolidation to hazy focal infiltrate to diffuse bilateral interstitial opacities (Fig. 33-1). Although chest radiography is the "gold standard" for the diagnosis of CAP, its exact performance characteristics are unknown and it is clearly not 100% sensitive or specific. The utility of the chest radiograph can be limited by patient body habitus, underlying lung disease, or dehydration. Computed tomography (CT) scanning, while not recommended for routine use, can identify pulmonary consolidation in patients with a normal or equivocal chest radiograph in whom pneumonia is suspected.[12] Limitations in the performance of the chest radiograph have resulted in an interest in the diagnostic performance of serologic markers of infection such as C-reactive protein (CRP), procalcitonin, and soluble triggering receptor expressed on myeloid cells (s-TREM). Preliminary evidence suggests that these inflammatory markers may ultimately prove useful in differentiating infectious from noninfectious pulmonary processes, but regular use of these new tests cannot currently be recommended.

Additional diagnostic tests in patients with community-acquired pneumonia are often done to help identify a specific microbiologic agent once the diagnosis of CAP is made; these include blood cultures, sputum Gram stain and culture, and tests directed at particular etiologies, such as the pneumococcal and legionella urinary antigens. Unfortunately, the presenting symptoms, signs, and basic laboratory findings (including the chest radiograph) cannot be reliably used to predict the etiologic pathogen or to distinguish "typical" (e.g., *S. Pneumoniae*, *H. influenzae*, *M. catarrhalis*, etc.) from "atypical" organisms (*Chlamydia* spp., *Mycoplasma pneumoniae*, *Legionella* spp.).

Two sets of blood cultures should be performed *prior to antibiotic administration* in all patients with suspected community-acquired pneumonia.[9–11] It is estimated that blood cultures will be positive for pathogenic organisms in 5–10% of cases and in up to 25% of cases of CAP caused by *S. pneumoniae*. Isolation of bacteria from blood cultures in CAP is a very specific way to identify a causative organism and subsequently narrow therapy. Obtaining blood cultures within 24 hours of admission is associated with 10% lower odds of 30-day mortality in patients with CAP.[13] Moreover, obtaining blood cultures prior to antibiotic administration is a national quality indicator. Blood cultures can also help in prognosis, as bacteremia in CAP is associated with a higher mortality.

Because the sensitivity of blood cultures is generally low for all patients admitted to the hospital with CAP, some groups have argued to obtain blood cultures only in those with severe pneumonia, as they are more likely to be bacteremic. One study risk-stratified patients in a testing algorithm and were able to increase the overall identification of bacteremia with fewer overall cultures.[14] National quality indicators do not currently reflect "targeting" of blood cultures; it remains the standard of care, therefore, to obtain blood cultures prior to antibiotics in all patients with suspected CAP.

Substantial controversy surrounds the utility of routine sputum Gram stain and culture in patients admitted to the hospital with CAP. Sputum collection is a relatively simple and inexpensive procedure that can potentially identify pathogenic organisms and have an impact on both initial and long-term antibiotic therapy. However, sputum samples in general have low sensitivity, specificity, and positive predictive value; for example, the positive predictive value of finding *S. pneumoniae* on sputum Gram stain is only 30–50%.[9] Furthermore, the utility of sputum testing is also limited practically; in one study, 30% of patients could not produce an adequate sputum specimen, and up to 30% had received prior antibiotic therapy, substantially reducing the yield.[15] While the diagnostic performance of sputum analysis is not optimal, the high rate of antibiotic resistance among common community isolates (e.g., *S. pneumoniae*), and the increasing prevalence of infecting organisms not targeted by routine empiric therapy (methicillin-resistant *Staphylococcus aureus*—MRSA) have made isolation of potential causative pathogens increasingly important. Most expert guidelines recommend obtaining sputum for Gram stain and culture *if* the patient is producing purulent sputum *and* has not received prior antibiotic therapy.[9,11] Practically, all experts would agree that specimens must be collected early, must be immediately transported to the laboratory, and should be "good" specimens with >25 polymorphonucleacytes and less than 10 squamous cells per high powered field. Gram stain and culture results should be interpreted in the specific clinical context, and antibiotic choices targeted appropriately.

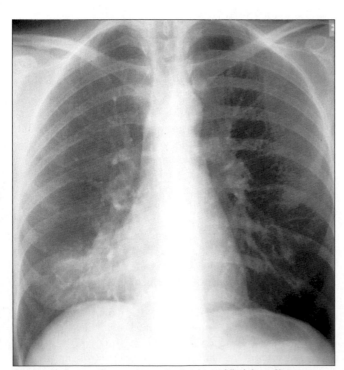

Figure 33-1 • Chest radiograph of right middle lobe infiltrate in a patient with CAP.

Alternative Options

The pneumococcal urinary antigen assay is a relatively sensitive (50–80%) and highly specific (~90%) test for the detection of pneumococcal pneumonia, when compared with conventional diagnostic methods.[16] The test is simple, convenient, rapid (~15 minutes), and, with its high specificity, may allow for more focused antimicrobial therapy early in management. The need to culture an organism to determine antibiotic sensitivities, however, requires that blood and sputum analysis still be performed in addition to urinary antigen testing. For patients with suspected *Legionella* pneumonia (primarily critically ill and immunocompromised patients, or in association with regional outbreaks), the urinary *Legionella* antigen assay is the test of choice, which detects 80–95% of community-acquired cases of Legionnaires' disease with a specificity of 90%.[16] Specific diagnostic tests targeting other organisms, such as *Mycobacterium tuberculosis* or *Pneumocystis jiroreci*, should be employed in the appropriate clinical setting.

PROGNOSIS/ADMISSION DECISION

Once the diagnosis of CAP has been made, the initial site of treatment, whether in the hospital or the home, must be determined. The hospitalization decision should be based on three factors: (1) calculation of the Pneumonia Severity Index (PSI), (2) evaluation of home treatment safety, and (3) physician clinical judgment. The PSI, or Pneumonia Outcomes Research Team (PORT) score, is a validated prediction rule that quantifies mortality and allows for risk stratification of patients with CAP.[1] The PSI combines clinical history, physical examination, and laboratory data at the time of admission to divide patients into five risk classes and to estimate 30-day mortality (Fig. 33-2). Thirty-day mortality ranged from 0.1% in patients in risk class I to 27.0% in risk class V.

Based on the estimated prognosis, in the absence of concerns about home safety or comorbidities, patients in risk classes I, II, and III should be managed at home. Many prospective trials have shown that implementation of PSI significantly increases the number of low-risk patients who are managed outside of the hos-

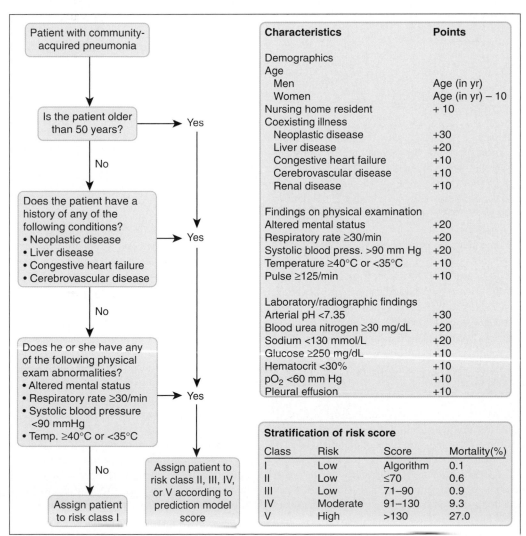

Figure 33-2 • Pneumonia Severity Index (PSI): Validated prediction tool to estimate prognosis and aid in admission decisions in patients with community-acquired pneumonia (CAP). The score is calculated by adding the patient's age (in years for men or in (years—10) for women) plus the points for each applicable characteristic. Adapted from Halm EA, Teirstein AS. Management of community-acquired pneumonia. N Engl J Med 2002; 347(25):2039–2045. With permission. Copyright © 2002. Massachusetts Medical Society. All rights reserved.

Figure 33-3 • A practical decision tree using the PSI to aid in the admission decision. Adapted from Halm EA, Teirstein AS. Management of community-acquired pneumonia. N Engl J Med. 2002; 347(25):2039–2045. With permission. Copyright © Massachusetts Medical Society. All rights reserved.

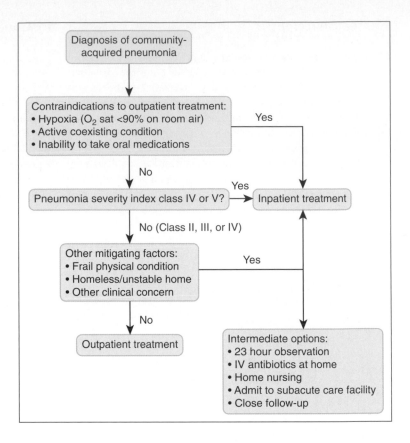

pital with no differences in quality of life, complications, readmissions, or short-term mortality. Most guidelines for the management of CAP recommend utilization of the PSI to help determine the initial site of treatment, with the caveat that using the prediction rule should never supersede clinical judgment in the admission decision.[9–11,16] A practical decision tree for the use of the PSI is shown in Figure 33-3.

There are no reliable prediction rules for deciding on the need for intensive care unit admission. Hemodynamic instability requiring resuscitation and monitoring or respiratory failure requiring ventilatory support are clear indications for ICU admission. Additional variables such as tachypnea (respiratory rate ≥30), altered mental status, multilobar disease, and azotemia are associated with severe CAP and should prompt consideration of ICU admission, especially when two or more variables coexist.[10]

POSTDISCHARGE

The overall 30-day mortality for patients hospitalized with CAP ranges from 5% to 30% and depends on multiple factors, including the severity of the pneumonia and individual patient comorbidities as delineated by the PSI. In elderly patients, hospitalization for CAP portends a poor long-term prognosis. A large, matched case-control study of a Medicare database compared patients hospitalized for pneumonia versus other diagnoses and found the one-year mortality for patients with CAP was nearly 40%, compared to 29% in patients with other diagnoses.[17] The notable high 1-year mortality rates can be important for prognostication, medical decision-making, and counseling patients and families.

MANAGEMENT

Treatment

Initial Treatment

Once the admission decision is made and the initial diagnostic tests are completed (including blood and sputum cultures), patients with presumed CAP should receive necessary supportive care (O_2, intravenous fluids, etc.) and prompt antimicrobial therapy. Antibiotics should be administered within 4 hours of arrival in patients with suspected CAP, as this may be associated with decreased inhospital and 30-day mortality.[18,19] Multiple organizations (JCAHO, Center for Medicare Services [CMS], etc.) have made delivery of antibiotics in less than 4 hours a hospital quality measure.

Despite our diagnostic tests, the specific agent causing CAP remains unknown in up to 75% of patients admitted to the hospital. Therefore, *empiric, broad-spectrum antibiotics targeting the most probable pathogens should be initiated in all patients with suspected CAP.*

Because causative organisms cannot be predicted based on presenting symptoms and signs, empiric antibiotics in patients hospitalized with CAP must be directed at both typical and atypical organisms, and must treat the pathogens that most commonly cause CAP. Table 33-1 shows the most common causative agents in CAP in hospitalized patients divided by severity of illness.[20]

Many national organizations have published guidelines on the empiric treatment of CAP in hospitalized patients.[10,11,16] All guidelines are based on four fundamental treatment principles:

1. Antimicrobial therapy must treat all organisms that typically cause CAP (e.g., cover "typical" and "atypical" organisms).
2. Antibiotic resistance, including emerging drug-resistant *S. pneumoniae*, must be considered in antibiotic selection.
3. Comorbidities and risk factors for specific agents (e.g., *P. aeruginosa*) must be considered.
4. Antibiotic coverage should be narrowed if diagnostic tests yield a specific etiologic agent.

Table 33-2 displays a summary of expert guidelines for the treatment of CAP requiring hospitalization. A typical adult patient without additional risk factors should receive a parenteral extended-spectrum β-lactam plus either doxycycline or an advanced macrolide (*see* Table 33-2). Extended spectrum β-lactams include cefotaxime, ceftriaxone, ampicillin-sulbactam, or ertapenem. Evidence suggests that combining a macrolide with a cephalosporin confers a mortality benefit over a cephalosporin alone.[18] The cause of the mortality benefit is unclear. The benefit may be derived from the "atypical" coverage provided by macrolides, their anti-inflammatory properties, or "double" antibiotic coverage. Adding a second agent to a β-lactam, either doxycycline or a macrolide, remains the standard of care. A respiratory fluoroquinolone as a single agent can be used for patients with CAP without additional risk factors, but this is generally discouraged secondary to concerns about cost and increasing gram-negative rod fluoroquinolone resistance.

Patients hospitalized with severe CAP who require ICU-level care are at increased risk of *Legionella* spp. and drug-resistant *S. pneumoniae*, which must be reflected in their initial antibiotic therapy.[20] Patients with severe pneumonia should receive an intravenous extended-spectrum β-lactam plus either an intravenous macrolide or an intravenous respiratory fluoroquinolone.

All patients with severe CAP who are admitted to the intensive care unit (ICU) should be routinely screened for risk factors for *P. aeruginosa*. The known risk factors for pseudomonas infection are bronchiectasis, immunosuppression including >10 mg/day of prednisone, malnutrition, and treatment with broad-spectrum antibiotics in the last month.[10] Those at risk for *P. aeruginosa* or other resistant gram-negative rod infection should be treated with an antipseudomonal β-lactam plus an antipseudomonal fluoroquinolone. Many patients with severe CAP have risk factors for MRSA infection, including recent prolonged hospitalization, recent broad-spectrum antibiotics, and significant underlying lung disease, which should be considered in choosing initial antibiotic therapy.[21] Additionally, there have been reports of patients *without* underlying risk factors presenting with severe community-acquired MRSA pneumonia. If an institution's rate of methicillin resistance among *S. aureus* community isolates is

Table 33-1 Most Common Pathogens in community-Acquired Pneumonia by Site of Care

Non-ICU inpatients	ICU inpatients (severe)
S. pneumoniae	*S. pneumoniae*
M. pneumoniae	*Legionella* spp
C. pneumoniae	*H. influenzae*
H. influenzae	Gram-negative bacilli
Legionella spp	*S. aureus*
Aspiration	
Respiratory viruses	

From File TM. Community-acquired pneumonia. Lancet 2003; 362:1991–2001.

Table 33-2 Initial Empiric Antimicrobial Therapy in Immunocompetent Patients with Suspected Community-Acquired Pneumonia

Patient Group	Empiric antibiotic therapy
Inpatient, non-ICU	β-lactam[a] + *either* doxycycline *or* an advanced macrolide[b]
Severe β-lactam allergy[c]	Respiratory fluoroquinolone[d]
Inpatient, ICU	
No risk for *Pseudomonas*	β-lactam + *either* an advanced macrolide *or* a respiratory fluoroquinolone
Severe β-lactam allergy	Respiratory fluoroquinolone + clindamycin
Pseudomonas risk factors[e]	Antipseudomonal β-lactam[f] + an antipseudomonal fluoroquinolone[g]
Severe β-lactam allergy	Aztreonam + a respiratory fluoroquinolone
MRSA risk factors[h]	Add vancomycin to above regimens
From nursing home	See Chapter 34, Hospital-Acquired Pneumonia
Aspiration pneumonia	β-lactam or respiratory fluoroquinolone ± clindamycin[i]

a Cefotaxime, ceftriaxone, ampicillin-sulbactam, or ertapenem.

b Azithromycin or clarithromycin.

c Severe β-lactam allergy defined as anaphylactic shock, bronchospasm, and hives.

d Levofloxacin, moxifloxacin, gatifloxacin.

e Risk factors for pseudomonas include severe structural lung disease (e.g., bronchiectasis), broad-spectrum antibiotics or ICU hospitalization in the last 30 days, or immunosuppression (e.g. ≥10 mg/day prednisone).

f Piperacillin, piperacillin-tazobactam, imipenem, meropenem, cefepime.

g Ciprofloxacin.

h Risk factors for methicillin-resistant *Staphylococcus aureus* (MRSA) pneumonia include recent prolonged hospitalization, recent broad-spectrum antibiotics, significant underlying lung disease, and possibly high institutional prevalence of community MRSA isolates.

i If risk factors for anaerobic infection exist: alcoholism, poor dentition, pulmonary abscess, concern for empyema.

high (>15–20%), it may be appropriate to add initial empiric MRSA coverage for patients admitted to the ICU with CAP.[22]

Other patients will have unique risk factors and clinical presentations in which these empiric recommendations may need to be modified. Several studies indicate 5–15% of cases of CAP are aspiration pneumonia. Risk factors for aspiration events are: dysphagia, history of stroke, altered level of consciousness, poor dentition, and tube feeding, among others. Traditionally, aspiration pneumonia was felt to be secondary to oral anaerobes, but recent research suggests that gram-positive cocci and gram-negative rods are the predominant organisms.[23] Antibiotic therapy in patients with clear aspiration pneumonia should be directed at this microbiology with an extended-spectrum β-lactam (e.g., ceftriaxone) or a respiratory fluoroquinolone (e.g., levofloxacin, moxifloxacin, etc.). Anaerobic bacterial coverage can be added in patients with severe periodontal disease, alcoholism, concern for empyema, or evidence of aspiration with pulmonary abscess.[23]

Patients residing in long-term care facilities are at high risk for pneumonia. The microbiology of infections acquired in nursing facilities is similar to that in hospital-acquired cases.[24,25] As a result, patients who develop pneumonia in institutional settings such as nursing homes should be treated with broad-spectrum antibiotics, including coverage for MRSA (*see* Chapter 20 on nosocomial pneumonia for specifics).

Subsequent Treatment

Initial empiric antibiotic treatment should be modified based on the results of diagnostic testing. Although the specific etiologic agent is determined in only 25% of cases of CAP,[18] when it occurs antibiotic coverage should be narrowed to cover that particular organism with an antibiotic with adequate lung penetration. Evidence suggests clinicians often do not adjust or narrow antibiotics based on sensitivity results, potentially breeding resistant organisms.

Patients hospitalized with CAP usually improve quickly if they receive early, appropriate antibiotic therapy and supportive care. Excluding patients with severe CAP requiring intensive care unit admission, most patients resolve their tachycardia, tachypnea, and fever by day 2 or 3.[26] Recent practice experience, evidence, and published guidelines[11,16] all indicate that patients can safely be transitioned to oral antibiotics therapy earlier in their hospital course. Box 33-1 outlines criteria that can be used to identify patients who have had an adequate response to parenteral therapy and can be considered for a switch to oral antibiotics. If these criteria are met, patients have <1% chance of clinical deterioration necessitating ICU or transitional care unit admission.[26] When an etiologic organism is not identified, oral therapy should reflect a similar spectrum of coverage to the initial IV therapy. In some cases, this may require use of more than one oral agent. We have had success, however, transitioning patients initially treated with IV ceftriaxone + doxycycline to oral doxycycline monotherapy at discharge.[27]

There are no good randomized trials examining the optimal duration of treatment for CAP. Most practice guidelines recommend 7–10 days for patients with CAP requiring hospitalization, with 14 days for documented *M. pneumoniae* or *Chlamydia pneumonia*. Legionella is usually treated for 10–21 days. Patients with more virulent pathogens like *S. aureus* or *P. aeruginosa* or other suppurative complications should be treated for at least 14

Box 33-1 Criteria to identify clinically stable patients for potential switch to oral antibiotic therapy

Stable vital signs and clinical criteria for ≥24 hours

Temperature ≤37.8°C (100°F)

Heart rate ≤100 beats per minute

Respiratory rate ≤24 breaths per minute

Systolic blood pressure ≥90 mm Hg

Oxygen saturation (on room air) ≥90%

Ability to take oral medications

From File TM. Community-associated methicillin-resistant *Staphylococcus aureus*: not only a cause of skin infections, also a new cause of pneumonia. Curr Opin Infect Dis 2005; 18:123–123.

---

days.[9–11,16] In determining length of therapy, clinicians should use these durations of treatment as guides and always consider patient age and frailty, comorbid conditions, severity of illness, and hospital course to individualize therapy.

PREVENTION

Prevention of CAP has traditionally relied on vaccination with the polysaccharide pneumococcal pneumonia vaccine and the seasonal influenza vaccine. The vaccine for *S. pneumoniae* comprises the 23 serotypes that cause 85–90% of the invasive pneumococcal infections in the United States. Although the vaccine has not consistently prevented CAP or death in elderly patients or those with comorbidities in randomized trials, it likely prevents invasive pneumococcal infection.[28] National guidelines and the CDC recommend that the pneumococcal vaccine be given to all patients older than 65 years and those with chronic medical conditions.[9–11]

The seasonal influenza vaccine has clearly been shown to decrease influenza-related illness in elderly and high-risk patient populations. As well, in a meta-analysis and a large observational study of patients >65 years old, vaccination against influenza prevented pneumonia, hospitalization, and death.[29,30] Vaccination of health care workers may also confer a mortality benefit in elderly patients. The CDC recommends the influenza vaccine for all patients >50 years old, those with comorbidities and at high risk for influenza, and health care workers in the inpatient and outpatient setting.

Pneumococcal and influenza vaccination have traditionally been relegated to the outpatient setting. National guidelines and the CDC recommend vaccination of all eligible hospitalized patients. Vaccination is safe and effective in the setting of almost any medical illness, and both vaccines can be given simultaneously at the time of discharge.[30] Administration of the pneumococcal and influenza vaccines to patients hospitalized with CAP has become a Joint Commission on Accreditation of Healthcare Organizations (JCAHO) and CMS quality measure. Utilization of "standing orders" is the most effective means of ensuring vaccination.

Finally, in addition to vaccination, there is some evidence to suggest that tobacco smokers are at increased risk of invasive pneumococcal disease or pneumonia. Patients hospitalized (for all illnesses but for CAP in particular) should be counseled about smoking cessation and offered pharmacotherapy and outpatient follow-up.

DISCHARGE/FOLLOW-UP PLANS

Patients hospitalized for CAP can safely be discharged when they have reached clinical stability, are able to tolerate oral medications, have no other active comorbid conditions, and have safe, close, appropriate outpatient follow-up (Box 33-2). Clinical pathways employing these discharge criteria have shown them to be safe and effective in reducing the length of stay for CAP. Most importantly, patients should have met most if not all of the vital sign and clinical criteria noted in Box 33-1 in the criteria for switching to oral therapy. Patients with two or more abnormal vital signs ("instabilities") at the time of discharge are at high risk for readmission and mortality, but those with one or fewer generally have good outcomes.[31] Absent other clinical factors or extenuating circumstances (persistent hypoxia, poor functional status, etc.), most patients with CAP should reach clinical stability by day 3–4, be considered for a switch to oral therapy, and, if stable, discharged shortly thereafter.

When patients with CAP are discharged from the hospital, they should be counseled as to the expected course of recovery. Most importantly, patients and families must be informed that many of the symptoms of CAP may persist well after the hospitalization. In one study, up to 80% of patients reported persistent cough and fatigue 1 week after discharge, and up to 50% still had dyspnea and sputum production. In some, the cough can last for 4–6 weeks.[3]

All patients discharged after treatment of CAP should have follow-up with their outpatient provider. The physician responsible for their inpatient care should communicate directly with this provider and outline the hospital course, the discharge medications, and the duration of antibiotic therapy. There is no specific timeframe within which patients must be seen, but follow-up should be dictated by patient age, comorbidities, clinical stability at discharge, and degree of illness. The American Thoracic Society guidelines do recommend that patients with a substantial smoking history who are hospitalized with CAP have a follow-up chest radiograph 4–6 weeks after discharge to establish a radiographic baseline and exclude the possibility of underlying malignancy.[10]

Box 33-2 Criteria for Identifying Patients for Possible Discharge

Patients should meet clinical criteria in Box 33-1.

Able to tolerate oral medications (no need to observe for 24 hours on oral therapy).

Have no evidence of active comorbid conditions (myocardial ischemia, pulmonary edema, etc.).

Have a normal mental status (or have returned to their baseline).

Have safe, appropriate outpatient follow-up.

Key Points

- *Streptococcus pneumoniae* is the most common cause of CAP requiring hospitalization, while *Legionella pneumophila* is a common cause of severe CAP.

- The chest radiograph remains the gold standard in the diagnosis of CAP and should be supplemented by blood cultures sampled prior to antibiotic therapy and sputum for Gram stain and culture if a high-quality specimen can be rapidly processed.

- Once the diagnosis of CAP has been made, the Pneumonia Severity Index (PSI) should be used to optimize the location of treatment and provide prognostic information.

- Most patients with nonsevere CAP reach clinical stability in 2–3 days and should be considered for switch to oral therapy and discharge shortly thereafter.

- Patients should receive pneumococcal vaccination, influenza vaccination, and tobacco cessation counseling prior to discharge if eligible.

SUGGESTED READING

Fine MJ, et al. A prediction rule to identify low-risk patients with community-acquired pneumonia. N Engl J Med 1997; 336:243–250.

Halm EA, Teirstein AS. Management of community-acquired pneumonia. N Engl J Med 2002; 347(25):2039–2045.

Metlay JP, Fine MJ. Testing strategies in the initial management of patients with community-acquired pneumonia. Ann Intern Med 2003; 138:109–118.

Niederman MS, Mandell LA, Anzqueto A, et al. American Thoracic Society: Guidelines for the management of community-acquired pneumonia: Diagnosis, assessment of severity, antimicrobial therapy, and prevention. Am J Respir Crit Care Med 2001; 163:1730–1754.

British Thoracic Society. Guidelines for the management of community-acquired pneumonia in adults. Thorax 2001; 56(Suppl 4):IV1–64.

Mandell LA, et al. Guidelines from the Infectious Disease Society of America: Update of guidelines for the management of community-acquired pneumonia in immunocompetent adults Clin Infect Dis 2003; 37:1405–1433.

File TM. Community acquired pneumonia. Lancet 2003; 362:1991–2001.

Nichol KL, Nordin J, Mullooly J, et al. Influenza vaccination and reduction in hospitalizations for cardiac disease and stroke among the elderly. N Engl J Med 2003; 348:1322–1332.

CHAPTER THIRTY-FOUR

Nosocomial Pneumonia

Scott A. Flanders, MD

BACKGROUND

Nosocomial pneumonia (NP) is the leading cause of mortality among patients who die from hospital-acquired infections. Defined as pneumonia occurring 48 hours or more after hospital admission, NP also includes the subset of ventilator-associated pneumonia (VAP)—pneumonia developing 48–72 hours after initiation of mechanical ventilation. The incidence of NP is between 5 and 15 cases per 1,000 hospital admissions. Health care associated pneumonia (HCAP), part of the continuum of NP, describes an increasingly common proportion of pneumonia developing outside the hospital (Box 34-1).[1] People in a nursing home or assisted living setting typically are afflicted and at risk for antibiotic resistant organisms and should be approached similar to cases of nosocomial pneumonia rather than community-acquired pneumonia. Most of the data informing our diagnostic and treatment decisions about NP come from studies performed in mechanically ventilated patients and are extrapolated to make recommendations for nonventilated patients.

Mortality attributable to NP is debated, but may be as high as 30%. The presence of nosocomial pneumonia increases hospital length of stay an average of 7–10 days, and in the case of VAP, is estimated to cost between $10,000 and $40,000 per case.[2]

ASSESSMENT

Clinical Presentation

Signs and Symptoms

Nosocomial pneumonia is usually diagnosed based on clinical grounds. Typical symptoms and signs consist of fever, cough with sputum, and shortness of breath in the setting of hypoxia and a new infiltrate on chest radiograph (CXR). In the elderly, signs may be more subtle; and delirium, fever, or leukocytosis in the absence of cough should trigger its consideration. The likelihood of NP increases among patients with risk factors for microaspiration and oropharyngeal colonization or overgrowth with resistant organisms (Table 34-1).[3]

Differential Diagnosis

Prior to settling on a diagnosis of NP, alternative causes of fever, hypoxia, and pulmonary infiltrates should be considered. Impor-

tant etiologies include pulmonary embolus and pulmonary edema. Alternative sources of infection, such as urinary tract, skin and soft-tissue, and devices (i.e., central venous catheters) are common in hospitalized patients and should be ruled out before diagnosing nosocomial pneumonia.

Diagnosis

Diagnostic strategies for NP seek to confirm the diagnosis and identify an etiologic pathogen, thus allowing timely, effective, and streamlined antibiotic therapy. Unfortunately, no consensus exists on the best approach to diagnosing nosocomial pneumonia. After obtaining a complete blood count and blood cultures, you can choose between a clinical or microbiologic diagnostic approach to diagnosis. A clinical diagnosis relies on detection of a new or progressive radiographic infiltrate along with signs of infection such as fever, leukocytosis, or purulent sputum. Clinical diagnosis is sensitive but is likely to lead to antibiotic overuse. The microbiologic approach requires sampling of secretions from the respiratory tract and may reduce inappropriate antibiotic use, but takes longer and may not be available in all hospitals.

Preferred Studies

The microbiologic approach to diagnosis relies on the use of quantitative or semiquantitative cultures to create thresholds for antibiotic treatment. Bacterial cultures that demonstrate a level of growth above the thresholds described below warrant treatment, while those below it should trigger withholding or discontinuation of antibiotics.

Bronchoscopic Approaches: Bronchoalveolar lavage (BAL) with a cutoff of 10^4 organisms/mL or protected specimen brush (PSB) with a cutoff of 10^3 organisms/mL are felt to be the most specific diagnostic tests when performed prior to initiating antibiotics, or prior to changing antibiotics if a patient is already receiving them. In clinically stable patients, antibiotics can be safely discontinued if bacterial growth falls below these thresholds. If cultures are positive, antibiotic therapy should be tailored to target the organism identified. The bronchoscopic approach is favored in patients who are mechanically ventilated, develop their pneumonia late in the hospital stay (>5–7 days), are at risk for unusual pathogens, are failing therapy, or are suspected of having an alternative diagnosis.

Table 34-1 Risk Factors for Nosocomial Pneumonia

Impaired Host Defenses/Increased Aspiration

Endotracheal tubes	Supine positioning
Nasogastric tubes	Impaired mental status
Enteral feeding tubes	Sedation

Large Inoculum of Organisms

Bacterial colonization	Sinusitis
Gastric alkalinization (enteral feeds / H_2 blocker)	Malnutrition
Iatrogenic (forced hand ventilation)	Contaminated respiratory equipment

Overgrowth of Virulent Organisms

Prolonged antibiotic use	Comorbid illness
Iatrogenic (inadequate hand washing)	Frequent hospitalizations
Central venous lines	Prolonged hospital stays

Box 34-1 Risk Factors for Health Care–Associated Pneumonia

Receiving Home Therapy For:

- IV antibiotics

- Wound care

- Nursing care

Hospitalized ≥2 days in past 90 days

Residence in nursing home or long-term care facility

Hospital or dialysis clinic in past 30 days for:

- Dialysis

- Any IV therapy

Adapted from the 2005 ATS/IDSA Guideline for the Management of Adults with Hospital-Acquired, Ventilator-Associated, and Healthcare-Associated Pneumonia.

Nonbronchoscopic Approaches: Qualitative endotracheal aspirates (ETA) have been shown to be quite sensitive in ventilated patients, regularly identify organisms that may be subsequently found by BAL or PSB, and if negative, should result in withholding antibiotics. *Quantitative* endotracheal aspirates with a cutoff of 10^6 organisms/mL are often encouraged to reduce antibiotic overuse, but results should be interpreted cautiously, as they only have a sensitivity and specificity of about 75%.[1] Consideration should be given to withholding antibiotics in a clinically stable patient with a negative quantitative ETA if antibiotics have not been changed in the preceding 72 hours. Many intensive care units (ICUs) have begun to perform blinded sampling of lower respiratory tract secretions with suction catheters (blind PSB, blind mini-BAL). These techniques can be performed at all hours by trained respiratory therapists or nurses; they provide culture data similar to that of bronchoscopy, and may be safer and less costly than bronchoscopy. In general, nonbronchoscopic techniques are preferred in patients who are not mechanically ventilated. Sputum sampling, while easy to obtain, has not been well studied in NP. However, in patients in whom bronchoscopic or other non-bronchoscopic techniques are not feasible, sputum sampling may

be performed to identify potentially resistant organisms and help tailor therapy.

Alternative Options

Clinical Pulmonary Infection Score: Combining Clinical and Microbiologic Approaches

The clinical diagnosis of nosocomial pneumonia (new infiltrate + fever, leukocytosis, or purulent sputum) likely leads to antibiotic overuse, yet pursuing a bronchoscopic diagnosis is invasive, costly, and requires technical expertise. The quantitative ETA, blind PSB, and blind BAL discussed above are examples of some compromises that avoid the need for bronchoscopy, yet add microbiologic data in an attempt to prevent excess antibiotic therapy. Formally combining diagnostic approaches (clinical + microbiologic) may also be useful. One such option is the use of the clinical pulmonary infection score (CPIS), which combines clinical, radiographic, physiologic, and microbiologic data into a numerical result. Scores >6 have been shown to correlate well with quantitative BAL.[4] More recent studies, however, have suggested a lower specificity, which could still result in antibiotic overuse, but this approach remains more accurate than a general clinical approach. Using the CPIS serially at the time NP is suspected and again at 72 hours may be more useful. Patients with an initial low clinical suspicion for pneumonia (CPIS of 6 or less) could have antibiotics safely discontinued at 72 hours if the CPIS remains low.[5] Such a strategy may be useful in settings where more sophisticated diagnostic modalities are not available.

Multiple studies of biologic markers of infection have attempted to find a noninvasive, rapid, accurate means of determining who needs antibiotics for presumed NP. Unfortunately, the results have largely been disappointing. More recently, measurement of a soluble triggering receptor expressed on myeloid cells (sTREM-1) that is up-regulated in the setting of infection seems to improve our ability to diagnose NP accurately. Measurement of sTREM-1 was 98% sensitive and 90% specific for the diagnosis of pneumonia in mechanically ventilated patients.[6] While promising, more data are needed before this test can be recommended for routine use.

MANAGEMENT

Initial Treatment

Early initiation of *adequate* empiric antibiotic therapy (i.e., the antibiotics administered are shown to be active against all organisms isolated) is associated with improved survival compared to initial *inadequate* therapy.[1,7] Antibiotics should be started immediately after obtaining blood and sputum samples for culture and should not be withheld in the event of delay in diagnostic testing. The need to choose antibiotics quickly and expeditiously drives the use of broad-spectrum antibiotics. In an effort to avoid unnecessary overuse of broad-spectrum antibiotics, therapy should be based on risk for multidrug-resistant (MDR) pathogens. Identifying patients at low risk for MDR pathogens by clinical criteria allows for more narrow, but effective, antibiotic therapy. Low-risk patients include those who develop their pneumonia early in the hospitalization (<5–7 days), are not immunocompromised, have not had prior broad-spectrum antibiotics, and do not have risk factors for *HCAP* (*see* Box 34-1).[1,7] In these patients, antibiotics should target common community-acquired organisms (Table 34-2). Appropriate initial antibiotic therapy could include a third-generation cephalosporin or a beta-lactam/beta-lactamase inhibitor. In some communities or hospital wards, the incidence of methicillin-resistance among *Staphylococcus aureus* isolates (MRSA) and may be high enough to warrant initial empiric therapy with vancomycin or linezolid.

Unfortunately, today's increasingly complex hospitalized patients are unlikely to be "low risk," especially in intensive care units. Patients not meeting low risk criteria are considered to be at high risk for MDR pathogens (*see* Table 34-2). Initial empiric therapy needs to be broad, and it should include one antipseudomonal agent (cefepime or imipenem or beta-lactam/beta-lactamase inhibitor) ***plus*** a fluoroquinolone or aminoglycoside ***plus*** vancomycin or linezolid. The specific initial empiric therapy should be dictated by local resistance patterns, cost, and availability of preferred agents. When such broad-spectrum therapy is initiated, it becomes imperative that antibiotics be "deescalated" to limit antibiotic overuse. Deescalation therapy focuses on narrowing the antibiotic spectrum based on culture results, and on limiting the overall duration of therapy. Hospitalists should aim to accomplish such deescalation within 48–72 hours of initiating broad-spectrum antibiotics.

Subsequent Treatment

Patients started on initial empiric antibiotic therapy for presumed nosocomial pneumonia should be reassessed at 48–72 hours.

Specifically, cultures should be checked, and the clinical response to treatment evaluated. Figure 34-1 describes an algorithm for guiding treatment.[1] In patients who are clinically stable and have negative lower respiratory tract cultures, antibiotics can be stopped. Patients with positive cultures should have antibiotics tailored, or "deescalated" based on the organisms identified. In general, the most narrow-spectrum antibiotic that is active against the bacteria isolated should be used. The use of combination therapy for gram-negative organisms (two or more antibiotics active against a bacterial isolate) is widely practiced to achieve synergy, or to prevent the development of resistance. However, in the absence of neutropenia, combination therapy has not been shown to be superior to monotherapy,[8] and monotherapy is preferred. The isolation of MRSA from a respiratory sample should also result in use of monotherapy. Although some studies have suggested that linezolid may be superior to vancomycin for MRSA pneumonia, this finding needs validation in prospective randomized controlled trials.

A second component of deescalation is shortening the total duration of therapy. The CPIS may be used to shorten the duration of therapy in patients at low risk for pneumonia. Investigators at a Veterans Affairs medical center randomized patients suspected of having NP, but who had a CPIS score ≤6, to either treatment for 10–21 days, or short-course therapy. Patients receiving short-course therapy were reassessed at day 3, and if their CPIS score remained ≤6, antibiotics were stopped.[5] The short-course therapy group had no difference in mortality when compared to the standard treatment group, but had less antibiotic use, had shorter ICU stays, and was less likely to develop a superinfection or infection with a resistant organism. If the CPIS is not used, or if patients are felt to be at higher risk or convincingly demonstrated to have NP, a shorter course of therapy may still be preferred. A large randomized trial showed that 8 days of antibiotic therapy for patients with VAP resulted in similar clinical outcomes when compared to 15 days of therapy. Additionally, shorter duration antibiotic therapy was associated with lower likelihood of developing subsequent infections with multiresistant pathogens. A subset of patients in the 8-day treatment group infected with nonfermenting gram negative bacilli (e.g., *Pseudomonas aeruginosa*) did have a higher pulmonary infection recurrence rate, but due to aggressive surveillance, this did not translate into a higher mortality risk in this subset of patients.[9]

In summary, treatment of patients with suspected NP starts with immediate initiation of antibiotics and collection of respiratory secretions. While low-risk patients can receive narrower spectrum therapy, most patients will require broad initial empiric therapy. The antibiotic regimen, however, should be narrowed at

---

Table 34-2 Pathogens Associated with Nosocomial Pneumonia

Low-Risk Pathogens	High-Risk Pathogens
Streptococcus pneumoniae	*Pseudomonas aeruginosa*
Haemophilus influenzae	Methicillin-resistant *Staphylococcus aureus* (MRSA)
Methicillin-sensitive *Staphylococcus aureus* (MSSA)	*Acinetobacter* species
Escherichia coli	
Klebsiella pneumoniae	
Enterobacter species	

Figure 34-1 • Management of suspected nosocomial pneumonia. Adapted from the 2005 ATS/IDSA Guideline for the Management of Adults with Hospital-Acquired, Ventilator-Associated, and Healthcare-Associated Pneumonia.

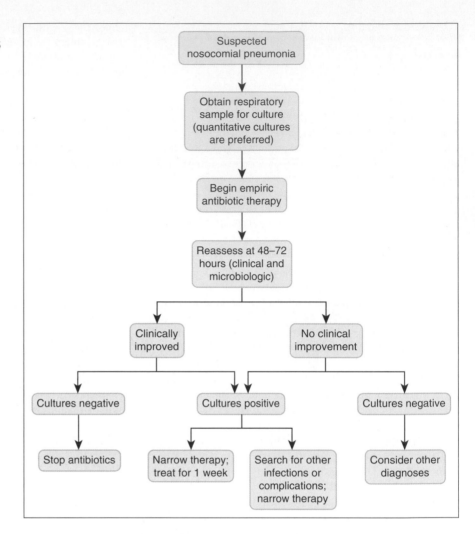

48–72 hours based on microbiologic results if the patient is improving. Overall treatment duration of 1 week is safe and effective with less chance of promoting growth of resistant organisms. In the subset of patients with pseudomonal infections, treatment of 1 week duration should be followed by active surveillance for recurrence, or alternatively, treatment can be extended to 2 weeks.

PROGNOSIS

Once treatment for NP is initiated, clinical improvement is usually seen by 48–72 hours. There is little support for following either microbiologic response (clearance of positive cultures) or the response by chest radiography. The chest radiograph often lags behind the clinical response, but a markedly worsening CXR (>50% increase in infiltrate) within the first 48 hours may indicate treatment failure. Clinical resolution as measured by temperature, white blood cell count, and oxygenation usually occurs by 6–7 days.[10] Failure of oxygenation to improve by 72 hours has been shown to be predictive of treatment failure.

The overall mortality in patients with NP is as high as 30–70%, largely due to severe comorbid disease in the at risk population. Higher mortality rates are seen in patients with VAP and resistant organisms. The mortality attributable to the episode of NP is about 30%, and it can be reduced to <15% with appropriate antibiotic therapy.[1]

PREVENTION

Preventive strategies are either directed at reducing the overall incidence of infectious complications in hospitalized patients, or they are specifically targeted at reducing the incidence of nosocomial pneumonia.[3] The majority of the data supporting preventive strategies are limited to patients in the ICU, and, in particular, patients receiving mechanical ventilation. However, many of the preventive principals can be extrapolated to the non-ICU population. The preventive strategies are highlighted in Table 34-3.

General Preventive Strategies

General preventive strategies aim to avoid contamination of patients with antimicrobial-resistant organisms that exist in hospitals, or mitigating the emergence of antimicrobial-resistant organisms in the first place. Preventing iatrogenic spread of resistant organisms depends on careful hand hygiene. Handwashing before and after patient contact reduces the incidence of nosocomial infection. Alcohol-based hand rinses placed at the bedside may actually be superior to soap and water and, in addition, improve compliance with hand hygiene.

Minimizing the use of indwelling devices (central lines, urinary catheters) also reduces the emergence of resistant organisms. When these devices are necessary, focusing on their timely removal is critical. The control of antibiotic use has been central to many preventive strategies. Prolonged or unnecessary use of

Table 34-3 Strategies Utilized to Prevent Nosocomial Pneumonia

Intervention	Process-Specific Issues	RECOMMENDATION LEVEL		
		Strongly Recommended	Recommended	Not Recommended
General Preventive Strategies				
Handwashing	Alcohol-based solution preferred	X		
Indwelling devices	Avoid if possible		X	
	Minimize duration		X	
Antibiotic rotation	Cycling (every 3 months) of empiric antibiotic regimens			X
Targeted Preventive Strategies				
Noninvasive ventilation	Best with CHF/COPD		X	
Orotracheal intubation	Favored over nasotracheal		X	
Semi-recumbent positioning	>30–45° head of bed elevation	X		
Subglottic secretion drainage	Need specialized endotracheal tube (use if MV > 3 days)		X	
Sucralfate use	Vs. other agents for stress ulcer prophylaxis			X
Avoid stress prophylaxis overuse	Limit to coagulopathy, respiratory failure >48 hours, or shock		X	
Selective digestive decontamination	Oral only			X
	Oral and IV			X
Ventilator circuit changes	Avoid routine changes		X	
Heat and moisture exchangers	Rather than heated humidifiers		X	
Reduce frequency of heat and moisture exchanger changes	Limited data		X	

CHF—congestive heart failure; COPD—chronic obstructive pulmonary disease; MV—mechanical ventilation

broad-spectrum antibiotics is strongly associated with development and colonization of resistant organisms. Strategies that focus on aggressive antibiotic deescalation (described above) are a key preventive tool. Some institutions have had success with antibiotic restriction or rotation, but long-term data on the effectiveness of these techniques are lacking.

Targeted Preventive Strategies

Preventive strategies to lower the incidence of NP focus on reducing risk factors for oropharyngeal or gastric colonization and subsequent aspiration of contaminated oropharyngeal or gastric secretions.[1,3,7,11]

Endotracheal intubation is one of the most important risk factors for NP in patients requiring ventilatory support. The use of noninvasive ventilation (NIV) or positive pressure-mask ventilation in selected groups of patients has been effective in preventing nosocomial pneumonia. Noninvasive ventilation has been most successful in patients with acute exacerbations of chronic obstructive pulmonary disease (COPD) and pulmonary edema secondary to congestive heart failure (CHF) and should be considered in appropriately selected patients. When intubation is required, the use of nasotracheal intubation should be avoided, due to higher rates of NP when compared to orotracheal intubation.

Supine positioning may contribute to the development of NP, likely due to an increased risk of gastric reflux and subsequent aspiration. Studies of semirecumbent positioning (elevation of the head of the bed >45 degrees) have shown less reflux, less aspiration, and in one recent randomized control trial, a significant reduction in the rate of VAP.[12] Elevation of the head of the bed is clearly indicated in mechanically ventilated patients and is also likely to benefit all patients at risk for aspiration and subsequent

NP, although this technique has not been well studied in nonventilated patients.

Subglottic secretion drainage (SSD) involves the removal of pooled secretions above the cuff of a specialized endotracheal tube that might otherwise leak into the lung. A meta-analysis of five studies evaluating this new technology showed significant reductions in the incidence of VAP. The use of SSD should be considered for use in patients requiring more than 3 days of mechanical ventilation.[13]

Medications used for stress ulcer prophylaxis that increase gastric pH—such as H_2 antagonists and antacids—allow for colonization of the upper gastrointestinal tract by potentially pathogenic organisms and therefore increase the risk for NP. The use of sucralfate instead of H_2 antagonists is felt to lead to less alkalinization of the stomach and less bacterial overgrowth. The ability of sucralfate to prevent nosocomial pneumonia, however, has not been well demonstrated, and its routine use is not recommended.[14] Instead, efforts should be targeted at limiting use of stress ulcer prophylaxis to populations at high risk for clinically significant bleeding, namely patients with coagulopathy and prolonged ventilatory failure. Most patients who are not in the ICU should not receive stress ulcer prophylaxis. The risk of NP related to use of proton pump inhibitors has not been well studied.

Selective digestive decontamination (SDD) involves sterilization of the oropharynx and gastrointestinal tract in mechanically ventilated patients in order to prevent aspiration of large numbers of potentially pathogenic organisms and subsequent VAP. Most evaluations of SDD have involved oral (and sometimes gastric) application of topical polymixin, aminoglycoside, and amphotericin. In many cases, short courses of IV antibiotics have been added. At least 10 meta-analyses have shown a reduction in the risk of VAP with the use of SDD. The addition of IV antibiotics may also provide a mortality benefit. However, the long-term risk for emergence of resistant organisms, and insufficient data on the cost-effectiveness of SDD prevent its recommendation for routine use.[14]

There are several preventive strategies targeted at reducing aspiration of contaminants in ventilator circuits, filters, and tubing. Recommended strategies, listed in Table 34-3 include avoidance of routine ventilator circuit changes (change the tubing only when visibly contaminated or for a new patient), use of heat and moisture exchangers rather than heated humidifiers, and reduction in the frequency of changes of the heat and moisture exchangers.[1,11,14]

DISCHARGE/FOLLOW-UP PLANS

Patients should be followed in the hospital until it is clear they are responding to therapy and clinically improving. There has been limited evaluation of strategies to rapidly transition patients to oral therapy. However, if patients are improving, are tolerating oral therapy, have a functional GI tract, and have an organism isolated that is sensitive to available oral antibiotics, the switch to oral therapy can be made. If no organism is isolated, but a patient definitely was felt to have NP, the oral antibiotics selected should have the same spectrum of activity as the previously administered IV antibiotics. In many cases, patients will have an infection with an organism that is only susceptible to IV antibiotics. These patients are likely to be ill enough to complete a full 1-week IV course in the hospital, but if they have no active comorbid illness and have improved, they can have a peripherally inserted central catheter (PICC) line placed (or other long-term IV access) and receive the remainder of their therapy at home or in another lower acuity setting.

In all patients who develop NP, reversible causes of aspiration should be sought, and in cases where multidrug resistant organisms are isolated, this should be reported to any facility to which a patient is being transferred or to the primary care physician or home nurse who will assume care after discharge.

Key Points

- In clinically stable patients suspected of having nosocomial pneumonia, antibiotics can be withheld when respiratory secretions show less than 10^4 organisms/mL by BAL or less than 10^3 organisms/mL by PSB.

- Early initiation of *adequate* empiric antibiotic therapy is associated with improved survival compared to initial *inadequate* therapy.

- At 48–72° initial empiric antibiotic regimens should be stopped if cultures are negative and the patient is stable, or they should be tailored to the narrowest possible regimen that adequately covers any isolated pathogen.

- Nosocomial pneumonia should be treated for a duration of 1 week (in the absence of nonfermenting gram-negative bacilli).

- Careful hand hygiene, elevation of the head of the bed, and avoidance of mechanical ventilation (with the use of noninvasive ventilation) are effective strategies at preventing nosocomial pneumonia.

SUGGESTED READING

Guidelines for the management of adults with hospital-acquired, ventilator-associated, and healthcare-associated pneumonia. Am J Respir Crit Care Med 2005; 171:388–416.

Chastre J, Fagon JY. Ventilator-associated pneumonia. Am J Respir Crit Care Med 2002; 165:867–903.

Collard HR, Saint S, Matthay MA. Prevention of ventilator-associated pneumonia: an evidence-based systematic review. Ann Intern Med 2003; 138:494–501.

Drakulovic MB, Torres A, Bauer TT, et al. Supine body position as a risk factor for nosocomial pneumonia in mechanically ventilated patients: a randomised trial. Lancet 1999; 354:1851–1858.

CHAPTER THIRTY-FIVE

Urinary Tract Infections

Carol E. Chenoweth, MD, and Sanjay Saint, MD, MPH

BACKGROUND

Urinary tract infections (UTI) account for over 7 million office visits per year, at a cost of over $1 billion. Approximately 40% of women will develop UTI at least once during their lifetime, and many of these women will have recurrent urinary tract infections. In addition, pyelonephritis accounts for 100,000 hospitalizations in the United States yearly. *Escherichia coli* is the predominant pathogen in uncomplicated community-acquired UTI in women, associated with approximately 90% of cases (Table 35-1). *Staphylococcus saprophyticus* is found in <10% of cases, and the majority of remaining infections are caused by other members of the Enterobacteriaceae family, such as *Klebsiella sp.*, *Proteus sp.*, or *Enterobacter sp.*[1] Resistant strains of gram-negative bacilli and enterococci are found more frequently in complicated UTI, as defined by symptoms >7 days, diabetes mellitus, immunosuppression, urologic structural or functional abnormality, presence of nephrolithiasis, presence of urinary catheter, or recent hospitalization. Treatment recommendations for uncomplicated cystitis and pyelonephritis are changing as resistance patterns in urinary *E. coli* isolates evolve.[2,3]

UTI is also the most frequently reported nosocomial infection, accounting for up to 40% of hospital-acquired infections. The vast majority of these infections are associated with urinary catheters, which are frequently associated with bacterial colonization and formation of biofilm. The microbial etiology of catheter-related UTI has changed over the past few decades, and varies by patient population. The most common pathogens associated with hospital-wide catheter-related UTI are the Enterobacteriaceae, including *Escherichia coli*, *Klebsiella sp.*, and *Enterobacter sp.* Other significant pathogens, which are more common in the ICU setting, include *Pseudomonas aeruginosa*, enterococci, and *Candida sp.*[4] Antimicrobial resistance in hospital pathogens has complicated treatment choices for nosocomial UTI.[5]

ASSESSMENT

Clinical Presentation

Prevalence and Presenting Signs and Symptoms

UTI presents in a spectrum of illness, from asymptomatic bacteriuria to uncomplicated cystitis to urosepsis. Lower tract infections are associated with symptoms related to irritation of the urethra and bladder (i.e., dysuria, frequency, urgency). Women presenting with one or more symptom of UTI have a probability of infection of about 50%. The combination of symptoms, such as dysuria and frequency without vaginal discharge, raise the probability of UTI to >90%.[6] Generally, UTI symptoms are of abrupt onset (<3 days); a longer or intermittent course of symptoms increases the likelihood of other causes besides UTI.

Patients with associated flank pain, abdominal pain, nausea, vomiting, fever, or chills should be suspected of having pyelonephritis. Patients with complicating factors and medical conditions are at increased risk for development of pyelonephritis or infection with resistant organisms. Complicating factors include underlying structural abnormalities of the urinary tract, diabetes mellitus, age >65, immunosuppression, pregnancy, recent hospitalization, or urologic tract manipulation. Differentiating complicated from uncomplicated UTI is important for evaluation and treatment.

Emphysematous pyelonephritis is a rare, life-threatening presentation of UTI that occurs in diabetic patients, and patients with papillary necrosis, renal obstruction, or other renal impairment.[7] In this condition, facultative anaerobes, such as *E. coli* or other Enterobacteriaceae, produce, cause, or result in an acute, necrotizing infection with gas formation. This condition requires early diagnosis, as the mortality rate is 40–50%, and immediate nephrectomy is required.[8] It should be considered in severely ill older diabetic patients, especially in the presence of chronic urinary infections or renovascular disease.[8]

Catheter-associated UTI also presents in a spectrum, from completely asymptomatic bacteriuria to overwhelming urosepsis associated with death.[9,10] Only 10–32% of catheterized patients with bacteriuria develop symptoms referable to the urinary tract. In a recent study of nosocomial catheter-related bacteriuria, approximately 90% of infections were asymptomatic.[10] There were no significant differences between patients with and without bacteriuria with respect to fever, dysuria, urgency, flank pain, or leukocytosis.[10]

Bacteremia, with or without sepsis syndrome, is an important complication of UTI. The urinary tract is the source of infection in 11–40% of nosocomial bacteremia.[4,11] However, in prospective studies of nosocomial bacteriuria, secondary bacteremia occurs only infrequently; 0.4–3.9% of patients with nosocomial UTI have associated bacteremia.[4,10] Bacteremia is less likely to occur with asymptomatic bacteriuria and is more likely to be

Table 35-1 Percentage of Major Pathogens Isolated from Urinary Tract Infections

	Uncomplicated UTI	Complicated UTI	Catheter Associated UTI ICU
Escherichia coli	70–95	21–54	17.5
Staphylococcus saprophyticus	5–10	—	—
Candida sp.	<1		15.8
Enterococci sp.	1–2	1–23	13.8
Pseudomonas aeruginosa	<1	2–19	11.0
Proteus sp.	1–2	1–10	—
Klebsiella sp.	1–2	2–17	6.2
Enterobacter sp.	<1	2–10	5.1

Adapted from: Hooten TM. The current management strategies for community-acquired urinary tract infection. Infect Dis Clinic North Am 2003; 17:303–332; *and* Chenoweth CE, Saint S. Infections associated with urinary catheters. In: Seifert H, Jansen B, Farr BM, eds. Catheter-Related Infections, 2nd Edition. Monticello, New York: Marcel Dekker, 2005. 551–584.

associated with major underlying disease and comorbidities.[10] Current research is underway to identify what factors predict urinary tract–related bacteremia in patients with nosocomial bacteriuria.

UTI in patients with spinal cord lesions may be particularly difficult to diagnose because of the patient's inability to sense localizing symptoms. Symptoms of UTI in these patients may include fever, chills, diaphoresis, abdominal discomfort, costovertebral angle tenderness, or increased muscle spasticity.[12]

Differential Diagnosis

Other infections of the abdomen may present similarly to UTI and should be included in the differential diagnosis. Pelvic inflammatory disease should be considered in all sexually active women with apparent UTI. Severe pain with radiation to the groin is uncommon in acute pyelonephritis and suggests the presence of renal calculi. Occasionally, renal pain may be felt in the epigastrium, extending to the lower abdominal quadrants. These findings may suggest gallbladder disease, diverticulitis, or appendicitis as part of the differential diagnosis.

Diagnosis

Preferred Studies

For uncomplicated UTI, the presence of pyuria on microscopic examination of unstained, centrifuged urine under 40× power has a sensitivity of approximately 95%, but a low specificity of 71%.[13] Pyuria in a clean-catch urine specimen may represent contamination from vaginal discharge. Apparent bacteriuria may similarly represent perineal or vaginal contamination.

Urinary dipstick analysis for leukocyte esterase, an indirect test for the presence of pyuria, is the least expensive and time intensive test. Leukocyte esterase test has a sensitivity of 75–96% and specificity of 94–98% for uncomplicated UTI.[14] Nitrite testing by dipstick is positive in the presence of bacteria that produce nitrate reductase, but can be confounded by consumption of ascorbic acid. Urinary dipstick is most accurate if both nitrite and leukocyte esterase are measured.[15]

While pyuria is considered an important indicator of UTI in the noncatheterized patient, pyuria is less strongly correlated with UTI in the catheterized patient. In a recent prospective study of catheterized patients, pyuria was most strongly associated with infection caused by gram-negative bacilli, while infections caused by coagulase-negative staphylococci, enterococci, or yeast produced much less pyuria. Urinary white blood count >5/high-power field had a specificity of 90% for predicting infections with >10^5 colony-forming units (CFU)/mL, but had a sensitivity of less than 37%.[16]

A quantitative urine culture yielding ≥10^2 CFU/mL is the most sensitive (95%) and specific (85%) test for diagnosing uncomplicated UTI; however, urine culture is rarely indicated in women with uncomplicated UTI. Culture should be obtained for those with suspected pyelonephritis, relapsing uncomplicated UTI, or any complicated UTI. For asymptomatic patients, 10^5 CFU/mL on quantitative culture is considered significant.[14] Cultures are also necessary for guiding subsequent therapy in complicated UTI. Blood cultures should be obtained in any severely ill patient suspected of possible bacteremia.

In patients with long-term indwelling urinary catheters, neither urinalysis nor urine cultures are reliable tests for diagnosing symptomatic UTI. Bacteriuria in this setting is chronic and universal, and cultures obtained from the catheter may not reflect bladder cultures. Fever and chills may be the only symptoms of catheter-related UTI in patients with long-term indwelling catheters.[4,9]

Alternative Options

Women with recurrent uncomplicated UTI, with two or more symptoms of lower UTI (see above), can be diagnosed accurately based on symptom presentation alone. Patient guideline and telephone management have been successful for treating recurrent UTI in this patient group.[6,14,17]

Prognosis

During Hospitalization

Patients with uncomplicated pyelonephritis have an overall excellent outcome. Each episode of nosocomial bacteriuria, however, is expected to cost an additional $676, while urinary catheter-related bacteremia increases costs by as much as $2,836 per episode.[18] In prospective studies of patients with catheter-related nosocomial UTI, a mortality rate of 14–19% was found in infected patients. Infected patients were nearly three times more likely to die during hospitalization than patients without such an infection, even after a multivariate analysis excluded 20 other

Table 35-2 Options for Empirical Treatment of Urinary Tract Infections in Hospitalized Patients

	Route	Antimicrobials	Duration
Uncomplicated pyelonephritis or mild to moderate infection	Oral	Ciprofloxacin (500 mg twice daily) Levofloxacin (250 mg daily) Gatifloxacin (400 mg daily)	7–14 days
Severe illness, possible bacteremia*	Intravenous	Piperacillin/tazobactam (3.375 g every 6 hr) Ticarcillin/clavulanic acid (3.1 g every 6 hr) Ampicillin (2 g every 6 hr) plus Gentamicin (5 mg/kg/day) Imipenem (2,500 mg every 6 hr) or Meropenem (1 g every 8 hr) Ciprofloxacin (400 mg every 12 hr)	14–21 days

*May switch to oral therapy after 2–3 days if patient becomes afebrile and tolerates oral intake.

variables.[19,20] The attributable case-fatality rate from UTI-related nosocomial bacteremia is approximately 12.7%.[4]

Beyond the health and financial burden of catheter-related infection, these devices cause substantial patient discomfort. In a prospective study, 42% of catheterized patients reported that their indwelling catheter was uncomfortable; 48% complained that it was painful, and 61% noted that it restricted their activities of daily living.[21] Two respondents provided unsolicited comments that their indwelling catheter "hurts like hell."[21] For some patients, urinary catheters operate as a physical restraint, tantamount to binding them to the bed, substantially and unnecessarily limiting their ability to function freely and with dignity. Indeed, we have even referred to the urinary catheter as a "one-point restraint."[22] Restricted activity not only reduces patient autonomy, it also promotes other nosocomial complications, such as venous thromboembolism and pressure ulcers.

MANAGEMENT

Treatment

Healthy women with uncomplicated cystitis or pyelonephritis can be safely managed on an outpatient basis with oral antibiotics.[13] Hospital admission with intravenous antibiotics is indicated for complicated UTI, including acutely toxic patients, pregnant women, immunocompromised patients, patients unable to take in oral fluids, or in those where compliance is a significant issue. The recommended course of therapy for acute pyelonephritis or mild complicated UTI is 2 weeks of a full-dose quinolone (Table 35-2). Oral ciprofloxacin is as effective as the intravenous formulation for the treatment of complicated UTI in patients who are able to take oral medications.[23] If bacteremia is present, initial parenteral therapy is recommended; patients may be switched to an oral quinolone as soon as they are able to tolerate oral therapy to complete a 14-day course.[23] Urine cultures should be collected prior to antibiotic therapy and sensitivities checked to guide therapy. Routine structural evaluation is rarely indicated for uncomplicated pyelonephritis.

Severely ill patients or catheterized patients who develop symptoms of bacteremia should be treated with intravenous antibiotics (see Table 35-2). Blood and urine cultures taken prior to instituting antibiotics may help with the subsequent selection of antimicrobial therapy. Empirical antimicrobials should be selected based on knowledge of organisms, previous resistance patterns from the patient, and from resistance patterns in the medical unit or geographic area.[4,7,9] While there are no adequate clinical studies to guide the length of therapy for catheter-related UTI, treatment for 7 to 21 days has been recommended. Early imaging to rule out obstruction, abscess, or other surgical emergencies is warranted in this patient population, especially those who do not respond as quickly as expected.[8,24]

Biofilms develop on long-term indwelling urinary catheters and allow bacteria to evade activity of antibiotics and normal immune mechanisms.[9] A recent prospective randomized controlled trial showed that subsequent bacteriuria was significantly lower in patients who received a new catheter prior to initiation of antibiotic therapy when compared to patients who had no catheter replacement.[25] In addition, patients who had their catheter exchanged became afebrile sooner, had improved clinical status at 72 hours, and had a lower rate of symptomatic clinical relapse 28 days after therapy. Therefore, a catheter should be replaced if it has been in place for more than a week at the time treatment of symptomatic UTI is initiated.

Once culture information is available, antibiotic management should be directed by susceptibilities of clinical isolates, using the narrowest spectrum, least toxic, and least expensive effective antimicrobial agent. Clinical response to treatment should be evaluated over a 2- to 3-day period. When the patient has had a clinical response and fever is decreasing, then parenteral therapy may be switched to oral therapy. If fever has not resolved after the third day of therapy, imaging of the urinary system should be performed to evaluate for obstruction, renal calculi, acute bacterial nephritis, or malacoplakia.[24,26]

Alternative Options

Screening and treatment of asymptomatic bacteriuria are warranted in only a few situations. The risk of complications from asymptomatic bacteriuria is low; treatment does not prevent bacteriuria from recurring, and treatment may select for resistant bacteria.[4,9–10,27] Treatment of asymptomatic bacteriuria is recommended for pregnant women, patients who will undergo genitourinary tract manipulation or instrumentation, or if bacteriuria persists for 48 hours after removal of a urinary catheter.[27]

Similarly, candiduria requires treatment in only select situations. In catheterized patients, candiduria frequently resolves without treatment if the catheter can be removed. Fluconazole treatment has been shown to clear candiduria short term; however, long-term clearance, especially in catheterized patients, was not achieved.[28] On the other hand, candiduria in a patient with local or constitutional symptoms or in a patient with diabetes, immunosuppression, or urologic abnormality deserves an aggressive approach. These patients require evaluation for disseminated candidiasis and may require systemic antifungal therapy.[29]

PREVENTION

Women with recurrent UTI, as defined as three or more episodes of UTI over the past 12 months or two UTIs in the past 6 months, may benefit from prophylactic antibiotics. Prophylactic cotrimoxazole, nitrofurantoin, or a quinolone, taken either daily or postcoitally, has been shown to reduce frequency of UTI in sexually active women.[13] Postcoital prophylaxis appears as effective as daily dosing. Patient-initiated treatment of uncomplicated recurrent urinary tract infection is another cost-effective method of managing recurrent urinary tract infection in adherent women.[17]

Since as many as 80% of nosocomial UTIs and 97% of UTIs in ICUs are associated with a urinary catheter, the best strategy for prevention is avoidance of urinary catheterization.[30] Nevertheless, urinary catheters are important for patients requiring drainage of anatomic or physiologic outlet obstruction, patients undergoing surgery of the genitourinary tract, patients requiring accurate urinary output measurements, and patients with sacral or perineal wounds (Table 35-3).[4,30]

Dr. Paul Beeson persuasively argued against routine use of indwelling urinary catheters in hospitalized patients almost five decades ago, making the "case against the catheter."[31] He urged:

Table 35-3 Appropriate Indications for Short-term Indwelling Urinary Catheter Use in Hospitalized Patients

Bladder outlet obstruction
- Temporary relief of anatomical or functional obstruction
- Longer-term drainage if surgical correction is not indicated

Monitoring of urine output required
- Frequent or urgent monitoring is needed, as for critically ill patients
- Patient is unable or unwilling to collect urine

Urinary incontinence (without obstruction)
- In presence of a sacral or perineal wound
- At patient request

During and after prolonged surgical procedures with general or spinal anesthesia.

From: Chenoweth CE, Saint S. Infections associated with urinary catheters. In: Seifert H, Jansen B, Farr BM, eds. Catheter-Related Infections, 2nd edition. Monticello, New York: Marcel Dekker, 2005. 551–584; and Saint S, Lipsky BA. Preventing catheter-related bacteriuria: Can we? Should we? How? Arch Intern Med 1999; 159:800–808.

"the decision to use this instrument should be made with the knowledge that it involves risk of producing a serious disease."[31] This advice remains relevant today. Regrettably, unjustified and excessively prolonged catheter use persists, despite clear evidence of its detrimental effects.

In recent prospective studies of catheterized patients, the decision for catheterization was judged to be inappropriate 21–50% of the time.[4,32,33] Among 202 hospitalized patients with a urinary catheter, the initial indication for its insertion was judged inappropriate 21% of the time.[33] More importantly, continued catheterization was judged inappropriate for almost half of patient-days.[33] In one study, 28% of health care providers were unaware that their patient had an indwelling urinary catheter. The level of unawareness increased with the level of training: 21% of medical students, 22% of interns, 28% of residents, and 38% of attending physicians were unaware of catheters in their patients. Unawareness was correlated with inappropriate catheter use.[32]

Given these disturbing findings, many investigators have examined whether or not a system-wide administrative intervention, similar to an antibiotic "stop-order" but designed to alert physicians to the catheter status of their patients, might help reduce inappropriate catheterization.[22] The initial results of urinary catheter reminders appear promising. Cornia et al.[34] evaluated a computerized reminder using a before-and-after crossover design that prompted physicians at the Seattle Veteran Affairs Medical Center either to remove or continue the urinary catheter 72 hours after catheter insertion. The computerized reminder shortened the duration of catheterization by 3 days (which represented an approximately 30% reduction in catheter days), while not affecting recatheterization rates.[34] The main impediment in using such a computerized reminder is that the vast majority of hospitals in the United States do not routinely use computerized physician order entry. Very recently, Huang et al.[35] evaluated a nurse-based reminder system in the adult intensive care units of a large Taiwanese hospital. The nursing staff were instructed to remind physicians to remove unnecessary urinary catheters 5 days after insertion. Using a before-and-after design, these investigators found that the intervention significantly reduced duration of catheterization (7 days versus 4.6 days; P < 0.001) and urinary tract infection (11.5 versus 8.3 per 1,000 catheter-days; P = 0.009)[35]. Finally, Saint et al.[36] completed a pilot study at the University of Michigan Medical Center in which a nurse-based reminder after 48 hours of catheterization significantly reduced the proportion of time patients were catheterized.

In those requiring indwelling catheters, the most important advance in the prevention of urinary catheter–related infection was the introduction of the closed catheter drainage system. Effective maintenance of a closed drainage system includes the use of sealed urinary catheter junction. Proper aseptic technique, including aseptic insertion and maintenance of the catheter and drainage bag, remains essential in preventing catheter-related UTI. Use of gloves and proper handwashing during insertion and manipulation of catheters are essential to prevent exogenous acquisition of hospital pathogens.[4,9,30] Several studies support the use of anti-infective urinary catheters as adjunct to the above proven methods of prevention in patient populations receiving indwelling catheterization for 2 to 10 days, including the critically ill.[18,37]

DISCHARGE/FOLLOW-UP PLANS

Patient Education

Patients should be instructed to call with recurrence of symptoms or fever. Standardized patient education for UTI should be given to women with uncomplicated UTI.

Outpatient Physician Communication

Most patients hospitalized with UTI will require follow-up of symptoms to ensure resolution. In patients with recurrent infections, ongoing symptoms, or other complicating factors, repeat urine culture is warranted at 2 weeks after completion of antibiotic therapy.

Key Points

- *E. coli* is the predominant cause of uncomplicated UTI, but other more resistant microorganisms are seen most frequently in complicated UTIs.

- Most nosocomial UTIs are associated with urinary catheters; the risk of infection increases with duration of catheterization.

- Urinary dipstick is accurate for diagnosis of uncomplicated urinary tract infection. Urine and blood cultures should be obtained to guide therapy in complicated UTI.

- Oral fluoroquinolones are appropriate therapy for most uncomplicated pyelonephritis. Intravenous antimicrobials should be instituted for severe illness or suspected urosepsis.

- Nosocomial UTIs may be prevented by measures aimed at avoiding use of or removal of urinary catheters, aseptic placement and care of urinary catheters, and closed drainage systems.

SUGGESTED READING

Nicolle LE, Bradley S, Colgan R, et al. Infectious Diseases Society Guidelines for the diagnosis and treatment of asymptomatic bacteriuria in adults. Clin Infect Dis 2005; 40:643–654.

Hurlbut TA III, Littenberg B. The diagnostic accuracy of rapid dipstick tests to predict urinary tract infection. Clin Infect Dis 2000; 30:152–156.

Saint S, Chenoweth CE. Biofilms and catheter-associated urinary tract infections. Infect Dis Clin North Am 2003; 17:411–432.

Hooten TM. The current management strategies for community-acquired urinary tract infection. Infect Dis Clinic North Am 2003; 17:303–332.

Bent S, Nallamothu BK, Simel DL, et al. Does this woman have an acute uncomplicated urinary tract infection? JAMA 2002; 287:2701–2710.

CHAPTER THIRTY-SIX

Skin and Soft Tissue Infections

Lakshmi K. Halasyamani, MD

BACKGROUND

Skin and soft tissue infections (SSTIs) are common inpatient problems managed by hospitalists. In the United States, approximately 330,000 patients are hospitalized annually for SSTIs.[1] They represent a common indication for antibiotic therapy and in some regions account for approximately 10% of hospitalizations.[2]

Specific populations at higher risk for SSTI include patients who use illicit intravenous drugs and those with impaired immune systems. Glucose intolerance and diabetes mellitus confer significant additional risk for the development and the severity of SSTI. SSTI account for the largest number of diabetes-related hospital bed days.[3]

ASSESSMENT

Presenting Signs and Symptoms

The Eron classification system assigns a numerical class rating to a constellation of patient-specific factors that include both historical and vital sign parameters.[4,5] The Eron classification system is summarized in Table 36-1.

Clinical evaluation of a patient with a SSTI requires a careful assessment and integration of historical and physical examination findings. Essential historical factors summarized in Box 36-1 include age, comorbid illness, immune status, medications, and exposures. Critical physical examination factors include both local as well as systemic manifestations of infection (Box 36-2). Two or more of any of the critical physical examination findings are associated with worse outcomes.[1] Signs unique to particular subsets of SSTI (such as osteomyelitis) are discussed in greater detail in the section on diagnosis (see below).

Differential Diagnosis

SSTIs encompass a broad continuum of infectious manifestations, from superficial infections of the dermis to deep infections involving tissue necrosis. Furthermore, SSTIs must be distinguished from noninfectious causes of skin erythema and ulceration. In particular, venous insufficiency, peripheral arterial disease, and vasculitis can mimic SSTI. Other important but less common causes of skin erythema and ulceration include collagen and fibromuscular disorders, chemical injury, and hemato-logic disorders leading to changes in blood viscosity.[6] Not all leg wounds represent infections, and their management is beyond the scope of this chapter.

Diagnosis

The diagnostic evaluation of a patient with an SSTI must be tailored to an individual's risk profile. Patients with Class 1 infections may need no further diagnostic testing, whereas patients with Class 4 infections may require extensive laboratory, radiologic, and microbiologic testing. Elements of the diagnostic evaluation for SSTIs are summarized in Box 36-3.[5]

Patients with diabetic skin infections represent an important subset of patients with SSTI due to the high rate of limb-threatening infections. Diabetes-induced limb amputations result in a 5-year mortality rate of 39–68%.[7] Peripheral neuropathy and neuroosteoarthritic deformities (Charcot joint) or limited joint mobility exacerbate severity of SSTI in patients with diabetes mellitus and can lead to the development of ulcerations and deeper wounds. Diabetic risk factors for foot ulceration and infection are summarized in Table 36-2.[1]

The PEDIS classification system provides a framework for grading the severity of diabetic wound infections and includes specific assessment of the wound along several dimensions: P = perfusion, E = extent, D = depth/tissue loss, I = infection, S = sensation. The PEDIS classification system in summarized in Table 36-3.[8]

Evaluation of diabetic foot infections with accompanying wounds must include a neurovascular evaluation. Peripheral sensation regarding soft touch and vibration can easily be assessed at the bedside quickly. If dorsalis pedis and posterior tibial pulses are palpable, arterial supply is generally adequate.[9] However, if peripheral pulses are not palpable, further vascular evaluation is necessary. The ankle-brachial index (ABI) is a noninvasive method of evaluating peripheral vascular perfusion. Values of 0.5–0.9 suggest mild-to-moderate peripheral vascular disease.[10] Values <0.5 suggest ischemia that will likely impair would healing.[11] Values >1.0 in patients with multiple risk factors for arterial calcification most likely are falsely elevated and will require measurement of ankle and toe pressures and/or assessment of waveforms. Ankle pressures should be >50 mm Hg, and toe pressures should be >30 mm Hg if peripheral perfusion is preserved.[12] In addition to ankle and toe pressures, dampened waveforms in the setting of a normal ABI suggest calcified vessels.

Table 36-1 Eron Classification System

Class	Patient Criteria
1	Afebrile and healthy, other than cellulitis
2	Febrile and ill-appearing, without unstable comorbidities
3	Toxic-appearing; ≥1 unstable comorbidities; or limb-threatening infection
4	Sepsis syndrome or life-threatening infection

From: Eron LJ, Lipsky BA, Low DE, et al. Managing skin and soft tissue infections: expert panel recommendations on key decision points. J Antimicrob Chemother 2003; 52 (Suppl):i3–i17.

Box 36-1 Summary of Essential Historical Factors

- Age
- Comorbidities
    - Glucose intolerance/DM
    - Chronic liver disease
    - Chronic renal disease
    - Vascular disease
    - Obesity
    - Malnutrition
- Immunocompromised
    - Neutropenia
    - Asplenia
    - Alcohol abuse
    - IV/SQ drug abuse
- Medications
    - Glucose intolerance/DM
    - Recent use of antimicrobials
    - Corticosteroids
- Exposures
    - Animals
    - Bites
    - Environmental/travel

DM—diabetes mellitus; IV/SQ—intravenous/subcutaneous

Box 36-2 Important Physical Examination Findings

- Local signs
    - Bullae
    - Hemorrhagic lesions
    - Anesthesia or pain out of proportion to the objective findings
    - Fluctuance
    - Crepitus
    - Wound odor
    - Color of wound drainage
- Systemic signs
    - Hypotension
    - Tachycardia
    - Temp <35°C or >40°C
    - Confusion or decreased level of consciousness

From Lipsky BA, Berdendt AR, Grunner HD, et al. Diagnosis and treatment of diabetic foot infection. Clin Inf Dis 2004; 39:885–910.

Box 36-3 Elements of the Diagnostic Evaluation

- Laboratory testing
    - CBC with differential
    - Electrolytes, BUN, creatinine
    - Creatine kinase
    - Serologic tests (streptozyme, anti-Dnase, anti-hyaluronidase) are generally not helpful
- Radiologic studies (to consider)
    - X-rays
    - Doppler examination
    - Ankle-Brachial Index (ABI)
    - MRI
    - Radionuclide scan
- Culture specimens
    - Tissue or bone specimens
    - Needle aspiration of fluid from leading edge of infection

Toenails should be inspected for the presence of onychomycosis, which is a risk factor for cellulitis.

Three subsets of SSTI require focused discussion regarding their diagnostic evaluation. These include deep soft tissue infections with or without sinus tracts, osteomyelitis, and necrotizing soft tissue infections.

Deep Soft Tissue Infection

Deep soft tissue infections require an assessment of the extent of infection. This evaluation can be done initially by probing the wound for the presence of a sinus tract. Probing pedal ulcers to bone has a positive predictive value of almost 90% that an accompanying osteomyelitis is present.[13] If the clinical examination is nondiagnostic, further evaluation can be completed with either computerized tomography or ultrasound. In addition to radio-logic evaluation, the wound must be cleansed and debrided, with a tissue specimen obtained from the debrided base. The tissue specimen must be sent for both aerobic and anaerobic culture. There is little utility in swabbing undebrided ulcers or wound drainage.[1,14,15]

Osteomyelitis

Osteomyelitis or a bone infection should be considered in the following settings:

- The ulcer is deep or extensive.
- The ulcer has not healed despite at least 6 weeks of appropriate care and off-loading.
- The ulcer overlies a bony prominence.
- The bone is either visible or easily palpated with a sterile blunt metal probe.
- The patient's erythrocyte sedimentation rate is >100.

Table 36-2 Diabetic Risk Factors for Foot Ulceration and Infection

Risk Factor	Mechanism of Injury
Peripheral motor neuropathy	Abnormal foot anatomy and biomechanics
Peripheral sensory neuropathy	Lack of protective sensation
Peripheral autonomic neuropathy	Deficient sweating leading to dry, cracking skin
Neuro-osteoarthritic deformities (Charcot joint) or limited joint mobility	Abnormal anatomy and biomechanics
Arterial insufficiency	Impaired tissue viability, wound healing, and neutrophil penetration
Hyperglycemia	Impaired neutrophil function and wound healing
Patient disabilities	Reduced vision, limited mobility
Patient adherence and self-management	Foot care, diet, and medication adherence
Health care system failures	Inadequate patient education, self-management tool development, and monitoring of self-management

From: Lipsky BA, Berendt AR, Gunner HD, et al. Diagnosis and treatment of diabetic foot infections. Clin Infect Dis 2004; 39:885–910.

Table 36-3 PEDIS Clinical Classification System

Clinical Manifestations	Infection Severity	PEDIS grade
Wound without sign of infection/inflammation	Uninfected	1
≥2 manifestations of inflammation (purulence erythema, pain, tenderness, warmth, or induration)	Mild	2
Cellulitis extends ≤2 cm around ulcer		
Infection limited to skin or SQ		
No systemic illness		
Infection as above with one or more of the following	Moderate	3
Cellulitis extending >2 cm		
Lymphangitic streaking		
Involvement of muscle, tendon, or bone		
Deep tissue abscess		
Gangrene		
Systemic involvement with signs of metabolic instability	Severe	4

From: International Working Group on the Diabetic Foot. International consensus on the diabetic foot (CD-ROM). Brussels: International Diabetes Foundation, May 2003.

Box 36-4 Risk Factors for Necrotizing Soft Tissue Infections

Age >50

Atherosclerosis

Burns

Cancer or other immunocompromised state

Chronic alcoholism

Corticosteroid use

Diabetes mellitus

Hypoalbuminemia

Intravenous drug use

Malnutrition

Obesity

Peripheral vascular disease

- The radiograph shows bony destruction.
- The patient has an unexplained elevated white blood cell count.

The evaluation of a possible osteomyelitis frequently includes both radiologic and microbiologic evaluation.[1,16] Plain radiographs are usually the first step in evaluating whether a wound infection may involve the underlying bone. Changes on plain radiographs typically appear after 30–50% of the bone is destroyed, which usually takes up to 2 weeks to appear. The classic triad on plain radiographs suggestive of osteomyelitis is demineralization, periosteal reaction, and bony destruction. When plain radiographs do not definitely establish the diagnosis of bony involvement of an SSTI, other radiologic modalities should be considered. These include both magnetic resonance imaging (MRI) and nuclear medicine scans.[17,18] MRI is the preferred modality of evaluation with high sensitivity and specificity in patients with likely infections.[1] Nuclear medicine scans may be used if the patient is ineligible for MRI but are limited because of their high sensitivity with low specificity.[1,18,19]

Bone biopsy should be considered when the diagnosis remains in doubt, or if the etiologic agent or antibiotic susceptibilities are not predictable. Bone biopsy should also be considered if the suspected lesion is in the mid or hind foot because these lesions are more difficult to treat medically and more frequently result in an above-the-ankle amputation.[1,20] Bone biopsy samples should consist of 2–3 specimens, with at least one sent for culture and one sent for histologic analysis.[21] There are no published reports of complications from foot bone biopsy procedures.[22,23] In patients with concomitant extensive soft tissue infections, the bone culture is more accurate for identification of etiologic agent than soft tissue specimens.[1]

Necrotizing Soft Tissue Infections

Necrotizing soft tissue infections represent a life-threatening subset of soft tissue infections. Many of the risk factors are similar to the risk factors for SSTI in general and are summarized in Box 36-4.[14] The clinical clues of pain that extends beyond the margins of apparent infection, pain that is out of proportion to the physical findings, or decreased pain or anesthesia at the apparent site of infection are frequently found in necrotizing soft tissue infections and should serve as red flags to the clinician caring for the patient.

Other findings unique to necrotizing soft tissue infections include the presence of tense edema, vesicles or bullae, and/or crepitus.

Tissue biopsy done at the time of wound debridement and surgical exploration is the gold standard for making the diagnosis of a necrotizing soft tissue infection. A white blood cell count above 20,000 is present in approximately 50% of patients. Plain radiographs demonstrate soft tissue gas in only 25% of the patients.[14] In studies of small series of patients, creatine kinase (CK) values have been elevated in patients with some necrotizing infections, such as those caused by *Vibrio vulnificus* and streptococcal infections leading to toxic shock syndrome, but the CK is not universally elevated with necrotizing infections.[24,25] Ultimately, to influence patient outcomes, the clinician must have a high clinical suspicion based on historical and physical examination findings.

MANAGEMENT

SSTIs are caused by a variety of bacteria, and the cause of the SSTI is often linked to an individual patient's history and risk factors. A summary of characteristic pathogens associated with specific risk factors is summarized in Table 36-4, and Table 36-5 summarizes recommended antibiotic therapy.

Table 36-4 Summary of Characteristic Pathogens with Specific Risk Factors

Risk Factor	Characteristic Pathogen(s)
Diabetes	
cellulitis	*S. aureus*, group B strep, anaerobes, gram-negative bacilli
Necrotizing infections	Polymicrobial—*S. epidermidis*, streptococci (including beta-hemolytic strep), enterococci, Enterobacteriaceae species (*E. coli, P. mirabilis, pneumoniae, P. aeruginosa*), *K. streptococci, Bacteroides/Prevotella* species anaerobic gram positive cocci *clostridium* species
	Single Pathogen—Group A strep or *S. pyogenes; S. aureus* (MSSA *and* MRSA); *C. perfringens*
Neutropenia	*P. aeruginosa*
Bite wounds	
Human	Oral flora (*Eikenella corrodens*)
Cat	*P. multocida*
Dog	*C. canimorsus, P. multocida*
Rat	*Streptobacillus moniloformis*
Animal contact	*Campylobacter spp.*
Reptile contact	*Salmonella spp.*
Hot tubs/loofah	*P. aeruginosa*
Fresh water	*Aeromonas hydrophilia*
Sea (or fish tank) water	*V. vulnificus, Mycobacterium marinum*
Drug abuse	
Intravenous	MRSA, *P. aeroginosa*
Subcutaneous	*E. corrodens*
Hospital nursing for one patient	ARSA

Methicillin resistant *S. aureus* (MRSA) is a frequent cause of SSTI and of particular concern for the hospitalist. With the emergence of community-associated MRSA (CA-MRSA), MRSA infections are no longer only the pathogen of the hospitalized patient. Persons with MRSA infections that meet all of the following criteria likely have CA-MRSA[26]:

- Diagnosis of MRSA made in the outpatient setting or by a positive culture within 48 hours of admission
- No medical history of MRSA infection or colonization
- No medical history in the past year of:
  Hospitalization
  Admission to a subacute facility or hospice
  Dialysis
  Surgery
- No permanent indwelling catheters or medical devices that pass through the skin into the body

Other epidemiologic risk factors associated with CA-MRSA include individuals in crowded conditions with skin-to-skin contact, such as sports teams, the military, prisons, or daycare centers; children, especially those under the age of 2; and intravenous drug users.[27-29] Although both Healthcare associated - MRSA and CA-MRSA are methicillin resistant, their specific manifestations may differ, with CA-MRSA often presenting as a boil or abscess. Both CA-MRSA and HA-MRSA can cause more serious infections such as bloodstream infections or pneumonia. Finally, the virulence factors found in CA-MRSA strains appear to be distinct from those of HA-MRSA and may be responsible for the observation that the SSTI associated with CA-MRSA leads to more focal infections such as abcesses.[30]

Antibiotic therapy is the backbone of most SSTIs, but without appropriate local care, antibiotics alone can be ineffective. Specific antibiotic choices are guided by clinical factors, culture and susceptibilities, local formularies, cost, medication adherence, and side effects. The decision to hospitalize a patient with a SSTI is often based on both patient-level (clinical assessment, risk factors, social support) and system-level (insurance coverage, ability to administer intravenous antibiotics 24 hr/day, every day) issues. Patients with SSTI on the face, perineum, or hand (or the result of a human bite) should usually be cared for in an inpatient or observation unit setting for at least 24 hours to assess response to therapy and need for further intervention.[31]

Twenty-two percent of patients with SSTI followed in the Outpatient Parenteral Antibiotic Therapy (OPAT) registry were switched to parenteral therapy after oral therapy failure.[32] However, whether that switch always warrants hospitalization depends on the patient- and system-level issues outlined previously.[32,33] Hospitalists can partner with outpatient primary care physicians in developing strategies for OPAT implementation within institutions and frequently facilitate the transition of patients from the hospital to the outpatient setting. For patients who require ongoing parenteral therapy, peripherally inserted central catheter (PICC) lines or longer peripheral intravenous lines that can remain in place for up to 2 weeks are frequently required for the ongoing delivery of antimicrobials. Hospitalists can help to spearhead strategies to optimize the inpatient and inpatient/outpatient transition management of patients with SSTI. Although not meant to be exclusive or exhaustive, Table 36-5 summarizes some common antibiotic regimens for patients requiring parenteral therapy. The timing of the switch from parenteral to enteral therapy should be guided by: clinical response,

Table 36-5 Parenteral Antibiotic Selection

Eron Infection Class*	Antimicrobial Agents	Comments
Class 2 Non-MRSA	Ceftriaxone (or clindamycin)	Once-daily dosing For patients allergic to PCN, Ceph
Class 3 Non-MRSA	Cefazolin Semi-synthetic penicillins Clindamycin	Can cause phlebitis; for patients allergic to PCN, Ceph
Community-associated MRSA	Clindamycin Quinolones Trimethoprim-sulfa Doxycycline or minocycline	If isolate is erythromycin-resistant, in vitro clindamycin resistance may develop during therapy; consult with microbiology laboratory prior to treatment; may be sensitive in vitro, but the potential for resistance limits the use of this class; if prescribed should strongly consider adding rifampin Isolates resistant to tetracycline in vitro but susceptible to doxycycline or minocycline may develop resistance when exposed to doxycycline or minocycline monotherapy
Health care–associated MRSA	Vancomycin Linezolid	Expensive; oral bioavailability almost 100%; hematologic toxicity
Class 2 Diabetic limb infections†	Ceftriaxone + metronidazole or Fluoroquinolones + clindamycin or Co-trimoxazole + metronidazole or Amp-sulbactam	 Easy oral conversion Easy oral conversion
Class 3 Diabetic Limb infections†	Ceftriaxone + metronidazole or Fluoroquinolones + clindamycin or Piperacillin/tazobactam or Semi-synthetic pcns + metronidazole	 Easy oral conversion Must be administered several times a day
Necrotizing infections†	Penicillin G + clindamycin or Ampicillin-sulbactam or Piperacillin-tazobactam	Clindamycin may be particularly useful for infections caused by CA-MRSA Streptococcal infections due to an antitoxin effect

*See Table 36-1.

†± Vancomycin depending on MRSA risk factors and institutional MRSA rates.

PCN—penicillin; Ceph—cephalosporin

From Enron LJ, Lipsky BA, Low DE, et al. Managing skin and soft tissue infections: Expert panel recommendations on key decision points. JAC 2002; 52(Suppl 1):113–117.

culture and sensitivity results, and the patient's ability to take and tolerate oral therapy. Most patients can be safely switched to oral agents after 3–4 days of intravenous therapy.[34–37] The use of prolonged parenteral therapy (after 3–4 days) does not correlate with better outcomes. In addition, data from OPAT suggest that if a patient has a prolonged parenteral course, oral therapy may not be warranted.[38]

One study compared a 5-day course of antimicrobial therapy with a 10-day course and found no difference in outcomes; however, almost a quarter of patients were ineligible for the short course option because of progressive symptoms and signs.[39] Most cases of SSTI are successfully treated after 1–2 weeks of therapy.[40] However, the following risk factors may suggest a need for prolonged therapy: accompanying tissue necrosis; an organism that is difficult to eradicate; immunocompromised patient (diabetes,

on corticosteroids); adverse local factors (lymphedema, morbid obesity, ischemia, chronic venous insufficiency).[40]

The duration of therapy for patients with osteomyelitis depends on whether the infected bone is resected and/or how much of the infected bone remains.[1] A guideline to antibiotic treatment duration is presented in Table 36-6. For patients with necrotizing soft tissue infections, antibiotics are necessary but alone are insufficient to eradicate the infection. A multidisciplinary approach, including wound debridement and surgical exploration, is critical.[14] Adjuvant therapy for SSTI should be considered in all patients but is critical in the management of infections with wounds and/or osteomyelitis. The affected limb must be elevated so that accompanying edema and swelling can resolve, leading to more effective delivery of antimicrobial agents to the infected area.[14]

Table 36-6 Summary of Antibiotic therapy for Osteomyelitis

Extent of Bone Infection	Route of Administration	Duration of Therapy
No residual infected bone (post amputation)	Parenteral or enteral	2–5 days
Residual infected soft tissue (but not bone)	Parenteral or enteral	2–4 weeks
Residual infected (but viable) bone	Initial parenteral and then consider switch to enteral*	4–6 weeks
No surgery; residual dead bone postoperatively	Initial parenteral and then consider switch to enteral*	≥3 months

*Duration of parenteral therapy depends on clinical response.

From: Lipsky BA, Berendt AR, Gunner HD, et al. Diagnosis and treatment of diabetic foot infections. Clin Infect Dis 2004; 39:885–910.

For patients with deep soft tissue infections, the need for vascular evaluation and surgical evaluation must be determined early on in the clinical evaluation. Wound care for non-necrotizing soft tissue infections should include debridement of dead and unhealthy tissue, which can be done with a sterile scalpel or scissors or with topical chemical debriding products. Wound dressings should allow daily inspection and encourage a moist wound-healing environment. The affected limb must be off-loaded so that the wound is not subject to more mechanical pressure. For patients with necrotizing soft tissue infections, surgical debridement is essential, and mortality increases as the time to debridement increases.[14]

Other treatments such as granulocyte-stimulating factors (G-CSFs) have been shown to have minimal impact on infection resolution but do decrease the need for operative procedures.[41-45] Hyperbaric oxygen is another adjuvant treatment option and which has also been shown in some studies to decrease the risk of major amputation for patients with deep infections, but is difficult to deliver, is not readily available, and requires further study for its targeted use.[46-48] At this time, routine use of hyperbaric oxygen is not recommended.[49] Intravenous immunoglobulin has also been used as adjuvant therapy to treat deep soft tissue infections, particularly in patients who may be poor surgical candidates or are unstable for surgery. Small case-control series have described its effectiveness in patients with streptococcal toxic shock syndrome.[50-52] However, there are no randomized control trials studying its efficacy or its role in the treatment of skin and soft tissue infections.

The treatment of osteomyelitis also frequently includes both medical and surgical management. In nonrandomized case series, medical therapy alone with prolonged courses (3–6 months) of antimicrobial therapy resulted in clinical success in 65–80% of the cases.[1] Although frequently amputation or removal of the infected bone is part of the treatment of osteomyelitis, medical therapy alone can be considered in the following situations: there is no acceptable surgical target; the patient has ischemia caused by irreparable vascular disease and the patient does not want amputation; the infection is confined to the forefoot with minimal soft tissue loss; the patient has excessive surgical risk.[1]

For all patients, appropriate nutrition and, when indicated, nutritional supplements are essential to wound healing; frequently, these are coordinated with the assistance and input of hospital-based nutrition experts. For patients with glucose intolerance, glycemic control, with target glucoses <200 should be achieved if possible. When serum glucose levels are consistently >200, neutrophil function becomes impaired.[53] If the SSTI leads to the patient becoming critically ill, studies by Van den Berghe and Krinsley have demonstrated that more aggressive glycemic control can lead to improved outcomes in some patient populations.[54,55] Whether more aggressive glycemic targets will lead to improved outcomes for patients who do not need intensive care remains to be determined.

PREVENTION AND FOLLOW-UP

Prevention of recurrent SSTI involves management of risk factors and comorbidities that can increase an individual's susceptibility to and/or the severity of SSTI. Some of the risk factors such as substance abuse and chronic disease require multidisciplinary team-based interventions with the patient as the most critical member of the team. For patients with glucose intolerance or diabetes mellitus who are at significantly increased risk for vascular compromise and worse outcomes, there must be careful attention to glycemic control, but also to foot-care issues such as the type of footwear and nail care.

Clinical management must be linked to educational interventions so that optimal patient self-management can be promoted and achieved. In addition, the communication between various members of the care team must be coordinated so that the patient's care is seamless and integrated. The transition from the hospital can be an especially vulnerable time for patients with ongoing active management of their SSTI, and both human and system factors must be aligned to mitigate the risk of the transition. There needs to be role clarity of the care team members, as well as a health system that helps to facilitate team-based care and follow-up.

Key Points

- SSTIs account for up to 10% of inpatient hospitalizations.

- The physical examination continues to remain the backbone of establishing the extent of infection.

- Community-associated MRSA SSTIs are increasingly common and typically present as boils or abscesses.

- A multidisciplinary team is essential in the management of patients with complex SSTI.

SUGGESTED READING

Eron LJ, Lipsky BA, Low DE, et al. Managing skin and soft tissue infections: expert panel recommendations on key decision points. J Antimicrob Chemother 2003; 52(Suppl):i3–i17.

DiNubile MJ, Lipsky BA. Complicated infections of skin and skin structures: when the infection is more than skin deep. J Antimicrob Ther 2004; 53(Suppl 2):ii37–ii50.

Swartz MN. Cellulitis. N Engl J Med 2004; 350:904–912.

Lipsky BA, Berendt AR, Gunner HD, et al. Diagnosis and treatment of diabetic foot infections. Clin Infect Dis2004; 39:885–910.

CHAPTER THIRTY-SEVEN

Acute Bacterial Meningitis

Christopher Kim, MD, MBA, and James C. Pile, MD, FACP

BACKGROUND

Acute bacterial meningitis is an inflammation of the meninges, resulting from bacterially mediated recruitment and activation of inflammatory cells in the cerebrospinal fluid (CSF). This can be a rapidly fatal disease if not identified and treated promptly. Incidence in the United States has been estimated at 2.4 cases/100,000 population caused by the five leading pathogens in 1995.[1] Outcomes remain suboptimal, despite advancements in prevention and therapy, with a reported mortality rate of 21% in one large study of adults with community-acquired meningitis.[2] The causes of bacterial meningitis vary by patient age and setting. In adults, the most commonly identified organisms in community-acquired cases are *Streptococcus pneumoniae* (40–50%), *Neisseria meningitidis* (14–37%), and *Listeria monocytogenes* (4–10%).[1–3] Table 37-1 lists the most common causes of bacterial meningitis in adults. In nosocomial bacterial meningitis, the most common etiologies are staphylococcal infections (both *Staphylococcus epidermidis* and *S. aureus*) and aerobic gram-negative bacilli (including *Pseudomonas aeruginosa*), with major risk factors including neurosurgical procedures and head trauma. Two important trends in bacterial meningitis have occurred in the past two decades. The first of these has been the precipitous decline of *Haemophilus influenzae* meningitis due to the widespread use of vaccination against *H. influenzae* type B,[1,3] and the other the emergence of antibiotic-resistant *S. pneumoniae*.[4]

ASSESSMENT

Clinical Presentation

Presenting Signs and Symptoms

Patients with bacterial meningitis typically appear very ill with rapid progression of illness, although some may present more subacutely with several days of symptoms. When the CSF is penetrated by an offending organism, an inflammatory reaction occurs with rapid accumulation of leukocytes within the CSF. The classic clinical presentation is the triad of fever, nuchal rigidity, and change in mental status; although only two thirds of patients present with all three of the findings.[3] A systematic review found a pooled sensitivity for the presence of all three components of the triad to be only 46%.[5] Although many patients will not present with all three findings, 95% will have two or more symptoms, and 99–100% at least one. Thus, if a patient presents without fever, nuchal rigidity, or mental status change, further evaluation for meningitis may not be needed.[5] Fever is consistently the most common presenting finding, present in 85–95% of patients at time of presentation, with an additional 4% developing fever within 24 hours of admission.[3,5] Nuchal rigidity alone had a sensitivity of 70% in the above systematic review, while that of change in mental status was 67%.[5]

Kernig's sign and Brudzinski's sign have been utilized in clinical settings for nearly a century; however, there has been minimal evaluation of their diagnostic utility. Kernig's sign is positive if a patient in the supine position with hips flexed at 90 degrees has resistance or pain in the lower back or posterior thigh during an attempt to extend the knee. Brudzinski's sign is present when passive flexion of the neck in a supine position results in flexion of the knees and hips. Brudzinski reported a sensitivity of 57% for Kernig's sign and a 97% sensitivity for Brudzinski's sign in 1909.[6] A recent study attempted to validate these results by evaluating a cohort of 297 patients with suspected meningitis. This study found both Kernig's sign and Brudzinski's sign had a sensitivity of 5% and specificity of 95%, with a positive predictive value of 27% and a negative predictive value of 72%;[7] however, only three patients in this study proved to have bacterial meningitis, limiting the study's applicability.

One of the most useful clinical bedside tests may be jolt accentuation of headache. In this test, the patient is asked to turn his/her head horizontally 2–3 times per second. Worsening headache constitutes a positive sign. A small study that looked at 34 patients with CSF pleocytosis demonstrated that the jolt accentuation of headache had 97% sensitivity and 60% specificity.[8] Patients with fever and headache who have negative jolt accentuation of headache thus appear to have a low likelihood of meningitis, although confirmatory studies have not been published to date.[5,8]

Other presentations of meningitis may include seizures, rash, focal neurologic deficits, nausea and vomiting, and signs of increased intracranial pressure (such as papilledema; decreased level of consciousness; sixth nerve palsies; decerebrate posturing; and Cushing's triad of hypertension, bradycardia, and irregular respiratory pattern). The sensitivities of these findings are low, and therefore their clinical utility in ruling out meningitis is limited.[5]

Differential Diagnosis

Patients presenting with signs and symptoms suggesting the possibility of acute bacterial meningitis merit a prompt and thorough evaluation. Infectious processes that may mimic bacterial meningitis include other infectious meningitides (viral—including enteroviral, arboviral [West Nile virus], herpes simplex virus and HIV), tuberculous, Lyme disease, syphilitic, fungal and parasitic, Rocky Mountain spotted fever, brain abscess, and epidural and subdural empyema. Non–central nervous system (CNS) infections, including pneumonia and urinary tract infection, may be mistaken for bacterial meningitis when accompanied by mental status changes. Noninfectious considerations include CNS bleed (e.g., subarachnoid hemorrhage), drug-induced aseptic meningitis, hematologic malignancy such as lymphomatous meningitis, and CNS vasculitis.

Diagnosis

Preferred Studies

A careful history and physical examination will identify patients with possible bacterial meningitis. Any patient deemed sufficiently likely to have bacterial meningitis should have a lumbar puncture (LP) performed for evaluation of the CSF. Only about

Table 37-1 Most Common Causes of Community Acquired Bacterial Meningitis by Patient Age

Age of Patient	Most Common Organisms
18–65 years	S. pneumoniae N. meningitidis H. influenzae L. monocytogenes
>65 years	S. pneumoniae L. monocytogenes

1 mL from each tube is necessary, unless special tests will be sent. A total of four tubes are collected for analysis. An opening pressure measurement may aid in the evaluation process and should be performed routinely. This should be done with the patient in the lateral recumbent position, as upright positioning artificially elevates the opening pressure. In one study, 39% of patients with bacterial meningitis had opening pressures in excess of 300 mm H_2O.[3] Cerebrospinal fluid should be sent for Gram stain and culture, protein and glucose, and cell count with differential. Table 37-2 outlines the CSF studies that should be routinely obtained and their expected normal values. Bacterial meningitis will typically have CSF findings of high protein (>500 mg/dL), low glucose (less than 45 mg/dL or <40% of serum glucose levels), and leukocytosis with a polymorphonuclear (PMN) predominance. Occasionally, aseptic meningitis can present with a PMN predominance, but this usually transforms to lymphocyte predominance within 8–24 hours.[9] There are also rare occasions when bacterial meningitis will have a "normal" cell count, differential, glucose, and protein values. If the clinical suspicion still remains very high for bacterial meningitis, despite normal CSF values, a repeat lumbar puncture should be performed 24 hours later.[10] Patients with bacterial meningitis who have recently been treated with antibiotics before their CSF can be analyzed will frequently have negative Gram stain and culture results. However, the other CSF analysis studies will often still be abnormal with a PMN leukocytosis, high protein, and low glucose levels, which should raise the clinical suspicion for bacterial meningitis. The clinician can then send the CSF for further diagnostic studies to evaluate for bacterial involvement. These studies are described in greater detail below. Patients with meningococcal meningitis may present with a petechial or purpuric rash, biopsy of which may demonstrate the organism. Other laboratory studies that should be obtained include blood cultures, complete blood count with platelets and differential (CBCPD), and basic chemistry labs.

Although CSF culture is the gold standard in the diagnosis of meningitis, other studies have utility in certain settings. Latex agglutination tests for bacterial antigens including S. pneumoniae, N. meningitidis, H. influenzae type B, group B streptococcus, and

Table 37-2 CSF Studies to Be Obtained and Their Expected Normal Values

LP Tube	Study	Expected Normal	Suggestive of Bacterial Meningitis
Tube #1: Gram stain and culture	Gram stain Culture	No organism Negative culture	Positive in 70% of cases Positive in 80% of cases
Tube #2: Protein and glucose	Protein Glucose Serum: CSF: serum glucose ratio	15–45 mg/dL 50–70 mg/dL >0.5	>500 mg/dL <45 mg/dL <0.4
Tube #3: Cell count and differential	WBC RBC	<5 WBC/μcL, lymphocytes or monocytes 0, unless traumatic LP	>10 WBC/μcL, predominantly PMNs. —
Tube #4: Any viral, fungal, or miscellaneous studies. This tube should be saved for any potential future studies.	—	—	—

E. coli are available, and they may be considered when bacterial meningitis is still suspected in patients with negative gram stain and culture results at 48 hours.[11] This occurs most commonly in patients who have received prior antibiotics. The latex agglutination test is highly specific for *S. pneumoniae* and *N. meningitidis* at nearly 100%; however, the sensitivity is 70–100% for *S. pneumoniae,* and only 50–93% for *N. meningitidis.* The limulus amebocyte lysate assay is a very sensitive test for gram-negative endotoxins (>90%), and it has a reported specificity of 85–100%. The polymerase chain reaction (PCR) test for bacterial pathogens from the CSF has been developed for some organisms, including *S. pneumoniae, N. meningitidis, H. influenzae* type B, and *Mycobacterium tuberculosis.* Although PCR appears to have promising capabilities, the test needs to undergo further testing and refinement before routine use in clinical practice. The utility of PCR may be greatest in identifying a viral cause, thus ruling out bacterial meningitis. Enteroviral PCR testing is highly sensitive and specific, and its use has been linked to a decreased length of stay and fewer interventions.[12] Many laboratories do not perform these alternative tests on site, however, and the time required to send to a reference laboratory may negate their usefulness.

The role of brain imaging prior to performing an LP has been an important issue for both patient safety and medical-legal reasons, largely due to the concern for precipitating uncal herniation by performing the LP (Fig. 37-1). Two large studies have looked at the clinical utility of obtaining a head CT prior to performing an LP.[13,14] Clinical features associated with an abnormal CT scan included: age >60; immunocompromised status; a history of CNS disease such as a mass lesion, stroke, or focal infection; a history of seizure within a week before presentation; and a focal neurologic abnormality (including altered level of consciousness, inability to answer two consecutive questions correctly or follow two consecutive commands, gaze palsy, abnormal visual fields, facial palsy, arm drift, leg drift, and abnormal language). The absence of these findings conferred a 97% negative predictive value of having an abnormal CT scan in these studies totaling 413 patients. In three patients who had none of these risk factors but nonetheless had a subsequent finding of an abnormal CT scan, LP was performed with no evidence of brain herniation. Thus, in a patient with none of these findings, available data suggest that an LP can be safely performed without obtaining a prior head CT scan.

The patients who underwent CT before LP waited 2 hours longer to get an LP, compared to those who did not get a CT scan; and antibiotic administration was delayed an average of 1 hour in the CT group.[14] The decision to obtain a CT scan prior to performing an LP should not delay the decision to administer the initial dose of antibiotic. The administration of a single dose of antibiotics should not alter the CSF findings significantly, provided LP is performed within about 4 hours of receiving antibiotics.

Algorithms

See Figure 37-2 for a diagnostic and treatment evaluation algorithm for suspected bacterial meningitis.

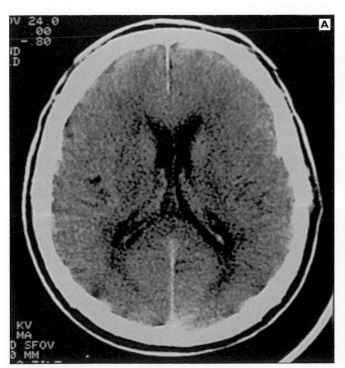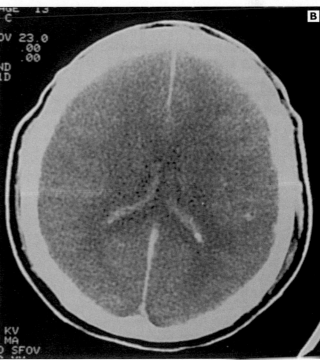

Figure 37-1 • Computed tomography (CT) scans of the head in a patient with pneumococcal meningitis. A, CT scan on presentation reveals moderate cortical atrophy. B, CT scan 3 days later reveals diffuse swelling of the cerebral hemispheres bilaterally, with effacement of the ventricular system. From: Mandell G, Bennett J, Dolin R. Mandell, Douglas, and Bennett's Principles and Practice of Infectious Diseases, ed 6, vol 2. Philadelphia: Churchill 2000; 1103.

Figure 37-2 • Algorithm for diagnostic evaluation and treatment of bacterial meningitis.

CT—computed tomography; CNS—central nervous system; CBCPD—complete blood count with platelet differential; CSF—cerebral spinal fluid

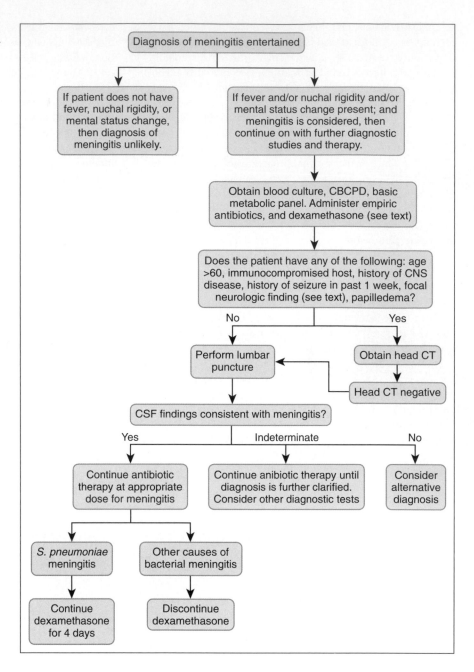

Prognosis

During Hospitalization

Prognosis is closely tied to the responsible organism, severity of disease at time of presentation, and rapidity of progression. Inhospital mortality rates related to meningitis in one large retrospective study were 25% for *S. pneumoniae*, 10% for *N. meningitidis*, and 21% for *L. monocytogenes*. Age >60, obtundation on admission, or development of seizures within 24 hours of admission was shown to confer an increased risk of mortality. Ninety-eight percent of the patients who died in this study had at least one of these risk factors. The overall inhospital mortality rate for community-acquired bacterial meningitis in this study was 25%. Twenty-one percent of patients developed neurologic deficits, and 9% had persistence of their neurologic symptoms at the time of discharge.[3] A population-based surveillance study reported mortality rates of 21% for *S. pneumoniae*, 15% for *L. monocytogenes*, and 3% for *N. meningitidis*, although both adult and pediatric patients were included.[1] Most recently, a large prospective study evaluating efficacy of dexamethasone in adults with bacterial meningitis reported an overall mortality of 15% for all types of bacterial meningitis in the control arm (no corticosteroids), with a 34% mortality for patients infected with *S. pneumoniae* in the control group.[15] Mortality rates for hospitalized patients who develop a single episode of nosocomial meningitis are estimated to be about 35%, and recurrent nosocomial infections have a mortality rate of about 16%.[3]

Table 37-3 Empiric Antibiotic Therapy by Age, and Most Common Bacteria in That Age Group

2–50 years: *S. pneumoniae*, *N. meningitidis*	Vancomycin 2–4 g/day IV divided every 6–12 hr + 3rd-generation cephalosporin (Ceftriaxone 2 g IV q 12 hr or cefotaxime 2 g IV q 6 hr)
>50 years: *S. pneumoniae*, *N. meningitidis*, *L. monocytogenes*	Vancomycin 2–4 g/day IV divided q 6–12 hr + 3rd generation cephalosporin (ceftriaxone 2 g IV q 12 hr or cefotaxime 2 g IV q 6 hr) + ampicillin 8–14 g/day IV or IM divided q 4–6 hr

Table 37-4 Empiric Antibiotic Coverage for Specific Predisposing Conditions and the Most Common Associated Organisms

Basilar skull fracture: *S. pneumoniae*, *H. influenzae*, group A beta-hemolytic strep	Vancomycin 2–4 g/day IV divided q 6–12 hr + 3rd generation cephalosporin (ceftriaxone 2 g IV q 12 hr or cefotaxime 2 g IV q 6 hr)
Penetrating trauma: *S. aureus*, coagulase negative staphylococci (CNS), gram-negative bacilli (GNB) (including *Pseudomonas*)	Vancomycin 2–4 g/day IV divided q 6–12 hr + cefepime 2 g IV q 8 hr or ceftazidime 2 g IV q 8 hr
Postneurosurgery: GNB (including *Pseudomonas*), CNS, *S. aureus*	Vancomycin 2–4 g/day IV divided q 6–12 hr + cefepime 2 g IV q 8 hr or ceftazidime 2 g IV q 8 hr
CSF Shunt: CNS, *S. aureus*, GNB (including *Pseudomonas*), *Propionibacterium acnes*	Vancomycin 2–4 g/day IV divided q 6–12 hr + cefepime 2 g IV q 8 hr or ceftazidime 2 g IV q 8 hr

Although delay in administration of antibiotics after presentation has long been suspected to lead to worse outcomes, this has been difficult to demonstrate conclusively. One study suggested an association only if rapid deterioration occurred before antibiotics were administered.[16] Outcomes are clearly worse if a patient suffers herniation as a result of increased intracranial pressure, or has other complications associated with meningitis such as vascular events, subdural effusion or abscess, and hydrocephalus.[3]

Postdischarge

The most common complications that develop after an episode of meningitis are neurologic. Potential persistent neurologic problems include hearing loss, cognitive impairment, seizures and focal neurologic symptoms including cranial nerve palsies. The most common neurologic complication postdischarge is hearing loss. In one study, 12% of patients treated with antibiotics for meningitis developed hearing loss at their 8-week follow-up. Subset analysis revealed that *S. pneumoniae* meningitis carried the highest rate of hearing loss, 21%.[15] Previous studies in children revealed similar rates of hearing loss. Hearing loss related to specific pathogens varied from 12% for *H. influenzae* (prior to the vaccine administration era) to 20% for *S. pneumoniae*.[17]

Persistent cognitive impairment after bacterial meningitis has been evaluated in a limited number of patients. Patients with pneumococcal meningitis who appeared to experience good recovery had significantly worse cognitive outcomes compared to controls, and an overall worse perception of their general health and quality of life as measured by a questionnaire performed 6–24 months after discharge.[18,19]

MANAGEMENT

Initial

When bacterial meningitis is suspected, the initial dose of antibiotic therapy should be given as soon as possible and at a dose adequate to penetrate the CSF. Since *S. pneumoniae* and *N. meningitidis* are the two most common organisms in younger adults, antibiotic therapy should be targeted to these organisms. With the development of increased resistance to penicillin and cephalosporins by *S. pneumoniae*, especially in the United States, initial therapy should consist of the combination of a third-generation cephalosporin and vancomycin. Ampicillin should be added in those patients at risk for *L. monocytogenes* infection (i.e., patients <3 months or >55 years of age, immunosuppressed, or pregnant). Table 37-3 lists recommended antibiotic therapy, based on the most common bacterial pathogens causing meningitis by age. For special conditions such as the postsurgical patient after a shunt placement, or a post-trauma patient, empiric coverage should expand to treat for possible staphylococcal infections and gram-negative infections, including *Pseudomonas*. Recommended therapy is vancomycin with ceftazidime. Table 37-4 lists recommended antibiotic therapy for specific predisposing conditions.

Subsequent

Once an offending organism has been identified either by Gram stain or culture, therapy should be tailored to that particular organism. Duration of therapy will vary, depending on the

Table 37-5 Specific Antibiotic Therapy, Dosages, and Recommended Duration Based on Isolated Organisms

S. pneumoniae:	Duration:
If PCN sensitive with MIC <0.1 mcg/mL: Penicillin G 50,000 units/kg IV/IM q 4 hr or ampicillin 8–14 g/day IV/IM divided every 4–6 hr	10–14 days
If MIC 0.1–1.0 mcg/mL: Ceftriaxone 2 g IV q 12 hr or cefotaxime 2 g IV q 6 hr	10–14 days
If MIC >1.0 mcg/mL: Vancomycin 2–4 g/day IV divided q 6–12 hr + ceftriaxone 2 g IV q 12 hr or cefotaxime 2 g IV q 6 hr	10–14 days
N. meningitidis:	Duration:
If MIC <0.1 mcg/mL: Penicillin G 1–2 million units IV/IM q 2 hr or continuous IV drip 20–30 million units/day	7 days
If MIC >0.1 mcg/mL: Ceftriaxone 2 g IV q 12 hr or cefotaxime 2 g IV q 6 hr	7 days
L. monocytogenes:	Duration:
Ampicillin 8–14 g/day IV/IM divided q 4–6 hr or penicillin G 15–20 million units/day IV/IM divided every 4–6 hr	At least 21 days
Streptococcus agalactiae (Group B Streptococcus):	Duration:
Ampicillin 8–14 g/day IV/IM divided every 4–6 hr or penicillin G 50,000 units/kg IV/IM q 4 hr	14–21 days
E. coli:	Duration:
Ceftriaxone 2 g IV q 12 hr or cefotaxime 2 g IV q 6 hr	21 days
Pseudomonas:	Duration:
Cefepime 2 g IV q 8 hr or ceftazidime 2 g IV q 8 hr	21 days
H. influenzae:	Duration:
Beta-lactamase negative: Ampicillin 8–14 g/day IV/IM divided every 4–6 hr	7 days
Beta-lactamase positive: Ceftriaxone 2 g IV q 12 hr or cefotaxime 2 g IV q 6 hr	7 days
S. aureus:	Duration:
MSSA: Nafcillin 2 g IV q 4 hr or oxacillin 2 g IV q 4 hr	14–28 days
MRSA: Vancomycin 2–4 g/day IV divided every 6–12 hr	14–28 days
Coagulase-negative staphylococcus:	Duration:
Vancomycin 2–4 g/day IV divided every 6–12 hr	14–28 days

MSSA—methicollin sensitive staphylococcus aure us; MRSA—methicollin resistant staphylococcus aureus; MIC—minimal inhibitory concentration

causative organism. (*See* Table 37-5 for recommendations on specific antibiotic therapy, dose, and duration based on isolated organism.) The decision to utilize a specific antibiotic therapy should be based on organism susceptibilities and the antibiotic's ability to penetrate the CSF. Treatment of bacterial meningitis should involve an antibiotic that has adequate bactericidal activity within the CSF for the offending organism. Because of their excellent CSF penetration, bactericidal activity with adequate minimal inhibitory concentration (MIC), and broad spectrum of activity against the most common causes of bacterial meningitis, the third-generation cephalosporins (ceftriaxone, cefotaxime) are most often used. Other antibiotics are added or substituted, based on specific circumstances.

For *S. pneumoniae* susceptible to penicillin, penicillin G and ampicillin remain the therapy of choice.[20] A third-generation cephalosporin may also be used if the MIC of the *S. pneumoniae* demonstrates susceptibility. However, with increasing prevalence of penicillin and cephalosporin-resistant *S. pneumoniae*, vancomycin may need to be used for isolates of *S. pneumoniae* where the MIC is >1 mcg/mL.[20] In these resistant strains of *S. pneumoniae*, however, vancomycin should not be used alone. A combination of ceftriaxone and vancomycin can be employed.[21] Serum vancomycin levels should be maintained in the range of 15–20 mcg/mL.[22] On the basis of experimental data, consideration may be given to the addition of rifampin to the regimen of vancomycin alone or in combination with ceftriaxone, provided the organism is susceptible to rifampin in patients with highly resistant strains of pneumococcal meningitis.

Neisseria meningitidis should be treated with a third-generation cephalosporin, although penicillin G or ampicillin may be used if the organism is fully sensitive. *Listeria* should be treated with ampicillin, probably with the addition of gentamicin; with trimethoprim/sulfamethoxazole an effective alternative in those with serious β-lactam allergy.[22]

Duration of therapy is based on the causative organism, and it varies from 7–21 days. Short courses of therapy with 7 days of antibiotics are sufficient for meningitis caused by *H. influenzae* and *N. meningitidis*. *S. pneumoniae* requires 10–14 days. Infection due to *Listeria* and gram-negative bacilli should be treated for 21 days.[20,22] Antibiotic therapy for bacterial meningitis should be given through the IV route for the full duration of treatment.

Adjunctive Therapy

The inflammatory reaction associated with meningitis is thought to be a major cause of morbidity and mortality associated with the disease.[22,23] Use of adjunctive steroids has been studied in patients with bacterial meningitis. Initial studies in children with meningitis showed benefit with use of adjunctive steroids along with antibiotics in treating meningitis.[17,24] In a recent landmark trial of adult patients with bacterial meningitis, treatment with adjunctive steroids in addition to antibiotics led to significant improvement in mortality and neurologic outcomes among those with pneumococcal disease.[15] In patients with meningococcal meningitis, there was a nonsignificant trend toward improved outcomes in mortality and neurologic complications. Adverse events were not increased in steroid treated patients compared to placebo groups.[25] Patients with suspected pneumococcal meningitis should receive adjunctive steroids with dexamethasone at a dose of 0.15 mg/kg q6h for 4 days. The first dose of dexamethasone should be given 10–20 minutes prior to or at the same time as the first dose of antibiotics. The use of corticosteroids appears to provide no benefit in patients who have already received a dose of antibiotics, and benefit in patients with meningitis due to organisms other than *S. pneumoniae* is unclear. Most authorities currently recommend withholding adjunctive dexamethasone in these patients whose meningitis is determined to be caused by bacterial pathogens other than *S. pneumoniae*. Although there are no randomized control trials to support this recommendation, most experts' recommendations are to initiate dexamethasone in all adults with suspected meningitis if antibiotics are to be administered, because the inciting pathogen is not always identifiable at initial evaluation.[15,17,22,25] In patients with pneumococcal meningitis resistant to penicillin and cephalosporins who receive vancomycin therapy, concern has been raised regarding the possibility that CSF penetration of vancomycin may be compromised if adjunctive steroids are administered. Current guidelines recommend, however, that patients with cephalosporin-resistant *S. pneumoniae* meningitis receive adjunctive steroids with appropriate antibiotic therapy. Other unanswered questions regarding the adjunctive use of corticosteroids include optimal duration of treatment, and their administration to immunosuppressed individuals.[26]

The need for a repeat LP should be based on the patient's clinical improvement. If the patient appears to be improving clinically, there is no need for a repeat LP. Repeat LP is recommended, however, in a patient with poor clinical response after 48 hours of antimicrobial therapy. Patients with a CNS shunt infection should have their CSF analyzed for improvement after shunt removal.[22] If a patient with bacterial meningitis does not appear to be improving after initiation of therapy, other considerations should include whether the empiric antibiotic therapy chosen is appropriate, whether antimicrobial resistance is present, and whether a complication of meningitis has developed.

PREVENTION

Some cases of bacterial meningitis can be prevented with the appropriate use of vaccination and by use of antibiotic chemoprophylaxis in high-risk situations. Currently available vaccines for bacterial meningitis include those targeting *S. pneumoniae*, *N. meningitidis*, and *H. influenzae*. The 23 polyvalent pneumococcal vaccine is recommended for all adults >65 years of age, or anyone older than 2 years of age with an immunocompromised state of health. The quadravalent meningococcal vaccine (serotypes A, C, Y, and W-135) is recommended for patients with functional asplenia, terminal complement deficiencies, those traveling to endemic areas of meningococcal meningitis, young adolescents ages 11–12, adolescents at high school entry age who have not been previously immunized and all college freshmen who will be living in dormitories. *H. influenzae* vaccine has changed the epidemiology of meningitis since its introduction, and it should be administered to all infants and children according to the recommended schedule.[1] It is currently not recommended for adults who have not received the vaccine as a child.

Antibiotic chemoprophylaxis has been recommended for close contacts of patients with certain types of bacterial meningitis. Currently, close contacts of patients with meningococcal meningitis and *H. influenzae* meningitis should be considered for chemoprophylaxis. Close contacts are defined as household members, day care contacts, or those with direct exposure to the patient's secretions (e.g., kissing). Health care workers at risk for meningococcal meningitis include only those directly exposed to the index patient's secretions, such as during mouth-to-mouth resuscitation, suctioning, or intubation. Chemoprophylaxis should occur as soon as exposure to the index case has been determined. There are several options for chemoprophylaxis against *N. meningitidis*. Rifampin may be used at a dose of 600 mg every 12 hours times 4 doses. Ciprofloxacin as a one-time dose of 500 mg orally is probably the regimen of choice in adults, due to its simplicity. Alternatively, ceftriaxone 250 mg intramuscularly once may be administered.[28] Rifampin and ciprofloxacin should not be used in pregnant patients due to risk of teratogenicity.

DISCHARGE/FOLLOW-UP PLANS

Completion of the duration of antibiotic therapy as directed is imperative. Complications from bacterial meningitis are rare after the first 3–4 days of appropriate therapy. Patients should follow up with their physicians after discharge from the hospital. Carefully selected patients may be considered as candidates to conclude their antibiotic therapy course as an outpatient; however, selection criteria should be quite stringent, and close physician follow-up is mandatory. Guidelines have been developed to aid in evaluation of patients for possible outpatient antibiotic therapy for bacterial meningitis.[22] These include:

1. Inpatient antibiotic therapy for at least 6 days
2. The absence of neurologic dysfunction, focal symptoms, or seizures
3. Afebrile for at least 24–48 hours in the hospital
4. Clinical improvement
5. Able to take PO fluids
6. Access to home health nursing for antibiotic administration
7. Reliable IV access
8. Prompt access to a physician
9. An established plan for follow-up laboratory testing and monitoring by health care personnel
10. Patient or family compliance with the program
11. A safe and reliable environment with access to telephone, utilities, and food

Short-term evaluation should focus on the complications that may have developed secondary to the meningitis (e.g., mental status changes, seizures, focal neurologic impairment, hearing loss). Long-term follow-up should focus on cognitive functioning, hearing assessment, and neuropsychiatric components of a patient's well-being.[15,18,19] Patients should be educated regarding the importance of follow-up with their physician as well as the need to monitor for recurrence of symptoms postdischarge.

Communication with the outpatient physician is critical in ensuring a smooth transition into outpatient therapy and follow-up. The details of the inpatient stay, antibiotic therapy and duration, imaging study results, details of any complications that may have developed during the hospital stay, and any follow-up imaging study recommended should all be relayed to the outpatient physician.

Key Points

- Bacterial meningitis can be a rapidly fatal disease; and it requires prompt recognition, diagnosis, and treatment.

- Two important trends that have emerged in bacterial meningitis have been (1) the precipitous decline of *Haemophilus influenzae* meningitis due to the widespread use of vaccination; and (2) the emergence of antibiotic resistant *Streptococcus pneumoniae*.

- The role of brain imaging prior to performing an LP is important from both a patient-safety and a medical-legal perspective. Clinical features associated with an abnormal CT scan include age >60; immunocompromised status; a history of CNS disease such as a mass lesion, stroke, or focal infection; a history of seizure within a week before presentation; and a focal neurologic abnormality. The absence of these findings conferred a 97% negative predictive value of having an abnormal CT scan in one large study of 413 patients.

- When bacterial meningitis is suspected, the initial dose of antibiotic should be administered as soon as possible, and it should not be delayed while waiting for LP or head CT results. In the United States, initial therapy should consist of the combination of a third-generation cephalosporin and vancomycin, with the addition of ampicillin in those patients at risk for *Listeria monocytogenes* infection.

- The inflammatory reaction associated with meningitis is thought to be a major cause of morbidity and mortality associated with the disease. Most experts recommend using dexamethasone as adjunctive therapy for patients suspected or confirmed to have pneumococcal meningitis. The first dose of dexamethasone should be given 10–20 minutes prior to or at the same time as the first dose of antibiotics.

SUGGESTED READING

Durand ML, Calderwood SB, Weber DJ, et al. Acute bacterial meningitis in adults: a review of 493 episodes. N Engl J Med 1993; 328(1):21–28.

Attia J, Hatala R, Cook DJ, et al. Does this adult patient have acute meningitis? JAMA 1999; 282(2):175–181.

Hasbun R, Abrahams J, Jekel J, et al. CT of the head before LP in adults with suspected meningitis. N Engl J Med 2001; 345(24):1727–1733.

de Gans J, van de Beek D. Dexamethasone in adults with bacterial meningitis. N Engl J Med 2002; 347(20):1549–1556.

Aronin SI, Peduzzi P, Quagliarello VJ. Community-acquired bacterial meningitis: risk stratification for adverse clinical outcome and effect of antibiotic timing. Ann Intern Med 1998; 129(11):862–869.

Quagliarello VJ, Scheld WM. Drug therapy: treatment of bacterial meningitis. N Engl J Med 1997; 336(10):708–716.

Tunkel AR, Hartman BJ, Kaplan SL, et al. Practice guidelines for the management of bacterial meningitis. Clin Infect Dis 2004; 39:1267–1284.

van de Beek D, de Gans J, McIntyre P, et al. Steroids in adults with acute bacterial meningitis: a systematic review. Lancet Infect Dis 2004;139—143.

Pile JC, Longworth DL. Should adults with suspected acute bacterial meningitis get adjunctive corticosteroids? Cleve Clin J Med 2005; 72:67–70.

CHAPTER THIRTY-EIGHT

Infective Endocarditis

Suzanne F. Bradley, MD

BACKGROUND

The precise epidemiology of infective endocarditis (IE) is not well understood due to referral bias, as many of these complicated infections are sent to tertiary medical centers for diagnosis and treatment. It is estimated that approximately 10,000–20,000 cases of IE or 5–7 cases per 100,000 person years are diagnosed in the United States each year.[1] If one considers that, on an annual basis, at least 250–500 cases of hospital-acquired bloodstream infection (BSI) occur per 100,000 person years in addition to all community- and health care-associated BSI, then IE is a relatively uncommon disease.

When IE does occur, substantial morbidity, cost, and mortality result. Endocarditis predominates in older adults and in men; most patients have predisposing valvular heart disease (Table 38-1). The number of cases due to rheumatic heart disease appears to have declined with an increase in prosthetic and degenerative valvular heart disease.[2,3] The most common causes of IE are bacterial, but the most prevalent genera and species vary with the population studied. Overall, *Streptococcus viridans* has generally been the most frequent pathogen, followed by *Staphylococcus aureus* and enterococci[1–3] (Table 38-2).

ASSESSMENT

Clinical Presentation

The clinical presentation of IE is quite variable and highly dependent upon microbial as well as host factors. The microbiologic cause of IE is also dependent upon a host's susceptibility and exposure to an organism and the propensity of that agent to cause infection. The initial history should focus on the acuity of the clinical presentation, presence of valvular predisposition, and exposure to pathogens that might cause IE in an appropriate clinical setting.

Prevalence

All microorganisms do not have the same capacity to cause IE in all hosts. Microorganisms have varying capacities, termed virulence, to cause damage to heart valves by direct invasion, elaboration of toxins, or induction of an acute inflammatory response (Fig. 38-1). Therefore, it is crucial that the clinician be aware of what infecting organisms cause IE and which patients are at greatest risk of acquiring those infections. For example, less virulent microorganisms (*Staphylococcus epidermidis* or coagulase-negative staphylococci, diphtheroids) that do not have the ability to invade tissues generally require the presence of a valvular abnormality or prosthetic device to establish an infection.[2,3]

In addition, all cardiac lesions are not at equal risk of developing IE.[2–4] Valvular lesions associated with high-pressure gradients, regurgitation, turbulence, and damage to vascular endothelium allow platelet aggregation and attachment of microorganisms. In the avascular environment within the vegetation, microorganisms freely replicate sequestered away from attack by phagocytic cells. Valvular prostheses and cardiac conditions associated with moderate-to-severe incidence of IE place patients at higher risk of infection with less virulent organisms (*see* Table 38-1). Thus, to assess IE risk and the likely causative organism, the clinician must determine if the patient has a prosthetic valve or prior history of a valvular abnormality that might increase risk of IE (*see* Table 38-2).

Moreover, some hosts are at greater risk of IE because they have greater exposure to a pathogen than other patients. Health care–related IE is associated with increased rates of bloodstream injection (BSI) following procedures and the use of devices. Intravenous drug users have similar risk of BSI related to needle use. Other causes of IE are related to exposures to pathogens found in specific environments, animal reservoirs, or insect vectors, or associated with certain comorbid conditions or procedure[5,6] (Table 38-3). If IE is suspected, a careful history may yield important clues to determine the possible organism(s) responsible for the infection.

Presenting Signs and Symptoms

In the patient with suspected IE, the history and physical examination should focus on the presence of nonspecific symptoms and signs of a systemic inflammatory illness as well as more specific symptoms and signs of valvular insufficiency and other complications.[7] IE due to more virulent organisms tends to have a shorter time (days to weeks) from introduction of infection to development of clinical symptoms and admission to hospital (acute IE) than less virulent microorganisms, where symptoms may persist for many weeks to months (subacute IE).

Table 38-1 Cardiac Conditions Associated with Increased Incidence of Infective Endocarditis (IE) and Poor Outcome

Risk level	Condition
High	Previous IE
	Valvular prostheses
	Unrepaired complex cyanotic congenital heart disease with pulmonary-systemic shunts
Moderate	Aortic valve—bicuspid, regurgitation, and stenosis
	Mitral valve—stenosis, prolapse with regurgitation or thickening
	Hypertrophic cardiomyopathy—obstructive with murmur
	Noncyanotic congenital cardiac defects (except ASD)
Low	Atrial septal defect (ASD)
	Mitral prolapse without above risk factors

Data from Danchin N, Duval X, Leport C. Prophylaxis of infective endocarditis: French recommendations 2002. Heart 2005; 91:715–718; and Antibacterial prophylaxis for dental, GI and GU procedures. Med Letter 2005; 47:59–60.

Table 38-2 Pathogens (%) That Cause Infective Endocarditis in Adults Based on Host Factors*

Host Factor	Streptococci	S. aureus	Enterococci	CNS	GNB	Fungi	Culture (−)	Diphtheroids	Polymicrobial HACEK Gr.
Native valves	31–65	30–40	5–8	4–8	4–10	1–3	3–10	5–7	1–2
IVDU	8	69	2	0	5	2	5	NA	9
Prosthetic valves									
Post surgery									
<2 months	0–1	20–24	5–10	30–47	0–15	0–10	0–27	5–7	2–4
2–12 months	7–10	10–15	10–15	30–35	2–4	10–15	3–7	2–5	4–7
>12 months	30–33	15–20	8–12	10–12	4–7	0–1	3–8	2–3	3–7

IVDU—intravenous drug user; CNS—coagulase negative staphylococci (e.g., *Staphylococcus epidermidis*); GNB—gram negative bacilli; HACEK Group—*Hemophilus* spp., *Actinobacillus* spp., *Cardiobacterium* spp., *Eikenella* spp., *Kingella* spp.; NA—Data not available from the studies cited.

*Data from Mylonakis E, Calderwood SB. Infective Endocarditis in adults. N Engl J Med 2001; 345:1318–1330; and Morellion P, Que Y-A. Infective endocarditis. Lancet 2004; 363:139–149.

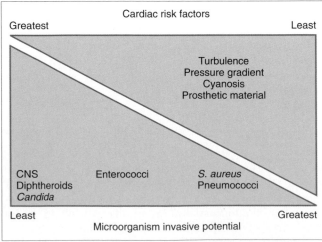

Figure 38-1 • Host factors and likelihood of infective endocarditis with various pathogens: a complex interplay between organism virulence and valvular abnormalities.

The clinical presentation of acute IE is typically more severe than those with subacute IE.[8,9] In acute IE, the onset of systemic symptoms of fever, rigors, and chills may be abrupt and associated with rapid development of signs of shock and organ failure. Rapid destruction of valves can lead to new-onset valvular insufficiency with quick progression to congestive heart failure.

In subacute IE, onset of symptoms, inflammatory signs, and development of organ dysfunction are much less dramatic. Patients may initially present with nonspecific symptoms of low-grade fever, sweats, chills, anorexia, and weight loss. Often, only when signs of valvular insufficiency or embolization occur is the diagnosis of IE suspected. An antibody response to the infection typically takes 2 or more weeks to occur, and therefore, manifestations of immune complex deposition, such as Roth spots or glomerulonephritis, are seen in patients with a subacute presentation.[7,10]

The clinical presentation may also depend upon the valves involved and whether clinical findings are manifested in the pulmonary or systemic circulation. Complications of right-sided IE

Table 38-3 Other Clinical Clues for the Diagnostic Cause of Infective Endocarditis

Risk factors	Microorganisms
Dental disease/recent procedures	Nutritionally variant streptococci (*Abiotrophia*)
	HACEK group
Depressed immunity	
Cellular function (e.g., transplants, pregnancy, aging)	*Legionella spp.* (endemic geographic areas)
	Listeria
AIDS	*Salmonella spp.*
Phagocytic/humoral function (e.g., cirrhosis, diabetes, AIDS)	*Staphococcus pneumoniae*
Devices	*Staphylococcus aureus*
	Coagulase-negative staphylococci
	Candida spp.
	Diphtheroids
Exposures-vectors/reservoirs	
Birds	Histoplasmosis
	Chlamydia pneumoniae
Dogs/cats	*Bartonella spp.*
	Coxiella burnetti (Q-fever)
Farm animals/animal products	*Brucella*
	Coxiella burnetti (Q-fever)
	Listeria spp.
	Salmonella spp.
Insects- body lice/fleas (common among homeless persons)	*Bartonella spp.*
Gastrointestinal symptoms/neoplasms/lesions	*Streptococcus bovis*
	Enterococci
	Trophreyma whipplei (with arthralgias, CNS symptoms)
Genitourinary disorders	Enterococci
	group B streptococci
Injectable medications	
Diabetes mellitus	*S. aureus*
	β-Hemolytic streptococci
Illicit drugs	*S. Aureus, Candida spp., Eikenella spp.*, other fungi
	Pseudomonas aeruginosa serotype 0111

Data from Baddour LM, Wilson WR, Bayer AS, et al. Infective endocarditis: diagnosis, antimicrobial therapy, and management of complications. A: Statement for healthcare professionals from the Committee on Rheumatic Fever, Endocarditis, and Kawasaki Disease, Council on Cardiovascular Disease in the Young, and the Councils on Clinical Cardiology, Stroke, and Cardiovascular Surgery and Anesthesia, American Heart Association. Circulation 2005; 111:e394–e433; and Albrich WC, Kraft C, Fisk T, et al. A mechanic with a bad valve: blood-culture-negative endocarditis. Lancet Inf Dis 2004; 4:777–784.

AIDS—Acquired Immunodeficiency Syndrome; IVDU—Intravenous Drug User; HACEK—*Hemophilus* spp., *Actinobacillus* spp., *Cardiobacterium* spp., *Eikenella* spp., *Kingellae* spp.; CNS—central nervous system.

typically result in pulmonary emboli and signs of right-sided heart failure. Embolic complications of left-sided IE can lead to arterial occlusion and abscess formation in virtually every organ system, including brain, gastrointestinal tract, kidney, and the musculoskeletal system as well as left-sided heart failure.[7] Physical findings and other diagnostic manifestations of IE are discussed further under Evidence for an Endocardial Source of Infection.

Differential Diagnosis

Any systemic inflammatory disease, infectious and noninfectious, may mimic the nonspecific signs and symptoms of IE. As already mentioned, BSIs are much more common than IE. Noninfectious diseases can be associated with embolic phenomena with signs and symptoms of inflammation. Fever commonly follows cerebrovascular events or emboli from cardiopulmonary sources due to hemorrhage or infarction. Autoimmune diseases or cardiac tumors involving the heart valve cause clinical syndromes identical to IE. Marantic endocarditis is associated with

neoplasms, particularly adenocarcinoma. Nonbacterial thrombotic endocarditis due to antiphospholipid syndrome and Libman-Sacks endocarditis due to systemic lupus erythematosus are uncommonly reported. Noninfectious causes of new valvular regurgitation, typically related to coronary artery disease, are frequent, and are generally not associated with fever or other stigmata of IE.[6]

Diagnosis

The diagnosis of IE should be considered if symptoms and signs consistent with infection are present, an organism is isolated that causes IE, and the appropriate predisposing risk factors are present that result in valvular infection. The diagnosis of IE is primarily a clinical diagnosis based on laboratory (histopathologic/microbiologic) evidence for infection and evidence for endocardial/valvular involvement (valvular dysfunction or evidence for an embolic source). These factors, discussed in more detail below, are the basis for the Duke Criteria commonly used for the diagnosis of IE[3,7,11] (Table 38-4).

Pathologic, microbiologic, or endocardial findings that are highly specific for the diagnosis of IE are termed major criteria. The diagnosis of definite IE is established by the presence of two major criteria or one major and three minor criteria. Less specific findings that are associated with IE, but can be seen with other diseases, are termed minor criteria. Minor criteria include risk factors for IE, fever, and other evidence for vascular involvement, immunologic phenomena, and microbiologic findings that are not sufficiently specific for IE to be major criteria. Definite IE can be established if all five minor criteria are met.

The diagnosis of possible IE remains even if only a few of the above criteria are present, unless the patient improves so rapidly with antibiotics that the diagnosis is unlikely, or a firm alternative diagnosis is established. Thus, the diagnosis of IE can be elusive and both under and over diagnosed. Early consultation with experts in the diagnosis and management of IE is strongly advised.

Pathologic and Microbiologic Evidence

The microbiologic diagnosis of IE is based primarily on culture of blood and by culture or histopathology of valvular tissue or peripheral emboli. Effective interpretation of blood cultures requires that multiple sets be drawn, appropriate volumes of blood be obtained for the culture system used, and sampling of blood be obtained at multiple intervals.[10,11] If three cultures of blood are negative, and culture negative IE is suspected clinically, serology based on exposure history or newer culture and DNA

Table 38-4 Modified Duke Criteria for the Diagnosis of Infective Endocarditis (IE)*

DIAGNOSIS

Definite IE	Pathologic or microbiologic evidence of vegetations, major emboli, or cardiac abscess
	2 major criteria
	1 major/3 minor criteria
	5 minor criteria
Possible IE	1 major/1 minor
	3 minor
Rejected	Resolved symptoms with ≤4 days of antibiotic treatment or alternative diagnosis established or no evidence at surgery or autopsy with ≤4 days antibiotic treatment or does not meet criteria for definite or possible IE

MAJOR CRITERIA

MICROBIOLOGY

Persistent Bacteremia
  Typical IE organisms (*Streptococcus viridans*, *S. bovis*, HACEK Group,
  community-acquired *S. aureus*, or enterococci without obvious focus.)
  ≥2/2 blood culture sets positive—obtained 12 hours apart (appropriate stable patients)
  ≥3/4 blood culture sets positive—obtained over 1–2 hours (appropriate unstable patients)
Positive serology for *Coxiella burnetti* (Q fever)

ENDOCARDIAL INVOLVEMENT

Physical Examination
  New valvular regurgitation
Echocardiogram

Prosthetic valves	New partial dehiscence, periannular abscess, or oscillating intracardiac mass on valve
Native valves	Clinical criteria for possible IE or suspected intracardiac abscess with discrete oscillating mass on valve, supporting structure, or in path of a regurgitant jet, resulting in likely endothelial damage; or presence of intracardiac abscess

MINOR CRITERIA

PREDISPOSITION
  IVDU
  Predisposing moderate- to high-risk cardiac conditions (See Table 38-1.)

FEVER ≥38°C (100.4°F)
VASCULAR FACTORS
  Arterial emboli, pulmonary infarcts, intracranial bleed. mycotic aneurysms, conjunctival petechiae, excludes other petechiae or splinter hemorrhages.
IMMUNOLOGIC FACTORS
  Glomerulonephritis (red cell casts), rheumatoid factor, Osler nodes, Roth spots.
MICROBIOLOGY
  Positive blood cultures that do not meet major criteria but exclude organisms that generally do not cause IE, e.g., single culture of coagulase-negative staphylococci.
  Other positive serology with organisms likely to cause IE.

Data from Morellion P, Que Y-A. Infective endocarditis. Lancet 2004; 363:139–149; Crawford MH, Durack DT. Clinical presentation of infective endocarditis. Cardiol Clin North Am 2003; 21:159–166; *and* Prendergast BD. Diagnostic criteria and problems in infective endocarditis. Heart 2004; 90:611–613.

*These criteria are a work in progress and recommendations regarding changes are ongoing.

HACEK—*Hemophilus* spp., *Actinobacillus* spp., *Cardiobacterium* spp., *Eikenella* spp., *Kingella* spp.; IVDU—Intravenous drug user; TEE—Transesophageal echocardiogram.

amplification diagnostic techniques such as polymerase chain reaction may be indicated[6,10,12] (Table 38-5).

Persistent isolation of an organism on blood culture is the hallmark of endovascular infection[10] (*see* Table 38-4). IE should be considered in any patient with repeated isolation of the same organism from multiple blood cultures obtained at different time intervals.

There are some organisms that are so characteristically associated with IE that the diagnosis should be always be considered, such as any patient with community-acquired *S. aureus* or enterococcal bloodstream infection without an obvious source. The diagnosis of IE should be particularly considered if uncommon organisms classically associated with IE are isolated, such as *S. viridans*, *S. bovis*, or members of the HACEK group (*Hemophilus* spp, *Actinobacillus*, *Cardiobacterium hominis*, *Eikenella corrodens*, or *Kingella kingae*).

For other organisms that are uncommon causes of IE, or are frequent contaminants, more evidence for persistence of bacteremia is reassuring, especially if predisposing valvular conditions are not present.[10] For example, coagulase-negative staphylococci or polymicrobial bacteremia are common causes of blood culture contamination and rarely cause native valve IE. Repeated isolation of the same organism(s) in three or more sets of blood cultures obtained at different times with identical antimicrobial susceptibilities increases the likelihood that true infection rather than contamination is present.

Culture-negative IE is uncommon, but should be considered if typical physical findings of IE such as peripheral emboli and new valvular dysfunction are evident but blood cultures are negative. Most cases of culture negative IE (~40%) are associated with prior treatment with antibiotics. Fortunately, only 5% of cases of IE are truly culture negative.

Evidence for an Endocardial Source of Infection

Indirect or direct evidence for endocardial or valvular involvement may be present on physical, laboratory, or radiologic examination. In the setting of suspected infection, the presence of a new regurgitant murmur is a major criterion for IE. Minor criteria or indirect evidence for valvular infection is provided by the presence of vascular or immunologic phenomena on physical examination (Janeway lesions, Osler nodes, Roth spots). Other minor criteria include presence of serum rheumatoid factor or glomerulonephritis (unexplained hematuria, red cell casts) in urine. Abscesses or infarcts suggestive of vascular phenomena may be seen on imaging studies.[7]

A positive echocardiograph suggests endocardial infection if the presumed vegetation has an appropriate appearance and is found in the proper location and in the appropriate clinical setting. A diagnostic intracardiac vegetation should be oscillating and located on a regurgitant valve, in the path of the regurgitant jet, or on supporting structures. New dehiscence or paravalvular

Table 38-5 Diagnostic Testing for Culture-Negative Infective Endocarditis (IE)

Diagnostic Approach	Organism(s)
Tissue Histopathology (valve/emboli)	
Acridine orange/Giemsa	Any bacterium
Gram stains (Brown Hopps/Brown-Brenn)	Gram-positive/gram-negative bacteria
Periodic acid–Schiff	Fungi, *Tropheryma whipplei*
Warthin-Starry	*Bartonella* spp.
Gimenez	*Coxiella burnettii*, *Legionella* spp.
Ziehl-Nielsen	Acid-fast bacilli
Kinyoun, Machiavello	*Chlamydia* spp.
Immunohistologic staining	*Bartonella* spp., *Chlamydia* spp., *C. burnettii*
	T. whipplei
Serology	*Bartonellae* spp., *Coxiella burnetti*, *Chlamydia* spp., *Mycoplasma* spp., *Brucella* spp., *Legionella* spp.
Culture Techniques	
Prolonged incubation	Extracellular or facultative intracellular organisms
	Abiotrophia spp., HACEK group, *Brucella* spp.
	Most grow within 5 days with current culture methods
Lysis centrifugation/subculture-specific media	If no growth within 5 days or specific growth requirements
	In patients with high clinical suspicion of IE
	Legionella spp., *Mycoplasma* spp., *Brucella* spp., *Mycobacteria* spp.
Tissue culture (shell vial)	Obligate intracellular organisms
	Bartonella spp., *C. burnetti*, *Chlamydia* spp., *T. whipplei*
Polymerase Chain Reaction (PCR)	
Broad-range PCR	Detects 16SrRNA present in all bacteria
Species-specific PCR (many under development)	*T. whipplei*, *C. burnettii*, *Bartonella* spp., *Chlamydia* spp., *Brucella* spp., *Legionella* spp., *Mycoplasma* spp., *Mycobacteria* spp.

Data from Albrich WC, Kraft C, Fisk T, et al. A mechanic with a bad valve: blood-culture-negative endocarditis. Lancet Inf Dis 2004; 4:777–784; Towns ML, Reller BL. Diagnostic methods: current best practices and guidelines for isolation of bacteria and fungi in infective endocarditis. Cardiol Clin North Am 2003; 21:197–205; and Houpikian P, Raoult D. Diagnostic methods: current best practices and guidelines for identification of difficult to culture pathogens in infective endocarditis. Cardiol Clin North Am 2003; 21:207–217.

* As an agent of bioterrorism, cultures for *Coxiella* are not routinely processed in most laboratories.

abscess suggests prosthetic valvular infection.[13] Not all patients with IE have a new murmur or abnormal echocardiograph; vegetations may take time to form, may be too small to visualize, or may not be evident after being embolized. Persistently positive blood cultures, in the absence of another source, suggest that an endocardial focus, such as IE, is still possible.

Preferred studies

Bloodstream infection is established by blood culture. Empiric treatment should be withheld until adequate culturing has been performed unless the patient is clinically unstable. In the absence of prior antibiotic therapy, two sets of blood cultures obtained 12 hours apart is sufficient to diagnose >95% of cases of IE.[3,10] If the patient is unstable, a total of 3–4 sets of blood cultures drawn from different sites over a 1–2 hour interval is an acceptable alternative to establish persistent bloodstream infection is present. In the patient with prior antimicrobial therapy, more blood cultures should be performed. Current blood culture methods are sufficient to detect nutritionally variant streptococci (*Abiotrophia*) and HACEK organisms after 5 days incubation.[6,10,12]

Echocardiography can be helpful to assist in the diagnosis of IE if not already established by microbiologic and clinical criteria. Duke Criteria that incorporate echocardiographic results diagnose 80% of confirmed cases of IE as opposed to ~50% diagnosed clinically by the Von Reyn/Beth Israel Criteria.[14] Use of transthoracic echocardiography (TTE) versus transesophageal echocardiography (TEE) should be based on risk for IE and clinical suspicion. Echocardiography is also performed in patients with known IE to obtain prognostic information and to detect complications that might alter management.[5,14]

TTE is noninvasive and less expensive than TEE; studies may be technically inadequate in 20% of adults who have chest wall abnormalities, obesity, or chronic obstructive pulmonary disease.[15] TEE should be performed initially in patients if they have conditions at high risk for IE, if there is moderate to high clinical suspicion for IE, or if imaging is likely to be difficult[4,5] (*see* Table 38-1). TEE based on clinical suspicion should be considered if there is a new unexplained regurgitant murmur or heart failure or stigmata of IE on examination. If the TEE is negative, patients should be restudied in 7–10 days if clinical suspicion remains high and there is no alternative diagnosis.

Proposed candidates for initial TTE are patients who have low-risk cardiac conditions and clinical suspicion for IE is low. A proposed definition for low clinical suspicion has included fever without stigmata of IE or previously described heart murmur. If large mobile vegetations, valvular insufficiency, paravalvular extension, or secondary ventricular insufficiency are found on TTE, then a TEE should be done to verify that IE is present and to assess for complications.[5]

A major area of controversy involves the need for TTE in all patients with BSI, given that IE is an uncommon infection.[15] Definitions for low clinical suspicion for IE have not been well established. In one study, patients with none or just one of the following risk factors, vascular/embolic phenomena, recent history of intravenous drug use or catheter, prosthetic valve, or positive blood cultures, had a <14% likelihood of having a positive TTE for IE[16] (*see* Chapter 20, Catheter-Related Bacteremia).

Another area of controversy is the recommendation for TEE in all patients with *S. aureus* bacteremia. IE may occur in 20–30%

of patients with *S. aureus* bacteremia. In studies at Duke, TEE was more effective than TTE or clinical examination in detecting IE compared with bacteremia alone; IE was associated with poorer prognosis as well.[17]

Alternative Options

TEE has been recommended to confirm the diagnosis of IE in patients at risk, to rule out complications that might require surgical intervention, and to obtain prognostic information. However, some patients with possible IE should be treated empirically with antibiotics alone without verification of the diagnosis by TEE. Typically, these patients are frail, have severe comorbid illness, and would not be candidates for surgery even if complications were found. The information obtained by TEE, associated with increased risk from anesthesia and aspiration, would not change the management of these patients.

Algorithm

A diagram outlining the evaluation and management of a patient with systemic febrile illness and possible IE is outlined in Figure 38-2.

Prognosis

Mortality from IE exceeds 20%.[18] Independent predictors for increased mortality include comorbid illness, moderate-to-severe

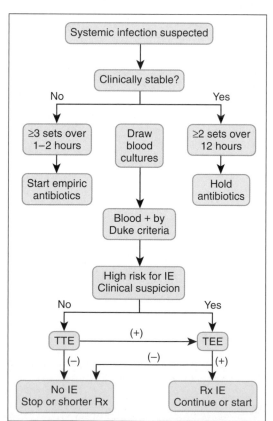

Figure 38-2 • A general approach to the patient with systemic infection and possible endocarditis. IE—infective endocarditis; TTE—transthoracic echocardiography; TEE—transesophageal echocardiography; Rx—treatment.

congestive heart failure, altered mental status, non–S. viridans etiology, and medical treatment without surgery.[19] In addition, up to 50% of patients with IE will have at least one complication of their IE.[20] Complications of IE may occur early in the course of infection or later, after antimicrobial treatment has been completed.

Successful outcome is dependent upon resolution of BSI, prevention of embolic complications, and preservation of valvular function. It is important for the clinician to monitor for and identify cardiac and distant complications of IE by initial and subsequent history and physical examinations.[14,20] Echocardiography may yield information regarding likelihood of embolization, local extension of infection, assessment of valvular and ventricular function, and need for surgical intervention that might alter management and outcome.[14,20]

Inadequately controlled infection leads to larger vegetations, with embolization to vital organs and structures. Embolization is identified most often in patients with left-sided IE (30–40%).[20] Most embolic complications occur prior to admission (75%) or during the first week of treatment (15%) and decline to 1% by 4 weeks.[18,21,22] The location, size, and shape of a vegetation may be associated with increased risk of embolization. Mitral valve lesions, particularly on the anterior mitral leaflet, are associated with greatest risk. Vegetations that are >1.0 cm or elongated are also more likely to embolize than smaller lesions.[18,20–22]

Following embolization, localized infection may ensue, causing abscess, infarct, or hemorrhage in many organs systems, including the central nervous (brain), reticuloendothelial (spleen), renal, and musculoskeletal systems (vertebral bodies, joints). Cerebral events occur in 20–40% of patients with left-sided valvular IE.[20,23] Manifestations include infarction (20–57%), meningitis (6–39%), and intracerebral hemorrhage (7–25%).[23] The prognosis of a patient with a cerebral event is poor if a valve replacement is required, due to the risks of immediate anticoagulation during surgery.[23,24]

In native valve IE, direct extension of infection into paravalvular structures and the conduction system leads to abscess and fistulae formation, infranodal conduction defects, and heart block.[20] The presence of infranodal conduction abnormalities or blocks on baseline electrocardiogram (ECG) is >80% specific for the presence of a paravalvular abscess in patients with IE.[24] In prosthetic valve IE, infection sown into the paravalvular ring may manifest as an abscess with dehiscence typically within 6 months of surgery. TEE is the most sensitive method to detect paravalvular abscess (>80%), a diagnosis that has >75% mortality without surgery.[20,24]

Failure to preserve valvular function leads to ventricular overload and development of congestive heart failure (CHF). A substantial decline in mortality due to CHF is seen in patients who undergo valvular replacement (10–35%) compared with medical therapy alone (55–85%).[21] Development of left-sided ventricular failure in a patient with IE is an urgent indication for repeat echocardiography and possible valvular replacement. Prompt surgery is needed for left ventricular failure unresponsive to 24 hours of aggressive medical management, aortic insufficiency, and infection with S. aureus.[10] Earlier intervention rather than duration of preoperative antimicrobial therapy plays the greatest role in improved surgical outcomes.[24]

Infection of distant cerebral or visceral blood vessels uncommonly can lead to mycotic aneurysms. Mycotic aneurysms may be suspected in patients with unexplained change in mental status or complaints of pain in the abdomen or an extremity. Many aneurysms are asymptomatic, improve with medical treatment alone, and do not bleed. The need for standard angiography or magnetic resonance imaging in all patients has not been established. Patients with subarachnoid bleed should be evaluated for surgical or noninvasive interventions.[21]

MANAGEMENT

Treatment

Preferred

Initial Antibiotic Treatment

When IE is suspected and after blood cultures are drawn, initial choice of empiric antibiotics typically is based on the most common bacterial causes such as S. viridans, S. aureus and enterococci. Empiric antibiotic choices may be further modified by the acuity of the illness, presence of other risk factors, and presence of prosthetic valves[20,25] (Table 38-6).

Subsequent Antibiotic Treatment

Subsequent antibiotic choices should be based on culture results, antimicrobial susceptibility testing, and recent guidelines from the American Heart Association in consultation with someone expert in the treatment of IE.[5] In-depth discussion of treatments for all possible causes of IE is beyond the scope of this chapter. Antibiotic choices for the treatment of IE should ideally be bactericidal with minimum toxicity and easily administered for prolonged periods of time. However, for some bacteria, aminoglycoside therapy is required, either because combination therapy results in bactericidal therapy or it shortens the duration of treatment. Most regimens will be intravenous, and placement of long-term venous access should be arranged after bacteremia has resolved (to avoid infection of the catheter).

The efficacy of antibiotic treatment is established by resolution of clinical symptoms and signs of infection as well as by clearance of BSI by multiple blood cultures performed over successive days. Documentation of clearance of BSI is particularly important, as persistence of fever and inflammation may not necessarily reflect antibiotic failure. In the absence of persistent BSI, repeat imaging should be done to ensure that fever is not due to abscesses that require surgical drainage. Persistent fever may also be due to autoimmune glomerulonephritis, hemorrhage and infarction from bland aseptic emboli, or drug fever.

Management of Complications

IE is a complex disease that requires early evaluation by many disciplines. Infectious diseases physicians can assist in the diagnostic evaluation, identification of complications, appropriate choice and duration of antimicrobial therapy, and determination of who should give the outpatient treatment and in what setting. Early consultation by cardiologists is also invaluable for echocardiographic assessment of valvular and ventricular functions and the integrity of the conduction system. Complications may require intervention by cardiothoracic surgeons, peripheral vascular surgeons, or neurosurgeons. In the patient with a cerebrovascular complication, the neurologist can assist with questions regarding optimal timing of valve surgery and anticoagulation issues.

Table 38-6 Initial Treatment of Suspected Infective Endocarditis

Drug	Dose	Rationale
Native Valves		
Acute presentation		
Vancomycin **plus:**	1 gm IV q 12 hr adjust by levels	− *Staphylococcus aureus* primary concern especially if no known valvular predisposition.
		− Prevalence of methicillin-resistance increasing.
Gentamicin[+]	3 mg/kg IV/IM q hr give in 2–3 divided doses	− Switch to naficllin or cefazolin if methicillin-susceptible *S. aureus* and no beta-lactam allergy.
		− Benefit of gentamicin beyond 3–5 days not established.
		− Vancomycin/gentamicin also active against enterococci
		− If ampicillin-susceptible enterococci, switch if not allergic and continue gentamicin for synergy.
Subacute or indolent presentation*		
Ampicillin **plus:**	2 g IV q 6 hours	− *Streptococcus viridans* primary concern especially if valvular predisposition.
Gentamicin[+]	3 mg/kg IV/IM per day give in 2–3 divided doses	− Verify PCN MIC <0.12 mcg/mL
		− Gentamicin reduces duration of ampicillin treatment
or:		− Ampicillin/gentamicin also active against susceptible
Ceftriaxone	2 g IV/IM q 24 hours	enterococci and culture negative bacteria.
Prosthetic Valves		
Any Presentation		
Vancomycin **plus:**	1 g IV q 12 adjust by levels	− Coagulase-negative staphylococci primary concern
		− Most isolates methicillin-resistant
Rifampin **plus:**	300 mg IV/PO TID	− Rifampin improved penetration into prostheses
		− *S. aureus*, streptococci, most enterococci also covered.
Gentamicin[†]	3 mg/kg per day IV/IM give in 2–3 divided doses	

Data from Baddour LM, Wilson WR, Bayer AS, et al. Infective endocarditis: diagnosis, antimicrobial therapy, and management of complications. A Statement for healthcare professionals from the Committee on Rheumatic Fever, Endocarditis, and Kawasaki Disease, Council on Cardiovascular Disease in the Young, and the Councils on Clinical Cardiology, Stroke, and Cardiovascular Surgery and Anesthesia, American Heart Association. Circulation 2005; 111:e394–e433; and Elliott TSJ, Foweraker J, Gould FK, et al. Guidelines for the antibiotic treatment of endocarditis in adults: report of the Working Party of the British Society for Antimicrobial Chemotherapy. J Antimicrob Chemother 2004; 54: 971–981.

*Unless beta-lactam allergic, then consider vancomycin + gentamicin as described above.

[†]Renal function may change rapidly with IE. For this reason, once daily aminoglycosides should be avoided or used with extreme caution.

Prevention

Patients with moderate- to high-risk cardiac conditions for IE should receive antibiotic prophylaxis as outlined in Tables 38-1 and 38-7. However, all guidelines recommend that the final decision regarding use of prophylaxis reside with the patient's individual physician.[4,26]

For optimum protection, timing of the first dose is important and differs with the route of administration. Patients must receive prophylaxis with oral agents 60 minutes and with intramuscular or intravenous agents 30 minutes prior to the procedure to achieve peak drug levels. More regimens rely on oral medications whenever possible; intravenous antibiotics are reserved for genitourinary and gastrointestinal procedures in patients at high risk, for patients allergic to oral medications, or those who cannot take medication by the oral route.[26]

The procedures are divided in to two groups based on the common associated cause of endocarditis (e.g., *S. viridans* [dental, esophageal, or upper respiratory tract] or enterococci [other gastrointestinal and genitourinary]).[26] Ultimately, prophylaxis has become a standard of care, even though no clinical trials have been or will be done to prove that prophylaxis prevents IE.[4,26]

DISCHARGE/FOLLOW-UP PLANS

Patient Education

Patients with IE may receive intravenous treatment at home, in an infusion center, or in an extended-care facility. Antibiotic treatment may last weeks to months, and post-treatment follow-up for 6–12 months to identify relapse of infection or complications is not uncommon. Patients treated as an outpatient must be able to comply with hygiene, catheter care, and frequent return visits. Some patients or their families may be required to have the skills to give infusions themselves. Patients and their families should be able to recognize signs of relapsing infection, complications of medications and intravenous catheters, and congestive heart failure. New or worsening symptoms should be reported promptly to the generalist as well as the physician coordinating antimicrobial therapy. Patients who are unable to comply should receive treatment in a supervised setting.

Outpatient Physician Communication

Outpatient follow-up should be coordinated with the generalist, infectious diseases specialist, cardiologist, and the surgical team.

Table 38-7 Antimicrobial Prophylaxis of Infective Endocarditis

Route	Antibiotic
Procedure—Dental, Esophageal, Upper Respiratory	
Oral (preferred)*	amoxicillin 2 g
Oral (penicillin-allergic)*	clindamycin 600 mg **or** cephalexin or equivalent 2 g **or** azithromycin or clarithromycin 500 mg
Parenteral (IM, IV) (preferred if NPO)[†]	ampicillin 2 g
Parenteral (IV) (penicillin-allergic and NPO)[†]	clindamycin 600 mg **or** cefazolin 1 g
Procedure—gastrointestinal (nonesophageal), genitourinary	
Oral (not if high risk condition)*	amoxicillin 2 g
Parenteral (IV) (preferred high-risk)[†]	ampicillin 2 g[§]
Parenteral (IV) (penicillin-allergic)[‡]	vancomycin 1 g above ± gentamicin 1.5 mg/kg (IV, IM) (preferred if high risk)[†]

Data from Danchin N, Duval X, Leport C. Prophylaxis of infective endocarditis: French recommendations 2002. Heart 2005; 91:715–718; *and* Antibacterial prophylaxis for dental, GI and GU procedures. Med Letter 2005; 47:59–60.

IV—intravenous; IM—intramuscular

*All oral medications should be given 60 minutes prior to the procedure

[†]All parenteral antibiotics should be given 30 minutes prior to the procedure except for vancomycin

[‡]Vancomycin should be started 60 minutes prior to the procedure and infused over that hour.

[§]Patients receiving IV ampicillin should have a second ampicillin dose (IV /IM) or oral amoxicillin 6 hours later.

Outpatient laboratory studies should be done at least on an every 1- to 2-week basis prior to the postdischarge visit to facilitate monitoring of antimicrobial therapy. Laboratory studies should include indicators of inflammation (complete blood count), renal complications (serum studies and urinalysis), and antibiotic levels (aminoglycosides, vancomycin). Erythrocyte sedimentation rate and/or C-reactive protein measurements obtained every 2–4 weeks can also provide useful evidence that the infection is resolving. The need for postdischarge echocardiography should be determined and scheduled as appropriate.

Key Points

- Infective endocarditis (IE) is a serious but relatively uncommon infection.

- Risk of IE is based upon the presence of predisposing valvular abnormalities and the likelihood that an organism will cause disease in that host.

- If IE is suspected, and the patient is clinically stable, antibiotic treatment should be held until appropriate cultures have been obtained.

- Echocardiography is useful to verify that vegetations are present and to identify complications that might alter management or prognosis.

- Treatment of IE is typically prolonged using of one or more intravenous antibiotics with cidal activity.

- Early involvement of consultants with expertise in management of antimicrobials and complications of IE is essential for successful treatment.

SUGGESTED READING

Mylonakis E, Calderwood SB. Infective Endocarditis in adults. N Engl J Med 2001; 345:13181330.

Morellion P, Que Y-A. Infective endocarditis. Lancet 2004; 363:139–149.

Prendergast BD. Diagnostic criteria and problems in infective endocarditis. Heart 2004; 90:611–613.

Baddour LM, Wilson WR, Bayer AS, et al. Infective endocarditis: diagnosis, antimicrobial therapy, and management of complications. A Statement for healthcare professionals from the Committee on Rheumatic Fever, Endocarditis, and Kawasaki Disease, Council on Cardiovascular Disease in the Young, and the Councils on Clinical Cardiology, Stroke, and Cardiovascular Surgery and Anesthesia, American Heart Association. Circulation 2005; 111:e394–e433.

Antibacterial prophylaxis for dental, GI and GU procedures. Med Letter 2005; 47:59–60.

CHAPTER THIRTY-NINE

Vascular Catheter-Related Infections

Carol E. Chenoweth, MD, and Sanjay Saint, MD, MPH

BACKGROUND

Intravascular catheters are ubiquitous and necessary devices in modern medical practice; over 150 million intravascular devices are used in hospitalized patients in the United States every year. The majority of catheters used are peripheral catheters, but over 5 million central venous catheters are placed each year. Central venous catheters include central temporary catheters; tunneled permanent catheters, such as dialysis and Hickman-type catheters; subcutaneous ports; and peripherally inserted central catheters (PICCs). While central venous catheters are often necessary, major risks are associated with their use. Infection is the most important complication, with 5% of central venous catheters becoming infected. There are an estimated 250,000 cases of catheter-related bloodstream infections (CR-BSI) in the United States annually, and 90% of those occur in the setting of a temporary central venous catheter (CVC).[1-3]

In short-term nontunneled central venous catheters, most infections arise from external colonization of the catheter, with organisms that originate from the skin at the catheter insertion site. Longer-dwelling catheters, including tunneled and cuffed catheters, are more likely to develop infection from intraluminal colonization of the catheter and catheter hub and from handling the catheter.[1,3] Therefore, it is not surprising that the microorganisms associated with intravascular catheters are most commonly skin organisms including, coagulase-negative staphylococci, coagulase-positive staphylococci, enterococci, and Candida species.[1,3,4] Rarely, contaminated infusion fluids may cause catheter or bloodstream infections.[1-3]

The attributable costs and morbidity due to an episode of catheter-related bloodstream infection is unclear, due to confounding. Specifically, patients with serious comorbidities or high illness severity are more likely not only to develop CR-BSI but also to have prolonged hospital stay and morbidity independent of infection status. Nevertheless, investigators estimate that each episode of CR-BSI prolongs a patient's hospital stay by several days.[1,3,5,6] Each CR-BSI is estimated to increase hospital costs by at least $7,000.[1,5-7] Estimated attributable mortality of CR-BSI varies, depending on the type of study performed, but has ranged from zero to 34%.[1,5-8] Thus, catheter infections are a major patient safety problem in hospitalized patients, leading to increased morbidity and health care costs.

ASSESSMENT

Clinical Presentation

Prevalence and Risk Factors

The incidence of nosocomial bloodstream infections increased over the past 3 decades, primarily related to a rise in the incidence of infections caused by coagulase-negative staphylococci, enterococci and Candida species (Table 39-1).[4,8-10] Most nosocomial bloodstream infections have been associated with central venous catheters.[1,3,8,10] Since most central lines are used in the intensive care unit (ICU) setting, most CR-BSI occur in ICUs. The incidence of CR-BSI varies depending on the ICU type; in data reported by the National Nosocomial Surveillance Infections Surveillance System, pooled mean CR-BSI rates were lowest in cardiothoracic ICUs (2.7 BSIs/1,000 central line-days) and highest in trauma ICUs (7.4 BSIs/1,000 central line-days).[11] Patients with large-gauge central catheters, such as extracorporeal membrane oxygenation catheters (18.8 BSIs/1,000 catheter-days) and dialysis catheters (up to 4.53 BSIs/1,000 patient-days), have even higher rates of infection.[12,13] Central venous catheters (primarily PICCs, tunneled catheters, and subcutaneous ports) used in the outpatient setting have much lower rates of infection, approximately 1 BSI/1,000 catheter-days.[14]

The type of intravascular catheter used is the most important risk factor for catheter infection. Peripheral intravascular catheters (PIV) are the most widely used catheter in hospitals, but are rarely associated with infection. CVCs, however, are associated with over 90% of all CR-BSI.[1-3] In some studies, multilumen central catheters have been associated with higher rates of infection, when compared to single lumen catheters. A recent meta-analysis, however, suggested that this risk is slight and may be offset by the improved convenience of multiple lumens in a critically ill patient.[15] Subcutaneously tunneled catheters and ports have lower rates of infection than nontunneled central catheters.[16] PICCs used in the outpatient setting have a very low rate of infection, but when used in high-risk hospitalized patients, the rate of infection approximates that of other temporary central venous catheters.[17] Catheters placed in lower extremities are more likely to become infected than catheters placed in upper extremities.[18] CVCs placed in the subclavian vein have lower rates of infection than those in the internal jugular or femoral

Table 39-1 Predominant Microbial Etiology of Catheter-Related Infections

Microorganism	% of cases
Coagulase-negative staphylococci	31–47
Coagulase-positive staphylococci	8–20
Enterococcus species	8–21
Candida species	9–11.5
Gram-negative organisms	14–25

Adapted from: Richards MJ, Edwards JR, Culver DH, et al. Nosocomial infections in combined medical-surgical intensive care units in the United States. Infect Control Hosp Epidemiol 2000; 21:510–5154; and Chaiyakunapruk N, Veenstra DL, Lipsky BA, et al. Chlorhexidine compared with povidone-iodine solution for vascular catheter-site care: a meta-analysis. Ann Intern Med 2002; 136:792–801; and Lark RL, Chenoweth CE, Saint S, et al. Four year prospective evaluation of nosocomial bacteremia: epidemiology, microbiology, and patient outcome. Diagn Microbiol Infect Dis 2000; 38:131–140; and Wisplinghoff H, Bischoff T, Tallent SM, et al. Nosocomial bloodstream infection in US hospitals: analysis of 24,179 cases from a prospective nationwide surveillance study. Clin Infect Dis 2004; 39:309–17.

Table 39-2 Factors Affecting Risk of Intravascular Catheter Infections

Increased Risk	Decreased Risk
Multilumen catheter	Tunneled catheter
Femoral or internal jugular site	Subclavian site
Valve-type needleless access devices	Peripherally inserted central catheter
Duration of catheterization	Antimicrobial catheter
Increased nurse to patient ratio	Experienced personnel, (i.e., intravascular catheter teams)
Total parenteral nutrition	
Host factors—neutropenia, burns, etc.	

sites.[3,16,18,19] Recently, certain valve-type needleless access devices used on intravenous lines have been shown to increase risk of catheter infections as well.[20]

Duration of catheterization is also a risk factor for infection; the cumulative risk of infection increases linearly with duration of catheter placement.[3,16,19] In addition, several studies have shown that catheters placed by experienced personnel, such as dedicated intravenous catheter teams, result in lower rates of infection. The risk of infection also increases when the nurse-to-patient ratio increases in intensive care, presumably due to inability to maintain aseptic practices with increased workload.[3,16,19] The use of total parenteral nutrition increases the risk of catheter infection, especially those associated with Candida species and coagulase-negative staphylococci. Finally, a number of host factors, including neutropenia, chemotherapy, human immunodeficiency virus (HIV) infection, infection at another site, and burned and nonintact skin have all been associated with increased risk of catheter infection (Table 39-2).[1–3,16,19]

Presenting signs and symptoms

Infections of intravascular catheters present in a spectrum of severity, from asymptomatic colonization of the catheter to sepsis syndrome associated with death. The presentation may vary, depending on the site of the infection and the microorganism causing the infection. An exit-site infection is defined as erythema or induration within 2 cm of the catheter insertion site, without the presence of purulence or concomitant bloodstream infection. A tunnel infection or clinical exit-site infection presents with local inflammatory signs (tenderness, erythema, or site induration) extending >2 cm from the catheter insertion along the subcutaneous tract of a tunneled catheter, with or without purulent drainage. In CR-BSI, the catheter is identified as the cause of bacteremia. CR-BSI are most often manifested by fever, without other identifiable infectious sources. Other signs and symptoms include hypothermia, rigors, hypotension, tachypnea, tachycardia, or mental status changes.[1,19]

Septic thrombophlebitis of a peripheral venous catheter presents with local signs of phlebitis and purulent drainage, associ-

ated with positive blood cultures. Septic thrombophlebitis related to a central catheter is not usually associated with local signs of infection or evidence of venous obstruction. Septic thrombophlebitis should be considered in any patient remaining febrile or with persistently positive blood cultures after removal of the offending catheter, despite appropriate antimicrobial therapy.[1,19] Endocarditis may arise from catheter-related bacteremia, especially those due to S. aureus, and it should also be considered in patients with persistently positive blood cultures (see chapter on endocarditis). In one study, 16 (23%) of 69 patients with CR-BSI due to S. aureus had evidence of endocarditis found on transesophageal echocardiography.[21] Finally, other sites may be secondarily seeded from catheter-related bacteremia, and clinicians must be attentive to clinical findings of secondary infections. Common secondary infections include septic joints, vertebral osteomyelitis, myositis, embolic skin lesions, and endophthalmitis. A careful retinal examination should be performed on all persons with intravascular catheter infections due to Candida species to rule out endophthalmitis.[22]

Differential Diagnosis

The differential diagnosis of local catheter infection, especially at a peripheral intravascular site, includes noninfectious phlebitis and thrombophlebitis. Other symptoms of catheter infection are nonspecific and could be associated with infections at other sites. In patients with intravascular catheters and fever, evaluation should include careful attention to other possible infectious causes of fever.

Diagnosis

Accurate and early diagnosis of CR-BSI is essential to guide management of infection. Clinical findings of catheter infection are neither sensitive nor specific.[1] Fever and chills are frequently present, but are nonspecific and associated with most other types of infection. On the contrary, localized signs of inflammation or purulence at the catheter site have a greater specificity for central venous catheter (CVC) infection, but lack sensitivity.[1,19]

Diagnosis of catheter-site infection can be made on the basis of clinical findings.

When evaluating a febrile patient with an intravascular catheter, two sets of blood cultures, one drawn from the line and one drawn from a peripheral site, are preferred.[1,23,24] Blood cultures that grow a known pathogen, such as *S. aureus* or *Candida* species, in the absence of another identified source, should be treated presumptively as a CR-BSI as outlined below. For common skin contaminants, such as coagulase-negative staphylococci, two blood cultures should be positive to confirm true infection. The studies below can be used for more definitive diagnosis of CR-BSI.[1,19]

Preferred Studies

Recently, the use of differential time to positivity has been used to accurately diagnose CR-BSIs in short- and long-term catheters.[23,24] This procedure involves simultaneous blood cultures drawn from a peripheral site and from a catheter. If the catheter-drawn blood culture turns positive >120 minutes before the peripheral culture, this is highly correlated with catheter infection (81% sensitivity and 92% specificity for short-term catheters; 93% sensitivity and 75% specificity for long-term catheters).[23] The use of paired quantitative blood cultures may increase the accuracy of diagnosis of CR-BSI; however, quantitative blood cultures are not readily available as routine tests in most standard microbiology laboratories.[24]

Septic thrombophlebitis should be considered in any patient who has persistently positive blood cultures after removal of the infected catheter. The diagnosis is made with noninvasive Doppler studies or venogram confirming vascular thrombus in the setting of repeatedly positive blood cultures.[1,19] Echocardiography is often used to assist in the diagnosis of endocarditis (*see* endocarditis, Chapter 38).

Alternative Options

Culture techniques of catheter segments can be used to diagnose catheter infection; however, these methods require removal of the catheter.[1,25] The semi-quantitative roll plate culture of a catheter segment is accurate for detecting infection in catheters inserted for <1 week.[25] However, for catheters in place for >1 week, intraluminal colonization of the catheter may be present and not identified by the roll plate method. Quantitative culture, which involves sonication of the catheter segment to dislodge intraluminal biofilm, has been used with high accuracy to diagnose infection in longer-dwelling catheters.[1,24] Acridine orange staining for visualization of microorganisms in a leukocyte cytospin test had high positive and negative predictive value in one study and may be a test that can be used routinely in the future.[1,24]

Prognosis

The effect of a catheter-related infection on mortality is unclear. The attributable mortality of a bloodstream infection related to a catheter has been as low as zero in some studies that match closely for severity of illness at the time of infection.[5-8] In these studies, catheter infections appear to be a marker of increased mortality and not causal. Other studies have found an attributable mortality as high as 34%.[1] Infections associated with coagulase-negative staphylococci appear to have a lower overall mortality (0.7%), while infections due to coagulase-positive staphylococci and *Candida* species have a significantly higher mortality rate than other organisms.[3,8] In all studies, hospital length of stay and costs are increased by a CR-BSI.

MANAGEMENT

Treatment

Preferred

Initial

Antimicrobial therapy for suspected intravascular infection is usually started empirically, while awaiting results of cultures and susceptibilities. Initial treatment will depend on the most likely pathogen (*see* Table 39-1), underlying patient risk factors (i.e., presence of neutropenia), and severity of infection. There are no randomized studies to support the empirical use of one antimicrobial over another. Since gram-positive bacteria are predominant infecting bacteria, vancomycin is recommended empirically in a hemodynamically stable patient with intravascular catheter infection. This is especially true in hospitals and countries with high rates of methicillin-resistant coagulase-positive and coagulase-negative staphylococci.[1] An antibiotic active against gram-negative bacilli, including *Pseudomonas* species, should be added in patients with hemodynamic instability or sepsis.[1] Empirical antifungal therapy should be considered for those patients at high risk for candidemia.[22]

In a recent study of risk factors for ineffective therapy for patients with bloodstream infection, health care–associated bloodstream infections were three times more likely than community-acquired bloodstream infections to be treated inadequately.[26] Hospitalization within 90 days was independently associated with ineffective therapy, likely due to colonization with resistant organisms during the preceding hospital stay.[26] Methicillin-resistant staphylococci and enterococci were associated with an increased likelihood of inappropriate therapy.[26] Therefore, previous hospitalizations and infectious histories should be considered when choosing empiric antimicrobial therapy.

Catheter removal is necessary for treatment of most catheter infections. This is especially important when treating *S. aureus*, gram-negative bacilli, and *Candida* species infections, in which metastatic spread of infection is most concerning.[1,22] In select patients who are only mildly ill, who have no evidence of metastatic infection or persistent bacteremia, and whose infecting organism is coagulase-negative staphylococci, the catheter may be retained. Infections of dialysis catheters present a unique problem and are addressed in detail in Chapter 50 (Messana et al.).

Subsequent

Subsequent therapy should be directed at the infecting organism, once culture and susceptibility results are available. In particular, vancomycin should be continued only for infections due to methicillin-resistant organisms or in patients with a β-lactam allergy.

There are few studies to support length of therapy for treatment of catheter-related infection. For treatment of coagulase-negative staphylococci, a less virulent organism, antibiotics may be discontinued after 5–7 days if the catheter is removed. For *S. aureus* CR-BSI, a transesophageal echocardiogram is recommended for evaluation for endocarditis.[1,21] In the absence of endocarditis, *S. aureus* bacteremia is treated by removal of the catheter and 14 days of parenteral antistaphylococcal antibiotics. Infections due to gram-negative bacilli may be treated with 10–14 days of effective parenteral therapy; oral quinolones, which achieve serum concentrations equivalent to parenteral dosing, may be used for therapy of susceptible gram-negative rods if the patient can tolerate oral medications. *Candida* infections should be treated for 14 days from the last positive blood culture.[1,22] Oral fluconazole may be used for treatment of susceptible *Candida* species.[22]

Metastatic infection complicating intravascular catheter infection may require longer treatment than uncomplicated catheter infection. Septic thrombophlebitis, endocarditis, or osteomyelitis is treated with at least 4–6 weeks of parenteral antibiotics (*see* Endocarditis, Chapter 38).[1,22] Treatment of peripheral septic thrombophlebitis may require excision of the infected peripheral vein if the patient does not respond rapidly to antibiotics. For central vein septic thrombophlebitis, heparin therapy should be used in addition to intravenous antibiotics.[1]

Alternative options

Several open trials of antibiotic lock therapy of tunneled catheter infections without removal of catheter have shown success in some settings.[1,27] This treatment involves filling the catheter with concentrated antibiotic and allowing antibiotic to dwell in the lumen for hours to days. Antibiotic locks have been most effective for treating infections due to coagulase-negative staphylococcus, and should be avoided with *S. aureus* infections.[1,27] Antibiotic locks, with or without concomitant parenteral antibiotics, have been successful when used for 10–14 days. Patients should be monitored after antibiotic completion for recurrence of symptoms associated with infection.

Prevention

Given the significant morbidity and mortality of catheter-related infections, prevention of catheter infection is paramount. One of the most important, yet often overlooked, preventive measures is to avoid placement of CVCs and to remove catheters when no longer necessary, because duration of catheterization increases the risk of catheter infection. Routine replacement of CVCs is not recommended; the risk of complication with new catheter placement far exceeded the benefit of decreased infection in one study.[28] Routine changing over a guidewire is not advisable, as the catheter tunnel site may be unknowingly colonized at the time of new catheter placement.[3,28]

Aseptic placement of central catheters is another essential preventive measure. Proper handwashing is critical before the procedure. Since most bacteria causing infection in temporary vascular catheters originate from the skin and track down the catheter to the blood extraluminally, catheter-site disinfection before and after insertion of the catheter is essential. Many studies have shown that chlorhexidine is superior to other disinfectants for site disinfection at the time of catheter placement.[7,29] Chlorhexidine is now the disinfectant recommended for all catheter placement procedures and for routine site cleansing during dressing changes.[3] Use of maximal sterile barriers (sterile gloves, sterile gown, mask, hair covering, with a full body drape) by personnel during placement of catheters has also been associated with decreased central catheter infections.[30,31] Maximal barrier precautions are recommended for placement of all central catheters, including PICC line placement.[3]

In addition, aseptic handling when accessing catheters is important to prevent intraluminal contamination of the line. Educational programs for all nurses and physicians on proper placement and care of catheters resulted in decreased catheter infections in a medical ICU.[32] Education of house staff on proper aseptic technique, including maximal barrier precautions, has also resulted in increased use of barriers and a decrease in bloodstream infections.[33] Antimicrobial catheters, impregnated with various antimicrobials, have been effective in reducing intravascular catheter infections, and may be considered when other prevention measures are not effective.[34–36] Box 39-1 outlines recommended insertion practices from the Centers for Disease Control (CDC) to prevent CR-BSI.[3]

Despite the fact that evidence-based guidelines for the prevention of intravascular catheter infections have been published, application of these practices have not been consistently applied across hospitals and ICUs.[37] A recent report from one surgical ICU showed that with strict adherence to the above evidence-based guidelines, including a checklist used at the time of insertion and empowering nurses to stop the CVC insertion if guidelines were not followed, the result was near elimination of CR-BSI in the ICU.[38]

DISCHARGE/FOLLOW-UP PLANS

Patient Education

Patients who are discharged with an intravascular catheter require careful instruction on catheter care. This should include reinforcement in the home by a visiting nurse for novices. Patients should be instructed to contact their physicians for onset of fever, catheter site erythema or swelling, or any catheter malfunction.

Box 39-1 CDC Recommended Practices for Insertion of Central Venous Catheters

Assess need for central venous catheter (CVC)

Do not routinely change CVCs

Ensure hand hygiene before insertion procedure

Subclavian is preferred site for CVC insertion

Use maximum sterile barriers (sterile gloves and gowns, mask, hair cover, full body drape) during insertion

Use chlorhexidine for skin disinfection

Antimicrobial CVCs in appropriate situations

Educate health care workers regarding: indications for intravascular catheter use, proper procedure for insertion, and maintenance of catheters

From: O'Grady NP, Alexander M, Dellinger EP, et al. Guidelines for the prevention of intravascular catheter-related infections. Clin Infect Dis 2002; 35:1281–1307.

Outpatient Physician Communication

Outpatient physicians should be notified of CR-BSI that occurred during a hospital stay so that they may monitor for signs or symptoms of recurrence or secondary infections. This information should include the infecting organism, duration of bacteremia, and whether the catheter was removed. Any associated secondary infections should be reported.

If a patient is discharged with an intravascular catheter, the type of catheter, site of the catheter, and expected duration of intravascular catheterization should be reported.

Key Points

- Intravascular catheters are essential for the care of hospitalized patients, but are associated with a significant risk of infection.

- Skin bacteria, coagulase-negative and coagulase-positive staphylococci, are the predominant causes of catheter-related bloodstream infection.

- Time-to-positivity of paired blood cultures is the most reliable method to diagnose CR-BSI in a febrile patient.

- Vancomycin is the most appropriate empirical therapy for catheter-related infections; removal of catheter is necessary for treatment, except in select situations.

- Adherence to recommended guidelines for insertion of central venous catheters can significantly decrease the risk of catheter-related infection.

SUGGESTED READING

Mermel LA, Farr BM, Sherertz RJ, et al. Guidelines for the management of intravascular catheter-related infections. Clin Infect Dis 2001; 32:1249–1272.

Mermel LA. Prevention of intravascular catheter-related infections. Ann Intern Med 2000; 132:391–402.

Safdar N, Fine JP, Maki DG. Meta-analysis: methods for diagnosing intravascular device-related bloodstream infection. Ann Intern Med 2005; 142:451–466.

Safdar N, Maki DG. Risk of catheter-related bloodstream infection with peripherally inserted central venous catheters used in hospitalized patients. Chest 2005; 128:489–495.

Fowler VG, Li J, Corey GR, et al. Role of echocardiography in the evaluation of patients with *Staphylococcus aureus* bacteremia: experience in 103 patients. J Am Coll Cardiol 1997; 30:1072–1078.

CHAPTER FORTY

Septic Arthritis

Vikas I. Parekh, MD, and James Riddell IV, MD

BACKGROUND

Infectious arthritis remains a common cause of acute arthritis in adults. If left untreated, it can result in rapid destruction of the joint and significant morbidity and mortality. Therefore, early recognition and treatment are essential. The incidence of bacterial arthritis varies depending on host factors such as underlying rheumatoid arthritis (RA) or the presence of prosthetic joints. In 1998, the Centers for Disease Control reported that there were an estimated 23,000 cases of infectious arthritis in the United States.[1] Of these cases, 39% were in patients over the age of 65, and the mean duration of hospitalization was about 7 days. The incidence of septic arthritis for native joints in the general adult population is estimated to be 5 to 10 per 100,000 but is upward of 30–70 per 100,000 in those with rheumatoid arthritis.[2–4] The rate of infection for prosthetic joints that is reported in the literature is highly variable. With modern operative techniques and routine use of antibiotic prophylaxis, the 10-year rate of infection has dropped considerably, although it should be noted that with increasing numbers of patients undergoing joint replacement surgery, the overall population level incidence of septic arthritis is increasing. Data from comprehensive joint replacement registries in Sweden suggest that the infection rate ranges from a 10-year rate of 0.4% for hips to 1.0% for knees in those without RA. The rate of infection in those with RA is nearly double that of the overall population.[5–7]

Infection of a joint is most often due to hematogenous spread of bacteria from other sites.[8] Synovial tissue has a very rich blood supply but no basement membrane, thus potentially predisposing it to blood-borne infections. Once bacteria enter the joint space, they trigger an acute inflammatory reaction that results in synovitis and sometimes rapid destruction of cartilage and bone. Direct inoculation of bacteria into the joint may occur in the setting of therapeutic joint injection or traumatic injuries such as animal bites. In prosthetic joints, the infection can also be related to seeding of the joint during the surgery itself or from a contiguous source such as a wound resulting in early postoperative infection.

Risk factors for infection include any condition that results in an abnormal joint, a higher risk for bacteremia or immunocompromise. Rheumatoid arthritis is likely the single largest risk factor for native joint disease, due to the presence of joint damage and inflammation as well as from immunosuppressive medication use.[2] Both osteoarthritis and trauma can predispose to septic joints. Other conditions that convey increased risk include diabetes, human immunodeficiency virus (HIV), malignancy, older age, organ transplantation, hemodialysis, and intravenous drug use.[9]

In addition to the comorbidities mentioned above, risk factors for prosthetic joint infection also relate in part to the location of the artificial joint and the nature of the prosthesis. Knees tend to have the highest rate of infection, whereas hips and shoulders tend to have the lowest rates.[5–7,10,11] Traditional cemented joints may have higher rates of infection than newer cement-less joints. This is thought to be related to the immunosuppressive effects of the polymethyl-methacrylate cement itself, which has been shown in experimental models to reduce leukocyte and complement function.[12,13]

The microbiology of septic arthritis has changed over time, especially as prosthetic joints become more common. *Staphylococcus aureus* is now the most common cause in adults, especially among those with RA or prosthetic joints. *Neisseria gonorrhoeae* remains common among young (<30 years of age), sexually active individuals, but the reported incidence varies widely depending on the patient population. Streptococci and gram-negative bacteria are the next most common pathogens in recent series (Table 40-1). Other pathogens vary, depending on the population, with gram-negative organisms, including *Pseudomonas aeruginosa*, possible in prosthetic joints and intravenous drug abuse (IVDA). Organisms generally considered nonpathogenic, such as diphtheroids and *Propionibacterium acnes*, have also been found to be causative agents in prosthetic joint infection.[3–5]

ASSESSMENT

Prevalence and Presenting Signs and Symptoms

Native Joint Disease

Nongonococcal, native joint infectious arthritis classically presents as the abrupt onset of a single hot, swollen, and painful joint. Systemic signs such as fever are also quite common and were seen in upward of 78% of patients.[14] While a monoarticular presentation is most common, up to 20% of patients can have polyarticular involvement usually involving two or three joints. Polyarticular involvement is especially common in those with underlying RA or systemic bacteremia (especially with S. aureus).[15] Disseminated gonococcal infection with septic arthritis is most often polyarticular and associated with a history of migratory joint pains, tenosynovitis, fever, and a typical rash. The genitourinary symptoms of gonorrhea (GC) are often absent.

On physical examination, the most common finding with infectious arthritis is a joint effusion with associated warmth, erythema, tenderness, and pain with both active and passive movement, often with restricted range of motion (Table 40-2). Involvement of the knee (Figs. 40-1, 40-2, 40-3) is the most common (55% of all cases), followed by ankles (10%), wrists (9%), shoulders (7%), and hips (5%).[2] The examination in disseminated gonococcal disease may often reveal diffuse tenosynovitis, especially of the hands and wrists, along with multiple painless macules and papules on the arms, legs, or trunk. Joint involvement is usually asymmetric, and the knees, elbows, wrists, and MCPs are commonly involved. This typical presentation occurs in about two-thirds of patients with disseminated GC. A minority may present later after this acute syndrome with monoarticular arthritis without tenosynovitis or skin lesions.[4]

Table 40-1 Basic Microbiology of Septic Arthritis

Acute Native Joint	Acute Prosthetic Joint	Chronic Arthritis
Staphylococcus aureus	Coagulase-negative Staphylococcus	Mycobacterium tuberculosis
Streptococcus sp.	Staphylococcus aureus	Atypical mycobacteria
N. gonorrhoeae	Gram negative bacilli	Fungi
Gram-negative bacilli	Enterococcus sp.	Lyme disease
Anaerobes	Anaerobes	Brucella

Table 40-2 Prevalence of Signs and Symptoms for Native Joint Septic Arthritis

Symptom	Frequency (%)
Joint pain	80–95
Limited range of motion	80–95
Joint swelling	80–90
Fever	40–80
Polyarticular involvement	10–20

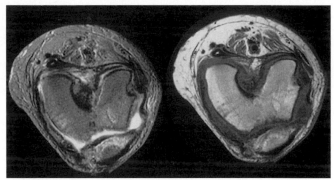

Figure 40-2 • MRI scan of right knee of a patient who has *Staphylococcus aureus* septic arthritis. Note the soft tissue inflammation and a joint effusion. From Cohen J, Powderly WG. Infectious Diseases, (2nd Edition) 2-Volume Set. Mosby, 2004.

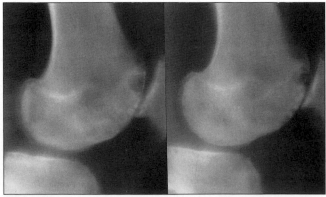

Figure 40-1 • Tomogram of right knee of a patient who has *Staphylococcus aureus* septic arthritis and periarticular osteomyelitis. Note the mixed sclerosis and lytic changes suggestive of osteomyelitis. From: Cohen J, Powderly WG. Infectious Diseases, (2nd Edition) 2-Volume Set. Mosby, 2004.

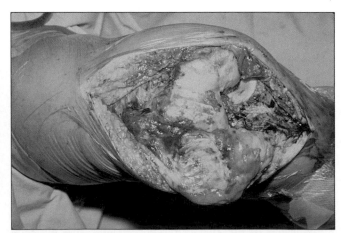

Figure 40-3 • Intraoperative photograph of right knee of a patient who has *Staphylococcus aureus* septic arthritis. Note the damaged joint and dark brown, boggy and hyperemic synovium. From Cohen J, Powderly WG. Infectious Diseases, (2nd Edition) 2-Volume Set. Mosby, 2004.

Table 40-3 Prevalence of Signs and Symptoms of Prosthetic Joint Septic Arthritis	
Symptom	Frequency (%)
Joint pain	80–95
Joint swelling	35–45
Fever	20–45
Sinus tract drainage	20–35

Prosthetic Joint Infections

Prosthetic joint infections have a more variable clinical presentation, but it is often helpful to think of them in terms of early infection (<3 weeks from surgery) and late infection (>3 weeks). Early infections are more likely to present with acute joint pain, effusion, and warmth, especially when caused by more virulent organisms such as *S. aureus*.[4,11] In late infections or early infection caused by less virulent bacteria, the signs of systemic infection such as fevers are absent (<50%). Mild progressive pain in the joint is often present and tends to be the dominant symptom. In some instances, a draining sinus tract to the skin often through the incision may be apparent on examination (Table 40-3). A separate focus of infection besides the joint itself is usually absent.

Differential Diagnosis

Given the significant morbidity and mortality associated with untreated septic arthritis, it should always be considered at the top of the differential for any presentation of acute monoarthritis. In addition, an infected prosthetic joint should be considered in any patient with an artificial joint who has new joint complaints or any systemic symptoms or signs of infection such as bacteremia. Septic bursitis can at times be confused with arthritis, but generally passive joint range of motion is preserved and is relatively painless. The presentation of other inflammatory, noninfectious arthritis is similar to that of joint infection. These include acute RA, gout, and pseudogout. It should be noted, however, that both acute gout and pseudogout can occur concomitantly with septic arthritis, and so the mere presence of joint crystal or other signs of gout or pseudogout should not be considered to exclude infection. Other possibilities include Lyme disease, Reiter's syndrome, and reactive arthritis associated with inflammatory bowel disease (IBD) or ankylosing spondylitis. Presence of extra-articular findings such as diarrhea (IBD), mouth ulcers (Reiter's, Behçet's), or skin changes such as erythema nodosum (sarcoid, Behçet's, IBD) may be helpful. Lyme disease occurs in specific endemic areas and is often diagnosed by serologies. Polyarticular involvement is more often noninfectious, although endocarditis or staphylococcal bacteremia can present with multiple involved joints, especially in the setting of underlying joint disease such as RA. Polyarticular arthritis can be associated with rheumatic fever, as well as viral causes. Chronic monoarticular arthritis can also be infectious in origin, and potential pathogens include *M. tuberculosis*, atypical mycobacteria, fungi, *Ureaplasma urealyticum*, and *Mycoplasma hominis*.

Diagnosis

Preferred Studies

Diagnostic arthrocentesis is mandatory in any patient suspected of having septic arthritis. The gold standard for diagnosis is a positive culture of joint fluid for a pathogen known to cause infectious arthritis, but culture results can often take several days to return. Therefore, the clinician relies on other data that are quickly obtained, primarily the synovial fluid white blood cell (WBC) count and differential, and Gram stain.

Native Joints

Synovial fluid WBC count and differential, in addition to Gram stain and culture, remain the mainstays of early diagnosis. All cultures and diagnostic studies should be obtained prior to the initiation of empiric antibiotic therapy to increase the diagnostic yield. While no single WBC count or differential establishes the diagnosis, there are generally accepted ranges that make the diagnosis of a septic joint more likely. Cell counts >20,000/μL are suggestive of infection, although both gout and pseudogout can produce results in this range (Figure 40-4). Generally, >75% neutrophils (PMNs) is also considered more suggestive of a septic etiology.

Sensitivity and specificity for a synovial WBC count >20,000 have been estimated at about 85% each in one study. A differential count >75% PMNs has been described to have a sensitivity of 75% but a specificity of 92% for infection.[16] It is important to note, however, that wide ranges of synovial WBC counts have been reported and can be as low as 2,000.

Synovial fluid glucose levels may also be helpful with glucose <25 mg/dL suggestive of infection, but it is generally less informative than the WBC and differential. Synovial protein levels, while sometimes ordered, are not felt to be helpful diagnostically.[16]

Gram stain is positive in about 75% of patients who have staphylococcal infections and about 50% of all infections. Recent antibiotic use will reduce these yields. Culture of synovial fluid is reported to be up to 90% sensitive in nongonococcal disease, but is much lower in gonococcal disease.[4,14] In suspected gonococcal infection, cultures of other sites such as the genitourinary tract, rectum, and throat should be obtained and can be positive in up to 80% of cases. Blood cultures are positive in up to 30% of patients, reflecting the high rate of association between bacteremia and septic arthritis. The role of polymerase chain reaction (PCR) for the detection of infectious organisms is still undefined, but it may be helpful in tuberculosis (TB). In the setting of HIV disease, chronic arthritis caused by atypical mycobacteria or TB may be extremely difficult to diagnose. Synovial biopsy with culture of tissue and special stains on formalin fixed tissue samples is critical to establishing a diagnosis.

Radiographs, although often ordered, are generally unhelpful in the ultimate diagnosis in native joints since specific changes such as periosteal erosions do not occur until after weeks of infection. Computed tomography (CT) and magnetic resonance imaging (MRI) may be more helpful in the diagnosis of adjacent osteomyelitis (MRI) or soft tissue abscesses (both modalities) but are not considered routine studies. Radionucleotide scans are sometimes helpful in difficult-to-diagnose cases or in determining if specific joints may be involved; however, they are sometimes negative in early disease and can be falsely positive in the setting

Figure 40-4 • Diagnostic algorithm for native joint septic arthritis.

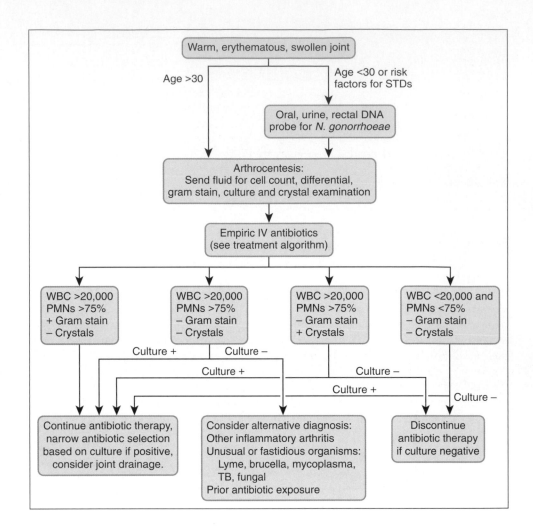

of underlying joint disease such as RA or severe osteoarthritis (OA).

Prosthetic Joints

Infection in prosthetic joints is often more difficult to diagnose. Although the gold standard remains a positive culture from synovial fluid, diagnosis is much more challenging. Cultures may be positive in less than half the cases often due to concomitant antibiotic use.[11] In addition, certain organisms that are typically felt to be contaminants in most settings, such as diptheroids, may indeed be pathogens in prosthetic joints. Orthopedics consultation for arthrocentesis is strongly suggested if there is a clinical suspicion of an infected prosthetic joint.

Synovial WBC counts are often only mildly elevated compared to native joint disease. A recent study described a sensitivity of 94% for a WBC > 1,700/μL and a sensitivity of 97% for >65% PMNs. This study was in patients without underlying inflammatory joint diseases.[17] Measures of inflammation such as ESR and C-reactive protein (CRP) are generally not felt to be useful in native joint disease, but their utility in prosthetic joint infection is felt to be better, especially if baseline ESR and CRP levels are available. Studies have shown that postoperatively CRP levels are initially elevated but then return to normal within weeks. Thus, an elevated CRP coupled with some evidence of joint inflammation is considered highly suggestive of infection.[18]

Radiographs of the joint may demonstrate new subperiosteal bone growth and transcortical sinus tracts which are very spe-cific for infection; however, other findings such as migration of the implant or periprosthetic osteolysis are not as useful since they can be seen in noninfectious conditions as well. Nuclear bone scans using technetium-99 are often positive in the absence of infection and are of limited utility. CT and MRI have not been widely studied and, again, are useful for potentially diagnosing abscess or osteomyelitis; however, their use is not routine.

PROGNOSIS

Although some individuals with septic arthritis recover without any residual deficits, others may be left with persistent symptoms. In many series, up to 50% of adults were left with some limitation of motion or persistent pain. Poor outcomes were more common in the elderly, those with RA, those with hip or ankle infection, and those who start treatment >7 days after the start of symptoms. In addition, nonresponders who fail to sterilize the joint within a week are more like to suffer morbidity and have higher mortality.[3,4,10,19] The organism that caused the infection is also predictive of outcome. S.aureus is associated with poor outcomes, while gonococcus and pneumococcus are associated with better outcomes. Overall mortality rates remain high, despite modern therapy, with reported average of 10–15%. Mortality is more often than not related to the bacteremia that caused the septic arthritis and is higher in those with comorbid illnesses. Polyarticular septic arthritis with S. aureus in RA is associated with the highest mortality rates, perhaps as high as 50%.

MANAGEMENT

Antibiotic Selection

Treatment for septic arthritis includes the prompt initiation of intravenous antibiotics after synovial cultures and blood cultures have been obtained, and in most cases, some form of joint drainage. Empiric antibiotic therapy is often guided by initial gram stain results as well as consideration of host factors (Table 40-4 and Figure 40-5).

Native Joints

In patients with a negative Gram stain, reasonable empiric therapy should be directed against the common pathogens, with staphylococcus and streptococcus the most commonly found. All patients with a suspicion of an infected joint should be hospitalized for intravenous (IV) antibiotic therapy, pending further diagnostic evaluation and final culture results. Initial therapy may thus include a third-generation cephalosporin. In instances where MRSA is prevalent in the community or likely because of host risk factors, vancomycin should be used empirically until culture results are known.

In special populations, empiric therapy may need to be broadened to cover other organisms. IVDA is associated with gram-negative organisms, including pseudomonas, so often an anti-pseudomonal β-lactam is used in combination with vancomycin. If the patient has a risk factor for MRSA such as indwelling line, end-stage renal disease (ESRD), or recent hospital stay, then vancomycin should be used. Other populations,

Table 40-4 Empiric Treatment of Adult Native Joint Septic Arthritis

Gram Stain and Clinical Scenario	Antibiotic and dosage (normal renal function)
Gram-positive cocci with no risk factors for MRSA*	Nafcillin/oxacillin 2 g q4 hr IV
Gram-positive cocci with risk factor for MRSA*	Vancomycin 1 g q12 hr IV
Gram-negative bacilli with no risk factors for resistant organisms**	Ceftriaxone 1 g q24 hr IV
Gram-negative bacilli with risk factor for resistant organisms**	Anti-pseudomonal β-lactam such as: Cefepime 2 g q12 hr IV or Piperacillin-tazobactam 3.375 g q6 hr IV
Gram stain negative	Regimen for gram-positive cocci plus regimen for gram-negative bacilli as above dependent on risk factors

*Risk Factors for MRSA include: previous MRSA infection, ESRD, recent hospitalization, and indwelling vascular catheters. In some communities, all patients with gram-positive cocci should receive empiric vancomycin.

**Risk Factors for resistant gram-negative organisms include: IVDA, immunosuppression, and prior resistant gram-negative infection.

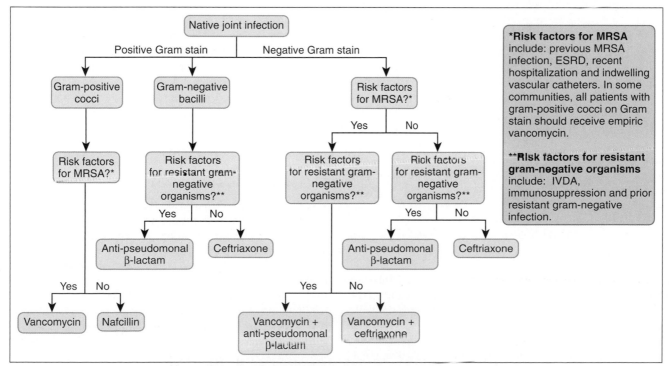

Figure 40-5 • Initial treatment of suspected native joint septic arthritis.

such as athletes, are now being found to be at risk for infection with MRSA. Also, in unusual cases such as direct inoculation of the joint by animal bites, *Pasteurella* is a consideration, and a penicillin/β-lactamase combination should be used.

Ultimately, final antibiotic choices should be guided by culture and sensitivity results. Duration of therapy has not been clearly studied and varies according to local practice, the underlying host comorbidities, response to treatment, and the organism identified. Most experts agree that treatment should include at least 2–4 weeks of IV antibiotics. Longer courses of therapy are suggested for particularly virulent organisms such as *Pseudomonas*. In addition, a minimum of 4–6 weeks is suggested in those patients with documented *S. aureus* bacteremia and a septic joint (evaluation to rule out concomitant infectious endocarditis and other metastatic infection is also important in these cases).

Prosthetic Joints

It is even more important to isolate a pathogen in cases of prosthetic joint infections, given the wide array of bacteria that have been implicated and the polymicrobial nature of these infections. While awaiting culture results, empiric therapy usually would include vancomycin combined with broad gram-negative coverage such as an antipseudomonal β-lactam.

Joint Drainage

Joint drainage has always been considered a critical part of the treatment for septic arthritis of native joints. Controversy exists, however, over both the method of drainage (surgical vs needle) and the indications for repeated drainage of the joint. Drainage can be accomplished either via arthrocentesis or surgically, most commonly via arthroscopic incision and drainage procedures.

Generally, septic arthritis of the shoulder, hip, and knees is considered an indication for surgical drainage. For other joints, initial needle drainage and close monitoring for reaccumulation and response to therapy would be a reasonable plan in the absence of osteomyleitis, abscess, or loculation.[4,21] If there is significant reaccumulation or lack of response to antibiotic therapy (generally within 48 hours), then surgical drainage should be considered in any joint. Unfortunately, there are no well-controlled randomized trials comparing the method of drainage, and often local practice will dictate the method of drainage. Early orthopedic consultation is suggested, especially in native joint disease of the shoulder, knee, or hip and in all cases of prosthetic joint infection where surgical treatment (if possible) is the accepted standard of care, regardless of joint location.

Surgical Management of Prosthetic Joint Infection

Prosthetic joint infections pose many management challenges. Standard practice would suggest early consultation with orthopedics and infectious diseases specialists. Generally, definitive therapy will require a one- or two-stage hardware exchange procedure in order to completely eradicate the infection. Some authorities support performing debridement and antibiotic treatment with retention of the prosthesis if the infection occurs in the immediate postoperative period.[11,22] A full discussion of the surgical management of prosthetic joint infections is beyond the scope of this chapter; however, it is important for the inpatient physician to understand the basic principles that underlie management of this common, frequently difficult-to-treat condition.

Eradication of the infection with drainage and antibiotics alone is often unsuccessful, due to the development of biofilm on the prosthetic material. Studies of antibiotic therapy and debridement alone have been conducted mainly in early postoperative infection (<3 months from surgery) where the duration of clinical symptoms is fairly short (<3 weeks) and the soft tissue and prosthesis are in good condition and stable. In these cases, IV antibiotic therapy for at least 2 weeks followed by oral therapy for a total of at least 3 months is suggested and has been reasonably successful. When the duration of the signs or symptoms of the infection is greater than 3 weeks, even in the early postoperative period, retention of the implant is not recommended. In these cases, either a one-stage or two-stage procedure involving resection and reimplantation of the prosthetic device is suggested. In the United States, two-stage procedures are generally favored over one-stage procedures, which are more common in Europe. A one-stage procedure involves irrigation and drainage followed by IV antibiotic therapy for several weeks followed by resection and reimplantation of the prosthesis in the same procedure. Success rates in some studies have been as high as 85–95%, but these studies have generally been limited to patients without significant comorbidities and with joint soft tissue that is in good condition.[11,22–24] A two-stage procedure, where resection of the prosthesis and insertion of an antibiotic impregnated spacer are followed by a prolonged interval of time with IV antibiotic administration before reimplantation, is generally felt to be more successful than one-stage procedures and is mandatory in any case where the soft tissue of the joint is not in good condition. Reported success rates are 90% or greater.[11,22,25,26]

In the instances where resection and a one- or two-stage procedure is not deemed a viable option because of significant patient comorbidities, treatment with IV antibiotics followed by chronic oral antibiotic suppressive therapy is advocated. Rates of breakthrough infection are high if oral suppressive medication is not used with an infected retained prosthesis, and sometimes patients require recurrent courses of IV therapy if breakthrough occurs on their suppressive regimen.

PREVENTION

The prevention of septic arthritis focuses primarily on the role of antimicrobial prophylaxis in patients with prosthetic joints. Currently, there is no defined preventive strategy for native joint disease. In artificial joints, there is no clear consensus on the use of antibiotic prophylaxis during routine invasive procedures that might result in bacteremia, although some organizations do suggest prophylaxis in high-risk individuals such as those with RA, immunosuppression, diabetes, recent joint replacement, or prior infected prosthesis.[11,27] Obviously, the rapid recognition of bacteremia and appropriate treatment is critical in preventing seeding of the artificial joint itself.

DISCHARGE/FOLLOW-UP PLANS

The postdischarge course of septic arthritis varies between native and prosthetic joint disease. For prosthetic infections, most patients are discharged on a prolonged course of antibiotics, often IV therapy followed by oral therapy. Close follow-up with an infectious disease and orthopedic specialist is usually required. Improvement is gradual, although most patients are improved at discharge. In cases of prosthetic joint infection when resection of the hardware is performed, patients will require immobilization of the involved limb. Clear instructions to seek immediate attention if symptoms reoccur or worsen should be given to all patients.

Native joint arthritis is often treated with a 2–4 week course of antibiotic therapy. Response to therapy varies, and those with underlying inflammatory arthritis or those who had late treatment may suffer considerable long-term disability.

Patient Education

Patients should be aware that they should see gradual improvement in symptoms over time but that many may not recover full joint function or may have persistent joint pain. Patients will often need to minimize weight bearing and may only be able to perform passive range of motion prior to more active exercises. They should understand the importance of finishing all antibiotics and close follow-up after discharge, especially in prosthetic joint disease. Those discharged on IV antibiotics should be instructed in appropriate peripherally inserted central catheter (PICC) line care and handling and of warning signs of PICC related complications such as deep venous thrombosis (DVT) or line sepsis. In addition, all patients should be made aware of the complications of prolonged antibiotic therapy, including the risk of *Clostridium difficile* colitis as well as the risk of toxicity from the drug itself, including allergic reactions which may be delayed in onset.

Those with prosthetic joint disease with plans for a two-stage resection should be made aware of the need for a prolonged interval between resection and implantation during which they will have limited use of the involved joint. Some patients who are unable to manage their activities of daily living during this time may require nursing home placement. Rehabilitation after discharge can be a lengthy process, and many patients, especially the elderly or those with underlying joint disorders, may benefit from inpatient rehabilitation programs.

Outpatient Physician Communication

Many patients with septic arthritis, especially prosthetic joint disease, will have a complicated postdischarge plan that may involve multiple visits to multiple specialists. Coordination among providers is paramount, especially among infectious disease, orthopedics, and the primary care physician. It is important to understand which provider will take responsibility for management of antibiotic therapy and the PICC line, and to have open lines of communication in case of problems. It is vital that the inpatient physician establish the various roles for each provider and arrange follow-up prior to discharge home.

Key Points

- *Staphylococcus aureus* is the most common etiology of septic arthritis in adults.

- Rheumatoid arthritis is a major risk factor for septic arthritis.

- No single WBC count or WBC differential can establish the diagnosis of septic arthritis, although synovial WBC counts >20,000/μL are highly suggestive of infection.

- Blood cultures are positive in up to 30% of patients, with septic arthritis reflecting the high association between bacteremia and joint infection.

- Septic arthritis has significant morbidity, with up to 50% of adults suffering residual deficits. Outcomes are worse in the elderly, those with RA, and those who have delays in initial treatment.

- Prosthetic joint infections require early consultation with orthopedics and infectious disease specialists.

SUGGESTED READING

Goldenberg D. Septic arthritis. Lancet 1998; 351:197–202.

Zimmerli W, Trampuz A, Ochsner P. Prosthetic-joint infections. N Engl J Med 2004; 351:1645–1654.

Goldberg DL, Reed JI. Bacterial arthritis. N Engl J Med 1985; 312:764–771.

Shmerling RH, Delbano TL, Tosteson AN, et al. Synovial fluid tests: what should be ordered? JAMA 1990; 264:1009–1014.

Lentino JR. Prosthetic joint infections: bane of orthopedists, challenge for infectious disease specialists. Clin Infect Diseases 2003; 36:1157–1161.

American Academy of Orthopaedic Surgeons. Antibiotic prophylaxis for dental patients with total joint replacements. Document no. 1014. www.aaos.org/wordhtml/papers/advistmt/1014.htm (last accessed 3/8/2005).

CHAPTER FORTY-ONE

HIV and AIDS

Daniel R. Kaul, MD, and Powel Kazanjian, MD

BACKGROUND

In the United States, approximately 1 million people are infected with the human immunodeficiency virus (HIV). Of these individuals, it is estimated that 25% have not been diagnosed.[1] With the advent of highly active antiretroviral therapy (HAART), the frequency of hospital admission among patients with HIV/AIDS has dramatically declined.[2] Most patients with diagnosed HIV infection admitted to the hospital for complications of their disease are either unable or unwilling to take HAART, or have multidrug-resistant virus that no longer responds to HAART. In patients with unrecognized HIV infection, admission with opportunistic infections may be the initial manifestation of their disease. The signs and symptoms of undiagnosed HIV infection, the typical presentation and management of opportunistic infections (OI), and the complications and drug interactions of HAART should be familiar to physicians involved in the care of the hospitalized patient.

ASSESSMENT

Clinical Presentation

Presenting Signs and Symptoms and Differential Diagnosis

Recognizing HIV Infection

Acute HIV Infection Patients with acute HIV infection develop a nonspecific syndrome characterized by fevers, chills, myalgias, lymphadenopathy, and rash (Fig. 41-1). Acute retroviral syndrome is clinically indistinguishable from infection with Epstein Barr virus (i.e., mononucleosis), acute cytomegalovirus, influenza, and other viral infections; and therefore a high degree of suspicion is required to make the diagnosis. Unfortunately, while up to 85% of patients will present to the health care system, the correct diagnosis is made in only 25% of cases.[3] As patients are highly infectious early in the course of infection, rapid diagnosis is critical from a public health standpoint and relies on health care providers considering acute HIV in any patient with recent risk factors for infection.

Chronic HIV Infection HIV infection or the associated opportunistic infections may involve almost any organ system (Table 41-1). As one quarter of HIV-infected patients in the United States have not been diagnosed, it is critical that physicians consider HIV infection in the differential diagnosis of a variety of major or seemingly incidental clinical findings. Invasive pneumococcal disease is 10- to 100-fold more common in AIDS patients, and its diagnosis should prompt HIV testing if any risk factors are present.[4] HIV testing should be included in the workup of otherwise unexplained thrombocytopenia, anemia, or neutropenia. HIV may directly affect virtually any organ, and as such, a new diagnosis of otherwise unexplained cardiomyopathy nephropathy or dementia should prompt consideration of performing an HIV serology.

Importance of Immune Status

The risk of a particular opportunistic infection is highly dependent on the degree of immune compromise. For example, disseminated *Mycobacterium avium complex* (MAC) seldom occurs in patients with CD4+ cell counts >75 cells/mm. Thus, the immune status of the patients as measured by the CD4+ count is essential in formulating a differential diagnosis (Table 41-2). In contrast, the HIV RNA viral load is primarily useful in assessing response to treatment and predicting the rate of decline of the CD4+ cell count.

Respiratory Symptoms

When an HIV-infected patient develops acute onset of fever, productive cough, and lobar infiltrate, bacterial pneumonia caused by *Streptococcus pneumoniae* or *Haemophilus influenzae* is the most likely diagnosis. However, when a patient who has a CD4+ cell count <200 cells/mm^3 presents with a subacute onset of nonproductive cough, fever, and crackles auscultated at the lung bases, the most likely diagnosis is *Pneumocystis jiroveci* pneumonia (PCP), even when the chest x-ray is normal or reveals a pattern other than the classic bilateral interstitial perihilar pattern (Fig. 41-2). Variant patterns of PCP on the chest x-ray include lobar infiltrate, cavitation, pneumothorax, and even pleural effusion. Many other opportunistic infections, malignancies, and inflammatory conditions may mimic PCP (Table 41-3). Tuberculosis may present with atypical noncavitary pulmonary lesions in HIV-infected patients, and the immunosuppression associated with HIV increases the chance of reactivation of latent tuberculosis infection. Thus, it is often necessary to place HIV-infected patients admitted to hospital in respiratory isolation until tuberculosis can be ruled out.

Neurologic Symptoms

The most common central nervous system (CNS) disorders in patients with AIDS that result in hospital admission are cryptococcal meningitis, cerebral toxoplasmosis, primary B cell lymphoma, and progressive multifocal leukoencephalopathy (PML). The clinical presentations of these illnesses are variable, and they overlap; for example, headache and fever are absent in 15% of cases of cryptococcosis, and meningismus is present in only 30% of cases (Box 41-1).[5] In general, patients with mass lesions in the brain (i.e., most cases of toxoplasmosis and lymphoma) are more likely to present with new-onset seizure than are patients with cryptococcal meningitis. PML typically presents with hyper-reflexia, gait disturbance, and cognitive changes. Many other fungal, mycobacterial, and viral pathogens (e.g., histoplasmosis,

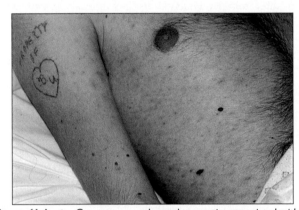

Figure 41-1 • Cutaneous maculopapular eruption associated with acute HIV infection. From: Morse SA, Ballard RC, Holmes KK, et al. Atlas of Sexually Transmitted Diseases and AIDS, 3rd Edition. St. Louis, Mosby, 2003.

tuberculosis, cytomegalovirus [CMV]) may result in mass lesions or meningitis in the late-stage HIV-infected patient.

Gastrointestinal Symptoms

Diarrhea is frequent in patients with AIDS, and the most common causes of chronic diarrhea in AIDS patients include *Cryptosporidia*, MAC, *Microsporidia* species, CMV, and medications (generally protease inhibitors).[6] Esophageal disease is also

Table 41-1 Conditions Common in HIV Infection

Consider HIV testing	
Hematologic/oncologic	Unexplained thrombocytopenia, anemia, neutropenia Generalized lymphadenopathy Lymphoma Seminoma
Neurologic	Cognitive decline in a younger patient Unexplained peripheral neuropathy
Pulmonary	Recurrent pneumonia Streptococcal pneumonia Pulmonary hypertension
Dermatologic	Atypical/recurrent herpes zoster Kaposi's sarcoma Severe oral herpes simplex virus Bacillary angiomatosis
Oropharynx	Oropharyngeal candidiasis Oral hairy leukoplakia Severe apthous ulcers Kaposi's sarcoma Lymphoma
HIV "opathy" (organ dysfunction in atypical setting)	Nephropathy (African American) Cardiomyopathy

Table 41-2 Risk of HIV Associated Conditions Stratified by CD4 Count

CD4+ LYMPHOCYTE COUNT		
<100 cells/(cells/µL)	<200 (cells/µL)	>200 (cells/µL)
Disseminated MAC	*Pneumocystis* pneumonia	Herpes zoster
CMV disease	PML	Tuberculosis
Retinitis	Endemic fungi	Lymphoma
GI tract disease	Histoplasmosis	Bacterial pneumonia
Meningoencephalitis	Coccidiomycosis (if exposure hx)	
Toxoplasmosis	HIV-related organ dysfunction	
Chronic diarrhea	Cardiomyopathy	
Cryptosporidiosis	Dementia	
Microsporidiosis	Nephropathy	
MAC	Neuropathy	
Cryptococcosis		
EBV-related CNS		
Lymphoma		

MAC—*Mycobacterium avium complex*; CMV—*cytomegalovirus*; PML—progressive multifocal leucoencenhalopathy; GI—gastrointestinal; EBV—Epstein-Barr virus; CNS—central nervous system.

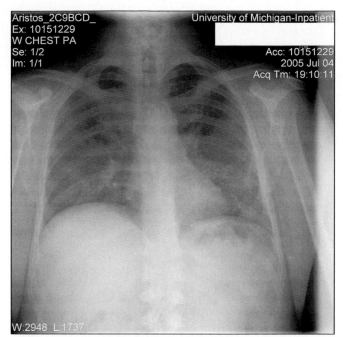

Aristos_2C9BCD_
Ex: 10151229
W CHEST PA
Se: 1/2
Im: 1/1

University of Michigan-Inpatient

Acc: 10151229
2005 Jul 04
Acq Tm: 19:10:11

W:2948 L:1737

Figure 41-2 • Typical interstitial and alveolar infiltrates of *Pneumocystis jiroveci* pneumonia.

common in patients with AIDS. *Candida* typically causes dysphagia, and oropharyngeal lesions are usually present; whereas herpes simplex virus (HSV), CMV, and aphthous ulcers generally present with odynophagia. Pathogens such as *Cryptosporidium, Microsporidium,* and CMV are associated with a cholangiopathy presenting with right upper quadrant pain in patients with late-stage HIV infection.[7]

Fever of Unknown Origin

Fever of unknown origin (FUO)—temperature above 38°C persisting for >3 weeks as an outpatient or 3 days as an inpatient without a discovered source—is frequent in the late stages of HIV infection. This symptom is uncommonly caused by HIV itself and is more often a result of drug reactions, malignancies (e.g., lymphoma), or opportunistic infections associated with advanced HIV infection (*P. jiroveci, M. avium, M. tuberculosis, H. capsulatum,* CMV, or *Cryptococcus neoformans*).[8] Furthermore, accompanying clinical features of opportunistic infections causing prolonged fever often overlap with those associated with drug reactions (cytopenias and elevation of liver enzyme tests).

Medication-Related Symptoms/Immune Reconstitution Syndrome

Adverse events caused by HAART may result in hospital admission (Table 41-4). Lactic acidosis—caused by mitochondrial toxicity of nucleoside reverse transcriptase inhibitors—is most commonly caused by stavudine or didanosine and may present with vague abdominal complaints, pancreatitis, and neuropathy.[9] A serum lactate is the best diagnostic test, and antiretrovirals should be discontinued if the diagnosis is made. Abacavir hypersensitivity syndrome occurs in approximately 5% of treated

Table 41-3 Conditions That May Be Mistaken for or Accompany *Pneumocystis jiroveci* Infections

Bacteria	Fungi	Parasites	Viruses	Other
Streptococcus pneumoniae	*Cryptococcus neoformans*	*Toxoplasma gondii*	*Cytomegalovirus*	Kaposi's sarcoma
Haemophilus influenzae	*Histoplasma capsulatum*	*Strongyloides stercoralis*	*Herpes simplex*	Lymphoma
Staphylococcus aureus	*Aspergillus* species	*Cryptosporidium*	*Adenovirus*	Drug toxicity
Myobacterium tuberculosis				Lymphoid interstitial pneumonitis
Pseudomonas aeruginosa				

Table 41-4 HAART Adverse Events That May Result in Hospital Admission

Drug	Adverse Event
Non-nucleoside reverse transcriptase inhibitors (nevirapine, efavirenz, delavirdine)	Rash, fever; rarely will progress to Stevens-Johnson syndrome Severe hepatitis (nevirapine)
Nucleoside reverse transcriptase inhibitors (zidovudine, stavudine, didanosine, abacavir, tenofovir, lamivudine, emtricitabine)	Lactic acidosis (stavudine > didanosine > others) Anemia (zidovudine) Fanconi's syndrome (tenofovir) Hypersensitivity reaction (abacavir)

patients and presents as a combination of fever, rash, and flu-like symptoms. Deaths have occurred on rechallenge or when the drug was continued in severe cases; however, premature discontinuation in unclear cases should be avoided, as the drug cannot be restarted.

Immune reconstitution inflammatory syndrome (IRIS) occurs in up to 25% of patients treated with HAART and is characterized by clinical manifestations of a previously asymptomatic infection as the immune system becomes able to mount an inflammatory response. In addition, recognized treated infections may clinically worsen with the addition of HAART. Any infection may prompt IRIS, but mycobacterial (e.g., MAC), fungal, and viral pathogens (e.g., CMV retinitis) have been reported most frequently.[10] Occasionally, treatment with glucocorticoids is required.

DIAGNOSIS

Acute HIV Infection

The absence of risk factors for acquiring HIV infection in the 8 weeks preceding the development of symptoms largely excludes the diagnosis. Seroconversion has generally not occurred when symptoms of acute infection develop, and a direct test for HIV (i.e., a quantitative HIV ribonucleic acid polymerase chain reaction [PCR]) is required to make the diagnosis, although these tests are not FDA approved for this purpose. Viral load is generally very high in acute retroviral syndrome, and false positive tests (less than 10,000 copies/mL) have been reported.[11] A diagnosis of acute HIV infection by molecular testing requires later serologic confirmation.

Chronic HIV Infection

Standard serologic testing is a two-stage procedure. An enzyme-linked immunosorbent assay (ELISA) screening test, if positive, must be confirmed by a more specific immunoblot (i.e., Western blot). False positive Western blots are exceedingly rare. Indeterminate tests (positive ELISA, equivocal Western blot) commonly do not represent true HIV infection, but may occur during seroconversion. A repeat test in 3–6 months will resolve the issue. If earlier results are needed, a quantitative or qualitative PCR for HIV RNA or DNA may be helpful, but false positives do occur.

Respiratory Symptoms

Patients who present with acute-onset cough, fever, lobar infiltrate on chest film, and shortness of breath should be treated for bacterial pneumonia and generally do not require bronchoscopy. Severely immunosuppressed patients (CD4+ < 200 cells/μL) with a subacute presentation require evaluation for *P. jiroveci* pneumonia. Nebulizer-induced sputum examined by monoclonal antibody staining or PCR is often positive, but a negative test does not rule out *P. jirovcei*. If induced sputum is nondiagnostic, bronchoscopy with bronchoalveolar lavage (BAL) should be performed. In the setting of an abnormal chest radiograph, transbronchial biopsies should be done to evaluate for the diagnoses in Table 41-3. Even in patients treated for PCP, the sensitivity of a BAL is excellent, and a negative monoclonal antibody

or PCR virtually excludes the diagnosis. Pulmonary tuberculosis is more common in the HIV-infected population and may present atypically (e.g., without cavitary disease), and isolation and evaluation (acid fast smear on BAL or sputum) are reasonable in patients with a subacute presentation and no alternative diagnosis.

Neurologic Symptoms

If neurologic symptoms are subacute, focal neurologic findings are present (e.g., hemiparesis, hemisensory loss, visual field defects, aphasia, or focal seizure), or if meningismus is absent, the patient should first undergo imaging of the brain with computed tomography (CT) or magnetic resonance imaging (MRI). MRI is more sensitive for disease processes such as PML or HIV dementia. Further evaluation of patients with multiple ring enhancing lesions depends on the *Toxoplasma* serology. Patients with a positive serology and multiple lesions may be treated empirically and reassessed for radiological response after 3 weeks of treatment. If the serology is negative or if only a single lesion is seen on MRI, brain biopsy should be performed, given the many possible causes (e.g., lymphoma, tuberculoma, pyogenic brain abscess, cryptococcoma, histoplasmoma). A lumbar puncture should be performed if CNS imaging does not reveal a diagnostic finding and the patient has no risk for developing uncal herniation. A positive cerebrospinal fluid (CSF) cryptococcal antigen will diagnose cryptococcal meningitis; if this is negative and pleocytosis is present, CSF should be sent for mycobacterial, fungal, Venereal Disease Research Laboratory (VDRL) slide test, and viral studies. CSF should be reserved for possible future studies (e.g., EBV PCR for CNS lymphoma or PCR for JC virus for PML).

Gastrointestinal Symptoms

Diarrhea that persists for >5 days with or without fever should be evaluated with three sequential stool examinations for ova and parasites, including a modified acid-fast stain for *Cryptosporidium parvum* and a modified trichrome stain for *Microsporidium* species. If these evaluations, routine cultures for enteric pathogens, and assay for *C. difficile* are negative and diarrhea persists, the patient should undergo colonoscopy with biopsy to search for potentially treatable causes of colitis, such as *Cytomegalovirus*, MAC, Kaposi's sarcoma, and lymphoma.

Patients with dysphagia who have oropharyngeal candidiasis generally can be empirically treated with fluconazole 200 mg orally daily. Odynophagia or failure to respond to empiric treatment mandates esophagogastroduodenoscopy (EGD), usually with biopsy and cultures. AIDS cholangiopathy, in which liver function tests suggest a cholestatic process, is best diagnosed by endoscopic retrograde cholangiography (ERCP) with brushings or biopsy for microbiologic diagnosis.

Fever of Unknown Origin

Employ a stepwise approach to the diagnosis of fever of unknown origin when the initial evaluation (chest radiology, liver function tests, blood cultures) of HIV-infected patients does not reveal an etiology. Appropriate initial tests include lysis-centrifugation blood cultures for fungi and mycobacteria, a serum cryptococcal antigen, studies for endemic fungi (e.g., serologies and urine histoplasma antigen in the midwest, coccidiomycosis serologies in the desert southwest), induced sputum for PCP, and retinal examination for CMV disease (if CD4 < 100 cells/μL). If these additional tests still do not produce a diagnosis, further studies include CT of chest, abdomen, and pelvis (lymphoma, other causes of lymphadenopathy), lumbar puncture, and bone marrow biopsy.

PROGNOSIS

In the HAART era, even patients with late-stage HIV infection and multiple AIDS-defining conditions may respond to treatment. Thus, aggressive treatment of opportunistic infections or malignancies is generally indicated. Previously "untreatable" conditions such as HIV dementia, CNS lymphoma, and PML may respond remarkably well to HAART. Some patients develop multidrug-resistant virus, and while HAART may slow the progression of disease in these cases, less aggressive care may be indicated in selected situations.

MANAGEMENT

Treatment

Respiratory

Given the high rate of infection with *Pseudomonas aeruginosa*,[12] patients with CD4+ cell counts <200 cells/μL and bacterial pneumonia should be treated with an antibiotic with antipseudomonal activity (e.g., cefepime 1 g IV every 8 hours or piperacillin/tazobactam 4.0 g IV every 6 hours) until culture results are available.

First-line treatment for *P. jiroveci* pneumonia is trimethoprim/sulfamethoxazole 15 mg/kg (of the trimethoprim component) divided every 8 hours. Up to 50% of AIDS patients are intolerant of high-dose sulfa agents[13]; alternative regimens are listed in Box 41-2. For patients with severe disease (pO_2 <70 mm Hg or A-a gradient >35 mm Hg), adjunctive corticosteroids (prednisone: 40 mg b.i.d. day 1–5, 40 mg daily day 6–10, 20 mg daily day 11–21) prevents early deterioration of oxygenation by reducing inflammation associated with lysis of *P. jiroveci*. The duration of therapy is 21 days, and after clinical improvement, patients may be switched to an oral regimen (*see* Box 41-2).

Neurological

First-line therapy for acute CNS toxoplasmosis is pyrimethamine 200 mg loading dose and then 50 mg/day orally in combination with sulfadiazine: 6 g/day in four divided oral doses and folinic acid 10–25 mg/day. Up to 40% of patients are unable to tolerate this regimen, with rash and hematologic side effects most common. Crystalluria, radiolucent stones, and renal failure can also occur with high-dose sulfonamides. Clindamycin may be substituted for the sulfadiazine as a second-line agent 900 mg IV every 8 hours or 450 mg orally 4 times a day. Corticosteroids should be added if significant edema is present (e.g., dexamethasone 4–6 mg every 6 hours). Radiologic and clinical response should occur within 2–3 weeks.

Box 41-2 Treatment of *Pneumocystis* Pneumonia (Requiring Hospitalization)

First line*

Trimethoprim/sulfamethoxazole (15 mg/kg/day) in three divided doses

(oral to complete therapy; two double-strength tablets 3 times a day)

Second line*

Trimethoprim (5 mg/kg/day IV q8h) + dapsone (100 mg/day PO)

or

Clindamycin (900 mg IV q8h) + primaquine (30 mg/day PO)

(Clindamycin may changed to 300–450 mg three times a day orally to complete therapy after discharge)

or

Pentamidine (4 mg/kg IV q24h)[†] (no oral formulation)

*All regimens are 21 days in duration.
[†]Nephrotoxicity, hypotension, hypo/hyperglycemia.

Increased intracranial pressure occurs frequently in patients with Cryptococcal meningitis as the organism's gelatinous capsule interferes with CSF reabsorption. Opening pressure should be measured in all patients, and outcomes are improved in patients with CSF pressures >200 cm H_2O with repeat (daily) large-volume taps to decrease pressure.[14] Induction therapy for Cryptococcal meningitis in AIDS patients consists of amphotericin deoxycholate 0.7–1 mg/kg IV daily in combination with flucytosine 100 mg/kg orally in four divided doses. Flucytosine hematologic toxicity may occur when clearance of the drug is decreased by amphotericin-induced renal toxicity. Liposomal preparations of amphotericin (e.g., Ambisome 4 mg/kg IV q24h) may be substituted for amphotericin deoxycholate, as they are less nephrotoxic.[5] After 2 weeks of treatment, a repeat lumbar puncture should be performed; if fungal culture does not grow *Cryptococcus* and the patient has improved, treatment may be changed to fluconazole 400 mg orally once a day. Follow-up cryptococcal antigens are not useful in the acute stage of treatment; India ink smear may show nonviable fungal forms that do not indicate treatment failure.

Gastrointestinal

Management of chronic diarrhea in the AIDS patient is challenging. Cryptosporidium, essentially untreatable in the pre-HAART era, resolves with immune reconstitution. Paromomycin 500–1,000 mg twice a day may speed clearance in patients successfully treated with HAART. CMV colitis generally requires intravenous ganciclovir (5 mg/kg b.i.d. for 2 weeks); oral valganciclovir is an option for patients able to absorb oral medications. Duration of therapy depends upon response; serum PCR for CMV may be helpful in determining duration of therapy. Bacterial pathogens are generally treated similar to HIV negative patients; salmonella, however, requires ongoing suppression to prevent recurrence. Treatment of AIDS cholangiopathy depends on the organism isolated; ERCP-guided biliary sphincterotomy may relieve symptoms if papillary stenosis is present.

Fever of Unknown Origin

Treatment in the patient with FUO is supportive until identification of the cause of fever. The treatment for some of the more common pathogens identified in an FUO workup are outlined below. Disseminated histoplasmosis is treated with amphotericin deoxycholate 0.7 mg/kg IV daily; patients may be switched to itraconazole 200 mg orally twice a day on discharge from the hospital if clinically improving.[15] Response to therapy can be monitored using the urine *Histoplasma* antigen. Disseminated MAC is best treated with the combination of clarithromycin 500 mg orally twice a day and ethambutol 15–20 mg/kg orally daily.

Drug Interactions

Protease inhibitors (PI), particularly ritonavir, are inhibitors of the P450 CYP3A4 isoenzyme and are metabolized by that enzyme. Non-nucleoside reverse transcriptase inhibitors (NNRTI) are metabolized by the same enzyme and may act as inducers, inhibitors, or both. Drugs that induce the P450 system (e.g., rifampin, phenobarbital) should generally be avoided, as they will result in reduced PI or NNRTI levels. Drug metabolized by these enzymes (e.g., most HMG Co-A reductase inhibitors, midazolam) may have marked increases or decreases in their levels when combined with PI or NNRTI. A partial list of drug interactions is available at http://aidsinfo.nih.gov/guidelines/.[16]

Occupational Exposure

Over 500,000 occupational needlestick injuries occur annually in the United States. Five thousand of these are estimated to be from an HIV-positive source. The risk of contracting HIV infection from a needlestick injury is estimated to be 0.3%; factors that increase the risk are open lumen needles, deep injury, visible blood on the device, and needle used in artery or vein. Mucosal exposures carry a lower risk 0.09%; exposure to nonbloody fluid (with the exception of CSF, ascitic fluid, and pleural fluid) is not considered to present an infectious risk. Skin exposures only carry risk if a break in the skin is present. Case control studies indicate that postexposure prophylaxis (PEP) with antiretroviral therapy reduces the risk of transmission by 80%. If possible, PEP should be given within 2 hours, but may be effective as late a week after the exposure.[17] An algorithm for occupational exposure is available at www.cdc.gov/mmwr/indrr_2001.html.

DISCHARGE/FOLLOW-UP PLANS

HAART may have been discontinued during hospitalization if a patient was not able to take oral medication. If no medication side effect (e.g., nevirapine-induced hepatotoxicity) prompted the admission, it is generally appropriate to restart HAART on discharge from the hospital. Mycobacterial or fungal cultures may take as long as 8 weeks to mature; primary care providers should be alerted to ensure appropriate follow-up on these results.

Key Points

- Acute HIV infection may present with a mononucleosis-like illness, and a direct test for HIV RNA or DNA (e.g., PCR for HIV RNA) is required to make the diagnosis.

- A wide variety of clinical conditions, including invasive pneumococcal disease and unexplained cytopenias, should prompt consideration of testing for HIV.

- HIV-infected patients with fever of unknown origin often have more than one cause of fever.

- Antiretroviral agents may result in life-threatening toxicities that result in hospitalization and are difficult to recognize. These include abacavir hypersensitivity syndrome, nucleoside-induced mitochondrial toxicity with lactic acidosis, and tenofovir-induced Fanconi's syndrome.

- Empiric treatment and diagnostic workup in HIV-infected patients are highly dependent on the status of the patient's immune system as measured by the CD4+ cell count.

SUGGESTED READING

Glynn M, Rhodes P. Estimated HIV prevalence in the United States at the end of 2003. In: National HIV Prevention Conference, 2005. Atlanta, 2005.

Kassutto S, Rosenberg ES. Primary HIV type 1 infection. Clin Infect Dis 2004; 38:1447–1453.

Saag MS, Graybill RJ, Larsen RA, et al. Practice guidelines for the management of cryptococcal disease. Infectious Diseases Society of America. Clin Infect Dis 2000; 30(4):710–718.

Yusuf TE, Baron TH. AIDS Cholangiopathy. Curr Treat Options Gastroenterol 2004; 7:111–117.

Hirsch HH, Kaufmann G, Sendi P, et al. Immune reconstitution in HIV infected patients. Clin Infect Dis 2005; 38:1159–1166.

Afessa B, Green B. Bacterial pneumonia in hospitalized patients with HIV infection: the Pulmonary Complications, ICU Support, and Prognostic Factors of Hospitalized Patients with HIV (PIP) Study. Chest 2000; 117(4):1017–1022.

Graybill JR, Sobel J, Saag M, et al. Diagnosis and management of increased intracranial pressure in patients with AIDS and cryptococcal meningitis. The NIAID Mycoses Study Group and AIDS Cooperative Treatment Groups. Clin Infect Dis 2000; 30(1):47–54.

(DHHS) PoCPfToHI. Guidelines for the use of antiretroviral agents for adults and adolescents. In: Department of Health and Human Services, 2004.

CDC. Updated U.S. public health service guidelines for the management of occupational exposures to HBV, HCV, and HIV and recommendations for postexposure prophylaxis. MMWR: Recommend Rep 2001; 50 RR 11.

CHAPTER FORTY-TWO

Bioterrorism

James C. Pile, MD, FACP

INTRODUCTION

The use of biologic agents, or biologicals, either in the context of warfare or as agents of terror, has been contemplated seriously for nearly a century. This chapter will focus on the employment of biologicals as potential vehicles for terrorism, with the realization that there is a great deal of overlap with their potential use in a military setting.

Biological weapons are potentially attractive to nation-states as well as terrorist groups because they are both relatively inexpensive and fairly simple to produce. One estimate suggested that a bioweapons laboratory of moderate sophistication could be implemented at a cost of only several hundred thousand dollars—well within the means of many terrorist groups.[1] Many agents have been proposed as candidates for use as biological weapons, although some are clearly more plausible than others in this regard. Effective biological weapons are generally developed to fulfill certain criteria, including causing high morbidity and mortality; being amenable to mass production; possessing stability in aerosol form; and being dispersible as 1–5 micron particles. The ideal bioweapon would also be transmissible in person-to-person fashion and have no effective vaccine or treatment.[2] The Centers for Disease Control and Prevention (CDC) has designated agents most likely to be successfully used as biological weapons as "Category A" and others thought to be possible but less likely candidates as "Category B" (Table 42-1). Those Category A diseases generally considered most likely to be utilized as bioweapons (smallpox, anthrax, botulism, and plague) are of most relevance to the inpatient physician and will be addressed below.

ASSESSMENT

Few North American physicians have seen clinical cases involving diseases on the CDC's Category A list, and in fact many infectious diseases specialists have never cared for a patient with any of these illnesses. As the timely recognition of a bioterrorist attack will most likely hinge on rapid and accurate identification of a rare disease as it did with the anthrax attacks in 2001, the importance of preparation by clinicians likely to encounter these patients early on (emergency physicians, hospitalists, and infectious disease specialists) is of critical importance. The ability to provisionally distinguish between smallpox and its imitators, or to suspect the correct diagnosis of anthrax in a very ill, febrile

patient with a widened mediastinum, cannot be overstressed. As was the case with the recent anthrax attacks, disease occurring in the milieu of bioterrorism may present in ways quite different than those classically presented in medical texts, and clinicians need to be cognizant of the fact that both epidemiological and purely clinical aspects of disease presentation may be novel if encountered in this context.[3] In any suspected bioterror-related illness, the hospital's epidemiologist as well as local and state public health officials must be promptly involved, with the CDC available for backup.

Clinical Presentation

Smallpox

Of all diseases potentially linked to bioterrorism, smallpox is perhaps the most feared—for reasons that include its lethality, contagiousness, tendency to disfigure survivors, and eradication from the world as a natural disease. Historically, smallpox caused the most illness during the winter and early spring in temperate climates, due to prolonged survival and transmissibility of the variola virus during periods of low temperature and humidity. Disease was typically spread via droplets, although on occasion the virus was capable of spread by aerosolization, in which case contagiousness was dramatically heightened.

Disease typically manifested after an incubation period averaging 10–14 days (range, 7–17) with a severe prodrome that included fever frequently in excess of 40°C, severe malaise, headache, backache, abdominal pain, nausea, and vomiting. Rash began after several days of prodrome, and evidence suggests that contagiousness coincided with the appearance of rash, not onset of prodrome.[4] The rash of smallpox was somewhat nondescript initially, beginning in the oropharynx and on the face and arms, with subsequent spread to the legs and trunk. Lesions turned from macular-papular to vesicular within 1–2 days, and then became pustular (Figs. 42-1 and 42-2). Patients typically remained febrile and severely ill for approximately 2 weeks after the appearance of exanthem and were contagious for 7–10 days after the appearance of rash. The World Health Organization categorized smallpox into 1 of 5 clinical types: ordinary, modified (mild disease in the previously vaccinated), hemorrhagic, flat, and variola sine eruptione (influenza-like illness without exanthem occurring in some of those previously immunized).[5] The hemorrhagic and flat forms of smallpox were often difficult to cor-

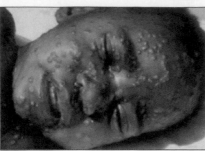

Figure 42-1 • Smallpox. Note the uniform stage of development of the vesicles. From: Swartz MH. Textbook of Physical Diagnosis, 5th Edition—History and Examination with STUDENT CONSULT Access. Copyright 2006.

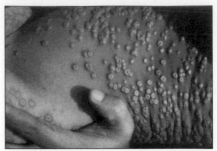

Figure 42-2 • Smallpox. Note the umbilicated lesions on the trunk. From: Swartz MH. Textbook of Physical Diagnosis, 5th Edition—History and Examination with STUDENT CONSULT Access. Copyright 2006.

Table 42-1 Potential Biological Agents of Concern as Possible Bioweapons

Category A	Category B
Variola (smallpox)	Coxiella burnetii (Q fever)
Bacillus anthracis (anthrax)	Brucella (brucellosis)
Yersinia pestis (plague)	Burkholderia mallei (glanders)
Clostridium botulinum (botulinum toxin)	Burkholderia pseudomallei (meliodosis)
Francisella tularensis (tularemia)	Alphaviruses (encephalitis)
Filoviruses and Arenaviruses (viral hemorrhagic fevers)	Rickettsia prowazekii (typhus) Toxins (Ricin, etc.)
	Chlamydia psittaci (psittacosis)
	Food safety threats (Salmonella, etc.)
	Water safety threats (Vibrio cholerae, etc.)

Adapted from the CDC's Public Health Assessment of Potential Biological Terrorism Agents.

Table 42-2 Distinguishing Characteristics of Smallpox and Chickenpox

Smallpox	Chickenpox
Lesions in same stage of development in given body area	Lesions in different stages of development ("crops")
Lesions 4–6 mm in diameter	Lesions 2–4 mm in diameter
Centrifugal distribution (bulk of lesions located peripherally)	Centripedal distribution (bulk of lesions centrally located)
Palms and soles typically involved	Palms and soles rarely involved
Lesions umbilicated	Lesions nonumbilicated
Lesions firm and deeply seated	Lesions soft and superficial
More lesions on back than abdomen	More lesions on abdomen than back
Severe prodrome	Mild prodrome

rectly identify, and they carried both an extremely high mortality rate as well as a markedly elevated risk of person-to-person transmission. The former, typically occurring in pregnant individuals, was characterized by an especially severe prodrome, followed by generalized erythema that soon progressed to petechiae, purpura, and disseminated intravascular coagulopathy (DIC). The flat (malignant) form of smallpox was likewise marked by a severe prodrome, with rash failing to progress to pustules, but rather becoming confluent and "velvety."[4]

The differential diagnosis of smallpox, which is potentially of critical importance to hospitalists and other physicians likely to find themselves on the frontlines of a smallpox outbreak, included varicella (chickenpox), generalized vaccinia (after smallpox vaccination), monkeypox, Norwegian scabies, drug reactions, molluscum contagiosum, disseminated herpesvirus infections, enteroviral infection, and erythema multiforme. The differential diagnosis of hemorrhagic smallpox would include meningococcemia, DIC, acute leukemia, and a variety of hemorrhagic fevers. Although a well-publicized case of disseminated herpes simplex virus 2 recently caused consternation when the CDC was asked to urgently investigate the possibility of smallpox,[6] historically, the disease that was by far most often confused with smallpox was varicella. A number of features help to distinguish the two diseases (Table 42-2), although these characteristics need to be examined as a whole, as there may be some overlap between the two illnesses. For example, a recent study of varicella suggested that the prodrome of the two diseases might be confused in a minority of cases.[7] An extremely useful interactive web-based tool entitled "Evaluate a Rash Illness Suspicious for Smallpox" is available through the CDC at www.bt.cdc.gov/agent/smallpox/diagnosis/riskalgorithm/index.asp; it helps to categorize the risk that a particular rash represents smallpox as high, medium, or low and includes accompanying instructions on how to proceed. Photographs depicting the stages of smallpox are available on the World Health Organization's website, www.who.int/emc/diseases/smallpox/slideset.

Anthrax

Anthrax, a disease described since antiquity, is caused by the large gram-positive "boxcar shaped" rod *Bacillus anthracis,* and causes three distinct forms of disease. Two of these, inhalational and cutaneous disease, are likely to occur after an intentional release of *B. anthracis,* with the third, gastrointestinal disease, less likely to be encountered in this setting.

Although it was long known in the animal hide industry, where it was known as "woolsorter's disease," most of what is known regarding inhalational anthrax stems from two biowarfare/bioterror incidents (Sverdlovsk, USSR in 1979 and the 2001 US attacks). Inhalational disease results after the deposition of aerosolized *B. anthracis* into alveoli, where spores are ingested by macrophages and transported to regional lymphatics. Spore germination then leads to a complex cascade that includes elaboration of two specific toxins, with production of cytokines, including TNF-alpha and IL-1, and subsequent clinical disease. After an incubation period that appears to average 4–5 days but may be considerably longer[8,9] disease begins as a nonspecific influenza-like illness, with fever and malaise lasting up to several days (Table 42-3). Patients then begin to rapidly deteriorate, with death seemingly inevitable unless appropriate treatment is instituted promptly. An analysis of the initial 10 inhalational cases from 2001 revealed fever, chills, and malaise in all patients; cough in 9; nausea and/or vomiting in 9; dyspnea in 8; chest pain in 7; and profound diaphoresis in 7. All presented with abnormal chest radiographs (although only 7 showed mediastinal widening initially); all eventually developed pleural effusions, and 7 of 9 had clearly elevated transaminases.[10] Of the 11 total inhalational cases, 6 patients survived, all of whom presented before the onset of fulminant disease. Contrary to prior experience with inhalational anthrax, 8 of 11 patients showed evidence of parenchymal lung involvement.[9] Meningitis occurs in a substantial percentage of patients with disseminated anthrax. A possible predilection of inhalational anthrax for older individuals had been suggested previously,[11] and the youngest patient with this form of the disease in the 2001 attacks was 43 years old.[10]

Cutaneous anthrax is much more common than inhalational disease in the natural setting, although the incidence of the two forms in the 2001 attacks was equivalent (11 cases). The cutaneous form of the disease was felt in the past to require a break in the skin,[11] although the 2001 cases have left this in question. Disease begins as a papular lesion that quickly ulcerates and then forms a characteristic black eschar (Figs. 42-3 and 42-4). The lesion is surrounded by edema, which may be profound enough to lead to airway compromise in cases involving the head and neck. Fever, malaise, headache, and regional lymphadenopathy are common, with systemic dissemination of disease in 5–20% of cases. The differential diagnosis of cutaneous anthrax includes streptococcal disease, ecthyma gangrenosum, tularemia, the bite

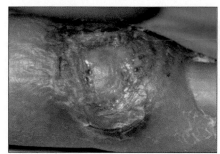

Figure 42-3 • Intentional anthrax (exposure secondary to bioterrorism) partially treated. From: Swartz MH. Textbook of Physical Diagnosis, 5th Edition—History and Examination with STUDENT CONSULT Access. Copyright 2006.

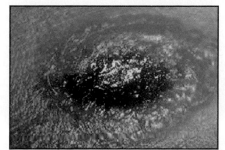

Figure 42-4 • Anthrax. Note the black eschar. From: Swartz MH. Textbook of Physical Diagnosis, 5th Edition—History and Examination with STUDENT CONSULT Access. Copyright 2006.

Table 42-3 Distinguishing Characteristics of Inhalational Anthrax and Influenza

	Anthrax	Influenza
Fever	Likely	Likely
Subjective fever/chills	Likely	Likely
Cough	Likely	Likely
Dyspnea	Likely	Unlikely
Chest pain	Likely	Unlikely
Myalgias	Moderately Likely	Likely
Rhinorrhea	Unlikely	Likely
Nausea/vomiting	Likely	Unlikely
Sore throat	Unlikely	Likely
Neurologic abnormalities	Moderately likely	Unlikely
Abnormal lung examination	Likely	Unlikely
Abnormal chest radiograph	Likely	Unlikely
Elevated transaminases	Likely	Unlikely

of *Loxosceles* genus spiders (e.g., brown recluse spider), plague, and rickettsial disease. The appearance of a fully developed lesion should be very suggestive to the prepared clinician, however. Cutaneous anthrax images may be viewed at www.bt.cdc.gov/agent/anthrax/anthrax-images/cutaneous.asp.

Botulism

Botulism, a disease mediated by a neurotoxin produced by *Clostridium botulinum*, continues to occur sporadically through contamination of foodstuffs. Botulinum toxin is purportedly the most lethal known substance, with 1 g capable of causing 1 million deaths under ideal circumstances. Iraq successfully weaponized botulinum toxin in the late 1980s and early 1990s, with a peak stockpile of 20,000 L, enough to eradicate the global population multiple times over.[12] Clinically, disease occurs in three forms, with similar illness resulting from all: wound, infant, and ingestion botulism. Seven toxin types are produced by *C. botulinum* strains, designated A–G, with types A, B, E and F causing naturally occurring human disease. Inhalational disease is not found naturally, but primate models suggest this as a feasible route for intentional infection.[12] Botulinum toxin exerts its effects through irreversible inhibition of release of acetylcholine from neuromuscular junctions and begins with bulbar symptoms that include multiple cranial nerve deficits. Disease is characterized by acute onset, absence of fever, symmetry, normal mental status, a lack of sensory changes, and a descending presentation. Specific manifestations include diplopia, ptosis, blurred vision, dysarthria, dysphonia, dysphagia, dry mouth, and generalized weakness. Illness frequently progresses to respiratory failure, as a result of inability to maintain the upper airway as well as diaphragmatic and intercostal muscle weakness. The differential diagnosis of botulism includes myasthenia gravis, the Miller-Fischer variant of Guillain-Barré, tick paralysis, brainstem stroke, Lambert-Eaton syndrome, inflammatory myopathies, organophosphate poisoning, magnesium or other toxicities, and conversion syndromes.[12,13] The diagnosis of botulism, it must be stressed, is primarily clinical (see below).

Plague

Plague, best known as the cause of the "Black Death" which decimated Europe in the fourteenth century, is caused by a gram-negative bacillus, *Yersinia pestis*. Naturally occurring disease typically manifests as bubonic plague, with the bite of an infected flea followed by development of intensely painful regional lymphadenopathy, the "bubo." Pneumonic plague is much less common, but occurs in perhaps 5% of natural cases, and has a mortality rate of approximately 50%.[14] Pneumonic plague is, however, the form of disease that would be seen following an intentional aerosol release of *Y. pestis*, and disease behavior in this setting would probably involve surprises. In the natural setting, pneumonic plague exhibits symptom onset after an incubation of 2–4 days, with high fever, malaise, and sputum that is frequently either watery or bloody. A variety of gastrointestinal manifestations including nausea and vomiting, diarrhea, and abdominal pain are frequent concomitants. Untreated disease progresses in fulminant fashion, with complications of gram-negative septicemia including DIC and acute renal failure occurring commonly. Meningitis may be seen in some cases. Chest radiographs show a variety of infiltrative patterns, and laboratory studies often show liver function abnormalities in addition to evidence of consumptive coagulopathy and azotemia. The differential diagnosis of pneumonic plague includes, in addition to more common

etiologies of community-acquired pneumonia, SARS, influenza, and inhalational anthrax.[15]

Diagnosis

Smallpox

The web-based tool described in the smallpox clinical presentation section is an excellent starting point in the evaluation of any individual with possible smallpox. The hospital epidemiologist and at least the local public health department should also be notified immediately, with the patient placed in respiratory and contact isolation, in a negative pressure room. Specimens (ideally the contents of an unroofed lesion) should be placed in a sealed vacutainer tube, placed into another secured container, and shipped as expeditiously as possible to a biosafety level-4 laboratory *with the assistance of state/local health officials*. Techniques capable of detecting presence of a poxvirus with a high level of specificity (but not capable, for example, of distinguishing smallpox from monkeypox) include electron microscopy for the presence of characteristic large, brick-shaped virions, and H and E (Haematoxylin and Easin) staining for pathognomonic cytoplasmic inclusions (Guarnieri bodies). Polymerase chain reaction (PCR) is available at the CDC and the United States Army Medical Research Institute for Infectious Diseases (USAMRIID). A real-time (Light Cycler) PCR assay for smallpox has been developed.[15]

Anthrax

The importance of an appropriate degree of clinical suspicion and communication of this to the microbiology laboratory, along with notification of the hospital epidemiologist and public health officials, cannot be overemphasized. Recent experience points out that in the absence of antibiotic therapy, *B. anthracis* is easily isolated from blood cultures.[9] Most microbiology laboratories should now be able to make a preliminary diagnosis of *B. anthracis*, with definitive identification available via reference laboratories. PCR and immunohistochemistry (IHC) staining are useful confirmatory techniques, and they may be particularly helpful in establishing a diagnosis when prior antibiotics have sterilized blood or pleural fluid cultures.[10] In the setting of cutaneous disease, culture of the lesion will readily yield *B. anthracis*. PCR and IHC are helpful if antibiotic administration has resulted in nondiagnostic Gram stain and culture.[8]

Botulism

Botulism is largely a clinical diagnosis and must be suspected *and treated* on the basis of a consistent clinical presentation. When botulism is suspected, the public health system must be notified, and definitive diagnostic techniques may be implemented, with the realization that confirmation of the clinical suspicion will be delayed. Testing for botulinum toxin is available at state and other reference laboratories, with blood, stool, and possible culprit foods appropriate for analysis. The gold standard remains the mouse bioassay, which may take up to 4 days to complete[16]; ELISA for toxin may also be obtained in some reference laboratories. Toxin has been reported to remain present in stools for up to 1 month after symptom onset, and stool cultures may also remain positive for *C. botulinum* for some time as well.[16]

Plague

While the presentation of multiple previously healthy patients with severe community-acquired pneumonia should raise the possibility of plague, particularly in association with hemoptysis, a definitive diagnosis will be made via the laboratory. While Gram stain may show characteristic bipolar staining, this is best appreciated with Giemsa, Wright, or Wayson's stains. Automated systems may correctly identify *Y. pestis,* although misidentification is common.[17] As with other Category A pathogens, definitive identification may be made by laboratories in the Laboratory Response Network for Bioterrorism (LRN). Identification via direct fluorescent antibody staining of the organism's capsule is available in a limited number of reference laboratories.[18]

Prognosis

Smallpox

Historically, mortality rates varied with the type of smallpox, which in turn was partially dependent on prior vaccination status as well as the status of a patient's immune system. The hemorrhagic form of the disease was uniformly fatal, while flat smallpox resulted in death in the majority of cases. "Typical" disease in those not previously vaccinated carried a mortality frequently reported to be in the vicinity of 30%. Successful vaccination provided solid immunity against disease for several years and likely conferred some degree of protection for much longer. One study of cases imported into Europe over a 20-year period found a mortality rate of 52% in those never vaccinated, compared to 11% in those vaccinated >20 years before contracting disease.[19] As immunity continues to wane in contemporary populations, suggestion has been made that reintroduction of smallpox might lead to devastation akin to that previously seen in Native American populations.[20] Conversely, essentially all experience with smallpox predated the advent of modern critical care medicine, and conceivably mortality would be lower than in the past.

Anthrax

Although inhalational anthrax was felt in the past to be invariably fatal, more recent experience in Sverdlovsk and the United States has shown that timely antibiotic administration and supportive care are often effective. In the 2001 attacks, eight patients sought medical care before the onset of fulminant illness, and the six patients in this group treated on the day of presentation with an antibiotic(s) active against *B. anthracis* all survived. Conversely, all of the individuals in that series with advanced illness at the time of presentation failed to survive.[10] Historical data suggest a mortality of 5–20% for untreated cutaneous anthrax, which may be reduced to <1% with appropriate antibiotic administration.[11]

Botulism

The mortality of botulism, which was approximately 25% in the 1950s, fell to 6% in the 1990s[12] as a result of both antitoxin use and improvements in supportive care, particularly mechanical ventilation. When intubation is required, patients with botulism will require ventilatory support for an average of 58 days with type A, or 26 days with type B.[13]

Plague

Untreated pneumonic plague has a mortality approaching 100%. Although prompt administration of appropriate antibiotics may be expected to reduce this substantially, any bioterror incident involving successful dissemination of aerosolized *Y. pestis* would be expected to cause many deaths. Substantial morbidity would

also be expected, given the propensity of plague to lead to digital/limb necrosis, the source of the "Black Death" appellation.

MANAGEMENT

Smallpox

Treatment of smallpox was strictly supportive. Varicella immune globulin has been successfully employed in the setting of vaccine complications but appears to have no utility against smallpox itself. Cidofovir has activity against the virus in vitro, as well as against other poxviruses in animal models, and would likely be used in the event of a smallpox introduction, although its renal toxicity and fairly complex administration are drawbacks. The drug has reportedly been modified to an orally bioavailable form, with significantly enhanced activity against variola.[20] Vaccination clearly provides the most effective protective strategy against smallpox, provided it can be successfully administered prior to or immediately (within 3 days) after exposure. Cogent arguments both for and against widespread preemptive smallpox immunization have been proposed,[21,22] with a consensus at present to limit immunization to the military and a select number of other individuals most likely to have early involvement with a smallpox outbreak. Although smallpox vaccination carries some risk of complications, including progressive vaccinia, postvaccinial encephalitis, and eczema vaccinatum, recent mass immunization involving the military has demonstrated the current vaccine to be generally well tolerated. The single surprise from recent experience with the vaccine was the unexpected occurrence of cases of myopericarditis.[20,23]

Anthrax

Much of what is known regarding treatment of anthrax derives from primate studies, along with analysis of the 2001 cases, and to a lesser extent from what is known of the Sverdlovsk outbreak. Naturally occurring *B. anthracis* is susceptible to penicillin, doxycycline, and ciprofloxacin, and all three agents have FDA approval for the treatment of inhalational anthrax. Other antibiotics with in vitro activity include first-generation cephalosporins, clindamycin, imipenem, rifampin, vancomycin, aminoglycosides, and linezolid.[8] The CDC has recommended the use of intravenous ciprofloxacin or doxycycline in conjunction with one or more additional agents from the above list for the treatment of inhalational disease. For cutaneous disease, oral ciprofloxacin or doxycycline may be used, unless systemic toxicity or head/neck disease is present, in which case treatment should be as for inhalational disease. In the setting of a bioterrorist attack, duration of treatment of either inhalational or cutaneous disease should be 60 days, to cover the possibility of ungerminated, inhaled spores.[8] A succinct approach to the patient with suspected inhalational anthrax may be found in Table 42-4.

Botulism

The mainstays of treatment for botulism are prompt administration of antitoxin and supportive care. Essentially, all disease occurring naturally in North America is type A, B, or E, and the antitoxin available through the CDC is a trivalent product targeting these. Conceivably, a terrorist attack might use a type other than these, and USAMRIID has a heptavalent product that would be available

Table 42-4 Proposed Staging of Inhalational Anthrax

Stage	Comments
1: Asymptomatic	Usually <1 week and rarely >1 month
2: Early— prodromal	Nonspecific malaise, myalgias, low-grade fever, mild headache, nausea, general "flu-like" prodromal illness.
3: Intermediate– progressive	Blood cultures are positive in <24 hours; mediastinal adenopathy present; pleural effusions that are often hemorrhagic, large, and require repeated drainage. Findings may include high fever, dyspnea, confusion or syncope, increasing nausea/vomiting. Patients in this stage can still be cured with appropriate antibiotics and intensive support.
4: Late–fulminant	Respiratory failure requiring intubation, meningitis, end-organ hypoperfusion ("shock"). Cure currently less likely in this stage. Future therapies for this stage may require inhibitors of both anthrax toxin and systemic inflammatory response mediators, in addition to antibiotics and intensive care.

This proposed staging system incorporates information from historic "early" and "late" stages with new timing of microbiologic and radiologic information (i.e., an "intermediate–progressive stage") from the 11 patients in the 2001 bioterrorism attacks.

under an investigational new drug (IND) protocol.[12] The antitoxins are equine derived and are associated with a significant rate of hypersensitivity reactions. One vial of antitoxin is generally sufficient for treatment and is probably most efficacious if administered within 24 hours of symptom onset.[16] Supportive care frequently involves not only mechanical ventilation, but also treatment of the dysautonomic symptoms that may accompany illness.

Plague

Prompt administration of appropriate antibiotics will be the cornerstone of any response to a bioterrorist-induced outbreak of plague. Streptomycin and gentamicin have the best track record in the treatment of plague, and the Civilian Working Group for Biodefense has recommended the use of either agent in the event of a contained (i.e., limited numbers of casualties) outbreak; with intravenous doxycycline (100 mg bid or 200 mg once daily) or ciprofloxacin (400 mg b.i.d.) as alternatives.[17] The same group has recommended orally administered doxycycline (100 mg b.i.d.) or ciprofloxacin (500 mg b.i.d.) in the event of an outbreak that outstrips ability to treat all patients with intravenous agents. The Working Group also recommends oral antibiotic prophylaxis for those having close contact (2 meters or less) with pneumonic plague patients, with patients remaining in respiratory isolation for at least 48 hours after antibiotic initiation.

CONCLUSION

While the likelihood of further successful bioterrorism attacks on the United States is uncertain, the events of September 11, 2001

and the anthrax attacks of the following month left no question that groups exist with the willingness to use any of these agents against western nations. In addition, little doubt remains that many of the key scientists from the former Soviet Union's massive biowarfare program have taken their expertise to the highest bidders. In light of this, the need for hospitalists, emergency physicians, and infectious disease specialists to recognize likely clinical syndromes resulting from a bioterrorism attack, and to know where to turn for assistance, are unfortunate facts of life. Early recognition of an attack may be expected to save lives, and particularly in the case of smallpox, may significantly limit the eventual size of an outbreak.

Key Points

- Timely recognition of a bioterrorist attack will depend in large part on the preparedness of front-line providers, including emergency physicians and hospitalists.

- Disease syndromes encountered in a bioterrorism scenario may present in epidemiologically and clinically novel fashion compared to natural presentation of the same disease. "Chance favors the prepared mind."

- Smallpox is most likely to be confused with varicella (chickenpox), but a variety of distinguishing characteristics help to distinguish the two illnesses, including a severe constitutional prodrome seen with smallpox but not varicella.

- Botulism is a clinical diagnosis, marked by descending weakness, prominent cranial neuropathies, clear sensorium, and absence of fever.

- Inhalational anthrax is not uniformly fatal as once felt, with early treatment with two or more CDC-recommended antibiotics appearing to markedly improve outcome.

- Infection control measures are critical in the event of a smallpox or pneumonic plague outbreak, to prevent person-to-person transmission.

SUGGESTED READING

Henderson DA, Borio LA. Bioterrorism: An overview. In: Mandell GL, Bennett JE, Dolin R, eds. Mandell, Douglas and Bennett's Principles and Practice of Infectious Diseases. Philadelphia: Elsevier Churchill Livingstone, 2005. 3591–3601.

Henderson DA, Inglesby TV, Bartlett JG, et al. Smallpox as a biological weapon. JAMA 1999; 281:2127–2137.

Inglesby TV, O'Toole T, Henderson DA, et al. Anthrax as a biological weapon, 2002: Updated recommendations for management. JAMA 2002; 287:2236–2252.

Jernigan JA, Stephens DS, Ashford DA, et al. Bioterrorism-related inhalational anthrax: The first 10 cases reported in the United States. Emerg Infect Dis 2001; 7:933–944.

Arnon SS, Schechter R, Inglesby TV, et al. Botulinum toxin as a biological weapon. JAMA 2001; 285:1059–1070.

Inglesby TV, Dennis DT, Henderson DA, et al. Plague as a biological weapon. JAMA 2000; 283:2281–2290.

CHAPTER FORTY-THREE

Fever in the Hospitalized Patient

Daniel R. Kaul, MD

BACKGROUND

Fever is a common occurrence in the hospitalized patient, and physicians who care for these patients face the challenging task of determining the etiology of fever, the appropriate workup, and the need for empiric antibiotic treatment. This chapter will focus on immunocompetent patients admitted to the hospital with nonfebrile illness who develop fever at least 48 hours after hospitalization; patients admitted with specific infections, the management of hospital-acquired infections, and fever in severely immunosuppressed patients are discussed elsewhere.

ASSESSMENT

Clinical Presentation

Prevalence and Presenting Signs and Symptoms

The threshold for "fever" varies with age. In general, an oral temperature of 38.0° C (100.4°F) is a reasonable and commonly used threshold. Subtract 0.4°C from rectal temperatures and add it to axillary temperatures. While convenient, tympanic membrane thermometers that do not directly contact the tympanic membrane may be unreliable.[1] Elderly and immunosuppressed patients may not be able to mount significant temperature elevations in the face of infectious or inflammatory conditions. In one study, patients admitted with pneumonia were found to have 0.15° C lower temperatures for each decade of age.[2] The absence of fever cannot be used to rule out infection; in a classic study, 15% of elderly bacteremic patients were afebrile.[3] Hypothermia, particularly in the septic patient, has a worse prognosis than clevated temperature.[4]

Depending on the type of hospital unit, hospital-acquired fever occurs in between 17% and 70% of patients, with fever much more common in intensive care unit (ICU) and postoperative patients.[5,6] Risk factors for hospital-acquired fever in the non-ICU setting include procedures such as indwelling urinary or intravascular catheters, congestive heart failure, fecal incontinence, and pressure ulcers.[7-9] In the ICU, higher severity of illness scores is associated with the development of fever.[4,5]

A meticulous review of the patient's hospital course and a careful history and physical examination are essential in evaluating a hospitalized patient with new-onset fever. Historical clues to the origin of fever may include pain in an extremity representing an early soft tissue infection or diarrhea suggesting infection with toxin-producing *Clostridium difficile*. Recent drug intoxication or transient delirium may be clues to an aspiration event. Spiking fever with chills occurring only during dialysis usually indicates an infection of the dialysis catheter. Physical examination should pay particular attention to current and previous intravenous access sites to assess for phlebitis or tunnel infections, rash suggestive of a drug reaction, or abdominal pain indicating pancreatitis. Patients with dementia or neurologic injuries should be carefully examined for evidence of an infected decubitus ulcer. Change in quantity or character of pulmonary secretions in an intubated patient suggests ventilator-associated pneumonia.

In the hospitalized patient, additional laboratory and radiologic information is likely to be available at the time of patient assessment, and this information may be useful in directing further investigations. In a patient started on phenytoin for new-onset seizures, elevated transaminase levels suggest a drug reaction as the cause of fever. Extreme elevations in white blood cell count in a patient with new-onset diarrhea and no known vascular disease likely represents *C. difficile*–associated diarrhea. In an elderly person with known vascular disease, this constellation of findings suggests ischemic colitis. In the setting of hospital-acquired fever, new-onset eosinophilia more often than not represents a drug reaction. An abdominal computed tomography scan done for another indication may reveal air space disease at the lung bases as an early clue to a hospital-acquired pneumonia. Thus, appropriate initial assessment of fever requires a careful review of the patient's hospital course and previous studies, as well as physical examination and history.

Differential Diagnosis

Fever is a nonspecific sign and may result from a great number of causes. It is often assumed that fever is most commonly infectious in origin; but only 50% of hospital-acquired fever in general medicine patients results from infection.[7,8,10] Common infectious and noninfectious causes of fever and associated findings or risk factors are presented in Table 43-1. The most frequent sites of infection include the lung, urinary tract, wounds, and bloodstream. Noninfectious causes of fever need to be given equal attention in the differential diagnosis. Given the fact that hospital patients are regularly started on new medications, the possibility of drug fever must be explored. Rash and eosinophilia are

Table 43-1 Common Causes of Hospital Acquired Fever

Infectious	Risk Factor/Associated Findings
Urinary tract infection	Indwelling urinary catheter
Wound infection	Recent surgery
Bacteremia/fungemia	Central venous access
Clostridium difficile diarrhea	Recent antibiotic use
Meningitis	Recent neurosurgical procedure
Sinusitis	Intubated ICU patient with nasogastric tube
Noninfectious	
Drug fever	Rash, eosinophilia
Postoperative	Duration less than 48 hours after surgery
Pancreatitis	Leukocytosis common.
Ischemic colitis	Patient with vascular disease
Myocardial infarction	Fever of brief duration
Alcohol withdrawal	Often associated with autonomic instability
Trauma	Most common in 48 hrs after event
Hematoma	Recent procedure or trauma
Pulmonary embolism	Immobility
Deep venous thrombosis	Usually low-grade fever
Superficial phlebitis	Intravenous catheter
CNS bleed	Subarachnoid or hemorrhagic CVA
Cervical quadriplegia	Impaired cooling
Malignancy	More common with hematologic malignancy or bulky tumor involving liver
Gout	Acute attack
Flair of rheumatic disease	RA, SLE, etc.
Acute sickle cell disease	Must be evaluated for infection

often associated with drug fever, but fever may be the only manifestation. Drug fever may be severe or mild, and it can be associated with chills and tachycardia. Fever may occur on initiation of the agent or after weeks of therapy. Any medication can cause a fever, but antibiotics and antiseizure medications are the most common culprits in the hospital setting.

Ischemia to any organ or tissue may result in fever-including bowel ischemia, myocardial infarction, pulmonary infarct following pulmonary embolism, or noninfected "dry" gangrene of the extremities. Leukocytosis regularly occurs in these conditions as well. Alcohol withdrawal may cause fevers, and patients with alcohol dependence are commonly admitted to the hospital for other reasons and may not be forthcoming regarding their history. In one study, 21% of patients admitted for alcohol withdrawal developed fever greater than 38° C, on average 2 days but as late as 8 days after admission.[11] Pancreatitis, particularly when necrotizing, may cause high fever and leukocytosis in the absence of infection. Atelectasis is often invoked as a cause of fever, but there is no convincing evidence to support this. Vascular causes of fever include deep venous thrombosis and superficial phlebitis; the latter will be obvious on physical exam. In intubated patients with prolonged ICU stays and nasogastric tubes, sinusitis is often invoked as a cause of fever; CT scanning and aspiration from the sinus are usually required to confirm this diagnosis.[12]

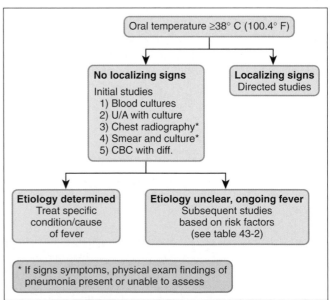

Figure 43-1 • Approach to the diagnosis of hospital-acquired fever.

Diagnosis

Directed Studies

Information obtained from the patient's history, physical examination, and laboratory studies must be integrated in making a decision regarding the need for further evaluation. A reflexive "pan culture" response to fever will result in unnecessary laboratory utilization and antibiotic use for positive cultures that merely reflect normal colonization. A general approach to diagnosis of fever in the hospitalized patient is presented in Figure 43-1. On a general medical ward, in approximately half of instances the cause of fever will be apparent on initial evaluation.[7] In these cases, further directed studies might include blood cultures for a patient with superficial catheter-associated phlebitis to rule out infection, or an abdominal CT in a patient with increasing abdominal pain 10 days after a colectomy. In many of these cases, localizing symptoms will provide a clear guide to appropriate studies.

Diagnosis Unclear—Initial Studies

The selection of diagnostic tests for the febrile patient without an obvious etiology or clear localizing signs or symptoms is challenging. Blood cultures are generally indicated and are mandatory if the patient has a central venous line. Urinalysis and urine cultures are routinely obtained in febrile hospitalized patients, but distinguishing urinary tract infection from colonization is very difficult in this population. The absence of pyuria in an immunocompetent patient by and large excludes infection, regardless of the culture results. Bacterial colonization rates approach 100% in patients with chronic indwelling urinary catheter. Although it is reasonable to obtain urinalysis and culture in patients with enigmatic fever, in the absence of signs or symptoms of cystitis or pyelonephritis, the attribution of fever to urinary tract infection becomes a diagnosis of exclusion. Chest radiography should be obtained in any patient with signs, symptoms, or physical examination findings suggestive of pneumonia, patients at high risk for pneumonia (e.g., quadriplegia), or patients whose clinical situation makes assessment of these findings difficult (e.g., dementia, intubated patients). As colonization of sputum with potential pathogens is very common in the hospital setting, sputum cultures cannot be used to diagnose pneumonia and should be obtained only if the above criteria for obtaining chest radiography are met. A complete blood count with differential should be obtained to assess white blood cell count, left shift, and eosinophil count.

Diagnosis Unclear—Subsequent Studies

If, after initial work up, fever continues and no cause is determined, continued observation and testing are necessary (Table 43-2). Risk factors are provided to help select studies most likely to be productive in an individual patient. Some diagnoses which would normally present no significant diagnostic dilemma may require further studies in particular hospitalized patients. For example, an elderly diabetic patient may have a gangrenous gallbladder and have no right upper quadrant pain. A patient with dementia at baseline may have had a subarachnoid hemorrhage with only subtle physical findings. In such patients, the threshold for obtaining diagnostic tests is lower. Blood cultures need not be repeated daily; they are most likely to be useful in patients at high risk for bacteremia (e.g., central venous access) or fungemia, as the yield for fungus is lower than for most bacteria. Fungal blood cultures are rarely required; their primary utility is in the diagnosis of histoplasmosis or uncommon molds. If the above suggested work up is unrevealing and fever continues, consultation from an infectious disease physician should be obtained if available.

Prognosis

Patients with hospital-acquired fever represent a heterogeneous group, and outcome in these patients largely depends on other factors. Prolonged fever, ischemic cause of fever, and fever in the ICU setting have been associated with increased mortality.[4,5,8] In addition, fever acquired in the hospital has been associated with a prolonged length of stay.[7,9] In cases of enigmatic fever that resolves without a cause being found, further work-up is rarely required.

MANAGEMENT

Treatment

When faced with fever in the hospitalized patient, clinicians must decide whether empiric treatment with antimicrobials is indicated. As only 50% of fever in the hospitalized patient is sec-

Table 43-2 Possible Further Testing for Enigmatic Fever

Test	Conditions	Risk Factors
AST, ALT, bilirubin, alkaline phosphatase	Drug-induced hepatitis or cholecystitis	Number of new medications history of cholelithiasis
Amylase, lipase	Pancreatitis	Trauma, abdominal surgery, ERCP*, medications
Venous Doppler ultrasound	Deep venous thrombosis	Surgery, immobility
Screening sinus CT	Sinusitis	Intubation, prolonged nasogastric tube, ICU setting
Contrast-enhanced abdominal CT	Abdominal abscess, colitis, splenic infarct or hemorrhage, biliary tract or gallbladder disease, lymphoma	Recent abdominal surgery, vascular disease (ischemic colitis), antibiotic use (C. difficile)
Brain CT	Subarachnoid hemorrhage, other CNS bleed, brain abscess	Dementia, trauma, recent neurosurgery, poor dentition
Lumbar puncture	Acute or chronic meningitis	Neurosurgery, CNS shunt

*Endoscopic retrograde cholangiopancreatography.

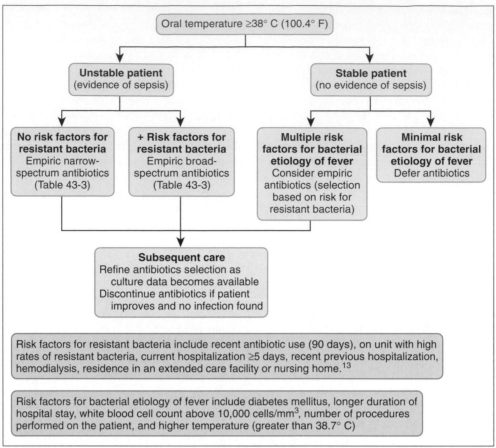

Figure 43-2 • Approach to the management of hospital-acquired fever without etiology after initial evaluation.

ondary to infection,[7,8,10] universal initiation of antibiotic therapy will result in substantial overuse of antibiotics; consequences of antibiotic overuse include increased resistance, antibiotic side effects such as rash and *C. difficile* diarrhea, and added pharmacy costs. On the other hand, in many infections that commonly cause fever such as hospital-acquired pneumonia, delayed initiation of appropriate antibiotic therapy results in worse patient outcomes. Figure 43-2 provides a general guideline to the management of these challenging patients.

In the subset of patients in which the cause of fever is not obvious on initial assessment, two major factors must be considered—the clinical stability of the patient and the probability that the fever is secondary to infection. The medical literature is limited, but in patients on a general medical ward, diabetes mellitus, longer duration of hospital stay, white blood cell count above 10,000 cells/mm^3, number of procedures performed on the patient, and higher temperature (greater than 38.7° C) have been identified as risk factors for bacterial etiology.[7,9] Patients who appear clinically stable and have limited risk factors for bacterial infection can generally be observed without antibiotic treatment while cultures mature. Patients who are clinically unstable (hypotension, tachypnea or tachycardia, mental status changes) or who have multiple risk factors for a bacterial etiology of their fever should generally be started on antibiotic therapy after cultures are obtained. For patients in whom antibiotic therapy is ini-

tiated, it is crucial to follow cultures and adjust or discontinue therapy as further culture and clinical data become available. Febrile patients who improve clinically rarely benefit from prolonged courses of antibiotics in the absence of the diagnosis of a specific infection.

Empiric Antibiotic Selection

For patients with infection from an obvious source, antibiotic selection is discussed elsewhere. Empiric treatment for unstable patients with suspected infections depends on the patient's risk factors for infection with highly resistant bacteria such as methicillin resistant *Staphlococcus aureus* (MRSA) or *Pseudomonas aeruginosa* (Table 43-3). Risk factors include current hospitalization of greater than 5 days, recent additional hospitalization, dialysis, recent antimicrobial therapy (past 3 months), or residence in a chronic care facility. Acquisition of infection in a unit with high rates of resistant bacteria should also be considered a risk factor.[13] For patients without the above risk factors, possible antibiotic choices include ampicillin/sulbactam (1.5–3 g IV every 6 hours), third generation cephalosporins (e.g., ceftriaxone 1 g IV every 24 hours), or a nonpseudomonal carbapenem (e.g., ertapenem 1 g IV every 24 hours). For patients with a significant allergy to beta-lactams, fluoroquinolones (e.g., levaquin 500–750 mg orally or IV every 24 hours) are reasonable alter-

Table 43-3 Empiric Antibiotic Options

Low Risk for Resistant Bacteria	High Risk for Resistant Bacteria
Ampicillin/sulbactam 1.5–3 g IV every 8 hours	Antipseudomonal penicillin e.g., piperacillin/tazobactam 3.375–4 g every 6 hours
Third-generation cephalosporin e.g., ceftriaxone 1 g IV every 24 hours	Third-or Fourth-generation cephalosporin e.g., cefepime or ceftazidime 1 g IV every 8 hours
Nonpseudomonal carbapenem ertapenem 1 g IV every 24 hours	Antipseudomonal carbapenem e.g., meropenem 1 g IV every 8 hours
Fluoroquinolone* e.g., levofloxacin 500–750 mg orally or IV every 24 hours	Fluoroquinolone* e.g., levofloxacin 500–750 mg orally or IV every 24 hours
	if unit or hospital with high MRSA rate add vancomycin 15–20 mg/kg IV every 12 hours

*option for beta-lactam allergic patients

natives. Treatment options for patients at higher risk of infection with resistant bacteria include piperacillin/tazobactam (3.375–4 g IV every 6 hours), cefepime (1 g IV every 8 hours), or ceftazidime (1 g IV every 8 hours). Antipseudomonal carbapenems (e.g., meropenem 1 g IV every 8 hours) should be reserved for situations when there is a high risk or resistance to other broad-spectrum antibiotics (e.g., during an outbreak of *Acinetobacter* infections). If the clinical situation indicates a high risk for MRSA (i.e., unit or hospital with high MRSA rates), addition of vancomycin (15 to 20 mg/kg IV every 12 hours) should be considered.

Considerable controversy surrounds the need for double coverage (usually a fluoroquinolone or aminoglycoside combined with a beta-lactam) for gram negative infections, particularly those involving *Pseudomonas aeruginosa*. Possible advantages of this strategy include synergistic activity, reduction in the development of resistance while on treatment, and broadening the spectrum of empiric antimicrobial coverage. A recent meta-analysis in non-immunocompromised patients showed that combination therapy resulted in increased toxicity without any benefit.[14] If local resistance patterns suggest that probable gram-negative pathogens are covered by a single agent, there is not convincing evidence to suggest an advantage to combination therapy with a fluoroquinolone or aminoglycoside for gram negative pathogens. If "double coverage" is initiated, one drug can likely be withdrawn after the responsible pathogen is identified and sensitivities are performed.

PREVENTION

Measures can be taken to reduce the incidence of nosocomial infection. Central venous catheters and indwelling urinary catheters should be not be used for convenience but only when a medical indication exists, and should be removed as soon as they are no longer required. Attention should be paid to infection control policies such as hand washing as well as widely available guidelines to reduce the risk of hospital-acquired pneumonia.[15]

Key Points

- Hospital-acquired fever is a common occurrence, and is often of noninfectious etiology.

- Drugs, ischemia to any tissue, alcohol withdrawal, pancreatitis, deep venous thrombosis, and superficial phlebitis are common noninfectious causes of fever.

- Hospital-acquired fever is often mistakenly attributed to urinary tract infection. In the absence of signs or symptoms of cystitis or pyelonephritis, urinary tract infection is a diagnosis of exclusion in the hospitalized patient.

- Empiric antibiotics may be deferred in stable patients with minimal risk factors for infectious etiology of fever.

- Selection of empiric antibiotics depends on an individual patient's risk factors for acquiring an infection with a resistant organism.

SUGGESTED READING

Bota DP, Ferreira FL, Melot C, et al. Body temperature alterations in the critically ill. Inten Care Med 2004; 30:811–816.

Circiumaru B, Baldock G, Cohen J. A prospective study of fever in the intensive care unit. Inten Care Med 1999; 25:668–673.

Arbo M, Fine MJ, Hanusa BH, et al. Fever of nosocomial origin: etiology, risk factors, and outcomes. Am J Med 1992; 95(5):505–512.

Trivalle C, Chassagne P, Bouaniche M, et al. Nosocomial febrile illness in the elderly: frequency, causes, and risk factors. Arch Intern Med 1998; 158(14):1560–1565.

Niederman, MS, Craven, DE (co-Chairs ATS and IDSA Official Statement). Guidelines for the management of adults with hospital-acquired, ventilator associated, and healthcare associated pneumonia. Am J Resp Crit Care Med 2005; 171:388–416.

Mical P, Benuri-Silbiger I, Soares-Weiser K, et al. Beta lactam monotherapy versus beta-lactam-aminoglycoside combination therapy for sepsis in immunocompetent patients: systematic review and meta-analysis of randomised trials. BMJ 2004; 328:668–682.

Section Five

Pulmonary

44 Chronic Obstructive Pulmonary Disease
Daniel D. Dressler, Alpesh N. Amin, Gerald Staton

45 Asthma
Michael P. Lukela, William F. Bria II

46 Pleural Disease: Pleural Effusion and Pneumothorax
Irene Krokos, Steven E. Gay

47 Interstitial Lung Disease
W. Bradley Fields, Kevin R. Flaherty

48 Pulmonary Hypertension
Jordan Messler, Allan Ramirez

CHAPTER FORTY-FOUR

Chronic Obstructive Pulmonary Disease

Daniel D. Dressler, MD, MSc, Alpesh N. Amin, MD, MBA, and Gerald Staton, MD

BACKGROUND

Chronic obstructive pulmonary disease (COPD) is characterized by airflow limitation that is not fully reversible. The airflow limitation is usually progressive and associated with an abnormal inflammatory response of the lungs to noxious particles or gases.[1] Chronic bronchitis and emphysema are underlying phenotypic features of COPD. Chronic bronchitis is defined clinically as cough and sputum production occurring for 3 months during 2 consecutive years.[2] Emphysema is characterized pathologically as destruction of alveoli, resulting in irreversible enlargement of the airways and loss of elastic recoil.[2] These phenotypic manifestations may be difficult to differentiate, as their symptoms often coexist, and many patients have both manifestations. An exacerbation of COPD is an event characterized by a change in the patient's baseline dyspnea, cough, and/or sputum beyond day-to-day variability necessitating a change in management.

Hospitalists frequently manage patients with COPD exacerbation or with chronic persistent COPD who present to the hospital for other reasons. This chapter outlines the clinical presentation, diagnosis, prognosis, and management of COPD in the hospital setting, with recommendations for effective transition to the outpatient setting.

ASSESSMENT

Clinical Presentation

Prevalence

According to the Third National Health and Nutrition Examination Survey (NHANES III), approximately 24 million adults in the United States have COPD.[3] This prevalence, however, is likely an underestimate, as early disease is often asymptomatic and unrecognized. Importantly, 70% of patients with COPD are <65 years old, therefore significantly affecting the workforce.[3] In the year 2000, COPD was responsible for an estimated 1.5 million emergency room visits and 726,000 hospitalizations.[3]

Pathogenesis

Inhalation of noxious stimuli, such as cigarette smoke, by patients with COPD activates inflammatory cells (e.g., macrophages, neutrophils, and T-lymphocytes), causing them to release cytokines and other mediators.[4,5] Airflow limitation results primarily from the slowly progressive structural changes that occur in the small airways and parenchyma.[6,7] Alterations characteristic of COPD include mucous gland hypertrophy, narrowing and fibrosis of the airways, destruction of the parenchyma, and changes in blood vessels (Fig. 44-1).[8–11] These pathologic features manifest as mucus hypersecretion, airflow limitation, hyperinflation, and abnormalities in gas exchange.[12]

Risk Factors

The most important risk factor for COPD is tobacco smoking (including cigarettes, pipes, and cigars), which accounts for 90% of cases.[1] COPD mortality is associated with total pack years, age at which the patient started smoking, and current smoking status. Other documented causes of COPD include secondhand smoke exposure, environmental and industrial pollutants, and chemicals.[1]

Less than 1% of COPD patients have α_1-antitrypsin deficiency, a known genetic defect that increases the risk of a progressive form of COPD. α_1-Antitrypsin deficiency should be considered in Caucasians with emphysema who have little tobacco exposure and COPD prior to age 50.[6,9]

Presenting Signs and Symptoms

COPD should be suspected in patients with symptoms of cough, sputum production, wheezing, or dyspnea on mild physical exertion (out of proportion to that expected for their age), and a history of exposure to risk factors.[13] Dyspnea is the most common presenting symptom and contributes substantially to disability associated with COPD.[1] Weight loss and anorexia are commonly associated with severe disease. Patients presenting with exacerbations of COPD may have features of increased dyspnea or cough with increased sputum production or change in sputum color. Other features may include wheezing, diminished air movement, other constitutional symptoms, or altered mentation.

Differential Diagnosis

COPD is sometimes misdiagnosed as asthma, particularly in women.[14] Although they have similar symptoms such as coughing and wheezing, COPD and asthma are distinct conditions with

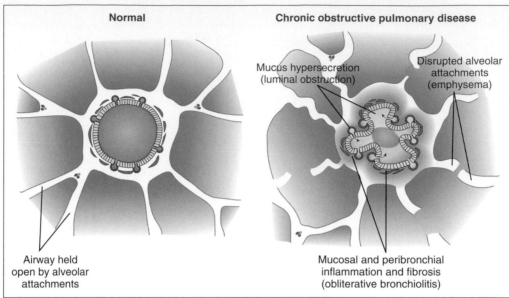

Figure 44-1 • In COPD, airflow limitation is due to a variable mixture of loss of alveolar attachments, obstruction of the airway due to inflammation, airway-wall fibrosis, and airway smooth muscle destruction, as well as luminal obstruction with mucus. Reprinted from: Barnes PJU. Chronic obstructive pulmonary disease. N Engl J Med 2000; 343:269–280.

Table 44-1 Differentiating COPD from Asthma

Feature	COPD	Asthma
Age of onset	Onset in older individuals	Onset at any age; younger individuals usually affected
Smoking	Significant history (20 daily/20 years)	Usually insignificant
Symptom presentation	Slowly progressive or chronic symptoms; dyspnea occurs during exercise	Exacerbations and remissions; symptoms occur at night or early in the morning; allergy, rhinitis, and/or eczema also present
Reversibility	Partial reversibility of symptoms	Airflow limitation largely reversible
Family history	Uncommon	Common
Inflammatory cells	Pulmonary alveolar macrophages, polymorphonuclear leukocytes, lymphocytes	Eosinophils, lymphocytes, mast cells

From: Global Initiative for Chronic Obstructive Lung Disease. Global Strategy for the Diagnosis, Management, and Prevention of Chronic Obstructive Pulmonary Disease. Updated 2005. Available at: http://www.goldcopd.com (accessed December 28, 2005); *and* Briggs DD. Chronic obstructive pulmonary disease overview: prevalence, pathogenesis, and treatment. J Manag Care Pharm 2004; 10:S3–S10.

differences in the underlying inflammatory process, natural history, and presentation (Table 44-1). However, uncontrolled asthma can eventually result in irreversible airway limitation, making it difficult to distinguish between patients with partially irreversible airflow due to asthma and patients with COPD who have partially reversible airflow obstruction with airway hyperreactivity.[6]

Other common conditions that may mimic or precipitate COPD exacerbations include pulmonary embolism, pneumonia, or congestive heart failure. Environmental irritants—such as smoke, smog, or occupational exposures—as well as viral or bacterial precipitants of tracheobronchitis may lead to COPD exacerbation. The most common bacterial precipitants include *Haemophilus influenzae*, Streptococcus pneumoniae, and Moraxella *catarrhalis*. A sizable minority (<10%) of bacteria-related COPD exacerbations are caused by atypical bacteria (*Mycoplasma* or *Chlamydia*). Patients with frequent hospitalizations may be at risk for *Pseudomonas aeruginosa* or other gram-negative enteric pathogens.

Diagnosis

Diagnosis of COPD is often made based on a history of progressive symptoms and a confirmatory spirometric test. Additionally, spirometry provides a measure of disease severity. Spirometry is not indicated in the evaluation of exacerbations of COPD unless the diagnosis of COPD is in question.

Spirometry measures the volume of air forcibly exhaled from the point of maximal inhalation (forced vital capacity [FVC]) and the volume of air exhaled during the first second of this maneuver (forced expiratory volume in 1 second [FEV_1]). A COPD diagnosis is made in the presence of a post-bronchodilator FEV_1 < 80% of the predicted value in combination with an FEV_1/FVC < 70%.[1,13]

FEV$_1$ is commonly used as a measure of disease severity. However, FEV$_1$ correlates poorly with the degree of dyspnea, inadequately reflects the rate of decline in patient health, and is less accurate than degree of dyspnea and health status scores in predicting risk of death.[13] In addition, FEV$_1$ does not adequately capture the systemic manifestations of COPD. Therefore, FEV$_1$ is no longer the only parameter used to assess disease severity. The GOLD guidelines pair FEV$_1$ with symptoms to classify disease severity from Stage 0 ("At Risk") to Stage IV ("Very Severe COPD") (Table 44-2).[1]

Exacerbations of COPD are diagnosed by history and examination findings consistent with increase in the patient's chronic symptoms of COPD. Specifically, patients may have an increase in wheezing, cough, sputum production, and shortness of breath, sometimes associated with constitutional symptoms.

Preferred Studies

Recommended diagnostic evaluation for patients admitted to the hospital for COPD exacerbation includes arterial blood gas, basic chemistry profile, complete blood count, and electrocardio-

gram, as abnormalities that may include hypoxia, hypercarbia, acidemia, electrolyte alterations, polycythemia, right heart strain, and multifocal atrial tachycardia may be detected. Of note, B-type natriuretic peptide (BNP) testing is effective at distinguishing an exacerbation due to heart failure from that caused by pulmonary disease.

Prognosis

During Hospitalization

COPD is a major cause of morbidity and mortality. Inpatient mortality ranges from 11–24% for intensive care unit (ICU) patients and 3–4% for non-ICU patients.

Postdischarge

In 2000, COPD was responsible for more than 120,000 deaths, making it the fourth leading cause of death in the United State.[3,15,16] COPD is also associated with an increasing mortality rate over the past 40 years.[10] In addition, COPD limits daily life activities, affects the patient's ability to work, and increases health care utilization.[16] The 1-year readmission rate for COPD patients is as high as 59%, and the 1-year postdischarge mortality rate is as high as 22%.[17-20]

MANAGEMENT

Criteria for Hospitalization

The GOLD and the American Thoracic Society/European Respiratory Society (ATS/ERS) guidelines provide criteria for hospitalization for treatment of acute exacerbation of COPD (Table 44-3).[1,6,13] Both the GOLD and ATS/ERS guidelines recommend hospital evaluation or admission for patients presenting with substantially increased dyspnea. Recognizing and treating significant comorbidities and determining need for ventilatory support for significant hypoxemia or respiratory acidosis are necessary in initial management.[1,22] Admission to the hospital should be based on the patient's current status, response to initial therapy, and

---

Table 44-2 Spirometric Classification of COPD Severity Based on Post-Bronchodilator FEV$_1$

Stage I: Mild	FEV$_1$/FVC < 0.70 FEV$_1$ ≥ 80% predicted
Stage II: Moderate	FEV$_1$/FVC < 0.70 50% ≤ FEV$_1$ < 80% predicted
Stage III: Severe	FEV$_1$/FVC < 0.70 30% ≤ FEV$_1$ < 50% predicted
Stage IV: Very Severe	FEV$_1$/FVC < 0.70 FEV$_1$ < 30% predicted or FEV$_1$ < 50% predicted plus chronic respiratory failure

COPD Diagnosis and Classification of Severity Reprinted from Global Initiative for Chronic Obstructive Lung Disease. Global Strategy for the Diagnosis, Management, and Prevention of Chronic Obstructive Palmonary Disease. Updated 2006. Available at: http://www.goldcopd.org. (Accessed March 5, 2007)

Table 44-3 Indications for Hospital Assessment or Admission for Exacerbations of COPD

GOLD Guidelines	ATS/ERS Guidelines
Marked increase in intensity of symptoms, such as sudden development of resting dyspnea	Presence of high-risk comorbid conditions, including pneumonia, cardiac arrhythmia, congestive heart failure,
Severe background COPD	diabetes mellitus, renal or liver failure
Onset of new physical signs (e.g., cyanosis, peripheral edema)	Inadequate response of symptoms to outpatient management
Failure of exacerbation to respond to initial medical management	Marked increase in dyspnea
Significant comorbidities	Inability to eat or sleep due to symptoms
Newly occurring arrhythmias	Worsening hypoxemia
Diagnostic uncertainty	Worsening hypercapnia
Older age	Change in mental status
Insufficient home support	Inability of the patient to care for herself or himself Uncertain diagnosis Inadequate home care

From: American Thoracic Society/European Respiratory Society Task Force. Standards for the Diagnosis and Management of Patients with COPD (Internet). Version 1.2. New York: American Thoracic Society; 2004 (updated 2005 September 8). Available from: http://www-test.thoracic.org/copd/; and Celli BR, MacNee W, and committee members. Standards for the diagnosis and treatment of patients with COPD: a summary of the ATS/ERS position paper. Eur Respir J 2004; 23:932–946; and Global Initiative for Chronic Obstructive Lung Disease. Global Strategy for the Diagnosis, Management, and Prevention of Chronic Obstructive Pulmonary Disease. Updated 2005. Available at: http://www.goldcopd.com (accessed December 28, 2005).

Table 44-4 Indications for ICU Admission of Patients with Exacerbations of COPD

GOLD Guidelines	ATS/ERS Guidelines
Severe dyspnea that responds inadequately to initial emergency therapy	Impending or actual respiratory failure
Confusion, lethargy, coma	Presence of other end-organ dysfunction, e.g.,
Persistent or worsening hypoxemia (PaO$_2$ <5.3 kPa, 40 mm Hg) and/or severe/worsening hypercapnia (PaCO$_2$ >8.0 kPa, 60 mm Hg) and/or severe/worsening respiratory acidosis (pH <7.25) despite supplemental oxygen and NIPPV	shock, renal, liver or neurological disturbance Hemodynamic instability

From: American Thoracic Society/European Respiratory Society Task Force. Standards for the Diagnosis and Management of Patients with COPD (Internet). Version 1.2. New York: American Thoracic Society; 2004 (updated 2005 September 8). Available from: http://www-test.thoracic.org/copd/; Celli BR, MacNee W, and committee members. Standards for the diagnosis and treatment of patients with COPD: a summary of the ATS/ERS position paper. *Eur Respir J.* 2004;23:932–946; Global Initiative for Chronic Obstructive Lung Disease. Global Strategy for the Diagnosis, Management, and Prevention of Chronic Obstructive Pulmonary Disease. Updated 2005. Available at: http://www.goldcopd.com (accessed December 28, 2005).
NIPPV—non-invasive positive pressure ventilation

the presence of comorbid conditions.[23] The GOLD and ATS/ERS guidelines suggest that patients who fail to respond to initial emergency therapy may require treatment in the ICU (Table 44-4). Other criteria for ICU admission include confusion; lethargy or coma; and worsening hypoxemia, hypercapnia, or respiratory acidosis.[1]

To determine the severity of an acute exacerbation, the clinician should consider the patient's past medical history, current symptoms, physical examination, prior lung function tests, current and prior arterial blood gas measurements, and other laboratory findings. Questions about past medical history and current symptoms should attempt to determine duration and severity of symptoms, frequency and severity of breathlessness and coughing episodes, sputum color and volume, effect on activities of daily living, previous exacerbations and hospitalizations for exacerbations, and episodes requiring ventilatory support.[1] Precipitating events include medication nonadherence, environmental exposures (e.g., pollutants, tobacco smoke), viral and bacterial infection of the tracheobronchial tree, fluid overload, thromboembolism, cardiac ischemia, aspiration, excessive sedation from medications, and bronchospasm.[24] However, the cause of approximately one third of severe exacerbations cannot be determined.[1]

Treatment

Although early diagnosis and proper management of COPD and its exacerbations may halt or even reverse symptoms, currently available medications do not modify the decline in lung function associated with the disease.

Preferred Initial Treatment

In the hospital setting, evidence-based pharmacologic management of acute exacerbations of COPD, supported by well-designed randomized controlled study evidence, includes the use of bronchodilators, antibiotics for patients with suspected bacterial infection, and corticosteroids. Additionally, oxygen therapy is used to relieve hypoxemia, and ventilatory support may be utilized in patients with evidence of respiratory failure. Typically, initial evaluation and treatment of acute exacerbation of COPD occur concomitantly. Figure 44-2 provides an assessment and treatment algorithm for patents admitted to the hospital for an acute exacerbation of COPD.

Bronchodilators

Inhaled bronchodilators are the cornerstone of therapy for acute exacerbations of COPD. β$_2$ agonists act by stimulating β$_2$ receptors on airway smooth muscle, increasing cyclic adenosine monophosphate, and thereby relaxing airway smooth muscle. Anticholinergic drugs bind to muscarinic receptors in human airways, blocking the effects of acetylcholine, producing preferential dilatation of the larger central airways, different from β$_2$ agonists, which tend to affect the peripheral airways.

Only short-acting bronchodilators are appropriate for treatment of acute exacerbations of COPD. Long-acting bronchodilators are used in outpatient management of patients with COPD.[4] In general, the onset of action of short-acting agents is approximately 10 minutes. Examples of short-acting β$_2$ agonists include albuterol and terbutaline. Importantly, the half-life of β$_2$ agonists can be shortened during acute exacerbations; thus, doses must be increased to three to four puffs per administration and as frequently as once every hour as necessary. Clinicians should be vigilant about detecting adverse sympathomimetic effects, such as tachycardia, arrhythmia, or hypokalemia.[24] Levalbuterol is a newer short-acting β$_2$ agonist that targets airway smooth muscle receptors (rather than cardiac muscle) more selectively than albuterol and may reduce the risk of tachycardia.[25] However, no treatment benefit has been demonstrated. The most commonly used short-acting anticholinergic is ipratropium, a nonselective muscarinic antagonist.

Recent meta-analyses found that inhaled β$_2$ agonists and anticholinergics are equally effective in patients with an acute exacerbation of COPD.[26,27] Both classes of agents have been shown to improve airflow during an acute exacerbation, providing a 15–29% increase in FEV$_1$ and FVC over 60–120 minutes.[28-31] Combination therapy with an anticholinergic and β$_2$ agonist can be used; however, the combination has not been judged in the guidelines to have clear superiority to maximal doses of either agent alone.[1,6] However, evidence suggests that the agents may act synergistically, and the use of combination therapy may be appropriate for an acute exacerbation of COPD.[1,6] In a meta-analysis, patients who received both a short-acting β$_2$ agonist and anticholinergic agent experienced shorter lengths of stay and larger increases in FEV$_1$ compared with patients receiving only one bronchodilator; however, there were no differences between groups in hospital admission rates.[27]

All inhaled bronchodilators can be administered via metered-dose inhalers (MDIs), and some (e.g., ipratropium, albuterol,

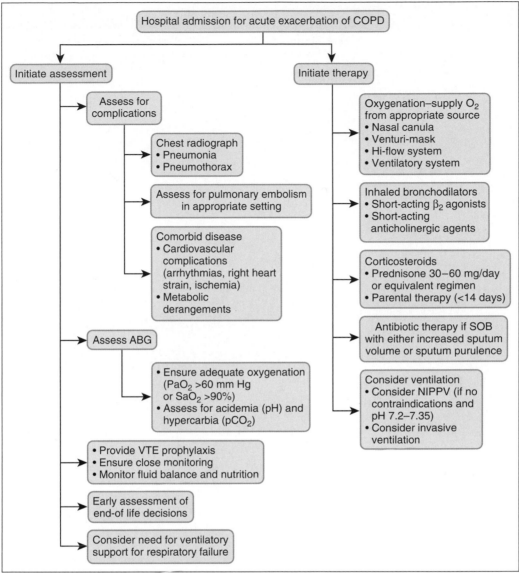

Figure 44-2 • Treatment algorithm for hospitalized patient with acute exacerbation of COPD.

COPD—chronic obstructive pulmonary disease; ABG—arterial blood gases; VTE—venous thromboembolism (deep vein thrombosis or pulmonary embolism); SOB—shortness of breath; NIPPV—non-invasive positive pressure ventilatioin

metaproterenol) are available by nebulization, which is useful for patients whose dyspnea or distress interferes with MDI administration. All patients receiving medication by MDI should use a spacer device and receive training in MDI use. There are no data to suggest that nebulization is superior to metered dose inhaler with spacer in cooperative patients.

Corticosteroids

Oral and intravenous corticosteroids should be used in addition to bronchodilator therapy for an acute exacerbation of COPD.[1,32] Data from randomized, controlled clinical trials suggest that improvements in airflow, gas exchange, and symptoms occur more quickly and treatment failure is decreased with systemic corticosteroids.[33–36] Although there are no clear recommendations on the duration of corticosteroid therapy, randomized control trial data suggest that a short course of treatment (e.g., 30–40 mg of prednisolone or prednisone for 10–14 days) is reasonable, especially considering that long-term therapy does not enhance efficacy and does increase adverse effects.[1] Additional

data suggest that a shorter course (i.e., 5–10 days) may be appropriate.[31,37] There is limited or no role for the use of inhaled glucocorticoids in the setting of acute exacerbations of COPD.

Oxygen

Oxygen is used in the management of COPD exacerbations to relieve hypoxemia (to achieve PaO_2 >8.0 kPa, 60 mm Hg or SaO_2 >90%) without causing respiratory suppression and associated CO_2 retention or acidosis.[23,1] Nasal prongs or Venturi masks can be used for oxygen delivery, with the latter allowing better control of the inspiratory fraction of oxygen (FiO_2).[23,1] Arterial blood gases should be monitored 30–60 minutes after initiation of oxygen therapy.[1]

Antibiotics

Studies report that bacterial infection plays a significant role in the etiology of acute exacerbations in about half of cases. Summary meta-analysis data confirm a significant symptom reduction when antimicrobials are prescribed empirically for

Table 44-5 Common Pathogens Associated with Acute Exacerbations of Chronic Bronchitis (AECB)

Category	Likely Pathogens	Antimicrobial Therapy
Uncomplicated AECB Age <65 years FEV$_1$ >50% predicted <4 Exacerbations/year No comorbid conditions	*Haemophilus influenzae* *Streptococcus pneumoniae* *Moraxella catarrhalis* *Haemophilus parainfluenzae* Virus *M. pneumoniae* *C. pneumoniae*	Macrolide* Ketolides[†] Doxycycline 2nd- or 3rd-generation cephalosporin Trimethoprim/sulfamethoxazole Respiratory quinolone[†]
Complicated AECB Age >65 years FEV$_1$ <50% predicted ≥4 Exacerbations/year Comorbid conditions	*H. influenzae* *S. pneumoniae* *M. catarrhalis* *H. parainfluenzae* virus *M. pneumoniae* *C. pneumoniae* Gram-negative enteric bacilli	Respiratory quinolone[†] 2nd-generation penicillin with beta-lactamase inhibitor (e.g., amoxicillin/clavulanate) 3rd-generation cephalosporin + macrolide or doxycycline
Complicated AECB at risk for *Pseudomonas aeruginosa* **infection** FEV$_1$ <35% predicted Recurrent courses of antibiotics or corticosteroids Bronchiectasis	*H. influenzae* *S. pneumoniae* *M. catarrhalis* *H. parainfluenzae* Viral *M. pneumoniae* *C. pneumoniae* Gram-negative enteric bacilli *P. aeruginosa*	Fluoroquinolone with anti-pseudomonal activity Anti-pseudomonal penicillin (e.g., piperacillin or ticarcillin) + macrolide

*In active smokers, *H. influenzae* infection is more prevalent, and azithromycin and clarithromycin demonstrate improved *in vitro* activity.

[†]Levofloxacin, moxifloxacin, gatifloxacin, gemifloxacin, and telithromycin have activity against penicillin-resistant *S. pneumoniae*.

Adapted from: Martinez FJ. Acute exacerbations of chronic bronchitis: therapeutic challenges and the disease free interval. Infect Med 2005; 22:217–228.

acute exacerbations of COPD.[38] Hospitalized patients appeared to benefit more than outpatients. Empiric antimicrobial therapy is recommended for all patients with suspected bacterial infection, with therapy targeted at the most common causal pathogens (i.e., *H. influenzae*, *S. pneumoniae*, and *M. catarrhalis*).[1] Criteria for the use of antimicrobial therapy in managing acute exacerbations include at least two of the following symptoms: increased dyspnea, increased sputum volume, and sputum purulence. In addition, the presence of sputum purulence alone and need for management in the ICU are reasonable indications for antibiotics.[39] Recommendations regarding antimicrobial selection are generally stratified on the basis of host factors or likely bacterial pathogens (Table 44-5).[1,39]

Ventilation

Mechanical ventilation includes invasive and noninvasive ventilation, and is used to support ventilation and/or oxygenation until the underlying cause of acute respiratory failure is treated and reversed.[13] In COPD, mechanical ventilation should be considered for patients with worsening or moderate to severe dyspnea with the use of accessory muscles and paradoxical abdominal motion, acute respiratory acidosis (pH <7.35), hypercapnia (PaCO$_2$ >7.0 kPa, 50 mm Hg), and respiratory frequency >30 breaths per minute.[1,13,31] Noninvasive ventilation is preferred over invasive ventilation whenever possible, as intubation is generally associated with higher morbidity, resulting from complications, and it may be more difficult to wean these patients from ventilation.[40,41]

Noninvasive positive-pressure ventilation (NIPPV) delivers air or a mixture of air and oxygen from a flow generator through a full facial or nasal mask. The goal of NIPPV is to reduce CO_2 by

unloading fatigued respiratory muscles and augmenting alveolar ventilation, stabilizing arterial pH. Patients undergoing NIPPV should be closely monitored for comfort and use of accessory muscles as well as signs of cyanosis, tachycardia, and tachypnea.[42] Arterial blood gas measurements are essential for assessment and should be obtained 30–60 minutes following initiation of NIPPV in order to monitor pH, PaCO$_2$, and PaO$_2$ response to intervention. Contraindications to the use of NIPPV are shown in Box 44-1. Patients requiring NIPPV should almost always be monitored initially in an ICU setting.

NIPPV has been shown to increase pH, reduce PaCO$_2$, and decrease the severity of breathlessness in the first 4 hours of treatment in patients with acute respiratory failure.[1] A meta-analysis of seven randomized, controlled clinical trials found that NIPPV with usual medical care significantly reduces mortality, endotracheal intubation, treatment failure, complications, and length of hospital stay in patients with respiratory failure resulting from an acute exacerbation of COPD.[43] It is recommended that NIPPV be considered early in the course of COPD exacerbations that require hospital admission and before severe acidosis ensues, to avoid the need for endotracheal intubation and to reduce mortality in patients with COPD.[43] Invasive ventilation should be considered in patients who fail NIPPV or patients with severe acidosis and hypercapnia or life-threatening hypoxemia.[13]

Alternative Treatment Options

While mucolytic, expectorant, and mucokinetic agents have been shown in some well-designed studies to improve symptom scores, other high-quality studies do not confirm such benefit, and these agents do not alter or shorten the course of exacerbation. Similarly, chest physiotherapy has not been shown to improve any clinical endpoints or FEV$_1$. Although some data suggest that methylxanthines, such as theophylline and aminophylline, improve diaphragmatic strength and fatiguability,[24,44] results from three randomized, controlled clinical trials showed that intravenous aminophylline in addition to an inhaled bronchodilator did not improve pulmonary function, provide clinical benefit, or decrease the risk of returning to the emergency room.[30,31,34,45] Guidelines indicate that theophylline may be considered in patients with severe exacerbations who are unrespon-

sive to other therapies.[1] However, if considering these agents, it is important to properly dose, and clinicians must monitor serum levels and signs of toxicity (e.g., nausea, arrhythmias, seizures).[24]

PREVENTION

Nonpharmacologic and pharmacologic interventions can help reduce the incidence of COPD exacerbations and hospitalizations (Fig. 44-3). Smoking cessation is the single most effective intervention to reduce the risk of developing COPD and halt its progression. Smoking cessation counseling should be provided prior to hospital discharge to all patients who smoke. Pharmacotherapies (e.g., nicotine patch, buprorion) for tobacco dependence may be offered to patients who desire such assistance with cessation and do not have contraindications to such therapy. Counseling regarding reduction of second-hand smoke, environmental pollutants, and occupational exposures may be beneficial as well.

Appropriate immunizations, including one-time pneumococcal vaccine (if not up to date) and annual influenza vaccine to reduce incidence or severity of respiratory illnesses should be offered during hospital stay of COPD patients. Influenza vaccination has been shown to reduce hospitalizations for pneumonia and exacerbations as well as mortality.

Other outpatient treatments for chronic COPD that help reduce exacerbations include the recommended step-wise approach to management of stable COPD based on clinical stage and chronic symptomatology (Fig. 44-3). Although currently available medications do not prevent the long-term decline in lung function in COPD, they reduce symptoms and complications.

Pulmonary rehabilitation utilizes a number of therapeutic modalities with the goal of improving quality of life and health status. A systematic review of six trials demonstrated a decreased

Box 44-1 Contraindications to NIPPV

- Cardiac or respiratory arrest
- Nonrespiratory organ failure
  - Severe encephalopathy (Glasgow score <10)
  - Severe upper gastrointestinal bleeding
  - Hemodynamic instability or unstable cardiac arrhythmia
- Facial surgery, trauma, or deformity
- Upper airway obstruction
- Inability to cooperate/protect the airway
- Inability to clear respiratory secretions
- High risk for aspiration
- Extreme obesity

Adapted from: Carrera M, Sala E, Cosio BG, et al. Hospital treatment of chronic obstructive pulmonary disease exacerbations: an evidence-based review. Arch Bronconeumol 2005; 41: 220–229; and International Consensus Conferences in Intensive Care Medicine: non-invasive positive pressure ventilation in acute respiratory failure. Am J Respir Crit Care Med 2001; 163: 283–291.

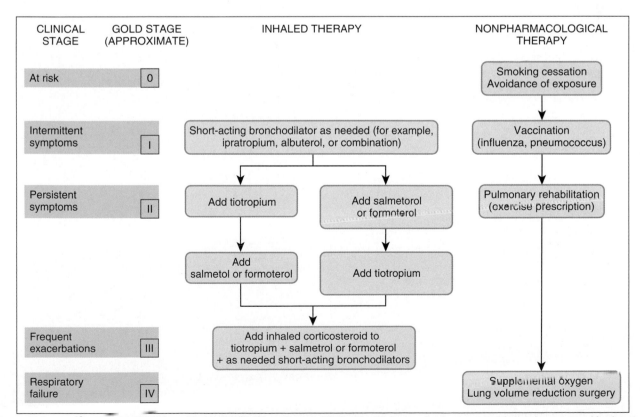

Figure 44-3 • Management Algorithm of Stable COPD. From: Cooper CB, Tashkin DP. Recent developments in inhaled therapy in stable chronic obstructive pulmonary disease. BMJ 2005; 330:640–644.

risk of subsequent hospital admissions and mortality.[46] Objective outcomes include decrease in respiratory symptoms, increase in exercise tolerance and functional activities, and reduction in anxiety and depression.[6]

Adequate prophylaxis against venous thromboembolism should be provided for most patients during hospitalization with COPD exacerbation, as mobility is frequently limited in this patient population.

DISCHARGE/FOLLOW-UP PLANS

Although the optimal length of hospital stay following an acute exacerbation of COPD has not been established, several discharge criteria have been developed to aid in the discharge decision-making process (Box 44-2). Importantly, patients should be clinically stable for at least a 12- to 24-hour period prior to discharge. Plans for follow-up, which should occur within 4–6 weeks after discharge or sooner if clinically warranted, must be established.[1] Simple postdischarge interventions, such as ensuring timely follow-up, decrease readmissions.[47]

The hospitalist's role in patient and family communication as well as outpatient physician communication to ensure optimal inpatient care and care transition includes all of the following:[48]

- Educate the patient and family about the natural history and prognosis of COPD.
- Communicate the importance of prevention measures such as smoking cessation and required follow-up care.
- Communicate with the patient and family regarding discharge medications, side effects, duration of therapy, dosing, and taper schedule.
- Ensure that patients receive training on proper inhaler techniques and use.

- Establish and maintain an open dialogue with the patient and/or family regarding care goals and limitations, including palliative care and end-of-life wishes.
- Address resuscitation status early during hospital stay.
- Collaborate with primary care physicians and emergency room physicians in admission decisions.
- Document treatment plan and discharge instructions, and communicate with outpatient clinician responsible for follow-up.
- Provide and coordinate resources for patients to ensure the safe transition from the hospital to arranged follow-up care.
- Develop educational modules, order sets, and/or pathways that facilitate use of evidence-based strategies for COPD management to improve outcomes.
- Lead efforts to educate staff on the importance of smoking cessation and other prevention measures so that they can help educate patients.

Box 44-2 Criteria for Hospital Discharge Following Acute Exacerbation of COPD

- Inhaled β_2 agonist therapy is required no more frequently than every 4 hours
- Patient, if previously ambulatory, is able to walk across room
- Patient is able to eat and sleep without frequent awakening by dyspnea
- Patient has been clinically stable for 12–24 hours
- Arterial blood gases have been stable for 12–24 hours
- Patient (or home caregiver) fully understands correct use of medication
- Follow-up and home care arrangements have been completed (e.g., visiting nurse, oxysen delivery, meal preparation)
- Patient, family, and physician are confident patient can manage successfully

From: Global Initiative for Chronic Obstructive Lung Disease. Global Strategy for the Diagnosis, Management, and Prevention of Chronic Obstructive Pulmonary Disease. Updated 2005. Available at: http://www.goldcopd.com (accessed March 5, 2007).

Key Points

- Less than 1% of COPD patients have α_1-antitrypsin deficiency, but it should be considered in Caucasians with emphysema who have little tobacco exposure and COPD prior to age 50.

- Spirometry is not indicated in the evaluation of exacerbations of COPD unless the diagnosis is of COPD is in question.

- Inpatient mortality ranges from 11–24% for intensive care unit (ICU) patients and 3–4% for non-ICU patients, and the 1-year post-discharge mortality rate is as high as 22%.

- The GOLD and ATS/ERS guidelines suggest that patients who fail to respond to initial emergency therapy may require treatment in the ICU.

- Inhaled short-acting bronchodilators are the cornerstone of therapy for acute exacerbations of COPD.

- Inhaled β_2 agonists and anticholinergics are equally effective, but patients who receive both a short-acting β_2 agonist and anticholinergic agent experience shorter lengths of stay and larger increases in FEV_1, compared with patients receiving only one bronchodilator.

- There are no data to suggest that nebulization is superior to metered dose inhaler with spacer in cooperative patients.

- Bacterial infection plays a significant role in the etiology of acute exacerbations in about half of cases, and significant symptom reduction results when antimicrobials are prescribed empirically for acute exacerbations of COPD.

- Noninvasive ventilation is preferred over invasive ventilation whenever possible, as intubation is generally associated with higher morbidity, resulting from complications.

- Smoking cessations is the single most effective intervention to reduce the risk of developing COPD and halt its progression, and cessation education should be provided prior to hospital discharge to all patients who smoke.

SUGGESTED READING

Almagro P, Calbo E, Ochoa de Echaguen A, et al. Mortality after hospitalization for COPD. Chest 2002; 121:1441–1448.

American Thoracic Society/European Respiratory Society Task Force. Standards for the Diagnosis and Management of Patients with COPD [Internet]. Version 1.2. New York: American Thoracic Society; 2004 [updated 2005 September 8]. Available from: http://www-test.thoracic.org/copd/.

Bach PB, Brown C, Gelfand SE, et al. Management of exacerbations of chronic obstructive pulmonary disease: a summary and appraisal of published evidence. Ann Intern Med 2001; 134:600–620.

Celli BR, MacNee W, and committee members. Standards for the diagnosis and treatment of patients with COPD: a summary of the ATS/ERS position paper. Eur Respir J 2004; 23:932–946.

Global Initiative for Chornic Obstructive Lung Disease. Global Strategy for the Diagnosis, Management, and Prevention of Chronic Obstructive Pulmonary Disease. Updated 2005. Available at: http://www.goldcopd.com (accessed December 28, 2005).

McCrory DC, Brown C, Gelfand SE, et al. Management of exacerbations of COPD: a summary and appraisal of the published evidence. Chest 2001; 119:1190–1209.

Mueller C, Scholer A, Laule-Kilian K, et al. Use of B-type natriuretic peptide in the evaluation and management of acute dyspnea. N Engl J Med 2004; 350:647–654.

Niewoehner DE. The role of systemic corticosteroids in acute exacerbation of chronic obstructive pulmonary disease. Am J Respir Med 2002; 1:243–248.

Pistoria M, Amin A, Dressler D, et al. Core competencies in hospital medicine. J Hosp Med 2006: 1 (S1): 14–15.

Saint S, Bent S, Vittinghoff E, et al. Antibiotics in chronic obstructive pulmonary disease exacerbations: a meta-analysis. JAMA 1995; 273:957–960.

Stoller JK. Acute exacerbations of chronic obstructive pulmonary disease. N Engl J Med.2002; 346:988–994.

CHAPTER FORTY-FIVE

Asthma

Michael P. Lukela, MD, and William F. Bria II, MD

BACKGROUND

Asthma is defined as a chronic inflammatory disorder of large and small airways associated with hyperresponsivenes, reversible airflow limitation, and respiratory symptoms. It is the most common lung disease in developed countries and affects approximately 14.9 million patients in the United States.[1,2] Each year, asthma exacerbations result in more than 1.5 million emergency department (ED) visits, 20–30% of which result in hospitalization.[3] Approximately 5,000 deaths are attributed to asthma annually.[1,2,4,5] In addition to its associated morbidity and mortality, health care expenditures related to asthma are estimated at 6 billion dollars per year.[1–3] Hospitalization and ED visits account for nearly 50% of these costs.

ASSESSMENT

Clinical Presentation

Approximately 50% of cases develop prior to age 10; an additional 30% develop prior to age 40.[1,2] Although the majority of cases are diagnosed during childhood or early adulthood, new cases may be identified in patients as late as the 7th or 8th decade of life. Typically, these patients are thought to have chronic obstructive pulmonary disease (COPD) based on their age alone, and it is only through careful review of their clinical history that it becomes apparent that the components of their disease are attributed to reversible airway obstruction consistent with asthma. During childhood, males are diagnosed with asthma twice as often as females; however, this ratio becomes equal by age 30. The classic triad of symptoms associated with acute asthma exacerbations is cough, dyspnea, or wheezing, although not all need to be present for the diagnosis to be made. Clinical history should focus on prior episodes, potential triggers, current medications, information regarding previous hospitalizations/ED visits, and prior need for intubation/mechanical ventilation. Key triggers to identify that promote acute exacerbations are exposure to tobacco, allergens (dust or cat dander), and environmental exposures (e.g., air or industrial pollution). Classification of asthma severity is based on the severity and frequency of symptoms and alterations in pulmonary function (Table 45-1).[1,3,6]

On physical examination, particular emphasis should be placed on accurate assessment of the patient's respiratory effort and overall appearance. The presence of labored respirations, accessory muscle use (e.g., sternocleidomastoid), and/or suprasternal/subcostal retractions are indicative of severe airflow obstruction. Tachypnea (respiratory rate >30 breaths/min), tachycardia (>120 beats/min), and pulsus paradoxus (>12 mm Hg) have previously been described as important signs suggesting a severe exacerbation in a patient with known asthma.[3,7–10] Auscultation of the chest will often demonstrate wheezing of varying pitch, quality, and intensity that occurs at different points during the respiratory cycle. The degree of wheezing does not necessarily correlate with disease severity and may be notably diminished or absent in patients with severe airflow limitation. Clubbing is not a feature of asthma and, if noted, should prompt the clinician to consider other etiologies such as interstitial lung disease or bronchiectasis as diagnostic possibilities.

Differential Diagnosis

Differentiation between asthma and other respiratory diseases may present a significant challenge, given the lack of specificity of patient symptoms and overlap of findings noted on physical examination. Accurate diagnosis may be more apparent in situations in which the patient has been previously diagnosed with asthma or has associated clinical features suggestive of atopy. The most common conditions that need to be differentiated from asthma in adolescents and adults include bronchiectasis, vocal cord dysfunction or paralysis, laryngeal edema, COPD, pulmonary embolus, and congestive heart failure (Table 45-2). Clinicians caring for patients with acute symptoms must discriminate between an acute flare of asthma and the conditions that mimic its presentation (Table 45-3).[1–3,6] An important condition to distinguish from acute asthma that may be overlooked is upper airway obstruction secondary to vocal cord dysfunction. Although its prevalence in patients admitted to the hospital is unknown, this condition has been estimated to occur in up to 10% of patients previously diagnosed with asthma. Risk factors for this condition are female gender, obesity, gastroesophageal reflux, and history of prior emotional/physical abuse. Symptoms arise from contraction of laryngeal muscles that result in adduction of the vocal cords. The physical examination is often notable for stridor or wheezing, most notable over the trachea, although sounds may be transmitted to the lung fields. Diagnosis may be confirmed by direct visualization under laryngoscopy or pul-

Table 45-1 Classification of Asthma Severity

Classification	CLINICAL FEATURES BEFORE TREATMENT		
	Symptoms	Nighttime Symptoms	Lung Function
Severe persistent	Continual symptoms Limited physical activity Frequent exacerbations	Frequent	FEV$_1$ or PEF ≤60% predicted PEF variability >30%

Moderate persistent	Daily symptoms
	Daily use of inhaled short-acting
	  beta$_2$-agonist
	Exacerbations affect activity
	Exacerbations ≥2 times a week;
	  may last days
		>1 time a week	FEV$_1$ or PEF >60–<80% predicted
			PEF variability >30%

Mild persistent	Symptoms >2 times a week but <1 time a day Exacerbations may affect activity	>2 times a month	FEV$_1$ or PEF ≥80% predicted PEF variability 20–30%

Mild intermittent	Symptoms ≤2 times a week
	Asymptomatic and normal PEF
	  between exacerbations
	Exacerbations brief (from a few hours
	  to a few days): Intensity may vary
		≤2 times a month	FEV$_1$ or PEF ≥80% predicted
			PEF variability <20%

FEV$_1$—time forced expiratory volume; PEF—peak expiratory flow rate; PEF variability—change in peak expiratory flow rate between two measurements.

From National Asthma Education and Prevention Program [NAEPP]. Clinical Practice Guidelines. Expert Panel Report 2: Guidelines for the diagnosis and management of asthma. NIH Publication No. 91-4051. Bethesda, MD: National Institutes of Health/National Heart Lung and Blood Institutes, July, 1997.

Table 45-2 Differential Diagnosis of Adult Asthma

Upper Airway	Lower Airway
Vocal cord dysfunction, paralysis	**Asthma**
Foreign body aspiration	COPD
Laryngotracheal mass	Bronchiectasis
Laryngeal or tracheal stenosis	Bronchiolitis obliterans
Tracheomalacia	Eosinophilic pneumonia
Airway edema (angioedema,	Cystic fibrosis
inhalation injury)	Lymphangitic
Retropharyngeal abscess	carcinomatosis
Systemic Vasculitis	**Miscellaneous**
Churg-Strauss	Pulmonary embolus
Wegener's granulomatosis	Congestive heart failure
Goodpasture's syndrome	Gastroesophageal reflux
	Medications (ACE
	inhibitors)
Psychogenic	
Psychogenic cough	
Anxiety	
Conversion disorders	
Emotional laryngeal	
wheezing	
Episodic laryngeal dyskinesia	

COPD—chronic obstructive pulmonary disease; ACE—angiotensin converting enzyme

monary functions tests/spirometry that demonstrates fixed limitation of inspiratory flow. Measurement of arterial oxygen tension via arterial blood gas (ABG) analysis shows a normal or narrow alveolar-arterial gradient in upper airway obstruction in contrast to a widened gradient observed in significant lower airway obstruction. Importantly, vocal dysfunction does not improve with bronchodilator therapy or local/systemic corticosteroids and, if given, may have deleterious effects. Likewise, the use of anxiolytics (e.g., benzodiazepines) may be helpful in treating flares of vocal cord dysfunction, but may precipitate significant respiratory depression in asthmatics.

Diagnosis

In conjunction with clinical evaluation, pulmonary function assessment is an integral component of the overall assessment to appropriately characterize the severity of an asthma exacerbation.[1,2,6] Physiologic abnormalities in airflow obstruction indicative of an acute asthma exacerbation are easily measured by peak expiratory flow rates (PEFR) or time forced expiratory volume (FEV$_1$). Predicted values differ according to the size and age of the patient and have been well described by the American Thoracic Society guidelines on pulmonary function test interpretation and standardization.[11,12] Generally, PEFR or FEV$_1$ values <50% of predicted or personal best indicate severe obstruction in the adolescent and adult population. Mild or moderate obstruction is characterized by PEFR greater than 80% or 50–80% of predicted (or personal best) values, respectively.[11,12] Oxygen saturation measured by pulse oximetry is helpful in assessing the degree of hypoxemia. Confirmation of hypoxemia or further assessment of airflow obstruction may be accomplished through ABG analysis, although this is usually not necessary unless patients demonstrate signs of impending respiratory failure. During the acute exacerbation, hypoxemia, hypercapnia, and metabolic alkalosis are often present. Hypercapnia, defined by PaCO$_2$ greater than 45 mm Hg, is present in approximately 17% of patients during a severe acute episode.[3] Chest radiographs often demonstrate clear lung fields with associated hyperinflation from air trapping. Less

Table 45-3 Common Mimics of Asthma

Condition	Clinical Features
Vocal cord dysfunction	Monomorphic wheezing, loudest at neck. Often with dysphonia and/or stridor. Fails to respond to bronchodilators, steroids. More commonly seen in women. Associated with obesity.
COPD	Prior history of smoking with dyspnea and productive cough. Irreversible airflow obstruction on spirometry. May overlap with asthma (see text).
Pulmonary edema	Prior history of CHF or cardiac dysfunction. Examination with elevated jugular venous pressure, S_3 gallop, abnormal lung examination (e.g., crackles), or peripheral edema.
Pulmonary embolus	Positive risk factors for thromboembolic disease. Signs of venous thrombosis. Dyspnea and/or hypoxemia without other explanation.
Bronchiectasis	History of recurrent pneumonia, underlying disorder leading to recurrent pulmonary infection (e.g., cystic fibrosis), productive cough, and/or fever. Chest x-ray or CT is usually diagnostic.
Lymphangitic carcinomatosis	Prior history or clinical features suggestive of malignancy. Chest x-ray with diffuse reticulonodular infiltrates and/or pleural effusion without evidence of pneumonia. CT or bronchoscopy is usually diagnostic.

COPD—chronic obstructive pulmonary disease

commonly, atelectasis or complications from an acute flare such as pneumothorax or pneumomediastinum may be present. Electrocardiograms may be useful in eliminating other causes that explain acute dyspnea. Sinus tachycardia is the most common finding during an acute asthma flare, but is very nonspecific. Right-axis deviation or evidence of right ventricular strain may also be seen, but if solely attributed to asthma, these changes should resolve within hours following treatment.

MANAGEMENT

Treatment of an acute asthma exacerbation should be implemented immediately after initial clinical and functional assessments have been made. The cornerstones of therapy are to alleviate hypoxemia and reversible airway obstruction (Fig. 45-1).

1. *Oxygen:* Hypoxemia is related to ventilation-perfusion (V/Q) mismatch. The goal of therapy is to maintain oxygen saturation >90% (>93% in children and pregnant patients).[1-3,13] There is some evidence that hyperoxia may be harmful for certain subgroups of patients. Higher oxygen levels may paradoxically cause an increase in $PaCO_2$ levels as a result of regional release of pulmonary vasoconstrictors leading to impaired gas exchange.[13] Most notable increases in hypercarbia secondary to hyperoxia occur in patients with a $PaCO_2$ >40 mm Hg prior to oxygen therapy. Routine humidification of supplemental oxygen is currently not recommended, although dehydration and dry air may induce bronchospasm during an acute flare that may be reversed with humidification.

2. *Beta agonists:* Short-acting beta-agonists are first-line therapy for acute asthma exacerbations.[1,2,6,14] Their mechanism of action is through β-receptor–mediated relaxation of airway smooth muscle, leading to increased airflow. Following initial administration, it should be noted that the alveolar-arterial oxygen gradient (A-a gradient) may at first increase (due to increased cardiac output) prior to bronchodilation. Long-acting β-adrenergic agonists such as salmeterol are not recommended for treatment of acute asthma flares.[1,2,6,15] Although there is no difference in efficacy comparing mixed β₁- and β₂-adrenergic agonists with selective β₂-adrenergic agonists, the latter are associated with fewer side effects such as tremor, tachycardia, tachyarrhythmia, and hypokalemia. In the United States, albuterol, bitolterol, pirbuterol, and tertbutaline are the most common selective β₂-adrenergic agonists used in clinical practice. Albuterol is the most commonly used. Its onset of action is within 5 minutes following administration, with a duration of action of approximately 6 hours. Levalbuterol, the R-isomer of albuterol, may be as efficacious as albuterol with fewer side effects. Bronchodilatory effects of β₂-adrenegic agonists are due to the pharmacologic activity of the R-isomer; the S-isomer is pharmacologically inert. Recent evidence suggests that the S-isomer may have physiologic activity, including proinflammatory and bronchoconstrictive effects on the airway. In addition, its longer half-life may result in accumulation with frequent dosing and may oppose the actions of the R-isomer over time.[3,15,16]

Administration of albuterol may be achieved through inhaled, oral, or intravenous routes (IV). Inhaled therapy is the most common and effective when balanced against systemic side effects.[3] Data are limited to demonstrate efficacy of IV or oral administration compared to inhaled therapy and should not be used routinely unless there are barriers that prevent successful administration of inhaled therapy. Administration of inhaled therapy may be provided through a nebulized mist or metered-dose inhaler (MDI) with a spacer device. Although there is no difference in efficacy between the two, the perception exists that nebulized mist is more successful in relieving symptoms. Much of this perception is due to the fact that the amount of albuterol provided via nebulized mist is significantly more than that delivered by a conventional MDI (2.5 mg per treatment versus 0.09 mg per puff). MDI therapy may provide medication more quickly (1–2 minutes) than nebulized therapy (10–15 minutes). Nebulized mist may have an advantage in clinical situations in which patients are not able to cooperate or correctly administer MDI therapy, such as in children, older patients, those with altered mental status, or severe exacerbations. Initial dosing for an acute asthma flare may be provided with an albuterol MDI with spacer device at four to six puffs (90 µg/puff) every 20–30 minutes for up to 1 hour.[1-3] Alternatively, nebulized mist therapy with 2.5–5 mg albuterol (0.5–1.0 ml of 0.5% albuterol solution combined with 1.5–2 mL isotonic saline) may be dosed at the same time interval. For severe exacerbations, continuous nebulized therapy may be used for up to 1 hour.

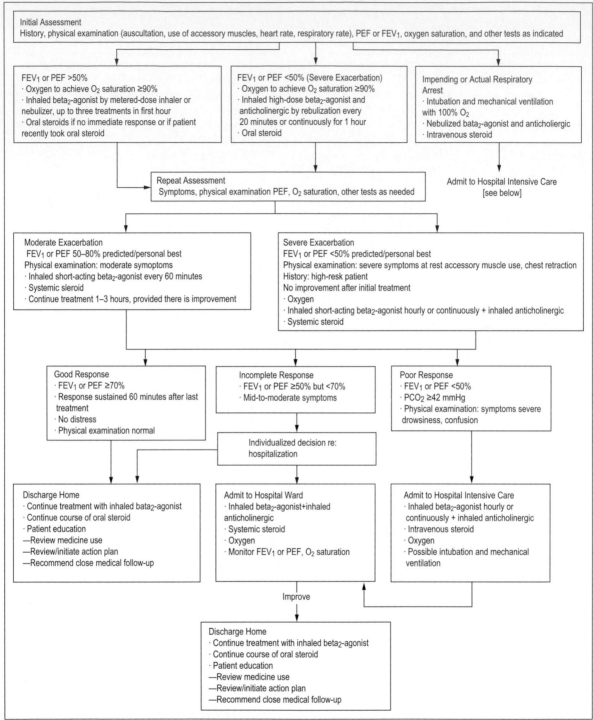

Initial Assessment
History, physical examination (auscultation, use of accessory muscles, heart rate, respiratory rate), PEF or FEV₁, oxygen saturation, and other tests as indicated

FEV₁ or PEF >50%
· Oxygen to achieve O₂ saturation ≥90%
· Inhaled beta₂-agonist by metered-dose inhaler or nebulizer, up to three treatments in first hour
· Oral steroids if no immediate response or if patient recently took oral steroid

FEV₁ or PEF <50% (Severe Exacerbation)
· Oxygen to achieve O₂ saturation ≥90%
· Inhaled high-dose beta₂-agonist and anticholinergic by rebulization every 20 minutes or continuously for 1 hour
· Oral steroid

Impending or Actual Respiratory Arrest
· Intubation and mechanical ventilation with 100% O₂
· Nebulized bata₂-agonist and anticholiergic
· Intravenous steroid

Repeat Assessment
Symptoms, physical examination PEF, O₂ saturation, other tests as needed

Admit to Hospital Intensive Care
[see below]

Moderate Exacerbation
FEV₁ or PEF 50–80% predicted/personal best
Physical examination: moderate symoptoms
· Inhaled short-acting beta₂-agonist every 60 minutes
· Systemic sleroid
· Continue treatment 1–3 hours, provided there is improvement

Severe Exacerbation
FEV₁ or PEF <50% predicted/personal best
Physical examination: severe symptoms at rest accessory muscle use, chest retraction
History: high-resk patient
No improvement after initial treatment
· Oxygen
· Inhaled short-acting beta₂-agonist hourly or continuously + inhaled anticholinergic
· Systemic steroid

Good Response
· FEV₁ or PEF ≥70%
· Response sustained 60 minutes after last treatment
· No distress
· Physical examination normal

Incomplete Response
· FEV₁ or PEF ≥50% but <70%
· Mid-to-moderate symptoms

Poor Response
· FEV₁ or PEF <50%
· PCO₂ ≥42 mmHg
· Physical examination: symptoms severe drowsiness, confusion

Individualized decision re: hospitalization

Discharge Home
· Continue treatment with inhaled bata₂-agonist
· Continue course of oral steroid
· Patient education
—Review medicine use
—Review/initiate action plan
—Recommend close medical follow-up

Admit to Hospital Ward
· Inhaled beta₂-agonist+inhaled anticholinergic
· Systemic steroid
· Oxygen
· Monitor FEV₁ or PEF, O₂ saturation

Admit to Hospital Intensive Care
· Inhaled beta₂-agonist hourly or continuously + inhaled anticholinergic
· Intravenous steroid
· Oxygen
· Possible intubation and mechanical ventilation

Improve

Discharge Home
· Continue treatment with inhaled beta₂-agonist
· Continue course of oral steroid
· Patient education
—Review medicine use
—Review/initiate action plan
—Recommend close medical follow-up

Figure 45-1 • Management of Asthma Exacerbations: Emergency Department and Hospital-Based Care. From National Asthma Education and Prevention Program [NAEPP]. Clinical Practice Guidelines. Expert Panel Report 2: Guidelines for the diagnosis and management of asthma. NIH Publication No. 91-4051. Bethesda, MD: National Institutes of Health/National Heart Lung and Blood Institutes, July, 1997.

3. *Anticholinergics:* Prior to the discovery of β-adrenergic agonists, atropine was the primary treatment for asthma and COPD. Side effects related to its anticholinergic properties limited its use until the development of derivatives that were not systemically absorbed. Currently, ipratropium bromide, oxitropium, and tiotropium are available for use; ipratropium bromide is most common. It exerts is pharmacologic effects by reversing vagally mediated bronchospasm. It does not appear to effect mucous secretion or ciliary movement. At higher dosages, salivary secretions may be decreased; however, anticholinergic systemic effects such as changes in intracocular tension, tachycardia, or urinary retention are not seen. Inhaled ipratropium bromide has an onset of action of approximately 3 minutes, with a peak effect of 1–2 hours. Its duration of action is 6 hours. At present, there is conflicting evidence to support widespread use of anticholinergics in the management of acute asthma.[1–3,6] It appears that they are less

effective when compared to β-adrenergic agonists alone, but may provide additive or synergistic benefits when used in combination. In recent studies of children and adults experiencing severe asthma exacerbations (FEV$_1$ <50%), improvement in lung function (PEFR variability), and reduction in hospital admission have been demonstrated in patients treated with combination therapy (multiple doses of ipratropium bromide and beta-agonists).[1–3] There is no clear evidence to support single- or multiple-dose therapy of inhaled anticholinergics in patients with mild or moderate acute asthma exacerbations. Currently, ipratropium bromide is the treatment of choice for bronchospasm due to beta-blocker medications. Dosage for an acute flare may be provided though an MDI with spacer device at 4 puffs (18 µg/puff) every 10–20 minutes for up to one hour. Alternatively, nebulized mist may be used to provide 500 µg per dose every 20 minutes for up to 1 hour.[1–3]

4. *Corticosteroids:* Corticosteroids are a cornerstone of therapy in the management of asthma and should be utilized in all patients admitted to the hospital for an acute flare.[1–3,17] Although not direct bronchodilators, corticosteroids provide an important role in reducing airway inflammation, speed resolution of airway obstruction, and prevent relapse of acute flares. Physiologic effects are not immediate and may take between 6 and 24 hours before a noticeable impact on pulmonary function is noted. Inhaled corticosteroids may have a complementary role in the treatment of acute flares with an earlier therapeutic effect (<3 hours).[3,18,19] Inhaled therapy likely achieves its therapeutic effects by inducing a topical response that decreases airway mucosal vasoconstriction. At present, there is no clear evidence to support the use of inhaled corticosteroids alone as treatment for an acute asthma flare. Corticosteroid therapy should be provided when insufficient response from bronchodilator therapy has been identified: FEV$_1$/PEFR <70% baseline after 1 hour of therapy or <10% improvement in FEV$_1$/PEFR following the first dose of β-agonist therapy.[1–3,17] Dosages for methylprednisolone, prednisone, or prednisolone usually range between 120 and 180 mg/day in three or four divided doses during the first 24–48 hours. As patients demonstrate response to therapy, the dosage of corticosteroids may then be decreased to approximately 60 mg daily. The bioavailability and efficacy of oral and intravenous therapy are nearly identical, so the method of administration should depend on the clinical scenario. At present, no convincing data exist to definitively support a particular method of tapering off corticosteroids. After conversion to an oral regimen, the dosage may be decreased by approximately 20% every 1–2 days over the following 7–12 days, depending on the patient's clinical response.

ADDITIONAL THERAPEUTIC CONSIDERATIONS

Heliox

As airway obstruction increases, airflow becomes turbulent, resulting in a functional increase in airway resistance. In addition, disruption of laminar airflow may impede the delivery of aerosolized particles to more distal airways, which may have an impact on the effectiveness of inhaled therapies designed to treat acute asthma flares. Through using a combination of a low-density, high-viscosity gas mixture of helium and oxygen (Heliox), laminar airflow may potentially be restored, resulting in

decreased airway resistance and improvement in pulmonary mechanics.[20–22] Heliox usually comprises a mixture of 80% helium and 20% oxygen. If the concentration of helium decreases below 70%, the gas mixture will be unlikely to provide significant benefit.[3] Although several small trials exist that demonstrate improvement in pulmonary function following treatment with Heliox, the overall evidence does not support routine administration of this combined gas mixture for patients with moderate to severe asthma exacerbations.

Magnesium sulfate

Magnesium was first used as a treatment for acute asthma in 1936. It is thought to act through inhibition of smooth muscle cell calcium channels, thereby blocking muscular contraction leading to bronchodilation.[2,23,24] Although several studies have investigated its clinical benefits, no convincing evidence exists for its routine use in the treatment of acute asthma.[23,24] Recent data from a randomized double-blind placebo-controlled trial demonstrated significant improvement in pulmonary function for patients receiving intravenous magnesium with severe asthma exacerbations (FEV$_1$ <25%). No benefit was noted in patients with an FEV$_1$ greater than 25%. In this study, magnesium sulfate was provided as a one-time dosage of 2 g intravenously in combination with standard therapy. Potential side effects include transient flushing, urticaria, lightheadedness, nausea, or burning at the site of intravenous administration.[25]

Leukotriene antagonists

Leukotrienes have been demonstrated to play an important role as mediators of inflammation and bronchoconstriction in patients with asthma.[1,2] Leukotriene-modifying drugs have an established role in the treatment of chronic asthma. Recent observations suggest that these agents may provide additive benefit when used with β-adrenergic agonists in the acute setting; however, additional studies are necessary to determine where these agents fit within routine therapy before their use in the acute setting can be endorsed.[1,2,26]

Theophylline

Methylxanthines such as theophylline and aminophylline are thought to act through inhibition of phosphodiesterases, resulting in bronchial smooth muscle relaxation. Acting alone, these agents are inferior to β-adrenergic agonists and do not confer additional benefit when used as part of combination of therapy. Side effects are common and include tremor, nausea, and tachyarrhythmia. In general, these agents should not be used in the treatment of acute asthma unless patients fail to respond to aggressive conventional therapy.[1,2]

Empiric Antimicrobial Therapy

Although infections are known to exacerbate bronchial asthma mediated through damage to airway epithelium and concomitant airway inflammation, the majority of infections are viral and will therefore not respond to antimicrobial therapy. If convincing evidence of bacterial infection exists (radiographic infiltrate, fever, dyspnea, cough, and purulent sputum with the presence of poly-

---

Box 45-1 Risk Factors Associated with Death from Asthma

Asthma History

Previous history of sudden or severe asthma exacerbations

Prior intubation from asthma

Prior admission to an intensive care unit

Two or more hospitalizations for asthma during the past year

Three or more emergency department visits for asthma during the past year

Hospitalization or emergency department visit during the past month

Poor perception of airflow obstruction or its severity

Medication Use

Use of >2 canisters per month of short-acting inhaled β-agonist

Current use or recent withdrawal from oral steroids

Miscellaneous factors

Presence of additional comorbidities (e.g., cardiovascular diseases or COPD)

Serious psychiatric disease, including depression

Psychosocial instability

Illicit drug use

Sensitivity to molds such as *Alternaria*

Low socioeconomic status and urban residence

COPD—chronic obstructive pulmonary disease

Box 45-2 Discharge Checklist for Patients Hospitalized with Acute Asthma Exacerbations

Clinical Readiness

FEV_1/PEFR >70% predicted or personal best

FEV_1/PEFR between 50–70% predicted and absence of warning signs for sudden death

Able to adequately perform and interpret peak flow meter

Has received education and teaching regarding disease, monitoring, and treatment, including proper usage of medications

Medications

Ensure that the patient has an adequate supply of medication until follow up appointment

Short acting β-agonist

Inhaled corticosteroid

Oral corticosteroid

Additional maintenance therapy (e.g., leukotriene antagonists)

Spacer devices for metered-dose inhalers, if appropriate

Teaching and supplies for nebulized mist treatments, if appropriate

Follow-up

Arrange follow-up appointment with primary care physician or asthma specialist within 3–5 days following discharge

Whenever possible directly contact follow-up physician regarding clinical course

Review asthma action plan with patient

---

morphonuclear leukocytes) empiric treatment may be warranted. In such cases, consideration of agents that cover atypical pathogens such as *Mycoplasma* or *Chlamydia pneumoniae* is recommended. In general, however, empiric antimicrobial therapy will not provide clinical benefit, and its routine use should be discouraged.[1,2]

INDICATIONS FOR HOSPITALIZATION

The need for hospitalization following initial treatment and evaluation in the ED is dependent on several factors: duration and severity of symptoms, degree of airflow obstruction as measured by FEV_1 or PEFR, comorbid conditions, response to therapy, ability to follow discharge instructions, and available resources to ensure adequate follow-up. Patients with an inadequate response to therapy (FEV_1 or PEFR <50% of baseline following initial therapy and/or severe symptoms) will need admission, with continued aggressive medical therapy.[1–3,8,9,27] Disposition for patients with an incomplete response to initial therapy (FEV_1 or PEFR 50–70% of baseline and/or persistent mild-to-moderate symptoms) should be determined based on clinical risk factors that place them at risk for outpatient treatment failure or death (Box 45-1). In general, patients with an adequate response to therapy with an FEV_1 or PEFR >70% of baseline sustained for 60 minutes following their last treatment are appropriate for discharge, provided that there

are no additional barriers that would prevent following an appropriate discharge care plan (Box 45-1 and 45-2).[9,28]

Use of severity classification scales may provide and highlight useful clinical information. Favorable response to initial therapy with improvement of FEV_1/PEFR at 30 minutes following treatment is the most reliable predictor for outcome. Poor prognostic factors include poor long-term control of asthma, FEV_1/PEFR <30% predicted, elevated $PaCO_2$, cyanosis, and lack of early response to therapy.[3,9,28,29]

During the first 24–48 hours of admission, continued reassessment of pulmonary functional status and response to therapy should be pursued. Although the treatment strategy of providing supplemental oxygen, bronchodilator therapy, and corticosteroids may not change, it should be noted that it may take up to 3–4 days before significant improvement in noted. Failure to respond to conventional therapy or inconsistencies in the clinical history/examination should prompt the clinician to consider other entities that may mimic asthma in the acute setting (*see* Table 45-3).[1–3,6]

INDICATIONS FOR ICU ADMISSION

Patients unresponsive to maximal conventional therapy are deemed to have *status asthmaticus*.[1,2,29] Clinical features may include altered levels of consciousness, upright posture,

Box 45-3. Asthma Action Plan

Name _____   **Date** _____

Current Asthma Medications

1. _____   5. _____
2. _____   6. _____
3. _____   7. _____
4. _____   8. _____

When to Monitor Peak Flow Numbers   **Important Peak Flow Numbers**

Morning, soon after waking up   Baseline _____

Before dinner

Before bed   _____ % baseline = _____

Before and 5–15 minutes after inhaled treatments

With increased asthma symptoms   _____ % baseline = _____

If your peak flow number drops below _____ or you notice:

Increased need for quick-relief medicine

Increased asthma symptoms after waking up

Awakening at night with asthma symptoms

Follow these steps:

Increase your quick-relief medicine

Take _____ puffs of _____   _____ times a day

Increase inhaled steroids

Take _____ puffs of _____   _____ times a day

Begin/increase treatment with oral steroids

Take _____ mg of _____ every a.m. _____ p.m. _____

Other _____

Call your doctor _____ or emergency room _____

If your peak flow number drops below _____ or you continue to get worse after increasing treatment according to the directions above, follow these treatment steps:

Begin/increase treatment with oral steroids

Take _____ mg of _____ every a.m. _____ p.m. _____

Other _____

Call your doctor _____ or emergency room _____

AT ANY TIME, CALL YOUR DOCTOR IF:

Quick-relief medicine are not last 4 hours, or

Your peak flow number falls below _____, or

Asthma symptoms worsen while you are taking oral steroids

If you cannot contact your doctor go directly to the Emergency Room

If you have questions please call:

_____   After hours   _____

Name   Phone   Name   Phone

Physician Signature _____   Date _____

Patient/Family Member Signature _____

diaphoresis, tachypnea (>30 breaths/min), accessory muscle use/fatigue, tachycardia (>120 beats/min), pulsus paradoxus (>15 mm Hg), hypoxia, or cyanosis. An FEV_1 <1.0 L/sec or PEFR <120 L/min is suggestive of severe obstruction. FEV1 <0.6 L/sec or PEFR <60 L/min heralds impending respiratory failure and must be addressed promptly.[3,5,9,28,30] Prior to clinical decompensation, it is imperative to identify these patients and transfer them immediately to an intensive care unit (ICU) setting. Depending on the clinical scenario, additional therapeutic options should be considered as adjuncts to conventional therapy. The decision to intubate is complex and should be approached carefully. Signs or symptoms indicative of impending respiratory failure such as altered mental status, progressive tachypnea, respiratory muscle fatigue, rising $PaCO_2$ or falling PaO_2 in spite of therapy, or hemodynamic instability should alert the physician to strongly consider intubation without delay;[29,30] however, it is imperative to have experienced clinicians with requisite airway management skills directly managing these patients, given its associated morbidity (due to increased risk of barotrauma) and mortality.

DISCHARGE FROM THE HOSPITAL

Preparation for discharge should begin shortly after patients have demonstrated clinical response to ensure adequate continued improvement after leaving the hospital and to prevent relapse of symptoms. In addition to improvement in symptoms, objective parameters such as oxygen saturation, heart rate, and tachypnea should be at or near baseline measurements. FEV_1/PEFR should ideally be >70% of predicted (or personal best) values, although carefully selected patients may be safely discharged with FEV_1/PEFR 50–70% predicted in the absence of clinical warning signs (*see* Box 45-1) and appropriate follow-up.[1–3] Hospitalization for an acute asthma flare should be seen as an opportunity to educate patients about their disease and for clinicians to be proactive in ensuring that patients are on appropriate medications, have adequate resources for disease management, and effective follow-up. Recent data support the concept of implementing asthma disease management programs in which patients are provided asthma education, medication teaching, and appropriate follow-up during hospitalization for an acute flare. These targeted interventions have demonstrated significant reductions in hospitalization, emergency department visits, unscheduled doctor visits, and cost savings. To accomplish this effectively, planning for discharge should occur early during the hospitalization. An asthma checklist should be used to ensure that a comprehensive care plan is established and communicated to the patient to optimize outcome.[1–3] In particular, it is important to review the patient's medication regimen, provide teaching for peak-flow monitoring,

referral for a follow-up medical appointment, and verbal and written instructions detailing a plan of action following discharge (Boxes 45-2 and 45-3). Follow-up should be within 3–5 days following discharge, and if possible, the patient's primary physician or office should be contacted directly prior to the patient's discharge. Additional recommendations regarding the transition to outpatient care can be found in the Michigan Quality Improvement Consortium guidelines at www.mqic.org.

Key Points

- Short-acting beta-agonists are first-line therapy for acute asthma exacerbations.

- Corticosteroids are a mainstay of therapy for acute asthma exacerbations requiring hospital admission.

- Empiric antimicrobial treatment of an asthma flare is not recommended.

- Measurement of time-forced expiratory volume (FEV_1) or peak expiratory flow (PEF) are useful parameters to characterize the severity of airflow limitation in acute asthma flares and to monitor improvement.

- Risk factors associated with death from asthma may be easily identified and play an important role in reducing morbidity and mortality.

SUGGESTED READING

Afessa B, Morales I, Cury JD. Clinical course and outcome of patients admitted to an ICU for status asthmaticus. Chest 2001; 120:1616–1621.

British Thoracic Society, et al. Guidelines on the management of asthma: management of acute asthma. Thorax 2003; 58:i32–i50.

Global strategy for asthma management and prevention. NIH Publication 02–3659, 2002. Available at: http://www.ginasthma.com.

National Asthma Education and Prevention Program. Expert panel report 2: Guidelines for the diagnosis and management of asthma. Bethesda, MD: National Institutes of Health, 1997; Publication No. 55–4051.

Rodrigo G, Rodrigo C. A new index for early prediction of hospitalization in patients with acute asthma. Am J Emerg Med 1997; 15:8–13.

Rodrigo G, Rodrigo C, Hall J. Acute asthma in adults. Chest 2004; 125:1081–1097.

CHAPTER FORTY-SIX

Pleural Disease: Pleural Effusion and Pneumothorax

Irene Krokos, MD, and Steven E. Gay, MD

BACKGROUND

Over 1 million people annually are diagnosed with pleural effusion. The incidence of pneumothorax varies between 1–7 cases per 100,000 persons per year, depending on the etiology of the pneumothorax and patient demographics. Patient characteristics (sex, age), presence of symptoms (dyspnea), and underlying comorbidities (emphysema, cancer, heart failure) directly influence the morbidity, mortality, length of stay, cost, and management.

ASSESSMENT

The pleural cavity is a dynamic environment, lined by mesothelial cells and influenced by hydrostatic and oncotic pressures, capillary permeability, and inflammatory mediators. As a potential space, it is occupied by a minimal amount of fluid (approximately 10 mL of fluid in each cavity) that helps facilitate the movement of the lungs during respiration.[1] This ultrafiltrate of plasma lubricates and separates the inner visceral layer of the pleura from the outer parietal layer. Over 2,400 mL of fluid per day is generated by the parietal layer, which is resorbed by the visceral layer.[2] In conditions such as congestive heart failure, infection, and malignancy, the delicate balance of fluid homeostasis is disrupted, and significant clinical pathology ensues as fluid accumulates, leading to pleural effusion.[3] Furthermore, the appearance of air within this space creates a pneumothorax that may also significantly compromise lung mechanics, leading to clinical signs and symptoms that are important to recognize.

Clinical Presentation

Pleural Effusion

The top three causes of pleural effusion in the United States are (1) congestive heart failure, (2) pneumonia, and (3) cancer (Table 46-1).[4] The most common symptom associated with pleural effusions is dyspnea; however, it is also the most nonspecific.[5] The patient with pleural effusion may complain of progressive dyspnea, chest pain or pressure, edema, fever, or cough.[2] Over half of patients with empyema have underlying diabetes, neoplasm, or alcoholism and can present with a more insidious onset

including weight loss, fever, leukocytosis, and anemia.[1] Parapneumonic effusions will be present in approximately 20–57% of hospital admissions for bacterial pneumonia.[3] Symptoms of hemoptysis, weight loss, malaise, and anorexia are highly concerning for malignant pathology. The most common finding in patients with pleural metastases is pleural effusion. A review of 1,783 cases found 36% of malignant effusions were a result of bronchogenic carcinoma, 25% breast cancer, 10% lymphoma, and 5% or less for ovarian and gastric carcinoma.[6] Furthermore, many patients will have additional clinical symptoms related to the primary malignancy that can provide clues as to the cause of an effusion, such as abdominal pain and bloating in patients with ovarian cancer.

Pneumothorax

Pneumothorax also presents with dyspnea and, commonly, pleuritic pain. If there is a prior history of pneumothorax elicited, the rate of recurrence after the first episode is 10%, and after the second episode up to 40%. Pneumothorax can be primary spontaneous (rupture of small subpleural blebs), secondary (from emphysema or asthma), traumatic, or iatrogenic. Primary spontaneous pneumothorax (PSP) is more frequent in males between the ages of 30 and 40 years, is common with approximately 10 cases per 100,000, and occurs slightly more often on the right side. Most episodes occur at rest, and 30% have recurrence on the ipsilateral side.[2] Secondary spontaneous pneumothorax (SSP) is the most common cause and usually a result of underlying emphysema, asthma, or infiltrative diseases such as idiopathic pulmonary fibrosis, sarcoidosis, eosinophilic granuloma, or lymphangioleiomyomatosis (LAM). LAM, a rare, idiopathic disease occurring in women of childbearing age, is characterized by smooth muscle proliferation in all parts of the lung and has the highest incidence of pneumothorax at 75%.[9]

Human Immunodeficiency Virus (HIV)

The patient with a history of HIV warrants special consideration for other causes of pleural effusion and pneumothorax. In the hospitalized patient with HIV, the rate of pleural effusion is 7–27%, and the rate for spontaneous pneumothorax is 1–2% with an increase to 4–12% in the setting of *Pneumocystis jiroveci* pneumonia.[10] In this population, cigarette smoking, injection drug use, therapy with aerosolized pentamidine, and pulmonary tuberculosis (TB) are other risk factors for pneumothorax.

Table 46-1 Causes of Pleural Effusion

Transudative
- CHF (#1 overall cause of pleural effusion)
- Cirrhosis
- Nephrosis
- Hepatic hydrothorax
- Urinothorax
- Pulmonary embolus*

Exudative
- Parapneumonic, empyema (#2 cause)
- Malignancy* (#3 cause)
  - Bronchogenic carcinoma (33% of malignant effusions)
  - Breast cancer (25%)
  - Gastric or esophageal cancer (5%)
  - Ovarian cancer (5%)
  - Mesothelioma (<5%)
- Pulmonary embolus or infarction*
- Collagen-vascular disease
- Tuberculosis
- Trauma
- Hemothorax
- Postcardiac injury
- Postcoronary artery bypass grafting
- Esophageal perforation
- Pancreatitis
- Drug-induced reactions
- Meig's syndrome
- Chylothorax

*Note: Can be exudative or transudative

Diagnosis

A thorough history and physical examination will often lead to the most likely cause of a pleural effusion or pneumothorax. A temporal description of symptoms, a pertinent past medical history of predisposing conditions, and specific findings on physical examination will also help guide the diagnostic workup.

Pleural Effusion

Physical Examination

The presence of pleural effusion can be elicited by dullness to percussion, diminished or absent breath sounds, and lack of fremitus in the affected area.[2] An elevated jugular venous pressure, peripheral edema, and third heart sound would suggest a cardiac etiology for the effusion. An enlarged and tender lower extremity may suggest deep venous thrombosis with pulmonary embolus and associated effusion. Fever and egophony would be consistent with pneumonia and parapneumonic effusion. Lymphadenopathy and hepatosplenomegaly may suggest a neoplastic process, and ascites may indicate the presence of hepatic hydrothorax.[4]

Chest Radiography

Chest radiography will demonstrate the effusion and may also identify associated pathology such as an infiltrate or mass. Pleural effusions become visible on posterior-anterior chest radiography at volumes of about 200 mL.[5] Blunting of the lateral costophrenic angle will occur if >200 to 500 mL of fluid is present. As more fluid accumulates, the hemidiaphragm is obscured, and the upper margin of the opacity becomes concave. Lateral decubitus films are more sensitive, as they can detect effu-

sion volumes as small as 50 mL, and are helpful in estimating if there is enough fluid to perform a throacentesis.[2,5] For example, if the distance between the outer border of the lung and the inner border of the chest wall is >10 mm, the ability to safely perform thoracentesis is higher and further imaging with ultrasound deemed unnecessary unless there is concern of a loculated effusion.[11] Computed tomographic (CT) imaging of the chest may aide in further identifying underlying parenchymal, mediastinal, or pleural disease if clinical suspicion warrants.

Thoracentesis

Thoracentesis is critical to guide diagnosis and treatment of a pleural effusion. Effusions are classified as either transudative or exudative. Transudative effusions evolve when there is an imbalance between hydrostatic and oncotic pressures. Examples include congestive heart failure (CHF), cirrhosis, and pulmonary embolus. In contrast, when local factors like inflammation, infection, or the presence of malignant cells in the pleural space result in the accumulation of fluid, exudates occur. The leading causes of exudates are pneumonia, cancer, and pulmonary embolus.[4] In one analysis, 42–77% of exudative effusions were secondary to malignancy.[12] Thus, this classification is important, as transudates do not typically necessitate further workup if they resolve, whereas exudates warrant a thorough evaluation if the etiology is not initially obvious.

Light's criteria developed in 1972 is the most sensitive classification system for differentiating transudates from exudates. Pleural effusions meeting any one of the following criteria are classified as exudates: (1) pleural fluid protein to serum protein ratio >0.5, or (2) pleural fluid LDH to serum LDH ratio >0.6, or (3) pleural fluid LDH more than two thirds the upper limit of normal serum LDH.[5,13]

In subsequent analyses, Light's criteria has shown a sensitivity of 98%, specificity of 77–83%, and accuracy of 93–95%.[11,14] It should be noted, however, that there is no single gold standard to establish the nature of an effusion, and so utilizing the underlying diagnosis as the gold standard in these studies introduces some bias into the laboratory investigations of pleural effusions.[15] Thus, given the higher sensitivity but lower specificity, some effusions that are actually transudates may be mistakenly classified as exudates when using Light's criteria. In this setting, it is useful to measure the serum-pleural fluid albumin gradient, and if it is >1.2 g/dL, the effusion is more likely a transudate and not an exudate. A common example is the false positive exudative appearance of effusions in CHF after treatment with diuretics. Using the albumin gradient in this situation helps to clarify the diagnosis and avoid further unnecessary costs and risks.[11,14] Further laboratory analysis of pleural fluid is usually performed when there is high clinical suspicion for a specific cause based on history and physical examination. For example, if there is concern of cancer, esophageal rupture, or lymphatic obstruction from tumor, then further testing with cell counts, amylase, and cholesterol can be considered, respectively. In addition to Light's criteria, the following tests may further clarify the cause of an effusion:

1. *Cell count and differential.* A predominance of neutrophils (>50%) suggests an acute process-like infection while mononuclear cells indicate a chronic process. Lymphocyte predominance can be seen with effusions in TB, cancer, or postcoronary bypass grafting. Eosinophilia (>10%) is caused

mostly by blood or air within the pleural space but can also be due to drugs, asbestos, and Churg-Strauss syndrome.

2. *Gram stain and culture.* Allows investigation for aerobes, anaerobes, fungi, and mycobacteria in the right clinical setting. Yield is increased with inoculation of blood culture bottles at the bedside, and mycobacteria are rarely positive unless there is a tuberculous empyema or the patient has AIDS.

3. *Glucose.* Low glucose levels are seen with infection, malignant effusion (usually <60 mg per 100 mL), and rheumatoid arthritis (<20–30 mg per 100 mL in 70–80% of cases). Care must be taken, though, in transporting the sample with preservative and also in comparing to a concurrent serum glucose.

4. *LDH.* LDH, in addition to its role in Light's criteria, correlates with the degree of pleural inflammation. Significantly increasing levels on repeated thoracentesis can indicate an active process and the need for a more aggressive pursuit of a diagnosis. However, it should be noted that pleural fluid LDH can rise slightly with repeated thoracenteses of a transudative effusion, and in patients with CHF on diuretics.[14]

5. *Cytology.* Three consecutive pleural fluid samples will identify malignant effusions with a sensitivity of 80%. Fluid tests positive 70% of the time in metastatic adenocarcinoma, 10% mesotheliomas, 20% squamous cell carcinomas, 25–50% lymphomas, and 25% sarcomas. For lymphomas, flow cytometry may be of further utility in identifying a clonal cell population.

6. *pH.* Like glucose and LDH, pH is an additional indicator of inflammation and when <7.20 indicates the need for drainage if empyema or parapneumonic effusion is suspected. In malignant effusions, a low pH can be associated with both a poor prognosis with an average survival of 30 days, and likely failure of pleurodesis.[4]

7. *Tumor markers.* Pleural fluid tumor markers such as CEA, CA125, CA15–3, and CA 19–9 are sometimes used to improve the rate of diagnosis; however, they should not be used as a definitive diagnostic modality.[3,16]

8. *Triglyceride levels.* A level >110 mg/dL is consistent with chylothorax that results from thoracic duct obstruction. This is differentiated from pseudochylothorax, where the level is <110 mg/dL, due to cell rupture that is commonly seen from chronic pleural effusions, rheumatoid arthritis, and tuberculosis (TB).[1]

9. *Creatinine.* If urinothorax is suspected, the pleural fluid creatinine will be greater than serum creatinine.

10. *Hematocrit.* Hemothorax will have a hematocrit >50% of peripheral blood. If <1%, then the blood in the pleural space is not significant. Bloody pleural fluid suggests malignancy, pulmonary embolus (PE), or trauma.[11]

Infection

In parapneumonic effusions, bacteria isolated are predominately *Streptococcus pneumoniae, Staphylococcus aureus,* and *Hemophilus influenzae.* The incidence of parapneumonic effusions with pneumococcal pneumonia is reported to be 29–57%.[17] Furthermore, 20% of atypical pneumonias can have pleural effusions, and frequent organisms isolated are *Mycoplasma pneumoniae* and also adenovirus and influenza.[2] There is a classification scheme for infected pleural fluid developed by Light that is a useful guide for therapy. In simple parapneumonic effusion, the appearance of the

pleural fluid is clear with normal pH, glucose, and LDH; and there is resolution with antibiotics alone, and no drainage is required. Complicated parapneumonic effusion has a clear-turbid appearance, pH < 7.3, low glucose, raised LDH, positive Gram stain or culture; antibiotics plus drainage is required for resolution. Finally, with empyema (pus in the pleural space), Gram stain or cultures are positive, and drainage is often surgically required for resolution, in addition to antibiotics.[5,18]

Human Immunodeficiency Virus (HIV)

The most common causes of effusions in HIV are parapneumonic, TB, and Kaposi's sarcoma (KS). With TB infection in non-HIV patients, there is pleural fluid lymphocytosis, elevation in adenosine deaminase (ADA) >40 units, and positive PCR testing for mycobacterial DNA.[1,4] However, with HIV infection, ADA false negatives are frequent, and the diagnosis of TB in HIV patients poses a diagnostic dilemma.[1] Furthermore, immunocompetent patients will have a positive PPD 70% of the time, versus 40% of HIV patients.

In the setting of parapneumonic effusions and HIV, the spectrum of organisms causing pneumonia parallels those found in immunocompetent individuals. However, HIV patients may have more frequent bacteremia and development of parapneumonic effusions and empyema. Advanced HIV disease can also predispose to *Pseudomonas aeruginosa* and *Rhodococcus equi,* which is associated with cavitary parenchymal lung disease.

Kaposi's sarcoma is associated with bilateral pleural effusions, focal airspace opacities, intrapulmonary nodules, and hilar lymphadenopathy, and can present without mucocutaneous involvement. The major goal is palliation, with median survival 2–10 months, although there have been some reports of regression with initiation of HAART.[10]

Other

Pleural effusions occur in 10–50% of patients with an acute pulmonary embolus. As such, PE should be considered in every patient with acute unilateral pleural effusion and no clear alternative diagnosis. The effusions associated with PE can be transudative or exudative, and they are usually small and occupy less than one third of the hemithorax.[17]

Drug-induced pleural disease and effusions are mediated by hypersensitivity reactions and direct toxic effects. At least 30 drugs are known to cause pleural disease. Pleural fluid eosinophilia >10% may provide a clue, and systemic eosinophilias may not always be present.[19,20]

Approach to Thoracentesis

There are no absolute contraindications to thoracentesis. Relative contraindications include bleeding diathesis, systemic anticoagulation, small volume fluid, mechanical ventilation, and cutaneous disease over the proposed puncture site.[22] It is recommended that the international normalized ratio (INR) be less than 1.6 and platelets >50 to minimize bleeding complications. Fresh frozen plasma and platelet transfusion may be considered, given the urgency of the procedure.

The best position for the patient undergoing thoracentesis is sitting up. Leaning forward is not advised, as fluid can shift anteriorly. With the patient sitting upright, the lung field is percussed and needle drainage attempt is usually made in the midscapular line one interspace below the upper limit of dullness percussed, but above the diaphragmatic reflection of the pleura.[2] The intercostal blood vessels run along the lower border of each rib, and in order to avoid injuring these, the thoracentesis needle should always be directed just over the top of the rib. It is recommended that prior to introduction of the thoracentesis needle, a smaller 22-gauge needle be used to ensure placement. A spinal needle may be required for patients with more subcutaneous tissue. Patients who are mechanically ventilated require an approach over the eighth rib at the mid to posterior axillary line. Ultrasound guidance should be used in all mechanically ventilated patients.

Complications from thoracentesis include bleeding, pneumothorax, and reexpansion pulmonary edema. Chest radiography is routinely performed after thoracentesis; however, studies suggest that it is usually not necessary unless air is obtained during thoracentesis; or symptoms of coughing, chest pain, or dyspnea develop during the thoracentesis; or tactile fremitus is lost over the superior aspect of the aspirated hemithorax. In one study, the incidence of pneumothorax was found to be 72% with one or more of these symptoms, and 1% without any symptoms. Reexpansion pulmonary edema is uncommon, even with removal of >1,000 ml of pleural fluid, as long as the procedure is terminated when symptoms of dyspnea or chest pain develop.[16] Most, however, would limit removal to 1,000–1,500 ml of fluid.

Pneumothorax complicates 12% of thoracenteses but requires treatment with a chest tube in less than 5% of cases.[22] Ultrasound-guided thoracentesis should be considered if there is physician inexperience, small effusion, or if the effusion is loculated or atypical.[16]

In certain instances, laboratory analysis of the pleural effusion may not reveal the specific etiology; and further invasive testing with thoracoscopy, needle biopsy, or open biopsy may be pursued. However, no diagnosis is established in 15–20% of patients, despite extensive evaluations.[3,4]

Pneumothorax

In patients with pneumothorax, the physical examination often reveals reduced chest expansion and breath sounds as well as hyper-resonance to percussion over the affected lung. Tension pneumothorax, in which the pressure of air trapped in the pleural space exceeds atmospheric pressure, can lead to tracheal deviation.[9] These patients are at risk of hemodynamic collapse. On chest radiograph, pneumothorax will present with lung collapse and air in the pleural space, with or without tracheal deviation.[2]

Prognosis

Prognosis will depend on the underlying disease process that is contributing to the effusion or pneumothorax. For example, with metastatic pleural effusions prognosis is poor, corresponding to advanced stage of neoplasm. Timeframe can be a few months in ovarian, stomach, and lung cancer, to several years in breast cancer. Survival in patients with malignant effusions is lower with a pleural fluid pH < 7.2, or a glucose <60 mg/dL.

MANAGEMENT AND TREATMENT

Pleural Effusion

The management of pleural effusions is dependent on the underlying disease process (Fig. 46-1). Initial thoracentesis is indicated for diagnostic purposes, but if there is significant dyspnea at rest, then therapeutic thoracentesis with removal of up to 1,500 ml of fluid is indicated.

Most transudates will resolve with treatment of the underlying disease. In CHF, 80% of patients have bilateral effusions, and 75% of these resolve within 48 hours after diuresis is started. However, if the effusions persist >3 days, then thoracentesis is indicated.[4]

Exudates related to infection may require appropriate antibiotic therapy with drainage and in some cases surgery. Malignancies may resolve with chemotherapy or radiation but are more likely to recur and be resistant to pleurodesis. Drug-induced effusions may resolve with withdrawal of the offending agent. Tuberculous effusions usually resolve spontaneously in 2–4 months in healthy individuals, but if left untreated, 65% will develop pulmonary or extrapulmonary TB within 5 years. Treatment consists of appropriate four-drug regimen for TB according to resistance patterns. In the acute setting, corticosteroids are advocated as an adjunct to hasten resolution of symptoms and absorption of pleural fluid and to prevent residual pleural thickening.[4,17] Treatment with broad-spectrum antibiotics with parapneumonic effusions that cover anaerobic and aerobic organisms is indicated until microbiologic results can guide therapy. If the fluid is loculated and drainage is difficult, intrapleural administration of fibrinolytics may be performed if other therapies have failed. Urokinase 250,000 units or streptokinase 100,000 units diluted in 30–60 mL of normal saline solution are instilled into the chest tube and then clamped for 1–2 hours. Thrombolytic therapy can be repeated daily for up to 2 weeks if drainage is adequate, but surgical drainage should be considered if using this method is not effective. There are no systemic side effects of bleeding associated with localized thrombolytic therapy.[1]

When chest tube placement is indicated for effusion, it should usually remain in place until <50–100 mL is drained per day and the lung has expanded. Pleuroperitoneal shunting may also be an option if the lung fails to reexpand. In the severe case of advanced empyema, decortication is often necessary. This is done by anesthesia with single lung intubation and removal of the fibrinous peel that has formed. Thrombolytic instillation is an option for nonoperative candidates.

With malignant effusions, treatment depends on the tumor type, and chemotherapy has been effective in lymphoma and breast carcinomas. Large symptomatic metastatic pleural effusions and >1 month life expectancy can be treated with pleurodesis with effectiveness of the sclerosing agent quoted as 82% with talc, 67% tetracycline, and 54% bleomycin.[2,23]

Pneumothorax

Most patients with an acute (<24 hours), asymptomatic presentation of a small (<15%) primary spontaneous pneumothorax can be managed by short period of observation (6–8 hours) and interval repeat chest x-ray. If the patient and pneumothorax are stable after this brief period of observation, the patient may be safely discharged with follow-up chest x-ray in 24–48 hours as an outpatient (Fig. 46-2).[8] However, patients with dyspnea or secondary spontaneous pneumothorax usually will require admission with catheter or chest tube drainage.

In tension pneumothorax, immediate decompression with needle thoracentesis through the second intercoastal space in the midclavicular line is indicated. In this instance, time should not

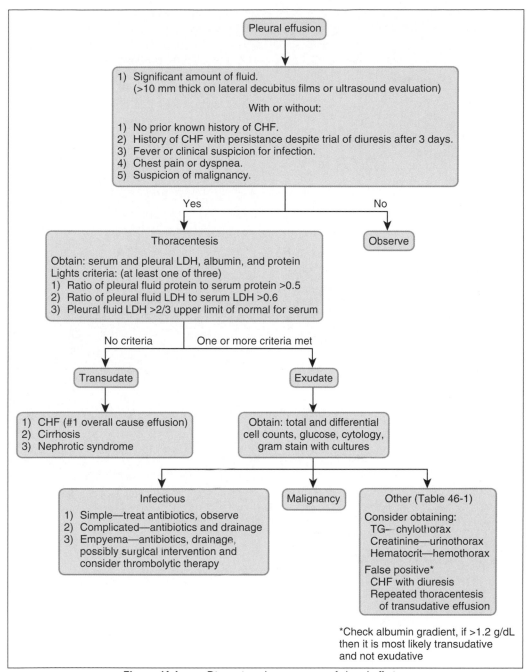

Figure 46-1 • Diagnosis and management of pleural effusion.

CHF—congestive heart failure; LDH—lactate dehydrogenase; TG—triglycerides

be wasted on confirmation by chest radiograph if the suspicion is strong.[2] Furthermore, in cases of associated hemothorax, such as from trauma, recent decompressed tension pneumothorax, patient on ventilator, or unsuccessful conservative management, chest tube drainage should be considered.[2]

Chest tubes are placed for a variety of conditions, including pneumothorax, parapneumonic effusion, empyema, recurrent symptomatic pleural effusions, and hemothorax. Chest tube is placed by blunt dissection in the fifth intercoastal space at the level of the nipple in the male or root of breast in the female, within the "triangle of safety" that is bordered by the pectoralis major superiorly, latissimus laterally, and the diaphragm inferiorly.[2] Upon insertion, the drain is connected to a one-way valve

system, and underwater seal is commonly used. Prophylactic antibiotics, usually a first-generation cephalosporin, are sometimes used in the setting of chest tube placement related to trauma and for no longer than 24 hours, although there are no established guidelines.[24]

Heimlich valves are another option for outpatient management of pneumothorax in selected patients.[2] Other options for persistent pneumothorax include pleurodesis through the chest tube using talc. Video-assisted thorascopic surgery (VATS) is another option. Flying personnel and divers are a special population where immediate recurrence prevention treatment should be considered even with the first episode of PSP, as pleurodesis is the cornerstone of recurrence and prevention treatment.[8]

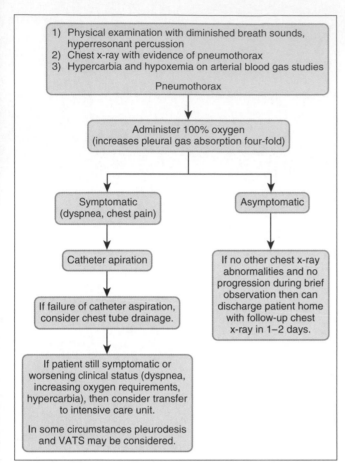

1) Physical examination with diminished breath sounds, hyperresonant percussion
2) Chest x-ray with evidence of pneumothorax
3) Hypercarbia and hypoxemia on arterial blood gas studies

Pneumothorax

↓

Administer 100% oxygen
(increases pleural gas absorption four-fold)

Symptomatic
(dyspnea, chest pain)

Asymptomatic

Catheter apiration

If no other chest x-ray abnormalities and no progression during brief observation then can discharge patient home with follow-up chest x-ray in 1–2 days.

If failure of catheter aspiration, consider chest tube drainage.

If patient still symptomatic or worsening clinical status (dyspnea, increasing oxygen requirements, hypercarbia), then consider transfer to intensive care unit.

In some circumstances pleurodesis and VATS may be considered.

Figure 46-2 • Diagnosis and management of pneumothorax.

DISCHARGE/FOLLOW-UP

Pleural Effusion

Discharge/follow-up will depend on the type of effusion and underlying etiology. For example, effusion related to CHF will require adjustments in diuretic therapy and monitoring of daily weights. Referrals to subspecialists may also be required for further treatment considerations and monitoring. All pending cultures and cytology results should be clearly communicated to the physician following up.

Pneumothorax

Activity recommendations after pneumothorax remain controversial. Certainly, patients with acute pneumothorax should not be subjected to air travel or scuba diving, as pneumothorax may

enlarge and compromise respiratory and circulatory function. After treatment, documentation of resolution of the pneumothorax is necessary, and some have advised postponing traveling for up to 6 weeks and considering alternative transportation for up to a year. Commercial airline and military personnel may require several months before returning to work. Athletes can usually return to their activities in 3–4 weeks, and scuba divers within 6 weeks.[25]

Key Points

- The evaluation of all pleural effusions of undetermined cause should include thoracentesis.

- Not all pleural effusions require immediate chest tube drainage; you should be certain of the cause of the effusion and how it will potentially respond to chest tube drainage prior to placement of a chest tube.

- It is important to understand the relative and absolute contraindications to thoracentesis to correctly determine if the procedure is warranted in specific clinical situations.

- Interventions on pneumothoraces and their timing are dependent on the patient's hemodynamic and respiratory stability or lack thereof.

- Long-term management of pleural effusions must be clearly tailored to the prognosis of both the patient and the ability to completely reverse or resolve the presence of the effusion. If a patient remains stable without comorbid complications from the effusion and is not experiencing significant respiratory compromise, a conservative approach can be considered.

SUGGESTED READINGS

Tarn AC, Lapworth R. Biochemical analysis of pleural fluid: what should we measure? Ann Clin Biochem 2001; 38(Pt 4):311–322.

Noppen, M. Management of primary spontaneous pneumothorax. Curr Opin Pulm Med 2003; 9(4):272–275.

Light RW. Diagnostic principles in pleural disease. Eur Respir J 1997; 10(2):476–481.

Rubins JB, Colice GL. Evaluating pleural effusions. How should you go about finding the cause? Postgrad Med 1999; 105(5):39–42, 45–48.

Antony VB, Loddenkemper R, et al. Management of malignant pleural effusions. Eur Respir J 2001; 18(2):402–419.

CHAPTER FORTY-SEVEN

Interstitial Lung Disease

W. Bradley Fields, MD, MS, and Kevin R. Flaherty, MD, MS

BACKGROUND

The lung interstitium is the space between the epithelial and endothelial basement membranes and serves as a connective matrix for the lung. The interstitium is the primary site of injury in interstitial lung diseases (ILD), also called diffuse parenchymal lung diseases. These disorders also affect the airspaces, peripheral airways, and vessels associated with the interstitium.[1] The pathogenesis of ILD is thought to involve an injury to the lung (environmental, autoimmune, drug-induced, infection) and an attempt to heal that injury. It is believed that the injury results in inflammation that over time leads to fibrosis and disruption of lung function. In some cases, the injury can be identified and treated with little loss of lung function. In other cases, the injury is idiopathic or the disease fails to respond to therapy, resulting in progressive loss of lung function and death. Key factors in the management of ILD include maintaining a high index of suspicion for the possibility of ILD, making a correct diagnosis, and in some cases initiating treatment. An exhaustive list of the causes and current treatment of each type of ILD is beyond the scope of this text. However, this chapter intends to introduce the hospital physician to a reasonable, systematic approach to the diagnosis of the various interstitial lung diseases. Treatment will also be discussed, with focus on those entities that have well-accepted or efficacious therapies.

ASSESSMENT

Clinical Presentation

Prevalence and Presenting Signs and Symptoms

Data are lacking regarding the overall prevalence of ILD due to the vast number of diseases. One estimate from England claimed ILD affected one in 3,500 people in 1990.[2] The most common symptoms of ILD are dyspnea and cough. Occasionally, patients will present with more specific features, such as fever or hemoptysis, alerting the clinician to the possibility of underlying infection or pulmonary hemorrhage syndromes. It is likely that the prevalence of ILD is underestimated, as the signs and symptoms are nonspecific and are often attributed to other, more common causes, such as cardiac disease, deconditioning, and aging.

Differential Diagnosis

The fact that cough and dyspnea are seen with so many diseases makes the differential diagnosis of ILD extremely broad. Examples of syndromes presenting with chest pain, dyspnea, or cough, with or without chest radiograph abnormalities, are listed in Box 47-1. Infection, obstructive lung diseases (such as COPD and asthma), collagen-vascular disease, malignancy, and cardiac disease all must be considered. Detailed history and physical are paramount to narrowing the differential diagnosis.

Diagnosis

General Considerations

Although the number of specific diseases that cause ILD is large, there are relatively few markers that confer strong specificity in diagnosis. There are also no validated criteria for the standard definition of an interstitial lung disease. Thus, clinicians must carefully utilize the tools at their disposal, including the history, physical, laboratory testing, imaging, and surgical biopsy, to attain the necessary information for accurate diagnosis.

The obvious starting point for the hospital physician is the patient's reason for admission. For patients with ILD, this will most likely include shortness of breath, cough, chest pain, and an abnormal chest radiograph. Occasionally, an abnormal laboratory value can prompt admission, such as eosinophilia, or hypoxemia noted on pulse oximetry or a resting arterial blood gas. Patients with pulmonary-renal syndromes may present with elevated creatinine, hematuria, or active urinary sediment. Patients with pulmonary hemorrhage syndromes may present with hemoptysis; however, the lack of hemoptysis does not exclude pulmonary hemorrhage.

The hospital physician should use the presenting signs and symptoms (see below) to place the patient into broad diagnostic categories (Box 47-2).[3] The broadest category includes "known causes" of ILD, such as environmental or drug exposures, collagen-vascular disease, and vasculitis. Also important are the "granulomatous causes," such as sarcoidosis and extrinsic allergic alveolitis (hypersensitivity pneumonia). The idiopathic interstitial pneumonias, neoplastic processes, and "rare or unknown causes," which include diseases such as pulmonary Langerhans' cell histiocytosis (also known as histiocytosis X or eosinophilic granulomatosis), complete the diagnostic framework.

Box 47-1 Differential Diagnosis of Interstitial Lung Disease

Acute or Worrisome Diagnoses:

Acute respiratory distress syndrome, diffuse alveolar hemorrhage, acute interstitial pneumonia (Hamman-Rich syndrome), severe infectious pneumonia

Cardiac:

Acute or chronic pulmonary edema due to cardiac failure, cardiac ischemia, pericarditis

Pulmonary/Thoracic:

Pulmonary hemorrhage, pneumothorax, bronchiectasis, chronic aspiration, primary or secondary pulmonary hypertension, acute or chronic asthma, chronic obstructive pulmonary disease, community-acquired pneumonia, atypical pneumonia—mycobacterial, viral, fungal, etc.

Renal:

Chronic uremia, uremic pericarditis, pulmonary-renal syndromes (systemic vasculitis, Wegener's granulomatosis, anti-GBM/Goodpasture's syndrome)

Collagen-Vascular Disease/Vasculitis:

Pleuritis or pericarditis from systemic lupus erythematosus, rheumatoid arthritis, mixed connective-tissue disease, polymyositis/dermatomyositis, Sjögren's syndrome, Behcet's disease, spondyloarthropathies

Neurological:

Neurocutaneous disorders including tuberous sclerosis and neurofibromatosis, myasthenia gravis, Lambert-Eaton syndrome, myotonic dystrophy, and other neuromuscular syndromes causing respiratory muscle fatigue

Malignancy:

Primary lung carcinoma, malignancy metastatic to lungs, lymphangitic carcinomatosis, primary pulmonary lymphoma

GBM—glomerular basement membrane

Box 47-2 Various Etiologies of Interstitial Lung Disease

Known Causes:

Inorganic Dusts:

Asbestosis, silicosis, berylliosis

Organic Dusts:

Fungi, spores, molds, parasites

Drugs:

Nitrofurantoin, sulfasalazine, aspirin, amiodarone, bleomycin, methotrexate, hydralazine, heroin, cocaine, talc

Connective tissue disorders:

Systemic sclerosis (scleroderma), rheumatoid arthritis, systemic lupus erythematosus, polymyositis, Sjögren's syndrome, ankylosing spondylitis, behcet's disease, inflammatory bowel disease

Vasculitis/Pulmonary-Renal Syndromes:

Wegener's granulomatosis, Goodpasture's syndrome, microscopic polyangiitis

Other:

Hypersensitivity pneumonitis, therapeutic radiation, amyloidosis, post bone marrow transplantation

Granulomatous Causes:

Sarcoidosis; some infections, including tuberculosis, histoplasmosis, blastomycosis, coccidiomycosis

Idiopathic Interstitial Pneumonias:

Usual interstitial pneumonia (UIP or IPF), desquamative interstitial pneumonia (DIP), nonspecific interstitial pneumonia (NSIP), respiratory bronchiolitis-associated interstitial lung disease (RBILD), lymphoid interstitial pneumonia (LIP), acute interstitial pneumonia (AIP), cryptogenic organizing pneumonia (COP, formerly BOOP)

Neoplastic:

Lymphoma, bronchioloalveolar cell carcinoma, lymphangitic spread of carcinoma

Unknown/Rare Causes:

Langerhans' cell histiocytosis (or eosinophilic granulomatosis or histiocytosis X), alveolar proteinosis, lymphangioleiomyomatosis (LAM), pulmonary eosinophilic pneumonia

Modified from: Travis WD, King TE, Bateman ED, et al. American Thoracic Society/European Respiratory Society International Multidisciplinary Consensus Classification of the Idiopathic Interstitial Pneumonias. Am J Respir Crit Care Med 2002; 165:277–304; and Cushley M, Davison A, du Bois R, et al. The diagnosis, assessment and treatment of diffuse parenchymal lung disease in adults. Thorax 1999; 54:1–28.

Sign/Symptom Acuity

To accurately categorize patients, physicians should first try to ascertain the acuity of the illness.[4] Acute symptom onset limits the differential diagnosis. A patient can decompensate from pneumonitis or the acute respiratory distress syndrome and require mechanical ventilation over a period of hours. Such early signs alert the clinician to serious conditions with a rapid progression, including diffuse alveolar hemorrhage, atypical infections such as viral or fungal pneumonia, tuberculosis, or *Pneumocystis jiroveci* pneumonia. Finally, a host of insults can cause acute inflammation of the lung parenchyma, known collectively as pneumonitis. These insults can include oral or gastric aspiration, chemical exposures, smoke inhalation, near drowning, or therapeutic chest radiation.

History

A detailed history is key to the accurate diagnosis of ILD and can often identify an etiology that when removed, results in improved pulmonary function. Potential environmental precipitants must be identified; thus, history should focus on exposures, both at home and work. As the exposure can precede symptom onset by years, past and present environments should be reviewed. Organic and inorganic dusts and other allergens may cause disease. Pet allergens, especially from birds, can cause a similar picture. Medications should also be carefully cataloged. Up-to-date information about drug-induced lung disease can be found at www.pneumotox.com. Heavy tobacco use is seen in the majority of patients with respiratory bronchiolitis-associated interstitial lung disease (RBILD), desquamative interstitial pneumonia (DIP), and pulmonary Langerhans' cell histiocytosis. Hypersensitivity pneumonitis is less likely in patients who smoke, but when present it is often more difficult to treat.[5]

Demographic information and symptoms may further facilitate categorization. Lymphangioleiomyomatosis (LAM) is seen almost exclusively in premenopausal women. Sarcoidosis is typically diagnosed in younger patients, whereas idiopathic pulmonary fibrosis is much more common in patients over age 50.[6] Constitutional symptoms such as fever, night sweats, or marked/rapid weight loss are atypical of *lung-specific* ILD, but may be seen in systemic syndromes, including infection, collagen-vascular disease, vasculitis, or malignancy.

Physical Examination

Few signs on the clinical examination implicate a specific ILD process. Fine inspiratory rales, also termed "dry rales" or "Velcro rales," are common in patients with idiopathic pulmonary fibrosis, while patients with sarcoid will often have a normal chest examination despite severe derangements in lung function. Perhaps the most useful function of the physical examination is to discover features such as skin rashes, joint swelling, or tenosynovitis that may point toward collagen-vascular disease or vasculitis, as these disorders are often more responsive to immunosuppressive therapy compared to idiopathic pulmonary fibrosis. Lymphadenopathy is an uncommon feature but may be seen in sarcoidosis, malignancy, or less commonly in connective tissue diseases.

Laboratory Data

Much like the history, physical examination, and pulmonary function testing, laboratory data, while clearly valuable in the evaluation of ILD, is rarely pathognomonic for a specific disease. Initial tests should include a complete blood count, comprehensive metabolic panel, and urinalysis. Other tests may be ordered, based on the clinician's suspicion for specific processes. Rheumatologic testing may be performed to evaluate for collagen-vascular diseases and would include antinuclear antibody (ANA), anti–double-stranded DNA, extractable nuclear antibodies, antibody to Scl-70 (scleroderma), rheumatoid factor, and antibody to Jo-1 (myositis-associated diseases). Inflammatory markers such as the erythrocyte sedimentation rate (ESR), C-reactive protein (CRP), and complement levels may also be abnormal. When suspicion for pulmonary vasculitis exists, antineutrophil cytoplasmic antibody (cANCA) and anti–glomerular basement membrane antibody should be drawn to evaluate for Wegener's granulomatosis and microscopic polyangiitis or Goodpasture's syndrome, respectively. The cANCA is positive in up to 90% of patients with Wegener's disease.[7] Elevated angiotensin–converting enzyme (ACE) levels are only variably present in 40–90% of cases of sarcoidosis[8]; thus, while often used to follow treatment or disease progression, the ACE level does not confer good sensitivity in diagnosis.

Pulmonary Function Testing

Physiologic tests of lung function are used as corroborative evidence in the diagnosis of interstitial lung disease. They are also used to follow disease progression and the efficacy of therapy. Pulmonary function studies are not useful in making a specific diagnosis or in distinguishing between different types of ILD. Most patients will manifest with a restrictive ventilatory defect and decreased gas transfer, although sarcoidosis and histiocytosis X may present with obstructive physiology.[9] Restriction is defined by a decrease in total lung capacity. This may also be reflected in spirometry with a reduction in the forced vital capacity (FVC) and relatively preserved forced expiration in 1 second (FEV$_1$). This typically gives a high ratio of FEV$_1$/FVC. However, coexisting obstructive disease such as chronic obstructive pulmonary disease or asthma can pseudo-normalize spirometry. Furthermore, poor effort or respiratory muscle weakness can falsely lower FVC, even if lung volumes are normal.

Impaired gas exchange is confirmed by finding a decrease in the diffusing capacity of carbon monoxide (D$_{LCO}$). Abnormalities in the D$_{LCO}$ may precede changes in lung volumes in ILD, especially early in the disease course.[1] Isolated reduction in the diffusing capacity of carbon monoxide can also be seen in pulmonary thromboembolic disease, heart failure, and in patients with mixed obstructive and restrictive ventilatory defects.

Chest Radiography

Patients with ILD typically have an abnormal chest x-ray and high-resolution computed tomography (HRCT) scan. However, a normal radiograph does not exclude the presence of ILD.[10] Findings on chest x-rays are usually nonspecific. Linear or reticular opacities are the most common. They are typically bilateral and frequently asymmetric. Some diseases, such as cryptogenic organizing pneumonia (COP), have both interstitial abnormalities and fluffy alveolar changes. Sarcoidosis can have many chest x-ray appearances, but bilateral hilar lymphadenopathy is evident in up to 75% of cases.[9]

High-Resolution Computed Tomography

High-resolution computed tomography (HRCT) has become the cornerstone in the diagnosis of ILD. By reducing section thickness to 1–2 mm and applying a different algorithm than employed in standard computed tomography, HRCT can accurately image lung architecture down to the secondary lobule.[11] This technology allows for higher sensitivity and specificity than chest radiography in the diagnosis of some ILD. The lack of a need for contrast further simplifies and increases the safety of this modality in the evaluation of patients with suspected ILD. Occasionally, defects on HRCT can be nearly pathognomonic for some interstitial disease processes (Box 47-3). In particular, hypersensitivity pneumonitis and sarcoidosis are often definitively diagnosed using HRCT scanning and bronchoscopy alone, without resorting to surgical lung biopsy.

The HRCT features of usual interstitial pneumonia (UIP or idiopathic pulmonary fibrosis, IPF) are becoming better recognized by radiologists and are used in many centers to diagnose this condition without biopsy. Changes include bibasilar and peripheral reticular infiltrates with honeycombing and a lack of predominance of ground glass infiltrate. A confident diagnosis of UIP/IPF can be made without a surgical lung biopsy when the correct clinical and typical HRCT features are present. This approach has been validated in several studies.[12–15] It should be noted, however, that these studies were performed at centers with expertise in HRCT and interstitial lung diseases. The accuracy of diagnosis

Box 47-3 Suspicious HRCT Appearances

- **Usual interstitial pneumonia (UIP):** Patchy changes mostly in a lower lobe, peripheral distribution. Septal thickening, reticular and honeycomb changes with traction bronchiectasis.

- **Sarcoidosis:** Dominate in mid and upper lung zones with micronodules in a bronchovascular and subpleural distribution. Often associated with lymph node enlargement.

- **Lymphangitic carcinoma:** Irregular septal thickening. Peribronchial cuffing. Thickening of fissures. No architectural distortion.

- **Hypersensitivity pneumonitis:** Ground glass opacification and poorly defined centrilobular micronodules. Air trapping on expiratory scans. Honeycombing can be present in later stages.

- **Pulmonary Langerhans' cell histiocytosis:** Cysts often of bizarre shape, usually associated with nodules. The lung bases are typically spared.

Modified from: Cushley M, Davison A, du Bois R, et al. The diagnosis, assessment and treatment of diffuse parenchymal lung disease in adults. Thorax 1999; 54:1–28.

may vary significantly at individual institutions, depending on the clinical and radiographic experience of their practitioners.

Bronchoscopy

Bronchoscopy has been part of the diagnostic armamentarium of pulmonary physicians for over 50 years. Bronchoalveolar lavage (BAL) is considered a safe and effective means of sampling the airspace for cellular changes. Transbronchial biopsy (TBBx) carries a slightly higher risk of pneumothorax and bleeding (<1% and <2%, respectively[16]), but it is also performed routinely and safely in most institutions. Despite continuing advancements in fiberoptic technology, bronchoscopy has a relatively limited role in the diagnosis of interstitial lung disease.

Bronchoalveolar lavage (BAL) can be used to obtain fluid from the alveolar spaces for cell counts, evaluation of malignancy, and culture. Alveolar white blood cell counts are largely nonspecific in ILD, with the exception of eosinophilia, where an eosinophil count >25% is highly suspicious for acute eosinophilic pneumonia. Other exceptions include malignancy and diffuse alveolar hemorrhage. Diffuse alveolar hemorrhage, which can be seen in pulmonary vasculitis syndromes and some collagen-vascular diseases, can be readily diagnosed with BAL. If repeated aliquots of fluid return with progressively more blood, this is highly suspicious for diffuse alveolar nemorrhage (DAH). In addition, BAL fluid in pulmonary alveolar proteinosis is commonly milky or cloudy in appearance, with visible material that settles to the bottom of the container.[17]

Tissue sampling in TBBx is typically too small for appropriate visualization of lung architecture to allow for a definitive diagnosis of ILD. An exception is sarcoidosis, where bronchoscopy and TBBx are very useful. A small, prospective study evaluated 13 consecutive patients with a clinical suspicion for sarcoidosis. Patients underwent BAL, TBBx, and transbronchial needle aspiration of lymph nodes. Sarcoidosis was diagnosed with 100%

sensitivity.[18] Though larger trials should be performed to validate this finding, this provides a rationale for using bronchoscopy as a standard approach to diagnosing sarcoidosis.

Surgical Lung Biopsy

When a diagnosis of ILD cannot be made through clinical, radiographic, and (if performed) bronchoscopic testing, a surgical lung biopsy should be considered. Whenever possible, a video-assisted thoracoscopic approach should be utilized, with some centers performing these procedures as an outpatient surgery.[19] Although often considered the gold standard in diagnosis, recent data suggest that utilizing an integrated approach between clinicians, radiologists, and pathologists results in higher diagnostic agreement compared to groups working in isolation.[20] This is critical, given the impact of diagnosis on subsequent treatment and prediction of prognosis.

Diagnosis—Interim Summary (Fig. 47-1)

The entire complement of skills at the clinician's disposal must be used to accurately and efficiently diagnose interstitial lung diseases. A stepwise or algorithmic approach should be used to effectively sift through the accumulating data.

- The history and physical examination should be used to first determine if an acute or potentially rapidly progressive form of ILD (acute respiratory distress syndrome, acute interstitial pneumonia, diffuse alveolar hemorrhage, severe infections requiring immediate attention, etc.) is present.

- Based on the initial evaluation and general laboratory data, the clinician should subsequently direct the evaluation toward the most suspicious category of interstitial lung disease.

- Chest radiography should be obtained in all patients. High-resolution computed tomography can be a useful adjunct in diagnosis. When interpreted by experienced personnel, HRCT can be highly accurate in diagnosing some forms of ILD, including sarcoidosis, lymphangitic carcinoma, hypersensitivity pneumonitis, and some forms of idiopathic interstitial pneumonia such as usual interstitial pneumonia/idiopathic pulmonary fibrosis.

- The most common abnormality seen with pulmonary function testing is a restrictive ventilatory defect with decreased gas transfer. However, normal pulmonary mechanics does not exclude ILD, and some diseases, such as sarcoid, can present with an obstructive pattern.

- Bronchoscopy is useful in establishing certain entities such as sarcoid, infection, malignancy, and hypersensitivity pneumonia.

- If the diagnosis remains in doubt after clinical, HRCT, and bronchoscopic evaluation, the benefit of a surgically procured biopsy should be weighed against the risks of the procedure for each patient.

Prognosis

The prognosis of interstitial lung disease is entirely dependent on the underlying etiology and response to therapy. In general, esosinophilic pneumonia, sarcoidosis, hypersensitivity pneumonitis (especially if an agent can be identified), and ILD associ-

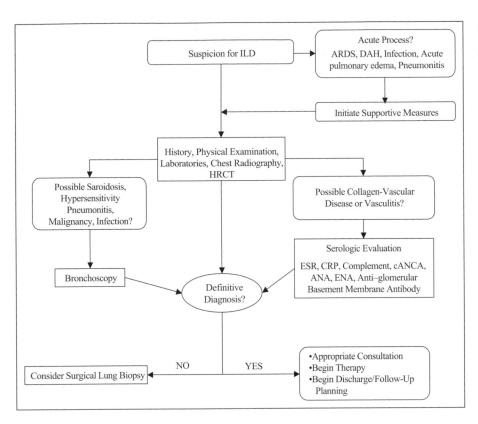

Figure 47-1 • ILD—interstitial lung disease; ARDS—acute respiratory distress syndrome; DAH—diffuse alveolar hemorrhage; HRC—high resolution chest computed tomography; ESR—erythrocyte sedimentation rate; CRP—c-reactive protein; cANCA—c antineutrophil cytoplasmic antibody; ANA—antinuclear antibody; ENA—extractable nuclear antibody

ated with collagen-vascular diseases[21] have a better prognosis when compared to idiopathic pulmonary fibrosis. In patients with idiopathic pulmonary fibrosis (IPF), those who show an initial course characterized by stability or improvement in pulmonary function have improved long-term survival.[22–24]

MANAGEMENT

Treatment

General Considerations

The treatment of interstitial lung disease (ILD) is as varied as the etiologic spectrum. Some treatments, such as allergen avoidance, are quite simple; other therapies, such as cyclophosphamide or plasmapheresis used in treating pulmonary vasculitis, are very sophisticated and require subspecialty care or an evaluation at a tertiary care institution. Once a firm diagnosis has been made, it is recommended that patients be evaluated by a pulmonologist to discuss therapeutic options. A thorough discussion of disease management for each cause of ILD is beyond the scope of this text. However, some general categories of ILD and a few specific syndromes will respond to treatment, and thus it is important to understand the management of these conditions.

Environmental Exposure

An extensive variety of organic and inorganic dusts can cause interstitial lung disease. Several medications can also cause a very similar picture. Avoidance of the offending agent is paramount to halting lung injury. Occasionally, this can result in some improvement of lung function when measured with spirometry

or D_{LCO}. More commonly, however, the changes are fixed and considered permanent. In some, lung function continues to decline, despite avoidance. In these patients, a trial of immunosuppressive treatment should be considered. Other known deleterious exposures should be minimized or avoided, including cigarette smoke.

Tobacco smoke is of particular interest in interstitial lung disease, as it can worsen nearly all processes if continued. Smoking cessation in these patients cannot be overemphasized. The interstitial processes DIP, respiratory bronchiolitis-associated interstitial lung disease, and pulmonary Langerhans' cell histiocytosis are clearly associated with heavy cigarette smoking. Langerhans' disease tends to show some improvement with smoking cessation. A trial of corticosteroids is commonly given and is considered a reasonable approach, although prospective studies are unavailable, due to the rarity of the disease.[25] Respiratory bronchiolitis and DIP are traditionally treated in a similar manner. Some contend that DIP is merely a more severe or later stage of respiratory bronchiolitis. Whereas respiratory bronchiolitis can resolve with smoking cessation, DIP is often progressive, despite conservative measures in addition to trials of steroids.[18]

Hypersensitivity pneumonitis (HP) is a specific type of allergen-mediated interstitial lung disease. Here, repeated exposure to an offending agent causes a brisk granulomatous inflammatory reaction in the alveoli and small airways. Disease prevalence is poorly understood, due to the intermittent nature of symptoms. Again, allergen identification and avoidance are the most important aspects of management. Occasionally, patients are required to vacate their residence or occupation to help control the symptoms. A short trial of corticosteroids is also frequently used, typically beginning at 1 mg/kg for a week followed by a relative decrease in steroid dose.[26] Despite these measures, recurrence or relapse is common.

Sarcoidosis

Patients with sarcoidosis can have a clinical course characterized by spontaneous remission (less common if the pulmonary parenchyma is involved), stability, or progressive disease. With symptomatic or progressive disease, a course of corticosteroids is considered first-line therapy. If the disease continues to progress or relapse, second-line cytotoxic therapy (such as methotrexate or azathioprine) is often considered. A minority of patients progress, despite aggressive treatment.

Alternative Therapies

Patients with ILD who have a progressively worsening course despite standard treatments may be considered for lung transplantation. It is still regarded as an experimental modality. Prognosis for patients and the natural history of their disease should be considered carefully; mortality for lung transplantation at experienced centers is only 50% at 5 years.[27] Transplantation should especially be entertained in patients with UIP, where median survival after diagnosis varies from 2.5 to 3.5 years. However, interstitial diseases with a better prognosis, including COP, sarcoidosis, and HP, should be scrutinized carefully.

PREVENTION

With the exception of smoking cessation and the avoidance of known toxic environmental exposures (such as silica, asbestos, etc.) there are no known ways to prevent the occurrence of ILD.

DISCHARGE/FOLLOW-UP PLANS

Patient Education

Interstitial lung diseases are complex disorders, often with complicated treatment regimens. Patients should understand the following prior to discharge:

- The name of their disease. If patient education materials regarding a specific disease are available, they should be administered.
- Treatment regimen and possible adverse reactions.
- Importance and methods for smoking cessation, if applicable.
- The importance for compliance with oxygen therapy, if applicable.
- The plan for follow-up and contact numbers for questions and concerns that arise prior to scheduled follow up. This should include relevant subspecialty contacts.

Outpatient Physician Communication

The majority of patients diagnosed with an ILD should be evaluated by a pulmonologist. This may be performed in either the inpatient or outpatient setting. If a patient is meeting a subspecialist as an outpatient for the first time, he or she should have all relevant data for the encounter, including laboratory results, any prior pulmonary function tests, and imaging. If treatment has been initiated, this should be communicated as well.

Key Points

- Interstitial lung disease comprises many different disorders defined by scarring of the lung connective matrix and airways. Prevalence, treatment, and prognosis are highly variable, depending on the specific process identified.

- Usual interstitial pneumonia (idiopathic pulmonary fibrosis) is one of the most common of the interstitial diseases. It responds poorly to treatment and has a dismal prognosis.

- Proper diagnosis is paramount to establishing appropriate therapy. This should be carried out in a systematic, algorithmic manner, using the history and physical examination, a focused laboratory evaluation, and appropriate imaging. In select patients, bronchoscopy and/or surgical lung biopsy should be considered.

- Treatment is based on the process identified. Smoking cessation must be emphasized in all patients. A trial of immunosuppression is commonly used.

- Pulmonary or rheumatologic subspeciality consultation (in patients with collagen-vascular diseases or vasculitis) should be sought in the majority of cases. In select patients refractory to standard therapy, an evaluation for lung transplantation may be entertained.

SUGGESTED READING

Cushley M, Davison A, du Bois R, et al. The diagnosis, assessment and treatment of diffuse parenchymal lung disease in adults. Thorax 1999; 54:1–28.

Travis WD, King TE, Bateman ED, et al. American Thoracic Society/European Respiratory Society International Multidisciplinary Consensus Classification of the idiopathic interstitial pneumonias. Am J Respir Crit Care Med 2002; 165:277–304.

Flaherty K, Martinez F. Diagnosing interstitial lung disease: a practical approach to a difficult problem. Clevel Clin J Med 2001; 68:33–34, 37–38, 40–41, 45–49.

King TE, Costabel U, Cordier JF, et al. Idiopathic pulmonary fibrosis: diagnosis and treatment. International Consensus Statement. Am J Respir Crit Care Med 2000; 161:646–664.

Lynch JP III, White E, Tazelaar H, et al. Wegener's granulomatosis: evolving concepts in treatment. Semin Respir Crit Care Med 2004; 25:491–521.

Costabel U. Sarcoidosis: clinical update. Eur Respir J 2001; 18:S56–S68.

Flaherty KR, Thwaite E, Kazerooni EA, et al. Radiological versus histological diagnosis in UIP and NSIP: survival implications. Thorax 2003; 58(2):143–148.

Hunninghake G, Lynch D, Galvin J, et al. Radiologic findings are strongly associated with a pathologic diagnosis of usual interstitial pneumonia. Chest 2003; 124:1215–1223.

Hunninghake G, Zimmerman M, Schwartz D, et al. Utility of a lung biopsy for the diagnosis of idiopathic pulmonary fibrosis. Am J Respir Crit Care Med 2001; 164(2):193–196.

Raghu G, Mageto Y, Lockhart D, et al. The accuracy of the clinical diagnosis of new-onset idiopathic pulmonary fibrosis and other interstitial lung disease: a prospective study. Chest 1999; 116:1168–1174.

Latsi PI, du Bois RM, Nicholson AG, et al. Fibrotic idiopathic interstitial pneumonia: the prognostic value of longitudinal functional trends. Am J Respir Crit Care Med 2003; 168(5):531–537.

Collard H, King T, Bartelson B, et al. Changes in clinical and physiologic variables predict survival in idiopathic pulmonary fibrosis. Am J Respir Crit Care Med 2003; 168(5):538–542.

Flaherty KR, Martinez FJ. Cigarette smoking in interstitial lung disease: concepts for the internist. Med Clin North Am 2004; 88:1643–1653.

CHAPTER FORTY-EIGHT

Pulmonary Hypertension

Jordan Messler, MD, and Allan Ramirez, MD

BACKGROUND

Pulmonary hypertension (PH) is caused by a wide range of diseases. Idiopathic pulmonary arterial hypertension (IPAH), formerly primary pulmonary hypertension, is a rare disease, affecting 1–2 people per million per year.[1] Conditions such as HIV infection, portal hypertension, and scleroderma can elevate pulmonary arterial pressures and create a disease state that mimics the pathophysiology of IPAH. These and other secondary causes of pulmonary hypertension are categorized based on similarities of pathophysiology, presentation, and treatment strategies.[2,3] The more recent classification includes five categories: (1) pulmonary arterial hypertension (PAH), which includes IPAH, (2) PH with left heart disease, (3) PH with lung disease or hypoxemia, (4) PH with chronic thromboembolic disease, and (5) disorders affecting the pulmonary vasculature, such as sarcoidosis[3] (Table 48-1). This chapter will focus on the first category, PAH. Conditions associated with PAH include collagen-vascular diseases, such as scleroderma and systemic lupus erythematosus, HIV, congenital cardiac disease, portopulmonary hypertension, and drug-related causes. IPAH includes familial, genetic, and sporadic forms of PH. This disparate group of etiologies leads to vascular lesions and pathophysiology virtually identical to IPAH. Pulmonary hypertension etiologies from left-heart dysfunction (Chapter 21), valvular disease (Chapter 27), thromboembolic disease (Chapter 29), and lung disease (Chapter 44) are reviewed elsewhere.

The initial diagnostic evaluation of patients with PH frequently occurs in the hospital setting, especially for those suffering from severe dyspnea, angina, or syncope. Thus, hospitalists admitting patients with these common complaints need to understand the diagnostic workup and management of PH, and coordinate treatment with the specialized care initiated by pulmonologists or cardiologists at referral centers.

Pathophysiology

The pulmonary vasculature must accommodate the entire cardiac output, and it accomplishes this with a high-flow, low-pressure system having low vascular resistance. Large increases in cardiac output, such as during exercise, do not result in appreciable changes in pulmonary artery pressure (PAP). However, in PH, structural changes occur in the arterioles, causing blood pressure dysregulation in the pulmonary vasculature. These changes are evidenced histologically by *in situ* thrombosis, vasoconstriction, and vessel wall remodeling, including intimal proliferation, medial hypertrophy, and smooth muscle hyperplasia.[4] Alterations in vasoactive compounds are implicated in these pathophysiologic changes, with measured elevations in thromboxane, endothelin, and serotonin levels and downregulation of prostacyclin and nitric oxide.[4] Available pharmacologic agents used to treat PAH work largely by shifting the imbalance of these factors.

At the physiologic level, these mechanisms cascade into an elevation of PAP, subsequent right ventricular dilation, increased right ventricular pressure, and right atrial pressure; and they end with eventual right heart failure (i.e., cor pulmonale).

ASSESSMENT

Clinical Presentation

Prevalence

The true prevalence of PAH depends on the associated underlying disease. For instance, IPAH occurs at a rate of 1–2 cases per million people,[1] whereas HIV-associated PAH occurs in approximately 1 per 200 HIV cases.[5] The familial form of PH accounts for about 6% of IPAH cases.[6] PAH occurs in about 15% of patients with systemic sclerosis.[7] Those with more than 3 months of previous exposure to anorectic agents, such as fenfluramine, dexfenfluramine, or phentermine, have a 23-fold increased likelihood of developing IPAH.[8] PAH occurs in approximately 1% of patients with cirrhosis,[9] and with a higher incidence among end-stage patients awaiting liver transplantation.[10]

History

Since treatable underlying causes of PH exist, a detailed social, work and family history are crucial, in particular to identify secondary causes of PH, for which treatment of the underlying condition would be indicated. Questions about cocaine use, HIV risk factors, drug treatment for obesity, and alcohol use or other risk factors for cirrhosis can help elucidate an underlying cause of PH. PH may be related to amphetamine use, pregnancy, thyroid disease, and cocaine. Contraceptives, estrogen, tobacco, and antidepressants are unlikely to be associated with PAH.[3]

Table 48-1 Clinical Classification of pulmonary hypertension

1. Pulmonary Arterial Hypertension
   a. Idopathic Pulmonary Hypertension
   b. Familial
   c. Associated with
      i. Collagen Vascular Disease
      ii. Portal Hypertension
      iii. Congenital Heart Disease
      iv. HIV infection
      v. Anorexigens
   d. Pulmonary Venous Hypertension
2. Pulmonary Hypertension with left heart disease
   a. Mitral valve disease
   b. Left ventricular dysfunction
3. Pulmonary Hypertension associated with disorders of the respiratory system and/or hypoxemia
   a. Parenchymal lung disease(COPD, ILD)
   b. Chronic alveolar hypoxemia
4. Pulmonary Hypertension due to chronic thrombotic and/or embolic disease
5. Miscellaneous
   a. Sarcoidosis, histocytosis X, lymphangiomatosis

ILD = interstitial lung disease, COPD = chronic obstructive pulmonary disease. Adapted from the Evian Clinical Classification. Simonneau et al. JACC 2004; 43:5S–12S.

Table 48-2 World Health Organization Classification of Functional Status of Patients with PH

Class I: No limitation of physical activity. Ordinary activity does not cause dyspnea, chest pain, or near syncope.

Class II: Slight limitation of physical activity. No symptoms at rest. Ordinary activity causes dyspnea, chest pain, or near syncope.

Class III: Marked limitation of physical activity. No symptoms at rest. Less than ordinary activity results in dyspnea, chest pain, or near syncope.

Class IV: Cannot carry out any activities without symptoms. Symptoms often present at rest. Patients may have signs of right heart failure.

Presenting Signs and Symptoms

The goal of evaluation is to identify patients with PH before they manifest more severe symptoms such as syncope. On average, symptoms arise 2 years before the diagnosis of PH is made.[6] Early symptoms include dyspnea, exertional dyspnea, angina, and fatigue. Later symptoms include syncope, exertional dizziness, edema, and anorexia. Dyspnea is the presenting symptom in 60% of patients.[6] Ten percent may present with Raynaud's, though not necessarily related to an underlying connective tissue disease.[6] As the disease progresses, symptoms of right heart failure will develop, such as anorexia, abdominal swelling, and lower extremity edema. The symptoms are classified according to systemic lupus erythematosus.

A thorough cardiac examination may elicit many of the findings of PH. Classically, examination of the neck veins reveals a prominent *a* wave in the presence of right ventricular hypertrophy and a prominent *v* wave with tricuspid regurgitation. In severe PH, cardiac examination can uncover a loud S_2, right-sided S_4, right-sided S_3, tricuspid regurgitant murmur, a left sternal border diastolic murmur of pulmonary insufficiency, and/or a widely split S_2.

Differential Diagnosis

As noted, multiple conditions can cause PH (*see* Table 48-1). Systemic signs can be clues for an underlying etiology. Dry cough, dysphagia, and Raynaud's suggest scleroderma. Physicians should look for signs of a modified version of the New York Heart Association classification for patients with congestive heart failure (Table 48-2), stigmata of chronic liver disease, evidence for deep venous thrombosis, underlying emphysema, congenital murmurs, and physical examination clues of HIV disease, such as thrush.

Diagnosis

Preferred Studies

While the evaluation may be conducted in the outpatient setting, patients presenting with severe enough symptoms, such as hypoxemia, commonly require admission and initial evaluation in the hospital. The standardized diagnosis of PH requires a mean PAP measurement of >25 mm Hg at rest or >30 mm Hg with exercise.[6,11] Simple noninvasive tests are helpful to screen for the presence of PH and can uncover clues to an underlying cause.

A chest x-ray may show a prominent pulmonary artery, enlarged right ventricle, and/or larger hilar vessels, as well as ruling out other pulmonary disorders[6] (Fig. 48-1). The electrocardiogram (ECG) may show right axis deviation, changes of right ventricular strain, and/or right atrial enlargement.

An echocardiogram helps support the diagnosis; assess the severity of tricuspid regurgitation and ventricular enlargement; and identify left-sided heart disease, valvular disease, or shunts as possible underlying causes of PH (Fig. 48-2). The measurement of the PAP by noninvasive means is the best indication for an echocardiogram. A systolic PAP more than 40 mm Hg at rest suggests the diagnosis of PH. The tricuspid regurgitation jet is measured to estimate the pulmonary artery systolic pressure. If tricuspid regurgitation is not identified by the echocardiogram, it is very unlikely that the patient has PH. However, mild PAH might be missed on echocardiogram, especially if not performed by an experienced echocardiographer.

If feasible in the dyspneic patient, pulmonary function tests will help identify other PH causes. Restrictive and obstructive diseases can easily be diagnosed, and normal spirometry would encourage a further workup for thromboembolic disease. In IPAH and in scleroderma, a low-diffusion capacity may be the only abnormality discovered.[6] If restrictive lung disease is found on spirometry, a high-resolution CT helps identify parenchymal lung disease. Additionally, a high-resolution CT will identify other underlying diseases such as emphysema. Thromboembolic disease can be identified with CT angiography. Ventilation perfusion scan may show segmental mismatches consistent with thromboembolic disease. An arterial blood gas measurement identifies the degree of hypoxemia and hypercapnia if other causes are present. A sleep study, sometimes obtainable in the hospital, should be undertaken if sleep apnea is suspected.

Serology

Serologic tests helpful in the search for systemic conditions include anti-nuclear antibody (ANA), antineutrophil cytoplasmic antibodies (ANCA), rheumatoid factor, HIV, thyroid stimulating hormone (TSH) and hepatitis serologies if liver enzymes are abnormal.

Invasive testing

The gold standard for diagnosis is a right heart catheterization (RHC) and should be performed in everyone with suspected PH, both to guide therapy and to determine the prognosis. Future therapy is determined in part by testing vasoreactivity with short-acting pulmonary vasodilators. Other indications for RHC include the inability to measure the tricuspid regurgitation jet, the need to perform a left heart catheterization, and to exclude a shunt.

Lung biopsy is rarely used for diagnosis, unless an unknown parenchymal disease needs to be evaluated.

Prognosis

Although PH is still an incurable disease, treatment may improve survival. Prognostic information can be determined by NYHA class, laboratory tests, and hemodynamic measurements. The history, examination findings, arterial blood gas measurements, and spirometry results have not been shown to predict survival. In IPAH, the mean age of diagnosis is 36,[6] with a mean survival of 2.5 to 3 years without treatment.[13] Class I or II patients survive almost twice as long as patients with class III or IV symptoms.[13] Elevated levels of troponin T have been shown to be a marker of worsened prognosis.[14] Additionally, findings on echocardiogram of septal shift, pericardial effusion, or increased right atrial size also are a marker for worse disease and outcomes.[15] The 6-minute walk, a simple test, may also provide useful prognostic information. A 2000 study showed a significantly higher mortality in patients who walked less than 332 meters during a 6-minute walk.[16]

Patients with scleroderma associated PH have worse outcomes than their IPAH counterparts.[17] These patients also have a mortality that is 2–3 times higher than IPAH patients with similar hemodynamics.[18]

MANAGEMENT

Treatment strategies are centered on the use of vasodilators, anticoagulation, and symptomatic management of right-sided heart failure. The vasodilator medications currently available for use in the treatment of PH include calcium channel blockers; the prostacyclin analogs epoprostenol, iloprost, and treprostinil; the endothelin receptor antagonist bosentan; and the phosphodiesterase inhibitor sildenafil (see Table 48-3).

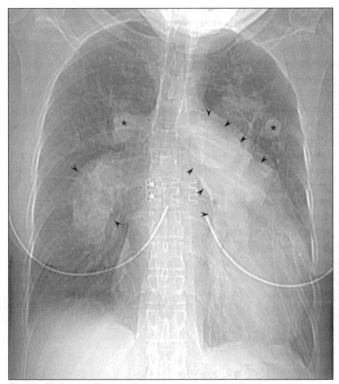

Figure 48-1 ● Chest radiograph of a woman with advanced pulmonary hypertension. There is cardiomegaly and massive enlargement of the right and left main pulmonary arteries (arrowheads). Note the bilateral upper lobe nodular opacities (*), which were confirmed as dilated pulmonary artery branches.

Figure 48-2 ● Echocardiogram. Left panel: subcostal view of the heart demonstrating right atrial dilatation and right ventricular hypertrophy and enlargement. Right panel: encroachment of the interventricular septum from the dilated right ventricle into the left ventricle, creating a D-shaped LV cavity. RA = right atrium, RV = right ventricle, LA = left atrium, LV = left ventricle.

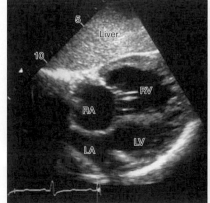
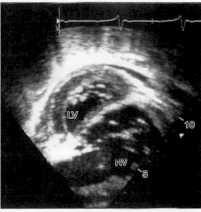

Determining the optimal medical management of patients with established pulmonary hypertension necessitates a vasodilator challenge. With a pulmonary artery catheter in place, adenosine, prostacyclin, or nitric oxide is administered, and changes in hemodynamics recorded. Patients are classified as responders if they have a reduction in mean PAP (mPAP) greater than 10 mm Hg and an absolute mPAP lower than 40 mm Hg during a right heart catheterization, without alteration in systemic blood pressure.[19,20] Overall, less than 10% of patients with IPAH respond to testing.[19]

The relevance of acute vasodilator testing is threefold. First, in terms of prognostication, responders have a 94% 5-year survival, compared to the 55% 5-year survival in nonresponders.[21] Secondly, vasoreactivity testing also determines those patients who experience adverse effects, such as oxygen desaturation or pulmonary edema, in whom the use of vasodilators would be contraindicated. Finally, a positive response to an acute vasodilator challenge identifies a subset of patients who may benefit from treatment with calcium channel blockers.

Calcium Channel Blockers

Calcium channel blockers, such as nifedipine and diltiazem, are used in high doses if patients are responders. Up to 26% of IPAH patients can have significant reductions in PAP with calcium channel blockers.[21] Even when used at doses higher than those used to treat systemic hypertension, calcium channel blockers clearly have much greater ease of use and fewer side effects than prostacyclin analogs.[21] Patients who do not meet the above criteria during vasoreactivity testing (i.e., nonresponders) are at greater risk for sudden death and symptomatic hypotension with the use of a calcium channel blocker. Thus, the empiric use of these agents in patients with pulmonary hypertension is strongly discouraged. With the development of safer oral agents for the treatment of PH (described below), the use of calcium channel blockers is probably best considered as adjunctive therapy.

Prostacyclin Analogs

Prostacyclin analogs have been used since the early 1980s. These short-acting medications appear to lower pulmonary vascular resistance by vasodilation, prevention of platelet aggregation, and inhibition of tissue remodeling.[22] These short-acting medications require continuous intravenous or frequent subcutaneous delivery. If epoprostenol is abruptly stopped, even for just seconds, the patient may suffer syncope or death. Epoprostenol, delivered intravenously, appears to have short-term benefit.[23] Additionally, a retrospective analysis provided demonstrable survival benefit independent of acute vasoreactivity, increasing the predicted 1-year survival from 58–85% and 5-year survival from 28–55%.[24]

Epoprostenol has also been shown to improve survival in patients with PAH from congenital heart disease,[25] portal hypertension,[26] and HIV.[27] Scleroderma patients have improvements in hemodynamic and exercise capacity, but no survival benefit with epoprostenol.[28] The only randomized trials have been in IPAH and PAH with scleroderma. The FDA has approved use of prostacyclin analogs for IPAH patients with class NYHA III or IV disease and PAH with scleroderma.[20]

A very expensive medicine, epoprostenol, costs over $100,000 per year and must be administered continuously. The most common side effect is jaw pain; hypotension, nausea, flushing, and headache are also frequently seen. Catheter-related sepsis has been reported at 0.1–0.6 cases per patient year.[24]

Table 48-3 Comparison of Medical Treatment

Treatment	Indication	Comments
Diuretics	Hypervolemia, symptoms of right-sided heart failure	Maintain euvolemia. Loop diuretics preferred. Spironolactone may be added for persistent hypokalemia.
Oxygen	Oxygen saturation <90%	
Warfarin	All patients with PAH who do not have a contraindication	Titrate to maintain normal saturation Target INR 1.5–2.5
Digoxin	Consider for cardiac index <2.0 l/min/m²	Some evidence for hemodynamic improvement.[33]
Calcium channel blockers	Consider only in patients who respond to a vasodilator challenge.	High doses may be needed.
Epoprostenol	FDA approved for NYHA class III or IV patients with IPAH and PAH with scleroderma. Benefit seen with patients with HIV, other CTD, and portopulmonary hypertension.	Prostacyclin analog. Continuous intravenous infusion. Cannot be abruptly stopped. Common side effects include: thrombocytopenia, nausea, flushing, jaw, and muscle pain.
Treprostinil	FDA approved for PAH patients in NYHA class II, III, or IV	Prostacyclin analog. Delivered via continuous intravenous or frequent subcutaneous infusion. Similar side effect profile as epoprostenol. High incidence of subcutaneous infusion site pain.
Bosentan	PAH patients with NYHA class III or IV symptoms.	Oral endothelin-1 receptor antagonist. Monthly monitoring of liver function tests required.
Sildenafil	Indicated for as early as class II symptoms	Phosphodiesterase-5 inhibitor. Oral agent. Improves 6 min walk.
Iloprost	Inhaled. PAH patients with NYHA class III or IV symptoms.	Prostacyclin analog, inhaled 6–9 times daily.

Treprostinil is also indicated for patients NYHA II, III, or IV heart failure. This prostacyclin analog can be administered subcutaneously or intravenously, and it has a longer half-life than epoprostenol. Treprostinil has been approved in the United States since 2002. Eighty percent of patients report pain at the site of subcutaneous infusion, a major reason for discontinuation.[29] Treprostinil is often used when oral medications are no longer beneficial[22] or when epoprostenol is contraindicated due to its complex delivery system.

Endothelin Receptor Antagonists

The endothelin receptor antagonist bosentan, another vasodilator, was approved in 2001 for patients with advanced PAH. The BREATH 1 study showed a clinical improvement in patients with NYHA III and IV heart failure symptoms, but demonstrated no mortality difference.[30] In a follow-up study of these patients over 2 years, the actual survival over 12 and 24 months was significantly improved as compared to the predicted survival from an NIH registry formula.[31] This oral agent is approved in the United States for patients with NYHA class III and IV heart failure.

Phosphodiesterase Inhibitors

Sildenafil, a phosphodiesterase-5 inhibitor, has recently been shown to improve exercise capacity in patients with PAH. A randomized, double-blinded trial, revealed benefit at 12 weeks in patients with NYHA II or III symptoms.[32]

Anticoagulants

Warfarin is a mainstay of treatment in PH. Among patients treated with warfarin, survival improved from 31–62% at 3 years in a retrospective analysis.[33] The supportive studies are largely retrospective or based on secondary outcomes in prospective studies.[21] Currently, warfarin is recommended for all patients with PAH, to a goal INR of 1.5–2.5.

Other Therapy

Right heart failure symptoms can be managed medically. Diuretics may aid in symptoms if volume overload is present. Renal function and electrolytes should be closely monitored. There is some evidence that digoxin treatment yields hemodynamic benefits.[34] The role of other inotropes, such as nesiritide, is unclear. Additionally, oxygen treatment is indicated if a patient's oxygen saturation is less than 90%.

Antiplatelet agents, β-blockers, hydralazine, and ACE-inhibitors have not been shown to have any role in PH.[35,36]

Alternative Options

Transplantation is indicated for patients with NYHA III or IV symptoms who are not responding to or cannot tolerate medical therapy. Epoprostenol continues to provide a bridge to transplant.[37]

Hospitalization

Patients with existing PH are generally hospitalized when they have right-sided heart failure, hypoxemia, or other severe symptoms of PH. The management of such patients requires the optimization of volume status as well as the exclusion or treatment of any acute medical condition that can increase myocardial demand, as in pulmonary embolism, sepsis, pneumonia, etc. Many patients are admitted to the hospital with infections related to the delivery system of the prostacyclin analogs. Additionally, secondary causes may warrant hospitalization, such as COPD exacerbation and thromboembolic disease management.

DISCHARGE/FOLLOW-UP PLANS

Patient Education

Fluid restriction to 2 L/day or less, as well as reduced sodium intake are recommended, especially as right-sided heart failure develops. Physical activity as tolerated, under the guidance of a physician, is recommended, though patients must be counseled on the avoidance of overexertion to the point of angina or near-syncope. Women of childbearing age with PH should be counseled to use birth control, because pregnancy could be life threatening.

Education regarding the delivery system for prostacyclin analogs is a crucial part of the discharge process. If an intravascular device or subcutaneous device is started, extensive coordination with nursing and the patient and family will need to occur.

Outpatient Physician Communication

Referral to a pulmonologist or cardiologist experienced in the care of patients with PH should occur early in the process. In addition, a multidisciplinary team approach is suggested to address adequately the medical, psychosocial, financial, and dietary implications of newly diagnosed PH to the patient.

Key Points

- PAH occurs in patients with idiopathic PAH as well as PAH from causes such as HIV, cirrhosis, scleroderma, anorexigens, and congenital heart disease.

- The seemingly disparate group of causes for PH has similar vascular pathophysiology: *in situ* thrombosis, vasoconstriction, and vessel wall remodeling.

- The standardized diagnosis of PH is an mPAP measurement of >25 mm Hg at rest or >30 mm Hg with exercise.

- An echocardiogram is an excellent noninvasive means for diagnosis, suggested by a systolic PAP >40 mm Hg at rest. If tricuspid regurgitation is not identified on the echocardiogram, it is very unlikely that the patient has PH.

- PAH is an incurable disease, often diagnosed late in its course. Treatment strategies need to be initiated early, aggressively, and in coordination with subspecialists. These treatment strategies are centered on the use of vasodilators, anticoagulation, and symptomatic management of right-sided heart failure.

SUGGESTED READING

Rubin LJ. Primary pulmonary hypertension. N Engl Med J 1997; 336:111–117.

Simonneau G, Galie N, Rubin LJ et al. Clinical classification of pulmonary hypertension. JACC 2004; 43:5S–12S.

Humbert M. Treatment of pulmonary arterial hypertension. N Engl Med J 2004; 351:1425–1436.

Rich S. Primary pulmonary hypertension: A national prospective study. Ann Intern Med 1987; 107:216–223.

Colle IO, Moreau R. Diagnosis of portopulmonary hypertension in candidates for liver transplantation: A prospective study. Hepatology 2003; 37:401–409.

Bossone E, Paciocco G, Iarussi D, et al. The prognostic role of the ECG in primary pulmonary hypertension. Chest 2002; 121:513–518.

McGoon M, Gutterman D, Steen V, et al. Screening, early detection, and diagnosis of pulmonary arterial hypertension: ACCP evidence-based clinical practice guidelines. Chest 2004; 126:14S–34S.

Galiè N, Torbicki A, Barst R, et al. Guidelines on diagnosis and treatment of pulmonary arterial hypertension: The task force on diagnosis and treatment of pulmonary arterial hypertension of the European Society of Cardiology. Eur Heart J 2004; 25:2243–2278.

Rubin LJ, Badesch DB. Evaluation and management of the patient with pulmonary arterial hypertension. Ann Intern Med 2005; 143:282–292.

Galiè, N, Ghofrani H, Torbicki A, et al. Sildenafil citrate therapy for pulmonary arterial hypertension. The Sildenafil Use in Pulmonary Arterial Hypertension (SUPER) Study Group, N Engl J Med 2005; 353:2148–2157.

Farber H. Pulmonary arterial hypertension. N Engl J Med 2004; 351:1655–1665.

Gaine S. Pulmonary hypertension. JAMA 2000; 284:3160–3168.

Section

6 Six

Nephrology

49 Acute Renal Failure
Gregory M. Bump, Rachel Fissell, William Fissell

50 Chronic Renal Failure and Dialysis
Uptal D. Patel, Joseph M. Messana

51 Hyponatremia and Hypernatremia
David H. Wesorick, Robert M. Centor

52 Other Electrolyte Disorders
David H. Wesorick

53 Acid-Base Disorders
David H. Wesorick, Robert M. Centor

CHAPTER FORTY-NINE

Acute Renal Failure

Gregory M. Bump, MD, Rachel Fissell, MD, MS, and William Fissell, MD

BACKGROUND

Acute renal failure (ARF) is common in the inpatient setting. Roughly 5% of hospitalizations[1,2] and 1–2% of surgeries are complicated by ARF.[3] Acute renal failure exists on a continuum from mild and easily reversible to severe and progressive requiring dialysis. In its severe form, ARF is associated with significant mortality, but even mild kidney injury is associated with increases in mortality. Although the term acute renal failure is often taken to imply acute tubular necrosis (ATN), ARF has many etiologies. Furthermore, the term ATN has fallen into disfavor in recognition of the complexity of renal response to injury, and the term Acute Kidney Injury (AKI) is gaining wider acceptance to describe tubular injury causing ARF. The objective of this chapter is to re-familiarize the internist with the evaluation of ARF and the identification of injury patterns requiring nephrology consultation and disease-specific intervention.

Although there is no widely accepted definition of ARF, a practical definition is any recent increase in serum creatinine above baseline by 0.5 mg/dL. A more rigorous research definition is an increase in serum creatinine for 2 weeks or less of 0.5 mg/dL in patients with a baseline serum creatinine of 2.5 mg/dl or less. In patients with an elevated baseline creatinine (2.5 mg/dL or greater), an increase of serum creatinine by 20% is recognized as clinically meaningful.[4] Elevations in creatinine are considered more specific than elevations in blood urea nitrogen (BUN).

When considering ARF, most practitioners adhere to the time-honored approach of classifying the causes of worsening renal function as prerenal, intrarenal and postrenal. Cohort analyses of ARF demonstrate that prerenal azotemia and ATN account for nearly 80% of all cases.[1,2,5] In hospitalized patients who develop ARF, ATN and prerenal azotemia are equally common.[4] This may represent publication bias, and in routine clinical practice prerenal azotemia is probably seen more frequently. In patients who present to the hospital with ARF (so-called community acquired ARF), prerenal azotemia and obstruction are the two most common etiologies.[6,7] In the following discussion, emphasis will be placed on the most common entities, on outlining standard workup and management for all patients, and on identifying red flags that indicate a need for more investigation. In addition, several rare conditions are presented, as the consequences of missing them may be grave.

ASSESSMENT

Clinical Presentation

Most patients with ARF are asymptomatic from their renal disease and are identified by abnormal serum chemistries. Initial symptoms when present are often referable to another organ system. Symptoms related to ARF may include shortness of breath from volume overload and pulmonary edema, lower extremity edema, or hypertension. Uremia refers to the clinical state associated with the accumulation of toxins and waste products normally removed by the kidney, as distinguished from azotemia, which is merely the presence of an elevated blood nitrogen level. Uremic symptoms include nausea, vomiting, malaise, poor appetite, confusion, asterixis, myoclonus, and pruritus. In advanced stages, uremic patients may develop obtundation, coma, seizures, and malignant arrhythmias from electrolyte derangements. Depending on the etiology of the ARF, patients may have flank pain from urinary tract obstruction, decreased urination, dysuria, hematuria, or dark urine caused by hemoglobinuria or myoglobinuria. Physical examination findings associated with individual etiologies of ARF are described below in the section on diagnosis.

Patients are often divided into nonoliguric renal failure (>400 cc of urine per day), oliguric renal failure (<400 cc of urine per day), or anuric renal failure (<100 cc of urine per day). Patients with oliguric renal failure have a worse prognosis compared to those with nonoliguric renal failure.[1,7,8] Although there is considerable overlap between causes of oliguric and nonoliguric renal failure, only a few conditions are associated with anuric renal failure (Box 49-1).

Diagnosis

Once acute renal failure has been identified, a detailed history and physical examination should be directed to discovery of events predisposing to acute kidney injury. Often, the history of present illness may be adequate to complete the diagnosis by itself: a new medicine, including ACE inhibitors, nonsteroidal anti-inflammatories (NSAIDs), and diuretics may produce prerenal azotemia. New antihypertensives may precipitate hypotension, while recent antibiotics may cause allergic interstitial

Box 49-1 Causes of Anuric Acute Renal Failure

Acute tubular necrosis (ATN)

Complete obstruction

Rapidly progressive glomerulonephritis (RPGN)

Vascular obstruction

nephritis. A history of immobility and poor access to food and water may guide the clinician to seek further evidence of hypovolemia. Recent contrast-enhanced imaging studies and cardiac catheterizations may precipitate renal dysfunction.

Physical examination should be conducted with a special emphasis on estimating extracellular fluid volume. Vitals should be measured seated and standing. Heart and lung sounds should be examined, and murmurs, gallops, rubs, and wheezes and rales sought and identified or excluded. Jugular veins should be inspected with the patient flat, at a 30-degree position, and while standing, lest jugular venous pressure be missed below the clavicle or above the angle of the jaw. Edema may lurk behind the sacrum, as well as in the extremities. Skin turgor is most specifically assessed on the anterior chest and abdominal walls.

Diagnostic studies at initial evaluation should include a dipstick urinalysis, which identifies proteinuria, glucosuria, urinary ketones, and hematuria. A microscopic urinalysis is used to identify pyuria, dysmorphic red blood cells (acanthocytes), and cellular casts. Serum chemistries should be inspected for the trend in BUN and creatinine. The complete blood count should be examined, with a special eye to evidence for hemolysis.

The initial evaluation of acute renal failure should include ultrasound imaging of the patient's kidneys. Except in extraordinary cases, this permits immediate diagnosis of obstructive "postrenal" causes of renal failure. The size of the kidneys will also provide valuable clues to the chronicity of the renal insufficiency. Bladder catheterization may assist in decompressing a urinary system and in measuring urinary output, but it is uncomfortable and places the patient at increased risk of infection.

If dipstick analysis of proteinuria is positive for moderate- to high-grade proteinuria, the amount of proteinuria should be quantified with a spot urinary protein/creatinine ratio. The spot protein/creatinine ratio has largely replaced 24-hour urinary protein measures. The interpretation of this test relies on estimation of the patient's baseline creatinine excretion, which is difficult when renal function is changing. Most patients produce around 20 mg creatinine per kg body weight, or 1–1.4 g of creatinine per day. In steady state, that 1–1.4 g is excreted in the urine and provides a benchmark by which excretion of other solutes in the urine may be quickly estimated. A spot protein/creatinine ratio of 1.0, for example, suggests that the patient excretes a gram of protein per gram of creatinine in his or her urine daily, or 1–1.4 g/day, an elevated value. The upper limit of normal for a urinary protein/creatinine ratio is 0.15, which corresponds to 150 mg protein excretion in a patient excreting 1.0 g of creatinine daily. In the acute renal failure setting, where serum creatinine is rising, urinary creatinine excretion is by definition lower than in steady state, and so a spot protein/creatinine ratio will overestimate actual 24-hour urine protein excretion. In the differential diagnosis of ARF, the spot protein/creatinine ratio is most useful in distinguishing massive (glomerular) proteinuria from low-level (0–2 g) levels of protein excretion that may be associated with tubular injury alone. When significant proteinuria exists, urine electrophoresis is often indicated to distinguish glomerular from tubular proteinuria, or to identify monoclonal antibodies in multiple myeloma when clinically suspected. Urinary electrolytes, including spot BUN, creatinine, and sodium, are often most helpful when measured early in the episode of ARF.

Obstructive Nephropathy

Obstructive nephropathy is common in community-acquired ARF and accounts for roughly 5–10% of the causes of ARF.[2,6] Frequently, obstructive ARF is due to prostatic disease, hence an increased incidence in older men.[6,7] Whether to obtain a renal ultrasound on every patient with ARF is a matter of expert opinion. Most renal ultrasounds are negative for obstruction and do not change management. However, missing obstruction can have drastic consequences. In patients from the community with ARF, obstruction should be ruled out quickly; in hospital-acquired ARF, obstruction is less commonly identified.

Obstruction of the urinary tract is divided into upper-tract disease, including the kidneys and ureters; and lower-tract disease, involving the bladder and urethra. ARF is uncommon in patients with upper-tract disease unless the causative process is bilateral, the patient has a solitary kidney, or the contralateral kidney is already injured from previous renal disease. Conversely, lower-tract disease commonly presents with ARF. Because urinary retention causes direct damage to renal tubule cells, patients with obstructive disease may have renal tubular acidosis (types 1 and 4), pyuria, hematuria, and tubular proteinuria (<1 g/day). Renal ultrasound is the screening test of choice for obstruction, with a sensitivity of 90% and a specificity of 80%. False negative results may occur in the first 1–3 days of obstruction, when the collecting system is relatively noncompliant or at any time when the collecting systems are encased by retroperitoneal tumor or fibrosis. While renal ultrasound is a useful screening test, it is not helpful for localizing the site of obstruction. Computed tomography is better suited to localize the site of obstruction. Postrenal, or obstructive, causes of azotemia are summarized in Table 49-1.

Prerenal Azotemia

In prerenal states, the kidneys are morphologically normal but receive inadequate perfusion. This may be due to an actual decrease in extracellular fluid volume, or a decrease in effective intra-vascular volume, classically seen in congestive heart failure and cirrhosis. The history and physical should be directed at distinguishing true hypovolemia from decreased effective arterial blood volume (EABV), and identifying the cause(s) of hypoperfusion. A history of decreased oral intake, emesis, diarrhea, increased solute loss through skin breakdown, fever, or tachypnea suggests true hypovolemia. Significant renal dysfunction at baseline predisposes to volume contraction, as renal concentrating function is impaired. Markedly elevated blood glucose can cause an osmotic diuresis and volume loss. Similarly, hypercalcemia impairs the ability of the kidney to concentrate urine, and this can lead to dehydration. Signs/symptoms of active infection should be elicited, as any infectious process may also be associ-

Table 49-1 Post Renal (Obstructive) Causes of Acute Renal Failure

Upper-tract disease

Intrarenal
  Stones
  Blood clots
  Papillary necrosis from nonsteroidal anti-inflammatories, cyclosporine, sickle cell, diabetes
  Malignancy—renal cell cancer or transitional cell cancer of renal pelvis
  Obstructed tubules from multiple myeloma (paraprotein casts), myoglobin from rhabdomyolysis, urate (crystal formation) from tumor lysis syndrome, methotrexate (crystal formation), anti-retroviral therapy (crystal formation)

Extrarenal
  Uterine enlargement from malignancy, fibroids
  Intra-abdominal abscesses from diverticulitis, appendicitis, Crohn's
  Intra-abdominal malignancy (ovarian, colon, lymphoma)
  Retroperitoneal fibrosis (idiopathic vs. malignant, radiation induced, medication related from methylsergide, β-blockers)
  Post surgical from scarring or inappropriate ligature of ureter

Lower-tract disease—More common cause of obstruction than upper-tract disease

Bladder
  Blood clots
  Transitional cell cancer of bladder
  Obstructing stone
  Acute urinary retention from medications (anticholinergics, opioids)
  Urinary retention from neurogenic bladder (multiple sclerosis, diabetes, spinal cord injury, CVA)

Bladder outlet
  Prostatic enlargement from cancer, benign prostatic hypertrophy (BPH), prostasitis
  Urethral stricture

Table 49-2 Causes of Prerenal Azotemia

Hypovolemia
  Emesis, decreased oral intake, diarrhea
  Burns
  Hemorrhage
  Third spacing (usually into the peritoneum)
  Solute diuresis from hyperglycemia
  Overly aggressive diuresis

Hypotension
  Sepsis
  Acute infection
  Myocardial infarction, cardiogenic shock, arrhythymia
  Pulmonary embolism
  Acute pancreatitis
  Overly aggressive blood pressure treatment

Decreased effective arterial blood volume (EABV)
  Congestive heart failure (CHF)
  Cardiac arrhythmias
  Cirrhosis
  Nephrotic syndrome
  Severe alcoholic hepatitis
  Severe acute hepatitis
  Nonsteroidal anti-inflammatories
  Intravenous contrast
  ACE inhibitors

ated with prerenal azotemia. Hypovolemic patients may be identified by physical findings of flat neck veins, decreased turgor, orthostatic hypotension, a weight below baseline, and a highly concentrated urine

Prerenal states arising from decreased EABV may manifest as extracellular fluid volume overload. Patients may have shortness of breath, cough, orthopnea, paroxysmal nocturnal dyspnea, chest pain, arrhythmia, lower-extremity edema, or ascites formation. Patients may have an elevated jugular venous pressure, S_3 or S_4, pulmonary crackles, hepatomegaly, ascites, or anasarca. Common causes include worsening congestive heart failure (CHF), arrhythmias that impair cardiac output, and cirrhosis. General causes of prerenal azotemia are summarized in Table 49-2.

The renal response to decreased perfusion is increased reabsorption of salt and water. Renal salt avidity may be assessed by calculating the fraction excretion of solutes that are reabsorbed in the tubule, including sodium and urea. The fractional excretion of sodium is calculated by comparing urinary and serum values of sodium and creatinine as follows:

$$FeNa\ (\%) = (Urine\ Na/Plasma\ Na)/(Plasma\ Cr/Urine\ Cr) \times 100$$

A FeNa of <1% is consistent with prerenal azotemia, while a FeNa of >1% is consistent with ATN.[11] A few caveats regarding FeNa interpretations merit comment. In chronic kidney disease, the baseline FeNa is approximately the same as the baseline creatinine. Thus, in a patient with a creatinine of 2.5, a FeNa of 1% represents a sodium avid kidney and prerenal physiology. Secondly, a low FeNa is not specific for prerenal azotemia. Several conditions (early ATN, acute glomerulonephritis, contrast nephropathy, hepatorenal syndrome, and pigment-induced tubular injury from rhabdomyolysis or hemolysis) unrelated to prerenal azotemia are also characterized by a low FeNa. A common dilemma when interpreting FeNa calculations is the recent use of loop diuretics. Loop diuretics given before urinary studies will elevate the urinary sodium, causing a falsely elevated FeNa. The fractional excretion of urea (FeUrea)

$$FeUrea\ (\%) = (Urine\ urea\ nitrogen/BUN)/(urine\ creatinine/plasma\ creatinine) \times 100$$

has been advocated as a better predictor of prerenal azotemia in patients treated with diuretics. A FeUrea of less than 35% has a positive predictive value of 98% for prerenal states.[12]

The urinalysis is central to distinguishing ARF etiologies. In patients with prerenal azotemia, the urinalysis is bland, and contains no white blood cells (WBC), no red blood cells (RBC), and minimal protein. Tests for leukocyte esterase and nitrates are also negative. Occasional hyaline casts may be present. Patients with a urinary tract infection causing prerenal azotemia are an exception. In patients with ATN, the urinalysis shows muddy brown granular casts with few RBCs, few WBCs and minimal protein (Fig. 49-1).

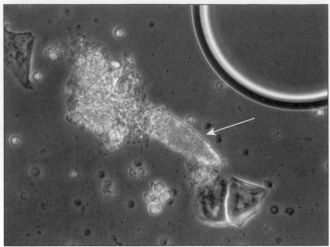

Figure 49-1 • Phase microscopy of a granular cast seen in acute tubular necrosis (ATN).

Box 49-2 Causes of ATN

Longstanding hypoperfusion from any cause

Sepsis

Post surgical—occurs in 1–2% of cardiac surgery and 10% of aneurysm repairs

—more common with long surgeries and large fluid shifts

Intravenous contrast

Aminoglycosides

Amphotericin B

High-dose acyclovir

Antiretrovirals (especially tenofovir)

Cisplatin

Pigment induced ATN

Myoglobinuria from rhabdomyolysis

Hemoglobinuria from intravascular hemolysis

Time-dependent trends in the BUN and creatinine elevations are also helpful in distinguishing prerenal azotemia from ATN. In ATN, the serum creatinine increases steadily by 0.5 mg/dL to 1.0 mg/dL per day in proportion to muscle mass. Older patients with less muscle mass may have slower increases. Daily creatinine fluctuations are more consistent with prerenal azotemia with variable kidney perfusion.

If prerenal azotemia is not identified by history and physical examination, and postrenal causes have been excluded by ultrasound, then intrarenal causes should be considered. Intrinsic renal diseases are subdivided into four categories: tubular disease, glomerular disease, vascular disease, and interstitial disease. ATN is the most common intrinsic renal disease. Predisposing factors for ATN are summarized in Box 49-2.

For many conditions, prerenal azotemia and ATN exist on a continuous spectrum, and persistent precipitants of prerenal azotemia can cause ATN. Consequently, distinguishing prerenal azotemia and ATN can be difficult. The presence of granular casts (Fig. 49-1) makes the diagnosis of ATN. The casts represent debris from injured cells that are shed into the urine. However, in the absence of characteristic granular casts, there is no gold standard test short of renal biopsy, and the distinction relies on integrating the clinical presentation with supporting laboratory data. A few clinical pearls:

1. Steadily decreasing weight and rising creatinine = prerenal azotemia. Rising weight and rising creatinine = ATN, cirrhosis, or CHF.
2. Prerenal azotemia is often associated with a metabolic alkalosis, whereas injury to the tubule commonly results in metabolic acidosis
3. Clinical uremia is less common in prerenal azotemia than ATN, as the tubular barrier to reabsorption of toxins is intact; many patients are awake and alert with BUNs >100 mg/dL from prerenal azotemia. ATN may be associated with altered mental status and uremia at much lower BUN levels.
4. Although caution is necessary in the individual application of the rule, the traditional guideline that the BUN/creatinine ratio is elevated to greater than 20:1 in prerenal azotemia and is closer to 10:1 in ATN can be helpful. Steroids, gastrointestinal bleed, starvation, and hematoma may elevate BUN out of proportion to creatinine.
5. Prerenal azotemia is associated with a concentrated urine Urine osmolality (U osm) > 500 or urine Specific gravity (SG) > 1.020. In ATN, the tubule is unable to concentrate the urine, and the urine osmolality is closer to serum (290–300 mOsm).

Prerenal azotemia, ATN, and obstruction account for nearly 90% of cases of ARF. A multitude of diseases account for the remaining 10% of cases.[1,5,6] The following diseases individually occur less commonly, but in certain circumstances they should be strongly considered.

Hepatorenal Syndrome

Hepatorenal syndrome (HRS) is a complication of liver failure. It is thought to arise from altered renal blood handling and is rapidly reversed by liver transplantation. HRS may be considered a state of profound prerenal azotemia and is characterized by the acute onset of oliguria, a very low urine sodium concentration (less than 10 mEq/L), a progressive rise in the plasma creatinine, and minimal proteinuria. The urine sediment is variable from patient to patient in liver failure, with HRS patients having a bland (empty) urine sediment. Patients with HRS are not responsive to volume expansion or withdrawal of diuretics.[13] HRS has a grave prognosis, and the only curative therapy is liver transplantation. There are limited data that a combination of octreotide and midodrine may temporize the disease course.[14]

Intrarenal (Vascular)

Vascular causes of ARF include renal artery emboli, renal artery dissection, atheroemboli syndrome, scleroderma, hemolytic-uremic syndrome (HUS), thrombotic thrombocytopenic purpura (TTP), disseminated intravascular coagulation (DIC), malignant hypertension, and renal vein thrombosis. Patients with renal artery embolization usually have evident risk factors for embolization, such as atrial fibrillation, left ventricle thrombus, or mitral valve disease. Vegetations from subacute bacterial endocarditis may also embolize to the kidney. In addition to creatinine elevations, patients with renal artery embolization may present with pain in the abdomen, back, or right upper quadrant. Fever, nausea, and vomiting affect roughly 50% of patients of renal artery embolization, and half of patients with renal artery embolization have hematuria or proteinuria.[15] A contrast CT demonstrates wedge-shaped defects, which do not enhance with contrast. In contrast, patients with atheroemboli lack pain and may present as mild elevations in BUN and creatinine. Renal atheroembolic disease typically has a stepwise progression, with a series of identifiable decrements in renal function over the course of several days to weeks. Typically, patients present days to weeks after a vascular procedure, with coronary angiography being the most frequent inciting event. The diagnosis is elusive and depends on clinical findings of azotemia with a known precipitant. Patients may have cyanotic digits, livedo reticularis, eosinophilia, and hypocomplementemia.[16] Urine eosinophilia is found with variable frequency. Renal vein thrombosis is usually a complication of the nephrotic syndrome and often presents as ARF with bloody urine and flank pain.

HUS, TTP, and DIC are a group of multisystem disorders known as thrombotic microangiopathies. These clinically similar syndromes all share ARF and microangiopathic hemolytic anemia. Thrombocytopenia and neurologic disease are common but not invariable in all three. The outcome is quite different between the disorders, and successful treatment requires urgent and aggressive therapy from the nephrologist, hematologist, and pathologist. Any patient with ARF and a microangiopathic hemolytic anemia that cannot be immediately explained by another cause should be seen by nephrology and hematology urgently.

Intrarenal (Glomerular)

Intrinsic glomerular diseases make up a small fraction of causes of ARF.[2,5] A full discussion of glomerular disease is outside the scope of this chapter. However, swift diagnosis and treatment of glomerulonephritis (GN) are imperative. Early treatment can save renal function and may mean the difference between mildly impaired renal function and ESRD. Because an acute GN requires urgent intervention if renal function is to be saved, a hospitalist should be able to identify the clinical features indicative of glomerular disease that prompt urgent nephrology consultation. Succinctly put, ARF accompanied by hematuria mandates a renal consultation if urologic disease (stones and tumors) have been excluded. Unlike prerenal disease, in which the urinalysis is bland, the urinary sediment in glomerular disease is abnormal. Two broad categories of glomerular disease merit discussion: GN (including rapidly progressive GN) and the nephrotic syndrome.

Rapidly progressive glomerulonephritis (RPGN) refers to the clinical setting of a nephritic syndrome (new hypertension and glomerular hematuria) accompanied by accelerated renal dysfunction. In GN, the urinary sediment contains red blood cells that have been deformed by passage through the glomerular capillary (Fig. 49-2). Red blood cell casts may also be present (Fig. 49-3) and are pathognomic of glomerular disease when seen. Patients with GN have variable degrees of proteinuria, ranging from trace amounts to several grams per day.

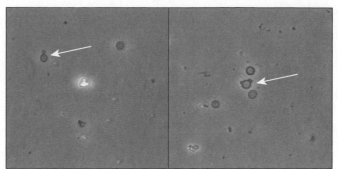

Figure 49-2 ● Phase microscopy of urinary sediment. Arrows indicate dysmorphic red blood cells (acanthocytes) seen in acute glomerubnephritis. Normal-appearing red blood cells are also seen.

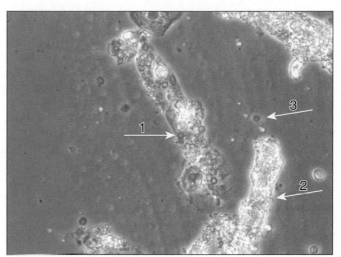

Figure 49-3 ● Phase microscopy of urinary sediment. Arrow 1 points to a red blood cell cast. For comparison, arrow 2 points to a granular cast, and arrow 3 points to an isolated red blood cell.

GN is frequently considered an autoimmune disorder, and rheumatologic diseases weigh heavily in the differential diagnosis. While awaiting the complete nephrologic consultation, insight may be gleaned from examination of serum complement levels, which may be depressed in immune-complex GN, including systemic lupus erythematosus, postinfectious GN, cryoglobulinemia, and membranoproliferative GN, but will be normal or nearly so in the pauci-immune vasculitidities (Wegener's granulomatosis, Churg-Strauss, polyarteritis nodosa), as well as IgA nephropathy, Goodpasture's, and the thrombotic microangiopathies (HUS and TTP). Table 49-3 contains a differential diagnosis for GN.

The nephrotic syndrome is characterized by edema, massive proteinuria of over 3 g per day (spot protein/creatinine ratio of 3.0 or higher), albuminuria, and hypoalbuminemia. Hyperlipidemia may also occur. The urinary sediment is characterized by massive proteinuria but few red or white blood cells. The nephrotic syndrome is caused by many conditions that manifest as three main histopathologic findings of minimal change

Table 49-3 Glomerular Diseases Causing ARF

Nephritic syndrome—Low complement
  Subacute bacterial endocarditis
  Lupus nephritis
  Membranoproliferative glomerulonephritis (MPGN)—
    usually hepatitis C related
  Cryoglobulinemia—usually hepatitis C related
  Post streptococcal, post infectious

Nephritic syndrome—normal complement levels
  Henoch-Schönlein purpura
  IgA nephropathy
  Wegener's granulomatosis, microscopic angitis, polyarteritis
    nodosa
  Anti–glomerular basement membrane (anti-GBM) disease
    (Goodpasture's syndrome)

Nephrotic Syndrome
  Minimal change disease—primary vs. secondary to
    lymphoma, nonsteroidal anti-inflammatories
  Membranous nephropathy—primary vs. secondary to SLE,
    malignancy, hepatitis B, C
  Focal segmental glomerulosclerosis—Primary vs. secondary
    to HIV, heroin, lithium
  Membranoproliferative glomerulonephritis (MPGN)
  Amyloid

disease, focal segmental glomerulosclerosis, or membranous disease (*see* Table 49-3).[19]

Intrarenal (Interstitial)

Acute interstitial nephritis (AIN) is a common cause of ARF and is one that should be recognized promptly. The majority of cases of AIN are medication related. Common culprits are penicillin derivatives, cephalosporins, sulfonamides, and NSAIDs.[20] The presentation of AIN may be days to weeks after the medication exposure, depending on whether the patient is naïve to the culprit drug. The classic triad of AIN is fever, rash, and eosinophilia. This triad is seen in only 10% of patients. Fever, eosinophilia, and rash occur individually in 27%, 23%, and 15% of AIN patients, respectively.[20] Consequently, a high index of suspicion is needed to detect AIN. Additional laboratory abnormalities may include eosinophiluria, a urinary sediment with pyuria, hematuria, red or white blood cell casts, tubular range proteinuria (less than 3 g/day), an elevated FeNa, or renal tubular acidosis. The sensitivity of eosinophiluria for diagnosing AIN is 65%, with a specificity of 85%.[21] The sensitivity of eosinophilia increases with multiple examinations of the urine. The diagnosis of AIN is usually clinically based. If the clinical picture is in question, renal biopsy may be indicated.

Intrarenal (Tubular)

Rhabdomyolysis is the rapid release of muscle enzymes into the circulation. Myoglobin precipitates in the kidney tubules, causing obstructive cast formation. Many conditions are associated with rhabdomyolysis, including trauma, seizures, medications, illicit drugs, alcohol, strenuous exercise, and hyperthermia. In all cases, an elevated creatinine kinase establishes the diagnosis.[22] Generally, the urinalysis will be positive for blood, while hematuria is absent on microscopy, as the urine dipstick does not distinguish myoglobin from hemoglobin. Rhabdomyolysis may cause a rapid rise in serum creatinine of more than 1 mg/dL/day.

Prognosis

The prognosis of ARF is dependent upon the underlying cause and severity. ATN carries a mortality risk of 10% upward to 90%, depending on the etiology.[23-25] Risk factors for death in ATN include advanced age, malignancy, and comorbidities such as diabetes and cardiac disease. The need for ICU-level care nearly doubles mortality from 37 to 70%.[26] Patients with nonoliguric ATN have a better prognosis than oliguric patients. The mortality from ATN from purely nephrotoxic agents (i.e., gentamicin or IV contrast) is lower than ATN from sepsis (10% vs. 30–50%). If patients survive an episode of ATN, the chances of renal recovery are good with over 50% of patients experiencing full recovery, 25% experiencing mild-to-moderate renal dysfunction, and 10% experiencing severe renal dysfunction.[27] In ICU-treated patients, the chances of renal recovery are lower.[28] The time course of ATN is variable and depends on the inciting cause, severity, and patient characteristics. Generally, renal recovery occurs in 1–2 weeks, with a fall in creatinine and increased urine output.

The prognosis of prerenal azotemia is much harder to quantify. Many cohort analyses of ARF excluded patients with purely prerenal azotemia not requiring hemodialysis. Moreover, the number of causes that manifest as prerenal azotemia are too broad to assign risk to this category. Recovery from obstructive ARF is directly related to the duration and severity of obstruction. Patients with relatively brief episodes of obstruction (<24 hours) have an excellent chance of renal recovery. After about 24 hours, obstruction causes progressive interstitial inflammation and scar formation. Over a matter of weeks to months, this progressive interstitial inflammation may progress to ESRD. The length of time needed for progression to irreversible damage in humans is unclear. Recovery from AIN is generally very good, with over half of patients recovering once the causative agent is discontinued.[29] The prognosis of nephritic and nephrotic syndrome is dependent on the underlying cause.

MANAGEMENT

Few treatment options for ATN other than supportive care are available. Treatments such as high-dose loop diuretics, "renal-dose" dopamine, atrial naturetic peptide, and invasive measures of central venous pressure have not proven effective in clinical trials to date. Given that nonoliguric ATN carries a better prognosis than oliguric ATN, clinicians may attempt to convert an oliguric patient to nonoliguric ATN with high doses of loop diuretics. Several trials have investigated this practice pattern and have been unable to demonstrate improvement in outcomes. In fact, one cohort analysis suggests this practice may actually increase mortality and delay renal recovery.[30] However, many patients are still treated with loop diuretics to ameliorate symptomatic pulmonary edema. The routine administration of high doses of loop diuretics to ATN patients is discouraged. The use of low-dose dopamine to treat ATN has also been clearly shown to lack efficacy.[31,32]

In the absence of effective therapies for ATN, prevention of additional renal injury is crucial. Nephrotoxic medications such as NSAIDs, ACE inhibitors, aminoglycosides, and radiocontrast dye should be avoided. All medications that are renally cleared should be dose adjusted. Hypotension should be corrected with intravenous fluids and vasopressor support if necessary. In general, mild-to-moderate degrees of hypertension are well tolerated and should not be treated aggressively. Hyperkalemia should be treated with potassium binders and renal replacement, if indicated. Given that patients with ATN frequently die of infection, invasive catheters should be minimized and infection aggressively treated. Indications for renal replacement therapy include intractable acidosis, hyperkalemia, volume overload, and uremic encephalopathy or pericarditis. Observational studies have not established whether outcomes are improved with traditional every-other-day hemodialysis, daily dialysis, or continuous low-flow hemofiltration. In clinical practice, patient characteristics such as disease severity, clinical stability, and resource availability dictate the frequency of dialysis.

The treatment of prerenal azotemia is determined by the underlying cause. Patients with volume contraction should receive intravenous fluids to normalize intravascular volume, while patients with edematous states may benefit from diuretic therapy, or vasodilatation and/or pressor support in congestive heart failure. Obstructive renal failure is treated with either percutaneously placed nephrostomy tubes, ureteral stents, Foley catheter drainage, or surgery, depending on the cause of obstruction. The treatment of AIN is to stop the offending agent. The role of steroids for AIN is controversial. In patients with AIN that is severe or does not respond to conservative therapy within 1–2 weeks, steroids may improve the clinical course.[21] Treatment of the nephritic and the nephrotic syndrome is generally determined in consultation with a nephrologist.

PREVENTION

The prevention of ARF in hospitalized patients undergoing tests and procedures with radiocontrast dye has been a focus of recent research. Most patients with contrast-induced nephropathy experience a transient increase in serum creatinine peaking 3 days after contrast administration and resolving within 1–2 weeks; rarely, patients require dialysis. Risk factors for contrast-induced nephropathy include advanced age, diabetes, heart failure, hypotension, a serum creatinine of 1.5 mg/dL or greater, or an estimated glomerular filtration less than 60 mL/min/ 1.73 m². A recent review[33] suggested stopping nonsteroidal anti-inflammatory medications, diuretics, and metformin for 24 hours prestudy and 48 hours poststudy. Additional fluids should be given for 12 hours prestudy and poststudy at 1 mL/kg/h IV. A single-center trial demonstrated improved protection using sodium bicarbonate versus sodium chloride, but confirmatory studies are awaited. The choice of anion (bicarbonate versus chloride) should be dictated by the clinical scenario, as the key to protection is volume expansion with sodium. The use of N-acetylcysteine remains controversial, and there is concern that the perception that N-acetylcysteine (NAC) is protective may decrease attention to saline volume expansion.

DISCHARGE AND FOLLOW-UP PLANS

Timing of follow-up is dependent on the severity and cause of ARF. For patients with mild elevations from a prerenal cause, follow-up in 1–2 weeks with a repeat creatinine and evaluation by a primary care physician is reasonable. For patients with more severe elevations in creatinine or severe ATN, follow-up with a repeat creatinine and evaluation by a nephrologist is preferred. For patients with nephritic or nephrotic syndrome or severe AIN nephrology, follow-up and management are essential. Follow-up of patients with obstructive causes generally occurs with a urologist.

Key Points

- Acute renal failure (ARF) is common in hospitalized patients. The differential diagnosis is broad and includes prerenal, intrarenal, and obstructive causes. The urinalysis is essential to distinguishing the cause.

- Prerenal azotemia is the most common cause of ARF seen in hospitalized patients and is characterized by a normal urinalysis and a concentrated urine. In patients with chronic kidney disease, the FeNa is close to serum creatinine. Thus, a FeNa of 1% in a patient with creatinine of 2.5 represents a concentrated urine and prerenal etiology.

- Proteinuria, hematuria, and cast formation are red flags suggesting a more serious cause than prerenal azotemia, and they warrant more investigation.

- ATN is the most common cause of intrarenal disease seen in hospitalized patients. Urine microscopy classically demonstrates granular casts. The mortality of ATN is significant. Renal recovery occurs over 1–2 weeks.

- Despite several recent trials on N-acetylcysteine, the best evidence supports volume expansion for the prevention of contrast-induced nephropathy.

SUGGESTED READING

Singri N, Ahya SN, Levin ML. Acute renal failure. JAMA 2003; 289(6):747–751.

Baker RJ, Pusey CD. The changing profile of acute tubulointerstitial nephritis. Nephrol Dialysis Transpl 2004; 19(1):8–11.

Mehta RL, Pascual MT, Soroko S, et al. Diuretics, mortality, and nonrecovery of renal function in acute renal failure. JAMA 2002; 288(20):2547–2553.

Barrett BJ, Parfrey PS. Clinical practice: Preventing nephropathy induced by contrast medium. N Engl J Med 2006; 354(4):379–386.

Vinen CS, Oliveira DB. Acute glomerulonephritis. Postgrad Med J 2003; 79(930):206–213; quiz 212–213.

Orth SR, Ritz E. The nephrotic syndrome. N Engl J Med 1998; 338(17):1202–1211.

CHAPTER FIFTY

Chronic Renal Failure and Dialysis

Uptal D. Patel, MD, and Joseph M. Messana, MD

BACKGROUND

Chronic Kidney Disease and End-Stage Renal Disease

Kidney disease is a worldwide public health problem associated with poor outcomes and high cost. In the United States, both the incidence and prevalence of chronic renal failure, or end-stage renal disease (ESRD), have doubled in the past decade and are expected to increase significantly in the future. Estimates of the incidence and prevalence of milder forms of kidney dysfunction, or chronic kidney disease (CKD), indicate that 11% of adults in the United States are affected.[1] Both CKD and ESRD are associated with increased hospitalizations, cardiovascular events, and death.[2] Hospitalizations are costly and occur relatively frequently in ESRD patients. Inpatient care accounts for a substantial portion (approximately 40%) of ESRD costs, which were $18 billion in 2000.[3,4] In addition, hospitalizations during later stages of CKD increase gradually as ESRD approaches, peaking in the 3 months immediately following the initiation of dialysis therapy.[5] Thus, inpatient care comprises an enormous share of direct medical costs and morbidity in ESRD patients. Approximately 50% of CKD/ESRD-related hospitalizations are the result of cardiovascular disease or infection. This chapter will summarize the practical aspects of diagnosis and management of common issues related to chronic renal failure and dialysis in the hospitalized patient.

Clinical Consequences of Chronic Kidney Disease

Adaptive changes compensate for metabolic impairments that occur as kidney function deteriorates. Yet, patients with glomerular filtration rate (GFR) below 25–30 mL/min/1.73 m^2 often develop abnormalities in volume homeostasis, medication metabolism, phosphorous excretion, vitamin D activation, potassium excretion, and erythropoeisis regulation. The limited compensatory mechanisms are perturbed or overwhelmed in patients with severely impaired kidney function when illnesses precipitate hospitalization or diagnostic and therapeutic tests are performed. Under the circumstances, hospitalized CKD/ESRD patients may then develop progressive anemia, volume overload, electrolyte disturbances, and overt uremic signs and symptoms (fatigue, anorexia, nausea, vomiting, pruritus, frequent hiccups, muscle twitching, dry skin, pericarditis, peripheral neuropathy, decreased alertness, drowsiness, somnolence, lethargy, confusion, delirium, and rarely, seizures or coma). Even if some reserve capacity remains in the diseased kidneys found in patients with CKD, relatively ineffective compensation is found for hospitalization-related metabolic demands.

Renal Replacement Therapy

Initiation of dialysis is indicated for patients with severely reduced GFR who develop associated uremic signs or symptoms, volume overload, electrolyte, or acid-base disturbances despite conservative measures. Intermittent hemodialysis, continuous renal replacement therapy (CRRT), and peritoneal dialysis are the renal substitution modalities that are available for hospitalized patients. Although a complete discussion of the relative merits of each renal substitution modality is beyond the scope of this work, a brief comparison is presented in Table 50-1. The ideal renal substitution modality for a specific clinical situation should be determined by an experienced nephrologist after carefully considering the prior dialysis history (if any), acute and chronic medical comorbidities, planned therapies and their side-effects, and available local dialysis resources. Each of the renal substitution therapies listed in Table 50-1 provides only a fraction of the average small solute clearance and volume removal otherwise provided by healthy kidneys. In addition, the instantaneous rate of clearance varies, particularly with intermittent renal substitution therapies, emphasizing the need to make coordinated medication dosing schedules, diagnostic test appointments, and dialysis treatment schedules.

Health care providers must be cognizant of a number of important management principles when caring for patients with CKD/ESRD. Medication dosing needs to be appropriately adjusted (including erythropoietin and darbepoetin) for reduced GFR; blood loss should be minimized by avoiding unnecessary phlebotomy; intravenous volume expansion with crystalloid should be used judiciously; supplementation of potassium should be given rarely, if ever; and appropriate dietary prescriptions and referral to a renal dietician should be arranged. These measures will facilitate volume and electrolyte homeostasis in hospitalized patients with CKD and ESRD. Although some hospitalized patients may benefit from maximizing caloric intake in the pres-

Table 50-1 Comparison of Dialysis Modality Choices in Hospitalized Patients

	Intermittent Hemodialysis	Continuous Renal Replacement Therapy	Peritoneal Dialysis
Access	AV fistula (preferred) Synthetic AV graft Percutaneous catheter	AV fistula (effect of extended cannulation not well studied) Synthetic graft (effect of extended cannulation not well studied) Percutaneous catheter	Intraperitoneal catheter
Anticoagulation	Low-dose systemic heparin Regional heparin, LMW heparin and citrate reported Can dialyze without anticoagulation but with increased thrombosis risk	Low-dose systemic heparin Regional citrate Can perform CRRT without anticoagulation but with increased thrombosis risk	None
Urea nitrogen clearance during treatment (mL/min)	200–275 mL/min	15–30 mL/min	6–15 mL/min
Urea nitrogen clearance—weekly average (mL/min)	10–15 mL/min	15–30 mL/min	8–9 mL/min
Fluid removal	Intermittent (48–72 hr interdialytic intervals for thrice weekly dialysis)	Continuous	Continuous with increased ultrafiltration intensity during periods of cycling PD (nightly for CCPD)
Medication dose adjustment[6]	Reduce dose for renally cleared medications If medication cleared by hemodialysis, may need to adjust timing for administration after HD or administer post-treatment supplement	Reduce dose for renally cleared medications. Specific kinetic data unavailable for some medications and clearance may vary by continuous technique used.	Reduce dose for renally cleared medications.

AV—anteriovenous; LMW—low molecular weight; HD—hemodialysis; CRRT—continuous renal replacement therapy; PD—peritoneal dialysis; CCPD—continuous cycling peritoneal dialysis.

ence of malnutrition, most require limits on phosphorous and potassium intake. Although each patient's diet should be individualized, common dietary restrictions in ESRD patients include low protein (<60 g/d), low potassium (<2 g/d), low sodium (<2 g/d), low phosphorous (<1 g/d), and fluid limitations between 1.5–2 L/d.

GENERAL INPATIENT MANAGEMENT

Prior to reviewing treatments for specific diagnoses, a review of general inpatient management for ESRD patients is warranted. If they are not already aware of the admission, the patients' nephrologists and dialysis unit should be informed, because they often have additional information in their own records (i.e., history of recent events or concerns, baseline parameters for weight and blood pressure, recent laboratory studies, medication changes, access history etc.) that may facilitate diagnosis and management.

Admission orders should include notifications to protect the vascular access of ESRD patients. For example, blood pressures should be measured in the contralateral arm to any vascular accesses to minimize risk of thrombosis. Intravenous catheters should be placed only for clear indications and, if needed, should be contralateral to the vascular access site; routine placement may unnecessarily limit future vascular access. If intravenous access is required ipsilateral to a vascular access, it should be placed as distal as possible. Careful monitoring for extravasation during infusion may help limit subsequent complications such as

venous sclerosis. Venipuncture for routine laboratory studies can be avoided by collecting blood at the beginning of hemodialysis (HD) sessions, deferring nonessential tests on nondialysis days. Volume status should be monitored by regularly weighing patients and recording all inputs and outputs.

The risk of nephrotoxicity of many medications in hospitalized patients is considerable. In addition, drug metabolism is dramatically altered in ESRD patients, requiring careful consideration of drug choice and dosing. Although a detailed review of the drugs requiring dosage adjustment is not feasible here, some general principles are outlined. First, consider whether dosing of the medications should be altered because of ESRD. Then, adjust drug doses if required; monitor drug levels and renal function; use the least nephrotoxic drug possible; keep up-to-date medication lists; and be aware of complementary medicines. If uncertain at any time, the appropriate information for dosing guidelines should be sought from readily available sources.[6]

When invasive diagnostic/therapeutic procedures or surgery are being considered in hospitalized patients on renal replacement therapy, careful coordination of care between the nephrologist, dialysis team, consultants, and hospital primary care team is necessary. The following questions should be considered: should dialysis be performed prior to or immediately after the planned procedure? Is anticoagulation for dialysis treatments contraindicated in the perioperative period? Will the procedure require a modality change (e.g., temporary conversion to intermittent hemodialysis after open laparotomy for peritoneal dialysis [PD] patients)? Will new medications be prescribed post procedure? Should the doses of medications be adjusted for low GFR (e.g., antibiotics, narcotic analgesics, some anticoagulants)?

SPECIFIC PRESENTING DISEASE CONSIDERATIONS

Cardiovascular events and infections are the most common precipitants of admission for patients with ESRD. Common cardiovascular diagnoses include congestive heart failure (CHF), coronary artery disease (CAD), and arrhythmias. The management of CAD and arrhythmia is generally similar in patients with and without renal disease and is detailed in Chapter 20. The most common conditions encountered in patients with ESRD include CHF, bacteremia/sepsis, hyperkalemia, peritonitis, and vascular access dysfunction.

ASSESSMENT—CHF/VOLUME OVERLOAD

Clinical Presentation

Prevalence and Presenting Signs and Symptoms

Volume overload may result from excessive interdialytic fluid accumulation or inadequate fluid removal at dialysis. It manifests with dyspnea, orthopnea, recumbent cough, anxiety, hypoxemia, worsened hypertension, elevated jugular venous pressure, dependent rales, pleural effusion, and dependent edema. In chronic dialysis patients, these findings are often most prominent immediately prior to dialysis since patients may not have received dialysis treatments for up to 72 hours.

Differential Diagnosis

Volume overload in a patient with ESRD is similar to a CHF exacerbation in a patient with normal renal function; thus, the differential diagnosis includes systolic and/or diastolic left ventricular (LV) dysfunction, valvular heart disease, arrhythmia, or myocardial dysfunction from ischemia. Additional considerations include acute anemia, pulmonary embolus, reversible causes of LV dysfunction (such as hyperkalemia or hypocalcemia), hypertensive urgency, and pneumonia.

DIAGNOSIS

Preferred Studies

All patients presenting with signs and symptoms of volume overload should have the following: electrocardiogram (EKG), chest x-ray (CXR), measurement of serum troponin concentrations, complete blood count (CBC) with differential, and serum, electrolytes. Echocardiography is generally reserved for patients in whom signs/symptoms persist after dialysis.

Alternative Options

If volume overload is not convincingly diagnosed after the initial diagnostic workup, alternative testing should be targeted at ruling out thromboembolic disease and would include ventilation-perfusion scanning or a chest computed tomography (CT) angiogram (see Chapter 27).

PROGNOSIS

During Hospitalization

If volume overload is unrelated to structural cardiopulmonary disease, prognosis for rapid recovery with dialysis is excellent, and early discharge may be anticipated. However, CHF due to other causes requires specific evaluation.

Postdischarge

For patients with ESRD diagnosed with CHF, an increased relative risk of mortality is present in the 6-month period postdischarge.[7,8]

MANAGEMENT

Treatment

Preferred

Early initiation of dialysis is the preferred treatment for CHF with symptoms from either volume overload or reversible LV dysfunction caused by electrolyte disorders related to renal failure (e.g., hyperkalemia and hypocalcemia). Supportive measures should be administered as clinically indicated until dialysis can be initiated. If clinical evidence supports other treatable diagnoses that may involve additional diagnostic testing or emergent therapeutic procedure (e.g., evolving anterior wall myocardial infarction (MI) with consideration of coronary artery catheterization), dialysis should be deferred until after the procedure or test.

Subsequent

In patients with symptomatic CHF related primarily to volume overload, more frequent dialysis treatments (even daily) may be useful during the hospitalization to progressively reduce total body volume and to define a new, lower target weight than had been previously achieved as an outpatient.

Alternative Options

Loop diuretics may be of some benefit in preventing volume overload in the minority of chronic dialysis patients who respond to these agents.

DISCHARGE/FOLLOW-UP PLANS

Patient Education

Continued patient education regarding adherence to dietary sodium and volume restrictions and antihypertensive medication is important.

Outpatient Physician Communication

Prior to discharge, the outpatient dialysis facility and patient's nephrologist should be contacted to review discharge diagnoses, medication changes, and the postdialysis target weight after the last treatment, in order to facilitate possible adjustment of target weight with subsequent outpatient dialysis treatments.

ASSESSMENT—BACTEREMIA/SEPSIS

Clinical Presentation

Prevalence and Presenting Signs and Symptoms

Nearly 25% of hospitalizations in patients with ESRD are related to infection, with vascular access–related bacteremia and pulmonary infections predominating.[7] Because of its contribution to overall patient morbidity and mortality, vascular access–related bacteremia/sepsis is presented in more detail in this section.

Patients with ESRD usually develop rigors and fever associated with major infection. Rigors and fever that develop during or shortly after the dialysis treatment are an important clue supporting the diagnosis of access-related bacteremia. Occasionally, the only symptoms associated with access-related bacteremia in dialysis patients are fatigue, malaise, or unexplained hypotension. In the absence of a metastatic infection, physical examination is often unremarkable or may only demonstrate signs of local infection around a percutaneous catheter insertion site or tunnel. A permanent vascular access (e.g., polytetrafluoroethylene [PTFE] grafts or anteriovenous [AV] fistulae) may also become infected and serve as a source for bacteremia. Thus, both catheters and permanent AV accesses may be the source for bacteremia in dialysis patients, despite absence of localized inflammatory signs.

Differential Diagnosis

Similar to patients with normal kidney function, a variety of infections can produce bacteremia and septicemia in patients with ESRD. Common sites of infection include the urinary tract, lungs, and intra-abdominal organs (e.g., acute cholecystitis, diverticulitis, etc.). In addition, access-related bacteremia may be complicated by secondary, metastatic infections. Sepsis in patients with a chronic vascular access for dialysis may present with signs and symptoms of a secondary infection site (e.g., endocarditis, paravertebral, iliopsoas or splenic abscess, septic arthritis), particularly when the primary infection involves aggressive organisms such as *Staphylococcus aureus*.

Diagnosis

Preferred Studies

In patients with suspected access-related bacteremia, two sets of blood cultures should be obtained from the vascular access during dialysis prior to initiating antibiotic treatment. Some clinicians also obtain blood cultures from peripheral vein sites in order to differentiate between access-related versus other causes of bacteremia. Untreated access-related bacteremia is often "high grade," typical of endovascular infections that lead to positive blood cultures from both the vascular access and peripheral blood.

Early removal of catheters in patients with access-related bacteremia is advocated by many centers and may provide diagnostic information in addition to potential therapeutic value. Initiation of appropriate antibiotic therapy often leads to resolution of fever and bacteremia within 24–36 hours after the removal of catheters in patients with catheter-related bacteremia that is uncomplicated by secondary infection. Secondary infection (e.g., septic phlebitis, endocarditis, metastatic abscess) should be suspected if clinical signs, symptoms, or bacteremia persist after catheter removal.

Prognosis

During Hospitalization

Vascular access–related bacteremia/ sepsis is a life-threatening disease and the second leading cause of death among patients with ESRD, accounting for nearly 25% of all deaths.[7,9] The majority of these episodes of bacteremia are related to access infection. Early and aggressive treatment is warranted to prevent metastatic infection.

MANAGEMENT

Treatment

Preferred

Ideally, treatment for access-related bacteremia should include early administration of parenteral bactericidal antibiotics and immediate removal of the endovascular source of infection (e.g., catheter, PTFE conduit, etc.). However, many nephrologists attempt antibiotic therapy without access removal to preserve access sites. In practice, maintenance of vascular access for dialysis is enigmatic since many patients have an extensive prior history of vascular access procedures, and some have limited potential access sites remaining. Definitive data are unavailable regarding the effectiveness of such salvage techniques in treating access-related bacteremia. Nonetheless, several recent studies highlight the risks of delayed resolution of bacteremia that include the development of metastatic infections.[11–13] In addition, consensus recommendations support removing infected devices early, particularly in unstable patients and those with persistent symptoms or bacteremia after 36 hours of initial antibiotic therapy.[14]

Initial

Broad-spectrum parenteral antibiotics should be administered to cover both gram-positive and gram-negative organisms. Specific antibiotic choices are influenced by local practice, antibiotic sensitivity patterns, and patient-specific patterns. Regardless, initial therapy should cover staphylococci, streptococci (including enterococci), and gram-negative enteric species. Appropriate dosing of antibiotics requires consideration of reduced clearance among ESRD patients as well as the potential for increased clearance during dialysis treatments, after which supplemental doses after treatments may be required.[6] Since *Staphylococcus* species account for 50–70% of access-related bacteremias in dialysis patients, typical initial antibiotic regimens must provide adequate coverage, which in many institutions now includes a drug with activity against methicillin-resistant Stophylococci.[10] Patients presenting with sepsis should have the infected access removed promptly, particularly if the access is a catheter. Early surgical removal of infected permanent vascular access should also be considered.

Subsequent

In stable patients who respond to initial antibiotics without immediate removal of the dialysis access, several management strategies have been advocated. Some centers attempt to treat catheter-associated bacteremia in stable patients without removal of the infected catheter with 3–4 weeks of antibiotic treatment. Surveillance blood cultures should be drawn at frequent intervals to document resolution of bacteremia. Others recommend more aggressive strategies designed to treat potential bacteria adherent to catheters, in conjunction with systemic antibiotics. Studies of intraluminal antibiotic-lock solutions have been mixed.[13] Still others advocate systemic antibiotic coverage and replacement of the infected catheter using guidewire techniques to reduce rates of recurrent bacteremia.[12,14]

Discharge/Follow-up Plans

Patients with access-related bacteremia can be discharged from the hospital when (1) the bacteremia has resolved, (2) the signs and symptoms of infection have improved, and (3) a plan has been made for continued administration of antibiotics. Often, the patients' outpatient dialysis facility and nephrologists can assist in ensuring completion of the antibiotic course and surveillance with blood cultures.

ASSESSMENT: HYPERKALEMIA

Clinical Presentation

Prevalence and Presenting Signs and Symptoms

Potassium homeostasis is complicated in ESRD patients since multiple factors contribute to individual serum potassium concentrations. Factors include reduced or absent clearance provided by the native kidneys, reduced and intermittent clearance by intermittent dialysis, transcellular potassium shifts by metabolic factors (e.g., altered insulin metabolism, adrenergic hormones, and Na-K ATPase function), additional potassium loads from increased potassium intake by mouth or IV, or decreased potassium excretion through stool. Thus, predialysis hyperkalemia is common in both inpatient and outpatient settings but is typically asymptomatic when serum levels are below 5.5 mEq/L. Serum potassium levels above 5.5 mEq/L can be associated with various signs and symptoms, but clinically important sequelae at any given potassium concentration are variable within and between patients. Symptoms associated with hyperkalemia include muscle weakness, paresthesias, and, less commonly, diarrhea and CHF symptoms. On examination, patients may exhibit bradycardia, hypotension, muscle weakness, and the appearance of volume overload without the hypertension that is typical in volume overload states. Classical EKG changes include peaked T-waves, diminished or absent P-waves, widened QRS, and bradycardia prior to cardiac arrest.

Differential Diagnosis

The weakness and hemodynamic consequences of hyperkalemia are similar to those seen in multiple other conditions, including myocardial infarction, hypovolemia, severe anemia, sepsis, and pulmonary embolus. Paresthesias also can be associated with hypocalcemia, severe hypomagnesemia, and hyperventilation.

Diagnosis

Preferred Studies

Freshly drawn blood is required for confirmation without prolonged venous occlusion during phlebotomy. If pseudohyper-

kalemia is suspected secondary to thrombocytosis, send a plasma potassium level. EKG may demonstrate the aforementioned changes, but a normal EKG does not exclude hyperkalemia. Furthermore, a normal EKG in the setting of potential hyperkalemia should not be used as a justification to defer appropriate treatment.

MANAGEMENT

Treatment

Preferred

Treatment of severe hyperkalemia in dialysis patients should be directed at removing potassium from the body since glomerular filtration and tubular secretion alone are no longer sufficient in dialysis patients. Urgent dialysis is required to remove the excess potassium. Alternatively, administration of sodium polystyrene resin, either orally with an osmotic cathartic or rectally with a suspension, can remove potassium in some clinical situations in which dialysis is not immediately available.

Initial

In patients with symptomatic hyperkalemia, emergent treatment of hyperkalemia is indicated. Calcium gluconate can rapidly antagonize the electrophysiologic effects of hyperkalemia on the heart, but this effect is temporary. Administration of calcium does not change the serum potassium concentration, and repeated doses may be required while more definitive treatment is being initiated. Intravenous insulin and dextrose temporarily lower serum potassium by stimulating intracellular uptake of potassium. The resultant decrease in potassium concentration achieved by this maneuver lasts less than 1–2 hours. High-dose, inhaled, beta-agonist sympathomimetic agents are also effective in temporarily shifting potassium intracellularly.[15] However, while these temporary measures above are being applied, dialysis or exchange resins should be used to provide definitive removal of the excess potassium from the patient.

Prevention

Prevention of hyperkalemia is possible in most patients with provision of adequate clearance of potassium through dialysis, appropriate dietary restriction of potassium-containing foods, prevention of severe hyperglycemia and/or insulin deficiency states, and careful review of medications for potassium content.

DISCHARGE/FOLLOW-UP PLANS

The patient's nephrologists should be notified about the presence of hyperkalemia and any dietary, medication, or dialysis regimen changes that were made during the hospitalization. Subsequently, predialysis serum potassium should be remeasured at treatments to ensure efficacy in prevention of recurrent hyperkalemia.

Patient Education

Patient education is central to prevention of hyperkalemia in patients with ESRD and can be facilitated by emphasizing the

Table 50-2 Intraperitoneal Antibiotic Dosing Recommendations for CAPD Patients Dosing of Drugs with Renal Clearance in Patients with Residual Renal Function (defined as >100 mL/day urine output): Dose Should Be Empirically Increased by 25%

	Intermittent (per exchange, once daily)	Continuous (mg/L, all exchanges)
Aminoglycosides		
Amikacin	2 mg/kg	LD 25, MD 12
Gentamicin	0.6 mg/kg	LD 8, MD 4
Cephalosporins		
Cefazolin	15 mg/kg	LD 500, MD 125
Cefepime	1 g	LD 500, MD 125
Ceftazidime	1,000–1,500 mg	LD 500, MD 125
Penicillins		
Nafcillin	ND	MD 125
Amoxicillin	ND	LD 250–500, MD 50
Others		
Ciprofloxacin	ND	LD 50, MD 25
Vancomycin	15–30 mg/kg every 5–7 days	LD 1000, MD 25
Aztreonam	ND	LD 1000, MD 250
Ampicillin/sulbactam	2 g every 12 hours	LD 1000, MD 100
Imipenem/cilastatin	1 g b.i.d.	LD 500, MD 200
Antifungals		
Amphotericin	NA	1.5

ND = no data; b.i.d. = two times per day; NA = not applicable; LD = loading dose, in mg; MD = maintenance dose, in mg.

Adapted from: Piraino B, Bailie GR, Bernardini J, et al. Peritoneal dialysis-related infections recommendations: 2005 Update. Perit Dial Int 2005; 25;107–131.

life-threatening potential of hyperkalemia and the benefits of adhering to a potassium-restricted diet.

ASSESSMENT—PERITONEAL DIALYSIS ASSOCIATED PERITONITIS

Clinical Presentation

Prevalence and Presenting Signs and Symptoms

Peritonitis develops frequently in patients performing PD, occurring once every 18–24 patient-months. The majority of peritonitis episodes are successfully treated; but refractory, recurrent, or frequent peritonitis episodes often result in technique failure and transfer to intermittent hemodialysis. The clinical presentation of peritonitis includes nausea, vomiting, abdominal pain, cloudy dialysis effluent, and sometimes fever. On examination, patients typically have signs of peritoneal irritation diffusely with guarding and rebound tenderness. A nonobstructive ileus is often present. Leukocytosis with left shift is common on assessment of blood tests. Some patients also develop inflammation at the PD catheter exit site or along the subcutaneous tunnel of the catheter.

Differential Diagnosis

The differential diagnosis of abdominal pain in a PD patient is broad and similar to that for nondialysis patients with diffuse peritonitis (see Chapter 58). In addition, intra-abdominal pathology (e.g., cholecystitis, appendicitis, diverticulitis) can result in transmigration of bowel fauna and contamination of the peritoneal dialysate, resulting in peritonitis that is characterized by polymicrobial growth (e.g., enteric gram-negative bacteria, anaerobes, and sometimes yeast).

Diagnosis

Laboratory assessment for peritonitis should occur prior to initiation of specific treatment and includes dialysate cell counts as well as Gram stain and cultures for aerobes, anaerobes, and yeast. Some centers culture dialysate for acid-fast bacilli (AFB), as both tuberculous and nontuberculous Mycobacterial species have been reported as pathogens in patients with peritonitis. Peritonitis is defined by an effluent white blood cell (WBC) count of >100 cells/mm^3 and should be suspected if >50% polymorphonuclear leucocytes (PMNs) are present on a differential count for WBCs. Cultures are positive in the majority of untreated cases, with 50–70% of bacterial isolates being gram-positive organisms. Most of the remaining isolates are usually gram-negative or polymicrobial, while <5% are yeast or fast-growing AFB.

Prognosis

PD-associated peritonitis is successfully treated in the majority of patients. A minority of cases require cessation of PD with removal of the peritoneal dialysis catheter if the peritonitis does not respond to appropriate antibiotics, or specific organisms associated with poor outcomes are identified (e.g., Pseudomonas species, yeast). Although often treated successfully with antibiotics alone, peritonitis is a serious infection with mortality rates up to 2.5%.[16] In addition to the need to convert to intermittent HD, other complications that may develop include sclerosing

Table 50-3 Intermittent Dosing of Antibiotics in Automated Peritoneal Dialysis

Drug	IP dose
Vancomycin	Loading dose 30 mg/kg IP in long dwell, repeat dosing 15 mg/kg IP in long dwell every 3–5 days, following levels
Cefazolin	20 mg/kg IP every day, in long day dwell
Tobramycin	Loading dose 1.5 mg/kg IP in long dwell, then 0.5 mg/kg IP each day in long day dwell
Fluconazole	200 mg IP in one exchange per day every 24–48 hours
Cefepime	1 g IP in one exchange per day

IP = intraperitoneal.

Adapted from: Piraino B, Bailie GR, Bernardini J, et al. Peritoneal dialysis-related infections recommendations: 2005 update. Perit Dial Int 2005; 25:107–111.

peritonitis, abdominal abscess, and recurrent or relapsing peritonitis.

MANAGEMENT

Treatment

Initial

Following collection of fluid for diagnostic testing, 2–3 rapid exchanges of dialysate often provide early pain relief. Patients should then receive parenteral antibiotics that provide coverage for both gram-positive and gram-negative organisms.[17] Specific regimens vary by center but often utilize either intraperitoneal (IP) cefazolin or vancomycin, and additionally, a second IP or oral antibiotic with gram-negative coverage (e.g., ceftazidime, aminoglycoside or fluoroquinolone) (see Tables 50-2 and 50-3 for specific dosing). Narcotic analgesics often provide pain relief; however, some patients will require hospitalization for pain control with intravenous medications or management of an ileus.

Subsequent

Antibiotic treatment regimens for peritonitis are usually narrowed after day 3–4 of therapy when dialysis effluent culture results become available. Successful antibiotic treatment of PD-associated peritonitis typically results in early symptomatic improvement in 2–3 days and resolution of cloudy dialysate and abdominal pain in 3–5 days. Removal of the PD catheter should be considered if clinical symptoms persist, if cultures of dialysis effluent remain positive, or if inflammation persists or worsens after 4–5 days.

DISCHARGE/FOLLOW-UP PLANS

Prior to discharge, the patient's dialysis facility should be contacted to arrange for continued antibiotic administration and follow-up assessment, including cell counts and cultures of the PD effluent. Treatment duration of 10–14 days is usually adequate for uncomplicated peritonitis, which responds rapidly to initial antibiotics.

Patient Education

Patient re-education regarding basic sterile technique can sometimes prevent recurrences of peritonitis since some episodes of peritonitis are the direct result of a failure of sterile technique with contamination of the luminal surface of the PD tubing.

Outpatient Physician Communication

Prior to discharge, the outpatient treating nephrologists should be contacted to confirm the duration of treatment, choice of antibiotics, and understanding of their responsibility for obtaining follow-up cultures and cell counts.

Key Points

- Among patients with CKD or ESRD, medication dosing needs to be appropriately adjusted for reduced glomerular filtration rate (GFR); blood loss should be minimized by avoiding unnecessary phlebotomy; intravenous volume expansion with crystalloid should be used judiciously; supplementation of potassium should be given rarely, if ever; and appropriate dietary prescriptions and referral to a renal dietician should be arranged.

- Although each patient's diet should be individualized, common dietary restrictions in ESRD patients include low protein (<60 g/d), low potassium (<2 g/d), low sodium (<2 g/d), low phosphorous (<1 g/d), and fluid limitations between 1.5–2 L/d.

- Prior to discharge, the outpatient dialysis facility and patient's nephrologist should be contacted to review discharge diagnoses, medication changes, and the postdialysis target weight after the last treatment in order to facilitate possible adjustment of target weight with subsequent outpatient dialysis treatments.

- Vascular access–related bacteremia/sepsis is a life-threatening disease and the second leading cause of death among patients with ESRD, warranting early and aggressive treatment to prevent metastatic infection.

- Symptomatic hyperkalemia requires emergent treatment with calcium gluconate, which can rapidly antagonize the electrophysiologic effects of hyperkalemia on the heart; however, this effect is temporary.

- Treatment of severe hyperkalemia in dialysis patients should be directed at removing potassium from the body since glomerular filtration and tubular secretion alone are no longer sufficient in dialysis patients—urgent dialysis is required to remove the excess potassium.

SUGGESTED READING

National Kidney Foundation. Clinical practice guidelines for chronic kidney disease: evaluation, classification, and stratification. Am J Kidney Dis 2002; 39(Suppl 1):S1–S266.

Go AS, Chertow GM, Fan D, et al. Chronic kidney disease and the risks of death, cardiovascular events, and hospitalization. N Engl J Med 2004; 351(13):1296–1305.

Mix TC, St. Peter WL, Ebben J, et al. Hospitalization during advancing chronic kidney disease. Am J Kidney Dis 2003; 42(5):972–981.

Aranoff GR, Berns JS, Brier ME, et al. Drug prescribing in renal failure: Dosing guidelines for adults. American College of Physicians, Philadelphia, 1999.

Allon M. Dialysis catheter-related bacteremia: Treatment and prophylaxis. Am J Kidney Dis 2004; 44(5):779–791.

Piraino B, Bailie GR, Bernardini J, et al. Peritoneal dialysis-related infections recommendations: 2005 update. Perit Dial Int 2005; 25(2):107–131.

CHAPTER FIFTY-ONE

Hyponatremia and Hypernatremia

David H. Wesorick, MD, and Robert M. Centor, MD

HYPONATREMIA

Background

Although hyponatremia and hypernatremia are recognized clinically as derangements of the serum sodium level, they actually represent defects of *water homeostasis*. Therefore, serum hyponatremia represents extracellular water excess, while serum hypernatremia represents a deficiency of extracellular water. Extracellular fluid volume is determined, in large part, by the amount of sodium in the extracellular space. However, hyponatremia and hypernatremia can occur in the presence of any of the states of sodium balance (hypovolemia, euvolemia, or hypervolemia). Since sodium is the major extracellular solute, derangements in serum sodium levels are of clinical concern because they often represent abnormalities in the osmolality of the extracellular fluid compartment, which can manifest clinically as neurologic dysfunction.

The clinical management of these disorders demands an understanding of the physiology of water homeostasis.[1,2] Serum hyperosmolality normally results in increased water intake (via the thirst mechanism) and increased levels of circulating antidiuretic hormone (ADH), which results in renal water retention. Conversely, serum hypo-osmolality normally results in decreased levels of circulating ADH, which enables renal excretion of water. Physiologic control of extracellular fluid volume (sodium balance, mainly via the renin-angiotensin-aldosterone system) and the control of extracellular osmolality (water balance, mainly via the ADH system) are not entirely separate. For example, hypovolemia (or ineffective circulating blood volume) also results in the secretion of ADH via stimulation of baroreceptors. Although this response does increase extracellular fluid volume, it does so at the expense of appropriate control of extracellular fluid osmolality, and complicates the clinical approach to hyponatremia.

Hyponatremia occurs in up to 6% of hospitalized patients.[24] Although many different disease processes can result in hyponatremia, most of these do so via a few common mechanisms. Most instances of hypo-osmolar hyponatremia are caused by the intake of water in excess of what can be excreted by the kidney. Although massive free water ingestions can overwhelm the excretory capacity of the normally functioning kidneys, more often, hyponatremia results from lesser ingestions of water coupled with either diminished renal function or excessive ADH effect.

Assessment

Clinical Presentation

Acute hyponatremia results in cerebral edema, which is often symptomatic. Chronic hyponatremia is more likely to be asymptomatic or only mildly symptomatic, with cerebral edema being less common secondary to neuronal adaptation (by lowering intracellular osmoles). The clinical presentation can range from early findings of nausea or malaise to more severe symptoms of headache, and altered mental status, including confusion, lethargy, and obtundation. The most severe effects of hyponatremia are coma with respiratory compromise and seizures, which usually occur in association with sodium levels less than 120 mEq/L, although symptoms can occur at higher sodium levels if the hyponatremia occurs rapidly.

In addition to elucidating these symptoms, a complete history in a hyponatremic patient should include a thorough medical history and review of systems emphasizing an assessment of volume status and recent water intake (including questions about nausea, vomiting, change in oral intake, diet, diarrhea or other fluid loss, blood loss, edema, or history of edematous states such as congestive heart failure, nephrosis, cirrhosis, or renal failure), an assessment of the patient's medications and drug history (including alcohol use and illicit drug use), and elucidation of possible pregnancy, signs of malignancy (weight loss, pain), or other pulmonary or neurologic disorders that might be associated with the syndrome of inappropriate ADH secretion.

The physical examination should include a complete neurologic examination, assessing the severity of neurologic compromise and ability of the patient to maintain the airway. The neurologic examination should also assess for signs of focal defects that might result from hyponatremia alone, but would also raise the question of an underlying primary neurologic defect (e.g., stroke, CNS neoplasm, etc.). In addition, signs of seizure might be recognized (signs of mouth, tongue, or other trauma). One critical aspect of the physical examination in the hyponatremia patient is the assessment of extracellular volume status. This should include an assessment of edema, jugular venous pressure, skin turgor, and resting and orthostatic vital signs.

Diagnosis/Differential Diagnosis

The diagnosis of hyponatremia is based on simple serum laboratory testing. Most of the diagnostic effort is, therefore, directed at characterizing the type of hyponatremia and its etiology. Table 51-1 presents the steps involved in the diagnosis of hyponatremia.[1,2,3]

Since sodium is the primary extracellular osmole, hyponatremia usually indicates a hypo-osmolar state. However, there are some instances when hyponatremia occurs in the setting of an elevated or normal serum osmolality. Pseudohyponatremia is the term used to describe the hyponatremia in these situations.

When pseudohyponatremia occurs in the setting of hyperosmolality, it is because of the presence of a nonsodium osmole. Hyperglycemia is the most common example of this. In hyperosmolar states caused by nonsodium osmoles, extracellular sodium levels decrease as water moves by osmosis out of the intracellular space. In the example of hyperglycemia, the fall in serum sodium is predictable. The commonly used formula is as follows: For every increment of 100 mg/dL that the plasma glucose rises above the normal level, the serum sodium measurement is expected to decrease by 1.6 mEq/L. More recent research suggests that this formula is accurate at plasma glucose levels <400 mg/dL, but that the conversion factor should be 2.4 mEq/L for each 100 mg/dL increment of glucose for plasma glucose levels >400 mg/dL.[4] It is important to recognize that patients with severe hyperglycemia can actually have a water deficit, despite a low serum sodium measurement, which may alter fluid management in these patients. Other causes of hyperosmolar pseudohyponatremia are listed in Table 51-1.

Table 51-1 A Stepwise Approach to the Diagnosis of Hyponatremia

Step 1. Measure serum osmolality to exclude pseudohyponatremia.
- Serum osmolality that is normal or high suggests pseudohyponatremia
  - In pseudohyponatremia, the serum osmolality can be high

    EXAMPLES: Hyperglycemia, administration of hypertonic mannitol, accumulation of maltose secondary to use of intravenous immunoglobulin in renal failure, radiocontrast administration in dialysis patients[8]

  - In pseudohyponatremia, the serum osmolality can be normal

    EXAMPLES: Hyperlipidemia or hyperproteinemia, administration of isotonic, non-sodium containing fluids (e.g., containing mannitol, glycine, sorbitol, etc.) including use as irrigants during surgery[#] (e.g., transurethral resection of the prostate, hysteroscopy)

- Serum osmolality that is low is consistent with hypo-osmolar hyponatremia (see below)

Step 2. Assess volume status and urine sodium concentration.
- Hypovolemia: Clinical signs of volume depletion, including tachycardia, hypotension, orthostatic vital signs, flat neck veins, decreased skin turgor, dry mucous membranes
  - In hypovolemia, the urine sodium can be low (<25 mEq/L) because of physiologic sodium avidity

    EXAMPLES: Diarrhea, third space fluid losses, blood loss, and other causes of hypovolemia not mentioned below

  - In hypovolemia, the urine sodium can be high (>40 mEq/L)

    EXAMPLES: Hypovolemia secondary to renal sodium losses, including ongoing diuretic effect (not usually seen with the thiazides), osmotic diuresis, mineralocorticoid deficiency, renal salt wasting related to intrinsic kidney disease (e.g., cystic diseases, analgesic nephropathy, obstructive uropathy) or cerebral salt wasting. Also high urine sodium can be an artifact of advanced renal failure or related to bicarbinaturia (resulting from upper gastrointestinal losses of acid such as vomiting or gastric drainage, or a proximal renal tubular acidosis).

- Hypervolemia: Clinical signs of volume overload, urine sodium usually <25 mEq/L (except in renal failure)

  EXAMPLES: States of ineffective circulating blood volume such as congestive heart failure or cirrhosis. Also nephrosis, renal failure.

- Euvolemia: See step 3

Step 3. In euvolemic hyponatremia, exclude hypothyroidism, adrenal insufficiency, and pregnancy with appropriate laboratory testing.

Step 4. Measure urine osmolality to exclude disorders associated with dilute urine.
- Urine osmolality < 100*

  EXAMPLES: Psychogenic polydipsia, iatrogenic water excess, low solute intake ("Beer drinker's potomania" or "tea and toast diet")

- Urine osmolality > 100: See step 5

Step 5. Suspect SIADH: Measure urine sodium (which is usually >40 mEq/L in SIADH) and serum uric acid (which is usually <4 mg/dL in SIADH).
- Common hospital disorders that stimulate ADH

  EXAMPLES: pain, surgery, severe nausea, emotional stress

- SIADH related to drugs or other conditions (see Table 51-2)

*Urine osmolality in these disorders may be higher in the presence of underlying kidney disease.

#Although the hyponatremia in these cases may be initially iso-osmolar, metabolism of the solute can result in a true water excess (true hyponatremia).

Pseudohyponatremia can also be associated with a normal serum osmolality. These cases are usually due to the administration of isotonic, nonsodium-containing fluids, or a laboratory artifact secondary to abnormal serum constituents. A patient might absorb a large amount of isotonic or slightly hypotonic fluid during a transurethral resection of the prostate or a hysteroscopy, in which these solutions are often used in large amounts for irrigation.[1,5,6] Although the initial serum osmolality in these cases will be normal, metabolism of the infused solute can lead to a true water excess. Iso-osmolar pseudohyponatremia can also result from cases of severe hyperlipidemia (usually hypertriglyceridemia) or paraproteinemia, in which the large volume of displaced plasma water results in the measurement of an artifactually low serum sodium. Modern analyzers often employ a direct, ion-specific electrode that eliminates this artifact, but there are still some laboratories that use older techniques (e.g., flame photometry or indirect electrodes) where this type of pseudohyponatremia still may occur.[7]

If the measured serum osmolality is low, then pseudohyponatremia is ruled out, and the evaluation can proceed.

When evaluating hypo-osmolar hyponatremia, assessment of the patient's volume status is very helpful in accurately classifying the etiology. Patients can be identified as hypervolemic, hypovolemic, or euvolemic by clinical assessment. The urine sodium helps to fine-tune this classification by assessing renal sodium avidity (*see* Table 51-1).

Hypovolemic Hyponatremia

Hypovolemic hypo-osmolar hyponatremia occurs as a result of the physiologic release of ADH in response to hypovolemia.

Hypovolemic hyponatremia can be further divided according to the concentration of sodium in the urine. Intravascular volume depletion causes renal sodium avidity and low urine sodium concentrations. However, there are some hypovolemic states that are accompanied by an elevated urine sodium.[1,9] Examples are listed in Table 51-1.

One disorder of renal sodium wasting deserves special mention. Cerebral salt wasting is a condition in which an intracranial process is thought to act as a stimulus (perhaps via release of a natriuretic substance) for renal wasting of sodium.[10,11] The syndrome has been described in association with intracranial hemorrhage, intracranial neoplasm, brain surgery (including transphenoidal), brain trauma, and tuberculous meningitis. Cerebral salt wasting causes renal sodium losses and results in volume depletion, which causes ADH release and hyponatremia. The hyponatremia in these cases is often wrongly attributed to the syndrome of inappropriate secretion of ADH (SIADH), which is also a common accompaniment of intracranial disease. In practice, the best distinguishing characteristic between these two disorders is the extracellular fluid volume, which should be normal (or slightly expanded) in SIADH, but depleted in cerebral salt wasting. The distinction is important because treatment for SIADH often includes fluid restriction while the treatment of cerebral salt wasting usually mandates aggressive administration of saline.

Hypervolemic Hyponatremia

Hypervolemic hypo-osmolar hyponatremia is, physiologically, very similar to hypovolemic hyponatremia. Patients with congestive heart failure and cirrhosis have ineffective circulating blood volume. In these cases, hyponatremia results from the activation of baroreceptors, and the subsequent release of ADH, just as described in the hypovolemic states. Hyponatremia can also been seen in nephrotic syndrome, even when the glomerular filtration rate is relatively maintained. Although the underfill theory, based on hypoalbuminemia, is a popular explanation for nephrosis-related hyponatremia, this may be an oversimplification.[12] Last, patients with significant renal failure can become hyponatremic by simply ingesting more water than can be excreted by their functioning renal tubules.

Euvolemic Hyponatremia

Euvolemic hypo-osmolar hyponatremia can be associated with a long list of disorders. Most of these relate to excess ingestion of water or excessive ADH affect.

In euvolemic hyponatremia, it is important to exclude hypothyroidism, adrenal insufficiency, and pregnancy with appropriate laboratory testing. Hypothyroidism, adrenal insufficiency, and pregnancy can all result in inappropriately increased levels of ADH, and a clinical syndrome that can be identical to the syndrome of inappropriate ADH (SIADH).

Low urine osmolality in the face of hyponatremia usually indicates a low ADH state and should alert the clinician to consider a few specific etiologies of the hyponatremia. Urine osmolality <100 mosm/kg, in the face of hyponatremia, should alert the clinician to a disorder caused by excess ingestion of water. Of note, the urine osmolality can be as high as 300 mosm/kg in these disorders if the patient has a significantly reduced glomerular filtration rate.

Psychogenic polydipsia occurs when psychiatric patients ingest large amounts of water that overwhelm the kidneys' excretory capacity. In patients with normal kidneys, it has been suggested that this requires the ingestion of over 20 L/day of water. However, as noted above, patients with significant kidney disease may be able to overwhelm the kidneys' excretory capacity by ingesting more modest amounts of water. Similarly, hypothalamic disorders affecting thirst (e.g., sarcoidosis), can also result in large water ingestions, even in the absence of psychiatric disease. In addition, the administration of excessive water can be iatrogenic. Alternatively, low urine osmolality might be indicative of very low solute intake, a phenomenon most commonly described in patients whose diets consist primarily of alcoholic beverages ("beer drinker's potomania"), or those with other types of low solute diets ("tea and toast").

If urine osmolality is >100 mosm/kg in a euvolemic patient (without severe underlying kidney disease), SiADH should be suspected.

SIADH is a syndrome caused by excess ADH effect. The excess ADH in SIADH is *not* released as a physiologic response to volume depletion or ineffective circulating blood volume. SIADH results from the ectopic production of ADH, or from increased secretion or effect of ADH. The physiologic effect of excess ADH is an inability to excrete water, resulting in hyponatremia and slight volume expansion. This slight volume expansion is thought to result in physiologic renal excretion of sodium and uric acid. Therefore, the classic laboratory profile of SIADH is a high urine osmolality, a high urine sodium (usually >40 mEq/L), and a low serum uric acid (usually <4 mg/dL). The many disorders associated with

Table 51-2 Medications and Conditions with Reported Associations with the Syndrome of Inappropriate ADH

Category	Examples
Drugs	Cytotoxic agents: intravenous cyclophosphamide, ifosfamide, vincristine, vinblastine Antipsychotic agents: thiothixene, thioridizine, haloperidol, fluphenazine Antidepressant agents: selective serotonin reuptake inhibitors (SSRIs), tricyclics, monoamine oxidase inhibitors Anticonvulsant agents: carbamazepine, oxcarbazepine Miscellaneous: bromocriptine, lorcainide, chlorpropamide, tolbutamide, NSAIDs, MDMA (ecstasy), exogenous ADH agonists, oxytocin, nicotine, narcotics, acetaminophen
Neoplasia	Small cell lung cancer, bronchogenic carcinoma, duodenal neoplasm, pancreatic neoplasm, thymic neoplasm, olfactory neuroblastoma, prolactinoma, carcinoma of the stomach, lymphoma, Ewing sarcoma, carcinoma of the bladder, prostate, or ureter, oropharyngeal tumors, Waldenström's macroglobulinemia
Pulmonary disorders	Pneumonia/abscess, tuberculosis, aspergillosis, acute respiratory failure, asthma, atelectasis, pneumothorax, positive pressure breathing, mesothelioma, cystic fibrosis
Neuropsychiatric disorders	CNS infections; CNS neoplasia; trauma; vascular processes, including vasculitis or thrombotic, embolic hemorrhagic disease; or temporal arteritis; psychosis; HIV infection; Guillain-Barré syndrome; acute intermittent porphyria; autonomic neuropathy; hypothalamic sarcoidosis; post-transphenoidal surgery; hydrocephalus; other inflammatory or demyelinating diseases
Miscellaneous	Postoperative state, severe nausea, pain, HIV infection, prolonged exercise

NSAIDs—nonsteroidal anti-inflammatory drugs; MDMA—methylenedioxymethamphetamine; ADH—anti-diuretic hormone; CNS—central nervous system; HIV—human immunodeficiency virus.

SIADH can be logically divided into three major categories: 1) SIADH stimulated by common inpatient disorders, 2) SIADH related to drugs, and 3) SIADH related to other conditions (*see* Tables 51-1 and 51-2).

SIADH can be seen in association with several conditions that are commonly encountered in hospitalized patients. Pain, surgery, severe nausea, and even emotional stress can result in exaggerated ADH effect.

In addition, there is a long list of medications that are felt to have a causal relationship with SIADH (*see* Table 51-2). A variety of antineoplastic agents, antipsychotic agents, antidepressant agents, and anticonvulsant agents have been reported to cause the syndrome. In addition, there are many other drug associations that fall outside of these categories. It is clear that some of the drugs listed in Table 51-2 cause SIADH only rarely, but a thorough review of a patient's medication list is essential in the evaluation of hyponatremia.

SIADH can also occur as a result of a variety of other medical conditions. Most of these are pulmonary or neuropsychiatric disorders, or neoplastic diseases (*see* Table 51-2). Some of these disorders are easily treatable or self-limited, whereas others represent situations where the SIADH becomes a chronic management issue.

Other Considerations

Some causes of hyponatremia deserve additional comments, either because they are particularly complex or because they do not fit neatly into the categories presented above.

Reset osmostat. In this poorly understood condition, the patient's osmostat seems to reset itself at a lower than normal level. These patients carefully maintain their serum osmolality in a narrow range, but do so to a lower set serum osmolality. These patients typically exhibit mild, chronic hyponatremia, and respond normally to water loads. Because of this, urine studies in patients with reset osmostat will be dependent on their recent ingestions. Reset osmostat is seen most commonly in association with psychosis, pregnancy, malnutrition, and quadriplegia.[1]

Thiazide diuretics. Although it has been hypothesized that thiazide diuretics cause hyponatremia, in part, by causing hypovolemia, the hypovolemia is often subclinical, and the patient can appear clinically euvolemic. Thiazide diuretics impair the dilution of tubular fluid in the ascending loop of Henle, and they may also result in excessive water ingestion in some patients. These factors likely explain the development of hyponatremia in those thiazide-treated patients who lack clinical evidence of hypovolemia.

Kidney disease. As noted above, decreased glomerular filtration rate impairs a patient's ability to excrete free water. Therefore, patients with underlying kidney disease can present with hyponatremia if they ingest more water than they can excrete, regardless of volume status.

Marathon runners. Hyponatremia is a recognized complication of marathon running. It appears that excessive water ingestion during the race is the primary cause.[22,23]

Preferred Studies

Table 51-3 summarizes the major studies that are often used in the evaluation of hyponatremic patients and offers an explanation of the utility and limitations of these studies. Urine chemistries always should be interpreted in the context of the quantity of sodium and water the patient has recently ingested and which medications the patient has taken, as well as the patient's underlying renal function. In addition to those tests in the table, other basic laboratory studies can be helpful, including BUN and creatinine (to assess renal function), other electrolytes (e.g., elevations of serum potassium may suggest adrenal disease), glucose level, liver studies (to assess hepatic synthetic function and detect hypoalbuminemia), and routine blood counts.

In cases in which volume depletion is a plausible explanation for a patient's hyponatremia, volume resuscitation is sometimes initiated empirically as a therapeutic trial. Although a rise in serum sodium in response to a therapeutic trial of volume expansion has

Table 51-3 Utility and Limitations of Some Initial Tests That Are Frequently Used for the Classification and Diagnosis of Hyponatremia

Test	Utility	Limitations
Serum osmolality	Allows identification of pseudohyponatremia as in Table 51-1.	—
Urine osmolality	Allows identification of hyponatremia secondary to excessive water ingestion or low solute intake (see Table 51-1). In these cases, absence of ADH results in dilute urine, with urine osmolality often <100 mosm/kg.	As with all urinary tests, results can be influenced by recent water, sodium, and medication ingestions. Renal function should also be considered in the interpretation (see text).
Urine sodium	An effective way to assess renal sodium avidity. Levels of <25 mEq/L suggest renal sodium avidity whereas levels >40 mEq/L suggest renal sodium excretion. Allows categorization of the hyponatremia as in Table 51-1.	As with all urinary tests, results can be influenced by recent water, sodium, and medication ingestions. Renal function should also be considered in the interpretation (see text).
Serum uric acid	Often <4 mg/dL in SIADH (and often >4 mg/dL in states of volume depletion)	Confounding disorders of uric acid metabolism.
Thyroid-stimulating hormone	Screens for thyroid disease	—
Morning cortisol level or stimulated cortisol level	Screens for adrenal insufficiency	—
Pregnancy testing	Screens for pregnancy	—
Chest radiography	Assesses for pulmonary disease	—

Table 51-4 A Stepwise Approach to the Management of Hyponatremia

Step 1. Immediately treat any life-threatening circumstances.
- Hemodynamically significant hypovolemia requires immediate volume resuscitation
- Ongoing seizures require pharmacologic therapy and efforts to protect the patient from mechanical trauma
- Respiratory failure requires respiratory support

Step 2. Decide if rapid, partial correction of the serum sodium is indicated.
- Rapid partial correction of the serum sodium is indicated in cases of severe, acute hyponatremia (serum sodium usually <120 mEq/L) accompanied by evidence of cerebral edema as indicated by:
  - Severe alterations of mental status
  - Seizures
  - Evidence of cerebral edema on imaging studies (e.g., brain computed tomography)

Step 3. If rapid partial correction of the serum sodium is indicated, this should be done according to the following guidelines:
- Do not correct the serum sodium concentration by more than 8 mEq/L in any 24-hour period. If rapid, partial correction is indicated, the serum sodium can be raised rapidly (e.g., raised by 2 mEq/L/hr to the target change of 8 mEq/L), but then further elevations should be avoided for the rest of that 24-hour period.
- Do not overcorrect the patient's serum sodium (i.e., to a level above the low normal range).
- Check the serum sodium frequently (e.g., every 2–3 hours) when actively correcting hyponatremia, because any calculation of the treatment effect provides only a rough estimate of the actual result.

Step 4. If rapid, partial correction of the serum sodium is not indicated, conservative management strategies targeting the underlying etiology of the hyponatremia should be employed. See Table 51-6.

been used as evidence for a volume depleted state, it is not clear that this reliably excludes other causes, such as SIADH.[14]

Prognosis

The prognosis of hyponatremia is directly linked to the underlying disorder. For example, hyponatremia related to volume depletion from a self-limited diarrheal illness is likely to have a good prognosis, while hyponatremia related to SIADH from a small cell lung cancer would have a poorer prognosis. In cases of acute, severe hyponatremia, the resulting cerebral edema can result in brain damage or death, mandating urgent treatment as outlined below. Premenopausal women appear to be at greater risk for irreversible neurologic damage secondary to severe hyponatremia.

Management

Treatment

A stepwise approach to treatment of hyponatremia is required and is summarized in Table 51-4.

First, any life-threatening circumstances must be aggressively managed. In cases of volume depletion resulting in hemodynamic instability, aggressive fluid resuscitation is critical, and it should supersede considerations about managing the serum sodium level. Similarly, patients with severely depressed mental status as a result of the hyponatremia should be managed in a unit capable of providing intensive care, including respiratory support, if needed. Patients having seizures should be treated with appropriate pharmacologic agents and closely observed. Severe mental status alterations and seizures are the two main indications for rapid partial correction of a patient's hyponatremia.

Next, the clinician must decide if rapid, partial correction of the serum sodium is indicated. The symptoms of acute hyponatremia are usually secondary to the presence of cerebral edema. Cerebral edema occurs when water moves, by osmosis, from the hypoosmolar extracellular space, into cells of the central nervous system (CNS). Because cerebral edema can result in irreversible brain damage and death, rapid, partial correction of the extracellular fluid osmolality is needed when significant cerebral edema is present.

Opposing tension, however, comes from the fact that rapid correction of the serum sodium can result in a devastating complication called osmotic demyelination of the central nervous system.[15] In this disorder, the osmotic changes associated with the rapid correction of hyponatremia are thought to result in demyelination of neurons, often affecting the pons. Because of this, the disorder is sometimes referred to as central pontine myelinolysis, although the CNS damage can also be extrapontine. The clinical syndrome can include pseudobalbar paralysis (including dysarthria and dysphagia), spastic quadriparesis, the "locked-in" syndrome, alterations of mental status or coma, and possible death. These symptoms are often irreversible and usually present several days after the rapid correction of hyponatremia.[16,17]

In addition to correcting the serum sodium too rapidly, other disorders also appear to be associated with osmotic demyelination, including alcoholism and liver transplantation.[16]

It is important to remember that symptomatic cerebral edema usually results from acute, severe hyponatremia. Correction of acute hyponatremia does not appear to be commonly associated with osmotic demyelination, even when done rapidly. In contrast, chronic hyponatremia is less likely to cause cerebral edema or symptoms because of neuronal adaptations that occur during the gradual development of hyponatremia. However, rapid correction of chronic hyponatremia is significantly more likely to result in osmotic demyelination.[18]

Therefore, rapid, partial correction of hyponatremia is generally believed to be indicated when severe hyponatremia (usually <120 mEq/L) is associated with signs of cerebral edema. These signs include severe alterations of mental status and seizures. Unfortunately, the chronicity of the hyponatremia may be difficult at times to ascertain clinically, as chronic hyponatremia can also cause neurologic symptoms, even without significant cerebral edema. Computed tomography of the brain can detect cerebral edema, which might justify more aggressive initial correction of the serum sodium in cases where the chronicity of the hyponatremia is in question.[18]

If rapid partial correction of the serum sodium is indicated, this should be done according to the guidelines in Table 51-4, to avoid osmotic demyelination. The precise rate of increase of the serum sodium can be debated. Most cases of osmotic demyelination have occurred with corrections of >12 mEq/L/24 hr (average

0.5 mEq/hr). In some cases, this complication occurred with corrections of only 10 mEq/L/24 hr, leading some authors to recommend a maximum correction of 8 mEq/L/24 hr (0.33 mEq/L/hr).[3,19] Therefore, a conservative recommendation would be to partly correct hyponatremia that is associated with signs of cerebral edema rapidly (e.g., 2 mEq/L/hr up to a goal of 8 mEq/L total), but to avoid further correction for the duration of that 24-hour period. This recommendation is based on the fact that this degree of correction is usually enough to eliminate the life-threatening aspects of the cerebral edema without resulting in demyelination of the CNS. Even seizures will usually abate with this degree of correction. If symptoms do not improve with this degree of correction, it is unclear if this limit should be exceeded.[3]

If a patient requires rapid, partial correction of the serum sodium, hypertonic saline (3%) is usually used. When outlining a strategy to elevate a hyponatremic patient's serum sodium, it is helpful to employ a simple calculation that can guide the management. This calculation can allow the clinician to estimate the amount of sodium that could be added to the extracellular fluid to correct the serum sodium to a higher value. Table 51-5 shows this calculation and a clinical example. It has already been noted that hyponatremia does not usually result from a simple deficit of sodium (which would result in hypovolemia), but rather an excess of extracellular water. Therefore, conceptually, it is better to think of this calculation as the amount of sodium that would correct the hyponatremia to a certain degree if it were distributed in the patient's excess extracellular water. The limitation of this calculation, of course, is that there is no clinically effective way of delivering sodium to the extracellular fluid without also delivering water as well. Since the formula in Table 51-5 assumes that no water is given with the sodium, it will be most accurate when more concentrated saline solutions are used (i.e., it will perform better with hypertonic saline than with normal saline). Any formula for calculating sodium requirements in hyponatremic patients should only be considered an estimate, and *frequent monitoring of the serum sodium is essential when attempting therapeutic corrections.*

If rapid, partial correction of the serum sodium is not indicated, conservative management strategies targeting the underlying etiology of the hyponatremia should be employed. Patients without signs of cerebral edema should *not* have their sodium levels rapidly corrected. In these patients, who are often chronically hyponatremic, the rapid correction of sodium is more likely to result in complications than benefit. Therefore, correction of hyponatremia is usually done slowly by attending to the underlying etiology. Table 51-6 allows comparison of all of the clinical interventions that will result in correction of the serum sodium.

Hypovolemic hyponatremia. Hypovolemic hyponatremia is treated with volume resuscitation. Most often, this is accomplished by administering normal saline, although sometimes the use of blood products is appropriate. Volume depletion that presents with hemodynamic instability requires rapid resuscitation, without regard to the serum sodium level. Lesser degrees of hypovolemia can also be treated with normal saline, but correction of the patient's volume status may result in rapid correction of the serum sodium, at a rate greater than desired. Some authors have suggested, when treating a patient whose hyponatremia is thought to be exclusively secondary to volume depletion, that the

Table 51-5 Calculation of the Theoretical Amount of Sodium That Could Be Administered to Affect a Desired Change in the Serum Sodium: Total Body Water (in Liters) × The Desired Change in Serum Sodium (in mEq/L) = The Amount of Sodium (in mEq) Needed to Correct the Hyponatremia

1. Calculate the patient's total body water content: TBW (in liters) = body weight in kg × n (n = 0.5 in elderly men and nonelderly women, 0.6 in nonelderly men, and 0.45 in elderly women).
2. Multiply this TBW by the change in serum sodium (in mEq/L) that is desired to estimate the total mEq of sodium that would need to be administered to achieve this change: Required mEq of sodium = TBW (in liters) × desired change in serum sodium (in mEq/L).
3. Recall the sodium content of commonly used intravenous fluids: normal saline = 154 mEq/L, 3% hypertonic saline = 514 mEq/L. Include potassium in the correction (see text).
4. Recognize the limitations of this calculation (see text).

Clinical Example:
How much saline solution might be given to a 50-kg patient who is having hyponatremia-related seizures to raise the serum sodium from 110 to 118?

TBW = 50 kg × 0.5 = 25 L

25 L × 8 mEq/L (change in serum sodium desired) = 200 mEq of sodium

This amount of sodium is contained in 389 mL of 3% hypertonic saline, which could be given over the desired time frame for the calculated change in serum sodium.

Table 51-6 Clinical Interventions to Raise a Patient's Serum Sodium Level, and the Clinical Settings in Which They Are Most Appropriately Used

Intervention	Most Appropriate Clinical Use	Notes/Caveats
Restrict ingestion of free water	Used alone for mild, asymptomatic cases. Also, often combined with the other interventions.	Although usually seen as a slow-acting intervention, in cases of polydipsia, this can result in rapid correction of hyponatremia.
Administer a loop diuretic	Treatment of choice for patients who are clinically hypervolemic. Also, often used in combination with other treatments (e.g., with saline solutions) to ensure at least partial excretion of the administered water. Mild-to-moderate hyponatremia in a hypervolemic patient may respond to loop diuretics combined with restricted ingestion of free water. In severe, symptomatic cases of hypervolemic or euvolemic hyponatremia, loop diuretics are often combined with hypertonic saline.	Loop diuretics result in a diuresis of fluid that is usually hypotonic to plasma.
Hemodialysis	Treatment of choice for patients with irreversible renal failure with severe or symptomatic hyponatremia.	Lack of immediate access to this intervention may limit its usefulness in some situations.
Intravenous normal saline	Treatment of choice for patients with clinical hypovolemia.	Correction of hypovolemia can result in rapid correction of hyponatremia (see text). Normal saline is *not recommended* for rapid treatment of euvolemic hyponatremia, when SIADH is a diagnostic consideration.
Hypertonic (3%) saline	The treatment of choice for most cases of euvolemic or hypervolemic, severely symptomatic (obtundation, seizures) hyponatremia. Hypertonic saline is often combined with a loop diuretic and restricted ingestion of free water.	The fastest-acting technique for correcting hyponatremia. Use requires a knowledgeable clinician and frequent monitoring of the serum sodium.

fluids be changed to hypotonic saline once there has been a partial correction in volume status and serum sodium level.[3] Even when using hypotonic fluids in this situation, a continued increase in serum sodium should be expected, as the correction of volume status removes the stimulus for ADH secretion and enables renal water excretion. The tonicity of the administered fluid can be altered, based on serial measurements of the serum sodium.

Hypervolemic hyponatremia. The mainstay of treatment of hyponatremia in the edematous states is water restriction, often combined with loop diuretics. Stringent water restrictions (<800 mL/day) may be required in these cases.

Euvolemic hyponatremia. The treatment of euvolemic hyponatremia is more dependent on an accurate diagnosis. When possible, disorders causing SIADH should be specifically treated, and offending medications stopped. Of course, hormone deficiencies should be corrected, when appropriate.

SIADH. SIADH can occur in situations in which the underlying cause is either untreatable or not rapidly correctable. In these cases, the clinician must formulate a long-term plan for the management of this water-retentive state. It has been suggested that the severity of the disorder can be estimated by the urine osmolality. That is, high urine osmolality typically results from higher levels of ADH activity, and this can be predictive of a more difficult management situation. Sometimes, water restriction alone can be successful, especially in those with relatively dilute urine. In other cases, a high-sodium, high-protein diet (to increase solute excretion, with water following obligatorily) combined with a loop diuretic will be required. Unfortunately, it is not uncommon for these patients to require additional measures to control their water balance, and medications including demeclocycline have been used for this purpose. Demeclocycline causes nephrogenic diabetes insipidus, which directly opposes the excessive ADH effect. Specific ADH antagonist drugs will likely provide a more rational treatment for SIADH in the future. Although not yet widely available, conivaptan is an ADH antagonist that has recently received FDA approval as a treatment for some types of hyponatremia.

Cerebral salt wasting. Most of these patients are volume depleted at the time of diagnosis, and aggressive resuscitation with normal saline may be required initially. Until the salt wasting resolves, patients may require treatment with oral salt supplementation or even fludrocortisone to maintain plasma volume. Although the natural history of cerebral salt wasting is uncertain, it appears that this syndrome is usually self-limited, often resolving after a period of weeks.

Other Considerations

Potassium. Potassium should be administered in cases in which hypokalemia accompanies the hyponatremia. When administering potassium in these situations, the clinician must realize that potassium will result in an elevation in the serum sodium that is nearly equal to that which would occur via the administration of an equal amount of sodium. This is because potassium causes a shift of sodium out of cells and water into cells, with the net effect of an increased extracellular sodium concentration.[3]

Prevention

The administration of hypotonic fluids to hospitalized patients can result in iatrogenic hyponatremia. This can be avoided by giving hypotonic saline to patients only after considering their ability to excrete a water load, and with periodic monitoring of the serum sodium.

Discharge/Follow-up Plans

A patient can be safely discharged from the hospital after an episode of hyponatremia if the serum sodium has been elevated

to a safe level and a plan has been formulated to maintain this. This decision-making is easiest when a clear diagnosis is made, and the process is reversible. In some cases, a definite diagnosis is not made, but the serum sodium corrects. In these cases, careful monitoring after discharge will be important. In other cases, a definite diagnosis might be made, but the process may not be immediately reversible. For example, if a patient is found to have SIADH related to a nonresectable lung cancer, a definite therapeutic strategy for maintaining adequate serum sodium levels will be critical, as will close follow-up and monitoring. In any case, physicians who are to follow up with a patient after discharge will need to be made aware of the diagnosis of the hyponatremia and the trend of the serum sodium in order to appropriately care for the patient.

HYPERNATREMIA

Background

Hypernatremia, in most cases, represents a deficiency of water in the extracellular fluid compartment, and always represents a state of extracellular hyperosmolality. Hypernatremia occurs when free water losses exceed free water intake. Even when excess water losses are present, patients will not become hypernatremic unless they fail to replace these losses. Failure to replace water losses only occurs if there is a defect in the thirst mechanism, or if access to water is somehow restricted. In any case, hypernatremia can result in neurologic dysfunction related to dehydration of cells in the central nervous system.

Assessment

Clinical Presentation

The severity of the presenting symptoms of hypernatremia depends more on the rapidity of the onset of the hypernatremia than the degree of the abnormality. Hypernatremia usually presents with symptoms of neurologic dysfunction. Mild symptoms may include weakness, difficulty concentrating, or irritability, but more severe symptoms can include severe mental status alterations, and even coma. Rapid increases in the serum sodium (acute) are more likely to cause symptoms than alterations that occur more gradually (chronic). In some cases, the severity of the cellular dehydration has even led to intracranial hemorrhage, presumably due to traction on the venous structures.[1,20]

A complete evaluation of the hypernatremic patient should include a careful history and physical examination, much as described above for the hyponatremic patient. Particular attention should be focused on assessing the patient's volume status and detecting any barriers to water ingestion or important fluid losses. In particular, polyuria, nocturia, and polydipsia suggest excessive renal water losses. Also, the clinician should be alert to clues that might suggest diabetes insipidus, such as neurologic signs or specific medications (*see* below).

Diagnosis/Differential Diagnosis

Like hyponatremia, the diagnosis of hypernatremia is based on simple laboratory testing. Most of the diagnostic effort is, therefore, directed at identifying the cause of the hypernatremia. Table 51-7 shows a summary of the major causes of hypernatremia.[1,20]

Table 51-7 The Major Causes of Hypernatremia

Inadequate water ingestion (always present)
- Barriers to obtaining or ingesting water:

  EXAMPLES: Disability (new or exacerbated), dementia, restraints, sedation, inadequate administration of water to patients who are dependent (e.g., failure to administer free water to an enterally fed, immobile patient)

- Lack of appropriate thirst response:

  EXAMPLES: Primary hypodipsia of the elderly or hypothalamic diseases (including neoplasia, sarcoidosis, or vascular disease)

Excessive water losses (present in some cases)
- Insensible losses via skin and respiratory tract (which can increase with fever, high ambient temperatures, burns, respiratory infections, etc.)
- Gastrointestinal (GI) losses:

  EXAMPLES: Vomiting, diarrhea (especially osmotic-type), others

- Renal losses:
  - Osmotic or postobstructive diuresis:

    EXAMPLES: Hyperglycemia, mannitol administration

  - Diabetes insipidus: (suspect if polyuria, polydipsia, or nocturia is prominent or if the urine osmolality is not maximally concentrated (urine osmolality <800 mosm/kg) in the setting of hypernatremia

Excessive ingestion or administration of sodium

  EXAMPLES: Iatrogenic (such as administration of hypertonic saline or concentrated sodium bicarbonate), excessive salt ingestion (rare), salt water drowning

---

Hypernatremia is virtually always caused by insufficient water intake (that does not adequately match ongoing water losses). Although some states of hypernatremia occur in the setting of excessive water loss, hypernatremia never occurs if the patient is able to ingest adequate water. For this reason, hypernatremia is most common in elderly or disabled patients, who are more often dependent on others to provide them with free water. Table 51-7 gives several examples of barriers to water ingestion. Sometimes, the inadequate water intake occurs because of an abnormality in the thirst mechanism (hypodipsia) that can be idiopathic or related to hypothalamic disease. Hypodipsia is most likely to be an important contributor to hypernatremia in those patients who have chronic hypernatremia, and who are not subject to other barriers to water ingestion.

Hypernatremia can also occur as a result of excessive water losses. Even under normal conditions, there are insensible losses via the skin (perspiration) and respiratory tract. However, these losses can be exacerbated by illness (see Table 51-7). Gastrointestinal disease can also result in water losses. In these cases, hypernatremia results if the water is lost in excess of solute, or if replacement of the lost fluid contains insufficient water. Water can also be lost via the kidney. Renal water losses can result from osmotic diuresis secondary to hyperglycemia or other osmotic agents, from postobstructive diuresis, or from diabetes insipidus. Chronic kidney disease results in a diminished ability to concentrate the urine, which can contribute to hypernatremia in patients with inadequate water intake. In most of these cases, the cause of the water loss is evident, and treatment is focused on the underlying disorder.

Diabetes insipidus (DI) is a disorder that results from the lack of circulating ADH secretion from the pituitary (central diabetes insipidus, CDI) or from renal resistance to the effect of ADH (nephrogenic diabetes insipidus, NDI). In either case, the absence of ADH effect results in an inability to concentrate the urine, leading to continuous renal water loss. CDI can be congenital,

Table 51-8 Major Causes of Diabetes Insipidus

Category	Examples
Central Diabetes Insipidus	
Neoplasm	Craniopharyngioma, germinoma, meningioma, pituitary neoplasm
Neurosurgery or head trauma	
Vascular events	Hemorrhagic or thromboembolic events
Granulomatous disease	Histiocytosis, sarcoidosis, tuberculosis
Autoimmune	Lymphocytic hypophysitis
Infectious	Meningitis, encephalitis
Congenital	
Idiopathic	
Nephrogenic Diabetes Insipidus	
Medications	Lithium, demeclocycline, cidofovir, foscarnet, streptozocin, amphotericin, cisplatin
Electrolyte abnormalities	Hypokalemia, hypercalcemia
Intrinsic renal disease	Polycystic disease, obstructive uropathy, sarcoidosis, amyloidosis
Congenital	
Gestational	

idiopathic, or can result from acquired disease of the neurohypophysis including neurosurgery, head trauma, ischemic or hemorrhagic neurologic insults, infections, neoplasm (especially craniopharyngioma and germinoma), granulomatous disease (including histiocytosis, sarcoidosis, and tuberculosis), autoimmunity, and others. NDI can also be congenital, but hospitalists are most often faced with acquired causes of NDI that can result from medications (lithium, demeclocycline, cidofivir, foscarnet, streptozocin, amphotericin, cisplatin), electrolyte abnormalities (hypokalemia, hypercalcemia), or some intrinsic renal diseases (e.g., polycystic disease, obstructive uropathy, sarcoidosis, amyloidosis). There is also a gestational form of DI. The causes of DI are summarized in Table 51-8.[2,21]

Of note, DI does *not* usually present with hypernatremia unless it is paired with a barrier to water intake or an additional cause of water loss. Rather, DI typically presents with polyuria, polydipsia (often craving cold water), and nocturia. DI patients with access to water will usually ingest enough water to avoid hypernatremia. In a patient hospitalized for hypernatremia, DI should be considered if the initial urine is not maximally concentrated (urine osmolality is less than 800 mosm/kg), in a patient with hyperosmolality, or if a history of polyuria, polydipsia, or nocturia is prominent and not explained by other factors.[2] A 24-hour urine collection can be useful when the diagnosis of DI is considered. A 24-hour urine volume >50 mL/kg body weight with a urine osmolality of less than or equal to 300 mosm/kg suggests DI, so long as hyperglycemia or intrinsic renal disease is not present.[2] The diagnosis of DI is usually made definitively by performing a water deprivation test.[2,21] In this test, the patient is asked to fast for a period of time. During the period of fasting, no water is ingested, causing serum osmolality to increase. If the serum osmolality rises, but the urine remains dilute, DI is diagnosed. ADH can also be measured in the hyperosmolar state, at which time it would be expected to be physiologically elevated. Administration of dDAVP can then help determine if the DI is central or nephrogenic. Water deprivation testing is typically performed with the assistance of an endocrinologist or nephrologist, after the initial correction of the patient's hypernatremia.

Hypernatremia resulting from the excessive ingestion of sodium is extremely rare, and it can be easily ruled out by a careful history. Similarly, iatrogenic hypernatremia secondary to excessive sodium administration is uncommon (*see* Table 51-7).

Preferred Studies

Most of the diagnosis of hypernatremia is based on history. As mentioned above, testing of the urine osmolality can help assess the renal concentrating ability, and testing of the serum potassium and calcium can identify obvious causes of NDI. A 24-hour urine collection with measurements of volume and osmolality and/or a water deprivation test are sometimes required when there is suspicion of DI.

Management

Treatment

The treatment of hypernatremia can be divided into efforts to treat the underlying cause and efforts to correct the hypernatremia.

Correction of the plasma hypernatremia will result in a decrease in the osmolality of the extracellular fluid. If done quickly, this will cause a rapid shift of water into cells of the central nervous system, and cerebral edema will ensue. This can result in alterations in mental status, seizures, and can even cause permanent neurologic damage or death. Therefore, analogous to the correction of hyponatremia, the correction of hypernatremia should be done slowly. The rate of correction should be no greater than 12 mEq/L/day.[1]

A hypernatremic patient's free water deficit can be calculated as:

$$\text{Free water deficit (in liters)} = \text{total body water (in liters)}$$
$$\times \{[\text{serum sodium (in mEq/L)}/140] - 1\}$$

where total body water (in liters) = the patient's weight in kilograms $\times$ n (n = 0.5 in elderly men and nonelderly women, 0.6 in nonelderly men, and 0.45 in elderly women).

Although free water can be given orally or enterally to some patients, it is often administered intravenously. Severe intravascular volume depletion (i.e., hemodynamically unstable) should be corrected with normal saline infusion before using hypotonic fluids to correct the free water deficit. Those patients with lesser degrees of volume depletion can be treated with hypotonic fluids containing some sodium (e.g., D5 $\frac{1}{4}$ normal saline) to administer both sodium and free water simultaneously. Those patients without clear signs of volume depletion can be treated with dextrose in water. In any case, the ongoing water losses, including those in the urine, should be considered when attempting to correct hypernatremia. To do this, it is reasonable to add 1,500–2,000 mL/day of water to the amount administered to account for expected water losses via the urine and insensible losses. However, the clinician must be acutely aware of the volume of ongoing water losses, and modify the amount of water that is administered accordingly.

CDI is typically treated, in consultation with an endocrinologist, with an ADH analog such as dDAVP. This medication can be titrated to control symptoms of polyuria and polydipsia. The dose of dDAVP can be delivered intranasally or parenterally. In hospitalized patients, it is often necessary to use the parenteral form to ensure accurate delivery of the drug, particularly in acute situations or those in which patient factors (e.g., altered mental status) might impede delivery via the nasal route.

Many of the causes of NDI are reversible, although those that are not can be treated with volume depletion (e.g., sodium restriction and thiazide diuretic agents) and mild protein restriction to help decrease urine output.

In the rare case of hypernatremia because of sodium overload, treatment should consist of the administration of free water along with sodium diuresis using a loop diuretic.

Prevention

At times, a hospital admission for hypernatremia can be an important sign of previously unrecognized or worsening disability. In these cases, discharge to a more supportive living environment can assure access to water.

Discharge/Follow-up Plans

After discharge, patients may require monitoring of their serum sodium, especially if a discrete cause for the hypernatremia is not apparent. Some hypodipsic elderly patients may require a "water prescription" to assure adequate daily intake.

Key Points

- A careful assessment of the patient's volume status, and a few simple laboratory tests (urine osmolality, urine sodium, and serum osmolarity) can help narrow an otherwise broad differential diagnosis in a patient with hyponatremia.

- When considering the diagnosis of SIADH, it is important to rule out hypothyroidism, adrenal insufficiency, and pregnancy, using appropriate laboratory testing.

- When therapeutically raising a patient's serum sodium level (e.g., by administering hypertonic saline), the sodium level should **not** be increased by more than 8 mEq/L in a 24-hour period to avoid the development of osmotic demyelination of the central nervous system.

- Hypernatremia is caused by inadequate replacement of water losses. The evaluation of a hypernatremic patient should include an investigation of barriers to water ingestion and excessive water losses.

- The majority of cased of hypernatremia are **not** related to diabetes insipidus. This disorder should be considered if polyuria, polydipsia, or nocturia are prominent, or if the urine osmolality is not maximally concentrated (urine osmolality <800 mosm/kg) in the setting of hypernatremia.

SUGGESTED READING

Rose BD, Post TW. Clinical Physiology of Acid-Base and Electrolyte Disorders, 5th ed. New York: McGraw-Hill, 2001.

Androgue HJ, Madias NE. Hyponatremia. N Engl J Med 2000; 342:1581–1589.

Palmer B. Hyponatremia in patients with central nervous system disease. Trends Endocrinol Metab 2003; 14:182–187.

Berl T. Treating hyponatremia: damned if we do and damned if we don't. Kidney International 1990; 37:1006–1018.

Androgue HJ, Madias NE. Hypernatremia. N Engl J Med 2000; 342:1493–1499.

CHAPTER FIFTY-TWO

Other Electrolyte Disorders

David H. Wesorick, MD

This chapter addresses the disorders of potassium and magnesium balance. Severe perturbations of these electrolytes can be life threatening; thus, the hospitalist must be able to quickly recognize and correct these imbalances. In most cases, these imbalances are expected manifestations of certain disease processes. However, in cases in which these abnormalities are unexpected or unexplained, the hospitalist must be able to recognize these abnormalities as diagnostic clues.

DISORDERS OF POTASSIUM BALANCE

Background

Most of the disorders of potassium balance can be understood in the context of a few simple physiologic principles. Potassium is ingested in the diet and is the major intracellular cation. In most cases, potassium is ingested in amounts greater than what would be needed to maintain potassium balance. The excretion of the excess potassium depends on the normal functioning of the kidney. Specifically, potassium excretion depends on the delivery of sufficient amounts of sodium to the distal tubule, where the sodium-potassium ATPase can then allow the exchange of sodium (to be retained) for potassium (to be excreted). This ATPase is stimulated by aldosterone. Aldosterone is, under normal conditions, released from the adrenal gland when stimulated either by an elevated serum potassium concentration or elevated levels of angiotensin II. The latter occurs as the result of increased activity of the renin-angiotensin-aldosterone system (RAAS). The physiologic steps of this system and potential perturbations of the system are summarized in Table 52-1. In general, conditions causing decreased activity of the RAAS can lead to hyperkalemia, whereas those conditions causing heightened activity of the RAAS can lead to hypokalemia[1-5] (see Table 52-1).

In addition to the renal excretion of potassium, serum potassium levels are also dependent on the relative amount of total body potassium that is contained in cells (as opposed to being free in the extracellular fluid). There are several clinical circumstances that will cause potassium to move into or out of cells, thereby affecting serum potassium levels. These are illustrated in Table 52-2 and discussed in more detail below.[1,2,4]

HYPERKALEMIA

Assessment

Clinical Presentation

Hyperkalemia most commonly causes muscle weakness and cardiac arrhythmias. The muscle weakness might only be perceived at very high levels of potassium, and it usually does not affect the respiratory muscles, or those muscles innervated by the cranial nerves. The electrocardiographic changes that occur with hyperkalemia progress as serum potassium rises and include early changes (peaked T-waves), later changes (diminished P-waves, and widening of the QRS complex), and preterminal changes (sine-wave pattern, ventricular fibrillation, asystole).[1] Serum potassium levels >7 mEq/L are most likely to cause cardiac arrhythmias, but there is variability in this threshold, since the sensitivity to hyperkalemia depends on a variety of other variables.

Diagnosis/Differential Diagnosis

There are many disorders that cause hyperkalemia, and these are summarized in Table 52-3. Of note, spuriously elevated serum potassium levels occur with some frequency, especially in the presence of a hemolyzed blood sample, as occurs in cases of difficult phlebotomy or poor handling of the blood specimen. Less commonly, spurious hyperkalemia can occur with extreme elevations of the leukocyte or platelet count because of shifting of potassium out of these blood elements.

Hyperkalemia occurs only rarely as the result of excess potassium intake, in the absence of other abnormalities. However, transfused blood is rich in potassium, and dietary salt substitutes sometimes contain potassium salts. Iatrogenic hyperkalemia can also result from the excess administration of potassium. Ingestion of excess potassium is more likely to result in hyperkalemia when it occurs in the presence of significant renal failure; however, ingestion of a normal quantity of dietary potassium does not cause hyperkalemia in patients with kidney disease until the disease is advanced and they become oliguric.[1]

Hyperkalemia can also occur in situations in which potassium moves out of cells into the extracellular space. The factors influencing the movement of potassium from cells into the extracellular space are summarized in Table 52-2. Insulin deficiency is an example of this phenomenon. One of insulin's effects on target

Table 52-1 The Renin-Angiotensin-Aldosterone System and Perturbations Affecting Potassium Balance

Steps in the Renin-Angiotensin-Aldosterone System	Perturbations Resulting in Decreased Activity (Hyperkalemia and Acidosis)	Perturbations Resulting in Increased Activity (Hypokalemia and Alkalosis)
1. Renin is released from juxtoglomerular cells in the kidney when stimulated by hypoperfusion or increased activity of the sympathetic nervous system.	• Medications causing hyporeninemia: beta-blockers, methyldopa, NSAID's (including COX-2 selective), cyclosporine, tacrolimus • Nephropathy causing hyporeninemia: diabetic, AIDs-related, lupus-related, acute glomerulonephritis	Conditions causing hyper-reninemia: volume depletion or other cause of renal underperfusion (e.g., CHF, cirrhosis), renal artery stenosis, malignant hypertension, scleroderma crisis, renal vasculitis, renin-secreting tumor
2. Angiotensin I is produced, as catalyzed by renin		
3. Angiotensin II is formed from angiotensin I, as catalyzed by ACE	• Medications inhibiting ACE: ACE inhibitors	
4. Aldosterone is released from the adrenal gland, as stimulated by angiotensin II (or directly by hyperkalemia)	• Medications decreasing aldosterone release: angiotensin receptor blockers, heparin (unfractionated or low-molecular-weight), ketoconazole • Primary adrenal failure • Congenital adrenal hyperplasia	• States of endogenous aldosterone excess: adrenal adenoma, adrenal hyperplasia, adrenal malignancy
5. Aldosterone acts in the collecting duct to stimulate the retention of sodium and the excretion of potassium and acid.	• Medications inhibiting the effect of aldosterone at the collecting duct: potassium-sparing diuretics (e.g., spironolactone, triamterene, amelioride), eplerenone, pentamidine, trimethoprim, cyclosporine, tacrolimus • Resistance to aldosterone: transplant rejection, obstructive uropathy, lupus nephropathy, amyloidosis, sickle cell anemia	• Aldosterone receptor stimulated by nonaldosterone hormone: Cushing's syndrome, glycyrrhizinic acid ingestion (in some licorice candy, chewing gum, chewing tobacco), or administration of fludrocortisone

ACE—angiotensin converting enzyme; NSAIDs—nonsteroidal anti-inflammatory drugs; COX-2—cyclooxygenase-2; CHF—congestive heart failure

Table 52-2 Factors Influencing the Shifting of Potassium into and out of Cells

Factors Promoting the Movement of Potassium out of Cells into the Extracelluar Space	Factors Promoting the Movement of Potassium into Cells from the Extracelluar Space
• Acidosis (nonorganic) • Elevated extracellular osmolarity (e.g., secondary to hyperglycemia, mannitol administration, etc.) • Insulin deficiency • Beta-adrenergic blockade • Medications: digoxin, succinylcholine • Hyperkalemic periodic paralysis • Massive cellular injury: Massive rhabdomyolysis (e.g., trauma), hemolysis, internal bleeding, tumor-lysis syndrome	• Alkalosis • Insulin action • Beta 2-adrenergic receptor stimulation (e.g., albuterol, epinephrine, pseudoephedrine, states of elevated endogenous catecholamines) • Medications: Beta-adrenergic agonists as above, methylxanthines (e.g., theophylline, caffeine), administration of vitamin B_{12} or folate when treating megaloblastic anemia, granulocyte-macrophage colony-stimulating factor for neutropenia • Hypokalemic periodic paralysis • Hypothermia

cells is to move potassium into the cell. In cases of severe insulin deficiency, such as occurs in diabetic ketoacidosis or hyperosmolar states, potassium moves out of cells, raising the serum potassium. For this reason, most patients presenting with these conditions are hyperkalemic, even though their total body stores of potassium are usually depleted (secondary to urinary losses resulting from the osmotic diuresis). In these cases, the administration of insulin results in the movement of potassium back into cells, which often results in hypokalemia if potassium supplements are not provided.

Similarly, conditions that result in the lysis of cells will cause the release of intracellular contents, including potassium. In this way, conditions such as massive rhabdomyolysis (e.g., traumatic), massive hemolysis, and tumor-lysis syndrome can raise the serum potassium. Many of these clinical situations can also lead to impairment of renal function, exacerbating the problem. Other examples of conditions causing hyperkalemia via cellular shifting of potassium are shown in Table 52-2. Digoxin and succinylcholine are examples of medications that can cause hyperkalemia by causing the movement of potassium out of cells.

Table 52-3 Causes of Hyperkalemia

Category	Examples
Spurious	Hemolysis of blood sample, extreme thrombocytosis or leukocytosis
Excessive intake of potassium (rare)	Blood transfusion, excessive potassium administration, overuse of potassium-containing salt substitutes
Shifting of potassium from inside cells to the extracellular space	See Table 52-2.
Renal retention secondary to low GFR	Renal failure, including that secondary to volume depletion
Renal retention secondary to hypoaldosteronism (type 4 renal tubular acidosis)	See Table 52-1.

GFR—glomerular filtration rate

Any condition that disrupts renal excretion of potassium can cause hyperkalemia. Severe reductions in the glomerular filtration rate will reduce potassium excretion. In addition, any condition that reduces the activity of the RAAS will also limit the renal excretion of potassium, leading to hyperkalemia in some cases. These conditions are summarized in Table 52-1. Spironolactone directly competes with aldosterone in the distal tubule, potentially causing hyperkalemia. A similar effect is seen with the other potassium-sparing diuretics, which inhibit apical sodium channels in the distal tubule.[3,5] Since these conditions also result in a metabolic acidosis (often called type 4 renal tubular acidosis), they are also discussed in the chapter on acid-base disturbances (see Chapter 53). Of note, some forms of type 1 RTA can also cause hyperkalemia. Hereditary causes of hyperkalemia are of less importance to hospitalists, and are not discussed here.

Preferred Studies

In most cases, the cause of hyperkalemia is apparent, and consideration of the causes of hyperkalemia (summarized in Table 52-3) will lead the clinician to the correct diagnosis, without extensive diagnostic testing. In all cases, a full panel of serum chemistries, including electrolytes, BUN, and creatinine, should be performed along with a complete blood count.

Sometimes, testing aimed at securing the diagnosis of other disorders that cause hyperkalemia can be useful. This testing might include the assessment of laboratory variables that might be affected by rhabdomyolysis (e.g., serum creatinine kinase concentrations), hemolysis (e.g., reticulocyte count, serum lactate dehydrogenase, bilirubin, or haptoglobin concentrations), or tumor-lysis (e.g., serum uric acid concentrations).

Clinical Approach

Patients with hyperkalemia should be assessed with a complete history and physical examination, including a careful medication inventory. These, in combination with the routine laboratory tests above, usually explain the patient's hyperkalemia, when the causes in Table 52-3 are carefully considered. Spurious hyperkalemia should always be considered, and high values should be confirmed with a repeat sample. Medications are an extremely frequent cause of hyperkalemia, as noted in Tables 52-1 and 52-2. Severe kidney failure is easily recognized with the use of standard laboratory testing. Most causes of potassium shifting out of cells are related to distinct and recognizable disorders, such as insulin deficiency states (see Table 52-2).

In the unusual case of hyperkalemia that is unexplained despite these considerations (especially if persistent and/or accompanied by normal anion gap metabolic acidosis), the clinician should again consider the possibility of hypoaldosteronism. This should prompt consideration of the many disorders that can cause decreased activity of the RAAS outlined in Table 52-1. In these cases, testing for primary adrenal insufficiency should be a priority, and it can be accomplished by measuring a morning serum cortisol concentration or a serum cortisol concentration after the administration of cosyntropin (stimulation testing). If primary adrenal failure is not present, an alternative cause of hypoaldosteronism is likely. Drugs are an extremely common cause of this syndrome, as summarized in Table 52-1. In the presence of a disorder in which such a deficiency might be expected (e.g., diabetic nephropathy), the diagnosis of hyporeninemic hypoaldosteronism is often made empirically.

Uncommonly, further testing is required to more completely elucidate the nature of the disorder and, in these cases, subspecialist consultation is appropriate. Measurement of urinary potassium that documents an unexpectedly low concentration of potassium in the urine can corroborate the clinical impression of hypoaldosteronism. A 24-hour urine sample with <150 mEq/day of potassium in the face of hyperkalemia or a transtubular potassium gradient (TTKG) of <10 in the face of hyperkalemia is suggestive of hypoaldosteronism.[1,6] The transtubular potassium gradient can be calculated from spot urine and serum samples as:

$$TTKG = \frac{\left(urine\ potassium \div \dfrac{urine\ osmolarity}{plasma\ osmolarity} \right)}{plasma\ potassium}$$

At times, direct assessment of the renin-angiotensin-aldosterone system (with paired plasma renin activity and aldosterone concentration) may be helpful as well. (This type of testing is described in greater detail below, in the hypokalemia section.)

Management

Treatment

The treatment of hyperkalemia depends on the severity of the abnormality and the degree to which the abnormality is compromising the patient. As a rule, serum potassium levels <6 mEq/L are not associated with severe manifestations, whereas levels >7 mEq/L are more likely to be significant. However, there is sig-

Table 52-4 Interventions for Reducing Serum Potassium Concentrations

Intervention	Notes/Caveats
Removal of potassium from the body	
Loop diuretics	Example: Intravenous furosemide Caveats: Depends on intact renal function, may not be appropriate if volume depletion is apparent or suspected
Potassium-binding resins	Example: Sodium polystyrene sulfonate, which can be given orally (15–30 g) or as an enema (30–50 g) Caveats: Requires functional gastrointestinal tract, slow-acting
Dialysis	
Intracellular shifting of potassium	
Beta-agonist therapy	Example: Albuterol, inhaled via a nebulizer or metered dose inhaler, 10–20 mg inhaled over 10 minutes or 0.5 mg given intravenously over 10 minutes Caveats: Tachycardia is a common side effect, and can be detrimental in patients with ischemic heart disease
Parenteral insulin	Example: 10 units of regular insulin intravenously, given with dextrose (e.g., 50 g of dextrose in a 50% solution intravenously) unless the patient is already hyperglycemic.
Parenteral sodium bicarbonate	Example: 50 mEq of sodium bicarbonate intravenously over 5 minutes Caveats: Weak efficacy data, probably not effective unless acidosis is present, can cause volume overload secondary to large salt load

nificant individual variation in the level of hyperkalemia that will cause manifestations. An electrocardiogram can provide information that is helpful in determining how urgently the hyperkalemia should be treated (see above under Clinical Presentation). However, the ECG is not a perfect predictor of the complications of hyperkalemia, and some recommend aggressive treatment for all patients with serum potassium concentrations >6 mEq/L.[7]

In cases of significant hyperkalemia, the initial focus of treatment is to protect the heart from the adverse effects of the hyperkalemia and to reduce the serum potassium to a safe level.[1,2,7]

The adverse electrical cardiac effects of hyperkalemia can be lessened by the parenteral administration of calcium salts. Calcium can be delivered as an ampule (10 mL of a 10% solution) of calcium gluconate, over a few minutes, intravenously. This can be repeated if there is no change in the electrocardiographic abnormalities. The protective effect of calcium occurs rapidly. Of note, this treatment should be avoided in cases of suspected digoxin toxicity, as hypercalcemia enhances the toxic effects of digoxin.

The serum potassium can be directly lowered by either removing potassium from the body (via the urine, gastrointestinal tract, or dialysis), or by causing some of the extracellular potassium to move into cells, thereby lowering the extracellular concentration. The available methods for decreasing the serum potassium are summarized in Table 52-4.[1,2,7]

Most commonly, potassium is removed from the body via the urine. This can be accomplished via the administration of loop diuretics, which will cause potassium wasting if the kidneys are functioning, especially if there is aldosterone acting at the collecting tubule (which will be present in most cases of hyperkalemia). The initial dose of loop diuretic should be chosen with the intent of causing a brisk diuresis.

Potassium can be removed from the body via other mechanisms as well. The oral or rectal administration of potassium-binding resins, such as sodium polystyrene sulfonate (Kayexelate), causes potassium to move into the stool, in exchange for sodium. The oral form is typically given with sorbitol to avoid constipation. This medication may not be appropriate for patients who will not tolerate the resulting sodium load (e.g., patients with volume overload, congestive heart failure, etc.). Also, colonic necrosis has been reported with the use of sodium polystyrene sulfonate, especially when administered rectally and with sorbitol. To avoid this complication, the rectal form is not recommended in patients with ileus (including postoperative ileus or critically ill patients), and sorbitol should not be coadministered when the medication is given via enema.[1,8]

In cases of severe renal failure, dialysis is the most reliable method for removing potassium from the body.

Since none of the methods for removing potassium from the body acts rapidly, it is common practice to transiently lower the serum potassium by causing potassium to shift into cells. Many of the methods for shifting potassium into cells take effect quite rapidly, allowing time for the more definitive removal of potassium by another method. One example is the use of intravenous insulin (e.g., 10 units of regular insulin). When used, it must be accompanied by the administration of dextrose (e.g., 50 g of dextrose in a 50% solution) unless the patient is already hyperglycemic. In patients presenting with hyperkalemia in the setting of insulin deficiency (with diabetic ketoacidosis or hyperosmolar hyperglycemia), the administration of insulin may result in a very rapid decrease in the serum potassium concentration. In many of these cases, the patient will be suffering from a total body depletion of potassium secondary to the ongoing osmotic diuresis. Therefore, these patients require close monitoring of their serum potassium and almost universally require potassium supplementation after the initiation of insulin therapy.

Table 52-4 lists several interventions for decreasing serum potassium concentration by shifting potassium into cells and offers some of the caveats to their use.[1,2,7]

Some disorders of hyperkalemia are chronic diseases that require a long-term management strategy. Some of the type 4 renal tubular acidoses are examples of such a situation. In cases of type 4 RTA, when the cause is not reversible, correction of the

Table 52-5 Causes of Hypokalemia

Category	Examples
Spurious (very rare)	Extreme leukocytosis, if blood is allowed to stand for long periods
Insufficient dietary intake of potassium (rare)	Extremely low potassium diets (e.g., tea and toast)
Nonrenal potassium losses	• Any gastrointestinal fluid losses including diarrhea • Perspiration
Shifting of potassium from outside of cells to the intracellular space	See Table 52-2.
Renal losses secondary to increased solute delivery to the distal nephron	Bicarbonaturia from vomiting or proximal renal tubular dysfunction (type 2 renal tubular acidosis), diuretics (e.g., loop, thiazide, acetazolamide), osmotic diuresis or other causes of polyuria, high-dose penicillin, aggressive saline administration
Renal losses secondary to hyperaldosteronism	See Table 52-1.
Other renal losses secondary to hypomagnesemia or the direct tubular effect of drugs	Aminoglycosides, amphotericin, foscarnet, cisplatin, and iphosphamide. Hypomagnesemia itself also causes renal wasting of potassium.

hyperkalemia can often be achieved by simply prescribing a low-potassium diet and a loop diuretic and removing any medications that might be exacerbating the hyperkalemia. Control of the serum potassium concentration often improves acid handling by the kidney and corrects the acidosis as well. Sometimes, however, these measures will fail to correct the hyperkalemia, the acidosis, or both. In these cases, alkali therapy such as oral sodium bicarbonate may be required as well.

Patients with medication-induced hyperkalemia should have the responsible agents held. However, there is a strong indication for the use of these medications in certain disorders (e.g., cyclosporine in renal transplantation, ACE inhibitors in congestive heart failure). Hyperkalemia is especially likely to occur with the use of medication when the glomerular filtration rate falls to less than 30 mL/minute. Often, these medications can be reinstituted if the appropriate measures are taken to control serum potassium. These measures might include the use of diuretics, administration of sodium bicarbonate in cases of acidosis (as discussed above), and a low-potassium diet.[3]

Patients with severe renal failure (with glomerular filtration rates <20 mL/min) should receive dietary education that will assist them in eating diets that are appropriately low in potassium.

HYPOKALEMIA

Background

Hypokalemia is an extremely common electrolyte abnormality in hospitalized patients. Hospitalists should recognize the common causes of hypokalemia and be facile at supplementing potassium to correct the deficiency when necessary.

Assessment

Clinical Presentation

Symptoms of hypokalemia are uncommon with serum concentrations >3 mEq/L. Severe hypokalemia can result in muscle weakness, and even the development of rhabdomyolysis, or intestinal ileus. Hypokalemia itself may induce renal abnormalities, including nephrogenic diabetes insipidus, and increased ammonia production, which may exacerbate encephalopathy

in patients with hepatic disease. A low serum potassium may predispose patients to cardiac arrhythmias, including sinus bradycardia, atrioventricular block, paroxysmal atrial or junctional tachycardia, and ventricular tachycardia or fibrillation. Hypokalemia also increases the cardiac toxicity of digoxin.

Electrocardiographic changes of hypokalemia include diminished T waves, accentuated U waves, prolongation of the PR interval, QRS widening, and ST segment depressions.

Diagnosis/Differential Diagnosis

The causes of hypokalemia are summarized in Table 52-5, and are commonly categorized with respect to the following precipitants: low potassium intake, potassium shifting into cells from the extracellular space, nonrenal losses, and renal losses.[1,2,4]

Spurious hypokalemia is rare, but can result if blood stands for a long period of time before the analysis is performed, with potassium shifting into blood cells. This is more likely to occur if there is an extreme elevation of the leukocyte count.

There are many conditions that cause potassium to shift into cells, and these are summarized in Table 52-2.

Nonrenal losses of potassium can occur when excess fluid is lost from the gastrointestinal tract or skin. Diarrhea is one of the most common causes of potassium loss. Also, excessive perspiring can result in the loss of potassium.

Renal losses of potassium are most likely to occur if there are *both* delivery of sodium to the distal nephron *and* an aldosterone effect there. However, it is useful to categorize these somewhat separately. The disorders that cause hypokalemia that are, at least in part, secondary to increase solute delivery to the distal nephron include bicarbonaturia (which occurs with the acid loss in vomiting or via proximal tubular dysfunction in the type 2 renal tubular acidoses), use of diuretics, osmotic diuresis (and other causes of polyuria), and large saline loads that occur with aggressive saline volume resuscitation.[1,2,4] The potassium wasting is especially prominent when sodium is delivered to the distal tubule along with a nonresorbable anion, such as bicarbonate or penicillin (in the case of high-dose penicillin therapy). Diuresis is most likely to cause hypokalemia when accompanied by hyperaldosteronism, for example, secondary to volume depletion, cirrhosis, or congestive heart failure. Urinary potassium wasting is also associated with a variety of drugs, including aminoglycosides, amphotericin, foscarnet, and cisplatin. These drugs cause direct

Table 52-6 Stepwise Approach to the Patient with Unexplained Hypokalemia

Unexplained hypokalemia exists if a cause is not identified after a complete history and physical examination, considering the etiologies in Table 52-5.

Step 1. Measure urinary potassium in a 24-hour urine collection or calculate the transtubular potassium gradient.
- If the daily 24-hour potassium excretion is <25 mEq or the TTKG is <2, consider the nonrenal causes in Table 52-5. If the 24-hour potassium excretion is >25 mEq or the TTKG is >2, consider the renal causes in Table 52-5, and go to step 2.

Step 2. If there is no clinical explanation for renal potassium loss, especially if it occurs concomitant with hypertension and/or metabolic alkalosis, consider a mineralocorticoid excess state.

Step 3. If mineralocorticoid excess is suspected, rule out glycyrrhizinic acid ingestion (see text) and measure 24-hour urine cortisol excretion and serum aldosterone concentration simultaneous with plasma renin activity.
- Elevated 24-hour urine cortisol suggests Cushing's syndrome
- Elevated aldosterone levels with suppressed plasma renin activity suggests primary hyperaldosteronism (see Table 52-1)
- Elevated renin levels with elevated aldosterone levels suggest a hyper-reninemic state (see Table 52-1)

tubular magnesium wasting, and hypomagnesemia of any cause will lead to urinary potassium wasting. Amphotericin also causes direct tubular potassium wasting. Type 1 renal tubular acidosis is classically associated with hypokalemia, and some acute leukemias appear to cause renal losses of potassium as well, via unclear mechanisms.[4] Several hereditary conditions cause hypokalemia, but these are not discussed here, as they are rarely diagnosed in adults.

Hyperaldosteronism can be primarily responsible for hypokalemia, as illustrated in Table 52-1. This table does not discuss congenital causes. A variety of common clinical conditions can result in secondary hyperaldosteronism. Conditions such as congestive heart failure, cirrhosis, and volume depletion result in elevated aldosterone concentrations in the serum, but often do not cause hypokalemia, as there is often a decrease in renal perfusion and the delivery of sodium to the distal tubule in these disorders. Although much less common than the other causes of hypokalemia described previously, primary states of mineralocorticoid excess are important to recognize when present. The presence of unexplained hypokalemia, especially if accompanied by hypertension that is resistant to treatment and/or metabolic alkalosis, should result in an evaluation for these disorders. Mineralocorticoid excess also causes a metabolic alkalosis, and the topic is discussed further in the acid-base chapter (Chapter 53).

Preferred Studies

Most cases of hypokalemia can be easily explained by a careful history and physical examination, without extensive laboratory testing. Laboratory testing for most patients with hypokalemia should include a basic chemistry profile (including basic electrolytes, a serum creatinine, and BUN), a serum magnesium level, and a complete blood count. Other testing is sometimes needed as outlined below.

Clinical Approach

Most cases of hypokalemia will be explained by potassium losses that are clinically apparent, such as renal losses secondary to diuretic medications or osmotic diuresis, or nonrenal losses, such as those that occur with gastrointestinal disease. Since medications are frequent causes of hypokalemia, a careful history in this regard is often fruitful.

Hypokalemia that is unexplained despite a careful history and physical examination warrants additional evaluation, even if the hypokalemia can be initially corrected with supplementation. Table 52-6 outlines a stepwise approach to the evaluation of unexplained hypokalemia. In these cases, it is important to consider the states of mineralocorticoid excess, particularly if the hypokalemia is accompanied by a metabolic alkalosis and/or hypertension. An assessment of urinary potassium excretion can be a useful initial step to guide the evaluation of these patients. This can be done by measuring the concentration of potassium in a 24-hour urine specimen (which should be <25 mEq/day if potassium depletion is secondary to nonrenal causes) or by calculation of the transtubular potassium gradient, described above (which should be <2 if potassium depletion is secondary to nonrenal causes)[1,6]

If a mineralocorticoid excess state is suspected, one should first exclude excessive licorice ingestion or Cushing's syndrome. Although not common in the United States, some licorice candy, chewing gum, and chewing tobacco contain glycyrrhizinic acid. This compound inhibits 11-beta hydroxysteroid dehydrogenase, which results in a state of effective mineralocorticoid excess.[9] Cushing's syndrome can be suggested by history and physical examination, and the history should also exclude exogenous steroid use. The measurement of cortisol in a 24-hour urine collection is an adequate screening test for glucocorticoid excess. In some cases, specific testing of the renin-angiotensin-aldosterone system may be necessary (see Table 52-6). Because of the complexities of interpreting plasma renin activity and aldosterone levels,[10,11] the consultative assistance of an endocrinologist or nephrologist may be especially helpful when performing functional assessments of the renin-angiotensin-aldosterone system. Since conditions of mineralocorticoid excess often result in metabolic alkalosis, the approach to these disorders is more thoroughly discussed in the chapter covering acid-base abnormalities (Chapter 53).

Management

Treatment

The initial treatment of hypokalemia should focus on correcting the serum potassium concentration, especially if the patient is experiencing adverse effects from the hypokalemia.

Potassium chloride is the potassium salt of choice for correcting hypokalemia, and it can be given via the oral or intravenous route.[1,4,12] Intravenous administration of potassium has some important limitations. Solutions containing concentrations of potassium chloride >60 mEq/L should not be delivered via a peripheral vein, as this can result in pain and sclerosis. Also, it is generally advised that potassium be administered at a rate not to exceed 20 mEq/hr. Taken together, these limitations suggest that the administration of large amounts of potassium chloride requires the administration of large volumes of fluid and are time limited. So, intravenous potassium repletion should be used when potassium levels are extremely low, when patients suffer the most severe manifestations of hypokalemia (e.g., cardiac arrhythmias, severe muscle weakness), or when the oral route is not an option. However, when possible, the repletion of potassium should be done via the oral route, usually over the course of several days.

It has been estimated that each 1 mEq/L decrease in the serum potassium value represents a total body potassium deficit of 200–400 mEq. However, serum potassium levels will begin to rise quickly with the initiation of therapy, and the total estimated deficit does not need to be supplemented immediately. In most cases, 40–100 mEq/day, given in divided, oral doses for several days, will correct the deficit.[12] Of course, this estimate assumes that there are not continued losses. Close monitoring of the serum potassium can help ensure that repletion is appropriate.

It appears that the adverse effects of hypokalemia are especially likely in patients with underlying organic heart disease, those taking digoxin, or those with significant hepatic dysfunction (in whom hypokalemia can cause encephalopathy). In these populations, it has been suggested that the serum potassium should be maintained above 4 mEq/L.[12]

Importantly, insulin and dextrose should not be given to most patients with severe hypokalemia, as both of these can cause an exacerbation of the hypokalemia. So, intravenous potassium chloride should not be mixed in a dextrose-containing solution for patients who are severely hypokalemic. Also, patients with diabetic emergencies (ketoacidosis or a hyperosmolar state) who are severely hypokalemic at presentation should *not* be given insulin as part of their initial treatment until potassium repletion has been initiated. Aggressive insulin treatment will further lower serum potassium in these patients, and it can result in life-threatening cardiac arrhythmias.

Hypomagnesemia must be corrected. Since hypomagnesemia causes significant renal potassium wasting, it may be impossible to correct a patient's hypokalemia with potassium supplements if hypomagnesemia goes unrecognized and untreated. Also, hypokalemia often occurs with metabolic alkalosis, and the patient's acid-base status should be addressed as discussed in the acid-base chapter.

Treatment of the underlying cause of the potassium deficiency is essential. Diuretic therapy is one of the most common causes of hypokalemia. In the hospitalized patient, aggressive diuresis is a common treatment modality that should be paired with empiric potassium supplementation in most cases. Although low-dose thiazides, used for hypertension, often do not require potassium supplementation, diuresis for conditions that are commonly associated with hyperaldosteronism (e.g., cirrhosis, congestive heart failure) usually requires at least low daily doses of potassium. Ultimately, the clinician must balance the effect of diuresis with the use of medications that can combat potassium loss (including potassium supplementation, potassium-sparing diuretics, eplerenone, ACE inhibitors, and angiotensin receptor blockers), all in the context of the patient's renal function.

In the case of a diarrheal illness, the volume of diarrhea should be reduced, if possible. Primary hyperaldosteronism is often treated in collaboration with an endocrinologist or nephrologist. Primary hyperaldosteronism secondary to adrenal adenoma or carcinoma can be surgically cured, while that resulting from bilateral adrenal hyperplasia is often treated medically, with potassium-sparing diuretics such as spironolactone, triamterene, or amiloride.

DISORDERS OF MAGNESIUM BALANCE

Hypermagnesemia is not commonly of clinical importance and is almost always caused by renal failure or the over administration or over ingestion of magnesium, and will not be discussed further. Hypomagnesemia is, on the other hand, commonly seen in hospitalized patients. Hypomagnesemia is, most commonly, the result of magnesium losses via the GI tract or kidneys. Hospitalists should recognize the situations in which hypomagnesemia is likely to be present and should be confident managing the disorder, when detected.

HYPOMAGNESEMIA

Background

Magnesium is highly filtered by the kidney. A normal kidney is able to resorb almost all of the filtered magnesium when stimulated to do so. Hypomagnesemia itself appears to be the primary stimulus for increasing magnesium reabsorption, which occurs primarily in the thick ascending limb of the loop of Henle.[2,13,14] Therefore, hypomagnesemia can occur as the result of failure of the kidney to resorb magnesium. This failure can occur secondary to increased tubular flow, tubular dysfunction (including that secondary to medications), or other metabolic abnormalities including hypercalcemia, hypokalemia, hypophosphatemia, or metabolic acidosis. There is not a significant storage pool of magnesium in the body. Therefore, alterations in intake and excretion can rapidly result in low serum concentrations of magnesium.

Assessment

Clinical Presentation

Hypomagnesemia is usually asymptomatic. Symptoms are more likely when the disorder is severe and can include neuromuscular dysfunction, cardiac arrhythmias, and other electrolyte abnormalities.[2,13] Neuromuscular symptoms can include weakness, fatigue, or irritability (including Trousseau's sign, Chvostek's sign, nystagmus, tetany, and seizures). Hypomagnesemia has a variety of cardiac effects. Modest hypomagnesemia can result in a widened QRS and peaked T waves on the electrocardiogram. More severe hypomagnesemia results in more prominent widening of the QRS and PR prolongation, and possibly ventricular arrhythmias. Ventricular arrhythmias, including ventricular tachycardia and ventricular fibrillation, are thought to be especially common in the setting of active cardiac ischemia. Torsades de pointes is the ventricular arrhythmia most closely associated with hypomagnesemia. Of note, hypomagnesemia also exacerbates digoxin toxicity.

Also of clinical importance is the effect of hypomagnesemia on the levels of other electrolytes. Hypomagnesemia actually causes hypokalemia (via renal potassium wasting) and hypocalcemia (via decreased release and effect of parathyroid hormone), a fact that must be remembered when treating either of these electrolyte disorders.

Diagnosis/Differential Diagnosis

The diagnosis of hypomagnesemia is typically based on routine laboratory measurement of the serum magnesium concentration. However, magnesium is, primarily, an intracellular cation, and the serum magnesium concentration is not a reliable predictor of intracellular magnesium levels. In addition, like calcium, serum magnesium levels decrease as the serum albumin decreases. However, assays for ionized magnesium levels are not widely available. Therefore, measurement of the serum magnesium concentration is, at best, a gross estimate of a patient's total-body magnesium stores.[13] Measurements of urine magnesium excretion can be helpful in assessing magnesium depletion. However, in practice, these measurements are not often performed, and clinicians are accustomed to estimating magnesium balance from measurements of serum magnesium concentrations, despite their shortcomings.

Once magnesium depletion is established, the clinician must determine the etiology of the deficiency. Box 52-1 shows the causes of hypomagnesemia.[2,13,15] Congenital causes are not discussed here.

In hospitalized patients, hypomagnesemia is often iatrogenic, related to intentional diuresis or other medications. Loop and thiazide diuretics can each cause hypomagnesemia. Hypomagnesemia is also exacerbated by hyperaldosteronism seen in common illnesses such as congestive heart failure and cirrhosis. Other conditions that are commonly associated with hypomagnesemia include severe hyperglycemia, diarrheal illnesses, pancreatitis, and hypercalcemia. Any gastrointestinal disease that causes malabsorption can result in hypomagnesemia. Steatorrhea results in saponification of magnesium and is particularly likely to cause the disorder.

Poor intake is not a common cause of hypomagnesemia, but it probably contributes to the hypomagnesemia seen in severely malnourished or alcoholic patients. The diet of the alcoholic patient is often low in magnesium, and alcohol is thought to result in renal magnesium wasting as well. Hypomagnesemia can also be seen in patients who are treated with parenteral nutrition, and it has been suggested that magnesium requirements increase in the parenterally nourished patient.[2,13]

Preferred Studies

If hypomagnesia is discovered, routine laboratory testing should include a serum potassium, calcium, creatinine, and bicarbonate levels in all patients.

Clinical Approach

A careful history and physical examination, along with the laboratory evaluations described above, will elucidate the cause of hypomagnesemia in most cases. Nonrenal causes of hypomagnesemia will usually be apparent, if sought (see Box 52-1). In patients without a clear nonrenal cause for the hypomagnesemia,

---

Box 52-1 Causes of Hypomagnesemia.

- **Renal losses**
  - Drug related
    - Diuretics (loop or thiazide)
    - Aminoglycosides
    - Amphotericin
    - Cisplatin
    - Calcineurin inhibitors (cyclosporine, tacrolimus)
    - Pentamidine
    - Foscarnet
  - Osmotic diuresis
    - Hyperglycemia
    - Volume expansion
  - Tubular dysfunction
    - Recovery from ATN, obstruction, transplantation
  - Other
    - Hypercalcemia (unless PTH also elevated), hypokalemia, hypophosphatemia, metabolic acidosis
    - Hyperaldosteronism (e.g., as seen in congestive heart failure)
- **Gastrointestinal losses**
  - Diarrhea or malabsorption (e.g., celiac disease, inflammatory bowel disease, Whipple's disease, chronic pancreatitis, short gut syndrome, etc.)
  - Gastric losses (only if extensive)
- **Skin losses (usually negligible)**
  - Burns
  - Toxic epidermal necrolysis
  - Miscellaneous
  - Hungry bone syndrome (after thyroidectomy for the treatment of hyperparathyroidism)
  - Pancreatitis
  - Poor intake (uncommon—most likely in alcoholism or parenteral nutrition)

ATN—acute tubular necrosis; PTH—parathyroid hormone

---

renal losses should be assumed. In these cases, diuretics or osmotic diuresis are the most common culprits, but other medications are also common causes in hospitalized patients (see Box 52-1). Of course, hypercalcemia, hypokalemia, hypophosphatemia, and metabolic acidosis are common conditions in hospitalized patients, and these may also contribute to hypomagnesemia when present.

Management

Treatment

Although hypomagnesemia is common, it is not entirely clear which patients with the disorder should be treated, or which treatment regimen is optimal.

Patients with underlying cardiac disease may be at risk of cardiac arrhythmias when hypomagnesemic. One study of patients with congestive heart failure showed that complex ventricular arrhythmias were more common in patients with lower serum magnesium levels, and confirmed that the administration of magnesium decreased the risk of the arrythmias.[17] However, another observational study was unable to show an association between hypomagnesemia and increased mortality over a longer period of time.[18] Although the prevention of hypomagnesemia in patients with cardiac disease is accepted as a standard therapeutic goal, the optimal serum magnesium concentration and the optimal replacement strategy in patients with heart failure are not certain.

In all cases, concomitant disorders of acid-base, potassium, phosphate, and calcium homeostasis should be treated. In patients who are receiving parenteral nourishment, adjustment in the magnesium concentration may be appropriate.

One to two grams of intravenous magnesium sulfate is recommended to be given as a bolus to patients who are experiencing torsades de pointes,[13] and a similar recommendation might be appropriate for patients who are experiencing other severe symptoms of hypomagnesemia, such as seizures. Patients with underlying cardiac disease, particularly those with cardiac ischemia, should also probably have magnesium deficits replaced promptly.

In asymptomatic patients, the optimal regimen for magnesium replacement is uncertain, and there are few scientific data and no clinical guidelines available. Some authors have recommended the administration of 8 g of magnesium sulfate intravenously in divided doses over the first 24 hours, decreasing to 4 g intravenously in divided doses per day for several days thereafter (continuing for a couple days beyond the correction of the serum concentration, to ensure repletion of intracellular levels).[2] However, rapid administration of magnesium intravenously is counterintuitive if one considers the physiology of magnesium homeostasis. Rapidly increasing the serum magnesium concentration will create a strong stimulus for renal magnesium wasting. Therefore, it is likely that most of the magnesium that is given in a rapid intravenous infusion is actually renally excreted, and therefore unable to correct the presumed intracellular deficit. This observation suggests that slower correction may be most effective.[2,13,16]

Oral treatment of magnesium deficiency results in slower correction, and therefore is theoretically advantageous in cases where magnesium repletion is less urgent, or when the hypomagnesemia is a chronic problem. There are several oral magnesium formulations available, and magnesium chloride is available in a slow-release formulation.[16]

Magnesium repletion can cause side effects. If repletion is overly aggressive, hypotension, atrioventricular block, and loss of deep tendon reflexes can occur.[2] Also, the administration of magnesium will result in a decrease in the serum concentration of ionized calcium. This is of importance in patients who are significantly hypocalcemic, in whom further decrement in calcium could result in symptomatic hypocalcemia. Also, when administering magnesium, the effects of the coadministered anion should be considered. Magnesium sulfate and magnesium gluconate contain nonresorbable anions that can cause hypokalemia, and magnesium oxide and magnesium hydroxide can result in systemic alkalosis.[2]

Chronic hypomagnesemia (e.g., that from needed diuretic treatment or secondary to needed drug therapy) is usually treated with chronic oral magnesium supplementation. Also, when renal magnesium losses are responsible for the hypomagnesemia, the addition of a potassium-sparing diuretic can decrease renal losses of magnesium.[2,13,16] This is especially helpful in patients who have chronic hypomagnesemia that is attributed to diuretic treatment.

Key Points

- An understanding of the basic physiology of the renin-angiotensin-aldosterone system is essential for understanding abnormalities of the serum potassium level.

- Hyperkalemia can be treated using a multimodal approach to achieve three main objectives:

  - Stabilization of the membrane of cardiac myocytes to avoid cardiac arrhythmia (via administration of intravenous calcium salts)

  - Shifting potassium from the extracellular space into cells to quickly reduce plasma levels (via administration of beta-agonist medications, insulin/dextrose, or sodium bicarbonate)

  - Removal of potassium from the body (via administration of diuretics or potassium binding resins, or via dialysis)

- Unexplained hypokalemia should prompt an evaluation for the causes of mineralocorticoid excess.

- Renal causes of hypokalemia can be distinguished from non-renal causes by measuring 24-hour urine potassium excretion or by calculating the transtubular potassium gradient.

- In hypokalemic patients, serum magnesium levels should always be measured. Hypomagnesium can cause hypokalemia, and hypokalemia may be difficult to correct until magnesium levels are corrected.

SUGGESTED READING

Rose BD, Post TW. Clinical Physiology of Acid-base and Electrolyte Disorders, 5th ed. New York; McGraw-Hill, 2001.

Palmer B. Managing hyperkalemia caused by inhibitors of the renin-angiotensin-aldosterone system. N Engl J Med 2004; 351:585–592.

Gennari FJ. Hypokalemia. N Engl J Med 1998; 339:451–458.

Halperin ML, Kamel KS. Potassium. Lancet 1998; 352:135–140.

Kim HJ, Han SW. Therapeutic approach to hyperkalemia. Nephron 2002; 92(Suppl 1):33–40.

Cohn JN, Kowey PR, Whelton PK, et al. New guidelines for potassium replacement in clinical practice. A contemporary review by the National Council on Potassium in Clinical Practice. Arch Intern Med 2000; 160:2429–2436.

CHAPTER FIFTY-THREE

Acid-Base Disorders

David H. Wesorick, MD, and Robert M. Centor, MD

Many medical conditions cause abnormalities of acid-base homeostasis. Often, the acid-base disturbance is not the primary clinical problem but, rather, a feature of the underlying disease process. Therefore, the diagnostic process for a wide range of disorders depends on recognition and accurate classification of the associated acid-base disturbances.

Acid-base homeostasis depends on the body's ability to buffer acute changes in pH and to eliminate excess acid or alkali. The respiratory system and the kidneys are the primary physiologic systems involved in acid-base homeostasis. Disorders can be generally divided into four categories:

1. Metabolic acidosis
2. Metabolic alkalosis
3. Respiratory acidosis
4. Respiratory alkalosis

GENERAL CLASSIFICATION

A patient's acid-base status provides important diagnostic information. Therefore, the clinician must be able to rapidly recognize and categorize acid-base disorders. Table 53-1 presents a stepwise approach to the evaluation of clinical acid-base disorders.[1,2]

The first step is to recognize the primary acid-base disturbance. Alkalemia (arterial blood pH >7.45) suggests that the primary disorder is an alkalosis, whereas acidemia (arterial blood pH <7.35) suggests that the primary disorder is an acidosis.

The second step is to compare the patient's data with the expected physiologic compensation. Table 53-1 summarizes the expected compensation for each of the individual acid-base disturbances. Analyzing the compensatory response allows the clinician to detect the presence of any concomitant disturbance ("mixed" disorders) and to judge the chronicity of the disorder. It should be noted that compensation is usually incomplete (i.e., it does not completely correct the pH) and that these formulae provide only estimates of the expected response.

The third step is to examine the anion gap. The anion gap can be calculated using the formula shown in Table 53-1. If this gap is significantly elevated, it suggests the presence of an anion gap acidosis. The normal anion gap is approximately 8–12, but there is significant variation of this value among individuals. When the anion gap is elevated, the clinician can gain additional information about the acid-base disturbance by comparing the degree of change in the anion gap to the degree of change in the serum bicarbonate, as shown in Table 53-1.

Using this simple process, a patient's acid-base status can be rapidly and accurately categorized. An example case is shown in Table 53-2.

METABOLIC ACIDOSIS

Background

Metabolic acidosis occurs as a consequence of a wide variety of clinical conditions. It is often initially recognized as a low serum bicarbonate concentration. Metabolic acidosis signifies an important underlying disorder that deserves further diagnostic and therapeutic attention.

Assessment

Clinical Presentation

Most of the presenting features of a metabolic acidosis are related to the nature of the underlying disorder (*see* Tables 53-3 and 53-4). Metabolic acidosis directly causes one classic physical finding: slow, deep breaths, called Kussmaul's respirations. Acidosis can lead to impairment of cardiac function and a decrease in vascular resistance, secondary to an attenuation of the usual response of these systems to catecholamines. Cardiovascular collapse can result. Acidosis also predisposes to cardiac arrhythmias. In addition, acidosis causes a shift of potassium out of cells, and can cause or exacerbate hyperkalemia. Mental status changes can also occur with severe acidosis.[1,4]

Differential Diagnosis

Once a metabolic acidosis is recognized, the diagnostic effort is turned to identifying the underlying disorder. Often, the underlying disorder is apparent, but sometimes further evaluation is needed. The first step in the differential diagnosis of a metabolic acidosis is to determine if there is an elevated serum anion gap (*see* Table 53-1).

Acidosis with an Elevated Anion Gap

The differential diagnosis of an acidosis associated with an elevated anion gap is shown in Table 53-3.[1,4] In these acidotic states, the anion gap is increased because of the accumulation of

Table 53-1 A Stepwise Approach to the Classification of Acid-Base Abnormalities

Step 1. Define the primary disorder.
- Use pH to determine the primary disorder (normal arterial blood pH = 7.35–7.45). pH >7.45 = alkalemia; pH <7.35 = acidemia.
- If an acid-base disturbance is suspected, but the pH is normal, make the best estimate of the primary disorder, considering the serum bicarbonate concentration, the pCO_2, the anion gap, and the clinical situation.

Step 2. Calculate the expected physiologic compensation to determine if there is a mixed acid-base disorder.
- For metabolic disorders, calculate the expected pCO_2: For metabolic acidosis: expected $pCO_2 = (1.5 \times [HCO_3]) + 8 \pm 2)$. For metabolic alkalosis: expected $pCO_2 = (0.9 \times [HCO_3]) + 9 \pm 2)$.
  - If the actual pCO_2 is higher than expected, consider a concomitant respiratory acidosis.
  - If the actual pCO_2 is lower than expected, consider a concomitant respiratory alkalosis.
- For respiratory disorders, calculate the expected serum bicarbonate: For respiratory acidosis: for every increase by 10 mm Hg in the pCO_2, serum bicarbonate concentration should increase by 1 mEq/L (acute) to 3.5 mEq/L (chronic). For respiratory alkalosis: For every decrease by 10 mm Hg in pCO_2, serum bicarbonate concentration should decrease by 2 mEq/L (acute) to 4 mEq/L (chronic).
  - If the actual serum bicarbonate concentration is higher than expected, consider a concomitant metabolic alkalosis.
  - If the actual serum bicarbonate concentration is lower than expected, consider a concomitant metabolic acidosis.

Step 3. Consider the anion gap.
- Calculate the anion gap $(AG = [Na] - ([Cl] + [HCO_3]))$: If elevated, this suggests an anion gap acidosis is present.
- If the anion gap is elevated, calculate the delta gap: for every 1 point increase in the anion gap (normal = 8–12), there should be a 1 mEq/l decrease in the serum bicarbonate concentration.
  - If the actual serum bicarbonate concentration is higher than expected, consider a concomitant metabolic alkalosis.
  - If the actual serum bicarbonate concentration is lower than expected, consider a concomitant normal anion gap acidosis.

Table 53-2 An Example Acid-Base Case, Illustrating the Stepwise Approach Shown in Table 53-1

Case: A 58-year-old schizophrenic man was brought to the hospital for strange behavior. Laboratory evaluation on the emergency department revealed the following: sodium 139, potassium 4.7, chloride 90, bicarbonate 14, creatinine 1.0, glucose 100, arterial blood gases: pH 7.49, pCO_2 15, pO_2 159 (on 2 L/min of O_2 by nasal canula).

Step 1. Define the primary disorder:
Arterial blood pH >7.45 = primary alkalosis. The low CO_2 suggests that this is a respiratory alkalosis.

Step 2. Calculate the expected physiologic compensation to determine if there is a mixed acid-base disorder:
The expected serum bicarbonate concentration for an acute respiratory alkalosis is 19. The actual serum bicarbonate concentration in this case is 14, suggesting that there is a concomitant metabolic acidosis.

Step 3. Consider the anion gap:
The anion gap is 35; therefore, there is an anion gap acidosis present. The anion gap is increased by 27 (assuming a normal of 8). However the serum bicarbonate is only decreased by 10 (assuming a normal of 24 mEq/L). The actual serum bicarbonate is therefore much higher than expected, suggesting a concomitant metabolic alkalosis.

Synthesis: This patient has a respiratory alkalosis, an anion gap metabolic acidosis, and a metabolic alkalosis.

Solution: This patient had a respiratory alkalosis and an anion gap acidosis, the classic acid-base findings associated with salicylate toxicity. However, in this case the toxicity was secondary to an overdose of Alka-Seltzer, which contains sodium bicarbonate (in addition to salicylate), resulting in the concomitant metabolic alkalosis.

anionic substances that are not normally present. The normal anion gap is approximately 8–12. Variations in the levels of normally occurring unmeasured cations (e.g., magnesium, calcium, immunoglobulins) and normally occurring unmeasured anions (e.g., albumin) will affect this range. The effect of the serum albumin concentration on the anion gap calculation is important. A useful clinical rule is that for every 1 mg/dL decrease in the serum albumin concentration from normal, the anion gap will decrease by approximately 2.5. Therefore, the anion gap in a patient with an organic acidosis and severe hypoalbuminemia might be somewhat lower than expected. Because of the variability of the normal anion gap and the many factors that affect this value, higher anion gaps are more likely to represent true organic acidosis. An anion gap >20 is often associated with an organic acidosis, whereas values less than this may not be. In one study, a demonstrable organic acidosis was present in 65% of all patients with an anion gap of 20–24, 80% of all patients with an anion gap of 25–29, and 100% of all patients with an anion gap of 30 or higher.[3] Most cases of anion gap acidosis are caused by the development of ketosis, the accumulation of lactate, intoxication with substances that raise the anion gap, or renal failure.

The disorders associated with ketosis can be recognized clinically via the detection of abnormally elevated level of urine or

Table 53-3 Common Disorders Causing Metabolic Acidosis, with an Elevated Anion Gap

Disorder (Accumulating Anions)	Clinical Features	Diagnosis	Notes
DISORDERS OF KETOSIS			
Diabetic ketoacidosis (ketones)	Known type 1 diabetes, or signs of diabetes (polyuria, polydipsia, polyphagia)	Triad of hyperglycemia, acidosis, and ketosis is suggestive	15% of patients with diabetic ketoacidosis present with glucose levels <350 mg/dL
Alcoholic ketoacidosis (ketones)	Known alcohol abuse, evidence of intoxication or withdrawal	Ketosis accompanied by appropriate history	
Starvation ketosis (ketones)	History of starvation or malnourishment		Usually mild and clinically less important
DISORDERS OF LACTIC ACID ACCUMULATION			
Lactic acidosis secondary to inadequate tissue oxygen delivery (lactate)	Multiple disorders, see "Notes"	Serum lactate level >4 mEq/L	Examples: Circulatory failure, hypoxemia, high-demand states (e.g., convulsive seizures), or localized tissue ischemia (e.g., bowel ischemia)
Lactic acidosis secondary to drugs (lactate)	Multiple disorders, see "Notes"	Serum lactate level >4 mEq/L	Examples: Metformin, zidovudine, stavudine
Lactic acidosis secondary to other disorders (lactate)	Multiple disorders, see "Notes"	Serum lactate level >4 mEq/L	Examples: Hypoglycemia, malignancy, liver disease, thiamine deficiency, carbon monoxide poisoning
DISORDERS WITH AN ELEVATED OSMOLAR GAP			
Ethylene glycol toxicity (glycolate, oxalate)	Alcoholic patient, often with low socioeconomic status, clinical presentation similar to alcohol intoxication, but ethanol level does not explain intoxication	UA may show oxalate crystals, osmolar gap often >25, urine may fluoresce under Wood's light (ultraviolet) if antifreeze was ingested, serum level is diagnostic	Ethylene glycol is found in "antifreeze"
Methanol toxicity (formate)	Alcoholic patient, often with low socioeconomic status, clinical presentation similar to alcohol intoxication and patient may also complain of blindness or visual disturbance, ethanol level does not explain intoxication	Osmolar gap often >25, serum level is diagnostic	Methanol is found in varnishes and shellacs
OTHER DISORDERS			
Advanced renal failure (phosphate, sulfate, urate, hippurate)	Acute or chronic renal failure		Renal failure can also be accompanied by a normal anion gap acidosis.
Salicylate toxicity (lactate, pyruvate, ketones)	Depressed or suicidal pts may deny ingestion, tinnitus may be present, can have hypotension	Usually no osmolar gap is present but ketones may be present and lactate may be slightly elevated as well; serum level is diagnostic	Respiratory alkalosis is the most common acid-base disturbance. Acidosis is uncommon alone.

UA—urinalysis

Table 53-4 Causes of Metabolic Acidosis Without an Anion Gap

Disorder	Clinical Features and Diagnosis	Notes
NONRENAL CAUSES		
Acid ingestion/iatrogenic		Rare. Causes include misallocation of amino acids in parenteral nutrition, massive administration of saline solutions.
Gastrointestinal bicarbonate loss	The cause is usually clinically apparent. While acidotic, urine pH <5.3, and urine anion gap negative (e.g., more negative than −20).	Common. Causes include diarrhea (including laxative-induced), external losses of pancreatic or small bowel fluids (e.g., pancreaticocutaneous fistula, pancreas transplants), or urinary to bowel diversions.
RENAL CAUSES		
Chronic kidney disease (before the development of an anion gap)	Usually apparent after standard testing.	
Type 2 RTA (proximal)	While acidotic, urine pH <5.3 (when serum bicarbonate concentration is below the resorptive threshold) and urine anion gap is usually negative. Glucosuria can be present in Fanconi's syndrome. Serum potassium is often low, but can be normal.	Associated diseases include: hereditary forms, multiple myeloma, light chain disease, other monoclonal gammopathies, amyloidosis, Wilson's disease, Sjögren's syndrome, hypocalcemia and vitamin D deficiency, and drugs (e.g., acetazolamide, outdated tetracycline, aminoglycosides, valproate, streptozocin, 6-mercaptopurine, iphosphamide, cidofovir, didanosine, lamivudine, stavudine).
Type I RTA (distal)	While acidotic, urine pH >5.3, urine anion gap positive (e.g., greater than −20). Serum potassium is usually low, but can be normal or elevated in some forms.	Associated diseases include: hereditary forms, hypergammaglobulinemia, cryoglobulinemia, amyloidosis, autoimmune diseases (systemic lupus,* Sjögren syndrome, rheumatoid arthritis, others), chronic pyelonephritis, renal transplant rejection,* obstructive uropathy,* sickle cell anemia,* disorders of hypercalcemia/nephrocalcinosis (e.g., hypervitaminosis D, hyperparathyroidism), drugs (e.g., amphotericin, lithium, iphosphamide, foscarnet)
Type 4 RTA (hyperkalemic)	While acidotic, urine pH <5.3, and urine anion gap positive (e.g., greater than −20). Serum potassium is often elevated.	Associated diseases include: mineralocorticoid deficiency (e.g., adrenal failure, congenital adrenal hyperplasia), nephropathies causing hyporeninemia (e.g., diabetic, lupus-related, AIDS-related, acute glomerulonephritis), chronic nephropathies causing mineralocorticoid resistance (transplant rejection, obstructive uropathy, sickle cell anemia, others), or drugs (e.g., beta-blockers, methyldopa, NSAIDs, ACE inhibitors/angiotensin II receptor blockers, heparin, potassium-sparing diuretics, trimethoprim, pentamidine, cyclosporine, tacrolimus).

*may be associated with hyperkalemia.

RTA—renal tubular acidosis; NSAIDs—nonsteroidal anti-inflammactory drugs; ACE—angiotensin converting enzyme

serum ketones. The nitroprusside test for ketones is commonly used and does not detect beta-hydroxybuterate, the predominant ketone in diabetic ketoacidosis (DKA), and therefore, it may underestimate the degree of ketosis. The presence of ethanol or lactate also favors the formation of beta-hydroxybuterate as the predominant ketone. Therefore, in cases of anion gap acidosis when a disorder of ketosis is suspected, the diagnosis should not be dismissed simply because of a negative nitroprusside test for ketones, especially if lactate or alcohol is also detected. In these cases, beta-hydroxybuterate can be measured directly. Of the disorders associated with ketosis, diabetic ketoacidosis is the most common, and is often easily recognized as the triad of hyperglycemia, ketosis, and an anion gap acidosis. Alcoholism and starvation can also result in ketosis, as outlined in Table 53-3.

Lactic acidosis occurs most commonly in hospitalized patients in association with a state of inadequate tissue oxygenation. Examples include states of circulatory failure, hypoxemia, high-demand states (e.g., convulsive seizures), or localized tissue ischemia (e.g., bowel ischemia). In these states, anaerobic metabolism results in lactate production. Measurement of a serum lactate level can corroborate the diagnosis when it is suspected and can uncover the diagnosis when it is not. Serum levels of lactate are normally <2 mEq/L and are most likely to be clinically important when >4 mEq/L.

Although less common, lactic acidosis can also occur in association with conditions that are *not* characterized by inadequate tissue oxygenation. Certain medications and a variety of other disorders can cause lactic acidosis (*see* Table 53-3).[1,5] These disorders should be considered when lactate levels are elevated and there is no clinical evidence of inadequate tissue oxygenation.

In the case of intoxication with ethylene glycol and methanol, the hallmark clinical finding (in addition to the elevated anion gap) is an elevated osmolar gap: Osmolar Gap = Measured serum osmolality – Calculated serum osmolality (The calculated serum osmolality = 2 [Na (in mEq/L)] + [glucose (in mg/dL)]/18 + [BUN (in mg/dL)]/2.8 + [alcohol (in mOsm/kg)]/4.6). An elevated osmolar gap suggests the presence of an unmeasured, osmotically active substance in the serum. Examples of such substances include methanol, ethylene glycol, isopropyl alcohol, mannitol, and radiocontrast. (Although isopropyl alcohol, mannitol, and radiocontrast can raise the osmolar gap, these substances do not usually raise the anion gap.) Also, although the normal osmolar gap is <15, significant ingestions will usually raise the osmolar gap to well over 25. In the case of methanol or ethylene glycol intoxication, serum levels are diagnostic. Other clinical features of these ingestions are detailed in Table 53-3.

The anion gap acidosis in the case of salicylate overdose is usually accompanied by a respiratory alkalosis. Recognition of this particular mixed acid-base disorder should prompt the physician to consider salicylate intoxication as a possible cause. Laboratory evaluation in these cases usually does not reveal an osmolar gap, but ketones and lactate can be present in modest amounts. Elevated serum salicylate levels are diagnostic. Some clinical features of salicylate toxicity are detailed in Table 53-3.

Advanced renal failure causes an elevated anion gap due to the retention of a variety of anionic compounds (phosphate, sulfate, urate, hippurate).

Consideration of the disorders in Table 53-3 will usually allow the clinician to explain an anion gap acidosis. Other rare causes of anion gap acidosis include paraldehyde, massive rhabdomyolysis, D-lactic acidosis (e.g., in the short bowel syndrome), isoniazid overdose, and toluene toxicity (e.g., secondary to glue sniffing).

Acidosis with a Normal Anion Gap

A different set of disorders should be considered when a metabolic acidosis presents without an elevated anion gap (Table 53-4).[1,2] In general, acidosis without an elevated anion gap occurs secondary to the ingestion of acid (rare), the gastrointestinal loss of bicarbonate (common), or as a result of renal tubular dysfunction associated with the renal tubular acidoses (RTAs).

Ingestion of excess acid is a rare cause of acidosis, but can occur with misappropriation of amino acids in parenteral nutrition. Also, rapid, massive infusions of normal saline can result in a dilutional or hyperchloremic acidosis, as the serum bicarbonate concentration declines proportionately to the added chloride (commonly seen after aggressive fluid resuscitation for DKA).

More commonly, normal anion gap acidoses occur as a result of gastrointestinal losses of bicarbonate, which can occur with diarrhea (including laxative induced), external losses of pancreatic or small bowel fluids (e.g., enterocutaneous or pancreaticocutaneous fistula, pancreas transplants), or urinary to bowel diversions. With the exception of surreptitious laxative abuse, these conditions are usually easily recognized.

Normal anion gap acidoses that are not explained by gastrointestinal bicarbonate losses are usually due to a renal cause of acidosis. Chronic kidney disease typically results in metabolic acidosis as the glomerular filtration rate (GFR) drops below 50 mL/min, and the acidosis becomes more severe as the GFR diminishes. Although end-stage renal disease typically results in an anion gap acidosis, earlier stages of kidney disease often result in an acidosis with a normal anion gap. The acidosis of renal failure occurs as the number of functional nephrons decrease, decreasing the renal production of ammonia available to buffer acid in the urine. Since this type of acidosis is not secondary to tubular dysfunction per se, it is not considered an RTA, although the clinical result is similar.

The RTAs are a group of disorders characterized by either failure of the proximal tubule to reabsorb bicarbonate (proximal, or type 2 RTAs), or failure of the distal tubule to acidify the urine (distal RTAs, type 1 or type 4 RTAs).[1] To some degree, the type of RTA (e.g., 1, 2, or 4) can be approximated by recognizing the clinical syndrome (*see* Table 53-4). It should be noted that each of the RTA types can be caused by a variety of molecular mechanisms, and each of them is associated with many disease processes. Table 53-4 outlines the types of RTA and lists some of the more common causes of each.[1,6–8]

Distinguishing the different types of RTAs can be done, roughly, using some simple clinical testing.[1] Urine pH provides a rough measurement of urine acidification, and the urine anion gap can provide a surrogate measure of ammonium excretion. Ammonia is the primary urinary buffer allowing secretion of protons in the collecting tubule. The urine anion gap is calculated as follows: [urine Na$^+$] + [urine K$^+$] – [urine Cl$^-$]. Secretion of ammonium (NH$_4^+$) requires secretion of chloride (Cl$^-$) for electroneutrality; therefore, in patients with normal renal tubular function, significant distal acid secretion with an ammonia buffer is usually accompanied by a negative urine anion gap (often more negative than –50 and usually more negative than –20), whereas a positive urine anion gap (more positive than –20) suggests an abnormally low ammonium excretion in the setting of acidosis.[2,7] Low urinary ammonium excretion is the result of either a failure to generate ammonia (as occurs with early renal failure) or a failure to move protons into the urine.

Type 2 (proximal) RTA occurs secondary to a proximal tubular defect that results in diminished ability to resorb bicarbonate. Sometimes, the bicarbonate wasting is a part of a more generalized proximal tubular dysfunction called Fanconi's syndrome, in which there is also urinary wasting of other molecules such as glucose, phosphate, urate, or amino acids. The increased delivery of solute to the distal tubule in type 2 RTA often results in hypokalemia, although serum potassium can be normal. In type 2 RTA, ammoniogenesis and distal acidification remain intact, allowing for an acidified urine and, usually, a negative urine anion gap. The proximal tubular wasting of bicarbonate diminishes at lower serum bicarbonate concentrations, such that the urine pH is often low (pH <5.3) when the patient's serum bicarbonate concentration is below the resorptive threshold. However, patients who are being treated with bicarbonate therapy will lose significant amounts of bicarbonate in their urine, causing an elevated urine pH. In fact, bicarbonate loading is a technique that is sometimes used to definitively diagnose a type 2 RTA. Some of the disorders that are associated with type 2 RTAs are listed in Table 53-4.

Type 1 RTAs occur secondary to tubular defects that disallow the acidification of the urine in the collecting tubule. In adults, these defects are often reversible with treatment of the underlying disease. In these disorders, acidosis can be quite severe (serum bicarbonate can be <10 mEq/L), urine pH is usually >5.3, and the urine anion gap is positive. Serum potassium can be low or normal. Some examples of the disorders associated with type 1 RTAs are listed in Table 53-4.

While type 1 and 2 RTAs are relatively uncommon in adults, type 4 RTAs are seen with some frequency. In type 4 RTA, aldosterone deficiency or resistance results in decreased acid and potassium secretion in the distal tubule. The resulting hyperkalemia has a significant effect on acid excretion. Hyperkalemia diminishes ammonia production, resulting in a positive urine anion gap.[1,9] However, type 4 RTA does not completely disallow acidification of the urine, and the urine pH is often <5.3 in the setting of acidosis. In these disorders, the acidosis may be relatively mild and clinically overshadowed by the hyperkalemia. Therefore, type 4 RTA can often be distinguished from type 1 RTA by the presence of hyperkalemia and a urine pH of less than 5.3 in the former. Any condition that impairs the release of renin, the release of aldosterone, or the action of aldosterone at the tubule can result in a type 4 RTA, and a patient with an unexplained type 4 RTA requires laboratory testing to rule out primary adrenal insufficiency or isolated aldosterone deficiency. Examples of disorders that are associated with type 4 RTA are listed in Table 53-4. These disorders are also discussed in Chapter 52 (other electrolyte abnormalities).

The complex physiology of these disorders creates a situation in which simple pattern recognition will not always lead to accurate classification. Detailed discussion of the complexities of the RTA's is beyond the scope of this chapter, but is available elsewhere.[6,7] Subspecialty consultation may be required if the type of RTA, or its clinical cause, is not clear.

Preferred Studies

In all cases of metabolic acidosis, a complete history and physical examination are critical to characterizing the patient's clinical problem, of which the acidosis is often only a single feature.

In anion gap acidosis, a few laboratory tests are helpful in most patients. Blood counts, a full metabolic profile including liver tests, and a urinalysis are indicated in all. Other frequently used tests include a measurement of serum osmolality (and calculation of the osmolar gap), an assessment of urine and/or serum ketones, a serum lactate level, and arterial blood gases. Other studies may be helpful in the right clinical setting and include measurement of the serum ethanol level, salicylate level, methanol level, ethylene glycol level, and examination of the urine for oxalate crystals or florescence under ultraviolet light. Using a rational combination of these tests, the clinician can almost always accurately determine the cause of the acidosis.

In normal anion gap acidosis, chronic kidney disease or gastrointestinal bicarbonate losses are the most common causes, and

are usually easily recognized. When an RTA is suspected, measurement of urine pH, urine anion gap, urine glucose, and serum potassium, can help the clinician begin to characterize the RTA, as shown Table 53-4.

Management

Treatment

Acidosis with an Elevated Anion Gap

Treatment of most forms of acidosis is aimed at correcting the underlying condition. In cases of acute acidosis, the role of alkali therapy is controversial. Studies of diabetic ketoacidosis, lactic acidosis, and cardiac arrest have not consistently shown improvement in outcomes with alkali therapy.[5,10] In addition, there are significant unintended consequences of alkali therapy, including volume overload, hypokalemia, and "overshoot alkalosis." More troubling are the theoretical physiologic disadvantages of alkali therapy, which include decreased cardiac output, the increased affinity for oxygen of hemoglobin with alkali therapy (theoretically worsening tissue ischemia), and the elevation of the partial pressure of carbon dioxide that may occur.[4,5,10] Despite the controversy, the judicious use of alkali therapy may be appropriate in situations of severe acidemia (pH <7.0)[1,4] if patients are experiencing the most severe consequences of acidosis. These consequences might include hemodynamic instability or cardiac arrhythmia. In addition, the therapeutic use of alkali is particularly appealing in cases where its use might lead to patient benefits beyond the correction of the acid-base status. Such conditions might include severe hyperkalemia (in which the alkali therapy will shift potassium into cells) and acidosis secondary to salicylate toxicity (in which the alkali therapy will assist with clearance of the toxin. See Chapter 88).[1,4] Also, methanol and ethylene glycol intoxications can result in severe acidosis, and the administration of bicarbonate is generally recommended to correct the acidosis in these situations. The treatment of methanol and ethylene glycol intoxication also includes specific therapies to remove the ingested substances (e.g., hemodialysis) and/or delay their conversion to toxic metabolites (e.g., alcohol dehydrogenase inhibitors). If used, acute alkali therapy mandates close monitoring of the acid-base status and the serum potassium concentration.

The alkalinizing agent of choice is sodium bicarbonate. This should be given as an isotonic (or slightly hypotonic) intravenous solution over minutes to hours unless clinical instability necessitates faster administration. It is a reasonable initial goal of therapy to raise the serum bicarbonate to approximately 10 mEq/L over a period of several hours. The ultimate goal is to raise the serum pH to the range of 7.2, a level considered high enough to limit the adverse effects of the acidosis.[4] The following formula can be used to calculate the amount of bicarbonate needed to raise the serum bicarbonate to 10 mEq/L: Body weight (in kg) × 0.5 (bicarbonate distribution) × bicarbonate gap (10 mEq/L − patient's bicarbonate level) = mEq of bicarbonate to administer. Calculations of this type are merely rough guides, and careful monitoring of the acid-base status is the only way to accurately achieve treatment goals when using alkali therapy.

Acidosis with a Normal Anion Gap

In chronic acidosis, treatment is generally advised to limit the long-term adverse effects, including loss of bone density. The acidosis of chronic kidney disease is routinely treated with oral alkali, and the National Kidney Foundation guidelines on the management of chronic kidney disease recommend titrating the dose to achieve a serum bicarbonate concentration of 22 mEq/L.[11] In chronic kidney disease, a dose of 0.5 mEq/kg/day is a reasonable starting dose to correct the acidosis. Sodium bicarbonate is often used, although sodium citrate can also be used, as long as the patient is not receiving aluminum-based phosphate binders (in which case citrate ingestion results in excessive aluminum absorption). In cases of type 4 RTA, when the cause is not reversible, correction of the hyperkalemia, using a low-potassium diet and a loop diuretic, often improves acid handling by the kidney. Sometimes, however, alkali therapy is required as well. Occasionally, patients with type 4 RTA may even require chronic treatment with potassium-binding resins to control serum potassium levels. Type 1 and 2 RTAs can also be treated with oral alkali, and type 2 RTA can require very large amounts of alkali to correct the acidosis.[1]

Discharge/Follow-up plans

In most cases, acute acidosis will have been corrected by the time of hospital discharge. Acidosis that is expected to be chronic and require long-term treatment will require close follow-up after discharge. Information about the cause of the acidosis and the treatment plan will need to be supplied to the outpatient physician.

METABOLIC ALKALOSIS

Background

Metabolic alkalosis occurs as a consequence of a wide variety of clinical conditions. It is usually initially recognized as an elevated serum bicarbonate concentration and can be confirmed as outlined in the initial section of this chapter. Metabolic alkalosis is usually an expected feature of a known underlying medical condition, but, occasionally, it can be a clue to an unsuspected diagnosis.

Assessment

Clinical Presentation

The clinical assessment, including a complete history and physical examination, will often result in an impression that explains the acid-base disturbance.

Severe alkalemia itself can result in neurologic symptoms, including mental status changes, seizures, and tetany. Alkalemia results in a decrease in the ionized calcium, which may also contribute to some of these symptoms. Alkalemia may also predispose the heart to arrhythmia and can decrease ventilatory drive, which can result in difficulty weaning patients from mechanical ventilators. Hypokalemia and hypomagnesemia may also develop as a consequence of increasing serum pH.

The history should focus on detecting gastrointestinal fluid loss and assessing medications (especially diuretics or alkali). The physical examination should focus on the assessment of extracellular volume status and blood pressure, and should detect any Cushingoid features.

Diagnosis/Differential Diagnosis

Metabolic alkalosis is usually recognized by an elevated serum bicarbonate concentration and can be further characterized as discussed in the first section of this chapter. Once detected, the major diagnostic effort relates to understanding the underlying cause of the alkalosis so that the appropriate treatment can be provided.

Metabolic alkalosis can be generated by excessive alkali input (uncommon) or acid loss. Acid losses commonly occur via losses of gastric fluid, but can also occur via the kidneys, especially secondary to the use of diuretics or excessive mineralocorticoid effect.

Volume depletion does not cause alkalosis in most patients. However, in those cases in which there is concomitant acid loss (e.g., vomiting), hypovolemia maintains the alkalosis by stimulating the release of aldosterone and by stimulating the resorption of bicarbonate by the kidney. Chloride depletion, which often accompanies volume depletion, contributes to the maintenance of the alkalosis. In addition, hypokalemia and hypomagnesemia work to maintain a state of metabolic alkalosis.[1,12]

Diuretic therapy is an especially potent cause of metabolic alkalosis, in that it can result in loss of hydrogen ions via the urine, volume and chloride depletion, hypokalemia, and hypomagnesemia. The volume depletion induced by diuretics stimulates aldosterone release while the effect of the diuretic results in continued delivery of solute to the distal tubule, resulting in further losses of acid and potassium.

Since there are so many factors that contribute to the maintenance of metabolic alkalosis, the approach to this condition requires attention to several variables. Table 53-5 shows a simple, stepwise approach to the etiologic diagnosis of metabolic alkalosis.[1,2]

First, it is important to rule out an iatrogenic cause of metabolic alkalosis (see Table 53-5). "Milk-alkali syndrome" is the name given to the excessive ingestion of the combination of alkali and calcium, which historically occurred as the result of the overuse of baking soda and milk to treat peptic diseases of the upper gastrointestinal tract. Today, this syndrome is more often an iatrogenic phenomenon that occurs in attempt to correct the acidosis and hypocalcemia of chronic kidney disease, usually using alkali therapy and calcium and vitamin D supplementation. A similar syndrome can occur in patients who overmedicate themselves with calcium supplements.

The next step is to assess the patient's intravascular volume status. If the patient is hypovolemic, gastric losses and urine losses secondary to diuretics are the most common causes. Of note, loss of *intestinal* fluids usually results in the development of a metabolic acidosis. However, occasionally, chronic losses (e.g., villous adenoma, laxative abuse) can result in a metabolic alkalosis. In most cases of metabolic alkalosis caused by fluid losses, the patient will appear volume depleted, and the cause of the syndrome will be clinically apparent. The urine sodium concentration is sometimes measured to assist in the assessment of intravascular volume. However, in states of metabolic alkalosis, the urine chloride is the preferred measurement. This is because renal excretion of bicarbonate will be high when the patient is alkalotic. Since sodium follows bicarbonate, the urine sodium can be falsely elevated, even when the patient is intravascularly volume depleted. Alkalotic patients suffering from volume depletion will have low urine chloride concentrations

Table 53-5 A Simple, Stepwise Approach to the Etiologic Diagnosis of Metabolic Alkalosis

Step 1. Rule out iatrogenic causes.
EXAMPLES: Administration of large amounts of citrated blood products, use of citrate anticoagulation, overadministration of alkali, or the milk-alkali syndrome

Step 2. Perform a detailed history and an assessment of intravascular volume status.
- Most patients will have signs of volume depletion and a clinical syndrome that will explain the metabolic alkalosis (urine chloride <25 mEq/L).
  EXAMPLES: Upper gastrointestinal fluid losses are common (e.g., vomiting), intestinal fluid losses are an uncommon cause (e.g., secondary to chronic laxative abuse or villous adenoma), volume depletion, diuretics (urine chloride may be >25 if diuretic effect continues or severe hypokalemia or chronic kidney disease are present), post–hypercapnic alkalosis
- If the patient lacks these features, continue as below.

Step 3. If the patient lacks clinical signs of volume depletion and has none of the disorders above, examine the patient's blood pressure, and measure the serum potassium concentration and a spot urine chloride concentration.
- Unexplained hypokalemia, significant hypertension, or urine chloride >40 (and not taking diuretics) should prompt consideration of mineralocorticoid excess.

Step 4. If mineralocorticoid excess is suspected, rule out glycyrrhizinic acid ingestion (see text), and measure 24-hour urine cortisol excretion, and serum aldosterone concentration simultaneous with plasma renin activity.
- Elevated 24-hour urine cortisol suggests Cushing's syndrome
- Elevated aldosterone levels with suppressed plasma renin activity suggests primary hyperaldosteronism
  EXAMPLES: adrenal adenoma or hyperplasia
- Elevated renin levels with elevated aldosterone levels suggest a hyper-reninemic state
  EXAMPLES: Volume depletion, renal underperfusion (e.g., congestive heart failure, cirrhosis), renal artery stenosis, malignant hypertension, scleroderma crisis, renal vasculitis, renin-secreting tumor

---

(<25 mEq/L), unless there is ongoing diuretic use, severe hypokalemia, or chronic kidney disease. Urine chloride concentrations >40 suggest that volume depletion may not be present.

Post–hypercapnic alkalosis occurs when a hypercarbic acidosis is rapidly corrected. Rapid correction of hypercarbia results in an alkalosis. Under normal circumstances, renal excretion of bicarbonate corrects this alkalosis, but hypoperfusion of the kidneys (e.g., hypovolemia, heart failure, etc.) and hypochloremia inhibit the normal excretion of bicarbonate.

In all, the group of disorders discussed above is referred to as the "chloride sensitive" metabolic alkaloses, as the administration of a chloride containing solution typically reverses the abnormality. If the patient does not appear to be volume depleted (or does not respond to sodium chloride administration), or the clinical picture is not consistent with these disorders, further evaluation is necessary.

In these situations, the possibility of a mineralocorticoid excess must be considered. Classically, a mineralocorticoid excess state will manifest with a syndrome of hypokalemic metabolic alkalosis with hypertension. Since hypertension is common in the general population and hypokalemia occurs frequently with several of the other cause of metabolic alkalosis, this syndrome is not at all pathognomonic for mineralocorticoid excess states. However, when hypokalemic alkalosis occurs in the setting of treatment-resistant hypertension or without an apparent cause, mineralocorticoid excess must be considered. Often, in these cases, the urine chloride is >40 mEq/L, as these patients are usually not volume or chloride depleted (the "chloride insensitive" metabolic alkaloses).

When a mineralocorticoid excess state is suspected, one should first exclude excessive licorice ingestion. Although not common in the United States, some licorice candy, chewing gum, and chewing tobacco contain glycyrrhizinic acid. This compound inhibits 11-β hydroxysteroid dehydrogenase, which results in a state of mineralocorticoid excess.[13] Cushing's syndrome should also be considered when mineralocorticoid excess is suspected. Cushing's syndrome can be suggested by history and physical examination, and the history should also exclude exogenous steroid use. The measurement of cortisol in a 24-hour urine collection is an adequate screening test for Cushing's syndrome. The congenital causes of mineralocorticoid excess are not discussed here.

Simultaneous measurement of the serum aldosterone level and the plasma renin activity can help to separate hyper-reninemic states from those of primary aldosteronism as in Table 53-5. Although calculation of the ratio of the plasma aldosterone concentration to the plasma renin activity is considered the test of choice to screen for primary hyperaldosteronism, the expected values and the test characteristics for this test are not well established.[14,15] Because of the complexities of testing the renin-aldosterone system, the consultative assistance of an endocrinologist or nephrologist may be helpful when performing these assessments. This evaluation is summarized in Table 53-5. Because they are often associated with hypokalemia, these disorders are also discussed in the hypokalemia section of Chapter 52 (Other Electrolyte Disorders).

Preferred Studies

In many cases, the cause of a patient's metabolic alkalosis can be ascertained via the history and physical examination. All patients with a metabolic alkalosis should have basic metabolic laboratory testing performed, including a measurement of the concentration of serum sodium, potassium, chloride, bicarbonate, creatinine, magnesium, and urine chloride.

Management

Treatment

In most cases of metabolic alkalosis, the cause is readily apparent, and in many cases it can be slowed or reversed. For example, vomiting can usually be slowed with the use of antiemetic medications. Most of the cases of metabolic alkalosis that are caused by acid, chloride, or volume loss can be remedied by the administration of a sodium chloride solution, with potassium supplementation, if needed. Even post–hypercapnic alkalosis usually responds to this treatment. Magnesium should also be supplemented, when necessary.[1,12]

Treatment of mineralocorticoid excess depends of the specifics of the underlying condition, but is often done in coordination with a subspecialist, as noted above.

Metabolic alkalosis that occurs as a result of the administration of diuretics can usually be limited by decreasing the intensity of this therapy. However, in some situations, the diuresis is therapeutically essential. For example, a patient with severe congestive heart failure might develop an alkalosis because of intensive diuretic use, but still have significant extracellular volume overload. In this case, the administration of sodium chloride would correct the alkalosis, but would also exacerbate the extracellular volume excess. In cases like these, the addition of a potassium-sparing diuretic (e.g., spironolactone, triamterene, or amelioride) can help to continue the diuresis with a lesser depletion of acid and potassium. More severe cases may require the addition of acetazolamide, which can more potently combat the alkalosis by forcing urinary excretion of bicarbonate. The situation can be even more difficult in those patients with underlying renal failure, and, at times, dialysis is required to correct the alkalosis.[12]

RESPIRATORY ACIDOSIS

Background

Respiratory acidosis occurs when ventilation is inadequate to eliminate the carbon dioxide that is generated via metabolism. Therefore, the discovery of respiratory acidosis must lead to an evaluation of reasons for respiratory insufficiency. This discussion will not focus on the diagnosis and treatment of the specific causes of respiratory failure (which can be found in other specific chapters).

Assessment

Clinical Presentation

Respiratory acidosis is typically discovered as a chronic finding in patients with known underlying lung disease, or in association with acute respiratory problems. Because respiratory acidosis results in the accumulation of carbon dioxide and often occurs in association with hypoxemia, it is often accompanied by mental status changes. Although the chronicity of the respiratory acidosis is sometimes unclear in patients with known underlying lung disease, the development of respiratory acidosis

in a patient who is in respiratory distress indicates impending respiratory failure, and should be recognized as a life-threatening condition.

Diagnosis/Differential Diagnosis

Acidemia, coupled with an elevated pCO_2, makes the diagnosis of respiratory acidosis. Chronic respiratory acidosis might be initially suspected in the setting of an elevated serum bicarbonate (occurring as compensation). Either of these findings can be further characterized as described in the opening section of this chapter.

Major causes of respiratory acidosis include central nervous system failure, failure of the diaphragm and respiratory neuromuscular system, or a pulmonary reason for respiratory failure, such as a disorder of diffusion or an obstructive ventilatory defect.[1]

Normally, the central nervous system provides a continuous drive to breathe. This can be interrupted by any central nervous system dysfunction that impairs ventilatory drive. In this way, sedative medications (including, but not limited to narcotics, benzodiazepines, and barbiturates) can cause this disorder. Although specific central nervous system lesions (e.g., tumor, trauma) are uncommon causes of respiratory acidosis, inadequate central respiratory drive does occur in central sleep apnea and the obesity-hypoventilation syndrome.

Neuromuscular disorders can also cause respiratory acidosis. Dysfunction of nerves or muscles involved in breathing can result in hypoventilation in myasthenia gravis, Guillain-Barré syndrome, amyotrophic lateral sclerosis, multiple sclerosis, spinal cord injury, and others. More generalized disorders such as hypothyroidism, hypophosphatemia, and other myopathic processes can also cause hypoventilation.

The diseases of airway obstruction (asthma, emphysema, other causes of bronchoconstriction, or disorders of the upper airway, including obstructive sleep apnea) classically result in a respiratory acidosis that can be chronic or acute.

Lastly, respiratory compromise from a wide variety of insults (e.g., pneumonia, acute respiratory distress syndrome (ARDS), pulmonary edema, pneumothorax, pleural disease, etc.) will result in respiratory acidosis secondary to inadequate gas exchange, if severe.

Preferred Studies

In most cases, respiratory acidosis is part of a clinical presentation in which the hypoventilation is expected or explainable. Chest radiography and spirometric testing will often lead to accurate classification of the respiratory failure. In cases where the cause of the respiratory acidosis is not clear despite a careful initial evaluation, further testing to rule out thyroid disease, myopathy (serum creatinine kinase), or neurologic disorders affecting respiratory drive (brain imaging, electromyography (EMG) testing, or other specialized testing) can be used to refine the diagnosis. Sleep studies can document sleep-related apnea.

Management

Treatment

Since respiratory acidosis represents respiratory failure, discussion of its treatment would span a large number of disorders. This discussion is beyond the scope of this chapter, but can be found in the specific chapters addressing these disorders.

RESPIRATORY ALKALOSIS

Background

Respiratory alkalosis is a disorder caused by hyperventilation. Unlike the causes of respiratory acidosis, which are quite intuitive, the disorders that cause hyperventilation are a more diverse and less easily categorized group.

Assessment

Clinical Presentation

Although not always the case, many patients presenting with respiratory alkalosis will actually appear hyperventilatory on close assessment. These patients may exhibit tachypnea or a pattern of deep breathing. Arterial blood gases should be drawn to evaluate the respiratory status in these patients.

Respiratory alkalosis is most likely to cause symptoms when it is acute, resulting in alkalemia. Symptoms can include light-headedness, mental status changes, paresthesias, and muscle spasms.

Diagnosis/Differential Diagnosis

Hyperventilation is usually driven by hypoxemia (as sensed in the carotid and aortic bodies) or the stimulation of mechanoreceptors in the lungs, and these phenomena can often not be distinguished. In addition, hyperventilation can be voluntary, psychiatric, caused by pain, or caused by a variety of disorders that stimulate the medullary respiratory center.[1]

A wide range of cardiopulmonary diseases can result in hypoxemia and the stimulation of mechanoreceptors in the thorax. Disorders such as pneumonia, pulmonary embolism, and interstitial lung diseases (fibrosis or edema) can cause respiratory alkalosis in this way. Hypotension and severe anemia also stimulate hyperventilation, probably via the carotid and aortic bodies.

Of course, patients can also hyperventilate volitionally, or because of psychological stimuli, such as anxiety. Sepsis, liver failure, pregnancy, neurologic insults (stroke, tumor, infection), and drugs (e.g., salicylate toxicity, methylxanthines, beta-agonists, progesterone) can also stimulate hyperventilation and should be systematically explored if a primary cardiopulmonary process is not obvious.[16]

Preferred Studies

Like those conditions causing respiratory acidosis, most of the conditions causing respiratory alkalosis present as part of a syndrome in which respiratory alkalosis is only one feature. A variety of specific tests might be performed to confirm suspected diagnoses.

Management

Treatment

Treatment of respiratory alkalosis is directed at the underlying disorder that is stimulating the hyperventilation.

Key Points

- Accurate classification of acid-base abnormalities can be accomplished by a stepwise approach in which the clinician estimates the primary disturbance, considers physiologic compensation, and calculates the anion gap and the delta gap.

- When an anion gap is present, this should prompt a search for the presence of unmeasured anions, which might include ketones, lactate, or ingested substances (e.g., salicylate, ethylene glycol, or methanol). Severe acute or chronic kidney disease can also be associated with an elevated anion gap.

- Type 4 RTA is the most common of the tubular acidoses and can be recognized clinically as the combination of an acidosis with a normal anion gap and hyperkalemia, in the absence of severe renal failure. This disorder is associated with a variety of common medications (e.g., beta-blockers, NSAIDs, ACE inhibitors/angiotensin II receptor blockers, heparin, potassium-sparing diuretics, trimethoprim, cyclosporine, tacrolimus) and disorders (e.g., diabetic nephropathy).

- The treatment of acute acidosis is aimed at appropriately treating the underlying disorder. Acute administration of alkali is only rarely needed and is usually reserved for cases of severe acidemia (e.g., pH <7.0) when patients are experiencing the most severe consequences of acidosis (e.g., hemodynamic instability, cardiac arrhythmia).

- Metabolic alkalosis is usually secondary to the excess administration of alkali or the loss of acid and/or volume (e.g., vomiting, diuretics). When the cause of a metabolic alkalosis is not apparent, the diagnosis of a mineralocorticoid excess state should be pursued.

SUGGESTED READING

Rose BD, Post TW. Clinical Physiology of Acid-Base and Electrolyte Disorders, 5th ed. New York: McGraw-Hill, 2001.

Gabow PA, Kaehny WD, Fennessey PV. Diagnostic importance of an increased serum anion gap. N Engl J Med 1980; 303:854–858.

Androgue HJ, Madias NE. Management of life threatening acid-base disorders. I. N Engl J Med 1998; 338:26–34.

Soriano JR. Renal tubular acidosis: the clinical entity. J Am Soc Nephrol 2002; 13:2160–2170.

Androgue HJ, Madias NE. Management of life threatening acid-base disorders. II. N Engl J Med 1998; 338:107–111.

Section

7 Seven

Gastroenterology

54 Upper Gastrointestinal Bleeding
Erica Brownfield, Marc D. Rosenberg

55 Acute Hepatitis
Nomi L. Traub

56 Cirrhosis and Its Complications
Vanitha Bala, Pratima Sharma, Frank A. Anania

57 Spontaneous Bacterial Peritonitis
Rangadham Nagarakanti

58 Acute Abdominal Emergencies
Mark G. Graham, Kris Kaulback

59 Inflammatory Bowel Disease
Cuckoo Choudhary

60 Gastroenteritis
Gretchen Diemer

61 Diarrhea and Clostridium difficile *Colitis*
Jeffrey Glasheen

CHAPTER FIFTY-FOUR

Upper Gastrointestinal Bleeding

Erica Brownfield, MD, FACP, and Marc D. Rosenberg, MS, MD

BACKGROUND

Acute upper gastrointestinal (GI) bleeding requires rapid assessment and treatment by a clinician. Early recognition is crucial to reduce morbidity and mortality. Defined as bleeding derived from a source proximal to the ligament of Trietz, upper GI bleeding typically presents with a history of hematemesis or melena, whereas hematochezia suggests a lower source. However, this maxim is not absolute, as patients with acute profuse upper GI bleeding can present with hematochezia, and melena can occur from bleeding sources in the small intestine or proximal colon.

Causes of upper GI bleeding are multiple, with nonspecific mucosal abnormalities, peptic ulcer disease, esophagitis, gastritis, and varices being the most common. Other common causes include Mallory-Weiss tears, arteriovenous malformations, and neoplasms.[1-3]

ASSESSMENT

Prevalence

The incidence of upper GI bleeding is approximately 100 cases per 100,000 people per year.[4] This translates to approximately 250,000–350,000 hospitalizations each year in the United States for acute upper GI bleeding. Bleeding from the upper GI tract is approximately four times as common as bleeding from the lower GI tract. Upper GI bleeding is twice as common in men than women and more common in the elderly.[5]

Clinical Presentation

History

A focused history should reveal risk factors for upper GI bleeding, comorbid conditions, medication use (both prescription and non-prescription), alcohol and illicit drug use, and symptomatology. As stated before, a history of hematemesis or melena suggests an upper GI source of bleeding; however, severe upper GI bleeding can result in hematochezia. A prior history of use of aspirin or nonsteroidal anti-inflammatory drugs should raise the suspicion of gastritis or ulcers. A history of alcohol abuse or cirrhosis suggests the possibility of variceal bleeding, portal hypertensive gastropathy, or gastritis. A history of vomiting, especially in an alcoholic, can suggest a Mallory-Weiss tear.

A systematic review[6] documented the incidence of presenting symptoms in patients with upper GI bleeding, as noted in Table 54-1. Melena, hematemesis, presyncope, and epigastric pain are most common.

Physical Examination

Initial physical examination should focus on hemodynamic stability and organ perfusion, signs of underlying comorbid conditions, and a careful abdominal and rectal examination. Measurement of vital signs with orthostatic measurements is essential in estimating the amount of intravascular volume loss, although this may not be as reliable in patients with chronic or recurrent bleeding. Resting tachycardia and a systolic blood pressure <100 mm Hg correlate to an estimated acute volume loss of 25% and >30%, respectively.

Laboratory and Other Studies

Specific blood tests should be obtained in patients with suspected acute upper GI bleeding. Hemoglobin with type and screen should be obtained initially in all patients, and serial hemoglobin values can help in identifying ongoing hemorrhage. It is important to consider that a drop in hemoglobin may not be seen until 24–72 hours after the start of bleeding; likewise, hemoglobin may continue to drop even once bleeding has stopped, especially with hydration. Coagulation studies should be obtained in all patients, as well as liver aminotransferase levels, blood urea nitrogen (BUN), creatinine, electrolytes, and albumin. An elevated BUN/creatinine ratio is often present with upper GI bleeding due to diminished renal perfusion. Coagulation abnormalities and low albumin can be markers of decreased synthetic function of the liver. Testing for *Helicobacter pylori* infection should be performed in those patients who are found to have peptic ulcer disease on upper endoscopy.

Differential Diagnosis

The broad differential diagnoses of upper GI bleeding include the most common causes of peptic ulcer disease, esophagitis, gastritis, varices, and nonspecific mucosal abnormalities. Clinicians should also consider Mallory-Weiss tears, arteriovenous malformations, and neoplasms. Less common sources include Cameron's lesions (ulcers in the sac of a hiatal hernia), Dieulafoy lesions (dilated aberrant submucosal vessels), traumatic or post-

Table 54-1 Presenting Symptoms in Upper GI Bleeding[6]

Symptom	Incidence (%)
Hematemesis	40–50
Melena	70–80
Hematochezia	15–20
Either hematochezia or melena	90–98
Presyncope	43.2
Epigastric pain	41
Heartburn	21
Dyspepsia	18
Syncope	14.4
Weight loss	12
Diffuse abdominal pain	10
Jaundice	5.2
Dysphagia	5

Box 54-1 Factors Associated with Poor Prognosis in Upper GI Bleeding

Age over 60

Markers of severe bleeding
- Red blood in nasogastric aspirate
- Red blood in stool
- Requirement for blood transfusion
- Use of anticoagulants
- Hemodynamic instability.

Comorbid conditions
- Active coronary artery disease
- Renal failure
- Congestive heart failure
- Active lung disease
- Sepsis
- Metastatic cancer
- Advanced liver disease

Bleeding etiology
- Varices
- Neoplasms
- Rendu-Osler-Weber syndrome

surgical causes such as aortoenteric fistulas, foreign body ingestion, and postsurgical anastomosis.

Diagnosis

Patients who present with suspected upper GI bleeding (except for patients assumed to have esophageal varices) should have a nasogastric tube lavage to help confirm the diagnosis and to assess the severity of bleeding. Lavage can also be helpful in removing residual blood and other gastric contents to aid in diagnosis. Silverstein et al.[7] found that 15.9% of patients with a clear aspirate, 29.9% with coffee-ground aspirate, and 48.2% with red blood aspirate had an active upper GI source of bleeding at the time of endoscopy. However, lavage without blood does not exclude an upper GI bleed, as it may miss up to 16% of actively bleeding lesions.[8] On the other hand, a lavage with a bilious aspirate suggests but does not guarantee that the bleeding is distal to the ligament of Treitz.[9] Identification of bleeding is a visual test, and guaiac testing of lavage fluid is not useful. Additionally, once performed the nasogastric (NG) tube should be removed for patient comfort and to prevent subsequent morbidity from the tube.

Upper endoscopy is the diagnostic modality of choice for acute upper GI bleeding and should be performed as quickly as possible to speed appropriate intervention. It is highly sensitive and specific for identifying bleeding lesions in the upper GI tract. All patients with acute upper GI bleeding should undergo upper endoscopy, unless the risks outweigh the benefits. Patients considered to be at high risk for complications (i.e., those within 30 days after myocardial infarction or very ill patients with an Apache II score >16) have higher complication rates; therefore, individual decisions need to be made regarding whether or not to proceed with endoscopy.[10] In all patients, endoscopy should only be done once hemodynamic stability, endotracheal intubation (if needed), and adequate monitoring in an intensive care unit setting have been achieved.

Angiography and radionuclide red blood cell scans detect active bleeding and can be useful if upper endoscopy does not reveal a source of bleeding or cannot reach the source for therapy.

Prognosis

Mortality rates from upper GI bleeding are 6–10% overall.[4] Despite advances in endoscopy and other minimally invasive procedures, the mortality figures are largely unchanged over the past 30 years, largely due to an aging patient population with an increasing prevalence of associated medical comorbidities.[6] Poor prognostic indicators such as being elderly, markers of severe bleeding, comorbidities, and certain causes are associated with higher mortality and are listed in Box 54-1. In the majority of fatal cases, death is caused by deterioration of underlying illnesses rather than by GI bleeding.[7]

Persistent or recurrent bleeding occurs in 5–30% of patients. Risk of rebleeding can be predicted by endoscopic characteristics of a lesion. Patients with oozing or pumping lesions and visible vessels on endoscopy have a higher risk of rebleeding and mortality rate than patients without active bleeding[8,11] (Fig. 54-1).

Prognostic factors should be used when determining hospital management and therapeutic options for patients.

MANAGEMENT

Treatment

Hemodynamic resuscitation and stabilization should be the first priorities in management. Two large-bore peripheral intravenous catheters or a central venous line should be placed for intra-

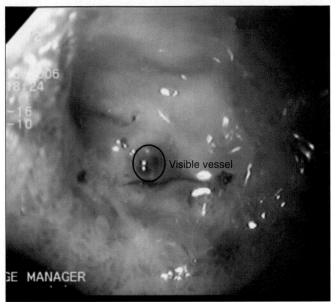

Figure 54-1 • Endoscopic picture of ulcer with visible blood vessel.

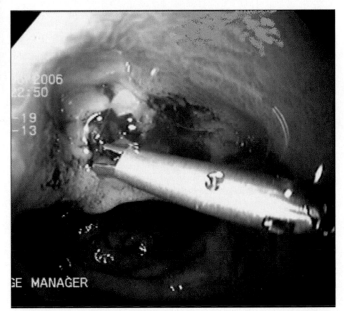

Figure 54-2 • Endoscopic picture of hemostasis being achieved with use of hemostatic clip on a bleeding ulcer.

venous access. In patients with massive hematemesis, endotracheal intubation should be considered to protect against aspiration. Intravenous fluids should be administered to maintain hemodynamic stability. Any patient who is hemodynamically unstable or who has varices should be admitted to an intensive care unit (ICU). ICU placement should also be considered for those patients with a high risk of rebleeding (i.e., visible vessel in a peptic ulcer).

Blood products should be given when necessary. As a general rule, in the setting of an acute GI bleed, young otherwise healthy adults should maintain a hematocrit of at least 20%; elderly patients and those with severe comorbidities (such as coronary artery disease) should maintain a hematocrit of at least 30% in order to maintain adequate oxygen delivery. Patients with a coagulopathy or thrombocytopenia should be given fresh frozen plasma and platelets, respectively.

Any modifiable factors that may have contributed to bleeding should be eliminated (i.e., aspirin, nonsteroidal antiinflammatory medications, anticoagulants, alcohol). Patients should be kept non per os (nothing by mouth) (NPO) until endoscopy.

Acid suppression with high-dose antisecretory therapy, with administration of proton pump inhibitors (PPI), significantly reduces the rate of rebleeding in patients with bleeding ulcers. This has not been shown with H_2 receptor antagonists.[12–14] Since peptic ulcer disease accounts for a large percentage of upper GI bleeds, it is reasonable to give a PPI while awaiting endoscopy. Of note, when given orally, PPIs are more effective with faster onset of action and raising of pH compared to intravenous administration and are far less expensive. However, if the patient needs to be NPO and endoscopy is imminent, intravenous administration is acceptable.

Octreotide, a somatostatin analog, may also be considered in treatment, as it has been shown to reduce the risk of rebleeding from variceal and nonvariceal causes.[15]

Consultation by a gastroenterologist is imperative in order to obtain both diagnostic and therapeutic upper endoscopy. Endoscopic therapy varies, depending on the findings, source of bleeding, availability of equipment, and the expertise of the endoscopist. If a bleeding lesion is identified, therapeutic endoscopy can achieve acute hemostasis and prevent recurrent bleeding in most patients.

Upper GI bleeding caused by peptic ulcer disease should be treated with antimicrobial agents targeted toward *H. pylori* when serologies are present. Antibiotic regimens are listed in Box 54-2. It is important to follow up on biopsy results of ulcers (Fig. 54-2).

Any patient who presents with significant upper GI bleeding (multiple blood transfusions required) or who remains refractory to endoscopic therapy should be managed in consultation with a surgeon. Patients who are not surgical candidates can be considered for angiography with embolization.

Secondary prophylactic measures are needed to decrease the risk of recurrent bleeding in patients with peptic ulcer disease and varices. Patients with these diagnoses should be discharged on antisecretory therapy and beta-blockers, respectively.

DISCHARGE/FOLLOW-UP PLANS

Repeat endoscopy with follow-up by a gastroenterologist should be arranged prior to discharge in any patient found to have a gastric ulcer. This is necessary in order to document healing of these lesions, as biopsy may be required of a nonhealing ulcer in order to exclude underlying malignancy. Patients found to be positive for *H. pylori*, should have follow-up studies such as stool antigen or breath test to document eradication. Patients with variceal bleeding will need close follow-up by a hepatologist.

Key Points

- Though hematemesis or melena suggests upper GI bleeding and hematochezia a lower source, acute profuse upper GI bleeding can present with hematochezia, and melena can occur from bleeding sources in the small intestine or proximal colon.

- Bleeding from the upper GI tract is about four times more frequent than bleeding from the lower GI tract, twice as common in men as women, and more common in the elderly.

- Resting tachycardia and a systolic blood pressure <100 mm Hg correlate with an estimated acute volume loss of 25% and >30%, respectively.

- Patients with suspected upper GI bleeding should undergo gastric lavage, recognizing that identification of bleeding is a visual test, and guaiac testing of lavage fluid is not useful. Once completed, the NG tube should be removed for patient comfort and to prevent subsequent morbidity from the tube.

- Upper endoscopy is the diagnostic modality of choice for acute upper GI bleeding and should be performed as quickly as possible to speed appropriate intervention. Persistent or recurrent bleeding occurs in 5–30% of patients and can be predicted by endoscopic characteristics of a lesion.

- Patients with upper GI bleeding require IV access (preferably two peripheral 18-gauge catheters or larger), volume resuscitation, and correction of coagulation abnormalities.

- In the majority of fatal cases, death is caused by deterioration of underlying illnesses rather than by GI bleeding.

SUGGESTED READING

Boonpongmanee S, Fleischer DE, Pezzullo JC, et al. The frequency of peptic ulcer as a cause of upper-GI bleeding is exaggerated. Gastrointest Endosc 2004; 59:788–794.

Fallah MA, Prakash C, Edmundowicz S. Acute gastrointestinal bleeding. Med Clin North Am 2000; 84(5):1183–1208.

Peter DJ, Dougherty JM. Evaluation of the patient with gastrointestinal bleeding: an evidence based approach. Emerg Med Clin North Am 1999; 17(1):239–261.

Cappell MS, Iacovone FM. Safety and efficacy of esophagogastroduodenoscopy after myocardial infarction. Am J Med 1999; 106:29–35.

Gisbert JP, Gonzalez L, Calvet X, et al. Proton pump inhibitors versus H2-antagonists: a meta-analysis of their efficacy in treating bleeding peptic ulcer. Aliment Pharmacol Ther 2001; 15:917–926.

Lau JY, Sung JJ, Lee KK, et al. Effect of intravenous omeprazole on recurrent bleeding after endoscopic treatment of bleeding peptic ulcers. N Engl J Med 2000; 343:310–316.

CHAPTER FIFTY-FIVE

Acute Hepatitis

Nomi L. Traub, MD

BACKGROUND

Patients admitted to the hospital with acute hepatitis comprise a group with diverse diagnoses. Challenges for the hospitalist include the establishment of the correct etiology for the hepatitis, identification of the subset of patients with acute liver failure, and rapid referral of suitable patients for liver transplantation.

Acute liver failure (ALF), a rare condition, involves the rapid development of hepatocellular dysfunction in a previously healthy individual. ALF is defined as coagulopathy (INR ≥1.5), with any degree of encephalopathy, in a patient without prior liver disease, whose illness is <26 weeks duration.[1] Chapter 56 reviews cirrhosis and liver failure in more detail. ALF tends to affect young people and has a high morbidity and mortality. The short-term survival, including patients undergoing transplantation, is currently about 65%.[2] In the United States, drug hepatotoxicity and viral hepatitis cause the majority of ALF. Poisonings, ischemia or vascular liver insults, pregnancy-related hepatitis, and malignant infiltration of the liver less commonly cause ALF. Wilson's disease and autoimmune hepatitis may be included as causes of ALF if these conditions have been recognized for <26 weeks. In most series of ALF cases, a sizable portion remains cryptogenic, despite meticulous evaluation.

Diagnosis-specific therapy is available for the minority of patients with ALF. For the majority, treatment focuses on prevention and management of a myriad of complications. These severely ill patients should be managed in an ICU, with early planning for transfer to a center with transplant capabilities.

ASSESSMENT

Clinical Presentation

Prevalence

While viral hepatitis used to be the most common cause of acute liver failure, more recent studies documented that acetaminophen overdose has become the most common cause (39%) in the United States.[3] Idiosyncratic drug reactions accounted for 13%, while viral hepatitis A and B were diagnosed as the etiology in 12%, and no cause was determined in 17%. About 2,000 persons per year in the United States suffer acute liver failure.

Acute viral hepatitis afflicts about 0.5–1% of the US population each year, but this annual incidence varies based on fluctuations in hepatitis A cases, given its infectious nature and propensity to epidemics. Among patients with viral-induced hepatitis, the etiology is hepatitis A in 48%, hepatitis B in 34%, hepatitis C in 15%, and unknown in about 3%.

Presenting Signs and Symptoms

Patients with acute hepatitis present with fairly nonspecific symptoms, including anorexia, nausea, vomiting, mild abdominal discomfort, diarrhea, malaise, myalgias, arthralgias, or fever. Many seek medical attention at the onset of jaundice. Assuming the clinician is aware of the aminotransferase elevation, the history should focus carefully on medication use, including over-the-counter medications and herbal preparations. Use of acetaminophen, in particular, should be discussed and quantified, as this is the most common cause of ALF in industrialized nations. In a recent study of ALF,[2] the majority of patients with acetaminophen toxicity had accidental overdose rather than overdose with suicidal intent. Alcohol use should also be documented. The clinician must review risk factors for viral hepatitis, including parenteral exposure, foreign travel, sexual practices, and ingestion of contaminated food or water. Table 55-1 lists the features of viral hepatitis. A family history of liver disease may suggest a genetic cause. Severe gastrointestinal symptoms such as abdominal cramps, nausea, vomiting, and diarrhea may point to mushroom poisoning.

Physical Examination

Stigmata of chronic liver disease, such as spider angiomata and palmar erythema, should be sought on physical examination. These findings make a diagnosis of ALF unlikely. Mental status assessment is crucial, as encephalopathy is a defining criterion for ALF. Thus, any finding of alteration in mentation should be documented in the medical record. Encephalopathy can range from subtle changes in affect and/or cognition (grade 1); to disorientation, drowsiness and confusion (grade 2); to marked somnolence and incoherence (grade 3); to frank coma (grade 4). Hepatomegaly and ascites may signify congestive heart failure, acute Budd-Chiari syndrome, or malignant infiltration.

Table 55-1 Features of Viral Hepatitis

Feature	HAV	HBV	HCV	HDV	HEV
Transmission	Common	Unlikely	No	No	Common
Fecal-oral	Rare	Common	Common	Common	No
Percutaneous sexual	No	Common	Rare	Rare	No
Incubation period (days)	15–50	28–180	14–160	Variable	15–60
Frequency of ALF pregnancy	0.1%	0.1–1%	Rare in U.S.	2–7.5%	0.5–3%; 25% in 3rd trimester
Diagnosis of acute infection	Anti-HAV IgM	HBs Ag Anti-HBc IgM	HCV RNA PCR	Anti-HDV IgM	Anti-HEV IgM

Diagnosis
Laboratory Testing

Initial laboratory testing should include aminotransferase levels, alkaline phosphatase, bilirubin, and prothrombin time/INR. Complete chemistries, complete blood count, and amylase and lipase levels may help narrow the differential diagnosis. Certain patterns of aminotransferase values offer valuable clues to the etiology of acute hepatitis. Generally, the ratio of aspartate aminotransferase (AST) to alanine aminotransferase (ALT) is ≤1 in acute liver injury. In alcoholic hepatitis, the AST/ALT is characteristically >2. An AST/ALT >4.0 is suggestive of fulminant Wilson's hepatitis in the appropriate clinical setting.[3] Marked elevations of aminotransferase levels (>2,000 units/L) occur almost exclusively with toxin- or drug-induced liver injury, ischemic insult, or acute viral hepatitis. Occasionally, patients with viral[4] or alcoholic[5] hepatitis display an atypical laboratory pattern, with an elevated alkaline phosphatase and bilirubin, and less remarkable transaminases. Hepatobiliary ultrasound may then be useful to exclude biliary tract pathology.

The American Association for the Study of Liver Diseases (AASLD) recommends an extensive set of laboratory tests (Box 55-1) if ALF is diagnosed.[1] Tests to evaluate the etiology of ALF include viral serologies, toxicology screen, acetaminophen level, pregnancy test, autoimmune markers, and a ceruloplasmin level in young patients. Additional tests are recommended to gauge the severity of ALF or assess feasibility of liver transplantation. Arterial pH should be measured, as a pH of <7.3 is associated with a poor prognosis in acetaminophen-related ALF.

After the history, physical, and basic laboratory tests, the clinician should be able to distinguish between severe hepatitis and ALF. Sepsis may mimic ALF, when the triad of jaundice, coagulopathy, and encephalopathy occur. Measurement of factor VIII levels may help distinguish sepsis from ALF, as factor VIII is not synthesized by the liver, and levels should be normal in ALF.[6] Once ALF is diagnosed, further testing to determine etiology should ensue.

Acetaminophen Toxicity

Acetaminophen causes dose-related hepatocyte injury, and most ingestions leading to ALF exceed 10 g/day. However, doses as low as 3–4 g/day can cause severe liver injury, particularly in patients with significant alcohol intake or starvation.[7] Since acetaminophen toxicity is the leading cause of ALF in the United States (39% in a recent series),[2] an acetaminophen level should always be drawn in cases of severe hepatitis. Low or absent levels do not completely rule out acetaminophen toxicity, particularly in cases

---

Box 55-1 Initial Laboratories in ALF

Prothrombin time/INR

Chemistries: sodium, potassium, chloride, bicarbonate, calcium, magnesium, phosphate, glucose, AST, ALT, alkaline phosphatase, GGT, total bilirubin, albumin, creatinine, blood urea nitrogen

Arterial blood gas

Arterial lactate

Complete blood count

Blood type and screen

Acetaminophen level

Toxicology screen

Viral hepatitis serologies: anti-HAV IgM, HBSAg, anti-HBc IgM, anti HEV[§], anti-HCV[*]

Ceruloplasmin level[#]

Pregnancy test

Ammonia (arterial if possible)

Autoimmune markers: ANA < ASMA, Immunoglobulin levels

HIV status[‡]

Amylase and lipase

---

[*]Done to recognize potential underlying infection
[#]Done only if Wilson's disease is a consideration (i.e., patients <40 years)
[‡]Implications for potential liver transplantation
[§]If clinically indicated
From Polson J, Lee WM. AASLD Position Paper: The management of acute liver failure. Hepatology 2005; 41:1179–1197.

---

of unintentional overdose, when the timing of ingestion may be remote or unknown. Recent data from the U.S. ALF Study Group reveal that unintentional overdose occurs more commonly than intentional overdose in ALF patients.[2] An additional clue to acetaminophen toxicity is an extraordinarily high aminotransferase level, often >4,000 units/L.[7]

Viral Hepatitis

Viral hepatitis is declining as a cause of ALF in the United States but is a common cause of ALF in other parts of the world. Currently, only 12% of ALF cases in the United States are caused by acute viral hepatitis.[8] In the United States, the majority of viral cases of ALF are caused by hepatitis B, followed by hepatitis A. Hepatitis C does not appear to be responsible for ALF in the United

States. Acute hepatitis D may occur in a hepatitis B–positive individual. Hepatitis E causes significant disease in countries where it is endemic, such as India, Pakistan, Mexico, and Russia, with pregnant women developing more severe illness.

In acute hepatitis A, anti–hepatitis A IgM is considered sensitive and specific for diagnosis. In acute hepatitis B, a positive hepatitis B surface antigen and/or anti–hepatitis B core IgM are diagnostic. For hepatitis C, one should obtain a hepatitis C virus RNA to diagnose acute infection. For hepatitis D coinfection, a positive anti–delta IgM antibody is used. For hepatitis E, a positive anti–hepatitis E virus IgM antibody is diagnostic (*see* Table 55-1). Rare viral causes include EBV, CMV, or HSV; and an IgM antibody against these viruses should be ordered to confirm the diagnosis.

Wilson's Disease

Wilson's disease is in the differential diagnosis of ALF in patients <45 years of age. Diagnostic tests for this uncommon cause of ALF include low ceruloplasmin levels, elevated serum and urinary copper levels, total bilirubin/alkaline phosphatase ratio >2.0,[3] slit lamp examination for Kayser-Fleischer rings, and hepatic copper levels from biopsy specimens.

Autoimmune Hepatitis

Autoantibodies such as antinuclear antibodies, anti–smooth muscle antibodies, and anti LKM (liver/kidney/microsome) type 1 antibodies are helpful for diagnosis if positive with a titer >1 : 80. Liver biopsy may be suggestive as well, if interface hepatitis and plasma cell infiltration are present.[9]

Budd-Chiari Syndrome

The clinician should suspect Budd-Chiari Syndrome in patients with hepatomegaly, ascites, and underlying hematologic or hypercoaguable conditions.

Diagnosis is confirmed with hepatic imaging (computed tomography, Doppler ultrasonography, venography, or magnetic resonance venography) which reveals acute hepatic vein thrombosis.

Malignant Infiltration

Diagnosis should be established by imaging and biopsy. Acute severe infiltration of the liver occurs with breast cancer, small cell lung cancer, lymphoma, and melanoma.[1]

There are no specific tests for mushroom poisoning, idiosyncratic drug toxicities, ischemic hepatitis, or pregnancy-related syndromes. Most idiosyncratic drug reactions occur within 6 months of drug initiation, and antibiotics, nonsteroidal anti-inflammatory agents, and anticonvulsants are often the culprits.[1] If the etiology of ALF remains obscure after initial evaluation, a liver biopsy via the transjugular approach may yield additional clues.

Prognosis

Accurate prognostication in ALF is crucial to avoid unnecessary transplantation and lifelong immunosuppression in patients likely to recover spontaneously, and to ensure transplantation for patients likely to expire without it. Unfortunately, no currently available prognostic scoring system adequately predicts outcome or the need for transplantation. The 2005 AASLD position paper on ALF does not recommend complete reliance on any scoring system.[1] The King's College Hospital criteria for identifying

---

Box 55-2 King's College Hospital Criteria for Liver Transplantation in ALF

Acetaminophen-induced ALF

pH <7.3 (irrespective of grade of encephalopathy)

or

Prothrombin time >100 seconds (INR 6.5) + serum creatinine >300 μmol/L (3.4 mg/dl) in patients with grade III or IV encephalopathy

Nonacetaminophen-induced ALF

Prothrombin time >100 seconds (INR 6.5) irrespective of grade of encephalopathy

Any 3 of the following, irrespective of grade of encephalopathy:

Age <10 or >40 years

Etiology—non A, non B hepatitis, halothane hepatitis, idiosyncratic drug reactions

Duration of jaundice before onset of encephalopathy >7 days

Prothrombin time >50 seconds (INR ≥3.5)

Serum bilirubin >300 μmol/L (17.5 mg/dL)

From: O'Grady JG, Alexander GJM, Hayllar KM, et al. Early indicators of prognosis in fulminant hepatic failure. Gastroenterology 1989; 97:439–455.

---

patients with a poor prognosis without liver transplantation are the most widely studied and utilized system[10] (Box 55-2). A recent meta-analysis of the King's criteria in acetaminophen-related ALF[11] concluded that the specifity was 92%, but the sensitivity was only 69%. The positive likelihood ratio was 12.33, and the negative likelihood ratio was 0.29. This indicates that the criteria are fairly insensitive and may miss patients requiring transplantation.

In the largest US study of ALF to date,[2] overall patient survival at 3 weeks was 67%; 43% of the patients recovered without transplantation. The most significant predictor of outcome was the apparent etiology of ALF. Patients with ALF due to acetaminophen, hepatitis A, shock liver, or pregnancy-related disease had a ≥50% transplant-free survival rate. Patients with all other etiologies (drugs other than acetaminophen, hepatitis B, autoimmune hepatitis, Wilson's disease, Budd-Chiari syndrome, cancer) or indeterminate cause had a <25% transplant-free survival rate. The grade of encephalopathy at admission also predicted outcome. Three-week transplant-free survival was 52% in patients presenting with grade I or II encephalopathy and 33% in patients presenting with grade III or IV encephalopathy. Survival rates for patients undergoing liver transplantation for ALF range from 50–75%.[6]

MANAGEMENT

Treatment

Patients with ALF should be transferred to the intensive care unit (ICU) for monitoring and treatment of complications. Factoring in etiology, grade of encephalopathy, and prognostic indicators, the clinician must rapidly decide whether transfer to a transplant facility is appropriate (Fig. 55-1). Early consultation with a trans-

Figure 55-1 • Algorithm for management of acute hepatitis.

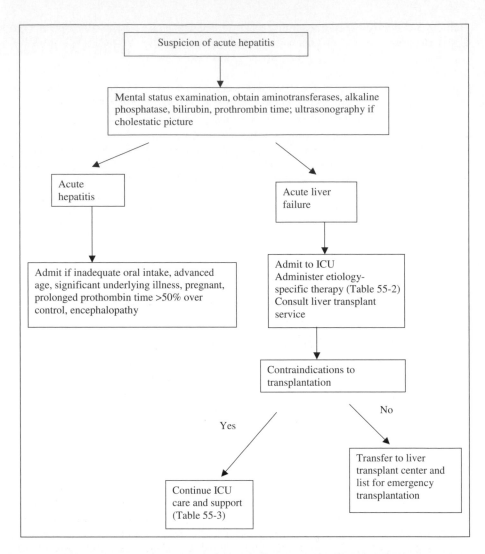

Table 55-2 Etiology-Specific Therapies to Consider in Acute Hepatitis

Condition	Therapy
Acetaminophen hepatotoxicity	Activated charcoal within 4 hours of ingestion; N-acetylcysteine 140 mg/kg, followed by 70 mg/kg q 4 h × 17 doses orally or via NGT[12]; IV form available with different dosing[13]
Hepatitis B	Lamivudine—no controlled trials
Wilson's disease	Reduce copper with albumin dialysis, plasmapheresis, hemofiltration[14] and list for transplant in ALF
Autoimmune hepatitis	Prednisone 30–60 mg/day ± azathioprine[15]; list for transplant if ALF
Acute fatty liver of pregnancy	Delivery
Budd-Chiari syndrome	Portal vein decompression[16]; list for transplant in ALF
Herpes simplex hepatitis	Acyclovir 15–30 mg/kg/day IV
Mushroom poisoning	Penicillin G 300,000–1 million units/kg/day Silibinin—commercially available as milk thistle in the United States. Not a licensed drug in United States.

plant facility is critical, as the risks of transport rise once encephalopathy worsens. ALF patients listed for transplant are considered as status 1 by the United Network for Organ Sharing (UNOS), denoting an urgent status.

Though much of the care of patients with acute hepatitis or ALF is supportive, there are several etiology-specific therapies that may be considered (Table 55-2). There is no specific therapy

generally recommended for hepatitis A or B, the most common causes of viral hepatitis in the United States. No antidotes exist for idiosyncratic drug hepatotoxicity. Ischemic liver injury is managed with cardiovascular support, and aminotransferase levels usually fall rapidly if the circulatory problem is stabilized.

Much of care of patients with ALF focuses on preventing complications and intervening when these occur (Table 55-3).

Table 55-3 Complications of ALF—Monitoring and Management

Complication	Monitoring	Management
Encephalopathy	Brain CT to rule out other causes of altered mental status	Avoid sedatives; lactulose may be helpful, intubate for grades III/IV
Cerebral edema	Intracranial pressure (ICP) monitoring	Elevate head of bed 30°; avoid stimulation, Valsalva, straining; treat seizures; hyperventilation lowers ICP but short-lived; mannitol for increased ICP; barbiturates; no steroids
Coagulopathy	Prothrombin time, platelet count, fibrin degradation products	Vitamin K 5–10 mg subcutaneously; replacement therapy for thrombocytopenia or prolonged prothrombin time only in the setting of hemorrhage or prior to invasive procedures
Infection	Periodic surveillance cultures for bacterial and fungal infection; chest radiograph	Prophylactic antibiotics controversial; low threshold for initiating antibiotics
Gastrointestinal bleeding	Coagulopathic, intubated patients are high risk; intragastric pH monitoring	Prophylactic H_2 blockers, proton pump inhibitors, sucralfate second line
Hypoglycemia	Frequent monitoring of glucose	Continuous infusion 5–10% dextrose solutions
Renal failure	Invasive hemodynamic monitoring to guide fluid management	Avoid nephrotoxic drugs; if dialysis required, continuous mode is recommended over intermittent mode[17]

DISCHARGE/FOLLOW-UP PLANS

There are limited data on the long-term outcome of patients who suffer acute liver failure. If there is no underlying liver disease, and liver function returns to normal, there are no specific measures to follow. Hepatotoxic medications and alcohol should be avoided during the recovery period. For patients with viral hepatitis, the primary care physician should assess the patient for chronicity of infection over the ensuing months.

Key Points

- Acetaminophen is the leading cause of acute liver failure in the United States, and all patients presenting with this clinical scenario should be queried about its use and tested; unintentional overdose occurs more commonly than intentional overdose.

- Mental status assessment in patients presenting with acute hepatitis is crucial, as encephalopathy is a defining criterion for acute liver failure.

- Marked elevations of aminotransferase levels (>2,000 units/L) occur almost exclusively with toxin- or drug-induced liver injury, ischemic insult, or acute viral hepatitis.

- Patients with acute liver failure should be evaluated for transfer to a center with transplant capability as soon as possible if this is an option.

SUGGESTED READING

Polson J, Lee WM. AASLD Position Paper: The management of acute liver failure. Hepatology 2005; 41:1179–1197.

Ostapowicz GA, Fontana RJ, Schiodt FV, et al. Results of a prospective study of acute liver failure at 17 tertiary care centers in the United States. Ann Intern Med 2002; 137:947–954.

Schiodt FV, Davern TJ, Shakil O, et al., and the ALF Study Group. Viral hepatitis-related acute liver failure. Am J Gastroenterol 2003; 98:448–453.

Czaja AJ, Freese DK. Diagnosis and treatment of autoimmune hepatitis. Hepatology 2002; 36:479–497.

Bailey B, Amre DK, Gaudreault P. Fulminant hepatic failure secondary to acetaminophen poisoning: a systematic review and meta-analysis of prognostic criteria determining the need for liver transplantation. Crit Care Med 2003; 31:299–305.

Roberts EA, Schilsky ML. AASLD Practice guidelines: a practice guideline on Wilson disease. Hepatology 2003; 37:1475–1492.

Czaja AJ. Treatment of autoimmune hepatitis. Semin Liv Disease 2002; 22:365–378.

CHAPTER FIFTY-SIX

Cirrhosis and Its Complications

Vanitha Bala, MD, Pratima Sharma, MD, and Frank A. Anania, MD, FACP

BACKGROUND

Cirrhosis represents the end stage of progressive hepatic disease interfering with normal function of the liver. It is characterized by fibrosis and distortion of the normal hepatic architecture into structurally abnormal nodules. Cirrhosis may lead to liver failure, requiring liver transplantation, the only curative option available for these patients. Alcoholic liver disease and hepatitis C are the most common causes of cirrhosis in the United States accounting for >40% of deaths from chronic liver disease. Cirrhosis and chronic liver disease are the 12th leading cause of death in United States in 2002, and accounted for 27,257 deaths and 360,000 hospital discharges according to the report from the National Center for Health Statistics. Up to 30-40% of cases are discovered during autopsy. The etiology of cirrhosis is varied, depending on the causes of the chronic liver disease (Table 56-1). A detailed history, combined with serologic and histologic evaluation, helps in determining the specific etiology.

This chapter reviews the common complications of cirrhosis and the approaches to their treatment.

ASSESSMENT

Clinical Presentation

Presenting Signs and Symptoms

The symptoms of chronic liver disease are nonspecific (Box 56-1), and a number of physical findings are described in patients with end-stage liver disease (Table 56-2).

LABORATORY TESTING

Abnormal liver function tests from laboratory testing as part of a routine physical examination are the presenting abnormality in most of the cases. The most common laboratory parameters classified as liver function tests include: enzyme tests (serum aminotransferases—ALT, AST, alkaline phosphatase, gamma glutamyl transpeptidase), tests of synthetic function (serum albumin concentration and prothrombin time), and the serum bilirubin, which reflects the transport capability of the liver. Patients with hepatocellular processes generally have disproportionate elevations in aminotransferases when compared to patients with a cholestatic process, where the alkaline phosphatase is commonly elevated. The serum bilirubin can be prominently elevated in both hepatocellular and cholestatic processes. A normal albumin suggests an acute process such as choledocholithiasis, while a low albumin suggests a chronic process such as cirrhosis. The failure of prothrombin time to correct with administration of vitamin K indicates advanced parenchymal liver disease. Ascites, variceal hemorrhage, spontaneous bacterial peritonitis (SBP), and hepatic encephalopathy, the complications of cirrhosis, may be the initial presentation in some patients.

COMPLICATIONS

The clinical course of patients with advanced liver disease is often complicated by a number of important sequelae resulting from **portal hypertension** (Box 56-2). The development of complications marks the transition from compensated to decompensated cirrhosis. **Ascites** results from sinusoidal hypertension and sodium retention secondary to arterial vasodilatation and activation of the neurohumoral system through rennin–angiotension–aldosterone and sympathetic nervous system activity.

Spontaneous bacterial peritonitis (SBP) most likely results from immunodeficiency secondary to depressed reticuloendothelial phagocytic activity and reduced complement levels, allowing translocation of gut bacteria into the peritoneal cavity. Gastroesophageal **varices** result from portal hypertension, and the hyperdynamic circulation in cirrhosis contributes to variceal growth and rupture. **Hepatic encephalopathy** results from accumulation of neurotoxins in the brain, due to hepatic insufficiency and portosystemic shunting. The **hepatorenal syndrome** results from hypovolemia and neurohumoral activation of potent vasoactive systems, leading to pronounced renal vasoconstriction and failure. Other complications include **hepatic hydrothorax** and **hepato-pulmonary syndrome.** The prevention and treatment of these complications improve the survival and quality of life in cirrhotic patients.

Portal Hypertension

Portal hypertension is a hemodynamic abnormality responsible for the most lethal complications of cirrhosis such as gastroesophageal varices, ascites, hepatorenal syndrome, and hepatic encephalopathy. It remains the most important cause of morbidity and mortality in patients with cirrhosis because of the

Table 56-1 Etiologies, Diagnostic Tests and Treatment of Chronic Liver Disease and Cirrhosis

Etiology		Diagnostic Tests	Treatment
Drugs and toxins	Alcohol Isoniazid Methotrexate Methyldopa Perhexilene maleate Pyrrolidizine alkaloids (venoocclusive disease)	LFTs	Abstention Identify the drugs and discontinue
Infections	Hepatitis B Hepatitis C	HBsAg, HbeAg, IgM anti—HBc, antHBs, Anti-HCV, confirmed by PCR for HCV RNA	Interferon/lamivudine, emtricitabine or adefovir Pegylated interferon/ribavirin
	Schistosomiasis Toxoplasmosis Brucellosis *Echinococcus*	ELISA Anti-toxoplasma IGg antibody titers Blood cultures, ELISA CT scan, ELISA	Praziquantel Pyrimethamine and sulfadiazine or clindamycin doxycycline and streptomycin or rifampicin surgery, protoscolidial agents (cetrimide, ethanol)
Autoimmune	Autoimmune hepatitis	Antinuclear, anti–smooth muscle antibodies, ANCA in type1 and anti-LKM-1 in type 2 Antimitochondrial antibodies	Corticosteroid, azathioprine Ursodiol, colchicine, methotrexate
	Primary biliary Cirrhosis		
Metabolic	Nonalcoholic Steatohepatitis Wilson's disease Hemochromatosis	LFTs and liver biopsy Serum ceruloplasmin, liver biopsy Iron studies, liver biopsy, genetic testing Serum AAT, phenotyping	Lifestyle modification Penicillamine, trientine, zinc Phlebotomy, deferoxamine IV augmentation therapy with AAT, transplant
	Alpha-1 antitrypsin deficiency Galactosemia Gauchers' disease Glycogen storage disease Tyrosinemia	RBC glactose-1 P concentration, urinary galactitol Glucocerebrosidase enzyme analysis in leukocytes Liver biopsy	Withdraw milk and milk products Enzyme replacement therapy, BM transplant Maintain physiologic glucose level, and Liver transplantation Withdraw dietary tyrosine
Biliary obstruction	Sclerosing cholangitis	ERCP	Endoscopic balloon dilation or stenting
Vascular	Chronic right heart failure Budd-Chiari syndrome Veno-occlusive disease	Right-side cardiac catheterization Ultrasound, MRI, venography	Diuretics Thrombolysis/TIPS/shunting/liver translantation
Cryptogenic	Cirrhosis without apparent cause	HLAB8 of DR3, liver biopsy with interface hepatitis	Corticosteroids

combined impact of these ominous complications. The normal portal pressure is up to 5 mm Hg, and complications occur when the portal pressure exceeds 12 mm Hg.

Ascites

Ascites is the pathologic consequence of fluid accumulation in the peritoneal cavity. Cirrhosis of the liver is the most common cause of ascites, accounting for nearly 85% of cases of ascites in United States.[1] Approximately 50% of patients with compensated cirrhosis develop ascites over a 10-year period.[2] Although the development of ascites is usually indicative of advanced liver disease, the clinical course of patients with cirrhosis and ascites

is highly variable. The initial evaluation of a patient with ascites should include a history, physical evaluation, and abdominal paracentesis with ascitic fluid analysis.

DIAGNOSIS

Paracentesis

Paracentesis should be performed in all patients with new-onset ascites and with clinical deterioration in patients with known ascites. Abdominal paracentesis with appropriate ascitic fluid analysis is probably the most efficient and cost-effective way to diagnose the etiology of ascites. Paracentesis is a safe procedure with few complications, even in patients with mild-to-moderate coagulopathy (defined as prothrombin time and partial pro-

Box 56-1 Common Symptoms of Liver Disease

Weakness

Disturbed sleep

Anorexia

Weight loss

Nausea

Vomiting

Muscle cramps

Eyelid lag

Jaundice

Abdominal pain

Fever

Menstrual irregularities

Loss of libido

Impotence

Sterility

Gynecomastia

Box 56-2 Complications of Cirrhosis

Ascites

Variceal hemorrhage

Spontaneous bacterial peritonitis

Hepatic encephalopathy

Hepatorenal syndrome

Hepatopulmonary syndrome

Hepatocellular carcinoma

include a cell count with differential, serum ascites albumin gradient (SAAG), and cultures. The SAAG is calculated by subtracting the ascitic fluid albumin from serum albumin, and it directly correlates with the portal pressure (see below).

Laboratory Testing

a. Appearance: Ascitic fluid is usually slight yellow and translucent. Turbidity of ascitic fluid suggests infection. Opalescent fluid indicates high triglyceride content. Milky fluid is seen with chylous ascites. Bloody ascitic fluid is commonly attributed to traumatic tap; however, 22% of cases of malignant ascites are bloody. A dark brown ascitic fluid with bilirubin concentrations greater than serum concentration usually indicates ruptured gallbladder or perforated duodenal ulcer.

b. Ascitic fluid testing: The initial laboratory ascitic fluid testing performed is cell count with differential, total protein concentration, and SAAG. If the results of the ascitic fluid testing are abnormal, further testing should be performed.

   i. *Cell count and differential:* Spontaneous bacterial peritonitis (SBP) is the most common cause of infection of the ascitic fluid in patients with cirrhosis. A polymorphonuclear neutrophil (PMN) count >250/μL suggests bacterial peritonitis and PMN count <250/μL with positive asctic fluid culture for single organism is indicative of monomicrobial non-neutrocytic bacterascites (MNB).

   ii. *Serum-ascites albumin gradient:* The SAAG is the single best test for the classification of ascites and identification of portal hypertension[1] (Table 56-3). An SAAG >1.1 g/dL suggests underlying portal hypertension with an accuracy of an approximately 97%; by contrast, a gradient of <1.1 g/dL suggests a nonportal hypertensive etiology.[1] If the specimens of serum and ascitic fluid are not drawn nearly simultaneously, the accuracy of the SAAG is reduced. Therefore, specimens of serum and ascitic fluid preferably should be obtained within the same hour.

   iii. *Cultures and gram stain:* Multiple prospective trials have revealed that inability to culture bacteria was largely due to insensitive technique and older methods. Inoculating blood culture bottles with 5–10 mL of ascitic fluid at patient's bedside will increase the sensitivity for detecting the bacterial growth above conventional methods. If PMN count is >250/μL and the ascitic fluid culture grows no bacteria, the diagnosis of culture-negative neutrocytic ascites (CNNA) is considered. *Escherichia coli*, streptococci, and Klebsiella are the most frequently isolated organisms in SBP.

Table 56-2 Signs of Liver Disease

Hepatomegaly	Physical Finding Description
Spider angiomata	Central arteriole surrounded by many smaller vessels
Palmar erythema	Mottled redness of hand palm
Muehrcke's nails	Paired transverse white bands
Terry nails	Discoloration of the nail except the distal edge
Clubbing	Change in the angle between the nail plate and the fold
Hypertrophic osteoarthropathy	Chronic proliferative periostitis of long bone
Dupuytren's contracture	Fibrosis of palmar fascia
Caput medusae	Collateral veins radiating from umbilicus
Ascites	Pathologic accumulation of fluid in the abdomen
Fetor hepaticus	Pungent odor to breath
Jaundice	Yellowish discoloration of sclera
Asterixis	Failure to actively maintain posture
Cruveilhier-Baumgarten murmur	Bruit auscultated in the epigastrium
Impaired glucose tolerance	Impairment in insulin secretion by beta cells of the pancreas and insulin resistance
Enlarged parotid gland	Secondary to fatty infiltration fibrosis and edema

thrombin time up to twice the midpoint of normal range). Prophylactic fresh frozen plasma and platelets should be used prior to diagnostic paracentesis only if there is evidence of coagulopathy with clinically evident fibrinolysis or disseminated intravascular coagulation (DIC). The initial ascitic fluid analysis should

Table 56-3 Classification of Ascites by the Serum Albumin-Ascites Gradient	
High Albumin Gradient with SAAG >1.1 g/dL	**Low Albumin Gradient with SAAG <1.1 g/dL**
Cirrhosis	Peritoneal carcinomatosis
Alcoholic hepatitis	Peritoneal tuberculosis
Congestive heart failure	Serositis
Massive hepatic metastasis	Pancreatitis
Constrictive pericarditis	Nephrotic syndrome
Budd-Chiari syndrome	

iv. *Total Protein:* Patients with ascitic protein value <1 gm/dL (low opsonin levels) are susceptible to SBP.

v. *Cytology:* The sensitivity rate for detecting peritoneal carcinomatosis by cytology is approximately 96.7% if three samples of ascitic fluid of 50 mL each are sent and processed promptly.

MANAGEMENT

Sodium Restriction

The mainstay of treatment of patients with ascites includes education regarding dietary sodium restriction (2,000 mg/day or 88 mmol/day) and oral diuretic therapy.[2] Weight change and fluid loss are directly related to sodium balance in patients with portal hypertensive–related ascites. Primary emphasis should be placed on sodium restriction and not fluid restriction. One of the important goals of the treatment is to increase the urinary excretion of sodium to >78 mmol per day.[2] Measurement of urinary sodium excretion is a helpful parameter in monitoring weight loss.[2] Patients who are excreting urine sodium >78 mmol per day and not losing weight should be counseled regarding dietary sodium restriction.[2]

Diuretics

Aldosterone antagonists (e.g., spironolactone) and loop diuretics are the most commonly used diuretics in the treatment of ascites. Increased aldosterone levels with subsequent sodium and water retention contribute to the development of ascites, so blockage of the aldosterone receptors is rational treatment.[2] Addition of loop diuretics has a synergistic effect with spironolactone and decreases the incidence of hyperkalemia. A successful beginning diuretic regimen consists of combined therapy with oral spironolactone at a dose of 100 mg and furosemide at 40 mg. The dose of both the diuretics can gradually be increased to a maximum dose of 400 mg of spironolactone per day along with 160 mg of furosemide per day, if weight loss and natriuresis are inadequate. Diuretics should be given as a single dose in the morning every day to optimize diuresis and minimize nocturia. For patients intolerant of the side effect of tender gynecomastia, amiloride or eplerenone can be tried. Approximately 90% of patients with cirrhotic ascites respond to sodium restriction and dual diuretic therapy. Patients with massive edema have no limit to daily weight loss as long as blood pressure is sufficient; however,

once the peripheral edema is resolved, the daily maximum weight loss is 0.5 kg/day.

Paracentesis

An initial large-volume paracentesis followed by strict dietary sodium restriction and diuretic therapy is appropriate treatment of patients with tense ascites. A prospective study demonstrated that paracentesis up to 5 L can be performed safely without postparacentesis colloid infusion, but large-volume paracentesis >5 L may need administration of intravenous albumin (8 g/L of fluid removed). The dose of the diuretics should be gradually titrated to increase urinary sodium excretion and achieve natriuresis and weight loss.

The commonly seen chronic hyponatremia in cirrhotic patients seldom causes morbidity. Rapid attempts to correct hyponatremia can lead to more complications than the hyponatremia itself. Cirrhotic patients do not usually have symptoms from hyponatremia until their sodium levels fall below 110 mmol/L, or until the decline in sodium is precipitous. Severe hyponatremia (serum sodium <120 mmol/L) in cirrhotic patients with ascites requires fluid restriction to about 1000 mL/24 hours.

Management of Refractory Ascites

Approximately 10% of patients with cirrhotic ascites suffer from refractory ascites, defined as fluid overload unresponsive to sodium-restricted diet and maximum recommended dose of diuretic regimen (400 mg per day of spironolactone and 160 mg per day furosemide), or ascites that recurs after therapeutic paracentesis. Patients with refractory ascites require expeditious liver transplant evaluation, given the poor prognosis of 50% dying within 6 months and 75% in a year.[1]

Patients with refractory ascites are at increased risk for developing hepatorenal syndrome (HRS) and have a poor prognosis. The treatment options for patients with refractory ascites include serial therapeutic paracentesis, transjugular intrahepatic portosystemic shunt (TIPS), peritoneovenous shunt, and liver transplantation.

Compared to diuretics alone, large-volume paracentesis (LVP) of greater than 5 L provides rapid resolution of symptoms, decreases the days of hospitalization, and has fewer complications. However, in 20% of ascitic patients, LVP is associated with postparacentesis circulatory dysfunction, characterized by hyponatremia, azotemia, and increase in plasma renin activity.[3] This may be prevented by administration of intravenous albumin (6 to 8 g/L of ascitic fluid removed) to improve the effective arterial volume along with large-volume paracentesis. Albumin is an important plasma protein responsible for generation of 70% of total plasma oncotic pressure, and it plays a major role in modulating the distribution of fluid in between compartments. Therefore, infusion of albumin will improve the low, effective arterial volume in cirrhosis.

Transjugular Intrahepatic Portosystemic Shunt (TIPS)

TIPS is a side-to-side portocaval shunt placed between the hepatic vein and an intrahepatic portal vein branch. Refractory ascites is one of the major indications for TIPS placement as a bridge to liver transplantation, and TIPS can mitigate the likelihood of bleeding from gastroesophageal varices. TIPS will effectively decrease the need for repeat large-volume paracentesis in patients with refractory ascites. Risks and benefits of TIPS should be discussed in detail with patient and family. Lactulose and diuretic therapy will probably still be required after the TIPS procedure. Unfortunately, TIPS is complicated by stenosis in about 75% of patients, as a result of thrombosis and pseudointimal hyperplasia within the hepatic vein. Doppler ultrasound is the most commonly used surveillance technique to identify TIPS stenosis. Repeat catheterization of the TIPS or upper endoscopy should be performed after a year of initial placement of TIPS. Hepatic encephalopathy is the most common complication and major cause for hospitalization after TIPS. Despite better control of ascites in patients who undergo TIPS as compared to LVP, there are currently no data that patient survival or quality of life are significantly improved by TIPS.

Spontaneous bacterial Peritonitis (SBP)

Spontaneous bacterial peritonitis (SBP) portends a 2-year survival of less than 50%. Impaired cellular immunity, defective leukocyte chemotaxis, hypocomplementemia, and impaired reticuloendothelial activity in cirrhotic patients predispose to virulent infections. Chapter 57 covers SBP in detail, but a brief review follows.

DIAGNOSIS

The criteria for a diagnosis of SBP includes: a positive ascitic fluid culture, or ascitic fluid absolute PMN count >250 cells/mm^3 without an evident intra-abdominal, or surgically treatable source of infection. *Escherichia coli*, klebsiella, and streptococci cause most episodes of SBP. Eighty-seven percent of patients with SBP are symptomatic at the time of diagnosis; however, the symptoms and signs of infection are subtle. Common symptoms are fever, abdominal pain, and mental status changes. Physical examination typically demonstrates subtle signs of chronic liver disease and abdominal tenderness. A high index of suspicion for SBP is necessary whenever a patient with cirrhotic ascites suddenly deteriorates with fever, worsening encephalopathy, or hepatic and renal dysfunction.

MANAGEMENT

Early diagnosis, prompt initiation of broad-spectrum antibiotics, and albumin infusion are the cornerstones for successful management of SBP. When the diagnosis of SBP is suspected, empiric antibiotic therapy should be given immediately after the ascitic fluid, blood, and urine samples are obtained for culture and analysis. Do not delay. Presence of fever, abdominal pain, change in mental status, and ascitic fluid PMN count >250 cells/mm^3 are sufficient indications for empiric therapy with antibiotics. If the initial clinical picture is unclear, initiate antibiotic therapy. If preliminary culture reveals no growth after 48 hours of antibiotic therapy, repeat paracentesis can be considered to assess the response of the PMN count to the therapy.

While awaiting susceptibility data, a broad-spectrum antibiotic should be initiated. In a controlled trial, cefotaxime has been shown to be superior to ampicillin in combination with tobramycin. Cefotaxime 2 g IV every 8 hours, or a similar third-generation cephalosporin, appears to be the drug of choice in the treatment of suspected SBP. Antibiotic therapy can be narrowed, depending on culture susceptibility results. Given the high incidence of nephrotoxicity with aminoglycosides, they should be avoided in patients with cirrhosis. Treatment with oral ofloxacin 400 mg twice a day in uncomplicated SBP with no shock or vomiting may be as effective as parenteral cefotaxime. The duration of therapy can be limited to 5 days in patients with dramatic response.

About 30% of patients SBP develop hepatorenal syndrome (HRS) and have a high mortality.[4] Intravenous albumin administration at a dose of 1.5 g/kg at diagnosis and 1 g/kg after 48 hours can prevent the development of HRS.

PROPHYLAXIS

SBP recurs in 70% of the patients after 1 year of the first episode; therefore, prophylactic antibiotic therapy is recommended for some patients to prevent recurrence and improve survival.[4] The risk of SBP is highest in cirrhotic patients with variceal hemorrhage, ascitic fluid protein concentration <1 g/dL, or a prior episode of SBP. Prophylactic maintenance therapy with oral administration of norfloxacin 400 mg daily has been reported to prevent SBP in patients with low ascites protein and prior episode of SBP. Intravenous antibiotics can be administered if the patient is actively bleeding.

Variceal Hemorrhage

This ominous complication of portal hypertension occurs in 25–40% of patients. The average lifetime risk of a first variceal bleed in patients with cirrhosis is 30%. Factors predicting the highest risk for first variceal bleed include large esophageal varices and "red wale markings," or raised red strenks visualized at endoscopy. Within 1 year after the initial bleed, 70% of patients experience a recurrent variceal bleed. The mortality rate of first variceal hemorrhage remains high, despite significant improvement in early diagnosis and treatment.

MANAGEMENT

Variceal hemorrhage is a life-threatening medical emergency, best managed in the intensive care unit with close consultation by a skilled gastroenterologist. Factors predictive of variceal hemorrhage are the degree of hepatocellular dysfunction, the portal pressure, and the presence of large varices.

Resuscitation

Two large-bore peripheral intravenous lines should be started for the restoration of the intravascular volume prior to any diagnostic tests. In patients with altered mental status, tracheal intubation should be considered to protect the airway.

Fresh frozen plasma and platelets should be transfused in patients with an INR >1.5 and platelets <50,000/mm.[3] The hematocrit is not a reliable indicator of the severity of acute bleeding because it requires 24–72 hours to equilibrate with extravascular volume. Of note, excess fluid administration can lead to rebound portal hypertension, resulting in exacerbation of variceal bleeding, and it should be avoided by close monitoring. Hypotension reduces portal pressure and bleeding. Prophylactic broad-spectrum antibiotics should be started to prevent spontaneous bacterial peritonitis. Emergency endoscopy of the upper gastrointestinal tract can then be performed and the most appropriate treatment modality chosen.

Pharmacotherapy

Vasopressin, somatostatin, and their analog are most studied.[5] Both somatostatin and vasopressin cause splanchnic vasoconstriction and thereby decrease the portal pressure and portal blood flow. Somatostatin and octreotide (a synthetic analog) do not induce systemic arterial vasoconstriction like vasopressin. When compared with other vasoactive drugs, octreotide was better than vasopressin and equivalent to terlipressin to control bleeding, and had less frequent and less severe side effects. Octreotide is administered intravenously as a continuous infusion of 50 mcg/hour for 5 days. The efficacy of octreotide as a single therapy is controversial. Results from a recent meta-analysis suggest that octreotide may improve the results of endoscopic therapy but has little or no effect if used alone.

Endoscopic Therapy

Endoscopic variceal band ligation in combination with vasoactive drugs is the preferred form of therapy for acute esophageal variceal bleeding. It is as effective as variceal sclerotherapy, which controls active hemorrhage in 80–90% of the patients, and is associated with lower complications and procedure related rebleeding rates. The combination of sclerotherapy with octreotide and vapreotide has been reported to be superior to sclerotherapy alone in terms of control of bleeding and reduction of treatment failures within 5 days.

Balloon Tamponade

The temporary measure of gastric or esophageal balloon tamponade stabilizes patients when medical and endoscopic therapies fail to control acute variceal bleeding, and more definitive procedures are being planned. Control of bleeding is successful in as many as 80–90% of cases, but rebleeding occurs in up to 50% when the balloons are deflated. Complications include upper airway obstruction, aspiration pneumonitis, esophageal ulceration, and asphyxia. Furthermore, significant perforation risk develops and may lead to high mortality if the balloons are inflated for prolonged periods of time.

TIPS and Shunt Surgery

The 10% of patients in whom rebleeding cannot be controlled with two endoscopic therapeutic sessions within 24 hours require evaluation for either TIPS or surgical shunt. An experienced surgeon with appreciation for preserving the portal vein by avoiding the hepatic hilum, which may be important in candidates for liver transplantation, should be involved in the care, or the patient should be transferred to a center with experience with liver failure patients. TIPS can be used in patients with Childs class B or C cirrhosis as a salvage therapy. TIPS is associated with hepatic encephalopathy in 30%, and stenosis in about 75% of patients by 6–12 months.

Primary Prophylaxis

Nonselective beta-blockers decrease portal pressure by splanchnic vasoconstriction and decreasing cardiac output. As the drugs of choice for primary prophylaxis to prevent variceal hemorrhage, propranolol (started at 10 mg three times daily) or nadolol (20 mg daily) are the two most commonly used. They should be titrated to achieve a 25% decrease in the resting heart rate while maintaining a rate >55 bpm. Hypotension, commonly seen in cirrhotic patients, will limit the use of these agents.

Secondary Prophylaxis

The risk of recurrent variceal bleed after the first episode is approximately 60% at 1 year.[6] Use of beta-blockers results in a significant reduction in the rate of variceal rebleeding and improvement in survival rates in patients with advanced liver disease. The risk of rebleeding is lowered with addition of variceal band ligation (30–42%). Significantly lower rebleeding rates were reported with TIPS (12–22%) and distal splenorenal shunt (11–31%). The frequency of hepatic encephalopathy in patients with TIPS placement was reported to be twice that of patients receiving beta-blockers alone.[7] The lowest bleeding rates were reported in patients who achieved the target reduction in hepatovenous pressure gradient (HVPG) below 12 mm Hg on drug therapy with beta-blockers and isosorbide-5-mononitrate (7–13%).[6]

Hepatic Encephalopathy

Hepatic encephalopathy (HE) is broadly defined as a disturbance in central nervous system function because of hepatic insufficiency reflecting the existence of a spectrum of neuropsychiatric manifestations related to a range of pathophysiologic mechanisms. These manifestations are present in acute as well as chronic liver failure and are potentially reversible.

DIAGNOSIS

Short-term memory loss, lack of concentration, sleep cycle reversal, and irritability in the early stages can profoundly affect the activities of daily living; more advanced disease with lethargy, stupor, or coma necessitates hospitalization and may be life threatening. Suspicion of HE in patients with chronic liver disease should prompt the search for precipitating factors and the other causes of change in mental status. Common precipitating factors include gastrointestinal bleeding, urinary tract infection, electrolyte abnormalities, renal failure, infection, recent placement of TIPS shunt, use of sedatives/hypnotics, development of hepatocellular carcinoma, and constipation. Other less likely causes of altered mental status, such as intracranial bleed or masses, hypoglycemia, and a postictal state, should also be considered. HE is a diagnosis of exclusion and a clinical diagnosis.

Although hyperammonemia is associated with HE, ammonia levels do not correlate with the level of encephalopathy. Venous ammonia levels are not reliable, and ammonia levels must be measured via arterial sampling for both diagnostic purpose and as general guide to the treatment. An electroencephalogram may be helpful in advanced stages to avoid erroneous diagnosis.

MANAGEMENT

The treatment goals for HE include supportive care, identification and removal of precipitating factors, reduction of nitrogenous load from the gut, and assessment of the need for long-term therapy (Fig. 56-1).

Nutritional Management

Protein restriction in patients with acute hepatic encephalopathy appears to have no salutary effect. Zinc, a cofactor of urea cycle enzymes, may be deficient in cirrhotic patients, especially if they are malnourished, and it should be supplemented

Ammonia Lowering Strategy

Nonabsorbable disaccharides such as lactulose are routinely used to decrease ammonia production in the gut. Lactulose increases the fecal nitrogen excretion by facilitation of the incorporation of ammonia into bacteria as well as a cathartic effect.[8] Lactulose administered orally reaches the cecum, where it is metabolized by the enteric bacteria, causing a fall in pH. This drop in pH leads to a metabolic shift in bacteria, favoring uptake and trapping of

ammonia. The dose of the lactulose is adjusted to produce two or three soft bowel movements daily.[8] Excess lactulose can provoke metabolic alkalosis, precipitating hepatic encephalopathy.

Antibiotics such as neomycin and metronidazole also lower blood ammonia, mainly by eradicating ammonia producing intestinal bacteria. However, neomycin and metronidazole are associated with significant adverse reactions such as ototoxicity, nephrotoxicity, and neurotoxicity, requiring careful renal, neurologic, and otologic monitoring.[8] Rifaximin is a synthetic antibiotic with a broad spectrum of antibacterial activity and a low rate of systemic absorption. The available evidence suggests a good tolerability profile in patients with hepatic encephalopathy, and the highest benefit/risk ratio in the overall treatment of HE.[9]

An alternative strategy for lowering blood ammonia is the stimulation of ammonia fixation. Under normal physiologic conditions, ammonia is removed by the formation of urea in periportal hepatocytes and by glutamine synthesis in perivenous hepatocytes, skeletal muscle, and brain. In cirrhosis, both urea cycle enzymes and glutamine synthetase activity are decreased in the liver. Strategies to stimulate residual urea cycle activities and/or glutamine synthesis have been tried over the last 20 years. L-ornithine–L-aspartate (OA) is one of the most successful agents used. Randomized controlled clinical trials with OA demonstrate significant ammonia lowering and concomitant improvement in psychometric testing. Benzoate is also effective in reducing blood ammonia both in patients with inherited urea cycle disorders and in cirrhotic patients.

Hepatorenal Syndrome

Acute renal failure is common in patients with cirrhosis, but its exact incidence is variable. Patients with cirrhosis are predisposed to acute renal failure following complications such as variceal bleeding or administration of nephrotoxic drugs such as nonsteroidal anti-inflammatory drugs, aminoglycosides, trimethoperim (TMP)-sulfamethoxazole, diltiazem, etc. In addition to usual causes of renal insufficiency, patients with cirrhosis develop a specific type of acute renal failure, HRS. A diagnosis of exclusion, hepatorenal syndrome (HRS) is an ominous complication of end-stage liver disease. Retrospective studies indicate that HRS is present in ~17% of patients admitted to the hospital with ascites and in >50% of cirrhotics who die from liver failure.

DIAGNOSIS

The hallmarks of HRS are reversible renal constriction and mild systemic hypotension. The kidneys are structurally normal, and, at least in the early part of the syndrome, tubular function is intact as reflected by avid sodium retention and oliguria. The cause of renal vasoconstriction is unknown but may involve both increased vasoconstrictor and decreased vasodilator factors predominantly involved in its pathogenesis. Two patterns of HRS are observed in clinical practice: type 1 and type 2. Type 1 HRS is an acute progressive form of HRS in severe liver disease, and it is associated with a poor prognosis with 80% mortality at 2 weeks. Type 2 HRS occurs in patients with diuretic resistant ascites. The course of renal failure is slow. It is also associated with poor prognosis, although better than type 1.

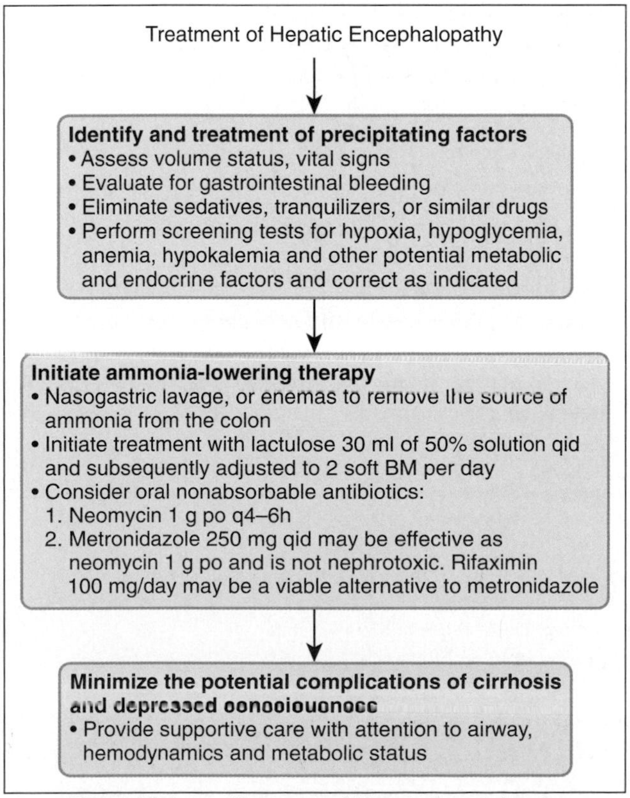

Figure 56-1 • Treatment of Hepatic Encephalopathy.

Treatment of Hepatic Encephalopathy

Identify and treatment of precipitating factors
- Assess volume status, vital signs
- Evaluate for gastrointestinal bleeding
- Eliminate sedatives, tranquilizers, or similar drugs
- Perform screening tests for hypoxia, hypoglycemia, anemia, hypokalemia and other potential metabolic and endocrine factors and correct as indicated

Initiate ammonia-lowering therapy
- Nasogastric lavage, or enemas to remove the source of ammonia from the colon
- Initiate treatment with lactulose 30 ml of 50% solution qid and subsequently adjusted to 2 soft BM per day
- Consider oral nonabsorbable antibiotics:
  1. Neomycin 1 g po q4–6h
  2. Metronidazole 250 mg qid may be effective as neomycin 1 g po and is not nephrotoxic. Rifaximin 100 mg/day may be a viable alternative to metronidazole

Minimize the potential complications of cirrhosis and depressed consciousness
- Provide supportive care with attention to airway, hemodynamics and metabolic status

MANAGEMENT

Although the best treatment for HRS is liver transplantation, patients with HRS who are transplanted have more complications and a higher inhospital mortality rate than those without. Systemic vasoconstrictor therapy may improve renal function in patients with HRS by increasing the effective arterial blood volume. Various nonrandomized retrospective studies have used the vasopressin analog, terlipressin, the vasoconstrictive agent noradrenaline, or midodrine with octreotide with some improvement in renal function. Nonrandomized studies suggest that TIPS may also improve renal function with HRS. Dialysis may be used for certain patients with HRS who progress to renal failure while awaiting renal transplantation.

Hepatic Hydrothorax

A pleural effusion can be detected on chest radiographs of as many as 13% of patients with cirrhosis.[10] The most common symptom of such a typically right-sided (85% of patients) hepatic hydrothorax is dyspnea without chest pain.

MANAGEMENT

Options include medical management of ascites and therapeutic thoracentesis, as well as paracentesis for the control of shortness of breath. Pleurodesis of the pleural space with chemical means such as talc, antibiotics, or chemotherapeutic agents almost always fails. TIPS has been successfully used to manage the symptoms of hepatic hydrothorax in the setting of marked ascites. Pleural-to-peritoneal and peritoneal-to-central venous shunts are associated with complications such as infection, disseminated intravascular coagulation, and failure to resolve effusions.

Hepatopulmonary Syndrome (HPS)

The triad of severe liver disease/portal hypertension, arterial blood deoxygenation, and intrapulmonary vascular dilatation characterizes HPS.[11] Occurring in 10% of patients with cirrhosis, HPS probably results from decreased hepatic clearance or increased hepatic production of cytokines and other vascular growth mediators that induce microvascular dilation of the pulmonary vasculature, resulting in intrapulmonary shunting and hypoxia. Severe hypoxemia with arterial PO_2 <60 mm Hg, with no signs of cardiovascular disease in cirrhotic patients, suggests hepatopulmonary syndrome.[12] Orthodeoxia is a characteristic clinical feature of patients with HPS. Orthodeoxia is a condition in which shortness of breath and hypoxia occur in the upright posture and are resolved with recumbency. In the upright position, blood pools in the dilated precapillary beds in the basal zones of the lung, resulting in increased intrapulmonary shunting and exacerbation of hypoxia. Contrast-enhanced echocardiography is the preferred screening test to detect shunts. Liver transplantation is the only effective therapeutic option.

Liver Transplantation

Liver transplantation is the only definitive treatment for many patients with end-stage liver disease. The Model of End Stage Liver Disease (MELD) is the clinical tool most widely used to estimate the mortality of patients awaiting liver transplantation. The United Network of Organ Sharing (UNOS) uses MELD scores for prioritizing organ allocation among patients with chronic liver disease who are awaiting liver transplantation. The MELD score was originally designed to predict the survival of patients undergoing TIPS; however, it was subsequently validated for use in patients with chronic liver disease.[13] The MELD score predicts patient mortality with adequate accuracy at different time periods. The laboratory parameters used in the MELD scoring system are the serum bilirubin, serum creatinine, and the INR. It is calculated according to the follow formula:

$$3.8 \times \log(e)(\text{bilirubin mg/dL}) + 11.2 \times \log(e)(\text{INR}) + 9.6\log(e)(\text{creatinine mg/dL})$$

Online calculators are available for calculating MELD scores. MELD scores ranging from 6 to 40 estimate a 3-month survival rate from 90–7%, respectively. Scores >40 predict mortality of 100% within 3 months.[14] Patients with severe liver disease without effective alternative therapy should be considered for liver transplantation. In critically ill patients, it is appropriate to begin specific therapy for the disease and to initiate evaluation for liver transplantation.

Cirrhotic patients should be referred for liver transplantation when they develop hepatic dysfunction (MELD >10) or when they experience the first episode of major complication such as ascites, variceal bleeding, or hepatic encephalopathy. The survival rates after liver transplantation in United States at 1, 3, and 5 years are 88%, 80%, and 75%, respectively. Patients with a MELD score of 15 or more are expected to achieve improved survival with liver transplantation.

CONCLUSION

The major goals of treating the cirrhotic patients include slowing or reversing the progression of liver disease, preventing the superimposed insults to the liver, and early detection and prevention of complications. Determining the appropriateness and optimal timing for liver transplant and transfer to a liver center with expertise in managing these patients will result in the best possible outcome for these patients.

SUGGESTED READING

Runyon BA. Management of adult patients with ascites due to cirrhosis. Hepatology 2004; 39(3):841–856.

Festi D, Vestito A, Mazzella G, et al. Management of hepatic encephalopathy: focus of antibiotic therapy. Digestion 2006; 73(Suppl 1):94–101. Epub 2006 Feb 8.

Krowka MJ. Hepatopulmonary syndromes. Gut 2000; 46:1–4.

CHAPTER FIFTY-SEVEN

Spontaneous Bacterial Peritonitis

Rangadham Nagarakanti, MD

BACKGROUND

Spontaneous bacterial peritonitis (SBP) is a bacterial infection of ascitic fluid in the absence of an apparent intra-abdominal source of infection (e.g., intestinal perforation, intra-abdominal abscess) or intra-abdominal inflammatory focus such as acute pancreatitis or cholecystitis. SBP among patients with liver cirrhosis most likely results from immunodeficiency secondary to depressed reticuloendothelial phagocytic activity and reduced complement levels, allowing translocation of gut bacteria into the peritoneal cavity.[1] Chapter 56 reviews liver cirrhosis and complications in addition to SBP.

ASSESSMENT

Clinical Presentation

Prevalence and Presenting Signs and Symptoms

A common complication among patients with advanced liver cirrhosis and ascites,[2,3] SBP occurs in about 15% of cirrhotic patients with ascites.[4] Development of SBP among hospitalized patients with chronic liver disease can be predicted based on the protein concentration of ascitic fluid. Patients with a total protein level <1 g/dL in their ascitic fluid had an incidence of 20%.[5] In one study, half of the episodes of SBP were evident on admission to the hospital, with the remaining 50% of patients developing SBP during the hospitalization.[6] Box 57-1 lists risk factors for SBP.

The typical features of SBP are described in Box 57-2. The most common symptoms are fever (69%), abdominal pain (59%), and altered mental status (54%). Patients with cirrhosis tend to be relatively hypothermic, and a temperature ≥37.8°C should be considered a fever. Patients with significant ascites and SBP will typically not have peritoneal signs such as rebound, and instead will simply have diffuse tenderness that is continuous in nature. Signs of altered mental status (AMS) may be quite mild and a very early sign. Asking family or friends if the patient seems "different" may elucidate such subtle changes and trigger early consideration of SBP. Patients usually do not present with the complete picture, and single elements of the typical presentation are more frequent, with isolated fever or abdominal pain being the most frequent presenting manifestations. Among patients with end-stage liver disease, clinical manifestations may be atypical and subtle.

Differential Diagnosis

SBP should be distinguished from secondary bacterial peritonitis due to intra-abdominal infection such as appendicitis, diverticulitis, or cholecystitis. Ascitic fluid in secondary bacterial peritonitis has elevated LDH, total protein >1 g/dL, and low glucose. Protein level increases in secondary peritonitis, but not in SBP. Patients with SBP have significantly lower total protein, albumin, and cholesterol levels in serum and ascites than patients without ascites infection.

The presence of multiple bacteria in cultures or on Gram stain is diagnostic of secondary bacterial peritonitis. Neutrophilic ascites is also seen in tuberculous ascites, pancreatic ascites, and peritoneal carcinoma, but the absolute neutrophil count is <50% of ascitic white cell count. Table 57-1 categorizes the different types of peritonitis based on ascitic fluid findings.

Ascitic fluid is usually slightly yellow and translucent. Turbidity of ascitic fluid suggests infection. Milky fluid is seen with chylous ascites. Bloody ascitic fluid is commonly attributed to a traumatic tap; however, 22% of cases of malignant ascites are bloody. A dark brown ascitic fluid with bilirubin concentrations greater than serum concentration usually indicates ruptured gallbladder or perforated duodenal ulcer.

Diagnosis

The clinical history and physical examination should provide sufficient information to consider the diagnosis, with subsequent laboratory tests helping to confirm SBP. Abdominal paracentesis is the gold standard test for diagnosis and should be performed as quickly as possible. A common fear is that patients having an elevated INR are at significant risk of hemorrhage, but this is unfounded at an INR of about ≤2. If there is significant risk of bleeding (e.g., evidence of coagulopathy with clinically evident fibrinolysis or disseminated intravascular coagulation), then fresh frozen plasma and/or platelets as needed should be given before the paracentesis.

The initial ascitic fluid analysis should include a cell count with differential, total protein, albumin, and cultures. Indications for paracentesis are listed in Box 57-3. Typical laboratory tests of the ascitic fluid are listed in Table 57-2. Most important is the cell count. Spontaneous bacterial peritonitis is defined as PMN count ≥250/mL in ascitic fluid. An alternative to manual counting is

Table 57-1 Types of Peritonitis based on Ascitic Fluid Findings

Type	Ascitic Fluid Findings
"Classical" SBP	PMNs >250 cells/mL with positive ascitic culture for single organism
Culture-negative SBP	PMNs >250 cells/mL with negative ascitic culture
Monomicrobial non-neutrocytic bacteriascites	PMNs <250 cells/mL with positive ascitic culture for single organism
Polymicrobial bacteriascites	PMNs <250 cells/mL and culture with multiple organisms
Secondary bacterial peritonitis	PMNs >250 cells/mL and culture with multiple organisms

Box 57-1 Risk Factors for SBP

- Total protein in ascitic fluid <1 g/dL
- Severe liver disease (Child-Pugh class C) with bilirubin >3.2 mg/dL[9]
- Esophageal variceal or gastrointestinal bleeding
- Urinary tract infection
- Previous spontaneous bacterial peritonitis
- Iatrogenic factors (e.g., urinary bladder and intravascular catheters)

Table 57-2 Analysis of Ascitic Fluid

Routine	Optional	Unusual
Total protein*	Gram stain	Cytology
Albumin*	Amylase	Acid-fast bacillus smear and culture
Cell count with WBC differential	Lactate dehydrogenase	Triglycerides
Culture in blood culture bottles	Glucose	

*Determined on initial diagnostic paracentesis only.

Box 57-2 Signs and Symptoms of SBP in Patients with Cirrhosis and Ascites

- Local signs of peritonitis (abdominal pain, vomiting, diarrhea, ileus)
- Systemic signs of infection (fever, leukocytosis, septic shock)
- Rapid renal function impairment without an apparent cause
- Change in mental status

Box 57-3 Indications for Diagnostic Paracentesis

- New onset of ascites
- Hospital admission in a patient with known ascites
- Clinical deterioration (e.g., onset of abdominal symptoms) in a patient with cirrhosis and ascites
- Azotemia
- Hepatic encephalopathy
- Gastrointestinal bleeding
- Deterioration in laboratory test values (e.g., leukocytosis)

the use of reactive strips for leukocyte esterase, which may provide a rapid bedside diagnosis of SBP.[5] Regardless, fluid should be sent to the lab for a formal cell count.

From 10–30% of patients with neutrophilic ascites have negative cultures. The sensitivity of ascitic fluid cultures can be increased by injecting 10 cc of the fluid into blood culture bottles as soon as it is collected. Fluid should also be submitted for Gram stain.

SBP is rarely caused by anaerobic organisms but is the result of monomicrobial aerobic bacteria. The most common organisms in 70% of the cases of SBP are gram-negative bacilli (*Escherichia coli, Klebsiella pneumoniae*), the remaining 30% are caused by gram-positive cocci (*Streptococcus pneumoniae*: 15%, *Enterococcus*: 6–10%).[8]

Prognosis

Mortality from SBP approaches 30%, with the majority of patients dying of severe liver disease, hepatorenal syndrome, or complications of portal hypertension. Therefore, early diagnosis and proper use of antibiotics according to culture and empirical antibiotics are important to reduce the mortality and improve prognosis.[10] Short-term prognosis of spontaneous bacterial peritonitis has improved in the past decades due to prompt diagnosis with the routine practice of diagnostic paracentesis, standardized

diagnostic criteria for ascitic fluid infection, and worldwide use of non-nephrotoxic, third-generation cephalosporins.[6,11] However, if treatment is not initiated before the patient develops signs of shock, mortality approaches 100%.

Although most episodes of spontaneous bacterial peritonitis are satisfactorily resolved when rapidly diagnosed and treated, a significant number of patients develop complications, such as hepatic encephalopathy, septic shock, and progressive renal failure, leading in some cases to an irreversible hepatorenal syndrome and death.[6] Despite the effectiveness of antibiotic therapy, the hospital mortality of patients with SBP is high. The outcomes in asymptomatic outpatients diagnosed with SBP while undergoing therapeutic paracentesis seem to be better than SBP occurring in hospitalized patients.[12]

The following factors statistically correlated with a higher death rate ($p < 0.05$) in chronic liver disease patients.[9]

- Child-Pugh class C
- Hepatic encephalopathy
- High peripheral blood leukocyte count ($\geq 12,000/mm^3$)
- Presence of renal dysfunction (serum creatinine level ≥ 2 mg/dL); Longer prothrombin time (INR ≥ 2.5)

Table 57-3 Options for Empiric Antibiotic Therapy for SBP

Drug	Dose	Route	Duration
Cefotaxime	2 g every 12 hours	Intravenous (IV)	5 days
Ceftriaxone	2 g every 24 hours	IV	5 days
Amoxicillin plus clavulanic acid	1 g/0.2 g every 6–8 hours; 500 mg/125 mg every 8 hours	IV; oral	2 days; 6–12 days
Ofloxacin[†]	400 mg every 12 hours	Oral	8 days

*Dose may need to be adjusted according to renal function.

[†]Only in patients without complications (i.e., sepsis, ileus, gastrointestinal bleeding, encephalopathy, or serum creatinine concentration >3 mg/dL) who have not received a quinolone prophylactically.

- Lower ascites protein level (<1 g/dL)
- Long history of liver disease
- Development of super infection in addition to SBP

MANAGEMENT

Treatment

Antibiotic therapy should be initiated as soon as the diagnosis of SBP is suspected, and after ascitic fluid has been collected and sent for cell count and culture. However, if the paracentesis must be postponed for any reason, this should not delay administration of antibiotics. Early empiric antibiotic therapy improves survival in SBP. Treatment for SBP should also be considered for patients with cirrhosis who present with variceal bleeding.

Third-generation cephalosporins (e.g., cefotaxime, ceftriaxone or ceftizoxime) are the initial antibiotics of choice, pending culture results. Other alternatives include ticarcillin/clavulanate, piperacillin/tazobactam, imipenem/meropenem, or a fluoroquinolone. Antibiotic options and dosing are listed in Table 57-3. Aminoglycosides should be avoided, as they provoke acute renal failure in up to 50% or more of patients. Shorter duration (5 days) of treatment appears to be as effective as a longer course (10 days) if the PMNs in the ascitic fluid drop below 250 after 48 hours of antibiotic therapy in a patient without other complications. Oral ofloxacin is as effective as intravenous antibiotics in uncomplicated spontaneous bacterial peritonitis.[14]

One of the most lethal complications of SBP is hepatorenal syndrome, which may develop in up to a third of cases. Administration of intravenous albumin appears to reduce the incidence of renal failure and mortality. It may accomplish this simply by volume expansion. One regimen is to give 1.5 g/kg at the time of diagnosis and another 1 g/kg after 48 hours.

PREVENTION

Once SBP occurs, the possibility of recurrence is high, and prevention of recurrent episodes is important, as the prognosis is poor.[13] Approximately 70% of patients surviving an episode of SBP will have another episode within 1 year. Prophylactic antibiotic treatment with either norfloxacin 400 mg/day or ciprofloxacin 750 mg/week or TMP/SMX one double-strength tablet daily should be considered in patients with a high risk of having infection (e.g., total protein in ascitic fluid of <1 g/dL).

Three specific groups of cirrhotic patients are known to benefit from SBP prophylaxis:

1. Those with gastrointestinal hemorrhage, independently of the presence or absence of ascites[14]
2. Low protein in the ascites fluid (ascites protein <1 g/dL)[12]
3. Previous episode of SBP

DISCHARGE/FOLLOW-UP PLANS

Given the underlying illness of liver cirrhosis, high risk of recurrence, and general poor prognosis of patients who have survived SBP, these patients require close follow-up with consultation by an experienced gastroenterologist or hepatologist. Patients with liver cirrhosis who have suffered an episode of SBP should also be scheduled for evaluation for possible liver transplantation.[16]

Patient and Family Education

Compliance with medications, especially any prophylactic antibiotics, should be emphasized, as well as close outpatient follow-up. Family members or significant others should be instructed to observe for fever, any changes in mental status, or gastrointestinal bleeding, and counseled to immediately seek care if these occur.

Key Points

- The most common symptoms on presentation with SBP are fever (69%), abdominal pain (59%), and altered mental status (54%).

- Patients with cirrhosis tend to be relatively hypothermic, and a temperature ≥37.8° C (100° F) should be considered a fever.

- The total protein level in ascitic fluid inversely correlates with the likelihood of SBP, with risk increasing dramatically at levels below 1 g/dL.

- The sensitivity of ascitic fluid cultures can be increased by injecting 10 mL of the fluid into blood culture bottles as soon as it is collected.

- Antibiotic therapy should be initiated as soon as the diagnosis of SBP is suspected.

SUGGESTED READING

Guarner C. Soriano G. Bacterial translocation and its consequences in patients with cirrhosis. Eur J Gastroenterol Hepatol 2005; 17(1):27–31.

Garcia-Tsao G. Milestones in liver disease, spontaneous bacterial peritonitis, a historical perspective. J Hepatol 2004; 41:522–527.

Sapey T, Mena E, Fort E, et al. Rapid diagnosis of spontaneous bacterial peritonitis with leukocyte esterase reagent strips in a European and in an American center. J Gastroenterol Hepatol 2005; 20(2):187–192.

Cholongitas E, Papatheodoridis GV, Lahanas A, et al. Increasing frequency of gram-positive bacteria in spontaneous bacterial peritonitis. Liver Int 2005; 25(1):57–61.

Frazee LA, Marinos AE, Rybarczyk AM, et al. Long-term prophylaxis of spontaneous bacterial peritonitis in patients with cirrhosis Ann Pharmacother 2005; 39:908–912.

Parsi MA, Atreja A, Zein NN. Spontaneous bacterial peritonitis: recent data on incidence and treatment. Cleve Clin J Med 2004; 71(7):569–576.

Rimola A, García-Tsao G, Navasa M, et al. and the International Ascites Club. Diagnosis, treatment and prophylaxis of spontaneous bacterial peritonitis: a consensus document. J Hepatol 2000; 32(1):142–153.

CHAPTER FIFTY-EIGHT

Acute Abdominal Emergencies

Mark G. Graham, MD, FACP, and Kris Kaulback, MD

BACKGROUND

The patient with acute abdominal pain represents an urgent challenge to the hospital-based physician. The differential diagnosis is very extensive (Table 58-1), and etiologies vary from benign and self-limited conditions to life-threatening emergencies requiring prompt diagnosis and treatment. In addition to a thorough history and physical examination, the clinician must consider factors such as patient age, sex, and risk factors for specific abdominal emergencies in order to identify the correct diagnosis in timely manner. An initial evaluation that includes rectal and pelvic examinations, urinalysis, and hemoccult testing will often yield a specific diagnosis. The ubiquitous availability and use of abdominal computed tomography (CT) in evaluation of patients presenting with acute abdominal pain certainly altered the classical approach and advanced diagnostic accuracy, and subsequently reduced in the frequency of exploratory surgery.

ASSESSMENT

Given that most hospitalized patients with abdominal pain are first evaluated in the emergency department, the American College of Emergency Physicians offers the following "expert consensus" guidelines to the approach to nontraumatic acute abdominal pain[1]:

- Patients with abdominal pain of undetermined etiology should have a diagnosis of undifferentiated abdominal pain (UDAP) rather than given a more specific diagnosis unsupported by history, physical, or laboratory findings.
- Discharged patients with UDAP should be given discharge instructions and follow-up.
- Do not restrict the differential diagnosis solely by the location of the pain.
- Do not use the presence or absence of fever to distinguish surgical from medical etiologies of abdominal pain.
- Among patients with UDAP assessment can include:
- Use of serial evaluations over several hours to improve the diagnostic accuracy in patients with unclear causes of abdominal pain
- Collection of a complete data set before reaching a differential diagnosis
- Performance of a stool analysis for occult blood in patients with abdominal pain

- Performance of a pelvic examination in female patients with abdominal pain

As previously noted, the use of abdominal CT is now often an essential aspect of evaluation. The American College of Radiology summary of the imaging approach in patients with acute abdominal pain and fever[2] favors CT scanning over plain radiographs or ultrasound in the initial evaluation process. CT scanning is the imaging method of choice in this setting for a number of reasons, as outlined in Box 58-1. Basically, it is superior to pure clinical examination (accuracy of 90–95% vs. 60–76%) and reduces both hospital admissions and exploratory surgery.

A standardized approach to the patient hospitalized with acute abdominal pain typically results in a specific diagnosis. Routine aspects of the history and physical are noted in Table 58-2. Five common acute abdominal emergencies are addressed in detail below. Clinical guidelines and the supporting evidence for them are provided.

APPENDICITIS

Assessment

Clinical Presentation

At 250,000 cases annually, acute appendicitis is one of the most common abdominal emergencies encountered in the United States. It occurs in all ages and both genders, but is most common in the second and third decades of life and occurs slightly more in men than women. The natural history of appendicitis begins with appendiceal inflammation and is followed by localized ischemic changes, perforation, and then diffuse peritonitis. The goal of therapy is prompt diagnosis and surgical removal of the appendix, prior to its rupture. Though retrospective analyses suggest that appendicitis presents with signs and symptoms including fever, anorexia, nausea, vomiting, right iliac fossa pain, right lower quadrant pain, abdominal tenderness, guarding, and peritoneal irritation, no single sign or symptom nor a combination thereof has been shown to be predictive of acute appendicitis with certainty.

Diagnosis

No single laboratory study or combination of studies is predictive of appendicitis. Common laboratory evaluation of patients presenting with acute abdominal pain is listed in Box 58-2. Although the white

Table 58-1 Differential Diagnosis of Acute Abdominal Pain by Location

RUQ	Epigastric	LUQ
Acute cholecystitis	Acute pancreatitis	Splenic infarction, rupture, enlargement, aneurysm
Biliary colic	Peptic ulcer disease	LLL pneumonia
Hepatic abscess	Ruptured AAA	
Retrocecal appendicitis		
RLL pneumonia		

RLQ	Diffuse	LLQ
Appendicitis	Peritonitis	Sigmoid diverticulitis
Ileitis	Acute pancreatitis	Perforated colon cancer
Meckel's diverticulitis	Sickle cell crisis	Left ectopic pregnancy
Cecal diverticulitis	Early appendicitis	Left tubo-ovarian abscess, torsion
Mesenteric adenitis	Mesenteric thrombosis	Left PID
Right ectopic pregnancy	Mesenteric ischemia	Endometriosis
Right tubo-ovarian abscess, torsion	Gastroenteritis	Mittelschmerz
Right PID	Ruptured AAA	Left urolithiasis
Endometriosis	Intestinal obstruction	Left pyelonephritis
Mittelschmerz		Incarcerated left inguinal hernia
Right urolithiasis		
Right pyelonephritis		
Incarcerated right inguinal hernia		

RUQ—Right Upper Quadrant; RLQ—Right Lower Quadrant; LUQ—Left Upper Quadrant; LLQ—Left Lower Quadrant; LLL—Left Lower Lobe; RLL—Right Lower Lobe; PID—Pelvic Inflammatory Disease; AAA—Abdominal Aortic Aneurysm

Table 58–2 Routine Components of the History and Physical for Abdominal Pain

History	Physical
Pain—location, radiation, quality	Vital Signs
Exacerbating and relieving factors	General appearance—icterus, jaundice?
Associated symptoms—especially nausea, vomiting and any remarkable stool complaints (e.g., constipation, diarrhea, hematochezia, melena)	Chest Abdomen—auscultation and palpation
NSAID use	Rectal examination, stool guaiac
Family history of abdominal disorders	Pelvic examination in women
Alcohol use	
Menstrual history in women	

Box 58-1 Advantages of CT Scanning Compared to Clinical Evaluation

- Results in 24% reduction of hospital admissions
- Superior to clinical evaluation with radiographs in diagnosing bowel obstruction, and can locate site of obstruction in 73–95% of cases
- Identifies "closed loop" obstruction (sensitivity 67%, specificity 82%)
- More sensitive in identifying intestinal ischemia/infarction than clinical evaluation and ultrasound (CT 65–86%, U/S 28%)
- Superior in the identification of myriad other problems, such as abscesses, phlegmon, fistulas, sinus tracts, extravasation from perforations, pseudomembranous colitis, and inflammatory bowel disease.

Box 58-2 Routine Laboratory Evaluation for Patients with Acute Abdominal Pain

- Complete blood count with differential
- Basic chemistries (electrolytes, BUN, creatinine, and glucose)
- Liver profile (AST, ALT, alkaline phosphatase, and bilirubin)
- Lipase
- Urinalysis
- Pregnancy test in women of childbearing potential

blood cell count is elevated in about 90% of patients, a normal count does not rule out appendicitis. Laboratory studies should also include β-HCG in females and urinalysis. Diagnostic imaging is not routinely recommended when there is a very high or very low pretest probability of appendicitis, but may be helpful in equivocal clinical presentations, though not flawless.[3,4] In such cases, CT scanning provides 94% sensitivity and 95% specificity. Corresponding values for ultrasound are 86% and 81%, respectively.

Prognosis

The prognosis and follow-up measures for appendicitis depend directly on how early in its course diagnosis and resection occur. When the appendix is removed prior to rupture, hospital confinement is typically 1–2 days. Postrupture diagnosis leads to lengthy hospitalizations and potentially serial interventions to evacuate abscesses from the peritoneal cavity. Discharge should not be contemplated until the patient is afebrile for at least 24 hours. The development of adhesions may lead to late problems with bowel obstruction.

Management

Preoperative Antibiotics

Wound infection is the most common source of morbidity after appendectomy. The infection rate varies from 6 to 50%, depending on timing of appendectomy and antibiotic coverage. Multiple studies have shown a reduction of infections with the use of pre-operative antibiotics; however, randomized, controlled clinical trials have failed to identify any specific antibiotic or combination of antibiotics as ideal in reducing infections rates. For non-perforated appendices, cefotetan 20 mg/kg given IV is recommended (retrospective analysis). For perforated appendicitis, ampicillin/sublactam (Unasyn) 75 mg/kg/dose q 6 hours with gentamicin 2.5 mg/kg q 8 hours OR piperacillin/tazobactam (Zosyn) 100 mg/kg/dose given alone q 6 hours is in common use (randomized controlled trial). For penicillin-allergic patients, with perforated appendicitis, an alternative regimen is metronidazole 500 mg IV q8 hours and a fluoroquinolone.

Pain Management

While historically some surgeons have advocated providing no pain medications prior to diagnosis, the available evidence suggests that appropriate use of analgesics in patients with acute abdominal pain effectively decreases pain and does not interfere with diagnosis or treatment.[5] Intravenous morphine (0.1–0.15 mg/kg) q 2 hours as needed is appropriate.

Operative Management

Appendectomy can be performed laparoscopically or by formal laparotomy. In either case, the following recommendations apply:

1. Administration of Zofran, pre-operatively to prevent post-operative emesis (small randomized controlled trial)
2. Delayed primary wound closure if peritonitis is present (small randomized controlled trial)
3. Individualized role of limited versus extensive peritoneal lavage by experienced surgeon
4. Decision for laparoscopic versus laparotomy approach considered "surgeon's choice" (large randomized controlled trial)
5. Routine intraoperative culture of peritoneal fluid not recommended
6. For nonperforated appendicitis, infiltration of wound at closure with local anesthetic to reduce post-operative pain

Pain Management

Begin feeding when anesthesia effects are resolved and ileus, if any, has resolved. Assess and treat pain as follows:

1. Pain assessment with age-appropriate, validated pain assessment tools
2. For severe pain, IV morphine (0.1–0.15 mg/kg) q 2 hours as needed
3. For mild-to-moderate pain, acetaminophen; and opiates for more severe pain
4. Following perforated appendix removal, use of patient-controlled anesthesia (PCA) pumps

Postoperative Antibiotics

For perforated appendicitis, use ampicillin/sublactam (Unasyn) along with gentamicin OR piperacillin/tazobactam (Zosyn), discontinuing same when patient is afebrile, eating, and without leukocytosis or left shift. For nonperforated appendicitis, it is recommended that one dose of cefotetan 20 mg/kg be given IV 12 hours post-operative.

Respiratory Care

Incentive spirometry is recommended to reduce complications of fever, atelectasis, pneumonia, and respiratory failure.

Discharge/Follow-up Plans

For nonperforated appendicitis, discharge can be considered when the patient has recovered from the anesthetic, is afebrile, tolerates diet, and achieves adequate pain control. For perforated appendix, it is recommended that discharge be considered when the patient is afebrile for 24 hours, tolerates diet, achieves adequate pain control on oral medications, and has a suitable home environment to assure postoperative antibiotic administration.

CHOLECYSTITIS

Assessment

Clinical Presentation

Though gallbladder disease occurs in all stages of adulthood and in both genders, it classically presents in patients with the five "F" risk factors; namely, fat, female, fertile, forty, positive family history. Acute cholecystitis typically presents with right upper quadrant or epigastric abdominal pain, radiating to the shoulder or back. The pain is steady and severe, and is associated with nausea, vomiting, and anorexia. Fatty food ingestion 1–6 hours prior to presentation is typical. Ten percent of cases are acalculous. Prolonged pain (>6 hours) suggests complete cystic duct obstruction. The physical examination is remarkable for an ill-appearing, febrile, tachycardic patient unwilling to move about due to marked peritoneal irritation. The abdominal examination is remarkable for voluntary and involuntary guarding, and a positive Murphy's sign in which deep palpation under the right costal margin over the gallbladder fossa elicits marked pain particularly during deep inspiration.

Differential diagnosis: simple biliary colic without infection, acute pancreatitis, appendicitis, acute hepatitis, peptic ulcer disease, right kidney disease or pyelonephritis, right lower lobe pneumonia, subdiaphragmatic abscess, hepatic abscess, Fitz-Hugh-Curtis perihepatitis, perforated viscus, and cardiac ischemia/injury.

Diagnosis

Acute cholecystitis should be suspected when a patient presenting with the above clinical picture is found to have gallstones on ultrasound or CT scanning of the abdomen, though absence of stones does not exclude the diagnosis and presence of stones does not confirm it. The diagnosis is confirmed when the clinical evaluation, laboratory tests, and imaging studies are considered together.[6] No single laboratory test or clinical finding is sufficiently accurate to rule in or rule out the diagnosis; however, Murphy's sign is the most powerful clinical finding, and a leukocytosis with left shift is the most important laboratory finding. Less consistent laboratory findings include elevations of transaminases, bilirubin, and amylase. Ultrasound evidence of stones in a patient with typical symptoms and signs of acute cholecystitis supports the diagnosis of same. Other sonographic findings include gallbladder wall thickening and a "sonographic" Murphy's sign. The sensitivity and specificity of ultrasound for acute cholecystitis are 84% and 95%, respectively.[7] CT scanning is also helpful in diagnosing acute cholecystitis, though if ultrasound is readily available, it is unnecessary.

Prognosis

Prompt diagnosis followed by antibiotics and cholecystectomy result in a good prognosis; the overall mortality rate is 3%, including high-risk patients. Undiagnosed, acute cholecystitis can progress to gallbladder gangrene (20%) and perforation (2%), with a high mortality. Other complications include cholecystoenteric fistula, gallstone pancreatitis, gallstone ileus, and emphysematous cholecystitis, all of which carry a substantially worse prognosis for complete recovery.[8]

Management

Treatment

The treatment of acute cholecystitis varies with the severity of the problem and the general health of the patient.[12] All patients should be admitted to the hospital and offered general supportive care and antibiotics. Supportive care measures include DVT prophylaxis, intravenous hydration, narcotic analgesia, and correction of electrolyte abnormalities, if any. Although acute cholecystitis is primarily an inflammatory condition, infection with *E. coli*, *Enterococcus*, *Klebsiella*, and *Enterobacter* is found in 22% of those with calculous cholecystitis and 46% of those with acalculous cholecystitis.[7] Although traditionally ampicillin (2 g IV q 4 hours) and gentamicin (weight, renal dosed) have been used, a beta-lactam/beta-lactamase inhibitor such as ampicillin/sulbactam (Unasyn) covers common offending organisms. Definitive therapy varies by the American Society of Anesthesiologist (ASA) rating of the patient's surgical risk.

Low-risk patients: ASA class I or II patients benefit from 24–48 hours of general supportive therapy, as described above, followed by laparoscopic or open cholecystectomy during the same hospitalization. Forestalling cholecystectomy to a separate hospitalization carries a small but unnecessary risk of death and peritonitis.[10]

High-risk patients: ASA class III, IV, and V patients have a surgical mortality of 5%–27% and are considered "high risk" for cholecystectomy. In these patients, prolonged stabilization with fluids and antibiotics is recommended, followed by consideration of nonsurgical options.[11] Those who do not recover, or those whose symptoms recur, are addressed with percutaneous cholecystostomy tube insertion and prolonged antibiotic courses. After stabilization, surgery can be reconsidered. For either low- or high-risk patients, a laparoscopic approach is usually feasible. The incidence of conversion to an open procedure is about 5%.[12]

Discharge/Follow-up Plans

These vary closely with the patient's ASA class. Postoperative wound care and follow-up are required. There is no defined role for prolonged antibiotics unless sepsis or abscess was discovered. Early ambulation is encouraged.

DIVERTICULITIS

Assessment

Clinical Presentation

Diverticular disease occurs in adults and increases with age. The majority of patients present with left lower quadrant pain (93–100%), fever, (57–100%), and leukocytosis (69–83%). Complicated acute diverticulitis may present with signs of marked peritoneal irritation or frank peritonitis. Useful initial examinations in evaluating the patient with abdominal pain suspected of having diverticulitis may include a complete blood count (CBC), urinalysis, and flat and upright abdominal radiographs. If the clinical picture is clear, no other tests are needed; the diagnosis of diverticulitis can be made on clinical grounds alone.

Differential diagnosis includes irritable bowel syndrome, inflammatory bowel disease, ischemic colitis, colon cancer, bowel obstruction, and gynecologic and urologic diseases.

Diagnosis

In cases in which the diagnosis is unclear, additional imaging is indicated. **CT scanning** with oral, rectal, and IV contrast is the preferred method for confirming the diagnosis of acute diverticulitis. Criteria include: (1) colonic wall thickening, (2) pericolic fat infiltration, (3) pericolic or distant abscesses, and (4) extraluminal air.

Because of the risk of barium extravasation through a perforated diverticulum, **barium enema** examination should be avoided. Such examination can be safely carried out after peritoneal signs are resolved. **Endoscopy** also should be avoided in the setting of acute diverticulitis because the insufflation or the instrument itself may cause perforation. **Water-soluble contrast enema** can be safely used when acute diverticulitis is suspected. Criteria for diagnosis confirmation include: (1) presence of diverticuli, (2) mass effect, (3) intramural mass, (4) sinus tract, and (5) extravasation of contrast material into peritoneum.

Prognosis

Following successful therapy for acute diverticulitis, 30–40% of patients will remain symptom-free, 30–40% will develop recurrent pain without evidence of infection, and 33% will develop a second attack. The prognosis worsens slightly after a second attack, with about 5% going on to develop many attacks. Nonetheless, most surgeons consider a second attack to be an indication for partial colectomy.

Management

Treatment

Simple acute diverticulitis is treated medically, but when complicated (25%) by abscess formation, extensive wall or distant abscess, perforation, sinus tract formation or obstruction, a surgical approach is indicated.[13]

Simple Diverticulitis/Medical management: Bowel rest or clear liquid diet and IV antibiotics result in complete resolution of infection in 70–100% of patients. Failure to improve should prompt imaging with a CT scan to identify evidence of a "complicated" case. Antibiotics should cover gram-negative rods and anaerobic organisms, such as *Bacteroides fragilis.* Acceptable antibiotic choices include: (1) a quinolone with metronidazole, (2) amoxicillin-clavulanic acid, or (3) sulfamethoxazole-trimethoprim with metronidazole. Antibiotics are continued for at least 5–7 days, or until all clinical features of the presentation have resolved.

Complicated Diverticulitis/Surgical Management: Acute diverticulitis with complications of perforation, obstruction, abscess formation, and peritonitis must be treated in the hospital setting. Intravenous hydration and broad-spectrum antibiotics are also required. The patient should be kept NPO until signs of resolution, after which a clear liquid diet may follow. Operative indications for diverticulitis are listed in Box 58-3.

Pre-operative measures for elective procedures: mechanical and antibiotic (neomycin) enemas are recommended. A sigmoid resection with primary anastomosis is performed.

Pre-operative measures for emergency procedures: If frank peritonitis with or without pneumoperitoneum is recognized, pursue IV fluid resuscitation. CT scanning is performed to identify abscesses, phlegmon, sinus tracts, or sites of obstruction. If abscesses can be drained by CT-guidance, such is performed, and colectomy is delayed.

PERITONITIS

Assessment

Clinical Presentation

Excluding the setting of obvious penetrating trauma, peritonitis most often occurs in connection with a perforated viscus. The hallmark physical finding indicative of a ruptured viscus is rebound abdominal tenderness. When present and localized, it is key to identifying the perforation site and diagnosis. When poorly localized, it is best described as a positive "shake" test, in which shaking the patient leads to severe discomfort. The patient is generally febrile and ill appearing, lying perfectly still to avoid pain provocation. Fever is generally present with a perforated viscus, regardless of location.

Diagnosis

The white blood cell (WBC) count is typically elevated with evidence of a leftward shift. Serum amylase and transaminase levels may be elevated. Pain localizes to the site of perforation early, but then becomes diffuse as the peritoneal cavity is soiled and inflamed. Days later, walled-off masses and phlegmon form in cases in which the diagnosis and/or surgical correction is delayed. Early after perforation, plain radiographs may demonstrate free air within the peritoneal cavity. Ultrasound and CT scanning are useful in identifying inflamed or ruptured appendices and phlegmon or abscesses due to a long-standing perforation. CT scanning is useful in identifying paracolonic abscesses early in the course of diverticular disease. Blood cultures do not provide additional clinically relevant information for patients with community-acquired intra-abdominal infections and are, therefore, not recommended.

Prognosis

The prognosis after viscus perforation is principally related to the timing of its discovery and repair. Long-standing perforations soil and inflame the peritoneal cavity, leading to abscess formation, adhesions, sepsis, and shock. In the case of inflammatory bowel disease, the prognosis is directly related to the patient's response to standard treatment.

Management

Treatment

The treatment of peritonitis includes repair of the source of infection and antibiotic therapy.[14] Bowel injuries due to penetrating, blunt, or iatrogenic trauma that are repaired within 12 hours and intraoperative contamination of the operative field by enteric contents under other circumstances should be treated with antibiotics for 24 hours or less. For acute perforations of the stomach, duodenum, and proximal jejunum in the absence of antacid therapy or malignancy, antibiotic therapy is also considered to be prophylactic. Similarly, acute appendicitis without evidence of gangrene, perforation, abscess, or peritonitis requires only prophylactic administration of inexpensive regimens active against facultative and obligate anaerobes.

Acute cholecystitis is often an inflammatory but not infectious disease. If infection is suspected on the basis of clinical and radiographic findings, urgent intervention may be indicated, and antimicrobial therapy should provide coverage against Enterobacteriaceae. Coverage against anaerobes is warranted in treatment of patients with previous bile duct-bowel anastomosis.

Antibiotics used for empirical treatment of community-acquired intra-abdominal infections should be active against enteric gram-negative aerobic and facultative bacilli and beta lactam-susceptible gram-positive cocci. Coverage against obligate anaerobic bacilli should be provided for distal small-bowel and colon-derived infections and for more proximal gastrointestinal perforations when obstruction is present. Routine coverage against *Enterococcus* is not necessary for patients with community-acquired intra-abdominal infections. Antimicrobial therapy for enterococci should be given when enterococci are recovered from patients with health care–associated infections. If a patient with diagnosed infection has previously been treated with an antibiotic, that patient should be treated as if he or she had a health care–associated infection. Agents that are used to treat nosocomial infections in the intensive care unit should not be routinely used to treat community-acquired infections.

For patients with mild to moderate community-acquired infections, agents that have a narrower spectrum of activity are preferable to more costly agents that have broader coverage against gram-negative organisms and/or greater risk of toxicity. Aminoglycosides have relatively narrow therapeutic ranges and are associated with ototoxicity and nephrotoxicity. Because of the availability of less toxic agents demonstrated to be of equal efficacy, aminoglycosides are not recommended for routine use in community-acquired intra-abdominal infections.

Completion of the antimicrobial course with oral forms of a quinolone plus metronidazole or with oral amoxicillin/clavulanic acid is acceptable for patients who are able to tolerate an oral diet.

Discharge/Follow-up Plans

In the case of perforation due to peptic ulcer disease, eradication of gastric acid with proton pump inhibitors is recommended. For diverticulitis, a prolonged course of antibiotics is advised. For viscus perforations in general, antibiotics may be recommended for several weeks for cases in which the peritoneal cavity was significantly soiled. In cases complicated by the development of phlegmon or wide-spread abscesses, additional procedures to evacuate necrotic or infected tissue may be necessary.

BOWEL OBSTRUCTION

Assessment

Clinical Presentation

Over one billion dollars were spent in a year on 300,000 hospitalizations and 800,000 hospital-confined days for bowel obstruction in the United States in the early 1990s.[15] Among adults, it primarily occurs in those with a past history of abdominal surgery. Fifteen per cent of abdominal surgeries are complicated by subsequent bowel obstructions, and 75% of bowel obstructions are attributed to adhesions. Hernias and cancer are less frequent causes.

The typical patient with intestinal obstruction presents with crampy, diffuse abdominal pain associated with profuse nausea/vomiting and dehydration. This can be complicated by third-spacing of fluids, bowel strangulation, and necrosis. Ten per cent of patients with obstruction develop strangulation,[16] presenting with localized abdominal tenderness. The diagnosis is largely a clinical one in which tachycardia due to pain and third-spacing of fluids is common. The abdomen is tender, distended, and firm. Bowel sounds may be increased or decreased.

Diagnosis

The WBC count and electrolytes are somewhat useful in monitoring for strangulation and dehydration, respectively. Radiography of the abdomen usually confirms the diagnosis. Erect abdominal radiographs may show air-fluid levels that are sometimes helpful in identifying the location of the obstruction. Supine radiographs are helpful in estimating the amount of distention. When clinical and radiographic evidence is clear, CT scanning is usually not needed in the diagnosis of obstructed bowel. However, in at least 20% of cases the diagnosis is equivocal, and CT scanning with oral contrast has replaced the small bowel follow-through study for confirming the diagnosis and locating the site of obstruction. The sensitivity and specificity of CT scan in the diagnosis of bowel obstruction are 93% and 100%, respectively, compared to 50% and 75% for radiographs.[16]

Prognosis

Patients suffering bowel obstruction without strangulation usually do well, though about half require surgery to correct it, and there is a high recurrence rate. The overall mortality rate is 5%.

Management

Treatment

The time-tested approach to the patient with intestinal obstruction is two-fold: (1) determine the degree of dehydration and metabolic derangement, and (2) address the need for and timing of operative intervention. Initial treatment includes keeping the patient NPO, providing intravenous hydration, and nasogastric decompression with a standard nasogastric tube to which low, intermittent suction is applied. Fluid and electrolyte abnormalities should be vigorously addressed. If there is no sign of improvement within 12–24 hours, surgical intervention is recommended. Earlier intervention is warranted if there is clinical evidence of strangulation. Laparoscopy appears to be a safe and effective alternative to laparotomy.

Discharge/Follow-up Plans

No special postoperative care is required for a simple intestinal obstruction that has resolved with nasogastric decompression. The patient should be advised of the high rate of recurrence. Patients presenting with repeated episodes of intestinal obstruction may benefit from procedures to lyse adhesions.

MESENTERIC ISCHEMIA

Assessment

Clinical Presentation

Mesenteric ischemia occurs in older people with cardiovascular disease, heart failure, cardiac dysrhythmias, diabetes, sepsis, and dehydration. Either arterial or venous occlusion of the mesenteric circulation can cause it. Arterial occlusion is due to atherosclerosis (25%) of the mesenteric arteries with or without dehydration, or by embolic disease (75%) from the heart due to low flow states or cardiac dysrhythmias. Mesenteric venous obstruction occurs in hypercoagulable states and low flow states. That 20–30% of mesenteric arterial occlusions are nonocclusive speaks to the multifactorial nature of the etiology.

Patients presenting with mesenteric ischemia have severe, colicky, diffuse abdominal pain, often associated with vomiting and diarrhea. The examination is frequently normal, though rectal examination may demonstrate guaiac-positive stool. Commonly observed physical findings include low-grade fever, diffuse abdominal tenderness, increased bowel sounds, and guaiac-positive stool.

Diagnosis

A pronounced leukocytosis is typically present. Elevations of serum amylase and CK are also common, as is evidence of metabolic acidosis. Plain radiographs are of limited value. CT scanning, magnetic resonance imaging (MRI), magnetic resonance angiogram (MRA), and standard angiography can identify specific abnormalities associated with ischemic bowel.

Prognosis

In large part due to the frail health of those at risk for mesenteric ischemia, the overall prognosis is poor. The mortality rate reaches up to 70%.

Management

Treatment

Diagnosis before infarction is the single most important factor to improve the otherwise dismal results. Initial therapy focuses on resuscitation to optimize blood pressure and correct cardiac arrhythmias. Relief of persistent vasoconstriction, which is the cause of nonocclusive mesenteric ischemia and occurs in association with occlusive forms of ischemia, is another important factor. If no evidence of thrombosis exists and peritoneal signs are present, laparotomy is indicated for bowel resection. If no peritoneal signs are present, an angiogram is performed. Normal, conservative therapy should be pursued, unless persistent peritoneal findings exist that mandate laparotomy.[18]

If thrombosis is suspected, the patient should be heparinized, assuming there are no persistent peritoneal findings. When thrombosis is evident and peritoneal findings are present, a laparotomy is recommended to remove thrombus or dead bowel. If a minor arterial occlusion or embolus is discovered, papaverine (which vasodilates mesenteric vessels during angiography) is infused while observing for peritoneal findings. Presence of peritoneal findings indicates laparotomy, while absence indicates observation and weaning of the papaverine. The discovery of a major thrombus or embolus indicates papaverine, embolectomy, and in some patients, thrombolytic therapy. Interventional radiologists can provide guidance and treatment in this situation.

Discharge/Follow-up Plans

This condition remits in about 30% of patients afflicted. Care is directed to ensure optimal hemodynamic status and to address specific risk factors peculiar to the patient. Long-term anticoagulation is indicated in those patients determined to have a hypercoagulable state.

Key Points

- CT scan is the optimal imaging approach to patients with acute abdominal pain and fever in the initial evaluation process, as it reduces both hospital admissions and exploratory surgery.

- No single sign or symptom nor a combination thereof has been shown to be predictive of acute appendicitis.

- Though gallbladder disease occurs in all stages of adulthood and in both genders, it classically presents in patients with the five "F" risk factors, namely, fat, female, fertile, forty, positive family history. A Murphy's sign is the most predictive clinical finding, and a leukocytosis with left shift is the most important laboratory finding.

- Simple acute diverticulitis is treated medically, but when complicated by abscess formation, extensive wall or distant abscess, perforation, sinus tract formation or obstruction, a surgical approach is indicated.

- The time-tested approach to the patient with intestinal obstruction includes treatment of dehydration and metabolic derangements, and addressing the need for and timing of operative intervention.

- Diagnosis before infarction is the single most important factor to improve the otherwise dismal outcome among patients with mesenteric ischemia.

SUGGESTED READING

American College of Emergency Physicians (ACEP). Clinical policy: critical issues for the initial evaluation and management of patients with a chief complaint of nontraumatic acute abdominal pain. Ann Emerg Med 2000; 36(4):406–415. www.guidelines.gov #2526.

American College of Radiology (ACR), Expert Panel on Gastrointestinal Imaging. Imaging evaluation of patients with acute abdominal pain and fever. Reston (VA): American College of Radiology (ACR); 2001; 4. (ACR appropriateness criteria). www.guidelines.gov #2484.

Terasawa T, Blackmore CC, Bent S, et al. Systematic review: computed tomography and ultrasonography to detect acute appendicitis in adults and adolescents. Ann Intern Med 2004; 141:537.

Flum DR, McClure TD, Morris A, et al. Misdiagnosis of appendicitis and the use of diagnostic imaging. J Am Coll Surg 2005; 201: 933.

Trowbridge, RL, Rutkowski NK, Shojania KG. Does this patient have acute cholecysytitis? JAMA 2003; 289:80.

Society for Surgery of the Alimentary Tract (SSAT). Treatment of gallstone and gallbladder disease. Manchester (MA): Society for Surgery of the Alimentary Tract (SSAT); 2003; 4. www.guidelines.gov #3756.

Practice parameters for the treatment of sigmoid diverticulitis. Standards Task Force. American Society of Colon and Rectal Surgeons. Dis Colon Rectum 2000; 43(3):289. www.guidelines.gov #1822.

Solomkin JS, Mazuski JE, Baron EJ, et al. Guidelines for the selection of anti-infective agents for complicated intra-abdominal infections. Clin Infect Dis 2003; 37(8):997–1005. www.guidelines.gov #3227.

American Gastroenterological Association Medical Position Statement: guidelines on intestinal ischemia. Gastroenterology 2000; 118(5):951–953. www.guidelines.gov #2295.

Terasawa T, Blackmore CC. Bent S, et al. Systematic review: computed tomography and ultrasonography to detect acute appendicitis in adults and adolescents. Ann Intern Med 2004; 141:537–546.

Janes SE, Meagher A, Frizelle FA. Management of diverticulitis. BMJ 2006; 332:271–275.

Oldenburg WA, Lau LL, Rodenberg TJ, et al. Acute mesenteric ischemia: a clinical review. Arch Intern Med 2004; 164:1054–1062.

CHAPTER FIFTY-NINE

Inflammatory Bowel Disease

Cuckoo Choudhary, MD

BACKGROUND

Inflammatory bowel disease (IBD) is a chronic, relapsing, inflammatory condition of the gastrointestinal tract affecting more than one million people worldwide. Though ulcerative colitis (UC) and Crohn's disease (CD) are the two most well-known forms of IBD, physicians should remember two other important forms of idiopathic IBD—the microscopic colitides, namely collagenous and lymphocytic colitis. Rates of hospitalization of both UC and CD rose from the early 1980s to the mid 1990s but have since been stable,[1] partially due to a better understanding and improving treatment of these illnesses.

In the last decade, especially more recently, our understanding of the etiology and pathogenesis of this enigmatic group of disorders has improved. We now know that IBD is not caused by a single agent. Genetic, environmental, infectious, and immunologic factors are all thought to play a role in the etiology and pathogenesis of IBD.[2] IBD is believed to develop due to altered gut immunity in a host that is genetically prone to develop the disease. Intestinal inflammation leads to disruption of its protective barrier, yielding exposure of the luminal bacteria to the mucosal immune system, which in turn activates pro-inflammatory pathways. In the genetically susceptible host, the fine balance between the pro- and anti-inflammatory pathways is lost. Thus, down-regulation of inflammation does not occur, leading to ongoing inflammation in the gut, and giving rise to disease symptoms.[3]

ASSESSMENT

Clinical Presentation

Prevalence and Presenting Signs and Symptoms

Crampy abdominal pain and diarrhea, worsened by eating, are the two most common symptoms of both UC and CD. The severity of diarrhea depends upon the extent and severity of the disease. The diarrhea in UC is almost always bloody; associated tenesmus and urgency is a rule—a feature indicating rectal involvement.[4]

The diarrhea in CD, on the other hand, is usually nonbloody, even when the colon is involved. Systemic symptoms such as anorexia, nausea, weight loss, fatigue, and fevers are more common in CD than UC. High fever in CD usually indicates a superimposed infectious colitis or the development of an intra-abdominal abscess.

Microscopic colitis, both lymphocytic and collagenous, usually presents with large-volume, nonbloody, watery diarrhea associated with abdominal pain. Collagenous colitis mainly affects middle-aged females; lymphocytic colitis, on the other hand, has an equal incidence in both sexes.[5]

The physical examination in UC is usually nonspecific and is characterized by mild abdominal distention and diffuse, mild tenderness. In severe forms of the disease, there may be diffuse tenderness with some guarding, and in such cases toxic megacolon needs to be considered. Though the physical examination of a patient with Crohn's colitis is similar to that of a patient with UC, involvement of the small bowel may give rise to additional physical findings. In patients who have terminal ileum or cecal involvement, there may be fullness or even a mass in the right lower quadrant. Ileocecal CD often mimics appendicitis, especially in the young presenting to the emergency room for the first time. In addition, perianal examination may detect important physical findings in patients with CD, thus mandating performance of a complete and thorough perianal examination in a patient with known or suspected IBD.

Tables 59-1 and 59-2 summarize the typical clinical features of UC and CD that bring a patient with IBD to the hospital and may therefore be seen by hospitalists on a regular basis. Detailed discussion of extraintestinal features of IBD are beyond the scope of this chapter, but Table 59-3 lists the more common ones that may be seen by the hospitalist.

Diagnosis and Laboratory Tests

IBD should always be in the differential diagnosis of a patient presenting with diarrhea, whether bloody or nonbloody, acute or chronic. The diagnostic tests performed on a patient admitted to the hospital depend not only on the overall clinical presentation and severity of illness, but also on whether he or she is known to have IBD or not. Routine blood tests include CBC, metabolic panel and hepatic profile. In addition, stool studies including culture should be performed to assess the possibility of infectious colitis in a patient presenting with diarrhea for the first time and superimposed infectious colitis in those carrying the diagnosis of IBD. Some important agents which cause infectious colitis that may mimic IBD are *Salmonella, Campylobacter jejuni, Clostridium diffi-*

Table 59-1 Symptoms of CD in Patient Coming to the ER/In the Hospital

Site of Disease	Symptoms	Physical examination
1. Terminal ileum/cecum	a) Colicky abdominal pain and diarrhea b) Acute RLQ pain mimicking appendicitis c) Partial SBO d) High grade SBO	Fullness in the right lower quadrant or tender mass in the RLQ
2. Colonic Crohn's	a) Severe diarrhea with blood in the stools and dehydration b) Weight loss and anemia c) Toxic megacolon (rare)	Diffuse abdominal tenderness; in case of toxic megacolon the abdomen is quiet
3. Crohn's of the upper gastrointestinal tract only (stomach and duodenum)	a) Severe upper abdominal pain not responding to treatment for PUD b) Early satiety, nausea, vomiting	Epigastric tenderness, signs of gastric outlet obstruction in those that have developed stricture of the duodenum
4. Crohn's of the jejunum and ileum only	a) Severe diarrhea with dehydration b) PSBO or high-grade SBO—either secondary to severe inflammation or stricture formation c) Fatigue due to severe anemia	Signs of dehydration, anemia together with those of SBO

5. Fistulizing disease
  a) Enterovaginal fistula
 	
  b) Enterovesicular or colovesicular fistula
	a) Foul-smelling vaginal discharge, frank stool per vagina, dyspareunia and pelvic pain
	b) Pneumaturia, fecaluria, or recurrent, polymicrobial UTI
		Thorough pelvic examination by gynecologists may or may not reveal the fistula

6. Perianal disease	Perianal abscess, fistula, fissures	Physical examination reveals fluctuant, tender, mass in the perianal area in case of abscess; single or multiple fistulous tract openings may be seen

PSBO—Partial small bowel obstruction; SBO—Small bowel obstruction.

Sources: Robert JR, Sachar DB, Greenstein AJ. Severe gastrointestinal hemorrhage in Crohn's disease. Ann Surg 1991; 203:207, and Aeberhard P, Berchtold W, Riedtmann HJ. Surgical recurrence of perforating and non-perforating Crohn's disease: a study of 101 surgically treated patients. Dis Colon Rectum 1996; 39:80; and Meyers H, Janowitz HD. Natural history of Crohn's disease: An analytic review of the placebo lesson. Gastroenetrology 1994; 87:1189.

Table 59-2 Symptoms of UC in Patients Coming to the ER/in the Hospital

Site of Disease	Symptoms	Physical findings
Proctitis only	a) Tenesmus with blood and mucus in the stool with/without diarrhea b) Constipation with mucus and blood in the stool/frank rectal bleeding	None except heme occult–positive stools on rectal examination
Proctosigmoiditis or left-sided colitis	a) Abdominal pain and diarrhea, usually with gross blood in the stool b) Significant rectal bleeding if disease is severe	Lower abdominal tenderness (left lower quadrant/ suprapubic); pallor in cases of significant bleeding
Pancolitis	a) Abdominal pain and diarrhea, usually with blood in the stool; severity of diarrhea may be greater b) Significant lower GI bleed if disease is severe	Diffuse abdominal tenderness, dehydration may be present; pallor in cases of severe bleeding
Toxic megacolon	Abdominal pain, fever, diarrhea may seem to have decreased	Toxic appearing patient, diffuse abdominal tenderness with rebound; absent bowel sounds if perforation has occurred

Sources: Both H, Torp-Pederson K, Kriener S, et al. Clinical manifestations of ulcerative colitis and Crohn's disease in a regional patient group. Scand J Gastroenterol 1983; 18: 987; and Rao SCC, Holdsworth CD, Read NW. Symptoms and stool pattern in patients with ulcerative colitis. Gut 1988; 29:342.

cile, and amoeba. Yersinia, which classically presents with right lower quadrant pain, is more likely to mimic CD than UC.

Flexible sigmoidoscopy remains a helpful diagnostic tool in a patient presenting with abdominal pain and bloody diarrhea. Not only does it help the physician visualize colonic mucosa and take biopsies, it is also helpful in differentiating IBD from ischemic colitis based on the pattern of distribution. In addition, in a patient with known IBD refractory to inpatient treatment and in whom surgery is being considered, performance of flexible sigmoidoscopy with biopsies can exclude superimposed viral causes of infectious colitis, such as cytomegalovirus, and Herpes simplex virus. Colonoscopy is not usually indicated in an acutely ill

Table 59-3 Common Extraintestinal Features of IBD

Systems	Manifestations	Parallels disease activity
Musculoskeletal[11,12]	Peripheral arthritis	Yes
	Sacroiliitis	No
	Ankylosing spondylitis	No
Dermatologic	Erythema nodosum	Yes
	Pyoderma gangrenosum	No
	Polyarteritis nodosa	No
	Perianal skin tags	No
	Metastatic Crohn's Disease	Yes
Ocular	Uveitis	No
	Iritis	No
	Episcleritis	Yes
	Scleritis	Yes
	Crohn's keratopathy	Yes
Hepatobiliary[13]	Primary sclerosing cholangitis	No
	Pericholangitis	No
	Fatty infiltration of the liver	No
	Autoimmune hepatitis	No
	Gallstones	Yes
Hematologic	Autoimmune hemolytic anemia	Yes
	Coagulation anomalies	Yes
	Increased risk of arterial and venous thrombosis	Yes
	Anaphylactoid purpura	No
Renal[14]	Nephrolithiasis	Yes
	Nephrotic syndrome	No
	Renal amyloidosis	No
	Retroperitoneal abscess	No

From: Greenstein AJ, Janowitz HD, Sachar DB. The extraintestinal complications of Crohn's disease and ulcerative colitis: a study of 700 patients. Medicine 1976; 55:401.

patient. Though barium enema is an important diagnostic aid in chronic IBD, both to know the extent and nature of the disease, it should not be performed in a patient presenting with a flare-up of IBD. Not only do colonoscopy and barium enema have an increased risk of perforation in a sick patient, but the bowel cleansing that precedes them may worsen the disease and even precipitate toxic megacolon. Similarly, a small bowel follow through usually is not indicated in the hospitalized patient, unless one has a strong suspicion of a patient with CD having multiple enteroenteric or enterocolonic fistulae.[15]

In a patient with suspected partial small bowel obstruction (SBO) or complete SBO, a flat plate and upright abdominal x-ray should be obtained for evaluation of possible free air, colonic dilatation, fecal contents, and thickness of small bowel loops. In most cases, a CT (computed tomography) scan of the abdomen and the pelvis follows to determine the level of intestinal obstruction, identify abscess(es), and also clarify the extent and severity of IBD.[16] A CT scan of the abdomen is also useful to diagnose fistulas. Importantly, if a perianal fistula is suspected in a patient with CD but the CT scan is negative, it is imperative to proceed to magnetic resonance imaging (MRI) of the pelvis.[17]

Many serologic markers exist for the diagnosis of IBD.[18] The two most widely studied markers for IBD are antineutrophil cytoplasmic antibody (pANCA with a perinuclear staining pattern) and anti-*Saccharomyces cerevisiae* antibody (ASCA).[19] However, their clinical value in patients presenting with IBD-like symptoms is very limited because of their low sensitivity. In addition, even among patients with IBD, these do not reliably distinguish between CD and UC.[20]

MANAGEMENT

Treatment

Treatment of a hospitalized patient with IBD depends upon the severity of the illness at the time of presentation along with; his or her current medications, compliance, precipitating factors, and other comorbidities. No definitive admission criteria exist for patients presenting with IBD.

The main goal of therapy in the hospital is to induce clinical remission and to identify factors that may have caused the flare-up. Such factors may include superimposed infection, recent use of medications such as antibiotics and NSAIDS, or 5-aminosalicylate class drugs that occasionally cause diarrhea. Bowel rest, intravenous fluids, and in some cases parenteral nutrition are an integral part of treatment, as most of these patients have a poor appetite and may be malnourished. Of note, the benefit of bowel rest in UC has not been proven effective in controlled trials, though this author has found it to be useful in selected cases.

Ulcerative Colitis

Currently most patients with UC having minor flares are managed as outpatients with oral/rectal steroids and different 5-aminosalicylate (5-ASA) preparations, depending upon the site of

Table 59-4 Different Oral 5- ASA Preparations Used in the Treatment of IBD

Drug	Formulation	Solubility	Site released	Indication
Asacol	Mesalamine	pH > 7	Terminal ileum (TI), colon	1) Ulcerative colitis 2) Crohn's colitis 3) Crohn's ileitis involving TI only
Pentasa	Mesalamine coated with ethylcellulose microgranules	Time released	Distal duodenum, jejunum, ileum, colon	1) Ulcerative colitis 2) Crohn's Disease involving distal duodenum, jejunum, ileum, colon
Dipentum	Olsalazine (two 5-ASA molecules bound by AZO bond)	Cleaved by colonic bacteria	Colon	1) Ulcerative colitis 2) Crohn's colitis
Colazol	Balsalazide (5-ASA + 4 aminobenzoyl beta alanine)	Cleaved by colonic bacteria	Colon	1) Ulcerative colitis 2) Crohn's colitis

their disease (Table 59-4). As a result, patients admitted to the hospital are usually acutely ill and have already failed a trial of oral steroids. Intravenous steroids, therefore, become the mainstay of therapy in hospitalized patients. Though the optimal dose of parenteral steroids still remains a matter of debate, most institutions use hydrocortisone 100 mg intravenously every 8 hours or 40 mg of solumedrol every 8 hours as their standard dose. In cases of severe, acute flares of UC, the addition of oral 5-aminosalicylates is not likely to improve the outcome and is not used initially. Once the patient starts improving clinically, usually in 3–5 days, oral 5-ASA preparations (mesalamine—Asacol or Pentasa) can be added.[22] An alternative to mesalamine is sulfasalazine, but it has more side effects and is less likely to be tolerated by the patient.[23] If the patient is known to have proctitis/left-sided disease only, and urgency was an important part of his or her symptoms before the flare, addition of mesalmine/hydrocortisone enemas at the time of discharge from the hospital is helpful in controlling symptoms. As the patient improves and starts tolerating liquids, the diet should be advanced to a lactose-free diet. An inpatient nutrition consult should be obtained, especially for patients with a relatively new diagnosis of IBD.

Treatment of UC varies, depending on the clinical scenario. For patients with UC who have been compliant with 5-ASA therapy, lack a precipitating factor, and have had few relapses within the past year, treatment requires consideration of efforts to induce remission after tapering steroids. The acute relapse should still be treated with intravenous steroids as mentioned above. Therapy with 6-mercaptopurine (MP)/azathioprine should be considered and initiated after discussion with the patient, and the consulting gastroenterologist. Potential side effects, including pancreatitis, leukopenia, effects of immunosuppression, and others, should be discussed in detail with the patient. The rationale for beginning this drug while the patient is still in the hospital is so that a therapeutic level of the drug in the serum is achieved by the time the patient is tapered off the corticosteroids. The clinical efficacy of 6MP and azathioprine as steroid sparing maintenance drugs has been well documented, though concerns do remain about the long- and short-term side effects of these agents.[24,25]

For patients unresponsive to a therapeutic approach of 5–7 days of bowel rest and intravenous steroids, intravenous cyclosporine may be tried. It is given as a continuous transfusion at the dose of 4 mg/kg/day. The dose needs to be adjusted with impaired renal function and in those with low serum cholesterol levels.[26]

Most of the data on cyclosporine involve achieving remission when combined with parenteral steroids followed by long-term therapy with 6MP/azathioprine. In this scenario, the patient would be discharged, after improving clinically, on a 3–6 month regimen of oral cyclosporine and azathioprine. Most experts recommend PCP prophylaxis with trimethoprim/sulfamethoxazole while the patient is on both cyclosporine and 6MP/azathioprine. Although cyclosporine may be beneficial over a short period, the short- and long-term risks should be weighed against the benefits of the drug. Infliximab, now FDA approved for UC, is another choice for inducing remission in a steroid refractory patient. It is given as an infusion at the dose of 5 mg/kg body weight over 2–3 hours. Careful monitoring of the patient is required during the infusion.[27]

While receiving pharmacologic therapy, patients should be monitored closely with regular assessment of vital signs and stool production (quality and quantity). CBC, ESR, CRP should be followed.

Crohn's Disease

Treatment options for CD, as in the case with UC, are rapidly evolving. Treatment of CD in hospitalized patients is divided into the common presentations discussed below.

Crohn's Colitis

The treatment of Crohn's colitis is very similar to UC, with a few differences.[28,29] Use of cyclosporine during flares has almost been abandoned, mainly due to the availability of infliximab (see below), which has been FDA approved for treatment of CD for almost a decade now.[30] Surgery, when performed in a patient with refractory Crohn's colitis, is different than that performed in UC. In addition, there is now an increasing trend to use intravenous antibiotics in combination with steroids or in lieu of steroids for both Crohn's ileitis and colitis. Antibiotics may be treating microperforations, bacterial overgrowth, or an unidentified infection. Ciprofloxacin and clarithromycin are used in ileitis, while metronidazole is preferred in ileocolitis and colitis.

Crohn's Ileitis

Patients with ileitis and ileocolitis comprise about two thirds of all patients with CD. Though the treatment of an acute exacerbation of Crohn's ileocolitis is similar to Crohn's colitis, budesonide is an alternative to intravenous hydrocortisone, especially in milder cases. Highly metabolized by the liver on first pass, it appears to have significantly fewer systemic side effects compared to hydrocortisone. Though more effective than mesalamine at inducing remission, it is slightly less effective than standard steroids. It is available in both oral and enema forms. A dose of 9 g per day is used to induce remission in CD.[32]

Treatment of SBO in Crohn's Disease

Small bowel obstruction in a patient with CD may be due to one of the following causes:
a) Active disease causing inflammation of the gut and resulting obstruction
b) Fibrostenotic stricture from the disease itself
c) Adhesions from prior surgery
d) Causes unrelated to CD

Initial management includes bowel rest, intravenous fluids, nasogastric tube suction, CT scan of the abdomen and pelvis, serial obstruction series, and a surgical consult. A surgical consult early in the hospital admission helps the patient establish a relationship with the surgeon, should the need for surgery arise. Intravenous steroids should be given in cases when the SBO is thought to be from inflammation from active disease. If the patient responds to conservative treatment, further treatment follows the standard approach described previously. Of note, this is one of the few instances that a SBFT is needed as an inpatient to see if the site of obstruction can be precisely identified, should symptoms recur.

Perianal Disease and IBD

Although perianal problems in patients with IBD are usually thought to be secondary to CD or indeterminate colitis, they have been described as occurring in patients with UC as well.[33] Depending upon the classification, 18–80% of patients with IBD will suffer from perianal complications at some time during the course of their illness. One may see hemorrhoidal disease, fissures, perianal skin tags, vulvar or rectovaginal fistulas, or perianal abscess. However, the more common perianal conditions seen in hospitalized patients are hemorrhoidal problems, anal fissures, anorectal abscesses, and rectovaginal fistulas.[34] Although hemorrhoids are common in the general population, patients with IBD have a higher incidence of hemorrhoids because of diarrhea associated with occurrence of hemorrhoids. They can cloud assessment when the bleeding from them is confused with an IBD flare. Treatment should be conservative and surgery avoided. However, surgical management of hemorrhoids in patients with UC is not as problematic as it is with CD.

Painless, acute fissures in IBD patients should be treated medically with stool softeners along with topical steroids, sitz baths, 0.25% lidocaine locally, or 5-ASA suppository. However, exam under anesthesia is needed if the fissure is painful or persistent to exclude perianal abscess. Once a perianal abscess is diagnosed, surgical consultation and drainage are required.[35] Antibiotics are only an adjunct to this definitive form of treatment.

Rectovaginal fistulae can occur in up to 5–10% of women with CD.[36] Most of these fistulae do not result in fecal incontinence; main symptoms are vaginal discharge and passage of gas through the vagina. Though surgical repair is the mainstay of therapy, antibiotics and immunomodulators should be used to induce remission of IBD prior to attempting repair.[37]

Infliximab and IBD

Infliximab is chimeric mouse/human monoclonal antibody to tumor necrosis factor (TNF) that is used both to induce and maintain remission in IBD. Though it was approved for the treatment of CD over a decade ago, FDA approval for UC is relatively recent. Infliximab is administered intravenously, at a dose of 5–10 mg/kg body weight over 2–3 hours. Recommended that dosing is three induction doses given at 0, 2, and 6 weeks; followed by maintenance dose every 8 weeks thereafter. Treatment guidelines are identical for both UC and CD. For a patient with IBD who has been refractory or dependent on corticosteroids and has either not responded to the immunomodulators or is unable to tolerate them, this represents an excellent therapeutic option.[30] Ideally, patients should be given their first infusion while still in the hospital; subsequent infusions can be given in the outpatient setting. Infliximab is effective in not only controlling the luminal disease in both CD and UC, but also severe forms of fistulizing and perianal CD. Remission rates may be as high as 30–40% in the first 4 weeks after the first dose of infliximab in patients with CD; an additional 30–40% of patients will report considerable improvement in their symptoms. Though the initial response rates of infliximab in the treatment of UC were not as promising, more recent data show better results.[27] Response rates are generally higher in younger patients and in those using concomitant immunomodulators.

Discharge/Follow-up Plans

Patients should follow up regularly with their primary care doctor. In addition, they should see a gastroenterologist who has both expertise and interest in managing IBD. Patients should be told that steroids are not meant to be taken on a chronic basis, and hence it is very important for them to follow up with their gastroenterologist on discharge from the hospital.

The initial physician–patient encounter, even in the hospital and thereafter in the office, is extremely important and should never be undermined. It often plays an important role in further follow-up with the physician and increases compliance with medications. Though IBD is mainly a disease of the young, it can affect any age-group. It is important for the physician to realize that the needs of the patients vary by age-group. Children with IBD do not have much understanding or interest in their disease and are happy as long as they feel well. Likewise, teenagers are mainly concerned about maintaining activities with their peers. They often exhibit denial that needs to be addressed, not only with the patient but also with his or her family. Young adults, the group that probably forms the largest number of IBD patients seen both in the hospital and in the office, are interested in career, dating, family, and sexual issues related to IBD. Though they seem most interested in education, it is important, if possible for the physician to meet with their significant other at the time of discharge from the hospital. Although older patients with IBD may be confident about dealing with their disease as a result of living with it for a long time, they have other issues that need to be discussed, including other illnesses and multiple medications.

In all IBD patients, it is important for the physician to clarify that though we may not know all the various causes of this disease, it is not psychosomatic, and is not caused by stress. It is also important to teach patients that the best way to prevent the relapse of IBD is by taking their medications regularly, even during periods when they may feel well.

The diagnosis of IBD may be associated with preconceived notions by the patient and family as well as be associated with social stigma. It is important for the discharging physician to reassure both the patient and the family that most patients with IBD are able to maintain a normal lifestyle. Patients may benefit from various IBD support groups in the area where they live. The Crohn's and Colitis Foundation of America (www.ccfa.org) has helpful resources. An organization of patients with IBD, physicians, and other medical professionals who are dedicated to treatment of IBD, it has more than 50 chapters across the country.

Key Points

- IBD should always be in the differential diagnosis of a patient presenting with diarrhea, whether bloody or nonbloody, acute or chronic.

- Patients with UC who present with diffuse abdominal tenderness and guarding should be evaluated for toxic megacolon.

- Colonoscopy and barium enema should be avoided in acutely ill patients with IBD, as they risk perforation, and the preparatory bowel cleansing may worsen the disease and even precipitate toxic megacolon.

- Intravenous steroids are a mainstay of therapy in hospitalized patients with a flare of UC. Patients with CD also may benefit from antibiotics.

- Painful or persistent anal fissures in patients with IBD require examination under anesthesia to exclude perianal abscess, which usually requires surgical intervention.

- Infliximab, a chimeric mouse/human monoclonal antibody to tumor necrosis factor (TNF), can both induce and maintain remission in IBD. Its use is targeted at patients who are refractory to steroids or require repeated steroid therapy.

SUGGESTED READING

Nabalamba A, Bernstein CN, Seko C. Inflammatory bowel disease: hospitalization. Health Rep 2004; 1594:25–40.

Melmed GY, Abreu MT. New insights into the pathogenesis of inflammatory bowel disease. Curr Gastroenterol Rep 2004; 6:474–481.

Hanauer SB, Present DH. The state of the art in the management of inflammatory bowel disease. Rev Gastroenterol Dis 2003; 3:81–92.

Kane SV, Bjorkman DJ. The efficacy of oral 5-ASAs in the treatment of active ulcerative colitis: a systematic review. Rev Gastroenterol Disord 2003; 3:210–218.

Armuzzi A, Lapascu A, Fedili P, et al. Infliximab in the treatment of moderate to severe glucocorticoid dependent ulcerative colitis: a randomized methylprednisolone controlled trial. Gastroenterology 2004; 126(Suppl 2):A–464.

CHAPTER SIXTY

Gastroenteritis

Gretchen Diemer, MD

BACKGROUND

There are over 200 million cases of infectious diarrhea in the United States each year. Most infectious agents are easily spread via person-to-person contact or through food or waterborne mechanisms and can cause severe illness in immunocompromised people. Acute diarrhea and gastroenteritis account for about 1–2% of all hospitalizations of adults in the United States. Gastroenteritis is a significant public health problem that is not limited only to developing countries. A targeted diagnostic and treatment approach to adults with gastroenteritis[1] is presented here.

ASSESSMENT

Clinical Presentation

Presenting Signs and Symptoms

Acute diarrhea is generally defined as more frequent stools with decreased form, lasting <14 days. Gastroenteritis often presents with other associated symptoms including nausea, vomiting, cramping, abdominal pain, bloating, tenesmus, and urgency. The diarrhea itself can span a broad range of presentations, including high volume and watery (suggesting small intestine involvement) to bloody or mucous-containing (suggesting invasive pathogens, particularly in the colon). Fever is often present as well.

Many patients never present to a physician and will recover without specific medical therapy. Patients requiring evaluation for their illness include those with copious, watery diarrhea and signs or symptoms of dehydration; those with bloody stools; those with fever; those with severe abdominal pain; those with prolonged illness; any patient over the age of 70; any patient who is immunocompromised such as patients with HIV; those with malnutrition or transplant; and those being treated with chemotherapy or immunosuppressive drugs.

In trying to elucidate the cause of the illness, a thorough history is crucial. Specific questions should include any food exposures (such as picnics, parties, or restaurants) and travel history, including developing countries or camping with exposure to fresh water. Exposure to children in day care and any sick contacts are important connections to make. Onset and duration of symptoms, and the quantity and quality of the diarrhea, should be documented. Sexual history is pertinent, as patients with HIV infection or those who practice anal receptive intercourse have additional infectious agents of which to be aware. History of recent hospitalizations or antibiotic use should be sought. Past medical history should be noted for comorbid illnesses and any factors suggesting immunosuppression. Review of systems should also include weight loss or any extraintestinal symptoms the patient is experiencing.

Attention should be paid to the patient's fluid status, noting dry mucous membranes or decreased skin turgor, and signs of orthostasis. A careful abdominal examination should be carried out, checking for tenderness, peritoneal signs, organomegaly, or masses. Note should be made of the patient's mental status as well, looking for signs of an altered sensorium.

Differential Diagnosis

The list of possible infectious agents is long. The list included here is not all inclusive, but it does contain the most commonly cited agents (Box 60-1).[2,3,5]

Viruses

The enteric viruses commonly present with nausea, vomiting, large-volume watery diarrhea, and sometimes fever. They can be foodborne or passed via a fecal–oral route. The incubation period for these viruses is short, typically 1–2 days from exposure to onset of symptoms, and symptoms last from 1 to 8 days. One exception is hepatitis A, which can present acutely with diarrhea, nausea, and abdominal pain, but is usually accompanied by jaundice, flu-like malaise, and marked abnormalities in liver function tests. Hepatitis A has an incubation period of 2–8 weeks, and symptoms can last 2–8 weeks.

Bacteria

Bacteria can be divided into two major categories: those causing disease by production of toxins, versus invasion by the bacteria themselves.

Preformed Toxins

Some toxins are preformed in the food. Patients generally have a sudden onset of nausea and vomiting several hours after exposure. Classic examples are enterotoxin from *Bacillus cereus* or *Staphylococcus aureus*. Improperly stored fried rice or potato salads are common culprits. Fortunately, these illnesses are very self-limited, lasting only 1–2 days. *Clostridium botulinum* makes a pre-

Box 60-1 Most Common Infectious Agents Causing Diarrhea[2]

Viruses
- Norwalk
- Rotavirus
- Enteric adenovirus
- Hepatitis A

Bacterial Toxins

Preformed
- *Clostridium botulinum*
- *Bacillus cereus*
- *Staphylococcus aureus*

Diarrheal
- *Shigella*
- Shiga toxin from *E. coli*
- *Clostridium perfringens*
- *Clostridium difficile*
- Enterotoxigenic *E. coli*
- *Vibrio cholera* toxin

Invasive Bacteria
- *Campylobacter*
- *Salmonella*
- *Yersinia*
- *Shigella*
- *E. coli*

Parasites
- *Cryptosporidium*
- *Microsporidia*
- *Giardia*
- *Entamoeba histolytica*

Box 60-2 Opportunistic Diarrheal Pathogens Commonly Seen in HIV-Infected Patients[7]

Cytomegalovirus

Mycobacterium avium complex

Cryptosporidium

Microsporidia

Cyclospora

Isospora

HIV enteropathy

Parasites

Parasites generally require a small inoculum and have a wide range of presentations, from voluminous watery stools seen with *Cryptosporidium* and *Microsporidia*, to bloating, smaller volume stools, or unexplained weight loss as is sometimes seen with *Giardia*, to bloody or watery stools and abdominal pain with *Entamoeba histolytica*. Environmental exposures (usually a contaminated water source) are a common alternative mode of infection with these organisms, in addition to the usual fecal–oral route.

Special Cases

Hospitalized Patients

Many patients develop diarrhea while in the hospital. *Clostridium difficile* is the cause in up to 20% of these patients, and the causes of the remainder are often never elucidated. Previous antibiotic use, which alters the normal bowel flora and allows the *C. difficile* bacteria to overgrow, is the biggest risk factor for developing colitis. The presentation of *C. difficile* infection ranges from asymptomatic carriers, to high fever with severe abdominal pain and diarrhea, to paralytic ileus and toxic megacolon with perforation. Chapter 61 is devoted to *C. difficile*–induced diarrhea and colitis.

Antibiotics themselves can cause diarrhea in the absence of *C. difficile* infection, and many systemic illnesses (such as pneumonia) can also have symptoms of diarrhea in their presentation.

HIV

Diarrhea occurs in up to 50% of AIDS patients in North America.[16] In addition to the usual agents described above, physicians must consider many additional infectious agents in patients infected with the HIV (Box 60-2). Disseminated cytomegalovirus (CMV) has a broad range of gastrointestinal presentations, including enteritis, colitis, colonic ulcers, appendicitis, and toxic megacolon. Up to 20% of AIDS patients with diarrhea will have CMV as a cause. Diagnosis usually requires a biopsy finding of classic cytomegalic inclusion cells surrounded by inflammation. *Mycobacterium avium* complex (MAC) can also cause a severe gastroenteritis (most commonly seen in patients with CD4 counts <100) with fever, weight loss, lymphadenopathy, and hepatosplenomegaly often accompanying the disseminated infection. Acid-fast stains of stool and biopsies or culture from stool or blood can assist with the diagnosis. *Cryptosporidium* and *Microsporidia* are more common in patients with HIV and can cause more severe disease in this population. *Cyclospora* infection is less common with the widespread use of trimethoprim/sulfamethoxazole prophylaxis but can cause a watery diarrhea accompanied by weight loss, anorexia, fatigue, bloating, and flatulence. Fever is also present. If left untreated, *Cyclospora* infection in AIDS patients

formed toxin that can cause nausea and diarrhea and can lead to a flaccid paralysis lasting days to months.

Diarrheal Toxins

Many bacteria, when ingested, make diarrheal toxins that cause disease by different mechanisms. These illnesses have a slightly longer incubation period than the preformed toxins, up to 24–72 hours for some. Shigella and Shiga toxin-producing *E. coli* can cause bloody diarrhea with a very small inoculum; *Clostridium perfringens* and *difficile* toxins cause enteritis and colitis with necrosis; enterotoxigenic *E. coli* and *Vibrio cholera* toxins cause a profound secretory diarrhea. Duration of symptoms is typically several days.

Invasive Bacteria

Bacteria that cause disease by invading the colonic wall typically have incubation periods of several days up to a week, and symptoms of diarrhea, cramping, bloody stool, or stool with mucous can last a week or more. Fever is more common with these bacteria. They include *Campylobacter*, *Salmonella* species, and *Yersinia*. *Shigella* and enterohemorrhagic *E. coli* can also be invasive.

will continue in a chronic fashion. Diagnosis is by identification of its acid-fast oocysts in fecal specimens and they can sometimes be confused with the smaller oocysts of Cryptosporidia. *Isospora* infection is similar to *Cryptosporidium* infection, with voluminous watery nonbloody stools, cramping abdominal pain, and nausea. The oocytes of *Isospora* can also be identified on acid-fast staining of fecal specimens. AIDS patients diagnosed with *Isospora* diarrhea require long-term suppressive therapy, as up to 50% of these patients will develop recurrent disease once therapy is discontinued. Finally, HIV itself can infect the enterocytes lining the colon and has been implicated as the cause of diarrhea when no other agent is identified. This syndrome can improve with highly active antiretroviral therapy (HAART).

The approach to diarrhea in HIV-infected patients requires an aggressive pursuit of diagnosis, including a low threshold for sigmoidoscopy, colonoscopy, and even upper endoscopy in HIV patients presenting with diarrhea. These tests can identify a causative agent in up to almost 40% of culture-negative diarrhea in patients with HIV infection. A lower CD4 count accompanied by weight loss, anemia, or hypoalbuminemia increases the chances that an organism will be identified on endoscopy.

Sexual Preference

Patients who practice anal receptive intercourse have an increased risk of proctitis caused by *Neisseria gonorrhea*, *Chlamydia trachomatis*, *Treponema pallidum*, and herpes simplex virus.

Day Care

Patients with exposure to children in day care may be at higher risk for *Shigella*, *Giardia*, and *Cryptosporidium*.

Noninfectious

Some patients with noninfectious causes may present with acute diarrheal illnesses. Diagnoses to consider include irritable bowel syndrome, inflammatory bowel diseases, laxative abuse, malabsorption, bacterial overgrowth, ischemic bowel, antibiotic side effects, carcinoid, radiation, and hyperthyroidism.

Diagnosis

Preferred Studies

A number of diagnostic tests should be considered by the hospitalist when evaluating a patient with gastroenteritis (Table 60-1). Stool specimens should be evaluated by microscopy for fecal leukocytes. These are commonly seen with inflammatory diarrhea and with invasive pathogens, including *Salmonella*, *Shigella*, *Campylobacter*, and *Yersinia*. They can be absent in some cases of enterohemorrhagic *E. coli*. Lactoferrin, a marker for fecal leukocytes, may be preferable because of its higher accuracy and the fact that it is less susceptible to the vagaries of specimen processing.

Stool specimens can be tested for *C. difficile* toxins A and B by ELISA (enzyme-linked immunosorbent assay) and have a sensitivity of 71–94% and a specificity of 92%–98%. If initially negative, tests should be repeated if there is significant clinical suspicion.

Stool Cultures

Stool cultures are often ordered but typically found to be positive in fewer than 2% of specimens, making them not worthwhile in all patients.[6] Culture the stool of patients who are febrile, patients who have bloody diarrhea, stools that contain leukocytes or lacto-

---

Table 60-1 Diagnostic Testing in Diarrhea

- Fecal leukocytes and lactoferrin
- *C. difficile* toxin
- Stool cultures — After 3 days in the hospital—target cultures only for patients with prior incomplete workup of diarrhea, age >65, significant comorbidities (ESRD, COPD, IBD, CVA, cirrhosis), neutropenia, immunosuppression, nosocomial outbreak.
- Ova & parasite
- Imaging (limited to suspicion of perforation or severe disease)—abdominal CT scan
- Sigmoidoscopy or colonoscopy

ESRD = End Stage Renal Disease; COPD = Chronic Obstructive Pulmonary Disease; IBD = Inflammatory Bowel Disease; CVA = Cerebrovascular Disease

---

ferrin, or those with severe or persistent diarrhea. Routine stool cultures include *Shigella*, *Salmonella*, *Campylobacter*, and *Yersinia*. Specific requests for other bacteria need to be made if there is a clinical suspicion for those agents. For example, a request for Shiga toxin-producing *E. coli* culture should be made in cases of bloody diarrhea, and a culture for *Vibrio* species should be made if there is a significant exposure to raw seafood or seawater. Cultures should also be ordered in situations of public health concern (e.g., contaminated food at a restaurant) or great potential for outbreaks (institutionalized patients, food service workers, day care attendees or workers).

"Three Day Rule"

Many patients develop diarrhea after being hospitalized. Routine cultures and evaluation for ova and parasites have an even lower rate of positivity if the patient has been hospitalized longer than 3 days. Following a modified 3 day rule increases the diagnostic yield of the studies without missing diagnoses and prevents unnecessary testing of these stools.[4] If a patient develops diarrhea after being in the hospital more than 3 days, order stool cultures only if:

- Incomplete workup of community-acquired diarrhea
- Age >65 with comorbidities including cirrhosis, ESRD, COPD, inflammatory bowel disease, hemiparesis after CVA, or leukemia
- Neutropenia
- HIV
- Immunosuppression
- Nosocomial outbreak
- Suspected nondiarrheal manifestation of enteric infection

Ova and Parasites

When clinical suspicion for parasites is high, special antigen testing or microscopic evaluation is warranted. These tests can often be negative in patients infected with these organisms, and multiple specimens may thus need to be submitted. Routine ova and parasite evaluation does not include *Cryptosporidium* or *Microsporidia*, so evaluation for them must be specifically requested when indicated.

Imaging

Routine imaging of patients with acute diarrhea has a low yield. Plain X-rays may show ileus or the "thumb printing" sign of edematous bowel. CT scans may reveal thickened bowel loops suggestive of colitis. Imaging studies should be ordered if there is a suspicion of bowel perforation or in patients who are severely ill. Barium enemas can be harmful in patients with acute inflammation of the colon and should be avoided.

Sigmoidoscopy/Colonoscopy

Direct visualization of the GI tract with endoscopy is not routinely indicated. Cases of bowel perforation with colonoscopy in patients with *C. difficile* colitis have been reported. When noninvasive means (i.e., stool testing) do not yield a diagnosis and clinically significant diarrhea persists, then direct visualization of the colon with sigmoidoscopy or colonoscopy should be considered. In rare cases, when a diagnosis is needed before stool studies return or there is an ileus preventing analysis of stool, sigmoidoscopy done by a skilled operator can be safely performed. Colonoscopy is indicated in cases with reasonable suspicion for noninfectious causes or if there is evidence of only proximal colonic involvement. There should be a low threshold for doing these tests in patients who have anal receptive intercourse or are infected with HIV, when routine evaluation of stool has not revealed the causative agent.[16]

MANAGEMENT

Treatment

Supportive care is the mainstay of therapy in cases of gastroenteritis.[1,2] Appropriate enteric isolation measures should be instituted for all hospitalized patients. Careful attention to fluid status is vital. The World Health Organization recommends an oral rehydration solution consisting of 3.5 g NaCl, 2.5 g NaCO$_3$, 1.5 g KCl, and 20 g of glucose per liter of fluid. Commercial preparations are available. Intravenous fluids and electrolyte replacement are standard treatments in the hospital setting. Cases in which the cause is a virus or preformed toxin currently have no treatment other than support.

Empiric Antibiotics

Empiric antibiotic use with a quinolone for 1 to 5 days is indicated for moderate-to-severe traveler's diarrhea. This has been shown to reduce symptoms from 3–5 days down to 1–2 days. Empiric therapy with a 3- to 5-day course of quinolones is also supported for patients with fever plus blood, leukocyte, or lactoferrin-positive diarrhea. Some evidence supports treating persistent diarrhea with a week of metronidazole 250 mg t.i.d. as empiric treatment for giardiasis.

Bacterial Infections

Where noted in Table 60-2, quinolone antibiotics include norfloxacin 400 mg b.i.d., ciprofloxacin 500 mg b.i.d., or ofloxacin 300 mg bid. Trimethoprim/sulfamethoxazole dosing is 160/800 b.i.d. All antibiotics are administered orally unless otherwise specified in Table 60-2.

Aeromonas

Aeromonas infections can be treated with trimethoprim/sulfamethoxazole or a fluoroquinolone for 3 days.

Campylobacter

Campylobacter infections should be treated with erythromycin 500 mg b.i.d. due to increasing resistance to quinolone antibiotics.[10]

Clostridium sp.

C. difficile infections should be treated with metronidazole 250 mg q.i.d. or 500 mg t.i.d. An alternative agent is oral vancomycin 125 mg q.i.d. The offending antibiotic should be withdrawn where possible. If not possible, treat until 1 week after antibiotic therapy completed. There is some evidence supporting the use of lactobacillus to repopulate normal colonic flora.

C. perfringens food poisoning caused by toxin A is a self-limited disease requiring no specific therapy. Cases of enteritis necroti-

---

Table 60-2 Antibiotic Therapy for Common Causes of Bacterial Diarrhea*

Bacteria	Antibiotic	Duration
Aeromonas	Trimethoprim/sulfamethoxazole Fluroquinolone	3 days
Campylobacter	Erythromycin 500 mg b.i.d.	5 days
Clostridium difficile	Metronidazole 250 mg q.i.d. or 500 mg t.i.d.	10 days or 1 week after offending agent withdrawn
E. coli O157H7	Should not be treated with antibiotics	
E. coli species other than Shiga-toxin producing	Trimethoprim/sulfamethoxazole Fluoroquinolone	3 days
Salmonella (nontyphi)	Treat only severe cases Trimethoprim/sulfamethoxazole Fluoroquinolone	5–7 days 14 days if immunocompromised
Shigella	Trimethoprim/sulfamethoxazole	3 days 7–10 day if immunocompromised
Vibrio (noncholera)	Fluoroquinolone	3–5 days
Vibrio cholera	Ciprofloxacin 1 g	One dose
Yersinia	Fluoroquinolone Ceftriaxone (in severe cases)	3–5 days

*Fluoroquinolone antibiotics include norfloxacin 400 mg b.i.d., ciprofloxacin 500 mg b.i.d., or ofloxacin 300 mg b.i.d. Trimethoprim/sulfamethoxazole dosing is 180/800 mg b.i.d.

cans caused by toxin C are rare but have high mortality and should be treated with broad spectrum antibiotics.[13]

E. coli

Shiga toxin–producing *E. coli* infections should not be treated with antibiotics.[8] There is some evidence that doing so may increase the chances of developing the hemolytic uremic syndrome and induce toxin production, and there is not evidence that it improves the course of illness.

Other species of *E. coli* can be treated with trimethoprim/sulfamethoxazole or a fluoroquinolone for 3 days.

Salmonella

Salmonella infection with non-typhi species does not usually require specific antimicrobial therapy. Antibiotics seem to prolong shedding of the bacteria in the stool. For those with the most severe disease, evidence of systemic toxicity, or comorbidities (including valvular heart disease, prostheses, malignancy, uremia, or severe atherosclerosis), a 5–7 day course of trimethoprim/sulfamethoxazole or quinolones can be initiated. Immunocompromised patients should be treated for 14 days. There are increasing reports of resistance to quinolone antibiotics. Other regimens include trimethoprim/sulfamethoxazole or ceftriaxone.

Shigella

Shigella infections originating in the United States should be treated with a 3-day course of trimethoprim/sulfamethoxazole 160 mg/800 mg b.i.d. Those acquired outside the United States should be treated with a quinolone for 3 days. Ceftriaxone and azithromycin have also been used. Immunocompromised patients should be treated for 7–10 days.[9]

Vibrio

Non–*cholera Vibrio* infections can be treated with 3–5 days of quinolones.

Vibrio cholera infections should be treated with aggressive oral rehydration, and patients may be given a one-time oral dose of ciprofloxacin 1 g.

Yersinia

Yersinia infections do not always require therapy but can be treated with 3–5 days of quinolones. Doxycycline, aminoglycosides, and trimethoprim/sulfamethoxazole have also been used. Severe cases may require ceftriaxone for 5 days.

Parasites

Cryptosporidium

Cryptosporidium infections, if severe, can be treated with paromomycin 500 mg t.i.d. for 7 days. Immunocompromised patients should be treated for 14–28 days (See Table 60-3).[14]

Entamoeba histolytica

E. histolytica infections can be treated with metronidazole 750 mg t.i.d. for 5–10 days. These infections also require a drug to treat the cysts to prevent relapse. Either diiodohydroxyquin 650 mg t.i.d. for 20 days, paromomycin 500 mg t.i.d. for 10 days, or diloxanide furoate 500 mg t.i.d. for 10 days can be used.

Giardia

Giardia can be treated with metronidazole 250 mg t.i.d. for 7 days.

Microsporidia

Microsporidia infections should be treated with albendazole 400 mg b.i.d. for 3 weeks, and highly active antiretroviral therapy should be initiated in those patients with AIDS.

Antimotility Agents

There are several medications that can help ease the symptoms of loose, frequent stools. Loperamide is commonly used. The first dose should be 4 mg, followed by 2 mg doses after each stool, up to 16 mg/24 hours. Atropine/diphenoxylate can also be used as an antidiarrheal agent, up to 2 tabs every 6 hours as needed. Antimotility agents should be avoided in cases of bloody diarrhea, in particular, Shiga toxin–producing *E. coli* and *C. difficile*.

PROGNOSIS

Most gastroenteritis and acute diarrheal illnesses are self-limited. Those who may have prolonged courses or complications are usually the very young, the very old, and those in immunocompromised states.

Complications

Hemolytic Uremic Syndrome (HUS)

Hemolytic uremic syndrome is seen in as many as 20% of Shiga toxin–producing *E. coli* infections.[15] It manifests itself with a microangiopathic hemolytic anemia, thrombocytopenia, acute renal failure, and often central nervous system symptoms such as

Table 60-3 Antibiotic Therapy for Common Causes of Parasitic Diarrheal Infections

Parasite	Agent	Duration
Cryptosporidium	Paromomycin 500 mg t.i.d.	7 days 14–28 days if immunocompromised
Entamoeba histolytica	Metronidazole 750 mg t.i.d.	5–10 days
	Also treat cyst phase with diiodohydroxyquin 650 mg t.i.d.	20 days
	or	
	Paromomycin 500 mg t.i.d.	10 days
	or	
	Diloxanide furoate 500 mg t.i.d.	10 days
Giardia	Metronidazole 250 mg t.i.d.	7 days
Microsporidia	Albendazole 400 mg b.i.d. and initiate highly active antiretroviral therapy in HIV/AIDS patients	21 days

altered mental status and seizures. It occurs 2–14 days after the onset of diarrhea. It is seen more commonly among patients with bloody diarrhea, fever, leukocytosis, the very young or old, and those treated with antibiotics or antimotility agents. A large range of severity is seen in affected patients, but about 50% of patients require hemodialysis with this complication, and about 75% will require red blood cell transfusions. HUS carries a 3–5% mortality rate, with another 5% of patients having severe sequelae, including long-term hemodialysis and permanent neurologic injury. Those patients with higher white blood cell counts, more severe diarrhea, early anuria, and age <2 years old tend to have more severe HUS.

Treatment for HUS is supportive. The gastroenteritis should not be treated with antibiotics or antimotility agents. Hemodialysis and supportive transfusions are the mainstay of therapy. Patients at high risk for developing this syndrome should be monitored closely. In some cases, plasmapheresis, administration of fresh frozen plasma, or intravenous immune globulin have also been tried, but remain unproven.

Toxic Megacolon

Toxic megacolon is a condition seen more frequently in inflammatory bowel disease, but it complicates some infectious diarrheal illnesses as well. It is defined as total or segmental colonic dilatation that is nonobstructive and accompanied by evidence of systemic toxicity. *C. difficile* is the most common inciting pathogen, but cases have been reported with *Salmonella*, *Shigella*, *Campylobacter*, and CMV colitis. Risk of developing this condition is increased with antimotility agents (including narcotics and anticholinergic drugs), hypokalemia, antidepressants, and barium enemas or colonoscopy. Hallmarks of the physical examination are abdominal distention and pain. The diarrhea often subsides due to the immotility that occurs. Plain X-rays of the abdomen show a dramatically dilated colon and occasionally free air in cases that have progressed to perforation. Surgery and GI consultation should be immediately obtained when suspected.

The initial treatment for toxic megacolon is medical, but 50% of cases require subtotal colectomy with ileostomy. The patient's stool should be tested for *C. difficile*, and broad-spectrum antibiotics (including IV and oral metronidazole or oral vancomycin) should be started. Patients should also receive stress ulcer prophylaxis and prophylaxis for deep vein thrombosis. The mortality rate in patients who develop this condition in association with *C. difficile* colitis is around 33% and is much higher in those who require surgery.

Guillain Barré Syndrome

Guillain Barré syndrome is a neurologic condition of acute inflammatory demyelinating polyradiculopathy with acute axonal degeneration. When it occurs, it usually follows an infectious illness, and *Campylobacter* infections are the most frequently seen.[17] Patients with symptomatic *Campylobacter* diarrhea are 100 times more likely than the general population to develop this syndrome. The postulated mechanism is an antibody that cross-reacts from the *Campylobacter* to the myelin sheath.

Onset of symptoms is typically 2–4 weeks after the infection has passed. Fine paresthesias develop in the fingers and toes, but the predominant finding is an ascending paralysis that can progress over hours to days. Physical examination is significant for muscular weakness and decreased reflexes, and 50% of patients will

have some autonomic dysfunction as well. It can progress to involve the respiratory muscles, and vital capacity should be followed in patients who are suspected to have this disease.

Diagnosis is via electrophysiologic testing. Treatment involves either plasmapheresis or intravenous immunoglobulin. Most patients recover complete function if they are supported through this illness.

PREVENTION

All of these causative organisms are transmitted via a fecal–oral route. Hand washing and food safety are the mainstays of prevention. Early notification of the local public health departments of suspected outbreaks can also prevent additional cases. Patients with *C. difficile* colitis in the hospital require appropriate isolation, or this can lead to outbreaks within a hospital. The hospital's director of infection control should be contacted.

DISCHARGE AND FOLLOW-UP

Patients need follow-up with their primary care providers (PCPs) within 1 week of discharge from the hospital. Recurrent diarrhea requires appropriate workup. Culture results should be communicated to the patient and his or her outpatient physician. Patients should be instructed to contact their PCP or return to the hospital if they have recurrent fever, diarrhea, or signs and symptoms of dehydration.

Health care workers, food handlers, and day care employees should have documented clearance of the offending organism before returning to work.

Key Points

- Enteric viruses have a short incubation period of 1–2 days and typically present with nausea; vomiting; large-volume, watery diarrhea; and sometimes fever.

- Patients who practice anal receptive intercourse have an increased risk of proctitis caused by *Neisseria gonorrhea*, *Chlamydia trachomatis*, *Treponema pallidum*, and herpes simplex virus.

- The approach to diarrhea in HIV-infected patients requires an aggressive pursuit of diagnosis, including a low threshold for sigmoidoscopy, colonoscopy, and even upper endoscopy in those presenting with diarrhea.

- Stool cultures should be performed in patients who are febrile, those who have bloody diarrhea, stools that contain leukocytes or lactoferrin, or those with severe or persistent diarrhea.

- Following a modified 3 day rule for hospitalized patients increases the diagnostic yield of stool cultures without missing diagnoses and prevents unnecessary testing.

- Antimotility agents should be avoided in cases of bloody diarrhea, in particular Shiga toxin–producing *E. coli*.

- Complications of gastroenteritis include HUS, toxic megacolon, and Guillain Barré syndrome.

SUGGESTED READING

Guerrant RL, Van Gilder T, Steiner TS, et al. Practice guidelines for the management of infectious diarrhea. Infectious Diseases Society of America. Clin Infect Dis 2001; 32:331–351.

Musher D, Musher B. Medical progress: contagious acute gastrointestinal infections. N Engl J Med 2004; 351:2417–2427.

Bauer T, Lalvani A, Fehrenbach J, et al. Derivation and validation of guidelines for stool cultures for enteropathogenic bacteria other than *clostridium difficile* in hospitalized adults. JAMA 2001; 285:313–319.

Diagnosis and management of foodborne illnesses: a primer for physicians. Morb Mortal Wkly Re 2001; 50(RR2)1–69.

Poutanen S, Simor A. *Clostridium difficile*-associated diarrhea in adults. Can Med Assoc J 2004; 171:51–58.

Chen X, Deithly J, Paya C, et al. Current concepts: cryptosporidiosis. N Engl J Med 2002; 346:1723–1731.

Cohen J, West AB, Bini EJ. Infectious diarrhea in human immunodeficiency virus. Gastroenterol Clin North Am 2001; 30:637–664.

CHAPTER SIXTY-ONE

Diarrhea and *Clostridium difficile* Colitis

Jeffrey Glasheen, MD

BACKGROUND

Diarrhea is a common symptom in the hospitalized patient; it can be present at the time of admission (community-acquired diarrhea) or develop 3 or more days into the patient's hospital course (hospital-acquired diarrhea). While community-acquired diarrhea (CAD) is most often infectious in nature, only 15% of hospital-acquired diarrhea (HAD) results from infectious sources, with most cases secondary to use of antibiotics.[1] In fact, diarrhea complicates up to 40% of the courses of antibiotics administered in the hospital. Fortunately, the vast majority of these episodes result in a rate-limited, benign course.

Antibiotics can elicit diarrhea through hypermotility, or osmotic or toxin-mediated mechanisms (Table 61-1). Increases, in motility leading to diarrhea are commonly seen with erythromycin and the beta-lactamase inhibitor clavulanate. This results from increases in gastric emptying (erythromycin) and intestinal transit time (clavulanate).[2] Osmotic diarrhea occurs when broad-spectrum antibiotics with good intestinal bioavailability reduce the normal bacterial flora responsible for carbohydrate fermentation and absorption, resulting in an increase distal osmotic load with subsequent diarrhea. More ominously, antibiotic-induced alterations in the intestinal flora can potentiate a toxin-mediated diarrhea through colonic overgrowth of *Clostridium difficile. C. difficile*, which causes diarrhea in 3–8% of all hospitalized patients, has now become the fourth most common nosocomial infection.[6-8]

The past two decades have seen a remarkable increase in the incidence of *C. difficile*–associated diarrhea (CDAD).[3-5] At the same time that we have noticed a disquieting increase in the number of cases of CDAD, evidence has appeared dispelling the myth that *C. difficile* merely produces a "nuisance" diarrhea. Hospital stays that are complicated by *C. difficile* infection result in an increased length of stay of 3.6 days and up to an additional $3,699 in hospital costs. Applying this last figure to all cases of CDAD results in an estimated cost to the health care system of $1.1 billion per annum.[9]

The major risk factors for developing CDAD, antibiotic use and hospitalization, have been known for some time, but our understanding of how these factors induce disease has recently undergone significant change.

Almost all cases of CDAD can be traced back to antibiotic use within the past month. While broad-spectrum antibiotics with good intestinal bioavailability most commonly induce disease, it is important to note that the use of any antibiotic can lead to CDAD (Table 61-2). Furthermore, the risk of becoming colonized with *C. difficile* is clearly tied to the length of hospital stay. While <1% of patients are colonized on admission to the hospital, the rate increases to 50% for those hospitalized for greater than 4 weeks (Table 61-3).[10] The traditional dogma posited that CDAD developed only in colonized patients who underwent treatment with an antibiotic that unfettered the bacteria, allowing it to cause disease. However, administering an antibiotic to a colonized patient seems less likely to produce CDAD than prescribing the same antibiotic to an uncolonized patient.[11]

Our current understanding of the mechanism by which patients develop CDAD requires a combination of three sequential events. First, the patient receives an antibiotic that alters his or her gut flora, thereby reducing innate defense mechanisms. Second, the patient with altered innate immunity is then exposed to *C. difficile*, which colonizes the gut. Last, the host's immune response is unable to contain this bacterial pathogen, which then releases toxin A and/or B, leading to mucosal injury and subsequent diarrhea (Table 61-1).

Recent reports document proliferation of a heretofore uncommon strain of *C. difficile* that is associated with epidemic outbreaks.[22,31,32] Traditional strains of *C. difficile* produce toxin A or B. This epidemic strain has a deletion of a regulatory gene, resulting in a 16–23 times increase in production of toxins A and B.[32,33] This, coupled with the emergence of a new binary toxin that is distinct from toxins A and B, is felt to result in the increased pathogenicity. Additionally, this new strain has a higher rate of cephalosporin and fluoroquinolone resistance. The clinical burden of this new strain is yet to be determined, but it likely plays a role in the increased incidence and severity of *C. difficile* infections seen throughout North America in the recent past.

Table 61-1 Mechanisms of Antibiotic-Associated Diarrhea

Hypermotility Diarrhea	Osmotic Diarrhea	*Clostridium difficile*–Associated Diarrhea
Antibiotics stimulate GI tract	Antibiotics reduce colonic bacterial flora	Antibiotics reduce colonic bacterial flora
↓	↓	↓
↓	Reduced bacterial carbohydrate fermentation	C. difficile colonization and overgrowth
↓	↓	↓
Increased transit to distal colon	Increased carbohydrate load to distal colon	C. difficile toxin production
	↓	↓
Hypermotility diarrhea	**Osmotic diarrhea**	**Toxin-mediated diarrhea**

Adapted with permission from Glasheen JJ. *Clostridium difficile*-associated diseases. Prim Care Case Rev 2003; 6:2–11.

Table 61-2 Strength of Association with *Clostridium difficile*–Associated Diarrhea

Low Risk	Intermediate Risk	High Risk
First generation cephalosporin	Second generation cephalosporin	Third generation cephalosporin
penicillin	anti-pseudomonal penicillins	quinolones
synthetic penicillins	aminoglycosides	clindamycin
vancomycin	metronidazole	
erythromycin	aminopenicillins	
tetracycline		

Adapted with permission from Glasheen JJ. *Clostridium difficile*-associated diseases. Prim Care Case Rev 2003; 6:2–11.

Table 61-3 Prevalence of *Clostridium difficile* Colonization Related to Hospital Length of Stay

Length of Stay	Prevalence (%)
<1 week	1
1–2 weeks	13
2–3 weeks	28
3–4 weeks	32
>4 weeks	50

Adapted from Clabots CR, Johnson S, Olson MM, et al. Acquisition of Clostridium difficile by hospitalized patients: evidence for colonized new admission as a source of infection. JID 1992; 166:561–567.

Table 61-4 Prevalence of Clinical Findings in *Clostridium difficile*–Associated Diarrhea

Finding	Prevalence (%)
Leukocytosis	50
Fever	28
Abdominal pain	22
Radiographic ileus	21
Toxic megacolon	3

Adapted from Gerding DN, Johnson S. *Clostridium difficile*. In: Infections of the Gastrointestinal Tract. Blaser MJ, Smith PD, Ravdin JI, et al. eds. Philadelphia, PA: Lippincott Williams and Wilkins, 2002. 763–784.

ASSESSMENT

Clinical Presentation

Prediction Rule

The presence of antibiotic use (within 30 days) along with either significant diarrhea (new onset of more than three partially formed or watery stools per 24 hour period) or abdominal pain is associated with a sensitivity and specificity for *C. difficile* of 86% and 45%, respectively. The use of this rule to identify low-risk patients (those without prior antibiotic use and either significant diarrhea or abdominal pain) has the potential to avert upward of 40% of *C. difficile* tests.[28]

Prevalence and Presenting Signs and Symptoms

C. difficile classically presents as diarrhea with associated fever, leukocytosis, and abdominal pain (Table 61-4). However the clin-ical spectrum of disease is broad and ranges from an asymptomatic carrier state to mild diarrhea and to the extreme of life-threatening pseudomembranous colitis (PMC). The difference in presentation is most likely related to the properties of the infecting bacterium and the host's immune response to the organism. It is well known that certain bacterial strains of *C. difficile*, such as those that produce toxin, are more virulent than others. Recent evidence suggests that the level of the host's IgG antibody response predicts disease expression, with more robust levels of antibody directed toward toxin A, resulting in less toxic disease.[7]

Asymptomatic Carriage

Fifteen to 25% of hospitalized patients become colonized with *C. difficile*, yet most will remain asymptomatic.[6,8] A prospective evaluation following 282 noncolonized patients found that 60 (21%) of the patients became colonized. However, only 9 became symptomatic, suggesting that approximately 85% of patients who become colonized do not develop symptomatic diarrhea.[12] Furthermore, compelling evidence exists that asymptomatic colonization at the time of hospital admission protects patients against overt diarrhea during their hospital stay.[11] It is hypothesized that exposure and containment of the organism (colonization) stimulate the host to acquire antibody-mediated immunity, which protects against colonization with more virulent *C. difficile* strains. Unfortunately, although these carriers do not develop diarrhea, they act as an important reservoir for bacterial shedding, playing a central role in continued disease transmission.

Clostridium difficile–Associated Diarrhea

Clostridium difficile–associated diarrhea classically presents within days to weeks of antibiotic use with profuse, foul smelling, semiformed stools. The diarrhea is often associated with low-grade fever and mild abdominal cramping. The physical examination may reveal mild lower quadrant abdominal pain but is most often normal. Leukocytosis is common and can often be the first and only sign of *C. difficile* infection. A recent study revealed that 58% of the evaluated cases of unexplained leukocytosis could be attributed to *C. difficile* after more in-depth questioning and stool sampling.[14]

Pseudomembranous Colitis (PMC)

As the most severe manifestation of *C. difficile*, pseudomembranous colitis (PMC) is most commonly seen in debilitated, intensive care unit (ICU) patients and is associated with poor outcomes[6] (Fig. 61-1). Patients classically present with voluminous, bloody diarrhea (5–20 episodes per day) and systemic findings such as fever, marked leukocytosis (as high as 40,000), nausea, and anorexia, as well as complaints of lower quadrant cramping abdominal pain that is often relieved with bowel movements. It is important to note that occasionally PMC can present with constipation rather than diarrhea. Such complaints are suggestive of intestinal ileus, which can progress to toxic megacolon and eventually perforation. This presentation appears to be more common in elderly, immunocompromised and (ICU) patients. Approximately 1–5% of patients with PMC will require

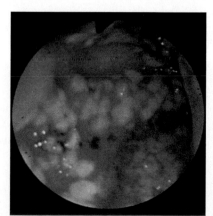

Figure 61-1 • Pseudomembranous colitis. Sigmoidoscopy or colonoscopy usually shows multiple yellow plaques and inflammatory changes and the diagnosis can be confirmed histologically. From: Forbes CD, Jackson WF. Color Atlas and Text of Clinical Medicine, 3 ed. Mosby, 2002.

surgical intervention, with an operative mortality approaching 50%.[3,4,6]

Differential Diagnosis

Other common causes of hospital-acquired diarrhea include antibiotics (e.g., erythromycin), other medications (e.g., metoclopramide, oral radiocontrast), gastrointestinal bleeding, enteral feedings, milk (secondary to lactose intolerance), and ischemic colitis. It is very uncommon for an immunocompetent patient hospitalized for more than 3 days to have a community-acquired cause of diarrhea, namely *Campylobacter, E. coli, Salmonella* or *Shigella*. As such, workup, including stool cultures, should not be directed at these organisms.

Diagnosis

General Factors

The diagnosis of *C. difficile*, as the name implies, can be difficult. This is in part due to clinician indifference toward asking about diarrhea symptoms but is complicated by the array of testing options and their less-than-optimal diagnostic capabilities.

The presence of semi-formed stools (versus watery), prolonged hospitalization (>15 days), symptoms occurring 6 or more days after commencing antibiotics, and recent cephalosporin antibiotic use have been shown to predict *C. difficile* over other causes of HAD.[15] Still, confirmation with a diagnostic test is required to definitively rule in the disease. Most of the available tests are aimed at detecting either the bacteria (stool culture, latex agglutination) or toxin (cytotoxin assay, enzyme assay). It is important to remember that it is the presence of the toxin, not the bacterium, that leads to the disease expression. Consequently, tests that identify the toxin tend to be more specific for the disease than those more sensitive tests that detect bacterial presence, but ultimately cannot differentiate colonization from infection (Table 61-5).

Specific Tests

Fecal Leukocytes

C. difficile does not typically cause an invasive diarrhea and is therefore not usually associated with inflammatory markers like fecal leukocytes or their by-product, lactoferrin. In fact, fecal leukocytes and lactoferrin are only present in approximately 50% and 60% of patients with CDAD, respectively. In terms of distinguishing the cause of diarrhea, this is not significantly different than the rates seen in other causes of HAD, and consequently, these tests should rarely be used in the work up of HAD.[16]

Stool Culture

Culturing the stool for *C. difficile* is a relatively sensitive test that lacks specificity, as the test only identifies the presence of the organism without differentiating between toxin and non-toxin-producing strains. Indeed, most patients with a positive culture will not develop the disease; rather, they will remain asymptomatic excretors. The high sensitivity of this test makes it most useful for ruling out disease and identifying carriers in an outbreak situation. Beyond those two scenarios, the poor specificity and long processing time (48–72 hours) severely limit the usefulness of this test.

Table 61-5 Diagnostic Capabilities of Tests Utilized in the Diagnosis of *Clostridium difficile*–Associated Diseases

Test	Sensitivity (%)	Specificity (%)	Comments
Endoscopy	51	100	Diagnostic of PMC, rapid result
Culture for *C. difficile*	89–100	84–100	Highly sensitive, time consuming
Latex agglutination	58–92	80–96	Moderate sen/spec, rapid result
Cytotoxin assay	67–100	85–100	Highly specific, time consuming
EIA toxin test	63–99	75–100	Highly specific, rapid result

Adapted from Gerding DN, Johnson S. *Clostridium difficile*. In: Infections of the Gastrointestinal Tract. Blaser MJ, Smith PD, Ravdin JI, et al. eds. Philadelphia, PA: Lippincott Williams and Wilkins, 2002. 763–784.

PMC = pseudomembranous colitis; EIA = enzyme immunoassay; sen = sensitivity; spec = specificity.

Latex Agglutination

Despite its rapid turn-around time, the latex agglutination test has fallen out of favor because of its low specificity and resultant high false positive rate. The test, aimed at detecting the enzyme glutamate dehydrogenase, does not differentiate between toxin and non–toxin-producing strains of *C. difficile*, other clostridial species or other bacteria such as peptostreptococcus.[16]

Cytotoxin Assay

The cytotoxin assay (an enzyme immunoassay) is considered the gold standard for detecting the *C. difficile* toxin. A positive test implies the presence of toxin B and occurs when the structure of a cultured cell is altered by the addition of toxin in a patient's stool. Normalization of the cultured cell after the addition of an antitoxin confirms the diagnosis.[16] The test is extremely sensitive for toxin-producing organisms (although it will not detect toxin A–producing organisms) but is limited by its time-consuming nature.

The enzyme immunoassay (EIA) provides reasonable sensitivity, specificity, and rapid results (usually less than 3 hours) and has become the most utilized test in the diagnosis of *C. difficile*. Several kits exist, with all of them directing an antibody toward toxin A, B or A and B, with the latter tests yielding the highest sensitivity. Many assays have specificities nearing 100% such that a positive test is virtually diagnostic for CDAD.[16] The sensitivity of the test can be improved by repeating the assay two or three times, thus raising the sensitivity from 72% to nearly 90% (three assays). Alternatively, coupling an EIA with a cytotoxin assay will raise the sensitivity to greater than 80% and even 90% with a second assay.[15]

Preferred Approach

One generally agreed upon approach is to order a stool culture (sensitive) and EIA toxin (specific) on a liquid stool.[1,17,18] If these tests are negative but the diagnosis is still suspected, repeating these tests may yield the diagnosis. If this second round of testing is again negative and the diagnosis is still suspected, then the options include repeat testing or empiric therapy for *C. difficile*. Many laboratories still employ the cytotoxin assay, which, as the gold standard for the presence of toxin, is a reliable alternative. However, the test can take days to produce a result, so empiric therapy should be considered while waiting for the results. In general, there is little role for fecal leukocyte and latex agglutination testing because they lack adequate sensitivity or specificity to aid in the diagnosis.

Prognosis

During Hospitalization

Traditionally, up to 85% of patients who acquired *C. difficile* remained asymptomatic with only 1–5% of patients suffering severe disease and the remaining 10–15% resolving their diarrhea within 1 week of effective treatment. However, recent reports show an increased incidence and morbidity of *C. difficile* that may be associated with a new epidemic toxin gene-variant strain.[31,32] One study reported an incidence of 22.5 cases per 1,000 admissions, with a 30-day mortality rate of 6.9%. Particularly concerning is the staggering rate of disease burden in the elderly. In patients over 90 years old, the incidence rose to 74.4 cases per 1,000 admissions with a mortality rate of 14%.[32]

Unfortunately, upwards of 20% of patients will develop a recurrence of CDAD.[18] This usually results from either a relapse with the same strain of *C. difficile* or a reinfection with a new strain. Unfortunately, patients who have relapsed once are more likely to, and often do, relapse a second time. Infection with *C. difficile* is associated with a remarkable amount of morbidity in terms of increased length of hospital stay, cost of care, and risk for acquiring other nosocomial infections. Still, the vast majority of patients with CDAD and PMC recover fully without long-term sequelae.

MANAGEMENT

Treatment

Stop Antibiotics

The role of antibiotics in the acquisition of CDAD is clear, making cessation of antibiotics one of the most important steps in disrupting the disease cycle. In fact, up to 25% of cases will require no further treatment after cessation of the inciting antibiotic. If antibiotics cannot be discontinued, then consideration should be given to substituting a less offensive antibiotic, such as vancomycin, metronidazole, or an antipseudomonal penicillin (piperacillin and ticarcillin).

Antibiotic Therapy

Antibiotic treatment should be considered in patients who have failed to improve within 2–3 days of antibiotic discontinuation, the elderly or immunocompromised, patients with significant comorbid or severe illnesses, and those patients in whom the instigating antibiotic must be continued.[6] Antiperistaltic agents, like loperamide and diphenoxylate with atropine, should be used with caution (or preferably avoided altogether), as their use has been associated with the development of toxic megacolon and perforation.[17]

If antibiotic treatment is warranted, both oral metronidazole and vancomycin are effective options, with similar cure rates approaching 95% (Table 61-6).[3] However, metronidazole has become the first-line therapy secondary to vancomycin's higher cost and the risk of developing vancomycin-resistant enterococcus. Vancomycin is indicated in patients with severe colitis or those who have failed two courses of metronidazole. Metronidazole can be dosed at 250–500 mg orally three to four times a day for 10–14 days. The oral vancomycin dose is 125 mg every 6 hours for 10–14 days. The use of intravenous antibiotics should be considered in patients who cannot take oral medications and those with adynamic ileus. Metronidazole, 500 mg intravenously, is the drug of choice, as intravenous vancomycin will not obtain adequate intestinal distribution. In the severely ill, adjunctive vancomycin enemas have been used with some success.[19]

C. difficile clearance and recurrence rates appear to be closely tied to the cumulative dose of the treating antibiotic, with higher doses associated with better clearance rates but also higher rates of recurrence. Thus, dosing regimens should be individualized based on the patient's underlying illness, severity of C. difficile, and overall risk of recurrence (higher if requiring continued hospitalization and antibiotics).

Cholestyramine

The use of cholestyramine, an anion-exchange resin that binds the toxin, has been advocated, especially in the treatment of recalcitrant C. difficile diarrhea. However, the resins also bind vancomycin (and should be staggered rather than dosed together) thus limiting the usefulness of this combination. Large-scale trials evaluating this therapy are limited, and therefore it cannot be recommended with confidence for routine use.

PREVENTION

Antibiotic Restriction

As the incidence of CDAD has sky-rocketed in recent years, investigators and infection control specialists have shown that altering antibiotic prescribing habits can greatly affect the incidence of C. difficile. The judicious use of antibiotics must be the cornerstone of any program aimed at reducing the burden of C. difficile. The incidence of C. difficile appears closely tied to the use of certain antibiotics such as clindamycin, cephalosporins, and the fluoroquinolones.[33] As such, success has been achieved through policies that restrict the use of high-risk antibiotics (Table 61-2). Most notably, programs aimed at reducing hospital use of clindamycin and cephalosporin antibiotics have yielded reductions in C. difficile rates.[20-24] There is some evidence to suggest that the antipseudomonal penicillins may be associated with less C. difficile secondary to less gastrointestinal penetration[25,26] This reduced gastrointestinal bioavailability may result in less alterations of the gut flora, which is felt to be a precursor to the acquisition of the bacteria. The data appear to indicate that, if deemed a suitable alternative, the use of either piperacillin/tazobactam or ticarcillin/clavulanate may reduce the risk of developing CDAD.

Barrier Precautions and Hand Hygiene

Other preventive methods such as disposable glove use and proper disinfection of rectal thermometers have also proven efficacious in reducing C. difficile transmission. Moreover, it is presumed that the traditional mainstays of infection control like hand washing, isolating infected patients, and properly disinfecting rooms are effective in reducing the hospital spread of the bacteria (Table 61-7). In the case of C. difficile outbreaks, this should be accomplished with vigorous washing with soap and water because alcohol-based waterless hand sanitizers do not kill C. difficile spores.

Probiotics

The use of probiotics, live microbial supplements that improve the host's gastrointestinal microbial balance, have been associated with a reduction in antibiotic-associated diarrhea.[29] Additionally, data support the use of probiotics in preventing recurrences of C. difficile in those patients undergoing antibiotic treatment. However, the data for probiotic use as primary prevention of C. difficile are less convincing and probiotics are not recommended for routine use.[30] Commonly used probiotics include Saccha-

Table 61-6 Summary of Randomized, Comparative Trials of Oral Therapy for Initial Episodes of _Clostridium difficile_–Associated Diarrhea

Antibiotic	Regimen	Cure (%)	Recurrence (%)	Mean days to Resolution
Metronidazole	250 mg qid × 10 days	95	5	2.4
	500 mg tid × 10 days	94	17	3.2
Vancomycin	125 mg qid × 5 days	75	?	<5
	125 mg qid × 7 days	86	33	4.2
	500 mg tid × 10 days	94	17	3.1
	500 mg qid × 10 days	100	15	2.6–3.6

? = not reported
qid = four times daily
tid = three times daily

Adapted from Gerding DN Johnson S. Clostridium difficile. In: Infections of the Gastrointestinal Tract. Blaser MJ, Smith PD, Ravdin JI, et al. eds. Philadelphia, PA: Lippincott Williams and Wilkins, 2002. 763–784.

Table 61-7 Methods for the Reducing Transmission of _Clostridium difficile_

Intervention	Efficacy
Barrier precautions:	
Glove use	Proven
Hand washing	Probable
Private rooms	Probable
Gowns	Untested
Proper cleaning/disinfection:	
Rectal thermometers	Proven
Endoscopes	Probable
Rooms	Possible
Commodes	Untested
Antimicrobial restriction:	
Clindamycin	Proven
Cephalosporins	Proven

Adapted from Gerding DN, Johnson S, Peterson LR, et al. Society for healthcare epidemiology of America position paper on _Clostridium difficile_-associated diarrhea and colitis. Infect Control Hosp Epidemiol 1995; 16:459–477.

romyces boulardii, Lactobacillus bulgaricus, L. casei, Bifidobacterium bifidum, B. longum, and _Enterococcus faecium._

DISCHARGE/FOLLOW-UP PLANS

Most patients with CDAD will improve within 3–4 days of therapy, with the majority enjoying full resolution of symptoms within a week.[16] However, 30% of successfully treated patients will continue to excrete _C. difficile_ asymptomatically without benefit from further antibiotic treatment. In fact, treating these asymptomatic patients with additional courses of antibiotics may increase their risk for future disease recurrences.[13] Consequently, sending a stool sample for a "test of cure" after a patient has been treated and is improving is not recommended.

Unfortunately, up to 20% of patients will suffer a recurrence of CDAD.[18] Recurrences are usually secondary to either a relapse of a dormant spore after cessation of an effective antibiotic or a reinfection with a different _C. difficile_ strain. Recurrences are almost never a result of metronidazole resistance and therefore should be treated with another course of this same antimicrobial. In fact, retreatment with another course of metronidazole has been shown to be 90% effective in eradicating _C. difficile_ recurrences.[16]

Although _C. difficile_ traditionally has been a hospital-acquired illness, outpatient cases have increased in proportion to reductions in hospital length of stay. In fact, in terms of overall bacterial etiology, _C. difficile_ trails only _Campylobacter jejuni_ as a cause of diarrhea.[6] It is therefore paramount that patients being discharged be instructed to follow up immediately with their primary care provider should they develop diarrhea, and that the provider be aware of the patient's hospital course and continued antibiotic use.

Patient Instruction

Instruct patients that the diarrhea may persist for up to a week and that they shoud drink plenty of fluids and look for signs of worsening disease such as fever, bloody stools, or increase in diar-

rhea. Patients also need to be aware that up to 1 in 5 patients will have a recurrence. As such, they should return to their primary care provider with recurrent diarrhea. However, if the diarrhea does not recur, no further testing is required.

The primary care provider (PCP) needs to be notified that the patient suffered from C. difficile induced diarrhea. As noted previously, the PCP should also be informed that subsequent testing is not indicated unless the patient redevelops symptoms. It is reasonable to also mention that possible recurrences could be treated with another course of metronidazole with a 90% likelihood of cure.

Key Points

- Diarrhea complicates up to 40% of treatment courses with hospital-administered antibiotics.

- Antibiotics can elicit diarrhea through hypermotility or osmotic- or toxin-mediated mechanisms.

- _C. difficile_ infection results in an increased length of stay of 3.6 days and additional hospital costs exceeding $3,500 case.

- The major risk factors for developing _C. difficile_ are antibiotic use and hospitalization.

- _Clostridium difficile_ classically presents as diarrhea with associated fever, leukocytosis, and abdominal pain.

- The recommended method of diagnosing _C. difficile_ requires stool to be sent for culture and an enzyme immunoassay for toxin. The diagnostic yield can be increased by sending two or more samples.

- Most patients with _C. difficile_ remain asymptomatic but can act as a reservoir for disease transmission. Recent reports show an increased incidence and morbidity associated with a new epidemic toxin gene-variant strain.

- The cornerstone of treatment is discontinuation of inciting antibiotics (if appropriate) and treatment with oral metronidazole or vancomycin.

SUGGESTED READING

Guerrant RL, Van Gilder T, Steiner TS. Practice guidelines for the management of infectious diarrhea. Clin Infect Dis 2001; 32:331–351.

Bartlett JG. Antibiotic-associated diarrhea. N Engl J Med 2002; 346:334–339.

Manabe YC, Vinetz JM, Moore RD, et al. _Clostridium difficile_ colitis: an efficient clinical approach to diagnosis. Ann Intern Med 1995; 123:835–840.

Johnson S, Gerding DN. _Clostridium difficile_-associated diarrhea. Clin Infect Dis 1998; 26:1027–1036.

Gerding DN, Johnson S, Peterson LR, et al. Society for healthcare epidemiology of America position paper on _Clostridium difficile_-associated diarrhea and colitis. Infect Control Hosp Epidemiol 1995; 16:459–477.

Glasheen JJ. *Clostridium difficile*-associated diseases. Prim Care Case Rev 2003; 6:2–11.

Katz DA, Lynch ME, Littenberg B. Clinical prediction rules to optimize cytotoxin testing for *Clostridium difficile* in hospitalized patients with diarrhea. Am J Med 1996; 100:487–495.

Probiotics in prevention of antibiotic associated diarrhoea: meta-analysis. BMJ 2002; 324:1361–1366.

Starr J. *Clostridium difficile* associated diarrhoea: diagnosis and treatment. BMJ 2005; 331:498–501.

Bartlett JG, Perl TM. The new *Clostridium difficile*: What does it mean? N Engl J Med 2005; 353:2503–2505.

Section

8 Eight

Endocrinology

62a Diabetic Ketoacidosis
Paul Cantey, Guillermo E. Umpierrez

62b Managing Diabetes Mellitus and Hyperglycemia
in Hospitalized Patients
Paul Cantey, Guillermo E. Umpierrez

63 Thyroid Disorders
Martin C. Were

64 Adrenal Insufficiency in Hospitalized Patients
Mahsheed Khajavi

65 Central Diabetes Insipdus Following Craniotomy
Kanchan Kamath

CHAPTER SIXTY-TWO A

Diabetic Ketoacidosis

Paul Cantey, MD, MPH and Guillermo E. Umpierrez, MD, FACP, FACE

BACKGROUND

Diabetic ketoacidosis (DKA) is the most common and serious acute complication of diabetes. Insulin deficiency and increased counter-regulatory hormones are the main underlying abnormalities leading to increased hepatic glucose production and reduced glucose uptake in peripheral tissues, resulting in hyperglycemia, and leading to increased lipolysis and ketogenesis, resulting in ketoacidosis. Clinical diagnosis is based on the finding of dehydration along with hyperglycemia, metabolic acidosis, and accumulation of ketone bodies. Treatment consists of insulin administration and adequate correction of the dehydration, hyperglycemia, ketoacidosis, and electrolyte deficits. In this chapter, we review and update recent advances in the epidemiology, diagnosis, and pathogenesis of DKA, and provide recommendations for its therapy based on the recent American Diabetes Association (ADA) guidelines for management of hyperglycemic crises.

Epidemiology

DKA is responsible for more than 100,000 hospital admissions and 500,000 hospital days per year in the United States, with substantial costs related to direct medical expenses and indirect costs. Recent epidemiologic studies in the United States and abroad have indicated that hospitalizations for DKA during the past two decades are increasing.[2,4] The increase in DKA admissions parallels the increase in the number of diabetic patients over the past two decades.[5,6]

In contrast to popular belief, DKA is more common in adults than in children.[7,8] In community-based studies, 45% of patients with DKA were older than 44 years and 26% older than 60 years.[1,2] Patients with type 2 diabetes may develop DKA under stressful conditions such as trauma, surgery, or infection. In addition, during the past decade, an increasing number of DKA cases without apparent precipitating cause have been reported among African Americans.[4,9,10] and other minority ethnic groups with type 2 diabetes.[11,12] Most adult patients with DKA have type 2 diabetes, since the majority of them are obese, have signs of insulin resistance and measurable insulin secretion, and have a low prevalence of autoimmune markers of β-cell destruction.[10,11,13–15]

Precipitating Causes

Table 62a-1 summarizes the results of various studies on precipitating factors for DKA. The most common precipitating factor for the development of DKA is infection, which accounts for 30–40% of all cases.[3,6,8,24] Urinary tract infection and pneumonia are the most common infectious precipitants of DKA.[4,25,26] Other acute conditions that may precipitate DKA include cerebrovascular accident, alcohol abuse, pancreatitis, pulmonary embolism, myocardial infarction, and trauma. Drugs that affect carbohydrate metabolism such as corticosteroids, thiazides, sympathomimetic agents (e.g., dobutamine and terbutaline), and pentamidine may also precipitate the development of DKA.[8]

Psychological issues and noncompliance are also known to be important factors, especially in patients with repeated episodes of DKA.[27] In a survey of 341 female patients with type 1 diabetes, psychological problems complicated by eating disorders were a contributing factor in 20% of recurrent episodes of ketoacidosis in young women. Noncompliance and poor compliance with therapy appear to be major precipitating causes for DKA in urban black and medically indigent patients.[4,6,28,29] The most common cause of DKA was stopping insulin therapy, which occurred in 60–85% of episodes. Reasons for stopping insulin included:[28] more than 50% of subjects stopped or reduced the dose of insulin because of lack of money or access to medical care; not knowing how to alter insulin dosage with changes in appetite, 21%; stopping insulin because of behavioral or psychological reasons, 14%; and stopping insulin because they did not know how to manage diabetes on sick days, 14%. In a different study, abuse of alcohol was reported in 35% and cocaine in 13% of patients with recurrent admissions for DKA.[4,30]

Pathogenesis

Diabetic ketoacidosis is a complex metabolic disturbance of carbohydrate, lipid, and protein metabolism, characterized by hyperglycemia, hyperketonemia, and metabolic acidosis. Ketoacidosis results from the lack of, or ineffectiveness of, insulin with concomitant elevation of counter-regulatory hormones (glucagon, catecholamine, cortisol, and growth hormone).[31–34]

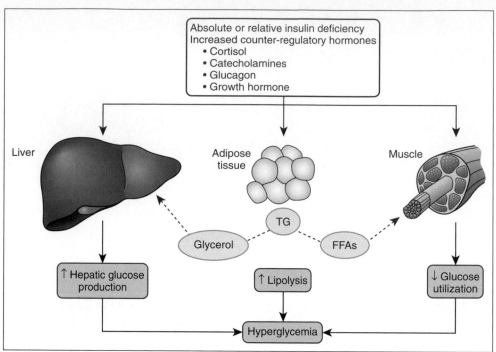

Figure 62A-1. • Increased glucose production in DKA. The combination of insulin deficiency and increased concentrations of counter-regulatory hormones (catecholamines, glucagon, cortisol, and growth hormone) results in increased hepatic glucose production and impaired glucose utilization in peripheral tissues.

Table 62A-1 Causes of DKA

Precipitating Cause	% of Admissions
Infection	30–40
Failure to take insulin	20–45*
New onset diabetes	15–25
Medical illnesses	10–20
Psychological problems	4–20**
Unknown	4–10

*Poor compliance with insulin therapy has been reported to be the most common precipitating causes for DKA in urban blacks and medically indigent patients.

**In young patients with type 1 diabetes.

The pathophysiologic basis for hyperglycemia in DKA is shown in Figure 62A-1. Hyperglycemia results from increased hepatic glucose production and impaired glucose utilization in peripheral tissues. The mechanisms that underlie the increased production of ketones in DKA are shown in Figure 62A-2. In addition, both hyperglycemia and high ketone levels cause an osmotic diuresis, leading to hypovolemia and decreased glomerular filtration rate; the latter further aggravates hyperglycemia.[8]

ASSESSMENT

Clinical Presentation

The clinical evaluation of patients with DKA consists of a prompt and careful medical history to assess the state of hydration and the presence of a potential precipitating event.[8] The clinical presentation usually develops rapidly, over a time span of <24 hours. Polyuria, polydipsia, and weight loss may be present for several days prior to the development of ketoacidosis, while vomiting and abdominal pain are frequently the presenting symptoms. Abdominal pain, sometimes mimicking an acute abdomen, is reported in 40–75% of cases of DKA.[41,42] The cause of the abdominal pain in most patients is not identified, but the pain spontaneously resolves after resolution of ketoacidosis.[42] The presence of abdominal pain in patients with DKA correlates with the severity of metabolic acidosis, but not with the initial blood glucose level or severity of dehydration. In a prospective study of 200 patients with hyperglycemic crises, abdominal pain was present in 86% of patients with serum bicarbonate ≤5 mmol/L, in 66% of patients with serum bicarbonate levels 5–10 mmol/L, in 36% of patients with bicarbonate levels 10–15 mmol/L, and in 13% of patients with bicarbonate levels 15–18 mmol/L.[42]

Mental status can vary from full alertness to profound lethargy; however, fewer than 20% of patients are hospitalized with loss of consciousness. In a recent study of 144 consecutive patients with DKA, 48% of patients were alert; 39% were lethargic, and only 13% were in a coma or unconscious[4] The mean total serum osmolality was 311 ± 3 mmol/kg in noncomatose patients and 345 ± 4 mmol/kg in comatose patients with DKA. Abnormalities in mental status correlate with increased morbidity and mortality.[1,3] Acidosis stimulates the medullary respiratory center, thereby resulting in deep Kussmaul respirations. Acetone may be noted by its characteristic fruity odor on the patient's breath. In spite of infection, which occurs in a considerable number of patients, the presence of fever is rare, as patients may present with hypothermia due to either vasodilatation of the skin or low fuel substrate levels. If a patient with DKA becomes

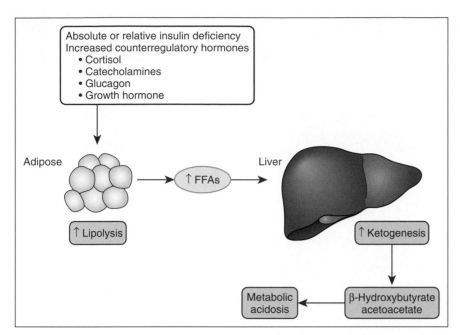

Figure 62A-2. ● Increased ketone body production in DKA. The combination of insulin deficiency and increased concentrations of catecholamines, cortisol, and growth hormone causes endogenous triglyceride breakdown (lipolysis) with subsequent release of large amounts of fatty acids into the circulation. Elevated FFAs are transported into the hepatic mitochondria, where they are oxidized to ketone bodies.

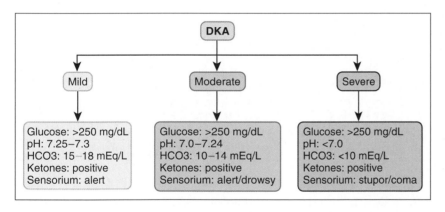

Figure 62A-3. ● Diagnostic criteria for DKA. The severity of DKA is classified as mild, moderate, or severe, based primarily on the severity of metabolic acidosis and the presence of altered mental status.

febrile, a vigorous search for an underlying infection must be undertaken.

DIAGNOSIS

Although the diagnosis of DKA can be suspected on clinical grounds, the confirmation is based on laboratory tests. The syndrome of DKA consists of the triad of hyperglycemia, ketosis, and acidemia. The initial laboratory evaluation should include determination of blood glucose, serum bicarbonate and electrolytes, venous pH, blood urinary nitrogen (BUN), creatinine, ketones, osmolality, and urinalysis as well as a complete blood count with differential and bacterial cultures as indicated.[8,43]

Recent ADA guidelines have provided three classification levels of DKA to outline different approaches to therapy depending on the degree of ketoacidosis.[43] The severity of DKA is classified as mild, moderate, or severe, based primarily on the severity of metabolic acidosis and the presence of altered mental status (Fig. 62A-3). The majority of patients with DKA present with mild metabolic acidosis.[4,44] Most patients presenting with DKA have a plasma glucose level of 14 mmol/L (250 mg/dL) or greater. The severity of metabolic acidosis bears little relationship to the degree of hyperglycemia, and cases of relative normoglycemic ketoacidosis (<13.8 mmol/L, 250 mg/dL) have been reported in ~10% of patients with DKA.[45,46] This phenomenon can occur during pregnancy, in patients with prolonged vomiting or prolonged starvation, and in those who present after receiving insulin. Similarly, relatively low glucose concentrations may occur in the presence of impaired gluconeogenesis, such as in patients with alcohol abuse or liver failure.

The key diagnostic feature is the elevation in circulating blood ketone concentration. In clinical practice, assessment of augmented ketonemia is usually performed by the nitroprusside reaction, which provides a semiquantitative estimation of acetoacetate and acetone levels. However, this reagent test can underestimate the severity of ketoacidosis because this assay does not recognize the presence of β hydroxybutyrate.[44,47] Rapid and specific enzymatic tests that measure β-hydroxybutyrate in capillary blood sample are now available and are preferable in establishing the diagnosis of ketoacidosis.

Table 62A-2 Treatment Protocol for the Use of Subcutaneous Rapid-Acting Insulin Analogs in Patients with Diabetic Ketoacidosis

Intravenous fluids:

1. 0.9% saline at 500–1,000 mL/hour for 2 hours
2. 0.45% saline at 250–500 mL/hour until blood glucose <13.8 mmol/L (250 mg/dL)
3. Dextrose 5% in 0.45% saline at 150–250 mL/hour until resolution of DKA

Potassium replacement:

1. If serum K^+ > 5.5 mmol/L, do not give K^+ but check serum K^+ every 2 hours
2. K^+ = 4–5.5 mmol/L, add 20 mmol of KCl to each liter of intravenous fluid
3. K^+ = 3–4 mmol/L, add 40 mmol of KCl to each liter of intravenous fluid
4. K^+ = <3 mmol/L, give 10–20 mmol of KCl per hour until serum K^+ >3 mmol/L, then add 40 mmol of KCl to each liter of intravenous fluid

Insulin Therapy:

1. **Subcutaneous insulin analogs (Aspart/Lispro) every hour (SC-1hr):**
   a) Initial dose SC: 0.3 unit/kg of body weight, followed by
   b) SC aspart insulin at 0.1 unit/kg every hour
   c) When blood glucose <13.8 mmol/L (200 mg/dL), change intravenous fluids to D$_5$% 0.45% saline and reduce aspart insulin to 0.05 unit/kg/hour to keep glucose ~11.1 mmol/L until resolution of DKA

2. **Subcutaneous insulin analogs (Aspart/Lispro) every 2 hours (SC-2hr):**
   a) Initial dose SC: 0.3 unit/kg of body weight, followed by
   b) SC aspart insulin at 0.2 units 1 hour later and every 2 hours
   c) When blood glucose <13.8 mmol/L (200 mg/dL), change intravenous fluids to D$_5$% 0.45% saline and reduce SC aspart to 0.1 unit/kg every 2 hours to keep glucose ~11.1 mmol/L (200 mg/dL) until resolution of DKA

3. **Laboratory:**
   a) *Admission:* Cell blood count with differential, complete metabolic profile, venous pH and serum β-hydroxybutyrate.
   b) *During treatment:* Basic metabolic profile (glucose, bicarbonate, potassium, chloride, urea, and creatinine), venous pH, phosphorus, and β-hydroxybutyrate at 2 hours, 4 hours, and every 4 hours until resolution of DKA.
   c) *Glucose by finger stick:* Check glucose every hour in patients receiving aspart insulin SC-1hr, and every 2 hours in patients receiving intravenous insulin or aspart insulin SC-2hr.

Accumulation of ketoacids usually results in an increased anion gap metabolic acidosis (Table 62A-2). The plasma anion gap is calculated by subtracting the major measured anions (chloride and bicarbonate) from the major measured cation (sodium). The normal anion gap has been historically reported to be 12 ± 2 mEq/L.[8] Most laboratories, however, currently measure sodium and chloride concentrations using ion-specific electrodes, which measure plasma chloride concentration 2–6 mEq/L higher than with prior methods.[50] Thus, the normal anion gap using the current methodology is between 7–9 mEq/L, and an anion gap >10–12 mEq/L indicates the presence of increased anion gap acidosis. Although most subjects with DKA present with a high anion gap acidosis, one study indicated that 46% of patients admitted with DKA had predominant anion gap acidosis; 43% had mixed anion gap acidosis and hyperchloremic metabolic acidosis, and 11% had hyperchloremic metabolic acidosis.[51]

The majority of patients with DKA present with leukocytosis. A leukocyte count >25,000 mm³ or the presence of >10% neutrophil bands is seldom seen in the absence of bacterial infection.[53] The admission serum sodium is usually low because of the osmotic flux of water from the intracellular to the extracellular space in the presence of hyperglycemia. An increase in serum sodium concentration in the presence of hyperglycemia indicates a rather profound degree of water loss. To assess the severity of sodium and water deficit, serum sodium may be corrected by adding 1.6 mg/dL to the measured serum sodium for each 100 mg/dL of glucose above 100 mg/dL.[26,31] Extreme hypertriglyceridemia, which may be present during the DKA due to impaired lipoprotein lipase activity, may cause lipemic serum with spurious lowering of serum sodium (pseudohyponatremia).

The admission serum potassium concentration is usually elevated in patients with DKA. These high levels occur because of a shift of potassium from the intracellular to the extracellular space due to acidemia, insulin deficiency, and hypertonicity. It is important to recognize, however, that total body potassium is low despite an even elevated potassium. The admission serum phosphate level may be normal or elevated because of metabolic acidosis. Dehydration also can lead to increases in total serum protein, albumin, amylase, and creatine phosphokinase concentration in patients with acute diabetic decompensation.

Differential Diagnosis

It should be remembered that not all patients who present with ketoacidosis have DKA. Patients with chronic ethanol abuse with a recent binge culminating in nausea, vomiting, and acute starvation may present with alcoholic ketoacidosis.[52] The key features that differentiates diabetic and alcohol-induced ketoacidosis is the concentration of blood glucose. While DKA is characterized by severe hyperglycemia, the presence of ketoacidosis without hyperglycemia in an alcoholic patient is virtually diagnostic of alcoholic ketoacidosis.[52] In addition, some patients with decreased food intake (<500 calories/day) for several days may present with starvation ketosis. However, a healthy subject is able to adapt to prolonged fasting by increasing ketone clearance by peripheral tissue (brain and muscle), and by enhancing the kidney's ability to excrete ammonia to compensate for the increased acid production.[31] Therefore, a patient with starvation ketosis rarely presents with a serum bicarbonate concentration less than 18 mEq/L.

Prognosis

Though DKA is the leading cause of mortality in children with type 1 diabetes mellitus, recent controlled studies in adult patients reported a mortality rate less than 5%, with higher mortality observed among elderly subjects and those with concomitant life-threatening illnesses.[8,16,17] Complications related to DKA are the most common cause of death in children, teenagers, and young adults with diabetes, accounting for approximately 50% of all deaths in diabetic individuals younger than 24 years of age.[18,19] In adults patients with diabetes, mortality increases substantially with age, reaching 20–40% in patients over 65–75 years old.[19,20,21] The major cause of death relates to the underlying medical illness (i.e., trauma, infection) that precipitated the ketoacidosis,[22] but in the younger patient, mortality is more likely to be due to the metabolic disarray.[23]

MANAGEMENT

Treatment

Successful treatment of DKA depends on prompt and adequate correction of dehydration, hyperglycemia, ketoacidosis, and electrolyte imbalances. Any comorbid precipitating event should be identified and treated appropriately. DKA is a serious medical emergency, and all patients must be admitted to the hospital; however, there are no guidelines determining the safety of treating patients in intensive care unit (ICU) or in non-ICU settings. Several studies have indicated no clear benefit of treating DKA patients in the ICU compared to step-down units or general medicine wards.[16,54,55] No differences in mortality rate or length of hospital stay were found in patients treated in an ICU compared to in a non-ICU setting; however, ICU care is associated with higher hospitalization cost.[16,54,55]

Increasing evidence indicates that ICU admission should not be dictated by the severity of hyperglycemia or metabolic acidosis but by the severity of intercurrent medical illness that led to metabolic decompensation.[55] Most patients with mild to moderate DKA, especially those who are alert and without associated precipitating cause other than noncompliance, may be safely managed in general medicine wards or intermediate care units, as long as there is a team of health care providers on site that is experienced in the management of DKA. In contrast, obtunded patients and those with critical illness as a precipitating cause for DKA (e.g., myocardial infarction, stroke, sepsis) require admission

to an ICU, where adequate nursing care and quick turnaround of laboratory tests results are available.

During therapy, capillary blood glucose should be determined every 1–2 hours at the bedside using a glucose meter; and blood should be drawn every 4 hours for determination of serum electrolytes, glucose, blood urea nitrogen, creatinine, magnesium, phosphorus, and venous pH. We do not recommend routine measurements of ketone levels during therapy. During treatment of DKA, the use of the nitroprusside test, which measures acetoacetate and acetone levels but fails to determine β-hydroxybutyrate concentration, should be avoided because the fall in acetoacetate lags behind the resolution of DKA. Admission chest X-ray, electrocardiogram, blood and urine cultures should only be performed if clinically indicated. Figure 62A-4 summarizes the ADA Position Statement algorithm for treatment of DKA.[43]

Fluid Therapy

The objective of initial fluid therapy is to expand intravascular volume and restore renal perfusion. In the absence of congestive heart failure or end-stage renal disease, infusion of isotonic saline (0.9% NaCl) at a rate of 500–1000 mL/hr during the first 2 hours is usually adequate. Patients with severe hypotension or hypovolemic shock may require a third or fourth liter of isotonic saline to restore normal blood pressure and tissue perfusion. After intravascular volume depletion has been corrected, the rate of normal saline infusion should be reduced to 250 mL/hr or changed to 0.45% saline, depending upon the serum sodium concentration. The free water deficit can be estimated, based on corrected serum sodium concentration, using the following equation: water deficit = (0.6)(body weight in kilograms) $\times$ $(1-$ [corrected sodium / $140])^{56}$. The goal is to replace half the estimated water deficit over a period of 12–24 hours.

Once the plasma glucose reaches 250 mg/dL, replacement fluids should contain 5–10% dextrose to allow continued insulin administration until ketonemia is controlled, while avoiding hypoglycemia.[43] An additional important aspect of fluid management in hyperglycemic states is to replace the volume of urinary losses. Failure to adjust fluid replacement for urinary losses may delay correction of electrolytes and water deficit.

Insulin Therapy

The cornerstone of DKA management is insulin therapy. It increases peripheral glucose utilization, decreases hepatic glucose production, inhibits the release of free fatty acid from adipose tissue, and decreases ketogenesis in the liver. Regular insulin given intravenously by continuous infusion remains the drug of choice. An initial intravenous bolus of regular insulin of 0.1 units/kg of body weight is followed by a continuous infusion of regular insulin at a dose of 0.1 units/kg per hour, until blood glucose levels reach 250 mg/dL.[8,26,43] At this time, dextrose should be added to intravenous fluids, and the insulin infusion rate is reduced to 0.05 units/kg per hour. Thereafter, the rate of insulin administration may need to be adjusted to maintain glucose levels at approximately 200 mg/dL. The infusion should be continued until ketoacidosis is resolved. In 144 patients with DKA treated with this protocol, serum glucose levels came into target range within 8 hours, with clearance of ketoacidosis occurring at a mean of 12 ± 2 hours. Compared to patients

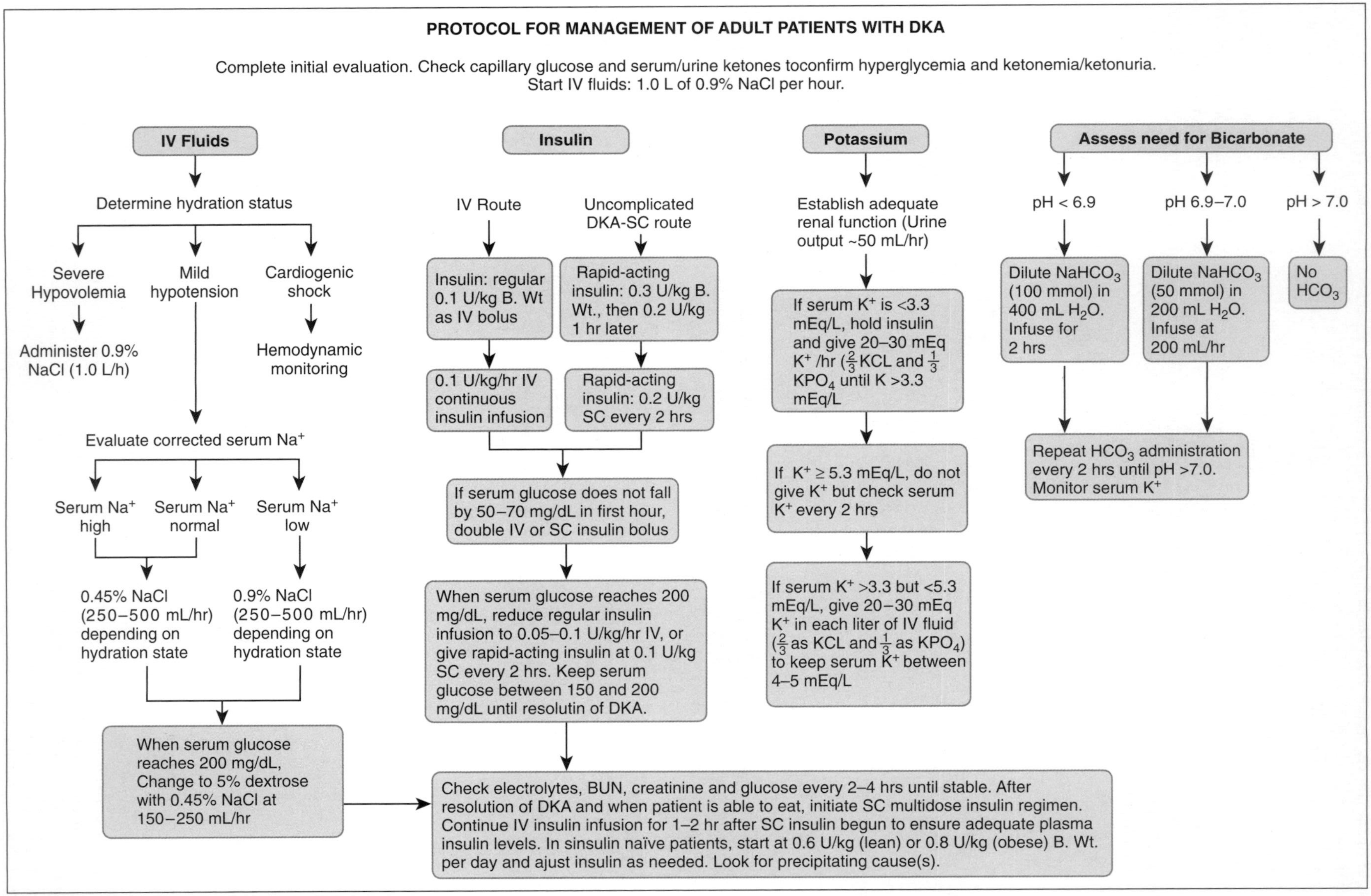

PROTOCOL FOR MANAGEMENT OF ADULT PATIENTS WITH DKA

Complete initial evaluation. Check capillary glucose and serum/urine ketones toconfirm hyperglycemia and ketonemia/ketonuria.
Start IV fluids: 1.0 L of 0.9% NaCl per hour.

IV Fluids

Determine hydration status

- Severe Hypovolemia → Administer 0.9% NaCl (1.0 L/h)
- Mild hypotension → Evaluate corrected serum Na⁺
- Cardiogenic shock → Hemodynamic monitoring

Evaluate corrected serum Na⁺

- Serum Na⁺ high → 0.45% NaCl (250–500 mL/hr) depending on hydration state
- Serum Na⁺ normal → 0.45% NaCl (250–500 mL/hr) depending on hydration state
- Serum Na⁺ low → 0.9% NaCl (250–500 mL/hr) depending on hydration state

When serum glucose reaches 200 mg/dL, Change to 5% dextrose with 0.45% NaCl at 150–250 mL/hr

Insulin

- IV Route → Insulin: regular 0.1 U/kg B. Wt as IV bolus → 0.1 U/kg/hr IV continuous insulin infusion
- Uncomplicated DKA-SC route → Rapid-acting insulin: 0.3 U/kg B. Wt., then 0.2 U/kg 1 hr later → Rapid-acting insulin: 0.2 U/kg SC every 2 hrs

If serum glucose does not fall by 50–70 mg/dL in first hour, double IV or SC insulin bolus

When serum glucose reaches 200 mg/dL, reduce regular insulin infusion to 0.05–0.1 U/kg/hr IV, or give rapid-acting insulin at 0.1 U/kg SC every 2 hrs. Keep serum glucose between 150 and 200 mg/dL until resolution of DKA.

Potassium

Establish adequate renal function (Urine output ~50 mL/hr)

If serum K⁺ is <3.3 mEq/L, hold insulin and give 20–30 mEq K⁺/hr ($\frac{2}{3}$ KCL and $\frac{1}{3}$ KPO₄ until K >3.3 mEq/L

If K⁺ ≥5.3 mEq/L, do not give K⁺ but check serum K⁺ every 2 hrs

If serum K⁺ >3.3 but <5.3 mEq/L, give 20–30 mEq K⁺ in each liter of IV fluid ($\frac{2}{3}$ as KCL and $\frac{1}{3}$ as KPO₄) to keep serum K⁺ between 4–5 mEq/L

Assess need for Bicarbonate

- pH < 6.9 → Dilute NaHCO₃ (100 mmol) in 400 mL H₂O. Infuse for 2 hrs
- pH 6.9–7.0 → Dilute NaHCO₃ (50 mmol) in 200 mL H₂O. Infuse at 200 mL/hr
- pH > 7.0 → No HCO₃

Repeat HCO₃ administration every 2 hrs until pH >7.0. Monitor serum K⁺

Check electrolytes, BUN, creatinine and glucose every 2–4 hrs until stable. After resolution of DKA and when patient is able to eat, initiate SC multidose insulin regimen. Continue IV insulin infusion for 1–2 hr after SC insulin begun to ensure adequate plasma insulin levels. In sinsulin naïve patients, start at 0.6 U/kg (lean) or 0.8 U/kg (obese) B. Wt. per day and ajust insulin as needed. Look for precipitating cause(s).

Figure 62A-4. ● Protocol for management of adult patients with DKA.
Adapted with permission from: Kitabchi AE, Umpierrez GE, Murphy MB, et al. Hyperglycemic crises in adult patients with diabetes: a consensus statement from the American Diabetes Association. Diabetes Care 2006; 29:2739–2748.

treated without a predefined protocol, this insulin adjustment protocol resulted in a <5% incidence of hypoglycemic events.[4]

Recent evidence indicates that new analogs of human insulin (aspart, lispro, glulisine) with a rapid onset of action may represent alternatives to the use of intravenous regular insulin in the treatment of DKA (see Table 62B-2).[59,60] We recently reported that treatment of patients with mild and moderate DKA with subcutaneous lispro and aspart insulin every 1–2 hours in non-ICU settings is as safe and effective as treatment with intravenous regular insulin in the ICU.[59,60] The rate of decline of blood glucose concentration and the mean duration of treatment until correction of ketoacidosis were similar among patients treated with rapidly acting subcutaneous insulin analogs every 1–2 hours when compared with intravenous regular insulin. We observed no significant differences in the length of hospital stay, in total amount of insulin administration until resolution of hyperglycemia or ketoacidosis, or in the number of hypoglycemic events among treatment groups.

Potassium

Despite a total body potassium deficit of ~3–5 mEq/kg of body weight, most patients with DKA have a serum potassium level at or above the upper limits of normal, due to concomitant acidosis on presentation.[61] With treatment of the DKA, serum potassium concentration invariably falls. Both insulin therapy and correction of acidosis decrease serum potassium levels by stimulating cellular potassium uptake in peripheral tissues.[31,61] Fluid administration also exerts a dilutional effect and increases urinary potassium excretion.

To prevent hypokalemia, we recommend replacement with intravenous potassium chloride (20 to 40 mEq/L) as soon as the serum potassium concentration is <5.5 mEq/L. The treatment goal is to maintain serum potassium levels within the normal range of 4 to 5 mEq/L. In some hyperglycemic patients with severe potassium deficiency, insulin administration may precipitate profound hypokalemia, which can induce life-threatening arrhythmias and respiratory muscle weakness. Thus, if the initial serum potassium is equal to or lower than 3.2 mEq/L, potassium replacement should begin immediately by an infusion of potassium chloride at a rate of 10–20 mEq per hour, and one may consider withholding insulin therapy until sufficient intravenous potassium replacement is given (1–2 hours).

Bicarbonate

Bicarbonate administration in patients with DKA remains controversial. Although severe metabolic acidosis can lead to impaired myocardial contractility, cerebral vasodilatation, and coma,[62,63] rapid alkalinization may result in hypokalemia, paradoxical central nervous system acidosis, and worsened intracellular acidosis with overshoot alkalosis.[8,64] Controlled and randomized studies have failed to show any benefit from bicarbonate therapy in patients with DKA and arterial pH between 6.9 and 7.1;[65,66] therefore, most experts in the field do not recommend administration of bicarbonate unless the admission pH is lower than <6.9.[43] In such patients, sodium bicarbonate should be administered in hypotonic fluid (44.6 mmol/L) every 2 hours until the pH is ≥7.0.[8] If the arterial pH is 7.0 or higher, no bicarbonate therapy is recommended.

Phosphate

Total body phosphate deficiency is universally present in patients with DKA, but its clinical relevance and the benefits of replacement therapy remain uncertain. Several studies have failed to show any beneficial effect of phosphate replacement on clinical outcome.[67,68] Furthermore, aggressive phosphate therapy is potentially hazardous, as indicated in case reports of children with DKA who developed hypocalcemia and tetany secondary to intravenous phosphate administration.[69] Theoretic advantages of phosphate therapy include prevention of respiratory depression and generation of erythrocyte 2,3-diphosphoglycerate. Because of these potential benefits, careful phosphate replacement may be indicated in patients with cardiac dysfunction, anemia, respiratory depression, and in those with serum phosphate concentration <1.0–1.5 mg/dL.[8]

Transition to Subcutaneous Insulin

Patients with DKA should be treated with continuous intravenous insulin until ketoacidosis is resolved. Criteria for resolution of ketoacidosis include a blood glucose <200 mg/dL, a serum bicarbonate level ≥18 mEq/L, and a venous pH >7.3.[4,8,70] To prevent recurrence of hyperglycemia and/or ketoacidosis during the transition period to subcutaneous insulin, it is important to allow an overlap of 1–2 hours between discontinuation of intravenous insulin and the administration of subcutaneous regular insulin.

If the patient is able to eat, split-dose therapy with both regular (short-acting) insulin and intermediate-acting insulin may be given. Patients with known diabetes may be given insulin at the dosage they were receiving before the onset of DKA. In patients with newly diagnosed diabetes, an initial total insulin dose of 0.6 units/kg/day is usually sufficient to achieve and maintain metabolic control. Obese subjects with DKA may require a higher initial insulin dose of 0.8 units/kg/day.[4,70] Two thirds of the total daily dose should be given in the morning and one third in the evening. Two thirds of each dose should be an intermediate-acting insulin with the remaining third as a short-acting insulin. If the patient is not able to eat, we prefer to continue the intravenous insulin infusion protocol. However, the patient could alternately receive subcutaneous regular insulin every 4 hours according to a sliding scale while an infusion of 5% dextrose in half-normal saline is given at a rate of 100–200 mL/h.

DISCHARGE/FOLLOW-UP PLANS

Patients with newly diagnosed diabetes benefit from education by a diabetes educator. Patients need to demonstrate comprehension of how to check their blood glucose and administer insulin to themselves. Precipitants of DKA such as noncompliance and psychological issues must be addressed prior to discharge from the hospital. Treatment of any complicating infections should be completed. All patients with diabetes require close follow-up with a physician experienced in the management of diabetes.

Key Points

- Most adult patients with DKA have type 2 diabetes, and hospitalizations for DKA are increasing as the number of patients with type 2 diabetes also grows.

- The most common reason that medically indigent patients with diabetes develop DKA is because they stop their insulin therapy secondary to lack of money or access to medical care.

- The most common precipitating factor for the development of DKA is infection, which accounts for 30–40% of all cases; and urinary tract infection and pneumonia are the most common infectious precipitants.

- Abdominal pain, sometimes mimicking an acute abdomen, is reported in 40–75% of cases of DKA. The presence of abdominal pain in patients with DKA correlates with the severity of metabolic acidosis. The etiology is not identified in most patients, but the pain spontaneously resolves after resolution of ketoacidosis.

- Abnormalities in mental status correlate with increased morbidity and mortality.

- To prevent hypokalemia, replace with intravenous potassium chloride (20–40 mEq/L) as soon as the serum potassium concentrations <5.5 mEq/L. For patients presenting with hypokalemia (K ≤ 3.2) and DKA, insulin administration may need to be delayed for 1 to 2 hours while potassium is given.

SUGGESTED READING

Newton CA, Raskin P. Diabetic ketoacidosis in type 1 and type 2 diabetes mellitus: clinical and biochemical differences. Arch Intern Med 2004; 164(17):1925–1931.

Kitabchi AE, Umpierrez GE, Murphy MB, et al. Management of hyperglycemic crises in patients with diabetes. Diabetes Care 2001; 24(1):131–153.

White NH. Management of diabetic ketoacidosis. Rev Endocr Metab Disord 2003; 4(4):343–353.

Maldonado MR, Chong ER, Oehl MA, et al. Economic impact of diabetic ketoacidosis in a multiethnic indigent population: analysis of costs based on the precipitating cause. Diabetes Care 2003; 26(4):1265–1269.

Kitabchi AE, Umpierrez GE, Murphy MB, et al. Hyperglycemic crises in diabetes. Diabetes Care 2004; 27(Suppl 1):S94-S102.

Freire AX, Umpierrez GE, Afessa B, et al. Predictors of intensive care unit and hospital length of stay in diabetic ketoacidosis. J Crit Care 2002; 17(4):207–211.

Umpierrez GE, Latif K, Stoever J, et al. Efficacy of subcutaneous insulin lispro versus continuous intravenous regular insulin for the treatment of patients with diabetic ketoacidosis. Am J Med 2004; 117(5):291–296.

Latif KA, Freire AX, Kitabchi AE, et al. The use of alkali therapy in severe diabetic ketoacidosis. Diabetes Care 2002; 25(11):2113–2114.

Umpierrez GE, Murphy MB, Kitabchi AE. Diabetic ketoacidosis and hyperglycemic hyperosmolar syndrome. Diabetes Spect 2002; 15:28–36.

CHAPTER SIXTY-TWO B

Managing Diabetes Mellitus and Hyperglycemia in Hospitalized Patients

Paul Cantey, MD, MPH, and Guillermo E. Umpierrez, MD, FACP, FACE

BACKGROUND

Hyperglycemia is a common finding in hospitalized patients with up to one third of hospitalized patients in an urban general hospital having hyperglycemia, defined as an elevated fasting glucose level >126 mg/dL or two or more random blood glucose levels >200 mg/dL.[10] Of note, about a third of patients may not have a prior diagnosis of diabetes. Increasing evidence from observational studies in hospitalized patients with and without a history of diabetes indicates that hyperglycemia is a predictor of poor outcome and increased mortality. Because hyperglycemia is perceived as a consequence of stress and acute illness, it is frequently overlooked, and rarely becomes a focus of care until blood glucose exceeds 200–250 mg/dL.

Several prospective, randomized trials demonstrated that intense glucose control with continuous insulin infusions in patients with acute critical illness reduces the risk of multiorgan failure and systemic infections and reduces mortality. Observational studies in noncritically ill patients admitted to general surgical and medical wards indicate that poor glycemic control is associated with poor outcome. However, there are no large interventional studies that have focused on the effect of optimal management of hyperglycemia on clinical outcomes in noncritically ill patients with diabetes. A common standard of care has been to hold a patient's diabetic medications and attempt to control blood sugars with sliding scale insulin—a practice documented to have limited therapeutic success and the potential to harm.

There remains some debate as to whether it is the correction of hyperglycemia or some other action of insulin that results in the benefits of tight glucose control with insulin. Cells that have passive uptake of glucose may become overloaded in the setting of hyperglycemia. This could cause direct toxicity or may act through intermediaries. Part of the toxicity may result from an increase in the production of reactive oxygen species via the oxidative phosphorylation pathway. Increased glucose as a substrate would result in the increased production of superoxide and peroxynitrites. Hypoperfusion-reperfusion injuries would add to the production of reactive oxygen species. Autopsy data reveal mitochondrial injury in tissues that acquire glucose through passive mechanisms in patients who died with stress hyperglycemia. Hyperglycemia has also been shown to result in the dysfunction of neutrophils, reducing their intracellular bacteriocidal and opsonic activity. Other effects may include nonenzymatic glycosylation of immunoglobins and inhibition of monocytic function. Evidence suggests that hyperglycemia may have direct toxicity in neurons, and insulin may have direct protective effects. Dyslipidemia occurs in the setting of critical illness and correlates with poor prognosis. Lipoproteins are involved in scavenging of endotoxins and may be involved in insulin's anti-inflammatory properties.[70] In this chapter we review current knowledge regarding the epidemiology, pathophysiology, and management of hyperglycemia in the critical care setting and in general medicine wards, particularly related to the medical conditions of acute myocardial infarction and stroke.

PATHOPHYSIOLOGY OF STRESS HYPERGLYCEMIA

Stress hyperglycemia is a well-known phenomenon. Acute stress results in a raised concentration of counter-regulatory hormones (catecholamines, cortisol, glucagons, and growth hormone) that promote pathways opposite to the action of insulin in the liver and peripheral tissues.[49–51] Both catecholamines and glucagon inhibit insulin-mediated glucose uptake in muscles and stimulate hepatic glucose production through increased glycogenolysis and gluconeogenesis. Catecholamine, cortisol, and growth hormone antagonize insulin action, which decreases peripheral glucose uptake. In addition, increased catecholamine and cytokines promote triglyceride breakdown (lipolysis) to free fatty acids (FFA).[28,52] Increased release of cytokines (i.e., tumor necrosis factor, interleukin-1, and interleukin-6) also contributes to insulin resistance through direct effects on insulin receptors. It is possible that the hyperglycemia associated with physiologic stress may reflect the strength of the counter-regulatory response.[5,6,36]

HYPERGLYCEMIA IN THE CRITICAL CARE SETTING

Hyperglycemia is a frequent manifestation of critical illness, resulting from the acute metabolic and hormonal changes associated with the response to injury and stress.[1,2] In the short term, hyperglycemia adversely affects fluid balance through glycosuria and dehydration, impairs immunologic response to infection, and promotes inflammation and endothelial dysfunction.[3–9] Increasing evidence suggests that in hospitalized patients with and without diabetes, the presence of hyperglycemia is associated with increased risk of complications and death.[10–15] Observational and prospective interventional studies among patients with critical illness, acute myocardial infarction, and stroke, and patients undergoing coronary bypass surgery suggest that aggressive glycemic control positively affects morbidity and mortality. Several interventional studies indicated that blood glucose control with intensive insulin therapy in patients with acute critical illness reduces the risk of multiorgan failure and systemic infections[16–18,67a] and decreases short- and long-term mortality.[11,14,17–19] The greatest benefit appears to be among patients after surgery, with less of an impact among patients hospitalized in an intensive care unit (ICU) for medical illnesses.

A retrospective analysis of 1,826 consecutive patients admitted to an ICU documented that the mean and maximum glucose values were significantly correlated with hospital mortality, and that mortality increased progressively as glucose values increased. The lowest hospital mortality (8.9%) occurred among patients with mean glucose values between 80 and 99 mg/dL, and the highest mortality (42.5%) was observed among patients with a mean glucose values exceeding 300 mg/dL.

In 2001, a large prospective, randomized nonblinded trial from Belgium studied the effect of intensive insulin therapy in 1,548 patients admitted to a surgical ICU.[16] In this study, subjects were randomized to tight control to a blood glucose level of 80–110 mg/dL (4.4–6.1 mmol/L) versus conventional control to a blood glucose of 180–200 mg/dL (10–11.1 mmol/L). Intensive glucose control significantly reduced mortality in the ICU from 8% to 4.6% (42% RRR). Other benefits found in the study included a 34% RRR of inhospital mortality, a 46% RRR of bloodstream infection, a 41% RRR of acute renal failure requiring dialysis, a 50% relative risk reduction (RRR) of blood transfusion, and a 44% RRR of ICU-related polyneuropathy. Most of the overall benefit of intensive therapy was attributable to its effects on patients who were in the ICU for more than 5 days, where a decrease in mortality from 20.2% to 10.6% (P = 0.005) was found. These investigators also showed that for each 20 mg/dL (1.1 mmol/L) of glucose levels above 100 mg/dL (5.5 mmol/L) the risk of ICU death was increased by 30%. A post hoc analysis of the data suggested that glucose control, not insulin dose, contributes more to the benefit of the intervention.[12] This landmark study was confirmed by additional research,[21] which demonstrated that intensive monitoring of ICU patients' blood glucose and treatment with continuous intravenous insulin to keep plasma glucose values lower than 140 mg/dL also reduced mortality.

HYPERGLYCEMIA AFTER CORONARY ARTERY BYPASS GRAFTING (CABG) SURGERY

Diabetes mellitus has been shown to be an independent risk factor for significant morbidity and mortality after coronary artery bypass grafting (CABG). Several studies have shown an increased rate of operative and postoperative complications and mortality among patients with diabetes.[22,23] Diabetic patients clearly had a significantly higher incidence of postoperative death and stroke,

and long-term mortality and need for revascularization.[24] Research using historical controls demonstrated reductions in mortality when diabetic patients were treated with continuous insulin infusion versus subcutaneous insulin and found an absolute risk reduction (ARR) of 2.8%.[17,25] Other research found that intensive blood glucose control reduced the risk of deep sternal infections by 64% (ARR 1.2%), saving $26,400 and 16 hospital days per infection prevented.[25] Tight control of blood glucose after CABG is now routine.

ACUTE MYOCARDIAL INFARCTION (AMI)

Coronary artery disease (CAD) is the major cause of morbidity and mortality in patients with diabetes.[26,27] CAD is usually more advanced at the time of diagnosis and has up to twice the morbidity and mortality related to acute myocardial infarction (AMI) compared to nondiabetic counterparts.[14,27–29] Up to 50% of patients with AMI have been recognized as having inpatient hyperglycemia.[14,28] Independent of a previous history of diabetes, the development of hyperglycemia in patients with acute coronary syndrome has been associated with an increased rate of complications and risk of death.[14,27,29–32] A recent meta-analysis of 15 studies that examined the relationship between hyperglycemia and the risks of inhospital mortality and congestive heart failure in patients with and without diabetes found that hyperglycemia resulted in increased risk of mortality for both groups.[14] In nondiabetic patients, risk of death appears to be increased at blood glucose levels >110–144 mg/dL (6.1–8.0 mmol/L), and risk of cardiogenic shock or congestive heart failure increased at blood glucose levels >144–180 mg/dL (8.0–10.0 mmol/L). In diabetic patients with AMI, the risk of death increased at blood glucose levels >180–198 mg/dL (10.0–11.0 mmol/L).

The Diabetes Insulin Glucose Infusion in Acute Myocardial Infarction (DIGAMI) study demonstrated that an aggressive intervention to control glucose levels significantly reduced morbidity and mortality in diabetic patients at 1 and 3.5 years.[13,33] In this prospective randomized trial, 620 patients with admission glucose values >198 mg/dL (>11 mmol/L) were randomized to either conventional diabetes care or intravenous glucose-insulin-potassium (GIK) infusion for 24 hours followed by intensive subcutaneous insulin therapy for at least 3 months. Patients in the control group attained a mean blood glucose of 210.6 mg/dL (11.7 mmol/L) at 24 hours and 162 mg/dL (9.0 mmol/L) by discharge. Patients in the intervention group attained mean blood glucose of 172.8 mg/dL (9.6 mmol/L) at 24 hours and 147.6 mg/dL (8.2 mmol/L) by discharge. The intervention group had a 0.5% greater decrease in A_1C at 1 year. Patients in the intervention arm had a 7.5% absolute risk reduction (ARR) of mortality at 1 year, with those patients at low cardiovascular risk and without prior insulin therapy receiving the most benefit—ARR 9.4%. This benefit increased to an ARR of mortality by 11% at 3.5 years.[34] Again, the greatest benefit was seen in the subgroup with low cardiovascular risk and no prior insulin therapy, with an ARR of 15% of death. Based on the positive and encouraging results of the initial DIGAMI study, the DIGAMI 2 study was designed to determine if the improved survival of post-AMI diabetic patients treated aggressively with insulin was due to improved glycemic control or to insulin therapy itself.[35] Unexpectedly, the trial failed to show that intravenous insulin-glucose infusion decreases mortality in diabetic patients post-AMI.[35]

What could account for differences in outcome between the DIGAMI studies? In DIGAMI 1, the patients had higher initial blood glucose, and those in the intervention arm achieved a significantly decreased glucose concentration both at short and long term. The overall change in HbA_1C levels in DIGAMI 1 was 1.4% in the intensively treated patients compared to a decrease of 0.5% in all three groups in DIGAMI 2. The ability of DIGAMI 2 to detect a difference among the three groups was reduced by an early termination of the study. The study as designed had a power of 85% to detect a difference; the final study had a power of only 50%. Analysis of the DIGAMI 2 study data; however, showed that fasting blood glucose remained an independent predictor of mortality in the study population. An increase in fasting blood glucose of 54 mg/dL (3 mmol/L) or HbA_1C of 2% resulted in a 20% increased risk of mortality. Taken in conjunction with the fact that the overall study mortality was only 18.4% at 2 years, considerably lower than the expected mortality of 22–23%, this indicates that glucose control in patients with acute coronary syndrome is important.[34–36]

The Clinical Trial of Reviparin and Metabolic Modulation in Acute Myocardial Infarction Treatment Evaluation (CREATE) Trial was designed to determine whether or not a glucose, insulin, and potassium (GIK) infusion decreased mortality in patients with AMI.[37] This randomized controlled trial conducted in 470 centers worldwide randomized 20,201 patients with STEMI who presented within 12 hours of symptom onset to receive GIK intravenous infusion for 24 hours plus usual care or to receive usual care alone. There was no difference in 7- or 30-day mortality. At 30 days, 9.7% and 10% of control and GIK treated patients died. There were no significant differences in cardiac arrest, cardiogenic shock, congestive heart failure, or reinfarction. The GIK treatment group did have a higher incidence of hyperkalemia, hypoglycemia, and phlebitis. Although no data were presented as to whether patients who presented with hyperglycemia benefited, prespecified subgroup analysis of diabetic patients with AMI demonstrated no benefit. The study, like several other trials, did find that patients with higher baseline glucose levels had a higher mortality. As the intervention group had a higher average glucose while receiving the infusion, any benefit may have been blunted by the hyperglycemia.

Taken together, the results of these trials suggest that glucose control is of critical importance to improving outcomes in patients with hyperglycemia at the time of acute myocardial infection. Insulin itself does not appear to provide the benefit. DIGAMI 2 suggests that any form of tight glucose control may be adequate; insulin drips may not be necessary.

STROKE

A relationship between admission plasma glucose concentration and inhospital mortality in patients with acute stroke has also been established.[39,45] Observational studies indicate that having diabetes mellitus increases the risk of stroke by approximately two- to three-fold.[39,46,47] The Framingham Study found that the incidence of stroke was 2.5 times higher in diabetic men and 3.6 times higher in women than in those without diabetes.[46] The prevalence of diabetes/hyperglycemia in patients with acute stroke varies from 20–50%,[19,38–40] with 5–20% having a previous history of diabetes.[19,38] A recent systematic review of studies reporting risk of mortality and/or functional recovery after stroke in relation to admission glucose found a significantly increased risk of poor outcome in patients with elevated glucose. The unadjusted risk of inhospital or 30-day mortality after ischemic or hemorrhagic stroke associated with admission glucose between 108 and 144 mg/dL (6–8 mmol/L) was 3.07 (95% CI 2.5–3.79) in nondiabetic patients and 1.30 (95% CI 0.49–3.43) in diabetic patients. Outcome for hemorrhagic strokes alone showed no relation to glucose level in diabetics or nondiabetics.[19,38] These findings are supported by studies showing higher mean admission glucose levels in nonsurvivors of stroke compared to survivors.[40] Other studies in the stroke literature reported that admission glucose levels and/or hemoglobin A_1C values correlate to stroke size, clinical severity, and functional recovery.[39,41,44,48]

There are no published randomized controlled trials that have examined whether or not strict glucose control in patients with acute stroke provides any short- or long-term benefit. The United Kingdom Glucose Insulin in Stroke Trial (GIST-UK) is currently underway. The trial compares glucose, insulin, potassium (GIK) infusion to saline infusion in patients with mild-to-moderate hyperglycemia during acute stroke. The initial pilot study, which included 53 patients, demonstrated that the infusion was safe, but found no difference in mortality.[44] The results of the ongoing study continue to suggest that the GIK infusion results in more rapid achievement of euglycemia (P < 0.01) and that the infusion is safe.[43] No definitive outcome data have been released.

MANAGEMENT

Although the exact mechanism of the detrimental effects of hyperglycemia is not fully understood, available data consistently demonstrate that inpatient hyperglycemia is associated with a poor outcome. Based on these observational and interventional studies, aggressive control of blood glucose is recommended in patients with critical illness.[6,12,61] A recent position statement of the American Association of Clinical Endocrinologists[65] recommended glycemic targets for hospitalized patients in the intensive care unit between 80–110 mg/dL, and in noncritical care settings a preprandial glucose goal <110 mg/dL and a random glucose <180 mg/dL. The current ADA ambulatory guideline for preprandial plasma glucose levels is 90–130 mg/dl. In the ICU, it is desirable to use a "trigger" glucose level of 140 mg/dL to prompt initiation of insulin replacement therapy, with the goal of achieving glucose levels as close to normal as possible, with avoidance of any symptomatic hypoglycemia or any blood glucose <70 mg/dL.[66] Recommendations for intravenous insulin therapy include prolonged fasting (>12 hours) in subjects with type 1 diabetes, and in subjects with type 1 or 2 diabetes during critical illness, before major surgical procedures after organ transplantation, diabetic ketoacidosis, total parenteral nutrition therapy, labor and delivery, myocardial infarc-

Box 62B-1 Recommended Blood Glucose Goals[2,6,11,14,16,17,21,29,34,61,65,66,72,73]

Non–Critical Care Setting

- Preprandial glucose <130 mg/dL

- Random glucose <180 mg/dL

Critical Care Units

- Glucose <110 mg/dl, in patients with:

- Prolonged fasting (>12 hours) in subjects with type 1 diabetes

- Critical illness

- Diabetic ketoacidosis

- Major surgical procedures

- Organ transplantation

- Total parenteral nutrition therapy

- Labor and delivery

- Myocardial infarction

- Acute cerebrovascular event

- Other illnesses requiring prompt glucose control

tion, and other illnesses requiring prompt glucose control (Box 62B-1).

Somewhat surprising results from a trial of intensive insulin therapy in a medical ICU[67a] indicated that attempts to achieve normoglycemia did not favorably affect mortality except among patients requiring 3 days or more in the ICU. However, morbidity was significantly reduced with prevention of renal failure, and some outcomes improved with accelerated weaning from mechanical ventilation and accelerated discharge from the ICU and the hospital. These results led to recommendations for a somewhat more conservative approach of giving insulin to achieve target glucose values of <150 mg/dL during the first 3 days of ICU care.[67b] If the patient requires continued critical care, then a goal of normoglycemia (80 to 110 mg/dL) is pursued.

Insulin Algorithms

Institutions around the world have reported a variety of insulin infusion algorithms that can be implemented by nursing staff.[38,39,41,53,56–58] These algorithms facilitate communication between physicians and nurses, achieve correction of hyperglycemia in a timely manner, provide a method to determine the insulin infusion rate required to maintain blood sugars within a defined the target range, include a rule for making temporary corrective increments or decrements of insulin infusion rate without under- or overcompensation, and allow for adjustment of the

maintenance rate as patient insulin sensitivity or carbohydrate intake changes.[61,67] In most insulin infusion protocols, orders to "titrate drip" are given to achieve a target blood glucose range using an established algorithm or by the application of mathematical rules by nursing staff. Physicians should keep in mind the risk of hypoglycemia, which is a frequent adverse effect of strict glucose control.[66,68] In the commonly encountered hospitalized patient with altered cognitive status due to the effects of age, illness, or psychotropic medications, the typical symptoms of impending hypoglycemia are not properly perceived. In the cardiac patient, hypoglycemia may result in excess catecholamine release that may aggravate myocardial ischemia or have proarrhythmogenic consequences.[69,70] Therefore, the risk/benefit ratio of strict glycemic control in all hospitalized patients must take into account the negative implications of more frequent hypoglycemic events.[66]

Glucose Management on the Hospital Ward

Increasing evidence indicates that glucose control is also important in diabetic patients with noncritical illness.[10,66] In such patients, however, no large prospective studies have focused on the optimal management or on the selection of various antidiabetic therapies available for the management of diabetic patients in general medicine services. A major concern of aggressively pursuing inhospital glucose control is the fear of hypoglycemia.[14,48–50] As a result, home diabetic medications are often held and replaced with sliding scale insulin, a practice that has not been proven effective for achieving euglycemia.[51–53]

Of the three primary categories of oral agents, secretagogues (sulfonylureas and meglitinides), biguanides, and thiazolidinediones, none have been systematically studied for inpatient use.[14,36] The major limitations to the use of these agents in the hospital setting are the slow onset of action and the inability to make rapid dose adjustments in response to changing inpatient needs. In addition, each agent has its own contraindications that may limit its use. A long-standing controversy regarding the vascular effects of sulfonylureas in patients with cardiac and cerebral ischemia exists. Data suggest that they may inhibit ischemic preconditioning and predispose to vascular events.[59–64] A large number of patients have one or more contraindications to the use of metformin upon admission, including congestive heart failure, renal dysfunction, or liver dysfunction.[65,66] Thiazolidinediones increase intravascular volume and may precipitate or worsen congestive heart failure and peripheral edema.[67–69]

Due to the limitations of oral agents, the use of insulin is preferable for blood glucose control in the hospital setting. In general, regular insulin by sliding scale as the sole form of glucose control should be avoided.[61,65,71] The use of a split-mixed regimen of intermediate (NPH) and short-acting regular insulin is effective and commonly used. Basal/bolus insulin coverage with the long-acting "basal" insulin glargine once daily and pre-meal rapid-acting insulin analogs (lispro, aspart, glulisine) also can be used to provide more physiologic insulin replacement, though inpatient studies are lacking. It is important to accept the fact that no single insulin regimen will meet the needs for all subjects with type 2 diabetes, and, more importantly, the quality of glucose control should be paramount, not necessarily the method by which this is achieved.

YALE INSULIN INFUSION PROTOCOL

The following insulin infusion protocol is intended for use in hyperglycemic adult patients in an ICU setting, but is not specifically tailored for those individuals with diabetic emergencies, such as diabetic ketoacidosis (DKA) or hyperglycemic hyperosmolar states (HHS). When the diagnoses are being considered, or if BG ≥ 500 mg/dL, an MD should be consulted for specific orders. Also, please notify an MD if the response to the insulin infusion is unusual or unexpected, or if any situation arises that is not adequately addressed by these guidelines.

Initiating an Insulin Infusion

1.) **Insulin infusion:** Mix 1 U Regular Human Insulin per 1 cc 0.9% NaCl. Administer via infusion pump (in increments of 0.5 U/hr).
2.) **Priming:** Flush 50 cc of infusion through all IV tubing before infusion begins (to saturate the insulin binding sites in the tubing).
3.) **Target blood glucose (BG) levels: 100–139 mg/dL**
4.) **Bolus and initial insulin infusion rate:** Divide initial BG level by 100, then round to nearest 0.5 U for bolus AND initial infusion rate.
   Examples: 1.) Initial BG = 325 mg/dL: 325 ÷ 100 = 3.25, round ↑ to 3.5: IV bolus 3.5 U + start infusion @ 3.5 U/hr.
   2.) Initial BG = 174 mg/dL: 174 ÷ 100 = 1.74, round ↓ to 1.5: IV bolus 1.5 U + start infusion @ 1.5 U/hr.

Blood Glucose (BG) Monitoring

1.) Check BG hourly until stable (3 consecutive values within target range). In hypotensive patients, capillary blood glucose (i.e., fingersticks) may be inaccurate and obtaining the blood sample from an indwelling vascular catheter is acceptable.
2.) Then check BG q 2 hours; once stable x 12–24 hours. BG checks can then be spaced to q 4 hours IF:
   a.) no significant change in clinical condition AND b.) no significant change in nutritional intake.
3.) If any of the following occur, consider the temporary resumption of hourly BG monitoring, until BG is again stable (2–3 consecutive BG values within target range:
   a.) any change in insulin infusion rate (i.e., BG out of target range)
   b.) significant changes in clinical condition
   c.) initiation or cessation of pressor or steroid therapy
   d.) initiation or cessation of renal replacement therapy (hemodialysis, CVVH, etc.)
   e.) initiation, cessation, or rate change of nutritional support (TPN, PPN, tube feedings, etc.)

Changing the Insulin Infusion Rate

If BG < 50 mg/dL: Give 1 amp (25 g) D50 IV; recheck BG q 15 minutes.
D/C Insulin Infusion ⇒ When BG ≥ 100 mg/dL, wait 1 hour, then restart insulin infusion at 50% of original rate.

If BG 50–74 mg/dL: If **symptomatic** (or unable to assess), give 1 amp (25 g) D50 IV; recheck BG q 15 minutes.
D/C Insulin Infusion If **asymptomatic**, give 1/2 Amp (12.5 g) D50 IV or 8 ounces juice; recheck BG q 15–30 minutes.
                          ⇒ When BG ≥ 100 mg/dL, wait 1 hour, then restart infusion at 75% of original rate.

If BG ≥ 75 mg/dL:
Step 1: Determine the **current BG level** - identifies a **column** in the table:

BG 75–99 mg/dL	BG 100–139 mg/dL	BG 140–199 mg/dL	BG ≥ 200 mg/dL

Step 2: Determine the **rate of change** from the prior BG level - identifies a **cell** in the table - then move right for **instructions**:
*(Note: If the last BG was measured 2–4 hrs before the current BG, calculate the **hourly** rate of change. Example: If the BG at 2PM was 150 mg/dL and the BG at 4PM is now 120 mg/dL, the total change over 2 hours is –30 mg/dL; however, the hourly change is –30 mg/dL ÷ 2 hours = –15 mg/dL/hr.)*

BG 75–99 mg/dL	BG 100–139 mg/dL	BG 140–199 mg/dL	BG ≥ 200 mg/dL	Instructions*
		BG ↑ by > 50 mg/dL/hr	BG ↑	↑ INFUSION by "2Δ"
	BG ↑ by > 25 mg/dL/hr	BG ↑ by > 50 mg/dL/hr *or* BG UNCHANGED	BG UNCHANGED *or* BG ↓ by 1–25 mg/dL/hr	↑ INFUSION by "Δ"
BG ↑	BG ↑ by 1–25 mg/dL/hr, BG UNCHANGED, *or* BG ↓ by 1–25 mg/dL/hr	BG ↓ by 1–50 mg/dL/hr	BG ↓ by 26–75 mg/dL/hr	NO INFUSION CHANGE
BG UNCHANGED, *or* BG ↓ by 1–25 mg/dL/hr	BG ↓ by 26–50 mg/dL/hr	BG ↓ by 51–75 mg/dL/hr	BG ↓ by 76–100 mg/dL/hr	↓ INFUSION by "Δ"
BG ↓ by > 25 mg/dL/hr *see below†*	BG ↓ by > 50 mg/dL/hr	BG ↓ by > 75 mg/dL/hr	BG ↓ by >100 mg/dL/hr	HOLD x 30 min, then ↓ INFUSION by "2Δ"

†D/C insulin infusion:
√BG q 30 min; when
BG ≥ 100 mg/dL, restart
infusion @ 75% of most
recent rate.

* Changes in infusion rate ("Δ") are determined by the current rate:

Current rate (U/hr)	Δ = Rate change (U/hr)	2Δ = 2X rate change (U/hr)
<3.0	0.5	1
3.0–6.0	1	2
6.5–9.5	1.5	3
10–14.5	2	4
15–19.5	3	6
20–24.5	4	8
≥25	≥5	10 (consult MD)

Figure 62b-1. • Yale Infusion Protocol. From: Goldberg PA, Siegel MD, Sherwin RS, et al. Implementation of a safe and effective insulin infusion protocol in a medical intensive care unit. Diabetes Care 2004; 27(2):461–467.

Key Points

- Hyperglycemia in the hospital is a predictor of worse outcomes and increased mortality.

- Up to one third of hospitalized patients are found to have hyperglycemia, even though a third of these will not have a previous diagnosis of diabetes.

- Several interventional studies indicated that blood glucose control with intensive insulin therapy in patients with acute critical illness reduces the risk of multiorgan failure and systemic infections, and decreases short- and long-term mortality, especially among postoperative patients.

- Lowering blood glucose to near physiologic levels appears to be the factor improving outcomes, not the insulin infusion itself.

- Control of blood glucose post-MI improves outcomes. However, glucose, insulin, potassium (GIK) infusions do not appear to affect mortality among patients post-MI.

- Physicians should **not** use "sliding scale" insulin alone to control patients' blood glucose in the hospital. Basal doses also need to be given.

SUGGESTED READING

Umpierrez GE, Isaacs SD, Bazargan N, et al. Hyperglycemia: an independent marker of in-hospital mortality in patients with undiagnosed diabetes. J Clin Endocrinol Metab 2002; 87(3):978–982.

Van den Berghe G, Wouters PJ, Bouillon R, et al. Outcome benefit of intensive insulin therapy in the critically ill: Insulin dose versus glycemic control. Crit Care Med 2003; 31(2):359–366.

Capes SE, Hunt D, Malmberg K, et al. Stress hyperglycaemia and increased risk of death after myocardial infarction in patients with and without diabetes: a systematic overview. Lancet 2000; 355(9206):773–778.

Clement S, Braithwaite SS, Magee MF, et al. Management of diabetes and hyperglycemia in hospitals. Diabetes Care 2004; 27(2):553–597.

Garber AJ, Moghissi ES, Bransome ED, Jr., et al. American College of Endocrinology position statement on inpatient diabetes and metabolic control. Endocr Pract. 2004; 10(Suppl 2):4–9.

Inzucchi SE, Rosenstock J. Counterpoint: inpatient glucose management: a premature call to arms? Diabetes Care 2005; 28(4):976–979.

Bode BW, Braithwaite SS, Steed RD, et al. Intravenous insulin infusion therapy: indications, methods, and transition to subcutaneous insulin therapy. Endocr Pract 2004; 10(Suppl 2):71–80.

Van den Berghe G, Wilmer A, Hermans G, et al. Intensive insulin therapy in the medical ICU. N Engl J Med 2006; 354:449–461.

Malhotra A. Intensive insulin in intensive care. N Engl J Med 2006; 354:516–518.

Gabriely I, Shamoon H. Hypoglycemia in diabetes: common, often unrecognized. Cleve Clin J Med 2004; 71(4):335–342.

Queale WS, Seidler AJ, Brancati FL. Glycemic control and sliding scale insulin use in medical inpatients with diabetes mellitus. Arch Intern Med 1997; 157(5):545–552.

Goldberg PA, Siegel MD, Sherwin RS, et al. Implementation of a safe and effective insulin infusion protocol in a medical intensive care unit. Diabetes Care 2004; 27(2):461–467.

Kitabchi AE, Umpierrez GE, Murphy MB, et al. Hyperglycemic crises in diabetes. Diabetes Care 2004; 27(Suppl 1):S94–S102.

Umpierrez GE, Smiley D, Kitabchi AE. Narrative review: ketosis-prone type 2 diabetes mellitus. Ann Intern Med 2006; 144:350–357.

Umpierrez GE, Maynard G. Glycemic chaos (not glycemic control) still the rule for inpatient care: how do we stop the insanity? J Hosp Med 2006; 3:141–143.

CHAPTER SIXTY-THREE

Thyroid Disorders

Martin C. Were, MD

BACKGROUND

Thyroid disorders are common; 5–10% of the general population, and almost 15% of women over 50 years of age, are hypothyroid. The prevalence of hyperthyroidism is approximately 1%, and it increases to 4–5% in older women.[1,2] A hospital-based study showed that 6% of patients had high serum T_3 concentrations at the time of admission.[3] Disorders of the thyroid can be the primary problem necessitating admission, as in the case of thyroid storm, supraventricular tachycardia from hyperthyroidism, or myxedema coma; or they can complicate the clinical condition for which the patient is being admitted. Many medications initiated during hospitalization affect thyroid hormone metabolism and might necessitate monitoring of thyroid function and possible adjustment of thyroid medications.

Physiology

Thyroxine (T_4) is the inactive form of thyroid hormone and is synthesized exclusively within the thyroid gland. It has a serum half-life of 8 days. Only 15–20% of triiodothyronine (T_3), the active form of thyroid hormone, is synthesized in the thyroid gland. The rest is mainly produced in the kidney and liver through the de-iodination of T_4. T_3 has a serum half-life of 1 to 1.5 days. In the serum, over 99% of T_3 and T_4 are bound by proteins—mainly by thyroxine-binding protein (70%), albumin (15–20%), and transthyretin (10–15%). During acute illness and with particular medications, (Table 63-1) the conversion of T_4 to T_3 can be down-regulated, and reverse T_3 (an inactive form of T_3 produced when the inner ring of T_4 gets de-iodinated) can be produced in relatively larger quantities[1] (Fig. 63-1).

Effect of Commonly Used Medications on Thyroid Function

All stages of thyroid hormone production from secretion, transportation, and metabolism can be influenced by medications commonly used in clinical practice[4] (Table 63-1). As a general rule, any interpretation of thyroid function tests should take into consideration the effects of the patient's medical regimen. Some medications relevant in the inpatient setting include:

Amiodarone—Can cause both hyper- and hypothyroidism, with an incidence of thyroid dysfunction of about 3.7% (as opposed to 0.4% in controls) after a minimum of 1 year of therapy with doses between 150 and 330 mg/day.[5] Amiodarone induces hypothyroidism by decreasing T_3 production and inhibiting the outer ring de-iodination of T_4, and it might also be directly toxic to follicular cells. Patients with underlying hypothyroidism (including occult hypothyroidism) can develop worsening hypothyroidism and goiter on amiodarone, and these changes may persist even after discontinuation of the medication. Hyperthyroidism can be caused by amiodarone via two mechanisms: (1) increased T_3 and T_4 synthesis (type I hyperthyroidism) because it provides a large iodine load[6]—more common in nodular or diffuse goiter, and (2) destructive thyroiditis (type II hyperthyroidism). Thyroid function tests should be checked before the initiation of amiodarone, and follow-up thyroid function tests should ideally be done after many weeks of amiodarone therapy. Tests performed within the first few weeks of starting amiodarone can be misleading, as some of the drug effects on thyroid hormone synthesis and metabolism are only transient. If a patient develops hypothyroidism while on amiodarone, thyroid hormone replacement should be initiated, and amiodarone should only be discontinued if it fails to correct the arrhythmia. The diagnosis and management of hyperthyroidism in the setting of amiodarone use are more involved, and the help of an endocrinologist should be solicited.

Glucocorticoids—These drugs decrease thyroid-stimulating hormone (TSH) secretion, decrease serum thyroid binding globulin (TBG) concentration, and decrease de-iodination of T_4 to T_3. In general, glucocorticoids cause short-term changes in thyroid function, and the effect of long-term glucocorticoid therapy on thyroid function is only slight.[7–10]

Dopamine—The need to test for thyroid function commonly arises in patients on dopamine infusions in an ICU. Patients receiving at least 1 mcg/kg/min of dopamine can have decreased TSH secretion, which over several days can lead to decreased thyroid hormone production. It is difficult to distinguish this decrease in thyroid hormone production from decreased production secondary to the underlying acute illness.[11,12]

Drugs that decrease T_4 absorption—Commonly used medications, including iron,[13] sucralfate,[14,15] aluminum-containing anti-acids,[16] and bile acid–binding resins (e.g., cholestyramine)[17] decrease the absorption of oral thyroxine (T_4) given for the treatment of hypothyroidism. These drugs should be given several hours before or after an oral thyroxine dose.

Table 63-1 Drugs That Influence Thyroid Function*

Drugs that decrease TSH secretion
Dopamine
Glucocorticoids
Octreotide

Drugs that alter thyroid hormone secretion
Decreased thyroid hormone secretion
Lithium
Iodide
Amiodarone
Aminoglutethimide
Increased thyroid hormone secretion
Iodide
Amiodarone

Drugs that decrease T_4 absorption
Cholestipol
Cholestyramine
Aluminum hydroxide
Ferrous sulfate
Sucralfate

Drugs that alter T_4 and T_3 transport in serum
Increased serum TBG concentration
Estrogens
Tamoxifen
Heroin
Methadone
Mitotane
Fluorouracil
Decreased serum TBG concentration
Androgens
Anabolic steroids (e.g., danazol)
Slow-release nicotinic acid
Glucocorticoids
Displacement from protein-binding sites
Furosemide
Fenclofenac
Mefenamic acid
Salicylates

Drugs that alter T_4 and T_3 metabolism
Increased hepatic metabolism
Phenobarbital
Rifampin
Phenytoin
Carbamazepine
Decreased T_4 5′-deiodinase activity
Propylthiouracil
Amiodarone
Beta-adrenergic-antagonist drugs
Glucocorticoids
Cytokines
Inteferon alfa
Interleukin-2

*TSH denotes thyrotropin, T_4 thyroxine, T_3 triiodothyronine, and TBG thyroxine-binding globulin.

From: Surks MI, Sievert R. Drugs and thyroid function. N Engl J Med 1995; 333:1691. Copyright 1995. Massachusetts Medical Society.

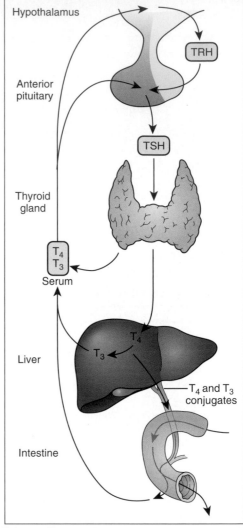

Figure 63-1 • The Hypothalamic-pituitary-thyroid axis and extra-thyroidal pathways of thyroid hormone metabolism. Triiodothyronine (T_3) and thyroxine (T_4) inhibit the secretion of thyrotropin (TSH) both directly and indirectly, by inhibiting the secretion of thyrotropin-releasing hormone (TRH). TSH stimulates the synthesis and secretion of T_4 and T_3 by the thyroid gland. T_4 is converted to T_3 in the liver (and many other tissues) by the action of T_4 monodeiodinases. Some of the T_4 and T_3 is conjugated with glucuronide and sulfate in the liver, excreted in the bile, and partially hydrolyzed in the intestine; the T_4 and T_3 formed there may be reabsorbed. Drug interaction can occur at any of these sites. From: Surks MI, Sievert R. Drugs and thyroid function. N Engl J Med 1995; 333:1691. Copyright 1995. Massachusetts Medical Society.

ASSESSMENT

Clinical Assessment

Prevalence and Presenting Signs and Symptoms

Clinical Manifestations of Hypothyroidism

While the clinical presentation of hypothyroidism is typically nonspecific, diagnostic laboratory testing with TSH and free T_4 levels is readily available. Manifestations of hypothyroidism can be divided into early and late clinical manifestations. Early signs

Table 63-2 Hypothyroid Clinical and Laboratory Findings

Cardiovascular:
   Rhythm abnormalities
   − Bradycardia
   − Premature ventricular beats
   − QT prolongation occasionally leading to torsade de pointes[18]
   Hypertension—diastolic with diminished pulse pressure[19]
   Heart failure
   Pericardial effusion—usually not hemodynamically significant[20]
   Edema—usually periorbital or non-pitting edema involving feet and hands

Hyponatremia
   − Occurs frequently, and thyroid function test should be part of hyponatremia work-up[21]
   − Mechanism of hyponatremia not clearly understood

Musculoskeletal:
   − Simple elevation of muscle enzymes without symptoms[22]
   − Myalgias with or without elevation of muscle enzymes
   − Myopathy:
      − Usually involving bilateral proximal muscles
      − Distinguished from polymyositis by coexisting symptoms of hypothyroidism like delayed DTR relaxation, normal EMG, and absence of inflammatory changes on biopsy[23]
   − Hoffmann's syndrome with muscle stiffness, cramps, and hypertrophy[24]
   − Rhabdomyolysis[25]

Myxedema Coma

Table 63-3 Hyperthyroid Clinical and Laboratory Findings

Cardiovascular:
   Atrial fibrillation
   − Present in 5%–15% of hyperthyroid patients[30]
   − Risk factors include male sex, coronary heart disease, increasing age, heart failure, and valvular heart disease[31]
   − Prevalence of atrial fibrillation similar with subclinical hyperthyroidism[32]
   Heart failure—if only secondary to hyperthyroidism, should disappear when hyperthyroidism is treated
   Angina or MI—Increased serum T3 concentration has been associated with 2.3-fold higher risk of angina and MI[33]

Neuromuscular:
   − Tremor/Tremulousness—most apparent with arms outstretched or when patient sticks out their tongue
   − Hyperactive deep tendon reflexes
   − Proximal muscle weakness and decreased muscle mass[34]
   − Hypokalemic Periodic paralysis (Thyrotoxic Periodic Paralysis)—especially in Asian men[35]

Thyroid Storm

and symptoms include fatigue, weakness, cold intolerance, weight gain, dry skin, and constipation due to decreased gut motility. Other symptoms include the classic clinical finding of delayed deep tendon reflexes, depression, goiter, infertility, menstrual irregularities (especially menorrhagia), coarse brittle hair, hypertension, and bradycardia. Hypothyroidism of several years' duration may produce a hoarse voice, slow speech, effusions (pleural, pericardial, or peritoneal), loss of the outer third of eyebrows, myxedema (nonpitting puffiness secondary to glycosaminoglycan infiltration of the skin), sleep apnea (secondary to macroglossia), preorbital puffiness, and hyperlipidemia (due to decreased lipid clearance).

Clinical manifestations of hypothyroidism with particular relevance in the inpatient setting are shown in Table 63-2.[18–25] These include cardiovascular alterations, musculoskeletal changes, and hyponatremia. Fortunately, these manifestations of hypothyroidism respond to correction of the thyroid dysfunction.

Myxedema coma, the most severe complication of hypothyroidism, usually presents with hypoventilation secondary to respiratory muscle weakness,[26] hypotension,[27] and hypothermia. Patients can also be hyponatremic due to decreased free water clearance as a result of inappropriate ADH secretion.[28] Myxedema coma is usually precipitated by trauma, infection, medications (e.g., narcotics or hypnotic agents), or exposure to cold in patients with severe hypothyroidism.[29]

Clinical Manifestations of Hyperthyroidism

Common symptoms of hyperthyroidism are somewhat the reverse of hypothyroidism and include weight loss, heat intolerance, sweating, difficulty sleeping, palpitations, tachycardia, and goiter. Less common symptoms include gynecomastia (in men), abdominal symptoms (nausea, vomiting, and pain), abnormal liver function tests (LFTs), menstrual irregularities, infertility, and difficulty concentrating. Among patients with hyperthyroidism due to a rapidly expanding goiter, dysphagia and tracheal obstruction are risks. Older patients can present with apathetic thyrotoxicosis with weight loss, difficulty sleeping, and decreased energy, the reverse of what is seen in younger patients with hyperthyroidism.

Hyperthyroid manifestations of particular importance in the inpatient setting are noted in Table 63-3.[30–35]

Thyroid Storm

Precipitating events for thyroid storm include infection (most common), surgery (thyroidal and nonthyroidal), therapy with radioactive iodine, withdrawal of antithyroidal medication, amiodarone therapy, administration of iodinated contrast dyes or ingestion of large stable iodine loads, exogenous thyroid hormone ingestion, hypoglycemia, congestive heart failure (CHF), diabetic ketoacidosis (DKA), toxemia of pregnancy, severe emotional stress, pulmonary embolism, cerebrovascular accident (CVA), acute trauma, bowel infarction, parturition and the immediate postpartum state, mania, tooth extraction, or vigorous palpation of the thyroid gland.[36]

Most common presenting symptoms of thyroid storm include: fever in association with excessive diaphoresis[37]; tachycardia (usually sinus, but supraventricular arrhythmias are also observed); CNS dysfunction ranging from agitation, restlessness, confusion, psychosis, and coma[38]; and GI disturbance including vomiting, diarrhea, obstruction, and acute abdomen.[39]

Box 63-1 Conditions That Might Necessitate Thyroid Function Testing in the Inpatient Setting

- Atrial fibrillation
- Bradycardia
- Pleural effusion of unknown etiology
- Heart failure
- Hyponatremia
- Myositis or abnormal muscle enzymes
- Other neuromuscular disorders
- Weight loss
- Dyslipidemia
- Suspected myxedema coma
- Suspected thyroid storm
- Hyperthermia of unknown etiology
- Hypertension
- Menstrual irregularities

Differential Diagnosis

Given the nonspecific nature of the clinical manifestations, thyroid dysfunction should be considered in the differential diagnosis of several conditions. Especially important in the inpatient setting are hyponatremia, hypothermia, hypotension, hypertension, depression, any supraventricular tachycardia and atrial fibrillation, pericardial effusion, heart failure, QT prolongation, and myopathy (See Box 63-1).

DIAGNOSTIC STUDIES

General Factors

Given that acute illness affects thyroid hormone synthesis, cautiously interpret thyroid function tests in the hospital setting. Screening of thyroid function is generally discouraged in the acutely ill patient, as changes in binding proteins, increased rT_3 production, central hypothyroidism, and medications can affect thyroid function tests. If thyroid function tests are necessary, both serum TSH and free T_4 values should be measured.[40–43] Indications for inpatient screening of thyroid function are listed in Box 63-1.

Thyroid disorders' diffuse effect on body physiology is revealed in other abnormal laboratory studies. Hypothyroidism is associated with hyponatremia, elevated lipid levels, and elevated creatine kinase (CK) levels. Hyperthyroidism is associated with abnormalities in liver function tests (LFTs) (particularly high serum alkaline phosphatase concentrations and, rarely, cholestasis) and with lipid study abnormalities (low serum total and high-density lipoprotein [HDL] cholesterol concentrations, and a low total cholesterol/HDL cholesterol ratio). These abnormalities usually correct with treatment of the thyroid disorder.

Specific Tests

Common thyroid tests are outlined in Table 63-4.

Algorithm

An approach to thyroid disorders is outlined in Figure 63-2.

Prognosis

In most cases, T_4 treatment reverses all symptoms of hypothyroidism. Untreated hypothyroidism can lead to myxedema coma with mortality as high as 30–60%.[45–47] Factors associated with poor prognosis in myxedema coma include hypothermia, bradycardia, and advanced age.[48] In adults, successful treatment generally reverses all symptoms of hypothyroidism. The mortality rate of untreated thyroid storm ranges from 20–30%. In thyroid storm, jaundice is associated with a poor prognosis.[49]

MANAGEMENT

Management of Hypothyroidism

The treatment goal of hypothyroidism is usually to restore euthyroid state, and this can be achieved with synthetic thyroxine T_4. The T_4 dose requirement in adults is approximately 1.6 mcg/kg, but it can vary widely and is usually correlated to lean-body mass.[51] Approximately 80% of oral T_4 is absorbed and converted peripherally into the active T_3 form.[50] Because of slight variability in the various T_4 formulations, patients should remain on the same brand in the hospital. The plasma half-life of T_4 is about 1 week, and thus, it takes about 6 weeks for a steady state to be achieved. Parenteral T_4 should only be given if a patient is unable take oral T_4 for 5–7 days. The dose should be about 80% of the patient's usual oral dose, as this is the fraction of the oral dose that is usually absorbed. Beginning thyroxine therapy without glucocorticoid therapy in patients who are adrenally insufficient can precipitate an acute adrenal crisis because the thyroxine may accelerate cortisol metabolism.

Overtreatment can cause subclinical hyperthyroidism complicated by atrial fibrillation and bone loss. Patients with coronary artery disease and elderly patients should receive lower initial doses (0.0125 to 0.025 mg daily) to avoid precipitating cardiac ischemia. Serum TSH levels should be measured 4–6 weeks after the initiation of therapy and after any dose changes. Once stable, serum TSH levels can be checked yearly. The goal serum TSH level should be between 0.5 and 3 mU per liter. Medications that affect thyroxine gastrointestinal absorption (e.g., iron sulfate and sucralfate) should be taken several hours after thyroxine dose. Treatment with a T_3 formulation is recommended only in situations where a patient with thyroid carcinoma needs radioiodine imaging and possible treatment, and treatment should be guided by an endocrinologist.

Women need more thyroid hormone during pregnancy, as higher estrogen levels increase serum TBG, and consequently the thyroxine dose might need adjustment.[52] Serum TSH should also be measured approximately 12 weeks after starting estrogen therapy in women receiving thyroxine therapy.

Table 63-4 Thyroid Function Tests

Test	Indication(s)	Comments
Serum TSH	Screening for suspected thyroid dysfunction.	Most sensitive test for detecting hypo- or hyperthyroidism, but can be misleading in pituitary disease (secondary)
Serum T_4 and T_3		Measures total serum concentrations, and is thus influenced by TBG and albumin levels.
Serum free T_4 (direct measurement)	Suspected thyroid dysfunction	An immunoassay not influenced by TBG. This is the preferred method of free T_4 measurement.
Free T_4 (thyroxine) index (FTI)	Suspected thyroid dysfunction	Less preferred method to measure free T_4. FTI = $(T_4/T_3RU)/100$. Calculation is poorly understood by clinicians, and can be inaccurate in many binding protein abnormalities.
T_3 resin uptake (T_3RU)	Suspected TBG abnormalities and for calculating FTI	Patient's serum (contains TBG) plus radio-labeled T_3 is added to insoluble resin that traps unbound radio-labeled T_3. The percent T_3 bound to the resin is reported as the resin uptake, and is inversely proportional to the TBG in patient's serum. I.E. $\downarrow T_3RU \approx \uparrow TBG$ and vice versa.
Serum free T_3	T_3 thyrotoxicosis	Limited utility
Reverse T_3		The inactive form of T_3. Can be increased in patients with sick euthyroid syndrome.
Serum thyroglobulin	A tumor marker for thyroid cancer (papillary and follicular)	Levels increased in subacute thyroiditis and variable in nodular thyroid disease
Serum thyroid stimulating immunoglobulin (TSI, anti-TSH receptor antibody)	Graves' disease in pregnancy, euthyroid ophthalmopathy	Not necessary to diagnose Graves' disease, is also expensive.
Antithyroid peroxidase antibodies (anti-TPO)	Suspected Hashimoto's (autoimmune) thyroiditis	Can predict development of overt hypothyroidism in patients whose TSH levels are between 5–10 μU/mL.
Radioactive iodine uptake (RAIU)	Biochemical Thyrotoxicosis	Useful in differentiating several causes of hyperthyroidism. Contraindicated in pregnancy and in breast-feeding women.

Adapted from: Evaluation of thyroid function. In: Wartofsky L, Ende J, Epstein, PE, eds. Medical Knowledge Self-Assessment Program (MKSAP) 13 Endocrinology and Metabolism. American College of Physicians, Philadelphia, PA, 2004. 45.

In patients with central hypothyroidism, it is imperative that pituitary-adrenal function be assessed by corticotropin stimulation test, before thyroxine therapy is initiated. In central hypothyroidism, the sufficiency of thyroxine treatment is monitored using symptoms and using serum T_4 levels, with the goal of maintaining levels in the upper normal range. There is no role of TSH measurement in monitoring effectiveness of treatment in central hypothyroidism.

In patients who have undergone thyroidectomy for thyroid cancer, the goal of treatment is not just to treat hypothyroidism, but also to prevent recurrence of thyroid cancer. TSH goal should be less than 0.01 mU/L if the patient has metastatic or inoperable disease, and 0.05 to 0.5 mU/L in most other cases.

Management of Myxedema Coma

Treatment of myxedema coma includes thyroid hormone replacement, supportive measures, and management of the precipitating process. Before treatment is initiated, measure TSH, free T_4, and cortisol levels.

Combination therapy is recommended with an initial dose of 200–300 mcg of intravenous (IV) T_4 depending on body weight, followed by daily 50–100 mcg IV T_4 until the patient can take oral thyroxine. T_3 is given at the same time, with an initial dose of 5–20 mcg followed by 2.5–10 mcg every 8 hours based on age and patient's cardiovascular risk, and it is continued until the patient is stable.[53] Patients might also need supportive measures, including mechanical ventilation, fluid repletion, and correction of any coexisting hypothermia and hyponatremia. High-dose steroids (e.g., hydrocortisone 100 mg IV every 8–12 hours for 2 days, then lower doses) should be given until adrenal insufficiency has been ruled out.

Management of Hyperthyroidism

The management of hyperthyroidism usually depends on the etiology. Hyperthyroidism with a high radioiodine uptake indicates *de novo* synthesis of hormone. These disorders can be treated with a thionamide, such as methimazole, which will interfere with thyroid hormone synthesis.

Hyperthyroidism with a low radioiodine uptake indicates either release of preformed hormone into the circulation due to inflammation and destruction of thyroid tissue (e.g., lymphocytic thyroiditis) or an extrathyroidal source of thyroid hormone. Thyroid

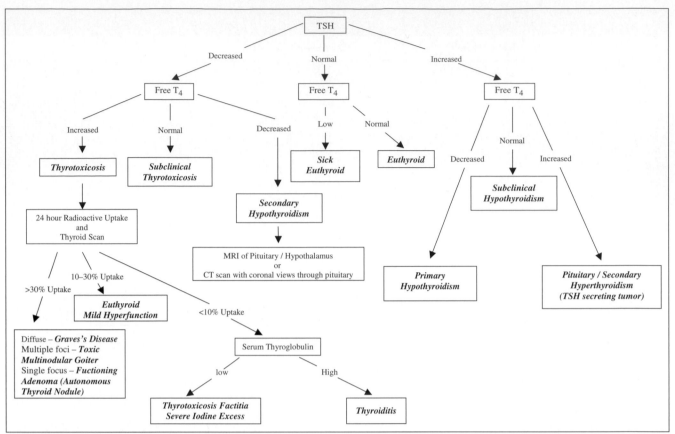

Figure 63-2 • Approach to thyroid disorders. Adapted from: Approach to Thyroid Disorders (figure). In: Sabatine MS, ed. Pocket Medicine. The Massachusetts General Hospital Handbook of Internal Medicine, Endocrinology. Philadelphia: Lippincott William & Wilkins, 2000.

hormone is not being actively synthesized when hyperthyroidism is due to thyroid inflammation; as a result, thionamide therapy is not useful in these disorders. Therapy consists of β-blockers for symptomatic control and anti-inflammatory drugs such as aspirin or nonsteroidal antiinflammatory drugs, or, in severe cases, prednisone.[54] Ipodate is also useful, as it blocks both the conversion of T_4 to T_3 and reduces the tissue effects of thyroid hormone.[55]

Hyperthyroid patients should be treated with β-blockers to ameliorate the β-andrenergic symptoms (palpitations, tachycardia, tremulousness, anxiety, and heat intolerance) associated with this condition.[56] Propranolol in high doses (above 160 mg/day), or the β1-selective agents, atenolol and metoprolol, are preferred.[57] There are questions about the use of β-blockers to treat hyperthyroidism during pregnancy, as one report demonstrated an increased risk of spontaneous abortion risk with treatment with propranolol and a thionamide versus a thionamide alone.[58]

Management of Thyroid Storm

Thyroid storm warrants an ICU admission, and treatment usually consists of several medications[59]:

- A **thionamide**, such as methimazole (MMI) or propylthiouracil (PTU) to block new hormone synthesis. Recommended doses are MMI 20–30 mg every 6 hours or PTU 200–250 mg every 4 hours.[60] Both medications can be given rectally.[60,61] PTU can also be given intravenously; a dose of 576 mg/day at 50 mg/mL has been used to attain euthyroidism.[62] While PTU blocks peripheral conversion of T_4 to T_3, if the patient is also being treated with an iodinated radiocontrast agent (see below) then the longer half-life of methimazole makes it preferable. Patients unable to take a thionamide or those who are allergic to iodinated radiocontrast agents can be treated with lithium bicarbonate at an initial oral dose of 300 mg every 6 hours, with titration to serum levels of around 1 mEq/L.[63]

- A **beta-blocker** to control the symptoms induced by increased adrenergic tone. Propanolol at an initial oral dose as a high as 80–120 mg every 6 hours can be given. IV administration of propranolol at an initial dose of 0.5–1 mg over 10 minutes with cardiac monitoring, then 1–3 mg (over 10 min) every several hours is used for those unable to take oral medications.[64] Esmolol, a short-acting beta-blocker, is used as an alternative regimen, especially in patients with relative contraindication to propanolol (asthma, CHF or DM). An IV loading dose of 250–500 mcg/kg over 10 minutes is given, followed by an infusion at 50–100 mcg/kg per min.[65]

- An **iodinated radiocontrast agent** to inhibit the peripheral conversion of T_4 to T_3. Iopanoic acid and other iodinated radiocontrast agents are currently not approved by the Food and Drug Administration for the management of thyroid storm. They have been used at an initial loading dose of 2 g IV, followed by 1 g IV daily, given at least an hour after thionamide administration to prevent the use of the iodine load for synthesis of new hormone.[66]

- An **iodine solution** to block the release of thyroid hormone through the Wolff-Chaikoff effect, where thyroid excess can cause hypothyroidism by inhibiting the organification of iodine and thus the synthesis of T_3 and T_4. The Wolff-Chaikoff effect is especially seen in patients with chronic autoimmune thyroiditis, or in those who have had partial thyroidectomy, radioiodine therapy, or with subacute thyroiditis from any etiology. Iodine solution regimens include Lugol's solution (30 drops PO daily in 3 or 4 divided doses) or a saturated solution of potassium iodide (SSKI) at 5–8 drops every 6 hours. Importantly, iodine should be administered at least an hour after thionamide administration; otherwise, it may be utilized for new thyroid hormone synthesis. IV sodium iodide (0.5–1 g IV every 12 hours) can also be used. Ten drops of Lugol's solution can be added to IV fluids, and given IV or rectally.[67,68]

- **Glucocorticoids** to reduce T_4 to T_3 conversion and possibly to treat any autoimmune process (e.g., Graves' disease). Hydrocortisone 100 mg intravenously every 8 hours is standard.

- **Supportive Care** is an integral part of thyroid storm management. Some patients require substantial amounts of fluids, while those with CHF might need diuresis and digoxin. Infections should be aggressively treated, and hyperpyrexia treated with acetaminophen as opposed to aspirin, which can increase serum free thyroxine (T_4) and triiodothyronine (T_3) concentrations by interfering with protein binding. If not contraindicated, anticoagulation should be initiated promptly in patients with atrial fibrillation.

PREVENTION

Both myxedema coma and thyroid storm can be avoided by aggressive management of a patient's thyroid disorder and of the aggravating factors. Other systemic complications of hypothyroidism and hyperthyroidism can also be prevented by treating the underlying thyroid disorder.

DISCHARGE/FOLLOW-UP PLANS

Chronic hyperthyroidism is associated with loss of bone density and increased fracture risk.[69,70] Thus, postdischarge, suppressive therapy for hyperthyroidism should be titrated to maintain a slightly low serum TSH concentration (e.g., between 0.1–0.5 mU/L).[71] Patients with hyperthyroidism should be on calcium supplementation and on inhibitors of bone resorption (e.g., bisphosphonates or calcitonin). Patients should be made aware of the risk of thyroid storm in the setting of aggravating factors.

Patients on levothyroxine treatment should have their TSH level monitored 4–6 weeks after dose changes or after initiation of medications that affect thyroid metabolism.

Key Points

- The serum half-life of T_4 is 8-days, and that of T_3 is 1–1.5 days. Thus, TSH levels should be checked about 4–6 weeks after initiation or change of therapy.

- Always think about how a patient's medical regimen will affect his or her thyroid hormone function, or how the regimen will alter the effectiveness of thyroid replacement therapy.

- Screening for thyroid dysfunction is generally discouraged in the acutely ill patient, but if there are strong indications for this, both TSH and free T_4 levels should be checked.

- Parenteral T_4 should only be given if a patient is unable take oral T_4 for 5–7 days. The dose should be about 80% of the patient's usual oral dose, as this is the fraction of the oral dose that is usually absorbed.

- Myxedema coma usually presents with hypoventilation, hypotension, hypothermia, and hyponatremia.

- Treatment of myxedema coma usually consists of thyroid hormone replacement (with both T_3 and T_4), high-dose steroids until adrenal insufficiency is ruled out, supportive measures, and management of the precipitating process.

- Thyroid storm usually presents with fever, tachycardia, CNS dysfunction, and GI disturbance.

- Treatment of thyroid storm usually consists of a thionamide, beta-blocker, an iodine solution, glucocorticoids, and supportive measures.

SUGGESTED READING

Wood AJ. Drugs and thyroid Function. N Engl J Med 1995; 333:1688–1694.

Klein I. Thyroid hormone and the cardiovascular system. Am J Med 1990; 88(6):631–637.

Fliers E, Wiersinga WM. Myxedema coma. Rev Endocr Metabol Disord 2003; 4:137–141.

Sarlis NJ, Gourgiotis L. Thyroid emergencies. Reviews in Endocrine & Metabolic Disorders 2003; 4:129–136.

Baloc Z, Carayon, P, Conte-Devolx B, et al. Laboratory medicine practice guidelines: Laboratory support for the diagnosis and monitoring of thyroid disease. Thyroid 2003; 13:3.

Wall CR. Myxedema coma: diagnosis and treatment. Am Fam Phycisian 2000; 62:2485–2490.

Tietgens ST, Leinung MC. Thyroid storm. Med Clin North Am 1995; 79:169–184.

CHAPTER SIXTY-FOUR

Adrenal Insufficiency in Hospitalized Patients

Mahsheed Khajavi, MD

BACKGROUND

Adrenal insufficiency increasingly must be considered in evaluating hospitalized patients. While primary disease is rare, the growing use of exogenous corticosteroids makes secondary adrenal insufficiency more prevalent. Acute adrenal insufficiency from any cause can mimic septic shock, with decreased peripheral vascular resistance and increased cardiac output.[1,2] Clinical assessment and diagnosis of adrenal insufficiency in acutely ill patients are difficult, with tremendous overlap between signs/symptoms suggestive of adrenal insufficiency and those of sepsis, cardiogenic shock, and volume depletion.[3] Hypotension refractory to catecholamines, diarrhea, vomiting, and alteration in mental status ranging from delirium to obtundation, as well as hypoglycemia, can be attributed to both sepsis and adrenal insufficiency.

Given recent research that supports the role of cortisol replacement when indicated to improve outcomes in critically ill patients,[4–6] it is essential that the inpatient clinician be aware of the possibility of adrenal insufficiency. This is especially important in three patient populations: (1) patients with known dysfunction and on steroid replacement therapy, (2) patients with other illnesses requiring chronic steroid use (e.g., autoimmune disorders and asthma), and (3) patients who have occult impaired adrenal reserve during critical illness, termed "relative adrenal insufficiency."

This chapter focuses on the diagnosis and treatment of adrenal insufficiency in hospitalized patients, and describes the clinical presentation of susceptible patients and studies done to determine appropriate diagnosis and therapeutic interventions.

PATHOPHYSIOLOGY

The glucocorticoids, including cortisol, are secreted from the adrenal cortex in humans. In healthy individuals, cortisol is secreted in response to adrenocorticotropic hormone (ACTH) from the pituitary gland. The neural control of pituitary ACTH secretion comes from corticotropin-releasing hormone (CRH) secreted by the hypothalamus. Both CRH and ACTH are subject to negative feedback by plasma cortisol levels.[7] This hypothalamic pituitary adrenal axis (HPA) is a major determinant of the host response to stress[8] (Fig. 64-1). Sepsis,[9,10] surgery,[11] anesthesia,[12–14] and certain trauma[15] result in heightened activation of the HPA axis. The result is a sustained increase in cortisol secretion. Cortisol is essential for the maintenance of vascular tone and permeability.[16–18] Cortisol concentrations also directly parallel the degree and extent of surgery and the severity of illness.[19–22]

Approximately 90% of circulating cortisol is bound to corticosteroid binding globulin, leaving 10% as bioavailable. The free hormone exerts its effect when it leaves the circulation and binds to intracellular receptors (glucocorticoid receptors).[23] In healthy individuals, cortisol is secreted in a diurnal mode with the highest levels in the morning and a gradual decline to an evening nadir. However, in patients with acute adrenal insufficiency, this pattern is lost, and ACTH levels are increased.[19,20]

Cortisol has a permissive effect on vascular tone by enhancing vascular responsiveness to vasopressors without a sustained effect when given alone.[24] Cortisol therefore has a vital role in the maintenance of vascular tone and permeability, and it is essential for circulatory stability. Cortisol also suppresses immunologic responses in a variety of ways. Cortisol decreases the accumulation and function of monocytes, lymphocytes, natural killer cells, macrophages, neutrophils, and eosinophils.[25,26]

ASSESSMENT

Diagnosis

Clinical Presentation

Acute adrenal insufficiency is characterized by hypotension refractory to both administration of adequate fluid resuscitation and vasopressor therapy.[3] In addition, it may be accompanied by increased or decreased cardiac output and persistent systemic inflammation.[27] Chronic adrenal insufficiency presents more insidiously, with constitutional symptoms such as fatigue, malaise, generalized weakness, and anorexia. Classically, patients complain of vague abdominal discomfort associated with nausea, possibly vomiting, and diarrhea.

Primary adrenal insufficiency is rare and is estimated to have a prevalence of 4–11 cases per 100,000. Primary hypoadrenalism is caused by adrenal disease (autoimmune, infectious, hemorrhagic, metastatic disease, and adrenalectomy). Secondary hypoadrenalism results from decreased ACTH production. This can be central (i.e., pituitary hypofunction) or, much more commonly, iatrogenic (as the result of glucocorticoid therapy). This

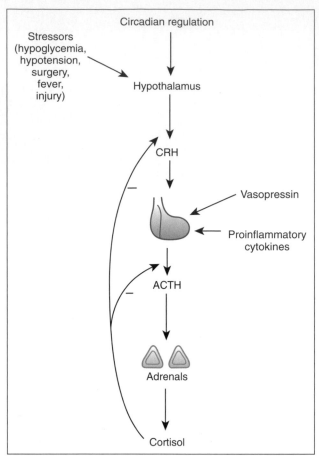

Figure 64-1 • Schematic outline of regulation of the HPA axis.

Box 64-1 Diagnosis of Adrenal Insufficiency

1) Cortisol level

   a. Morning level below 3 mcg/dL rules in disease

2) ACTH level (usually not rapidly available)*

   a. High level with low cortisol diagnoses primary adrenal insufficiency

   b. Low level with low due to pituitary or hypothalamic disease

3) ACTH Stimulation Test[†]

   a. Cosyntropin 250 mcg/dL IV bolus

   b. Measure cortisol 30 and 60 minutes later

   c. Cortisol <18 mcg/dL rules in adrenal insufficiency (95% specificity)

   d. Cortisol ≥18 mcg/dL rules out primary adrenal insufficiency (97.5% sensitivity)

4) Imaging

   a. Abdominal CT of the adrenal glands and possible biopsy for patients with primary adrenal insufficiency

   b. Pituitary CT or MRI for patients with secondary or tertiary adrenal insufficiency

*Must be drawn prior to glucocorticoid treatment.
[†]Dexamethasone is not measured in the assay and may be given prior to testing.
ACTH—adrenocorticotropic hormone; CT—computed tomography; MRI—magnetic resonance imaging

---

distinction is important because hypotension is always associated with primary adrenal insufficiency (on the basis of an inability to produce mineralocorticoids as well as glucocorticoids), but it occurs much less commonly with secondary hypoadrenalism. In the healthy individual who has secondary hypoadrenalism on the basis of exogenous steroid therapy, only ACTH is decreased, and, therefore, the renin–angiotensin axis is intact. Patients may not exhibit hypotension or other signs of acute adrenal insufficiency until such times when there is exposure to the stress of acute illness, anesthesia, or prolonged surgery.

Secondary hypoadrenalism caused by glucocorticoid therapy (intravenous, oral, inhaled, or topical) is much more common, given the large number of patients receiving these medications.[28] Interestingly, despite the number of patients on glucocorticoid therapy, steroid-induced adrenal crisis is rare among perioperative patients. Multiple well-documented case reports have been published,[29–31] but there has been no consensus regarding the time and duration of steroid use that increases the risk of adrenal failure; a tight correlation between chronic dose amount and existence of insufficiency on withdrawal does not appear to exist. Finally, the biochemical diagnostic criteria for adrenal failure are still a subject of controversy, and there are no exact data as to what adrenal response is appropriate in the critically ill patient.

There are no consistent data to delineate criteria for HPA suppression and identify patients at highest risk for adrenal insufficiency during the perioperative period. A subnormal response to ACTH (250 mcg) was found after only 3 days of supraphysiolog-

ical doses of prednisone;[32] at lower doses, HPA suppression was noted after 1 week to 1 month.[33,34] However, subnormal response to ACTH is not always associated with hypoadrenalism during anesthesia or surgery. It is possible that patients who undergo general anesthesia and surgery may have subnormal plasma cortisol responses to hypoglycemia or high dose ACTH but no differences in surgical outcomes when compared to controls.[35,36] Moreover, adrenal insufficiency is extremely low after routine surgery. Three large studies support this. Of the 11,311 patients who underwent urologic and cardiac procedures, only six patients (0.05%) were reported to have had adrenal insufficiency.[29,30] An even larger evaluation of 70,000 patients undergoing anesthesia found only nine patients who developed hypotension attributable to glucocorticoid insufficiency.[37]

Lastly, absence of a normal corticosteroid response to critical illness despite an anatomically intact HPA axis has been labeled "relative adrenal insufficiency." Consensus regarding the diagnostic criteria for this entity also is yet to be established.

Laboratory Testing

Diagnosing adrenal insufficiency requires demonstrating inappropriately low cortisol production as the first step (Box 64-1). Normally, cortisol levels are higher in the early morning (i.e., 6:00 a.m.), ranging from 10 to 20 mcg/dL. Thus, a morning level <3 mcg/dL diagnoses adrenal insufficiency, while results of 3 to 10 mcg/dL are suggestive. However, normal levels of cortisol levels follow the circadian rhythm of ACTH secretion and range from 3 to 10 mcg/dL by late afternoon (e.g., 4:00 p.m.) and then drop <5 mcg/dL an hour after typical sleep time onset. Unfortunately, while morning levels <5 mcg/dL have almost 100% specificity (i.e., levels <5 rule in adrenal insufficiency), sensitivity is only 36% (i.e., many patients with adrenal insufficiency will have levels >5). Sensitivity increases to 62% with a cut-off of 10 mcg/dL, but specificity drops to 77%.

Ideally, serum cortisol and ACTH could be measured simultaneously with immediate availability of results making diagnosis quick; but while results from cortisol testing are usually readily available, the ACTH laboratory assay is not. Patients with primary adrenal disease have inappropriately low cortisol levels and very high plasma ACTH. Adrenal insufficiency from pituitary (secondary) or hypothalamic (tertiary) disease correlates with low levels of both cortisol and ACTH. As an alternative, performance of a stimulation test with cosyntropin (synthetic ACTH) at any time of day can provide more rapid results. Serum cortisol should rise to 18 mcg/dL or higher 30 or 60 minutes after an IV bolus of 250 mcg of cosyntropin. Specificity is 95%, while sensitivity is 97.5% for primary adrenal insufficiency, but 57% for secondary. Thus, a muted response of cortisol to cosyntropin stimulation establishes the likely diagnosis of adrenal insufficiency, and a normal response rules out primary adrenal insufficiency. However, a normal response does not exclude the possibility of secondary adrenal insufficiency. Consultation with an endocrinologist is essential for more sophisticated testing of the HPA axis.

Relative Adrenal Insufficiency in Shock

Even among patients who have not been on chronic exogenous steroid therapy, severe illness can provoke a state of relative adrenal insufficiency in about half of patients in the intensive care unit (ICU) in shock. Patients with critical illness may have a blunted response to ACTH with little adrenal reserve. Alternatively, the adrenal gland may be maximally stimulated but still inadequate because of corticosteroid resistance at the tissue level. Studies consistently document increasing serum levels of cortisol and catecholamines with severity of illness.[8,38,39] The degree of HPA activation and subsequent plasma cortisol level is a direct function of illness severity.[8] Unfortunately, no definite laboratory diagnosis exists for relative adrenal insufficiency in septic shock.

As noted above, a serum cortisol of >18 in response to high-dose ACTH (250 mcg) was regarded as an appropriate adrenal response.[10] However, these values were based on concentrations determined using healthy and noncritically ill patients. Stress from illness elevates cytokines in the circulation, which stimulate the HPA axis. Cytokines can increase tissue cortisol levels by increasing cortisol receptor sensitivity and decreasing peripheral cortisol metabolism.[10,11] Conversely, cytokines in septic patients have been implicated in the direct inhibition of adrenal cortisol production.[42,43] Research also supports the hypothesis that although plasma cortisol levels are high, there is an attenuated effect of cortisol at local inflammatory sites.[44] Thus, patients can have high cortisol levels but a cortisol resistance syndrome.

In response to hypotension and severe illness, measured random cortisol levels are significantly higher than 18 mcg/dL in the vast majority of such patients, averaging 45–50 mcg/dL.[45,46] The rate of cortisol change in response to a cosyntropin stimulation test appears most predictive of relative adrenal insufficiency. A study of 189 patients meeting clinical criteria for septic shock found that a change in cortisol level of <9 mcg/dL after cosyntropin stimulation was an independent predictor of mortality. Of note, random cortisol levels of >34 mcg/dL in association with a

Box 64-2 Therapy for Adrenal Crisis

- Establish IV access and send blood for stat routine laboratories (i.e., electrolytes, glucose, BUN, Cr, and CBC), cortisol, and ACTH.
- Initiate therapy prior to test results becoming available.
- Infuse 2 to 3 L of normal saline of D_5NS rapidly to support blood pressure while monitoring the patient for volume overload.
- Administer dexamethasone 4 mg IV (preferred because it does not interfere with subsequent ACTH stimulation testing), or alternatively hydrocortisone 100 mg.
- Identify precipitating etiology, especially if infection present, and treat accordingly.
- Continue high-dose IV steroids for 1–3 days if precipitating illness resolving.
- Start mineralocorticoid (fludrocortisone, 100 mcg PO daily) when IV fluids stopped.

ACTH—adrenocorticotropic hormone; BUN—blood urea nitrogen; Cr—creatinine; CBC—complete blood count

cosyntropin stimulation response of ≤9 mcg/dL were associated with the highest mortality (82% at 28 days). Conversely, those patients with random cortisol level of <34 and a change in cortisol of >9 mcg/dL had the best outcomes, with a 26% mortality rate at 28 days.[44] Patients with cortisol levels >34 and cosyntropin response of >9 mcg/dL or cortisol level <34 and inadequate cosyntropin response of ≤9 mcg/dL had intermediate risk.

The above assays were performed using total serum cortisol levels. More recent literature indicates that serum-free cortisol levels may be more useful in determining relative adrenal insufficiency in critically ill patients. The measurement of serum-free cortisol appears significantly more accurate in determining actual adrenal function in patients who have hypoproteinemia, but further studies are needed to help define parameters for the measurement and predictive value of serum free cortisol.

MANAGEMENT

Treatment of adrenal insufficiency in hospitalized patients is dependent on the situation and can be categorized into patients with acute adrenal crisis, those in the perioperative setting, and patients with septic shock and relative adrenal insufficiency.

Adrenal Crisis

An adrenal crisis represents a true life-threatening emergency and situation requiring "stat" diagnosis and treatment (Box 64-2). Suspicion should be high when patients on chronic steroids present with hypotension unresponsive to IV fluids. After routine blood studies and initial diagnostic studies are sent as noted above (e.g., baseline cortisol), patients should be administered large volumes of saline and corticosteroids intravenously. IV fluids with dextrose (e.g., D_5NS) can be given if hypoglycemia is present or a concern. Dexamethasone (4 mg) is preferred, as it is long lasting and does not interfere with the ACTH stimulation test. Following completion of this test, hydrocortisone 100 mg IV every 6–8 hours can be given. Of note, treatment with mineralocorticoids is not helpful in the acute setting of an adrenal crisis because their effect requires several days to produce adequate sodium retention. Intravenous saline is adequate during this initial phase.

After initial treatment, efforts should focus on identifying the precipitating cause (e.g., infection) and rendering directed therapy. Upon stabilization of the patient, a cosyntropin stimulation test should be performed to confirm the diagnosis of adrenal insufficiency in patients not known to have disease. Once the diagnosis of adrenal insufficiency is confirmed, consultation with an endocrinologist is reasonable to help with subsequent testing to determine the exact cause.

For patients with known adrenal insufficiency, regardless of the cause, who are admitted to the hospital with intercurrent illness, supplementation with hydrocortisone should be considered. For "moderate" illness, a dose of 50 mg twice daily of hydrocortisone is recommended, and up to 100 mg IV every 8 hours may be given for "severe" illness. The dose of steroids can be rapidly tapered over 1–3 days back to maintenance doses as the patient recovers.

Perioperative or Pre-Procedure Treatment

For patients on chronic glucocorticoid therapy and at risk for this type of secondary adrenal insufficiency, physicians historically used large doses of steroids perioperatively and continued those doses for extended periods of time for fear of precipitating adrenal crisis. Subsequent studies did not support this approach.[47] Randomized, prospective trials of patients who had undergone abdominal and joint surgery concluded that patients who received the baseline preoperative dose of steroids had no increase in adverse outcomes and no evidence of acute adrenal insufficiency.[48] Not surprisingly, the risk of anesthesia and surgery parallels the duration and severity of the procedure as well as the severity of the underlying illness.

Based on these findings, recommendations for corticosteroid therapy in the perioperative setting indicate that:

- For minor procedures (i.e., local anesthesia), elective surgery in healthy patients, or most radiologic studies, maintenance corticosteroid therapy is recommended, and patients should continue taking their preoperative doses with no supplementation.
- For more "stressful" events such as endoscopy or arteriography, administration of one dose of 100 mg IV hydrocortisone immediately prior to the procedure and no subsequent supplementation is reasonable.
- For major surgery, 100 mg of hydrocortisone can be given IV just before anesthesia induction. Postoperatively, the same dose can be given q8 hours for one day and then rapidly tapered ($\frac{1}{2}$ dose decreased per day) back to the patient's maintenance level.

Relative Adrenal Insufficiency in Septic Shock

Hypotension refractory to adequate volume resuscitation and requiring vasopressors therapy is the most common clinical indicator of relative adrenal insufficiency.[7,46] A growing body of evidence suggests improved outcomes in some critically ill patients who receive low-dose steroid supplementation.[4-6,49-51] The results, however, depend upon the definition of adrenal insufficiency.

Initial enthusiasm for steroid use in sepsis began shortly after the introduction of steroids. Case reports in the 1950s

Box 64-3 Use of Corticosteroids in Septic Shock

- Patients with septic shock requiring vasopressors should undergo a high-dose (250 mcg) ACTH stimulation test with baseline cortisol and then 30- and 60-minute levels.
- Immediately following completion of the ACTH stimulation test, hydrocortisone 50–100 mg should be given IV and then 50 mg every 6 hours or 100 mg q 8 hours.
- Continue corticosteroids at full doses for 7 days if the maximum increase of serum cortisol is ≤9 mcg/dL after ACTH stimulation.
- Consider continuing corticosteroids for 7 days if there is a hemodynamic response to therapy with vasopressor withdrawal possible within 48 hours of starting steroid therapy.
- Discontinue corticosteroids in patients who demonstrate a serum cortisol increase of >9 mcg/dL following ACTH stimulation and no hemodynamic response to corticosteroid therapy.
- If the results of an ACTH stimulation testing are not be available within 48 hours, consider initiating corticosteroids in all patients with septic shock, with continuation versus discontinuation determined by clinical response.
- Fludrocortisone (50 mcg) can also be administered four times daily, but some experts believe this is unnecessary, as hydrocortisone may have sufficient mineralocorticoid activity.
- Patients on maintenance steroid therapy prior to the event of septic shock should be given stress dose steroids as indicated.

demonstrated improved outcomes in patients with sepsis who were treated with high-dose steroids. A study published in 1976 indicated a decrease in mortality rates when high-dose steroids were given to patients with septic shock.[52] Two subsequent large, multicenter trials published in 1987 demonstrated no benefit of steroids and suggested possible harm.[53,54] Use of steroids in patients with septic shock fell out of favor until reports in the 1990s indicated improved outcomes when lower doses of steroids were used.[55,56]

Then in 2002, Annane and colleagues published a large placebo-controlled clinical trial that enrolled 299 patients with septic shock from 19 medical ICUs in France.[4] Patients were randomized to receive placebo or 7 days of both hydrocortisone (50 mg IV every 6 hours) and fludrocortisone (50 mcg QID). The patients were further assigned to the categories of "non-responders" (ACTH-stimulated plasma cortisol increase of ≤9 mcg/dL) or "responders" (ACTH-stimulated plasma cortisol of >9 mcg/dL). A subsequent meta-analysis confirmed these results, with an absolute risk reduction in mortality at 28 days of about 10% when patients with septic shock received steroids. Of note, in the absence of vasopressor-dependent septic shock, there is no evidence to support the use of low-dose steroids.

Box 64-3 delineates the recommendations of the Surviving Sepsis Campaign Guideline Committee[57] for use of diagnostic studies and steroid treatment among patients with septic shock. There is no evidence to support the use of any particular steroid, but hydrocortisone is recommended. The rationale for this is three fold: (a) most well-designed studies used hydrocortisone; (b) hydrocortisone is equivalent to cortisol, and therefore there is no concern regarding metabolism of a precursor; and (c) hydrocortisone has mineralocorticoid activity while dexamethasone and methylprednisolone do not.

Currently, an ongoing international study (Corticosteroid Therapy of Septic Shock, CORTICUS) should help to develop a rational diagnostic testing system and recommendations for corticosteroid therapy in patients with septic shock. This study began in 2002 and is scheduled to be completed in 2007. Until those results are interpreted and published, low-dose corticosteroids given to catecholamine-dependent septic patients is reasonable and rational. Meanwhile, a recent analysis showed that 7-day treatment with the combination of low-dose hydrocortisone and fludrocortisone improved survival and reduced duration of mechanical ventilation among patients with septic shock and early Acute Respiratory Distress Syndrome (ARDS) if they also had documented relative adrenal insufficiency (i.e., cortisol response ≤9 mcg/dL to cosyntropin stimulation).[58]

DISCHARGE/FOLLOW-UP PLANS

All patients requiring steroid replacement for adrenal insufficiency while in the hospital will need outpatient follow-up. Those with primary adrenal insufficiency who require chronic steroid therapy will need follow-up with an endocrinologist as well as their primary care provider. Patients discharged on chronic steroid therapy require education to ensure they are alert to their increased susceptibility to infection (ranging from thrush to more serious infections) and that exposure to physiologic stress may indicate a need for higher doses of steroids. Use of a MedicAlert bracelet is recommended.

Key Points

- Acute adrenal insufficiency is characterized by hypotension refractory to both administration of adequate fluid resuscitation and vasopressor therapy.

- An adrenal crisis represents a true life-threatening emergency and situation requiring "stat" diagnosis and treatment with both intravenous saline and steroids.

- Patients with septic shock may have relative adrenal insufficiency and should undergo testing to confirm this, and hydrocortisone should be administered initially until test results guide subsequent treatment.

- Patients in septic shock who have a cortisol response of ≤9 mcg/dL to cosyntropin stimulation are considered "nonresponders" and benefit from hydrocortisone replacement therapy.

SUGGESTED READING

Rivers EP, Gaspari M, Abi Saad G, et al. Adrenal insufficiency in high risk surgical ICU patients. Chest 2001; 119:889–896.

Lamberts SWJ, Bruining HA, de Jong FH. Corticosteroid therapy in severe illness. N Engl J Med 1997; 337:1285–1292.

Streeten DHP. What test for hypothalamic-pituitary adrenocortical insufficiency? Lancet 1999; 354:179–180.

Annane D, Sebille V, Charpentier C, et al. Effect of treatment of treatment with low doses of hydrocortisone and fludrocortisone on mortality in patients with septic shock. JAMA 2002; 288:862–871.

Salem M, Tainish Jr. RE, Bromberg J, et al. Perioperative glucocorticoid coverage: A reassessment 42 years after emergence of a problem. Ann Surg 1994; 219:416–425.

Glowniak JV, Loriaux DL, A double-blind study of perioperative steroid requirements in secondary adrenal insufficiency. Surgery 1997; 121:123–129.

Annane D, Sebille V, Troche G, et al. A 3-level prognostic classification in septic shock based on cortisol levels and cortisol response to corticotropin. JAMA 2000; 283:1038–1045.

Hamrahian AH, Oseni TS, Arafah BM. Measurements of serum free cortisol in critically ill patients. N Engl J Med 2004; 350:1629–1638.

Annane DJ, Bellissant E, Bollaert PE, et al. Corticosteroids for severe sepsis and septic shock: a systemic review and meta-analysis. BMJ 2004; 329:480.

Minneci PC, Deans KJ, Banks SM, et al. Meta-analysis: the effects of steroids on survival and shock during sepsis depends on the dose. Ann Inern Med 2004; 141:47–56.

Dellinger RP, Carlet JM, Masur H, et al. Surviving sepsis campaign guidelines for management of severe sepsis and septic shock. Crit Care Med 2004; 32:858–873.

Annane D, Sebille V, Bellissant E. Ger-Inf-05 Study Group. Effect of low doses of corticosteroids in septic shock patients with or without early acute respiratory distress syndrome. Crit Care Med 2006; 34:22–30.

CHAPTER SIXTY-FIVE

Central Diabetes Insipidus Following Craniotomy

Kanchan Kamath, MD

BACKGROUND

Neurosurgery and trauma account for the vast majority of cases of central diabetes insipidus (DI) followed by primary or secondary neoplasms or infiltrative diseases such as Langerhan's cell histiocytosis, lymphocytic hypophysitis, sarcoidosis or a metastatic process that may affect either the hypothalamus or the posterior pituitary. Hypoxic or ischemic encephalopathy may also cause central DI. Transient postoperative DI occurs in approximately 12% of patients who have undergone intracranial sur-gery, with this being permanent in approximately 3% of these patients.[1] This chapter focuses on central DI. Chapter 51 provides a detailed review of the assessment and management of both hypo- and hypernatremia, including nephrogenic diabetes insipidus.

PATHOPHYSIOLOGY

Central DI is a metabolic disorder resulting from direct insult to the neurohypophysis. Postsurgical transient diabetes insipidus results from inflammatory edema around the hypothalamus or posterior pituitary and resolves with resolution of the edema. It may also be secondary to damage to the supraoptic and paraventricular neurons of the hypothalamus, the pituitary stalk, or the axon terminal in the posterior pituitary.[2] This, in turn, causes decreased secretion or impaired transportation of arginine vasopressin, the antidiuretic hormone (ADH). Arginine vasopressin is secreted by the supraoptic and paraventricular nuclei in the hypothalamus and transported via the neurons of the pituitary stalk to storage in the posterior pituitary.

A triphasic response may be noted in some cases after injury to the hypothalamus or the supraoptic hypophyseal tract. However, the relative frequency of these responses may vary, based on the size and involvement of the tumor excised, neurosurgical approach (transsphenoidal vs. craniotomy), and the extent of surgical injury.

1. Polyuric phase: Beginning within 24 hours and lasting over 4–5 days. This is secondary to ADH inhibition from hypothalamic dysfunction.
2. Antidiuretic phase: Lasts roughly from days 6–11 and is secondary to release of stored ADH from the disintegrating posterior pituitary. Excessive water intake can occur during this phase, giving a syndrome consistent with inappropriate ADH (SiADH).
3. Permanent DI: May or may not ensue, depending on the extent of neurohypophyseal injury.[3,4]

ASSESSMENT

Clinical Presentation/Diagnosis

If not treated, the clinical course of DI after neurosurgery can often be marred by complications from significant neurologic and cognitive disabilities secondary to abnormalities in water and sodium homeostasis. This is especially true in the early postsurgical phase, as patients are unable to compensate adequately for the water loss because of impaired cognition, and a coexisting hypodipsic state.

A neurosurgeon may seek internal medicine consultation for a patient to evaluate and manage hypernatremia and commensurate signs of hypovolemia such as tachycardia, postural hypotension, azotemia, hyperuricemia, and hypokalemia. This constellation of findings should steer an astute internist to consider DI, especially if polyuria is present.

The clinical hallmark of diabetes insipidus is the patient's inability to concentrate urine, yielding large volumes of dilute urine typically in excess of 3 L per day. This can lead to hyperosmolar, hypernatremic dehydration if the patient is unable to ingest adequate free water or there is inadequate concurrent IV fluid administration. The onset of polyuria from central DI is usually abrupt.

It is not a common practice in postsurgical patients to perform a formal water deprivation test to reach a diagnosis of diabetes insipidus. Instead, the diagnosis is ascertained clinically when the urine osmolality is inappropriately low relative to the serum osmolality. The clinical setting includes a high plasma osmolality >295 mmol/kg, an elevated serum sodium, and a urine osmolality of less than 300 mOsm/kg or a urine specific gravity of less than 1.010 (Table 65-1).

Administration of exogenous ADH can further distinguish between central and nephrogenic DI. The urine osmolality will rise at least by 50% or more in central DI after ADH initiation, but ADH will have minimal or no effect in the latter (See Figure 65-1).

Table 65-1 Principal Imbalances in Diabetes Insipidus

	Plasma	Urine
Intravascular Volume	Reduced	
Urine output	—	>200 mL/hr or >50 mL/kg/24hr
Sodium	>150 meq/L	<15 meq/L
Osmolality	>300 mOsm/L	<300 mOsm/L
Specific Gravity	—	<1.010

Early identification and treatment of patients with post-surgical DI optimize their potential for recovery and improve morbidity.

MANAGEMENT

Treatment

Acute management of postsurgical DI requires careful monitoring and balancing of fluid intake and output. In addition to fluid replacement, treatment is also aimed at decreasing urine output by antidiuretic hormone replacement[5] (Fig. 65-2).

In mild cases in which the patient is alert and can achieve ample fluid intake orally, it may be sufficient simply to allow free access to fluid with careful monitoring. More often, patients are not able to do this, due to underlying disease or the postoperative state.

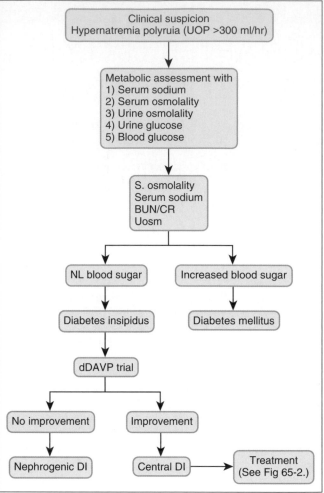

Figure 65-1 • Post Craniotomy DI Management and Treatment.

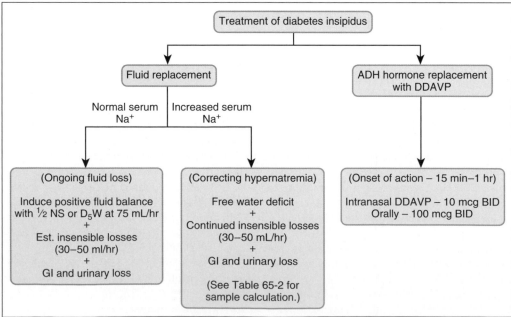

Figure 65-2 • Treatment.

Fluid Replacement

Two major components need to be addressed while replacing fluids.

Replacement of Urinary Loss

Each hour, the patient should receive maintenance fluids (preferably 1/2 normal saline; 0.45 NS) plus roughly three quarters of the previous hour's urinary fluid loss, with the cautions noted below. Though D_5W has been used for replacement, there is potential risk of severe and symptomatic hyperglycemia, especially at rates greater than 1000 mL/hr. This may occur even in the absence of diabetes mellitus. Marked glucosuria resulting from hyperglycemia can further complicate the picture, as this can lead to an osmotic diuresis that is ADH-resistant.

Given the potential for this approach to result in ever-increasing volumes of IV fluid administration, the clinician should monitor the patient closely for volume overload. Clinical judgment should be applied to ensure that the regimen is curtailed or adjusted once euvolemia is achieved. Electrolytes and blood glucose should be frequently monitored. Appropriate potassium replacement should also be undertaken. Insulin should be used to correct hyperglycemia as needed.

Correction of Hypernatremia

Hypernatremia is corrected by replacing the free water deficit. The following formula estimates the water required to return plasma sodium concentration to approximately 140 mEq/L.

Free water deficit = 0.5 body weight (kg) × ((Serum sodium −140)/140).

An allowance for continuing insensible losses (about 40 mL/hr) and gastrointestinal and urinary losses should also be added to the above. Close monitoring of the plasma sodium concentration is essential to confirm the desired rate of correction. Importantly, adjustment of the rate must be made, depending on the type of fluid used for replacement.[1,6] (See Table 65-2 for a sample calculation.)

Hormone Replacement

If the urine output in central DI is greater than 300 mL/hr, for greater than 2 hours consistently, the standard practice now is to replace the deficient hormone. Though there is little evidence on the long-term use of desmopressin (i.e., dDAVP – deamino-D arginine vasopressin) for central DI, limited studies do not suggest any long-term side effects or antibody formation with its use.[7] Intranasal desmopressin delivered by a nasal spray is now the treatment of choice. Though an oral form is available, its potency is 5–10% that of the nasal form, as it is poorly absorbed from the gut. Thus, a 0.1 mg tablet is equivalent to 2.5–5 mcg of the nasal spray.

The nasal formula is titrated upward in increments of 5 mcg until achieving a clinical response with resolution of the polyuria and hypernatremia. The daily maintenance dose thereafter is 5–20 mcg once or twice a day. For long-term management, it is

---

Table 65-2 Sample Calculation

70 kg patient s/p craniotomy POD #4
Plasma sodium concentration of 160 meq/L
(Rise of 30 meq/L over normal)
UOP – 3000 ml q 24° for past 48–72 hours.

Normal serum sodium = 140 meq/L

$$\text{Free water deficit (FWD)} = 0.5 \text{ body wt. (kg)} \times \frac{(\text{serum sodium} - 140)}{140}$$

$$= 0.5 \times 70 \times \frac{(160 - 140)}{140}$$

$$= 35 \times \frac{20}{140} = 4.9 \text{ L approx. } 5.0 \text{ L}$$

Therefore, FWD = 5.0 L

Sodium correction done over 48 to 72 hours.

$$\frac{\text{Total fluid replacement } (235 - 265\,\text{mL/hr})}{\text{Free water deflcit (if hypernatremic) i.e. } 70 - 100\,\text{mL/hr}}$$

If correction over 48 hours

$$\frac{5000 \text{ mL}}{48} = 104 \text{ mL/hr}$$

+

$$\text{Urinary losses/hr ie } \frac{3000 \text{ mL}}{24} = 125 \text{ mL/hr}$$

If correction over 72 hours

+

Insensible losses ie approximately 40 mL/hr

$$\frac{5000 \text{ mL}}{72} = 70 \text{ mL/hr}$$

Therefore, 70–100 mL/hr to correct free water deficit

recommended that the first dose usually be given in the evenings to control nocturia. The effectiveness of the evening dose may then determine the need to add a daytime dose.

Awareness of the potential risk of water retention and hyponatremia from desmopressin use is vital, especially in transient DI. Thus, close follow-up of these patients post discharge is essential for both electrolyte monitoring and titration of desmopressin.[7] Most cases will resolve spontaneously, and specific therapy can be discontinued within a week. Careful monitoring and free access to oral fluids should be ensured.

Alternatives

Other drugs have sometimes been used in conjunction with desmopressin, either to allay the cost, especially with long-term use, or to enhance the effect of the antidiuretic hormone.

1. Chlorpropamide: An oral hypoglycemic agent, it intensifies renal response to ADH.
   Usual dose: 125–250 mg, daily or BID.
   Side effect: hypoglycemia.
2. Carbamazepine: An anticonvulsant, it diminishes polyuria by enhancing the effects of ADH.
   Usual dose: 100–300 mg b.i.d.
3. Clofibrate: An antilipemic agent, it works similar to carbamazepine.
   Usual Dose: 500 mg q 6 hr.

These medications are generally reserved for cases that do not respond to the previous regimens.

DISCHARGE AND FOLLOW-UP

Fortunately, most individuals with transient postcranial surgery-related DI can self-regulate their fluid consumption to match their urine output once they have successfully been managed through the immediate acute post-operative. Intravascular osmotic pressures so strongly govern the perception of thirst that patients will correct any free water deficit if sufficient water is supplied and they are capable of accessing it.

However, it is important to develop a long-term management plan to prevent and minimize any episodes of electrolyte or fluid related mishaps. A practical method that a hospitalist can use to educate his or her patient and help achieve this goal would include:

- Patient education of day-to-day adjustment of fluid intake in accordance with body weight. This is imperative in patients suspected to be hypodipsic, as they are unable to regulate their fluid intake.
- Instructions on proper use of desmopressin (dDAVP) and also its potential complications such as edema and hyponatremia.
- Routine serial measurements of sodium is especially important in the early postdischarge phase. We recommend that the patient undergo lab testing post discharge within at least a week.

Key Points

- Transient postoperative diabetes insipidus (DI) occurs in approximately 12% of patients who have undergone CNS surgery, with this being permanent in approximately 3% of these patients.
- The clinical hallmark of diabetes insipidus is the patient's inability to concentrate urine, with production of a large volume of dilute urine.
- The onset of polyuria from central DI is usually abrupt, while it is more gradual in nephrogenic DI or polydipsia.
- If the urine output in central DI is greater than 300 mL/hr, for greater than 2 hours consistently, the deficient hormone (arginine vasopressin) should be replaced.

SUGGESTED READING

Vance ML. Perioperative management of patients undergoing pituitary surgery. Endocrinol Metab Clin North Am 2003; 32(2)355:365.

Thorton E, O'Kelley P, Tormey W, et al. Posterior pituitary dysfunction after traumatic brain injury. J Clin Endocrinol Metab 2004; 89(12):5987–5992.

Tommasino C. Fluids and the neurosurgical patient. Anesthesiol Clin North Am 2002; 20(2):329–346, vi.

Section

9 Nine

Oncology

66 Acute Complications of Therapeutic Agents Used in the Management of Cancer
Björn Holmström, Sheetal Desai

67 Anticoagulation in Cancer Patients
Kanchan Kamath

68 Cancer Emergencies: Fever and Neutropenia
Joan Cain, David Lawson

69 Cancer Emergencies: Hypercalcemia
Joan Cain, David Lawson

70 Cancer Emergencies: Hyperviscosity Syndromes
Asha Ramsakal, Darrin Beaupre

71 Cancer Emergency: Elevated Intracranial Pressure
Asha Ramsakal, Stephen G. Patterson

72 Cancer Emergencies: Spinal Cord Compression
Asha Ramsakal, Stephen G. Patterson

73 Cancer Emergencies: Tumor Lysis Syndrome
Asha Ramsakal, Stephen G. Patterson

74 Cancer Emergencies: Paraneoplastic Neurologic Syndromes
Kanchan Kamath

CHAPTER SIXTY-SIX

Acute Complications of Therapeutic Agents Used in the Management of Cancer

Björn Holmström, MD, and Sheetal Desai, Pharm D, BCOP

BACKGROUND

The treatment of patients with cancer includes a vast array of medications, including cytotoxic, immunomodulatory, and biologic agents. Their primary aim is to cause regression or slow the rate of growth of a tumor. Chemotherapy has its roots in the early 1940s with its first notable regressions of hematopoietic tumors, but it initially was plagued with high morbidity and mortality.

Although hospital specialists will unlikely initiate definitive cancer treatment, they should understand the common acute reactions and syndromes associated with the ever-expanding field of agents used in the treatment of cancer. Acute hypersensitivity reactions, subacute syndromes related to specific chemotherapeutic agents, and severe electrolyte abnormalities are the more common complications a hospitalist may be asked to manage. This chapter will focus on the usually urgent and unintended effects of commonly used agents that may require active involvement of the nononcologist hospital specialist. After an initial review of hypersensitivity reactions and causative chemotherapeutic agents, major system toxicity (pulmonary, cardiac, renal, neurologic) is reviewed.

Hypersensitivity Reactions

Nearly all therapeutic agents used in the treatment of cancer have the potential to produce hypersensitivity reactions (HSRs) and anaphylaxis (Table 66-1).[1] Chapter 81 reviews allergic reactions in more depth. Although the exact mechanism of action remains unknown for most of the anticancer agents, type I HSRs (IgE mediated) are observed most frequently in clinical practice, with anaphylactic (antibody response to a sensitizing antigen) or anaphylactoid reaction (no antigen sensitization required, different physiologic response mechanism). Although uncommon in general, high rates of HSRs have been described with certain agents such as L-asparaginase, monoclonal antibodies, taxanes, epidophyllotoxins, and carboplatin when compared to other commonly used agents.[2]

ASSESSMENT

Clinical Presentation

HSRs typically occur within minutes but can recur hours after the administration of a specific agent. Manifested by symptoms reflecting changes in the respiratory, cardiovascular, gastrointestinal, and dermatologic systems, HSRs can produce: shortness of breath (SOB) with or without wheezing resulting from bronchoconstriction and/or stridor with pharyngeal tissue angioedema; chest pain, tachycardia, dizziness, or diaphoresis from volume loss leading to vascular collapse or shock; nausea, vomiting, abdominal pain, and diarrhea; and significant pruritus with or without hives or wheals, angioedema of the face, swelling of the extremities, and generalized flushing.

Diagnosis

The diagnosis needs to be quickly established based only on clinical signs and symptoms, and the temporal relationship between the HSR and therapeutic agent given. Because cancer patients may be on a large number of medications, an acute reaction may be due to a recently added medication other than the current infusion. Such a possibility may not alter the acute management, but may provide important clues in the secondary prevention of recurrences. Differential diagnoses include reactive airway disease, pulmonary embolism, septicemia, bronchitis, tachyarrhythmias, side effects of new medications or myocardial ischemia. Categorizing HSRs into four grades based on the severity of symptoms helps with the diagnosis, prognosis, and treatment (Table 66-2).[3] Laboratory studies are not usually required and are rarely helpful, unless an alternative diagnosis is more likely.

Prognosis

The prognosis directly relates to the degree of the HSR. If intervention is quickly instituted, long-term sequelae are rare. On

Table 66-1 Hypersensitivity and Cytokine Release Reactions Caused by Therapeutic Agents Used in the Treatment of Cancer

Agent	Incidence %
L-Asparaginase	6–43
Rituximab	8–15
Trastuzumab	3–18
Alemtuzumab	30–40
Gemtuzumab	Unknown
Paclitaxel	2–4 (with premedication)
Docetaxel	2 (with premedication)
Etoposide	1–3
Teniposide	5–41
Carboplatin	12–27 (increased with >7 cycles)
Cisplatin	1
Oxaliplatin	Rare

Modified from Alley E, et al. Cutaneous toxicities of cancer therapy. Curr Opin Oncol 2002; 14:212.

Table 66-2 Grading of Hypersensitivity Reactions

Grade	Clinical Manifestations
0	None
1	Transient rash (not hives) or drug fever <38° C
2	Urticaria or drug fever ≥ 38° C or asymptomatic bronchospasm
3	Symptomatic bronchospasm, requiring parenteral medication +/− urticaria; allergy related-edema/angioedema
4	Anaphylaxis (hypotension, loss of consciousness, or respiratory distress)
5	Death

Data adapted from Cancer Therapy Evaluation Program, Common Terminology Criteria for Adverse Events, Ver 3.0, 12/12/2003.

occasion, patients require overnight monitoring or, in extreme situations of anaphylaxis, require critical care with positive-pressure ventilation and/or vasopressors if angioedema or shock occurs.

MANAGEMENT

Treatment

Prompt recognition of an HSR with immediate intervention is the key principle behind management. Nursing staff should be trained to seek immediate intervention when such a reaction occurs. The initial treatment is to stop the infusion of the offending agent with prompt clinical assessment including vital signs. The patient needs to be promptly evaluated because of the potential for quick progression to respiratory and circulatory failure. The patient should be placed supine and level of consciousness assessed. Table 66-3 summarizes a protocol for HSR treatment according to the grade of the reaction; such protocols await validation in clinical trials.

Grade 1 HSR usually subsides upon discontinuation of the offending agent. Current practice often includes administration of intravenous (IV) H_1-receptor antagonists if symptoms persist for more than a few minutes, though this is not strongly supported by the available evidence.

Grade 2 HSR requires more intensive therapy and monitoring with the use of an IV H_1-antagonist and nebulized short-acting beta-agonist if any signs of shortness of breath or wheezing are present.

Grade 3 and 4 HSRs require the use of IV H_1- and H_2-receptor antagonists along with volume expansion with crystalloids if hypotension is present. Epinephrine should be promptly given for patients with impending airway obstruction, progressive SOB, or hypotension because the drug maintains blood pressure, antagonizes the effect of released mediators, and inhibits future release of mediators from basophils and mast cells. IV access should be established, but epinephrine can be given intramuscularly (IM) without delay if needed. A nebulized short-acting beta-agonist should be initiated for any shortness of breath or wheezing, and nebulized racemic epinephrine may help reduce laryngeal swelling if present. The use of IV corticosteroids may prevent or control a late-phase response in grade 3 or 4 reactions but has no role in the acute setting.[1,4] In severe cases of HSRs, the patient should be transferred to the intensive care unit (ICU) for continuing treatment.

DISCHARGE

Once the acute event has subsided, the patient should be monitored for a minimum of 2 hours or as clinically indicated. The decision to restart treatment needs to be individualized based on the reaction, the drug given, and the cancer being treated. This decision is ultimately left to the patient and oncologist. Patients with mild-to-moderate reactions can sometimes be rechallenged by slowing down the infusion rate, or given intensive premedication with corticosteroids, H_1- and H_2-receptor antagonists. The patient can be discharged with close follow-up by the oncologist if the HSR resolves. The patient should be instructed about the symptoms of a delayed, biphasic HSR, including urticaria, wheezing, SOB, edema, or chest pain and should seek immediate medical attention if such symptoms occur.

Although it is common practice to treat patients with variable courses of corticosteroids following serious HSRs, this practice is of uncertain value. Certainly, a short course in well-selected patients is unlikely to carry serious risk, and the biologic plausibility of suppressing any lingering hypersensitivity for a few days has appeal. Nonetheless, the risks and benefits of such corticosteroid use should be carefully considered and not necessarily recommended for all patients.

Certain therapeutic agents pose an exceptional and specific risk of a hypersensitivity reaction. The specific attributes of these drugs including L-asparaginase, rituximab, trastuzumab, gemtuzumab, alemtuzumab, cetuximab, taxanes, epidophyllotoxins, and platinum drugs are discussed below.

SPECIFIC AGENTS

L-Asparaginase

Asparaginase is a unique chemotherapeutic agent that indirectly inhibits asparagine formation within leukemic cells (especially

Table 66-3 Hypersensitivity Treatment Protocol

No claims as to clinical efficacy, safety or appropriateness are made or intended. This table is intended solely as a conceptual model for readers' general information. Users should take all steps they deem necessary to confirm the clinical validity and sufficiency of this table in the clinical context of its intended usage, implementing whatever alterations they deem appropriate.

Caution: Findings and symptoms described in this protocol can be caused by conditions other than hypersensitivity reactions. This protocol is intended **solely for use in cases where the evaluating clinician determines that a hypersensitivity reaction is the likely cause** of the presenting symptoms and findings. It may not be appropriate in other clinical situations.

Call for urgent physician backup for any patient with pulse > 120, BP < 90/60, respiratory distress, T ≧ 40 degrees, chest pain, or marked alteration of mental status.

Do the following for Grade 4:
- Discontinue offending medication and call for urgent physician backup
- **IV Access**: epinephrine 1:10,000, 0.5 mg (5 ml) now (0.35 mg if weight <50 Kg), OR
- **No IV**: give epinephrine 1:1000, 0.5 mg IM (0.35 mg IM if weight <50 kg)
- Repeat epinephrine after 15 minutes if symptoms above persist, up to 3 doses
- Give diphenhydramine 50 mg IV (use 25 mg if patient weight is <50 Kg)
- Dexamethasone 8 mg IV once
- BP, pulse, respirations q 5 minutes for 30 minutes

Do the following for Grade 3:
- Discontinue offending medication and call for urgent physician backup
- If shortness of breath or signs of airway obstruction are present:
  - **IV Access**: epinephrine 1:10,000, 0.5 mg (5 ml) now (0.35 mg if weight <50 Kg)
  - **Or No IV**: give epinephrine 1:1000, 0.5 mg IM (0.35 mg if weight <50 kg)
- Give diphenhydramine 50 mg IV (use 25 mg if patient weight is <50 Kg)
- Dexamethasone 8 mg IV once
- BP, pulse, respirations q 5 minutes for 30 minutes
- Albuterol 0.35 ml per nebulizer if wheezing is present

Do the following for Grade 2:
- Discontinue offending medication
- Give diphenhydramine 50 mg IV (use 25 mg if patient weight is <50 Kg)
- Albuterol 0.35 ml by nebulizer if wheezing
- BP, pulse, respirations q 15 minutes for 60 minutes
- If symptoms subside, call primary oncologist or hematologist to determine whether infusion should be restarted
- If symptoms persist, call for physician backup

Do the following for Grade 1:
- Discontinue offending medication
- Give diphenhydramine 50 mg IV (use 25 mg if patient weight is <50 Kg)
- BP, pulse, respirations q 15 minutes for 60 minutes
- If symptoms subside, check with *prescribing* physician as to restarting infusion. If restarted, check BP, pulse and respirations q 5 minutes for first 15 minutes
- If symptoms recur (Grade 1) after second attempt, discontinue infusion and call prescribing physician

lymphoblasts), which depend upon an exogenous source of asparagine for survival. Asparaginase is available in three formulations: the original *Escherichia coli* (*E. coli*) derivative (Elspar); an *Erwinia chrysanthemi* (also known as *Erwinia carotovora*) derivative; and a form attached to polyethylene glycol (Pegaspargase, Oncaspar). Each dose incurs a 5–8% incidence of an HSR, but this can increase cumulatively to 33% by the fourth dose.[5] Serious anaphylactoid reactions occur in fewer than 10% of patients. Pegaspargase is the least immunogenic of the available formulations.[6–8] A history of atopy, prior use of drugs derived from *E. coli*, prior or infrequent drug exposure, IV administration and use without concomitant steroids, 6-mercaptopurine, and/or vincristine enhance the risk of asparaginase-induced HSRs.

Symptoms tend to occur within 30 minutes of an IV dose and usually more than 30–60 minutes after an IM dose, requiring patient observation for up to an hour after each dose. Despite various attempts to detect reactivity before a dose of asparaginase is administered, there is no reliable way to determine which patients will sustain an HSR. The manufacturer of the *E. coli* or

Erwinia preparations recommends the administration of a test dose; however, a negative test does not guarantee that an HSR will not occur.[5] Therefore, each dose of asparaginase that is administered should be treated as if it could cause a reaction, and staff needs to be prepared to manage this urgently.

General management is outlined under General Hypersensitivity reactions. If an HSR does occur, the hematologist/oncologist can switch to a different product; or if the therapy is felt to outweigh the risks of anaphylaxis, a desensitization protocol can be implemented.

Monoclonal Antibodies

Monoclonal antibodies (produced by a cloned population of cells) generally are well tolerated, with HSRs occurring anywhere from 3–40% (*see* Table 66-1). A variety of side effects do occur based on a number of factors, such as the specific target antigen or target cell, the rate of the monoclonal antibody infusion, and the total tumor cell burden. A few different toxicities have been identified with the administration of monoclonal antibodies. The first is an acute hypersensitivity or allergic reaction in which the symptoms can range from mild (urticaria, nausea, fever) to a more severe anaphylactoid reaction (bronchospasm, hypotension, tachycardia). Fortunately, true anaphylaxis is a rare complication.

The second symptom complex, known as the "cytokine release syndrome," is characterized by fever, rigors, nausea, and malaise, sometimes progressing to hypotension and bronchospasm. This syndrome occurs within hours of starting the infusion and is a result of the monoclonal antibodies binding to circulating leukemic or lymphoma cells. Symptoms are related to the removal of circulating target cells and are due to the release of various cytokines such as interleukins, interferons, and tumor necrosis factors. Since this reaction is evident primarily in a patient with a high number of circulating tumor cells, its incidence diminishes with subsequent infusions. Prophylactic diphenhydramine, acetaminophen, or corticosteroid administration does not prevent this reaction; therefore, a dose escalation approach with close monitoring has been recommended for patients with high peripheral blood tumor cell counts in order to minimize this toxicity.[9,10]

Rituximab (Rituxan)

Rituximab is a chimeric mouse/human anti-CD20 monoclonal antibody specific for CD20 antigen on B lymphocytes. It inhibits proliferation and induces apoptosis in some B-cell lymphomas as well as sensitizing cells to the effects of chemotherapy. Rituximab has three adverse effects that warrant a "black box" warning in the package insert: infusion reactions, tumor lysis syndrome, and mucocutaneous reactions. The manufacturer reports a 77%, 30%, and 14% frequency of a reaction with the first, fourth, and eighth infusions, respectively.

Reactions to the drug may include fever, chills, rigors, nausea, rhinitis, urticaria, pruritus, myalgias, headache, and asthenia that occur within the first 30 minutes to 2 hours of the first infusion in over 50% of patients.[10] Severe reactions may include hypotension, hypoxia, bronchospasm, and angioedema, which tend to occur in 10% of patients. Although these reactions have all the features of a type I HSR, they are generally related to fulminant cytokine (tumor necrosis factor and interleukin-6) release from the malignant lymphocytes in response to the therapeutic effect of the drug.

Because of the high rate of HSRs, the first infusion is initially administered at a rate of 50 mg/hour. If there is no evidence of hypersensitivity or cytokine release syndrome, the rate is increased by 50 mg/hour every 30 minutes to a maximum rate of 400 mg/hour. If the first infusion is well tolerated, subsequent infusions may be initiated at a rate of 100 mg/hour, increasing every 30 minutes by 100 mg/hour to a maximum of 400 mg/hour. Premedication with diphenhydramine (50 mg orally) and acetaminophen (650 mg orally) has become standard practice; however, it does not guarantee the prevention of a reaction.

Patients with non–life-threatening reactions are usually able to complete treatment after temporary discontinuation of infusion and reintroduction at a lower rate 30 to 45 minutes later (e.g., 50 mg/hour) with gradual increases per patient tolerance.[10,11] Patients with severe reactions should have the infusion stopped

and receive supportive therapy appropriate to the nature of the reaction.

Trastuzumab (Herceptin)

Trastuzumab is a recombinant DNA-derived humanized monoclonal antibody that inhibits proliferation of human tumor cells that overexpress human epidermal growth factor receptor 2 proteins (*HER2*); seen in some patients with breast cancer and other malignancies (e.g., ovarian, lung).[12] Trastuzumab monotherapy has been associated with hypersensitivity reactions at a frequency of approximately 40% increasing to 47% to 62% when used in combination with other cytotoxic agents.[13]

Symptomatically, fever and chills are common and occur in up to 40% of patients with the initial infusion while the incidence and severity subsides with continued therapy. Other symptoms reported during/after infusion include headache, nausea, vomiting, back pain, asthenia, rigors, dizziness, hypotension, and rash.

General management as outlined is recommended under General Hypersensitivity reactions. The infusion should be interrupted for any patient with dyspnea or clinically significant hypotension during administration.[14]

Gemtuzumab Ozogamicin (Mylotarg)

Gemtuzumab is a recombinant humanized anti-CD33 monoclonal antibody conjugated to the cytotoxic antibiotic calicheamicin. Gemtuzumab is indicated for use in patients with CD33+ AML in first relapse, ≥60 years of age, and not candidates for further chemotherapy. A postinfusion syndrome of fever (61%), chills (62%), and rigors is the most common nonhematologic adverse effect of gemtuzumab ozogamicin. Grade 3 or 4 infusion-related reactions, including chills, fever, and hypotension, occurred in approximately 30% of patients during the initial clinical studies and generally occurred at the end of the infusion and resolved within 2 to 4 hours. Infusion-related reactions were less common after the second dose, with only 12% of patients experiencing a grade 3 or 4 effect.[15,16]

The manufacturer recommends diphenhydramine 50 mg orally and acetaminophen 650 mg orally as premedications. A recent study at a single institution concluded that methylprednisolone 50 mg IV prior to the infusion and 1 hour into the infusion reduced gemtuzumab ozogamicin-related infusion reactions in patients with newly diagnosed or relapsed acute myelogenous leukemia.[16]

Alemtuzumab (Campath)

Alemtuzumab is a recombinant DNA–derived humanized monoclonal antibody directed against CD52 cell surface glycoproteins used primarily in the treatment of B-cell chronic lymphoycytic leukemia (CLL). Alemtuzumab is administered on a titration schedule based on patient tolerance of adverse infusion reactions, which tend to be frequent, due to high levels of cytokines in T lymphocytes. Infusion-related symptoms occur in the majority of patients during the first week of therapy, despite premedication, and include: rigors (90%), fever (85%), nausea (54%), vomiting (38%), fatigue, rash (33%), urticaria, and pruritus. Additional reactions included dyspnea (28%), hypotension (18%), and hypoxia (3%).

The manufacturer recommends pretreatment with acetaminophen (650 mg orally) and diphenhydramine (50 mg orally) prior to the first dose and at each dose escalation. Patients who develop severe reactions should also be pretreated with corticosteroids. Subcutaneous administration of alemtuzumab should be employed whenever possible, as it has been reported to have a decreased rate of infusion reactions.[17]

Cetuximab (Erbitux)

Cetuximab is a murine-human chimeric monoclonal antibody directed against epidermal growth factor receptor (EGFR); it is currently used primarily in gastrointestinal malignancies. Hypersensitivity, including urticaria and anaphylactoid reactions, has occurred during infusions with relatively high frequency (4–8%). Infusion-related reactions are reported to occur in approximately 3% of patients, with 90% of them being associated with the first infusion.[18] Severe reactions are manifested by the rapid onset of airway obstruction (bronchospasm, hoarseness), urticaria, and hypotension.

If a patient experiences a mild-to-moderate (grade 1 or 2) reaction, the infusion rate should be permanently reduced by 50%. Cetuximab should be permanently discontinued for any grade 3 or 4 reactions. Premedication with an H$_1$-antagonist (diphenhydramine 25–50 mg orally) is recommended along with a 1-hour observation period following the cetuximab infusion.

Taxanes

The taxanes, paclitaxel (Taxol) and docetaxel (Taxotere), are among the most widely used chemotherapeutic agents. Taxane plant derivatives promote microtubule assembly by enhancing the action of tubulin dimers, stabilizing existing microtubules, and inhibiting cell replication. HSRs were a major toxicity in the initial clinical trials, but the rate of severe reactions was reduced to less than 3% in subsequent trials using a three-drug prophylactic regimen of an antihistamine, a corticosteroid, and an H$_2$-receptor antagonist.

Abraxane is a nanoparticle albumin-bound formulation of paclitaxel, approved for use in metastatic breast cancer, which has eliminated the use of Cremophor as the vehicle. HSRs were not seen in a phase I study of this agent, despite the omission of any premedication. However, in a preliminary report of a phase III trial, a few hypersensitivity reactions were seen in patients receiving Abraxane without any premedication (4%), compared with 12% in patients receiving conventional paclitaxel including premedication.[19–21]

Epipodophyllotoxins

The epidophyllotoxins etoposide (VePesid) and teniposide (Vumon) are topoisomerase II inhibitors inhibiting DNA synthesis by causing DNA strand breaks. They are uncommonly associated with type I HSRs. The frequency increases with cumulative doses and is somewhat higher with teniposide.

Reactions generally occur during or shortly after drug infusion, implicating a possible solvent vehicle-induced reaction, but they can also develop following one or multiple doses of either agent, suggesting both immunologic and nonimmunologic mechanisms. Symptoms include hypotension, dyspnea, flushing, and chest tightness characteristic of histamine release, but can also occur if the infusion is administered too fast. In order to prevent hypotension, both drugs should be infused slowly over a period of 30–60 minutes, with continued medical observation for an additional 60 minutes.[22]

Platinum Drugs

Platinum-based anticancer drugs covalently bind to DNA and disrupt DNA functions by forming crosslinks. The incidence of HSRs with carboplatin (Paraplatin) rises significantly once patients have received six or more courses of therapy, (around 12% overall and 3–13% of patients treated with oxaliplatin (Eloxatin).[23,24] The true incidence of cisplatin (Platinol) reactions is unknown.

Reactions are generally characterized by an erythematous rash, urticaria, bronchospasm, and hypotension. Most patients who develop an HSR to carboplatin or cisplatin will react again if rechallenged. Treatment of an acute reaction includes stopping the infusion and following guidelines under general management of HSRs. Some patients have been successfully retreated following premedication with a corticosteroid and an H$_1$- and H$_2$-receptor antagonist, and the decision to continue or discontinue treatment must balance the potential for serious toxicity versus the clinical benefit to be achieved in an individual patient.[25]

PULMONARY TOXICITY

Cytotoxic agents can result in a variety of lung injuries, including diffuse alveolar damage, interstitial pneumonitis, pulmonary edema, pulmonary hemorrhage, eosinophilic lung disease, and bronchiolitis obliterans-organizing pneumonia (BOOP). Because the lungs are commonly the site of metastases and infection, differentiating between toxicities from cancer therapy and other common pulmonary complications can be challenging.[26] Agents commonly associated with pulmonary toxicity include bleomycin, methotrexate, all-*trans* retinoic acid, nitrosoureas, and busulfan.

Clinical Presentation

Patients with cytotoxin-induced pulmonary reactions often present with symptoms that are consistent with several other nonrelated illnesses, such as opportunistic infections, asthma, heart failure, pneumonia, worsening primary disease, or pulmonary fibrosis from other causes. Because pulmonary toxicity can occur at an unexpected time and present very subtly, the hospitalist must maintain a high degree of suspicion for possible chemotherapy-induced toxicity. The diagnosis is ultimately made by ruling out other disorders. Empiric treatment with corticosteroids should be undertaken with great caution in the absence of a diagnosis.

All the implicated agents can cause lung injury by different pathways, and thus present themselves both clinically and radiographically in a variety of ways. The history of timing of drug administration can assist in their detection. However, some agents have been reported to cause pulmonary injury months to years after exposure to the offending agent. Because pulmonary toxicity can occur even with small doses, dose accumulation is an inconsistent marker for development of pulmonary injury.

Diagnosis

A variety of radiographic appearances are seen with chemotherapy-induced pulmonary toxicity (e.g., pleural thickening or effusions, interstitial, alveolar, or mixed parenchymal patterns). Pulmonary function testing (PFT) is sensitive but not specific for lung injury related to agents used in the treatment of cancer. PFTs should only be used as an adjunct to clinical and laboratory findings. Typically, a restrictive pattern with reduction in the diffusing capacity to carbon monoxide (DLCO) is seen.

The primary technique used in the diagnosis of most presumptive cases of chemotherapy-associated lung injury is bronchoscopy with bronchoalveolar lavage (BAL). Although BAL's diagnostic yield for noninfectious interstitial diseases is low, its low rate of complications, ease, and availability makes the procedure the first step in evaluation. Lung biopsy is the gold standard, but because the procedure is invasive and associated with complications, the routine use of biopsy is precluded.[27]

Bleomycin (Blenoxane)

Bleomycin is a glycopeptide-antibiotic whose cytotoxic action relates to excising free bases after it binds to DNA and causing single strand breaks. The agent has been implicated in causing two distinct types of lung injury: hypersensitivity pneumonitis (HP) and pulmonary fibrosis. Bleomycin directly damages type I pneumocytes and the pulmonary capillary endothelium. The drug also stimulates inflammatory cells and releases proteolytic enzymes, causing further destruction of the lung parenchyma.[26] The incidence of bleomycin-induced pulmonary fibrosis is around 10% and can occur months to years after its administration. Risk factors for HP include combination use of bleomycin with other agents, advanced age, and IV route of administration. The incidence is higher in patients undergoing concomitant radiation, those treated for lymphomas, and in patients receiving >400-units cumulative dose.

HP presents with an acute or subacute onset of cough, dyspnea, and associated fever. The patient is usually tachypneic, and wheezes or crackles can be heard. Radiographs demonstrate bilateral diffuse infiltrates and patchy alveolar consolidation. PFTs exhibit restrictive defects with decreased diffusion. HP does not appear to be dose dependent and usually occurs during treatment. About 20% of bleomycin-induced pulmonary fibrosis patients are asymptomatic.

Treatment for HP includes withdrawal of the offending agent and supportive therapy including oxygen, bronchodilators, and steroids. Rechallenge with bleomycin does not necessarily cause recurrence of HP. Treatment for pulmonary fibrosis includes the use of steroids. However, the mortality rate is high, and patients are often left with residual lung injury.[28–30] Postoperative patients are at risk of developing acute respiratory distress syndrome (ARDS) related to use of intraoperative oxygen.[26]

Methotrexate

Methotrexate is a folic acid antagonist that reversibly inhibits dihydrofolate reductase. This inhibition interferes with the synthesis of DNA and cell reproduction. The incidence of pulmonary toxicity in patients receiving methotrexate is 5–10%. Hepatotoxicity and myelosuppression can also occur. Although pulmonary toxicity is not dose related, incidence is higher with more frequent treatments.[4] Patients generally present with fever, chills, malaise, headache, cough, and dyspnea within weeks of initiation of therapy. Peripheral eosinophilia is found in about 50% of cases, and a skin eruption is seen in up to 17% of patients. Chest x-ray (CXR) shows interstitial or alveolar infiltrates. The prognosis is good, with overall mortality around 10%. The toxicity usually regresses after cessation of the agent.[31,32]

All-*Trans* Retinoic Acid (ATRA) (Vesanoid)

ATRA is an agent that induces terminal differentiation of malignant cells into mature myeloid cells. The drug is commonly used to induce remissions in patients with acute promyelocytic leukemia (APL). A combination of fever, dyspnea, edema, hypotension, diffuse interstitial infiltrates, and pleural effusions occur in up to 26% of patients 2–47 days after initiating treatment (retinoic acid syndrome). These symptoms are most likely to occur in patients with high absolute blast counts. Pulmonary hemorrhage occurs occasionally as a complication of this syndrome. Treatment includes the use of high-dose corticosteroids (dexamethasone 10 mg IV q12 hr) and temporary discontinuation of ATRA therapy.[33,34]

Nitrosoureas

Nitrosoureas have unusually high activity against a broad spectrum of tumors. Their cytotoxic mechanism of action is thought to occur by liberating alkylating moieties. All of the nitrosureas, including carmustine (BiCNU) and lomustine (CeeNu), have been implicated in the development of pulmonary fibrosis.

Symptoms include cough, dyspnea, or acute respiratory failure. Carmustine has been implicated in three different syndromes: a) early-onset alveolitis and fibrosis, b) late-onset fibrosis, and c) as a contributing agent to bone marrow transplantation-induced pulmonary fibrosis. Appearance of toxicity appears to be greater in patients with chronic obstructive pulmonary disease and those receiving concomitant radiation and cyclophosphamide. The chest radiograph normally shows diffuse interstitial infiltrates. Corticosteroids have been used as primary treatment but with little known benefit.[35,36]

Busulfan (Myleran)

Busulfan is an alkylating agent that interferes with the normal function of DNA by alkylation and cross-linking the strands of DNA. Busulfan toxicity occurs at an approximate 4% incidence with no correlated risk factors. Symptoms can occur as soon as 6–8 weeks after therapy, but the usual course is presentation after a latency period of more than 3 years. Clinical and radiographic findings are similar to those seen with bleomycin toxicity.[26] Treatment involves discontinuing the drug and administering corticosteroids.

CARDIOVASCULAR COMPLICATIONS OF ANTICANCER AGENTS

Therapy for cancer is associated with a wide array of cardiac complications, including arrhythmias, cardiomyopathy, congestive heart failure, myocardial ischemia, pericardial disease, and even shock. Direct cellular damage, formation of free oxygen radicals, and the induction of immunogenic reactions with the presence of antigen presenting cells in the heart are the main mechanism of action thought to induce cardiac toxicities. Each drug has its own unique cardiac effects as well as the ability to exacerbate the effects of other drugs and interact with concomitant radiotherapy.[26,37] Agents commonly associated with cardiotoxicity include anthracyclines (e.g., doxorubicin), 5-fluorouracil, taxanes, trastuzumab, interleukin-2, interferon, cyclophosphamide, and ifosfamide.

Clinical Presentation

Patients typically present with acute chest pain, dyspnea, dizziness, palpitations, or cardiovascular collapse with syncope. Symptoms are typical for the underlining etiology, including: acute, substernal chest pain from myocardial ischemia or infarction; dyspnea from congestive heart failure (CHF), myocarditis or arrhythmias; palpitations from arrhythmias; pleuritic chest pain from pericarditis; syncope from arrhythmia or myocardial infarction (Table 66-4).[38]

Diagnosis

The diagnosis is established from the common complications seen with their respective chemotherapy drugs and constellation of sign, symptoms, and electrocardiographic (ECG) findings present. Diagnostic studies including electrolytes, ECG, cardiac enzymes, and chest radiograph (CXR) can greatly aid in making the diagnosis.

Treatment

Treatment includes stopping the mitigating anticancer agent and administering standard therapy for chest pain, pulmonary edema, myocardial infarction, or CHF.

Discharge

Once the acute event has subsided, the patient should be monitored for a minimum of 2 hours, or as clinically indicated. The decision to attempt to restart treatment needs to be individualized, based on the reaction, drug given, and cancer being treated. This decision is ultimately left to the patient and oncologist. The patient can be discharged with close follow-up by the oncologist if the patient is hemodynamically stable with no overt symptoms for cardiac dysfunction.

Anthracyclines

Anthracyclines inhibit DNA synthesis by forming a complex with DNA through intercalation between base pairs and inhibition of the uncoiling of the helix via topoisomerase II. The incidence of cardiac toxicity is greatest with doxorubicin (Adriamycin) followed by daunorubicin (Daunoxome), idarubicin (Idamycin), eprirubicin (Ellence), and least by mitoxantrone (Novantrone).

The most important cardiac toxicities are cardiomyopathy and left ventricular dysfunction, which develop chronically, usually within 1 year of exposure. A rare form of acute cardiac toxicity occurs immediately after treatment and is characterized by transient arrhythmias, pericarditis-myocarditis syndrome, or acute left ventricular failure. Risk factors include age, prior irradiation, underlying heart disease and concomitant administration of other chemotherapeutic agents.[39] The cumulative dose of the

Table 66-4 Cardiotoxicity Profiles of Chemotherapeutic Agents

	CHF/LV dysfunction	Hypertension	Hypotension	Arrhythmia	Pericarditis	Ischemia
Anthracyclines	+++					
Alkylating agents	++	++		++	+	
5-Fluorouracil			+			+
Paclitaxel	++		+	+		
Alemtuzumab	+		+++			
Bevacizumab	++	+++				
Cetuximab			+			
Rituximab			++	++		
Trastuzumab	++					
Interleukin-2			++++	++		
Interferon-alpha	+		+++			++
Imatinib	+++					
Etoposide			++			
Cisplatin	++	++++				++

CHF—congestive heart failure; LV dysfunction—left ventricular dysfunction
Relative frequency of specific adverse events: + indicate rare; ++ uncommon (1–5%); +++, common (6–10%); ++++, frequent (>10%). Adapted from: Yeh ET, Tong AT, Lenihan DJ, et al. Cardiovascular complications of cancer therapy diagnosis, pathogenesis, and management. Circulation 2004; 109:3122–3131.

drug appears to be the most important risk factor. The prevalence of cardiomyopathy rises in incidence to 4% with cumulative doses of 400–500 mg/m² and a steep rise in incidence to 36% with cumulative doses >600 mg/ m² when using doxorubicin. The damage results from direct myocardial injury from the release of free radicals.[40]

Echocardiography and radionuclide imaging are sensitive methods for diagnosing and following chemotherapy-induced cardiomyopathy. If confounding factors make the diagnosis questionable, then an endomyocardial biopsy might be necessary because it is the most specific test available.[40,41]

CHF caused by anthracyclines has a poor prognosis, and the only definitive therapy is cardiac transplantation. However, the prognosis can be altered with early recognition and treatment using conventional therapy for CHF.

Conventional treatment of heart failure using beta-blockers, angiotensin converting enzyme inhibitors, aldosterone antagonists, diuretics and/or digoxin provides promising results for doxorubicin-induced cardiomyopathy.[40,41] This approach is best for all other cases of anthracycline-induced damage as well.

5-Fluorouracil (Adrucil)

Fluorouracil is a pyrimidine antimetabolite that blocks methylation of deoxyuridylic acid by thymidylate synthetase inhibition, interferes with DNA synthesis, and inhibits the formation of RNA. This reaction creates a thymine deficiency resulting in cell death. Fluorouracil has been associated with a 2–10% incidence of cardiovascular complications. Risk factors for developing cardiac toxicity include preexisting coronary artery disease and concurrent radiotherapy.

The most common cardiac effect is ischemia, which typically occurs during first treatment with 5-fluorouracil (5-FU). The ischemia can manifest as angina pectoris extending to acute myocardial infarction. The incidence is as high as 4.5–10% of patients with a prior history of coronary artery disease. The mechanism of ischemia relates to coronary vasospasm, arterial vasoconstriction, or direct toxicity leading to abnormal myocardial function.

Prompt cessation of 5-FU and institution of anti-ischemic therapy usually reverses the ischemia. Thus, chest pain presenting in this setting should raise concerns about acute myocardial infarction. Standard cardiologic treatment guidelines apply. Unfortunately, measures to protect against 5-FU–induced cardiotoxicity are unavailable.[42–44]

Cyclophosphamide (Cytoxan) and Ifosfamide (Ifex)

Cyclophosphamide and ifosfamide are alkylating agents that prevent cell division by cross-linking DNA strands and thereby decreasing DNA synthesis. At low doses, the alkylating agents are generally well tolerated. However, high-dose cyclophosphamide used for bone marrow transplantation regimens has been associated with a broad spectrum of reactions.

These drugs can cause severe myocarditis, pericarditis, malignant arrhythmias, and congestive heart failure. The cumulative dose is most closely associated with myocardial injury (>100 mg/kg (2.5–4 g/m²) for cyclophosphamide and 1,000 mg/m² for ifosfamide). Autopsies have demonstrated increased cardiac weight with hemorrhagic myocardial necrosis. The mechanism of injury appears to be from direct myocyte injury. Ifosfamide has been shown to cause reversible myocardial dysfunction and arrhythmias.[26,46]

Interferon (Intron) and Interleukin-2 (Aldesleukin)

Interferon and interleukin-2 are biologic response modifiers used in a variety of tumor types, including renal cell carcinoma and metastatic melanoma. Interferon-induced cardiotoxicity usually manifests as arrhythmias, myocardial infarction, ischemia, cardiomyopathy, sudden death, atrioventricular block, and/or CHF. The main risk factor appears to be preexisting heart disease. Interleukin-2 has been associated with arrhythmias, myocardial ischemia, left ventricular dysfunction, hypotension, and reversible myocarditis. One of the more common side effects with this agent is capillary leak syndrome, which can result in hypotension, tachycardia, edema, hypoalbuminemia, and decreased systemic vascular resistance.[37]

Treatment as discussed above for hypersensitivity reactions can usually relieve these symptoms.

Taxanes

Paclitaxel has been associated with transient, asymptomatic bradyarrhythmias and atrioventricular block only evident with continuous ECG monitoring. These complications are more commonly seen in patients with existing cardiac abnormalities or in the presence of electrolyte imbalances.[38]

Trastuzumab

Cardiac toxicity associated with trastuzumab seems to be similar in scope to cardiac complications seen with anthracycline therapy. However, there appears to be no dose relation with cardiac side effects. Concomitant cardiotoxic chemotherapy, older age, and chest radiation appear to be independent risk factors. In clinical trials, the majority of patients who developed class III or IV CHF improved with standard medical therapy, suggesting a better prognosis than seen with anthracycline-associated cardiotoxicity.[12]

NEPHROTOXICITY

Several chemotherapy agents are nephrotoxic, causing acute or chronic renal failure or a specific renal lesion. Furthermore, the concomitant administration of anticancer, ancillary, and supportive care drugs cleared through the kidney becomes problematic when accumulation of drug yields more significant toxicity than usually seen in the patient with renal insufficiency. Prerenal failure is commonly seen secondary to dehydration from the nausea, vomiting, diarrhea, and/or anorexia resulting from cancer therapy. Intrinsic renal failure occurs with prolonged hypoperfusion, release of endogenous nephrotoxins, exposure to nephrotoxic agents, renovascular obstruction, and glomerular diseases. Acute tubular necrosis is the most common form of intrinsic renal failure typically seen with platinum-based drugs and methotrexate.[46]

ASSESSMENT

Clinical Presentation

Symptoms of acute renal failure are rare, unless the patient becomes uremic or develops severe electrolyte abnormalities. Signs of injury include electrolyte wasting, decreased glomerular filtration rate, renal tubular acidosis, and loss of urine concentrating ability.

Diagnosis

A thorough assessment of a patient's renal function is helpful in identifying patients at high risk of developing renal dysfunction, selecting appropriate drug dosages, and recognizing nephrotoxicity from anticancer agents. Not only does glomerular filtration decrease, but proximal and distal tubular dysfunction can occur as well.

Glomerular filtration rate can be estimated by utilizing serum creatinine and patient-specific parameters such as age, gender, and body size. However, this estimate is often inaccurate in patients with renal dysfunction. Proximal tubular function is evaluated by means of fractional excretion of glucose, uric acid, calcium, phosphorous, and magnesium. Urine osmolality and pH are used to evaluate distal tubular function. Together with urinalysis, the above tests provide a complete picture of the extent and location of kidney damage.[45]

MANAGEMENT

Renal dysfunction is a pathophysiologic effect of certain malignancies, such as renal cell carcinoma and multiple myeloma. Hyperviscosity syndrome (Chapter 70), hypercalcemia (Chapter 69), and tumor lysis syndrome (Chapter 73) can all result in acute renal failure.[47] These syndromes should be borne in mind when one is asked to manage renal dysfunction in the cancer patient. Only after such other causes are excluded should attention be focused on direct drug toxicities.

Cisplatin (Platinol)

Cisplatin-induced nephrotoxicity is both cumulative and dose related. An acute form of renal failure occurs primarily in patients who have not received adequate hydration during therapy. Cisplatin also induces several electrolyte disorders, the most prominent being hypomagnesemia, with subsequent hypokalemia and hypocalcemia.

The acute complication consists of azotemia with a rising serum blood urea nitrogen (BUN) and creatinine level. Symptoms of hypomagnesemia include dizziness, muscle weakness, tetany, paresthesias, and tremulousness. This disorder is generally dose related but can occur after a single treatment.

Management of acute nephrotoxicity requires either discontinuation or reduction in the dose. Dialysis is not an effective short-term treatment.[48] The magnesium deficit requires replacement, and patients can have persistent renal losses of magnesium for months or even years after they complete therapy with cisplatin.[49]

Ifosfamide (Ifex)

Ifosfamide can cause a proximal tubular defect, similar to Fanconi-like syndrome. Originally, this was thought to be due to large bolus dose administration, but has since been reported with fractioned dosing as well. Symptoms typically include fever, polyuria, polydipsia, muscle weakness, joint pain, hyperaminoaciduria, phosphate reabsorption impairment, and tubulopathy. The Fanconi-like syndrome appears to be reversible, once the medication is discontinued, with management being mainly supportive therapy.[50,51]

Methotrexate

Methotrexate is not usually nephrotoxic, although 90% of the drug is excreted unchanged in the urine. High doses ($1-12$ g/m^2) and long-term administration of conventional doses are situations when methotrexate can precipitate in the renal tubules and collecting ducts.[52] This occurs when the high concentrations exceed the solubility of methotrexate at pH 5.0. Therefore, adequate hydration and urinary alkalinization (to keep pH >7) should be administered to patients receiving high-dose therapy.

In the presence of renal insufficiency, the excretion of methotrexate is impaired, leading to prolonged exposure to high-serum methotrexate concentrations, resulting in greater bone marrow suppression and gastrointestinal side effects.

If renal failure is induced by methotrexate, the patient may be managed conservatively, unless uremia or other electrolyte disorders develop. Methotrexate is not a dialyzable compound.[53] Methotrexate-induced renal failure generally resolves within 2–3 weeks of drug discontinuation.

Aldesleukin (IL-2) (Proleukin)

Aldesleukin is a biologic response modifier primarily used in the treatment of renal cell cancer and metastatic melanoma. A major side effect of high-dose IV aldesleukin therapy (600,000 units every 8 hours for 14 doses) is capillary leak syndrome, leading to edema, plasma volume depletion, and a reversible fall in glomerular filtration rate.[54,55]

Therapy for renal failure secondary to IL-2 treatment is supportive. It is directed at maintaining intravascular volume and stabilizing hemodynamic parameters, as well as avoiding other potential nephrotoxic agents. Preventive measures include a strict selection of patients who are candidates for IL-2 therapy. Older patients, patients with underlying renal failure or hypertension, and patients taking nephrotoxic agents are at higher risk for complications such as capillary leak syndrome and prerenal azotemia. Signs of renal dysfunction tend to resolve within a week of drug withdrawal, and lasting tubular damage is unusual.

Common Acute Neurotoxic Complications

Common neurotoxic signs and syndromes can occur with nearly all chemotherapeutic agents with varying degrees from mild peripheral neuropathy to chemical meningitis and seizures. Three specific chemotherapeutic agents (methotrexate, cytosine arabinoside, and ifosfamide) require careful attention because of their heightened incidence of neurotoxic complications.

METHOTREXATE (RHEUMATREX)

When methotrexate is given intrathecally or in high doses, it is associated with a number of neurologic syndromes. Proposed mechanisms of methotrexate neurotoxicity include depletion of cerebral reduced folate, reduced cerebral protein, altered blood–brain barrier permeability, and impaired neurotransmitter synthesis. The risk of neurotoxicity increases with increasing total intrathecal (IT) methotrexate dose, prolonged elevated cerebrospinal (CSF) methotrexate levels, concurrent radiation therapy, or systemic high-dose methotrexate therapy.

Clinical Presentation

Acute methotrexate intrathecal toxicity includes acute chemical meningitis with fever, headache, nuchal rigidity, and CSF leukocytosis. Other acute complications include acute transverse myelopathy with paraplegia and transient radiculopathies. An acute stroke-like encephalopathy with seizures, confusion, hemiparesis, and coma may complicate high-dose intravenous methotrexate ($>1,000$ mg/m^2) in as many as 15% of patients.[56–58]

Prognosis

Neurotoxic complications are usually mild to moderate and begin within hours of IT administration but can last from 1 to 3 days. The syndrome resolves spontaneously and does not recur with subsequent therapy.

Treatment

Treatment requires immediate discontinuation of the offending drug and symptomatic treatment of its active complications. Once the patient is hemodynamically stable, then discharge with close follow-up is acceptable.

CYTOSINE ARABINOSIDE (ARA-C) (CYTOSAR)

Cytarabine (Ara-C) is an analog of pyrimidine nucleoside that inhibits DNA synthesis by inhibiting DNA polymerase and readily crossing the blood brain barrier. Typical IV doses of cytarabine at $100–200$ mg/m^2 rarely cause neurotoxicity, but when given in high dose regimens (>6 g/m^2 per course), almost half of the patients develop neurotoxicity.

Clinical Presentation

Symptoms typically begin 6 to 8 days after administration, depending on multiple risk factors: age over 55 years, hepatic and renal insufficiency, and dosages totaling >27 g/m^2. Symptoms can range from nystagmus and ataxia to confusion, somnolence, dysarthrias, seizures, or coma.[59,60]

Treatment/Prognosis

After discontinuation of the medication, most symptoms start to improve within 1 week and resolve completely within 2 weeks.

IFOSFAMIDE

Ifosfamide is an alkylating agent that can produce transient central neurotoxicities. The drug is metabolized by the liver to inactive metabolites, including chloroacetaldehyde, which is responsible for much of the neurotoxic side effects.

Clinical Presentation

Neurologic symptoms include transient seizures, somnolence, confusion, ataxia, malaise, and coma. Risk factors include infusion of the drug over 1 day versus 5 days, impaired renal and hepatic clearance, hypoalbuminemia, and low serum bicarbonate levels.

Treatment/Prognosis

IV methylene blue has been shown to reverse neurotoxicity at a dose of 50 mg using a 1–2% solution and can be repeated up to four times daily.[61]

MISCELLANEOUS

Hemorrhagic Cystitis

Acute, fulminant bladder hemorrhage usually is seen at tertiary care centers in which cancer patients are treated with alkylating agents such as cyclophosphamide and ifosfamide. One of the liver metabolites of these compounds is acrolein, a urotoxin that is suspected to be the cause for the cystitis. This complication occurs in 40–50% of patients treated with ifosfamide, 7–15% in patients treated with low-dose cyclophosphamide, and up to 40% of those receiving cyclophosphamide prior to bone marrow transplantation. In patients who develop hemorrhagic cystitis following bone marrow transplantation, the cause is usually not the chemotherapy but usually due to activation of BK virus, and in this instance, treatment is based on eradication of the virus itself.[63] Prevention of chemotherapeutically induced cystitis ideally will follow careful attention to adequate hydration and the prophylactic use of antitoxins, such as mesna.

Clinical Presentation

The complication is characterized by cystitis, severe dysuria, microscopic or gross hematuria, and urinary frequency.

Diagnosis

Hemorrhagic cystitis is usually an acute complication occurring hours to days following ifosfamide and cyclophosphamide administration, but it can also be a delayed side effect. Diagnosis is usually made after a thorough history is taken and a urinalysis obtained, which may be visually bloody or have microscopic red blood cells.

Treatment

The use of mesna (sodium-2 mercaptoethanesulfonate), a thiol compound that binds acrolein, greatly decreases the extent of hemorrhagic cystitis from ifosfamide administration. Mesna is given in a dosage equal to 20% of the ifosfamide dosage (weight/weight) at the time of ifosfamide administration and again at 4 and 8 hours after each dose of ifosfamide. If the use of mesna is unsuccessful, a large-bore bladder catheter is inserted, and saline bladder irrigation is done. Cystoscopy and fulguration may be required next. The use of mesna with cyclophosphamide is recommended only when high doses are used in combination with forced saline diuresis.[62–64]

Discharge

The patient can be discharged once the episode of cystitis is resolved and the patient is asymptomatic and stable.

Pulmonary Veno-occlusive Disease (PVOD)

Bleomycin, mitomycin-C, carmustine, and bone marrow transplantation (autologous and allogeneic), which commonly use very high doses of chemotherapeutic agents, have been reported to cause pulmonary venocclusive disease (PVOD).[65–67] This is a very rare condition with various risk factors and elucidated causes, but little or no formal studies.

Clinical Presentation

Patients present with dyspnea on exertion, lethargy, and nonproductive cough. Pulmonary hypertension can result in chest pain, cyanosis, and exertional syncope. The extensive and diffuse occlusion of pulmonary veins by fibrous tissue is the classic pathologic hallmark of PVOD. Radiographically, pleural effusions are more commonly seen in PVOD versus pulmonary hypertension. Ground glass opacities and septal thickening can be seen on computed tomographic (CT) scans.

Diagnosis

Definitive diagnosis can only be made by surgical lung biopsy. Because the current therapy of PVOD is not very efficacious, the risks of surgical biopsy in these patients need to be weighed very carefully. Diagnosis by transbronchial biopsy cannot be done.

Prognosis and Treatment

Prognosis is often poor. Treatment of PVOD includes discontinuation of the agent in question. Treatment with various agents such as vasodilators, immunosuppressive agents, and oxygen therapy has been tried with little success.[65–67] At present, lung transplantation is the only curative therapy for PVOD; however, the average waiting times in many parts of the United States exceed the life expectancy of patients with PVOD.[69]

Discharge

The patient can be discharged with close outpatient follow-up when hemodynamically stable.

Key Points

- Nearly all therapeutic agents used in the treatment of cancer have the potential to produce HSRs and anaphylaxis, especially L-asparaginase, monoclonal antibodies, taxanes, epidophyllotoxins, and carboplatin.

- Nursing staff should be trained to seek immediate intervention when an HSR reaction occurs, because the patient needs prompt evaluation, given the risk for quick progression to respiratory and circulatory failure.

- Agents commonly associated with pulmonary toxicity include bleomycin, methotrexate, all-*trans* retinoic acid, nitrosoureas, and busulfan. Physicians are challenged to differentiate between lung toxicity and effects of metastases and infection.

- The primary technique used in the diagnosis of most presumptive cases of chemotherapy-associated lung injury is bronchoscopy with bronchoalveolar lavage (BAL).

- Agents commonly associated with cardiotoxicity include anthracyclines (e.g., doxorubicin), 5-fluorouracil, taxanes, trastuzumab, interleukin-2, interferon, cyclophosphamide, and ifosfamide. Cardiomyopathy and left ventricular dysfunction usually develop chronically within 1 year of exposure.

- Acute tubular necrosis is the most common form of intrinsic renal failure typically seen with platinum-based drugs and methotrexate. Prerenal failure is commonly seen secondary to dehydration from the nausea, vomiting, diarrhea, and/or anorexia resulting from cancer therapy.

SUGGESTED READING

Alley E, Green R, Schuchter. Cutaneous toxicties of cancer therapy. Curr Opin Oncol 2002; 14:212–216.

Giles FJ, Cortes JE, Halliburton TA, et al. Intravenous corticosteroids to reduce gemtuzumab ozogamicin infusion reactions. Ann Pharmacother 2003; 37:1182–1184.

Shanholtz C. Acute life-threatening toxicity of cancer treatment. Crit Care Clinics 2001; 17(3):483–502.

Yeh ET, Tong AT, Lenihan DJ et al. Cardiovascular complications of cancer therapy diagnosis, pathogenesis, and management. Circulation. 2004; 109:312 3131.

Singal PK, Iliskovic N. Doxorubicin-induced cardiomyopathy. N Engl J Med 1998; 339(13):900–905.

Schimmel KJ, Richel DJ, van den Brink RBA, et al. Cardiotoxicity of cytotoxic drugs. Cancer Treat Rev 2004; 30:181–191.

Kintzel PE. Anticancer drug-induced kidney disorders. Drug Safety 2001; 24(1):19–38.

Neurotoxic complications of chemotherapy in patients with cancer: clinical signs and optimal management. Drugs 2003; 63(15):1549–1563.

Pelgrim, J, De Vos F, Van den Brande J, et al. Methylene blue in the treatment and prevention of ifosfamide-induced encephalopathy: report of 12 cases and a review of the literature. Br J Cancer 2000; 82(2):291–294.

Holcomb BW, Loyd JE, Ely W, et al. Pulmonary veno-occlusive disease. Chest 2000; 118(6):1671–1679.

CHAPTER SIXTY-SEVEN

Anticoagulation in Cancer Patients

Kanchan Kamath, MD

BACKGROUND

Clinical thromboembolism is the second leading cause of death in patients with overt neoplasms.[1] The incidence is even higher in certain cancers of the pancreas, breast, lung, ovary, brain, and the gastrointestinal (GI) tract. Lung cancer accounts for the largest number of thromboembolic occurrences by virtue of its prevalence.[2]

Trousseau first recognized the association between cancer and thrombosis more than a hundred years ago.[3] Cancer can cause a broad array of hemostatic abnormalities, ranging from abnormal coagulation tests with no clinical manifestations to massive thromboembolism. Trousseau's syndrome, idiopathic deep venous thrombosis (DVT), arterial thrombosis, disseminated intravascular coagulation (DIC), marantic endocarditis, and microangiopathic hemolytic anemia (MAHA) are but a few examples of how dysregulation of the hemostatic machinery presents itself in patients with cancer. Tumors can also lead to thrombosis through external vascular compression or from direct invasion of a blood vessel itself.

Cancer treatments also add to the risk of thrombotic events. Concomitant rise in thrombotic complications is noted with high-dose chemotherapy regimens, cancer-related surgery, and bone marrow transplantation.[4] Two well-known chemotherapeutic regimens, l-asparaginase and tamoxifen, used in the treatment of acute lymphocytic leukemia and breast cancer, respectively, are especially notorious for augmenting the risk of thrombosis. Placement of long-term central venous catheters (CVC) used for chemotherapy is another risk factor for upper extremity DVT.

Additionally, if patients with cancer develop venous thromboembolism (VTE), they have a much higher risk of recurrence of VTE than patients without cancer who experience VTE. The MEDPAR study, conducted between 1988 to 1990 involving 8 million hospitalized Medicare patients, demonstrated that patients with a diagnosis of VTE and malignancy have a greater than three-fold risk of recurrent thromboembolic disease and related death than patients with VTE and no underlying cancer.[5]

The principles of diagnosis and management of VTE are reviewed in more detail in Chapters 26 and 27. In this chapter, we focus on selected elements of thromboembolism that are unique or atypical in the patient with cancer.

PATHOPHYSIOLOGY

Though intense attention has been bestowed upon the mechanisms associated with the pathogenesis of cancer, there remains much to be learned about the pathophysiology of the prothrombotic state in malignancy, despite its being a major complication.

Several mechanisms explain at least some aspects of the prothrombotic state of malignancy. Abnormalities in each of the three components of Virchow's triad—venous stasis, vessel wall injury, abnormal blood constituents—predispose cancer patients to having a hypercoagulable state (Table 67-1). The prothrombotic nature of the tumor cells, along with the morbidity associated with cancer such as infections, presence of long-term indwelling catheters, surgery, and decreased activity, also plays a synergistic role. In addition, normal host tissue may display prothrombotic behavior in response to the tumor.

ASSESSMENT

Clinical Presentation/Diagnosis

Manifestations of a prothrombotic state can precede the diagnosis of cancer by several months to years. While thromboembolism by itself in the absence of abnormal clinical or routine laboratory findings has not been shown to warrant further evaluation for malignant disease, the clinician should be alert to signs and symptoms of malignancy, such as weight loss or persistent unrelated pain which, in this setting, may impart a greater degree of suspicion for coexisting malignancy than otherwise. Data on the use of aggressive diagnostic approaches such as tumor markers, upper endoscopy, and computed tomography (CT) scans for cancer screening in patients with a remote idiopathic DVT, have failed to show any survival benefit. A thorough history and physical examination including prostate examination, fecal occult blood tests, routine blood tests, urinalysis, chest radiography, and prostate specific antigen testing as clinically appropriate should be considered, followed by more aggressive investigation only if the results are abnormal.[4]

As in patients without cancer, the signs and symptoms of thromboembolic disease among patients with cancer are related to the site of the thrombus, its local effects, and its distant

Table 67-1 Virchow's Triad in Cancer

Blood component abnormality	Impaired platelet aggregation and activation	Surge of procoagulant factors	Depletion of anticoagulants and fibrinolytics.
Blood vessel abnormality	Endothelial damage and dysfunction	Increase in angiogenesis (?)	Normal anticoagulant Function loss
Blood flow abnormality	Increase viscocity	Increase in stasis	

embolization. In essence, its presentation is not clearly different from that seen in noncancer patients. Axillo-subclavian venous thrombosis may be seen more commonly among patients with cancer because of the use of peripherally inserted central catheters (PICC). It is often asymptomatic and causes no local symptoms. However, it can also be suggested by nonspecific neck and shoulder discomfort and unilateral upper extremity edema, which worsens with exercise. Clinical suspicion should also rise with presence of dilated veins on the anterior chest wall in an otherwise asymptomatic individual with a CVC.

Though less commonly encountered, thromboembolic disease can also present as pulmonary embolism, migratory superficial thrombophlebitis (Trousseau's syndrome), DIC, or thrombotic microangiopathy.

The ambiguity of the presentation, therefore, underscores the need for careful clinical surveillance of patients with venous thromboembolism. Evidence-based strategies often call for clinical risk stratification for thromboembolic disease when determining the optimal diagnostic strategy.[6] In the presence of known cancer, it is therefore plausible to presume a high risk for VTE, despite the absence of classic predictors such as prolonged immobility, obesity, and previous DVT.

Diagnosis

Given the previous factors, timely diagnosis and appropriate treatment are particularly significant in the cancer patient. The same approach used to diagnose DVT in patients without cancer is appropriate for those with malignancy (*see* Chapter 26).

Duplex venous ultrasonography, which is a combination of venous imaging with compression maneuver, is the most common noninvasive test used in the diagnosis of deep venous thrombosis. The positive predictive value of this test approaches 95%, especially for proximal DVTs in both upper and lower extremities. It is the screening tool of choice because of its high sensitivity (>95%) and specificity (>95%), and also its ease of execution.[7] Additional modes of imagining, such as contrast venography or magnetic resonance imaging (MRI), are available diagnostic alternatives should the clinical suspicion for a calf thrombosis be high and the Doppler test negative. This is particularly true in cancer patients in whom the probability of finding a clot is intermediate to high. MRI is especially useful for suspected thrombosis of the superior and inferior vena cavae and of the pelvic region.

MANAGEMENT

Treatment

Prevention of pulmonary embolism is the most important goal for treating DVT with anticoagulation. Approximately 50% of proximal DVTs can lead to pulmonary emboli in untreated patients. Treatment goals also include relieving symptoms and preventing embolization and recurrence, which is more common among patients with cancer.

Anticoagulants inhibit thrombus propagation by activating the endogenous lytic system. Several pharmacologic agents are available; however, the most widely used are still unfractionated heparin, low-molecular-weight heparin, and warfarin. All are efficacious in the treatment of thromboembolism as proven by several large prospective clinical trials and confirmed by meta-analysis.[6] Another class of anticoagulant, hirudin, obtained from medicinal leeches, is presently undergoing trials for use as an anticoagulant, especially in patients in whom other forms have failed. In contrast to heparin, hirudin is a direct inactivator of thrombin entrapped within established clots. Of note, its use in thromboembolic events related to malignancy has not been explored.

With our growing repository of antithrombotic agents and the complexities associated with their use, choosing the most appropriate regimen may bewilder clinicians. Thus, cost, convenience, safety, and efficacy all play a compelling role in those myriad situations where the use of an appropriate anticoagulation regimen is warranted.

Treatment Strategies in Cancer-Related VTE

In cancer patients, the management of thromboembolim is similar to that in noncancer patients; however, certain differences do exist in the choice of treatment modality. Patients with cancer have a substantially higher risk of recurrent thromboembolism and hemorrhagic complications. This is because treatment with oral anticoagulants may be suboptimal in patients with cancer, given the effects of chemotherapy-related drug interactions, malnutrition, and liver dysfunction. Moreover, treatment-related problems such as thrombocytopenia or placement of a central line may necessitate interruption of anticoagulation in these patients.[7]

In September 2004, the seventh ACCP Consensus Conference on Antithrombotic Therapy published updated recommendations for anticoagulation in patients with thromboembolic disease. The problem inherent in any anticoagulant therapy is the risk of hemorrhage. The risk of hemorrhage is closely related to the intensity and duration of treatment. Other factors that predispose to hemorrhagic complications include poor compliance with anticoagulation regimen, peripheral vascular disease, cerebrovascular accidents, and advanced age. Bleeding often occurs at the site of the anatomic cancer lesion. Thus, the treatment selected should be carefully considered, keeping in mind the risk of bleeding versus the benefits of therapy.

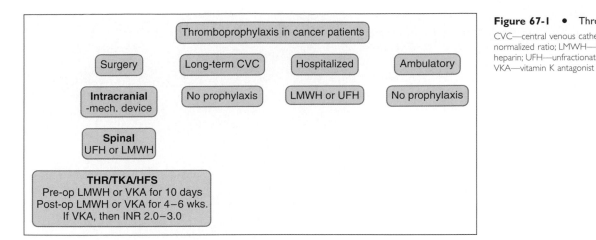

Figure 67-1 • Thrombophrophylaxis.
CVC—central venous catheter; INR—internation normalized ratio; LMWH—low molecular weight heparin; UFH—unfractionated heparin; VKA—vitamin K antagonist

---

Box 67-1 Treatment of Deep Venous Thrombosis in Cancer

Lovenox 1.5 mg/kg Sc q daily X 4–5 days.

Or

Lovenox 1.0 mg/kg Sc BID X 4–5 days.

+ Coumadin 5–10 mg PO q daily.

Check PT/INR In 4–5 days

If therapeutic (2.0–3.0), then discontinue lovenox.

Continue anticoagulation For 3–6 months.

Hospitalized and Ambulatory Cancer Patients

In patients with malignancy, initiating treatment with low-molecular-weight heparin (LMWH), though more expensive than unfractionated heparin (UFH), appears superior, especially given consideration of all expenses, including hospital admission, laboratory monitoring, and nursing needs. In addition, recent evidence based on a multicenter trial suggests long-term use of LMWH to be more effective than warfarin in preventing recurrences of VTE in patients with cancer, without an associated increased risk of bleeding.[8]

The optimum length of anticoagulation treatment remains controversial and should be determined by weighing the risks of bleeding with the risks of recurrence of VTE and its associated complications. Minimal duration of anticoagulation for DVTs has traditionally been for at least 3 months. Indefinite treatment should be strongly considered in advanced cancer and in patients with history of recurrent thromboembolic disease, provided the risk of bleeding is not high.

The role of prophylaxis in the medical oncology setting remains unclear. The prevention of VTE in hospitalized oncology patients is paramount, especially when they have additional risk factors for this complication. If these patients are undergoing surgery, aggressive prophylaxis for VTE is recommended according to the revised Chest guidelines (Fig. 67-1). Clinical trials in cancer surgery patients have proven that continuation of prophylaxis with LMWH for at least 3 weeks postdischarge reduces the risk of late DVTs.

Catheter-Related VTE

Though enough convincing data are now available on treatment strategies for lower extremity DVT, the same is not true for upper extremity DVTs. Upper extremity venous thromboses are usually a result of long-term CVC placement. The treatment options for catheter-related DVT vary from simple observation to anticoagulation to removal of the stimulus (i.e., catheter) to more invasive approaches such as fibrinolysis and surgery. Extrapolating from data gathered from different retrospective studies on treatment strategies for venous thrombosis, the risk of morbidity from embolization, even with an upper extremity DVT, is significant among patients with a procoagulant state (e.g., cancer). Thus, confronting it as aggressively as a lower extremity thrombosis becomes vital.[9]

Thus, management of cancer patients with an upper extremity DVT is guided by the same treatment principles as lower extremity DVT. Understandably, the risk of long-term obstruction or that of a distant emboli is smaller with upper extremity DVT; however, the looming hypercoagulable state warrants a more aggressive treatment approach.

The type and intensity of anticoagulation for catheter-induced upper extremity DVT remains the same as for DVT of the leg (Box 67-1). Most commonly, the initial dose of warfarin is between 5 mg and 10 mg, based on the patient's weight, age, nutritional status, and use of other medical regimens that are metabolized by the CYP 450 system. This can later be adjusted to achieve an INR of 2.0 to 3.0 in the postoperative period.

Though one randomized controlled trial with breast cancer patients did show a significant lower incidence of DVT in patients on a prophylactic dose of 1 mg warfarin, subsequent trials have not been able to repeat these results. Moreover, there was an increased risk of bleeding. This topic, therefore, remains controversial, and the 2004 Chest recommendations dissuade the use of any prophylactic measures of anticoagulation for upper extremity DVT.

Patients with CNS Malignancy

Despite the long held belief that brain malignancy precluded anticoagulation, treatment with warfarin to maintain an INR between 2.0 and 3.0 appears reasonably safe and is recommended for treatment of venous thromboembolism in patients with primary or secondary CNS malignancy.[10,11] Exceptions include tumors that have clearly sustained previous internal hemorrhage, impending neurosurgery, and presence of bleeding. The theoretic risk of tumor hemorrhage may warrant maintaining an INR at the lower end of the normal range, though evidence is lacking.

Though the risk of tumor-associated intracranial hemorrhage is a legitimate concern, several retrospective studies suggest that this risk is not significantly increased outside the perioperative period with oral anticoagulation if it is carefully managed with close monitoring. There is not enough evidence to support the use of LMWH for prophylaxis or therapy in patients with primary or secondary brain neoplasm alone, except perioperatively when the benefit far exceeds the risk, or as indicated by unrelated risk factors.

SUMMARY

In summary, the approach to prophylaxis, diagnosis, and management of VTE among patients with cancer should be adjusted based on a number of factors. Cancer markedly increases the incidence of VTE (and thus the pretest probability) by poorly understood, complex, direct effects on the coagulation cascade. Patients with cancer require prolonged duration of therapy if diagnosed with VTE because of the increased risk of recurrence. Cancer can compromise the stability of patients' intake and body weight and thus affect dosing of anticoagulants. The astute clinician will keep a low diagnostic threshold, pursue an aggressive diagnostic strategy, and make LMWH readily available, both acutely for VTE and for long-term maintenance in selected patients.

Key Points

- Clinical thromboembolism is the second leading cause of death in patients with known cancer.

- Cancer treatments add to the risk of thrombotic events. Specific chemotherapeutic agents (L-asparaginase and tamoxifen), surgery, bone marrow transplantation, and placement of long-term CVCs used for chemotherapy all can add to the risk.

- Thromboembolism in the absence of abnormal routine laboratory or clinical findings has not been shown to warrant further evaluation for malignant disease.

- Long-term use of LMWH appears to be more effective than warfarin in preventing recurrences of VTE in patients with cancer, without an associated increased risk of bleeding.

SUGGESTED READING

Rickles, FR, Edwards, RL. Activation of blood coagulation in cancer: Trousseau's syndrome revisited. Blood 1983; 62:14.

Otten HM, Mathijssen J, ten Cate H; et al. Symptomatic venous thromboembolism in cancer patients treated with chemotherapy: an underestimated phenomenon. Arch Intern Med 2004; 164(2):190–194.

Hyers TM, Agnelli G, Hull RD, et al. Antithrombotic therapy for venous thromboembolic disease. Chest 2001;119S(Suppl): 176S–193S.

Hutten BA, Prins MH, Gent M, et al. Incidence of recurrent thromboembolic and bleeding complications among patients with venous thromboembolism in relation to both malignancy and achieved international normalized ratio: a retrospective analysis. J Clin Oncol 2000;1 8:3078–3083.

Lee AYY, Levine MN, Baker RI, et al. Low-molecular-weight heparin versus a coumarin for the prevention of recurrent venous thromboembolism in patients with cancer. N Engl J Med 2003; 349:146–153.

CHAPTER SIXTY-EIGHT

Cancer Emergencies: Fever and Neutropenia

Joan Cain, MD, and David Lawson, MD

BACKGROUND

Neutropenic fever is defined by the National Comprehensive Cancer Network (NCCN) and the Infectious Diseases Society of America (IDSA)[1] as a temperature >38°C for more than 1 hour or a single temperature of 38.3°C in the setting of an absolute neutrophil count of <500 or <1,000 with a predicted nadir of less than 500. If appropriate treatment is not instituted in a timely manner, mortality rates may reach 70% in 24–48 hours. Neutropenia as a result of chemotherapy usually presents 7–14 days after treatment. Predisposing factors to neutropenic fever include a rapid decline in absolute neutrophil count, duration of neutropenia >7–10 days, leukemia induction; disruption of mucosal, mucociliary and cutaneous barriers; implanted devices; and comorbid illnesses.

The etiology of neutropenic fever is an infection in 60–80% of cases. However, it is important always to consider other causes of fever, such as pulmonary embolus or drug fevers. The infecting organism is most commonly bacterial, but can be fungal or viral. According to the IDSA guidelines, gram-positive bacteria account for 60–70% of infections. Of increasing concern are antibiotic-resistant organisms such as methicillin-resistant *Staphylococcus. aureus* (MRSA) or vancomycin-resistant *Enterococcus* (VRE).

ASSESSMENT

Clinical Presentation

Prevalence

Widespread use of prophylactic granulocyte or granulocyte-macrophage colony-stimulating-factors has decreased the incidence of admissions for febrile neutropenia, but in some series as many as 10% of solid-tumor patients will have at least one such admission. Prolonged neutropenia is an expected consequence of treatment of acute leukemia and of any bone marrow transplant regimen. Risk factors include prior radiation to areas of active bone marrow and prior chemotherapy.

Presenting Signs and Symptoms

Signs of infection in neutropenic patients are usually subtle, given the decreased ability to mount an immune response. However, fevers are still a relatively common early presenting complaint. However, one should always remember that septic patients may be hypothermic. History and physical examination should be thorough and directed at common sites of infection such as sinuses, nasopharynx, bronchi and lungs, alimentary tract, skin, and indwelling lines. Digital rectal examinations are usually avoided to reduce the risk of examination-induced bacteremia and perirectal abscess. Mucositis and areas of skin breakdown should be noted through visual inspection.

Diagnosis

Two sets of blood cultures should be obtained, with at least one set from any existing vascular access device. Bacteremia is found in up to 25% of patients. Additionally, urinalysis, urine cultures, and chest x-rays should be performed. It is important to note that urinalysis and chest x-ray may be negative, even in the presence of urinary tract or pulmonary infection because of the absence of neutrophils.

Prognosis

Without treatment, the estimated mortality is up to 70% in the first 24–48 hours. With appropriate treatment, almost all patients will survive, unless the neutropenia is prolonged past 7–10 days.

MANAGEMENT

Treatment

Initial Therapy

When an outpatient with neutropenic fever first presents, the first decision is whether the patient requires admission. Patients can be stratified into low- and high-risk groups.[3] The two major factors contributing to risk for outpatients are: (1) serious independent comorbidities, and (2) uncontrolled cancer. Patients who do not have any of these characteristics are classified as low risk with a 5% incidence of serious complications. On the other hand, among patients with these risk factors, or those who are inpatients when they become febrile, 34% will have serious medical complications. Therefore, it is reasonable to manage low-risk

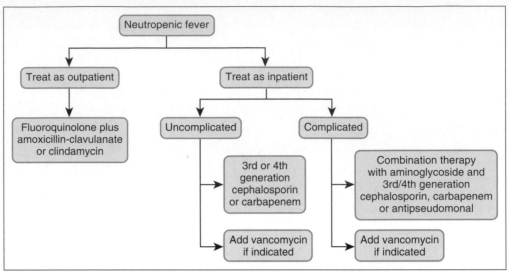

Figure 68-1 • Initial Treatment Scheme for neutropenic fever.

patients as outpatients if they are reliable for follow-up and the institution has the capability of providing adequate follow-up.

The antibiotic choice should be tailored to each institution's pattern of antibiotic resistance (Fig. 68-1). For outpatients, IDSA guidelines recommend a fluoroquinolone plus amoxicillin-clavulanate. Clindamycin may be substituted for penicillin-allergic patients. For inpatients, combination drug therapy has not been shown to be more efficacious than monotherapy according to IDSA. Monotherapy with a third- or fourth-generation cephalosporin such as ceftazidime or a carbapenem such as meropenem could be considered in uncomplicated neutropenic patients. Combination therapy should be considered in more complicated cases, such as septic shock. Combination therapy has the advantage of decreased emergence of antibiotic resistance and can be synergistic in some infections. Combination therapy usually consists of an aminoglycoside such as gentamicin and either an antipseudomonal carboxy-penicillin such as piperacillin-tazobactam, anti-pseudomonal cephalosporin such as ceftazidime, or anti-pseudomonal carbapenem such as meropenem. If the patient is unable to tolerate an aminoglycoside because of renal impairment, then aztreonam is a suitable alternative. The addition of vancomycin should be considered if there are concerns about a line infection, history of MRSA colonization, or skin lesions.

According to NCCN guidelines, empiric antivirals such as acyclovir should be started if there are skin or mucous membrane lesions suspicious for herpes simplex. Also, patients with hematologic malignancies have been shown to have a more favorable febrile response when placed on prophylactic or empiric acyclovir.[4]

Subsequent Therapy

If an etiology for the fever is found, then the antibiotic regimen should be adjusted accordingly. If vancomycin was added empirically, it should be discontinued if cultures are negative. For a documented infection, the antibiotics should be continued as indicated by the source (e.g., cellulitis should be treated for 7–14

days, but bacterial pneumonia should be treated 14–21 days); in stable patients, this can be on an outpatient basis once the neutrophil count is >500.

If no documented infection is found, then empiric treatment should be continued until the absolute neutrophil count is >500. IDSA guidelines suggest that antibiotics can be changed to the oral route after 2 days if the patient remains stable. If the patient's fever persists >5 days and no cause is found, then consideration should be given to changing the patient's antibiotics. Vancomycin could be added if the patient was not started on this initially. If the patient's neutropenia is expected to be protracted, then antifungals are usually added, given the increased risk of fungal infections in patients with prolonged neutropenia. NCCN recommends starting with fluconazole, but it does not have activity against mold. Therefore, if the patient remains febrile despite being on fluconazole, the clinician could consider changing to an agent with activity against mold, such as aspergillus. The agents voriconazole and caspofungin have been shown to have similar efficacy and improved side-effect profiles when compared to amphotericin.[5,6]

Addition of Granulocyte Colony-Stimulating Factors

Once neutropenia has developed, neither mortality benefit nor reduction in hospital stay has been demonstrated for these agents. Empiric use may be considered in patients who are critically ill or in whom prolonged neutropenia (>7 days) is expected.

PREVENTION

The only agents effective in prevention of neutropenia are the colony-stimulating factors mentioned previously. Some physicians empirically start patients on antibiotics prior to the period of expected neutropenia. Patients frequently want to know if nutritional factors can reduce the incidence of neutropenia, but this does not appear to be the case generally, although known vitamin deficiencies (e.g., B_{12}) should of course be corrected

DISCHARGE/FOLLOW-UP PLANS

Stable, reliable patients with no documented cause of infection may be discharged on no further therapy when afebrile and having an absolute neutrophil count >500. Patients with documented source of infection may also be discharged when stable and afebrile with neutrophils >500, but therapy should be continued as indicated by the cause of the infection. Patients without complicating issues such as organ dysfunction (e.g. renal failure) or other major co-morbidities may be seen in follow-up when chemotherapy is scheduled to resume, as recurrence of neutropenia during the same cycle would be rare. Patients continuing treatment may need to be monitored for drug toxicity (e.g., nephrotoxicity of gentamicin).

Patient Education

Patients being treated in the outpatient setting must be cautioned to call with worsening fever or any signs of clinical deterioration. Once the period of neutropenia has resolved, further patient education is dependent on next steps in cancer treatment.

Outpatient Physician Communication

The treating oncologist should be aware of the admission and any complications, as it may affect treatment decisions about the next cycle of chemotherapy. It is very important that the treating oncologist be aware of patients' continuing antibiotic therapy so that drug toxicity can be monitored.

Key Points

- Untreated patients with fever and absolute neutrophil count <500 have a mortality of up to 70% in 24 hours; therefore, appropriate treatment must be initiated promptly.

- Patients with no significant comorbidities and no active cancer (e.g., adjuvant treatment) and reliable support may be treated as outpatients.

- Although physical examination must be thorough, digital rectal examinations are usually contraindicated because of risk of causing bacteremia and possible development of perirectal abscesses.

- Some tests such as chest X-ray and urinalysis may be deceptively normal because of the absence of neutrophils.

- Vancomycin and antivirals should be used as initial therapy only in carefully defined instances.

- Once patients are neutropenic, use of colony-stimulating factors is of no value unless the period of neutropenia is expected to be greater than 7 days (e.g., a known drug overdose or marrow ablative therapy).

SUGGESTED READING

National Comprehensive Cancer Network Practice Guidelines—Fever and neutropenia. www.nccn.org.

Hughes WT, Armstrong D, Bodey GP, Bow EJ, Brown AE, Calandra T, Feld R, Pizzo PA, Rolston KV, Shenep JL, Young LS. 2002 Guidelines for the use of antimicrobial agents in neutropenic patients with cancer. Clinical Infectious Diseases 2002; 34:730–751.

Talcott JA, Finberg R, Mayer RJ, Goldman L. The medical course of cancer patients with fever and neutropenia: clinical identification of a low-risk subgroup at presentation. Arch Intern Med 1988; 148:2561–2568.

Baglin TP, Gray JJ, Marcus RE, Wreghitt TG. Antibiotic resistant fever associated with herpes simplex virus infection in neutropenic patients with haematological malignancy. J Clin Pathol 1989; 42:1255–1258.

Walsh Tj, Pappas P, Winston DJ, Lazarus HM, Petersen F, Raffali J, et al. Voriconazole compared with liposomal amphotericin B for empiric antifungal therapy in patients with neutropenia and persistent fevers. N Engl J Med 2002; 346:225–234.

Walsh TJ, Teppler H, Donowitz GR, Maertans JA, Baden LR, et al. Caspofungin versus liposomal amphotericin B for empiric antifungal therapy in patients with persistent fever and neutropenia. N Engl J Med 2004; 351(14):1391–1402.

CHAPTER SIXTY-NINE

Cancer Emergencies: Hypercalcemia

Joan Cain, MD, and David Lawson, MD

BACKGROUND

Hypercalcemia is seen in up to 20–30% of patients with advanced cancer. The incidence is probably decreasing due to standard preventive therapy with bisphosphonates to reduce skeletal complications. The most common malignancies that cause hypercalcemia are breast, lung, renal, and multiple myeloma. Hypercalcemia is also seen frequently in patients with squamous cell carcinomas of any organ.

The pathophysiologic etiologies for hypercalcemia of malignancy are multifactorial. Although there are several mechanisms of hypercalcemia associated with cancer, they all share the characteristic of osteoclast activation. Among patients with lytic bone lesions (e.g., myeloma), the etiology is usually increased secretion of locally acting factors that increase osteoclast activity causing bone resorption. A second cause is excretion of parathyroid hormone–related protein or actual parathyroid hormone into the bloodstream, both of which cause bone resorption and decreased renal excretion of calcium and may cause hypercalcemia in the absence of clinically detectable cancer bone involvement. Finally, a malignant tumor can secrete the active form of vitamin D (1, 25-dihydroxyvitamin D), which increases osteoclast activity and intestinal absorption of calcium. This is most commonly seen in patients with lymphoma. However, not all episodes of hypercalcemia in a cancer patient are cancer related. Therefore, other possible alternatives should be investigated as well. The most common cause of hypercalcemia other than the tumor itself is hyperparathyroidism.

ASSESSMENT

Clinical Presentation

Prevalence and Risk Factors

The most common risk factors are advanced cancers of the types listed previously. Immobility and presence of bone metastases are contributing factors. In some patients, concurrent medications such as hydrochlorothiazide may play a role. Although review of older literature indicated that up to 20–30% of patients with advanced cancer will develop hypercalcemia, usually as a preterminal event, the increasing use of bisphosphonates is likely decreasing the incidence of this complication.

Presenting Signs and Symptoms

Most clinical signs are nonspecific. Patients most commonly present complaining of constipation or abdominal pain, bony pain, anorexia, fatigue, and lethargy progressing to coma. Since these symptoms are also common among patients with advanced malignancy, a high index of suspicion is needed, especially with tumors commonly associated with hypercalcemia. Many of these patients will also have renal dysfunction at presentation. Of note, symptoms are not necessarily proportional to the degree of hypercalcemia, as chronicity also plays a role.

Differential Diagnosis

The most common causes of hypercalcemia include primary hyperparathyroidism, malignancy-related hypercalcemia, pseudo-hypercalcemia (hyperproteinemic states, including calcium-binding globulins in myeloma), sarcoidosis, hyperthyroidism, and medications (thiazide diuretics, lithium). Less common etiologies include Zollinger-Ellison syndrome, milk alkali syndrome, Paget's disease, Addison's disease, excessive vitamin A or D, and familial hypocalciuric hypercalcemia. However, in the context of known cancer and the absence of a strong clinical suspicion for an alternative cause, it can usually be safely assumed that cancer is the underlying cause without extensive diagnostic evaluation. Some, however, advocate routine measurement of parathyroid hormone levels as part of the diagnostic work-up.

Diagnosis

First, an elevated calcium level should be confirmed to rule out a spurious laboratory value. Once confirmed, additional diagnostic evaluation may include checking total protein levels to rule out a hyperproteinemic state causing pseudo-hypercalcemia. Additionally, one should attempt to determine for how long the hypercalcemia has been present. Persistent, asymptomatic hypercalcemia may indicate a longer standing disease process, such as familial hypocalciuric hypercalcemia. A normal calcium in the presence of decreased serum albumin concentration may also represent hypercalcemia. Formulas may assist in estimating the degree of hypercalcemia in the face of decreased albumin, but actual measurement of free calcium is more accurate. The degree of hyper-

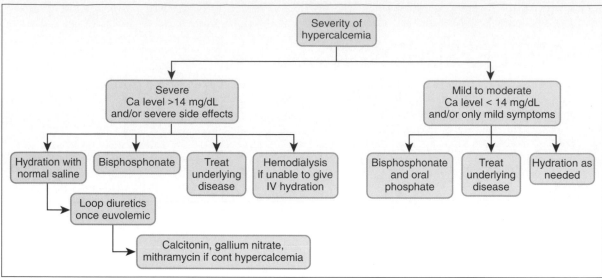

Figure 69-1 • Treatment algorithm for hypercalcemia of malignancy.

calcemia can help in diagnosis as well. Primary hyperparathyroidism rarely elevates serum calcium concentration to greater than 11 mg/dL, whereas markedly elevated calcium levels (greater than 13 mg/dL) are commonly a result of malignancies.

Laboratory Studies

Measuring intact parathyroid hormone (PTH) level is useful, given that hyperparathyroidism is common, and patients with malignancies seem to have a higher incidence of hyperparathyroidism than the general population.

Serum phosphate concentration is usually low in hyperparathyroidism and malignancy, due to inhibition of phosphate absorption at the proximal tubule. Phosphate is elevated in granulomatous disease, hypervitaminosis D, hyperthyroidism, and milk-alkali syndrome.

Urinary calcium is usually increased or high-normal in hyperparathyroidism and malignancy. Urinary calcium is low in milk-alkali syndrome, where a resultant metabolic alkalosis increases calcium reabsorption; thiazide diuretic use, which increases reabsorption of calcium at the distal tubule; and familial hypocalciuric hypercalcemia.

PTH–related protein is elevated in some patients with hypercalcemia of malignancy. In hypervitaminosis D, the inactive form (calcidiol) is elevated. There is no feedback regulation of this metabolite, so the liver continues to make the calcidiol as more vitamin D is presented to it. The active form (calcitriol) is elevated in granulomatous diseases caused by peripheral conversion to this metabolite and in hyperparathyroidism, which causes increased conversion to calcitriol in the kidney.

Prognosis

Hypercalcemia associated with malignancy represents an ominous sign since it indicates advanced disease. Approximately 50% of patients with hypercalcemia die within 30 days of diagnosis.[2] It may, however, be the presenting sign of a treatable

malignancy (e.g., myeloma). Prognosis is generally that of the underlying cancer, unless severe renal insufficiency is present.

MANAGEMENT

Treatment

Management depends on the severity of the hypercalcemia, availability of treatment for the underlying disease, and goals of treatment. It usually includes disease-specific measures as well as direct measures aimed at reducing the calcium level. The risks of hypercalcemia include respiratory arrest, altered mental status, and severe dehydration leading to acute renal failure, cardiac arrhythmias, and nephrolithiasis. If there is no effective treatment for the underlying disease, any improvement in serum calcium concentration and symptomatology is likely short lived. In the setting of untreatable cancer and recurrent hypercalcemia, end-of-life discussions should be undertaken with the patient and family, with consideration of not treating the increased calcium at all.

Initial Therapy

Patients should be stratified into those with severe hypercalcemia (usually defined as a calcium level greater than 14 mg/dL and/or severe side effects) and those with mild-to-moderate hypercalcemia (calcium level less than 14 mg/dL and only mild symptoms) (Fig. 69-1).

For severe hypercalcemia, the mainstay of treatment is hydration with normal saline, since hypercalcemia, regardless of the cause, induces progressive dehydration by causing a water-concentrating defect in the kidney. Once the patient is sufficiently rehydrated, one can consider adding a loop diuretic to increase renal excretion of calcium by blocking calcium reabsorption in the loop of Henle.

In the setting of hypercalcemia secondary to a malignancy, bisphosphonates are also used to decrease calcium levels by decreasing osteoclast activity. The bisphosphonates usually take effect within 2–4 days, with nadir calcium concentrations not seen until about 7 days. Thus, they should be initiated immediately once diagnosis of the hypercalcemia is made. There are several different bisphosphonates, and until recently no clear difference in efficacy between the different subclasses was apparent. However, a systematic review demonstrated that zoledronic acid (Zometa) and pamidronate (Aredia) were more effective than other bisphosphonates in both normalizing calcium levels and doubling the median duration of normocalcemia. The American Society of Oncology (ASCO) recommends zoledronic acid 4 mg delivered intravenously over >15 minutes or pamidronate 90 mg given over 2 hours. Possible side effects include azotemia, but ASCO does not recommend the use of reduced doses of bisphosphonates for patients with creatinine levels >3 mg per deciliter. ASCO does recommend that the duration of infusion not be shortened, however. Oral phosphates may also be given as tolerated. Intravenous phosphates are rarely indicated, but may be life saving in a patient with refractory arrhythmia.

For mild-to-moderate asymptomatic hypercalcemia, focusing on treating the underlying disease is the appropriate course of action. Additionally, oral phosphate and a high-salt diet can be used to decrease the serum calcium concentration. Oral phosphate combines with calcium in the gut, which decreases absorption. The high-salt diet induces volume expansion with resultant increased urinary calcium excretion. Practically speaking, however, most patients with hypercalcemia associated with malignancy will also need treatment with bisphosphonates. Many of these patients can be treated in the outpatient setting.

Subsequent Therapy

For patients with hypercalcemia to whom hydration and/or bisphosphonates cannot be given safely (renal failure, congestive heart failure), dialysis should be considered. For these patients, and for patients who are refractory to hydration and bisphosphonates, calcitonin may also be used; maximal response occurs within 12–24 hours, but the reductions are small and transient. Gallium nitrate can be used for both PTH-related and non-PTH related hypercalcemia. It works directly on osteoclasts to decrease bone resorption. Disadvantages are its nephrotoxicity and the need for a continuous infusion over 5 days. Mithramycin was widely used before bisphosphonates were available and may be considered in patients refractory to these agents.

PREVENTION

Prophylactic bisphosphonates have been given to patients with cancer metastatic to bone. One study showed a 50% reduction in the incidence of severe hypercalcemia when prophylactic pamidronate was given to women with breast cancer and at least one lytic bone lesion.

DISCHARGE/FOLLOW-UP PLANS

Discharge is likely driven more by symptoms, hydration status and ability of the patient to take adequate fluids (including intravenous supplementation in the clinic or by home health agencies), and therapeutic goals (further treatment of the malignancy versus hospice or palliative care only) than by the actual serum calcium concentration. Follow-up is dependent on these same criteria, but almost always the patient should have serum calcium rechecked in a week or less unless the patient elects hospice care.

Patient Education

Patients should be given an indication of underlying prognosis. Hypercalcemia in a patient who has been treated with multiple agents, or in a patient with a malignancy for which there are no good treatment options, is frequently an ominous sign. On the other hand, some patients may have hypercalcemia as the presenting sign of a treatable cancer (e.g., myeloma). A clear understanding of where the patient is in the natural course of his or her disease will drive most of the decisions that need to be made.

Patients not referred to hospice should be aware of the need for careful monitoring of serum calcium concentration and early reporting of symptoms suggesting recurrence of hypercalcemia.

Outpatient Physician Communication

A medical oncologist caring for the patient should be involved in any hospice decisions. If the patient is not a candidate for hospice, the hospitalist must ensure appropriate communication with the medical oncologist who will be following the patient this; consists primarily of ensuring careful follow-up.

Key Points

- Hypercalcemia may occur in up to 20–30% of patients with advanced cancer, primarily among patients with multiple myeloma or breast, lung, renal, and squamous cell carcinomas.

- Patients with hypercalcemia associated with cancer typically present with nonspecific symptoms that often afflict cancer patients without hypercalcemia, for example, constipation or abdominal pain, bony pain, anorexia, fatigue, or lethargy.

- Presence of hypercalcemia frequently, but not always, portends a poor prognosis. Treatment decisions are heavily influenced by availability of treatment for the underlying malignancy.

- Although there are several mechanisms of hypercalcemia associated with cancer, they all share the characteristic of osteoclast activation.

- The mainstays of treatment are hydration and bisphosphonates.

SUGGESTED READING

Farr, HW. Primary hyperparathyroidism and cancer. Am J Surg 1973; 126:539.

Ralston SH. Cancer-associated hypercalcemia: morbidity and mortality: clinical experience in 126 treated patients. Ann Intern Med 1990; 112:499–504.

Binstock ML. Effect of calcitonin and glucocorticoids in combination on the hypercalcemia of malignancy. Ann Intern Med 1980; 93:269–272.

Hortobagyi, et al. Efficacy of pamidronate in reducing skeletal complications in patients with breast cancer and lytic bone lesions. N Engl J Med 1996; 335(24):1785–1791.

Saunders Y. Systematic review of bisphosphonates for hypercalcaemia of malignancy. Palliat Med 2004; 18:418–431.

Stewart A. Hypercalcemia associated with cancer. N Engl J Med 2005; 352:373–379.

CHAPTER SEVENTY

Cancer Emergencies: Hyperviscosity Syndromes

Asha Ramsakal, DO, and Darrin Beaupre, MD, PhD

BACKGROUND

Hyperviscosity syndromes classically arise from elevated levels of compounds with high molecular weights, such as proteins. In cancer patients, these are invariably immunoglobulins, either (1) IgM (a pentamer) in Waldenström's macroglobulinemia, or (2) smaller IgA (a dimer), IgG (a monomer) or kappa light chains in multiple myeloma.[1]

ASSESSMENT

Clinical Presentation

Symptoms in the patient's history and his or her associated physical examination findings can be subdivided according to the four major physiologic processes described in Figure 70-1 (Pathophysiology of Hyperviscosity Syndromes). Clinical signs and symptoms seem to correlate but do not exhibit a linear relationship with the serum viscosity (measured in centipoises, C). One study documented the presence of clinical signs and symptoms in 0%, 67%, and 75% of patients with serum viscosities of <3, >3 and >4 centipoises respectively.[2]

Diagnosis

The physician should consider the diagnosis of hyperviscosity syndrome when a patient presents with unexplained neurologic symptoms such as visual change or headache in the setting of a concomitant immunoglobulin-producing hematologic condition. The diagnosis of hyperviscosity is based on a combination of the presenting clinical manifestations (see Fig. 70-1) and associated laboratory abnormalities. A viscosity of 4 centipoises or greater as measured by the Ostwald viscosimeter is considered consistent with the diagnosis. (Normal is 1.4–1.8 C)

Prognosis

Data on prognosis are limited, but at least in Waldenström's macroglobulinemia the presence of serum hyperviscosity does not appear to significantly affect overall survival.[3]

MANAGEMENT

Criteria for treatment are based primarily on the severity of signs and symptoms rather than the degree of hyperviscosity. The preferred therapy is plasma exchange, as the only randomized trial comparing plasma exchange to cascade filtration (plasmapheresis) revealed a superior decrease in serum viscosity in patients with Waldenström's macroglobulinemia.[4] Plasma exchange can reduce platelets; and it depletes albumin, coagulation factors, and complement, thus potentially affecting coagulability, depending on the volume of exchange. Emergency plasma exchange is needed for severe neurologic changes such as seizures, lethargy, or coma.[5] In practical terms, it is important to remember that red blood cell transfusion of anemic patients can increase serum viscosity, leading to catastrophic complications in the presence of hyperviscosity. Therefore, transfusion should be deferred unless absolutely required.

From the hospitalist perspective, the primary effort should be directed at expediting initiation of plasma exchange in collaboration with hematology consultants. Preliminary measures such as hydration and steroids provide temporizing benefit. Exchange of one plasma volume with saline and 5% albumin can be performed daily until resolution of symptoms and normalization of serum viscosity.[5,6] Obtaining serum quantitative immunoglobulins before and after exchange will help determine the frequency and length of exchange. IgA and IgG hyperviscosity syndromes may require an increased quantity and frequency of plasma exchange, since these smaller molecules occupy both the intra- and extravascular spaces and extravascular stores shift intravascularly after exchange.[7] Plasma exchange does not alter the course of the underlying plasma cell dyscrasia. Thus, these patients require immediate consultation by a hematologist or oncologist and intervention with chemotherapy, steroids, or other disease-modifying agents.

DISCHARGE/FOLLOW-UP

Patients can be safely discharged after successful management. Regular postdischarge serum viscosity measurements should be arranged, since cessation of plasma exchange without an adequate treatment response of the underlying disease is associated with recurrence of hyperviscosity syndrome in a few

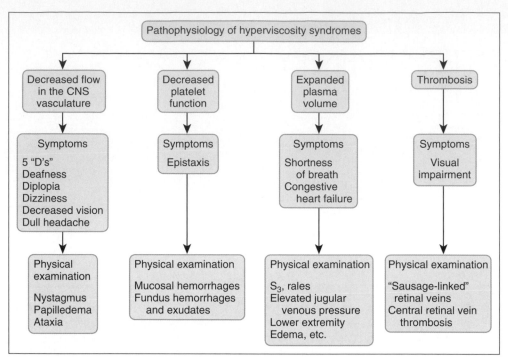

Figure 70-1 • Pathophysiology of hyperviscosity syndromes.

weeks.[8] Close follow-up of quantitative immunoglobulins can also be useful, since the offending paraprotein should remain significantly decreased after effective management. Certain symptoms of hyperviscosity may be irreversible and include hearing loss.

Key Points

- Clinical signs and symptoms seem to correlate but do not exhibit a linear relationship with the serum viscosity (measured in centipoises).

- Consider the diagnosis of hyperviscosity syndrome when a patient presents with unexplained neurologic symptoms such as visual change or headache in the setting of a concomitant immunoglobulin-producing hematologic condition.

- Preferred therapy is plasma exchange.

- Avoid red blood cell transfusion of anemic patients who also have hyperviscosity syndrome, as this can increase serum viscosity leading to catastrophic complications.

- Regular postdischarge serum viscosity measurements should be arranged, since cessation of plasma exchange without adequate treatment of the underlying disease is associated with recurrence of hyperviscosity syndrome in a few weeks.

SUGGESTED READING

Carter PW, Cohen HJ, Crawford J. Hyperviscosity syndrome in association with kappa light chain myeloma. Am J Med 1989; 86:591.

Crawford J, Cox EB, Cohen HJ. Evaluation of hyperviscosity in monoclonal gammopathies. Am J Med 1985; 79:13.

Facon T, Brouillard M, Duhamel A, et al. Prognostic factors in Waldenström's macroglobulinemia: a report of 167 cases. J Clin Oncol 1993; 11:1553.

Hoffkes HG, Heemann UW, Teschendorf C, et al. Hyperviscosity syndrome: efficacy and comparison of plasma exchange by plasma separation and cascade filtration in patients with immunocytoma of Waldenström's type. Clin Nephrol 1995, 43:335–338.

Drew, MJ. Plasmapheresis in the dysproteinemias. Ther Apher 2002; 6:45.

Siami GA, Siami FS. Plasmapheresis and paraproteinemia: cryoprotein-induced diseases, monoclonal gammopathy, Waldenström's macroglobulinemia, hyperviscosity syndrome, multiple myeloma, light chain disease, and amyloidosis. Ther Apheres; 1999; 3(1):8–19.

CHAPTER SEVENTY-ONE

Cancer Emergency: Elevated Intracranial Pressure

Asha Ramsakal, DO, and Stephen G. Patterson, MD

BACKGROUND

The brain is easily prone to increased intracranial pressure since its volume is limited by the nonexpansile cranium. Diverse etiologies can produce increased intracranial pressure (ICP) in cancer patients. These may be directly related to the cancer itself (e.g., vasogenic edema, hemorrhage, cerebrospinal obstruction) or to associated conditions (e.g., infections, abscesses, thrombotic states, and coagulopathies). Whereas increased ICP in cancer patients occurs most commonly due to brain metastases from melanoma and lung cancer,[1] cerebral hemorrhage causing increased ICP is most commonly associated with melanoma, choriocarcinoma, renal cell carcinoma, and papillary thyroid cancer.[2] Large mass lesions or tumor burdens (e.g., leukostasis with acute leukemias or leptomeningeal carcinomatosis) can directly impede cerebrospinal fluid (CSF) flow from the aqueduct of Sylvius or foramen of Monro. CSF obstruction may also occur from infections such as *Cryptococcus, Aspergillus, Candida, Listeria,* and herpes simplex virus, not uncommon among cancer patients, causing focal swelling. Additionally, ICP can be increased by cancer-induced hypercoagulopathy, causing sinus venous thrombosis. At the other end of the spectrum, some cancer patients are susceptible to cerebral hemorrhage as the cause of increased ICP, because of coagulopathies from anticoagulation for venous thromboembolism, thrombocytopenia after chemotherapy, or propensity to spontaneous bleeding (e.g., promyelocytic leukemia).

ASSESSMENT

Clinical Presentation

Symptoms

The most common presenting symptom of acute elevation of ICP is headache. Clinical clues supportive of headache being secondary to increased ICP include a history of the headache being worse in the morning (after lying supine all night) or changing with position (i.e., worse bending over and less with upright posture). Nausea and vomiting associated with headache support its being secondary to increased ICP. With increasing ICP, symptoms progress to depressed level of consciousness, lethargy, and coma.

Signs

The signs of elevated ICP may include the ocular findings of papilledema. Early on, elevation of ICP causes lack of venous pulsations of the optic disc, while later, the margin of the optic disc becomes blurred. Spontaneous periorbital bruising has been reported in 50% of patients.[3] Cranial nerve VI palsies may also be seen. The Kocher-Cushing triad consists of hypopnea, hypertension, and bradycardia probably secondary to brainstem compression and mandates urgent intervention.[4] In general, both symptoms and signs have limited accuracy in the diagnosis of elevated ICP.

Diagnosis

While the diagnosis of increased ICP may be suggested by a thorough history and physical examination, the gold standard is measurement of the intracranial pressure (ICP). The normal ICP in an adult is <15 mm Hg, while >20 mm Hg is considered pathologic; measurement currently requires an invasive not risk-free procedure.

The use of computed tomography (CT) scans is typically the first step in the diagnosis of increased ICP, but is less accurate than direct measurement. In a prospective study of 753 patients, 10–15% developed obvious elevated ICP during their hospitalization, despite initial CT scans negative for midline shifts or mass lesions.[5] However, this study involved patients with traumatic brain injury, and data on cancer patients are lacking. Hence, although findings that suggest increased ICP invariably generate imaging studies such as CT scanning, such studies, even when a mass is present, do not necessarily correlate with increased ICP.

MRI with gadolinium can better distinguish among infectious, neoplastic, and ischemic etiologies of increased ICP, and thus can inform treatment strategies. Among cancer patients suspected of ICP and intracranial pathology, MRI is the imaging modality of choice.

MANAGEMENT

The role of the hospitalist in the management of elevated ICP is to stabilize the patient medically, while facilitating prompt neuro-oncologic, radio-oncologic, and neurosurgical evaluation. Medical interventions and therapies have one primary goal—reduction of ICP. The intensity of immediate care varies with the clinical presentation. Measures may include:

A. Medical interventions
1. Elevation of head and upper trunk to facilitate gravity assisted cerebral venous drainage
2. If the patient is clinically unstable necessitating intubation, adequate sedation and mechanical hyperventilation to keep pCO_2 25–30 mm Hg are recommended. Hypocapnea stimulates cerebral vasoconstriction, theoretically reducing temporarily the increase in intracranial pressure.

B. Medical therapies
1. Fluids: Isotonic fluids such as 0.9% normal saline are recommended to maintain euvolemic iso- and hyperosmolality. The goal is to keep the cerebral perfusion pressure (CPP) 60–75 mm Hg. CPP equals mean arterial pressure (MAP) – ICP.[6] This has been associated with better outcomes in traumatic brain injury patients. Its applicability to cancer patients is not known.
2. Intravenous mannitol is recommended in medically unstable patients to promote osmotic diuresis. A dose of 20–25% at 0.75–1 g/kg IV initially, then 0.25–0.5 g/kg q3–6 h is recommended by most experts. This should be discontinued if the serum osmolality exceeds 300.
3. Corticosteroids are indicated if the elevated ICP is due to tumor-induced vasogenic edema. Dexamethasone 6–10 mg IV q6h is the usual dose. Steroids have no role in elevated ICP from tumor-induced hemorrhage, infarction, CSF flow obstruction, or ischemia.

Signs and symptoms that suggest herniation, such as stupor, coma, pupillary dilation, loss of oculocephalic reflexes, Cheyne-Stokes breathing, or hypotension, warrant immediate neurosurgical evaluation and possible intervention.

Concomitant treatment of the underlying cancer-induced condition is warranted. Mass lesions may need surgical intervention and/or radiation therapy, hematomas evacuated, abscesses and infections treated with appropriate antibiotics, dural venous sinus thrombosis treated with anticoagulation, and coagulopathies corrected with fresh frozen plasma and vitamin K.

Key Points

- The most common cause of increased ICP in cancer patients is brain metastases from melanoma or lung cancer.

- MRI with gadolinium best distinguishes among infectious, neoplastic, and ischemic causes of increased ICP, and thus is the imaging modality of choice among cancer patients suspected of ICP and intracranial pathology as it informs the approach to therapy.

- Steroids have no role in elevated ICP from tumor-induced hemorrhage, infarction, CSF flow obstruction, or ischemia.

SUGGESTED READING

Lassman AB, DeAngelis LM. Brain metastases. Neurol Clin 2003; 21:1.

Cushing HW. Some experimental and clinical observations concerning states of increasing intracranial tension. Am J Med Sci 1902; 124:375.

Rosner, MJ, Rosner, SD, Johnson, AH. Cerebral perfusion pressure: management protocol and clinical results. J Neurosurg 1995; 83:949.

CHAPTER SEVENTY-TWO

Cancer Emergencies: Spinal Cord Compression

Asha Ramsakal, DO, and Stephen G. Patterson, MD

BACKGROUND

Spinal cord compression (SCC) results from tumor invasion of the epidural space and subsequent compression of the thecal sac, which surrounds the spinal cord. By far the majority of cases of SCC are due to metastatic tumors seeded hematogenously.[1] The most common tumors producing SCC are prostate, breast, and lung; although multiple myeloma, plasmacytoma, lymphoma, and renal cell cancer have been described. The most common location of metastatic SCC is the thoracic spine.[2] SCC occurs in 5–10% of cancer patients.

ASSESSMENT

Clinical Presentation

Prevalence and Presenting Signs and Symptoms

Symptoms develop sequentially as back pain, weakness, numbness, and paresthesias, and then bowel and bladder dysfunction. Back pain is certainly the most common presenting symptom.[3] Classically, the pain is aggravated by sneezing, coughing, the Valsalva maneuver, or supine posture (alleviated by spinal flexion). If the nerve root is also involved, the back pain will typically be radicular in nature and lancinating.

Weakness is the most common motor disturbance at the time of diagnosis and occurs after back pain but before sensory symptoms.[4] Sensory symptoms are less common and are expressed as ascending numbness and paresthesias. Bowel and bladder dysfunction are a late manifestation yet interestingly are present in as many as 50% of patients at the time of diagnosis.[5] Common presenting symptoms are urinary hesitancy and a feeling of "incomplete" voiding.

Presenting Signs

Back pain may be associated with tenderness to percussion of the involved vertebra. Radicular pain can be diagnosed by the Lesegue test (pain reproduced by passive raising of the ipsilateral painful leg) or the crossed straight leg raising test (pain reproduced by passive raising of the contralateral pain-free leg).

Motor signs present as decreased muscle strength, then ataxia followed by paresis. Areas caudad to the lesion exhibit symmetric weakness, hyperreflexia, and upgoing plantar responses. Spastic-

ity may be present. Cervical SCC will produce quadriplegia, while thoracic SCC will produce paraplegia.

Sensory signs occur at one to five levels caudad to the lesion.[2]

Bowel and bladder dysfunction may present as decreased anal sphincter tone and a significant (>150 cc urine) postvoid residual due to overflow urinary incontinence.

Differential Diagnosis

The diagnosis of SCC is a true emergency as intervention needs to occur as rapidly as possible to prevent permanent neurologic damage. Table 72-1 lists the differential diagnosis for spinal cord compression.

Diagnosis

MRI of the spine is the most sensitive modality to detect thecal sac compression and preferred as the initial diagnostic test.[6] Computed tomography (CT) myelography should be considered as second option when MRI is not available or is contraindicated. MRI is more sensitive than CT myelography, does not involve lumbar puncture, and is not limited by coagulopathies, thrombocytopenia, or large, potentially hemorrhagic brain metastases.

Plain films and bone scans are inferior to MRI and CT myelography. In a small series of 24 patients, the initial radiation treatment fields created on the basis of x-ray findings were inadequate in 69% of patients and had to be altered based on subsequent CT myelography results.[7]

Prognosis

Even though the median survival after diagnosis of SCC is 6 months, this ranges from 3–16 months, depending on the presence of good prognostic indicators such as ambulatory patients and radiosensitivity of tumors (lymphomas, multiple myeloma, breast, and prostate).[8] SCC from lung cancer has a poor prognosis.

MANAGEMENT

The current standard of care includes concomitant steroids plus radiation and possibly surgery. The goals are reversal of neuro-

Table 72-1 Differential Diagnosis of Spinal Cord Compression

Syndromes	Symptoms	Motor	Sensory	Other
EXTRINSIC				
A. Cauda equina Syndrome	Bowel/bladder incontinence	Distal lower extremity weakness Unilateral hyporeflexia	Saddle paresthesias	Should lead to an increased suspicion of leptomeningeal carcinomatosis
B. Nerve root compression	No bowel/bladder incontinence	Deep tendon reflexes unaffected	Painful unilateral Polyneuropathy	
INTRINSIC				
A. Brown-Séquard syndrome	No bowel or bladder incontinence	Ipsilateral weakness	Contralateral absence of pain and temperature sensation Ipsilateral loss of proprioception	Signs and symptoms distal to the lesion
B. Metastatic disease				Signs and symptoms dependent on location.
C. Myelitis (autoimmune or infections)	Back pain Bowel or bladder incontinence	Bilateral leg weakness	Paresthesias	Multiple sclerosis Lupus Mycoplasma Herpes zoster Herpes simplex Virus I

logic sequela, adequate pain control, and accessory care such as prophylactic anticoagulation, peptic ulcer and hyperglycemic prophylaxis, and an adequate bowel regimen.

Steroids

Commonly asked questions are: What is the evidence? High dose or low dose? Oral or IV? Immediate initiation of steroids is recommended when SCC is suspected, even though there is limited evidence of efficacy and there are no randomized clinical trials. High-dose dexamethasone (96 mg IV followed by 24 mg q6h × 3 days, then tapered over 10 days to stopping usage) was associated with improved ability to ambulate at the end of therapy compared to a group treated without steroids; there were also increased side effects in the steroid treatment group.[9] A small study of 77 patients with SCC received either dexamethasone 10 mg IV or 100 mg IV followed by 16 mg daily orally, with no statistically significant difference in pain control or neurologic outcome.[10] Most experts recommend dexamethasone 10 mg IV or orally once, then 4 mg orally every 6 hours, tapered over a 2–3 week course.

Radiation

Radiation is the treatment of choice in most centers. Some experts recommend a total of 30–40 Gy,[11] with or without surgery.

Surgery

A recent randomized trial comparing radical surgical resection followed by radiation compared to radiation alone revealed promising results. There was a fourfold longer duration of ambulation with surgery plus radiation. Hence, this should be considered for all patients who meet surgical criteria.[12]

Key Points

- The most common tumors producing spinal cord compression are prostate, breast, and lung.

- Weakness is the most common motor disturbance at the time of diagnosis and occurs after back pain but before sensory symptoms.

- MRI of the spine is the most sensitive modality to detect thecal sac compression[6]; CT myelography should be considered as second option when MRI is not available or is contraindicated.

- Steroids and radiation are standard therapy, but surgery may be an increasingly important option.

SUGGESTED READING

Levack P, Graham J, Collie D, et al. Don't wait for a sensory level—listen to the symptoms: a prospective audit of the delays in diagnosis of malignant cord compression. Clin Oncol (R Coll Radiol) 2002; 14:472.

Loblaw DA, Laperriere, NJ. Emergency treatment of malignant extradural spinal cord compression: An evidence-based guideline. J Clin Oncol 1998; 16:1613.

Rades D, Fehlauer F, Stalpers LJ, et al. A prospective evaluation of two radiotherapy schedules with 10 vs 20 fractions for the treatment of metastatic spinal cord compression: final results of a multicenter study. Cancer 2004; 101:2687.

Patchell R, Tibbs PA, Regine WF, et al. A randomized trial of direct decompressive surgical resection in the treatment of spinal cord compression caused by metastatis. Proc Am Soc Clin Oncol 2003; 22:1.

CHAPTER SEVENTY-THREE

Cancer Emergencies: Tumor Lysis Syndrome

Asha Ramsakal, DO, and Stephen G. Patterson, MD

BACKGROUND

Tumor lysis syndrome (TLS) occurs as a sequelae to spontaneous or treatment-induced cell death, typically in the setting of poorly differentiated, highly proliferative, treatment-sensitive, high tumor burden myelolymphoproliferative disorders such as Burkitt's lymphoma and acute leukemias. However, it can also occur spontaneously and in solid tumors. This clinical syndrome develops when excessive electrolytes and metabolites released with cell death overcome the kidney's ability to maintain homeostasis. The subsequent hyperkalemia, hyperuricemia, hypocalcemia, hyperphosphatemia, and renal failure can be life threatening.

ASSESSMENT

Clinical Presentation

Presenting Signs and Symptoms

Recognition depends on finding key laboratory abnormalities in the appropriate clinical setting. The clinical presentation encompasses a broad spectrum, ranging from asymptomatic electrolyte and metabolite abnormalities, to nonspecific constitutional symptoms such as nausea, vomiting, mental status changes, to specific signs and symptoms of the particular metabolic complication, to sudden cardiac arrest from hyperkalemia.

Hyperkalemia is often the first sign of TLS and the most life threatening. The patient's symptoms may include nausea, vomiting, diarrhea, muscle cramps, paresthesias, chest pain, and palpitations. Signs are mainly electrocardiographic. Hyperkalemia often presents in the sequence of peaked T waves, QRS widening followed by flattened P waves, then progression to the classic "sine" wave, malignant ventricular arrhythmias, and finally cardiac arrest.

The most common metabolic abnormality is hyperuricemia, which presents as uremia, acute renal failure, and an elevated anion gap metabolic acidosis. Signs and symptoms include nausea, vomiting, mental status changes, flank pain (urate nephrolithiasis), chest pain (uremic pericarditis), seizures, edema, oliguria/anuria, and noncardiogenic pulmonary edema.

If the patient presents with neuromuscular manifestations such as muscle cramps, paresthesias, and tetany, acute hypocalcemia (from the precipitation of calcium phosphate during TLS)[1] should be suspected. Other symptoms may include mental status changes and seizures. Signs such as Trousseau's (induction of carpopedal spasm by keeping the blood pressure cuff >10 mm Hg above the systolic blood pressure for 3 minutes) and Chvostek's (induction of ipsilateral facial spasms by tapping on the facial nerve) are dramatic when present but of unknown sensitivity and specificity. Hypotension and electrocardiographic changes such as QT prolongation are other signs of hypocalcemia.

Patients with hyperphosphatemia are often asymptomatic initially but then develop acute renal failure (with the concomitant signs and symptoms discussed previously) as renal calcium phosphate deposition occurs during TLS.

Differential Diagnosis

The wide array of clinical manifestations above often warrants consideration of other causes of acute renal failure:

1. Rhabdomyolysis: History of classic drugs (ethanol, cocaine, "statins," for example), seizures, strenuous exercise, diffuse myalgias, markedly elevated creatinine kinase, elevated aldolase, myoglobinuria, and discordant blood/red cell ratio in the microscopic urinalysis
2. Direct nephrotoxicity from chemotherapeutic, IV contrast, or antimicrobial agents: Oliguric or anuric acute tubular necrosis, urine analysis with pigmented muddy brown casts and isothenuria
3. Ischemic injury: History of renal hypoperfusion as in shock (cardiogenic, septic, etc.) hypovolemia, or related to major surgery
4. Urinary tract obstruction from tumor

Diagnosis

Evaluation generally includes a complete blood count, comprehensive metabolic panel, uric acid, and urinalysis. Selected patients may need a creatinine kinase, urine drug screen, and serum ethanol level. Patients with large tumor burdens and very high levels of uric acid (>15 mg/dL) who develop acute renal failure should be strongly suspected of having TLS.

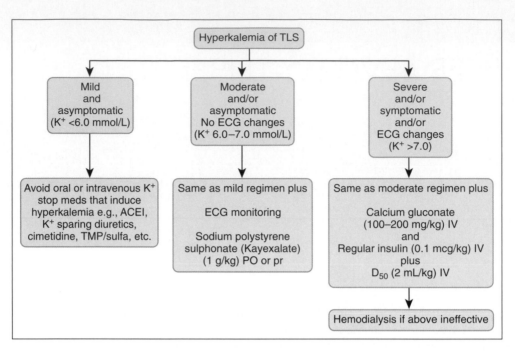

Figure 73-1 • Approach to hyperkalemia in TLS.

Classification

A recently proposed classification system appears quite clinically relevant.[2] This classification defines TLS as Laboratory TLS (LTLS) and Clinical TLS (CTLS). LTLS is defined as two or more abnormal serum levels of uric acid, potassium, phosphate, and calcium within 3 days before and 7 days after initiation of chemotherapy as described below:

1. Uric acid >8.0 mg/dL or 25% increase from baseline
2. Potassium >6.0 mEq/L or 25% increase from baseline
3. Phosphorus >4.5 mg/dL or 25% increase from baseline
4. Calcium <7 mg/dL or 25% decrease from baseline

CTLS, which is of most relevance to hospitalists, is defined as LTLS plus one or more of the following:

1. Creatinine >1.5 times the upper limit of normal (ULN)
2. Cardiac arrhythmia or sudden death
3. Seizure

Prognosis

Prognosis from the acute syndrome appears favorable once early recognition and treatment are instituted. There appears to be a higher mortality among solid tumors, perhaps related to delayed recognition. Patients with acute myeloid leukemia, acute lymphocytic leukemia, and non-Hodgkin's lymphoma who develop TLS have an overall hospital mortality of 17.5% compared to 0.9% for all patients.[4] Once the syndrome has resolved, there is no evidence to suggest long-term sequelae.

MANAGEMENT

The management of TLS involves a combination of prevention and treatment of the individual metabolic complications. Algorithms in Figures 73–1, 73–2 and 73–3 outline the approach to hyperkalemia, hyperuricemia, and hypocalcemia and hypophosphatemia, respectively. The management of hyperkalemia, hypocalcemia, and hyperphosphatemia is similar to their management as described in detail in Chapter 52. The prophylactic treatment of hyperuricemia prior to chemotherapy markedly diminishes the risk of TLS. Oral administration of allopurinol at least 2 days prior to chemotherapy or radiation treatment of a cancer with high cell turnover should be combined with intravenous hydration with normal saline. Furosemide or mannitol can also be given to ensure a high flow of urine, ideally >100 mL/hr/m^2 body surface area. Alkalinization does not seem to have much effect if sufficient hydration with diuresis is achieved.

PREVENTION

The old adage "prevention is better than cure" holds true for TLS. Allopurinol prophylaxis is recommended for patients who fit the criteria mentioned above in the "hyperuricemia of TLS" algorithm. Allopurinol prophylaxis prior to antitumor treatment has significantly reduced the development of urate nephropathy, which was as high as 10% in treated acute lymphoblastic leukemia.[7] Rasburicase is a recombinant urate oxidase enzyme (Elitek) that facilitates degradation of uric acid. Prophylaxis is recommended for patients with Bukitt's lymphoma and leukemias with WBC counts >50,000. Its use is also reasonable when renal function may be impaired by involvement of the kidney with tumor.

DISCHARGE/FOLLOW-UP PLANS

Patients can be discharged once signs and symptoms dissipate and metabolic/electrolyte abnormalities resolve with laboratory

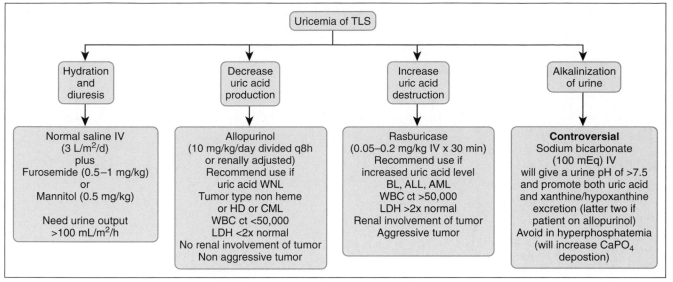

Figure 73-2 • Approach to hyperuricemia in TLS.

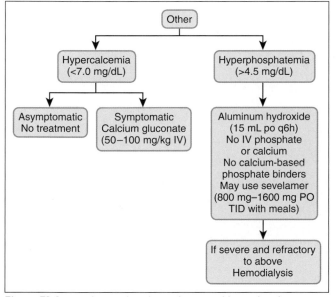

Figure 73-3 • Approach to hypocalcemia and hyperphosphatemia in TLS.

values in the normal range. Electrolytes, uric acid, phosphate, calcium, and LDH should be rechecked in the outpatient setting, probably within one week.

Patient Education

Patients should be counseled to call their physician for recurrent or new signs and symptoms as noted above.

Outpatient Physician Communication

The outpatient physician should be alerted to monitor renal function, uric acid levels, and allopurinol tolerance in particular.

Key Points

• TLS typically occurs in patients with tumors having high cell turnover, but can also occur spontaneously and in solid tumors.

• Hyperkalemia is often the first sign of tumor lysis syndrome and the most life threatening.

• There appears to be a higher mortality among patients with solid tumors and tumor lysis syndrome, perhaps related to delayed recognition.

• Prophylaxis of hyperuricemia, hydration, and diuresis are the primary approaches to treatment.

SUGGESTED READING

Cairo MS, Bishop M. Tumour lysis syndrome: new therapeutic strategies and classification. Brit J Haematol 2004; 127(1):3–11.

Hande KR, Garrow GC. Acute tumor lysis syndrome in patients with high-grade non-Hodgkin's lymphoma. Am J Med 1993; 94:133–139.

Annemans L, Moeremans K, Lamotte M, et al. Pan-European multicentre economic evaluation of recombinant urate oxidase (rasburicase) in prevention and treatment of hyperuricaemia and tumour lysis syndrome in haematological cancer patients. Support Care Cancer 2003; 11:249.

CHAPTER SEVENTY-FOUR

Cancer Emergencies: Paraneoplastic Neurologic Syndromes

Kanchan Kamath, MD

BACKGROUND

Paraneoplastic neurologic syndrome (PNNS) is a specific neurologic disorder often associated with an indolent malignancy. However, its effects remain remote from the site of primary neoplasm and its metastases. More often than not, neurologic symptoms push the patient to seek care, yielding the cancer diagnosis. The syndrome is believed to be secondary to immune mechanisms and not due to the direct effects of the tumor itself or due to other related causes from the tumor, such as nutritional deficits, infections, or the side effects of radiation or chemotherapy. The symptoms associated with PNNS result from damage to any part of the nervous system, ranging from cerebral cortex to neuromuscular junction and muscle (Table 74-1).

Though this chapter concentrates on paraneoplastic syndrome affecting the nervous system, paraneoplastic syndromes can also affect most other organs and tissues, as noted with cancer cachexia, hypercalcemia, Cushing's syndrome, and Trousseau's syndrome. The hospitalist in centers with large cancer practices may encounter paraneoplastic syndromes prior to their definitive diagnosis; familiarity with them can prevent delay, inappropriate diagnostic tests and treatment, and misdiagnosis.

Pathogenesis

Although not well understood, the pathogenesis of paraneoplastic syndromes relates to proteins secreted by the tumor that mimic a normal hormone or interfere with its function, or trigger an immune response. Currently, the most common model of pathogenesis is immunogenic; most or all of PNNS is believed to be immune mediated. This is either related to secretion of antibodies by the tumor itself or secondary to ectopic expression of a neural antigen by the tumor. The antibodies and cytotoxic T-cells associated with the tumor antigen cross the blood–brain barrier and act on the neuronal tissue expressing the same antigens as the tumor.[2,3] The combination of an occult malignancy and disabling neurologic symptoms suggest immune-mediated eradication of tumor cells and thus a more limited disease distribution, combined with autoimmune nervous system degeneration.

The pathogenesis of paraneoplastic antibodies has been conclusively shown for four syndromes in which injection of the affected patients' IgG, but not control IgG, into mice replicated the neurologic symptoms:

1) Lambert-Eaton myasthenic syndrome (LEMS): p/q gated calcium channel antibodies.[4]
2) Myasthenia gravis: Acetylcholine receptor antibodies.[5]
3) Autonomic neuropathy: Ganglionic acetylcholine receptor antibodies.[6]
4) Isaac's syndrome (neuromyotonia): Voltage-gated potassium channel antibodies.[7]

ASSESSMENT

Clinical Presentation

In general, symptomatic paraneoplastic syndromes are rare, affecting approximately 0.01% of patients with cancer. Exceptions to this include Lambert-Eaton myasthenia syndrome (LEMS) and myasthenia gravis (MG). The former is seen in 3% of the patients with small cell lung cancer, and the latter affects approximately 15% of all patients with thymoma.[3]

Demyelinating peripheral neuropathy is another PNNS; it notably affects about 50% of patients with the rare osteosclerotic form of plasmacytoma known as POEMS syndrome (polyneuropathy, organomegaly, endocrinopathy, M protein, and skin changes).

Any part of the nervous system can be affected and at different levels. That is, PNNS may affect a certain area of the nervous system as in limbic encephalitis or may affect a single cell type (e.g., Purkinje's cells of the cerebellum). Or it may involve multiple levels of the nervous system such as in encephalomyeloradiculitis. Thus, the clinical features of PNNS may markedly vary, depending on the area and extent of involvement.

The neurologic signs and symptoms often present even before the cancer has been identified. Though the onset of symptoms can be insidious and the patient may fluctuate between periods of exacerbations, it is important to be aware that PNNS can rapidly progress, causing severe disability and may sometimes even be fatal. Given the variable temporal relationship of a PNNS to its associated neoplasm, a high index of suspicion, the exclusion of other causes of neurologic deficit, and the demonstration of specific paraneoplastic antibodies are needed to garner a definite diagnosis.

Recognition of PNNS by the physician entails recognizing seemingly unexplained neurologic symptoms in a patient with known or suspected malignancy. Table 74-1 outlines charac-

Table 74-1 PNNS: Its Associated Antibodies and Symptoms

Symptoms	Syndrome	AB Target	Commonly Associated Cancer
BRAIN			
1. Mental status change, seizures	Limbic encephalitis	Hu	SCLCA, breast, colon, testicular, bladder
2. Cerebellar and ocular symptoms	Brainstem encephalitis or cerebellar degeneration	Hu Or Yo	SCLCA, ovary, uterus, hodgkin's
3. Involuntary eye movements, ataxia	Opsoclonus-myoclonus	Hu	Lung, breast In Children: neuroblastoma
SPINAL CORD			
1. Weakness, sensory loss at the spinal level, bladder incontinence	Necrotizing myelopathy	Unknown	SCLCA, lymphoma
PERIPHERAL NERVE			
1. Diffuse asymmetric sensory loss, pain, and ataxia	Sensory neuronopathy	Hu	SCLCA (>90%), prostate, breast, and ovary
2. Fasciculations, muscle stiffness, cramps, generalized weakness	Neuromyotonia (Isaac's)	Ab to K^+ channels	Thymoma, SCLCA, Hodgkin's
3. Polyneuropathy, lymphadenopathy, hepatosplenomegaly, endocrinopathy, skin hyperpigmentation	POEMS/osteosclerotic Myeloma	unknown	Multiple myeloma, Castleman's
NEUROMUSCULAR JUNCTION.			
1. Increasing fatigue with exercise of the affected muscle and improves with rest Also, ptosis, diplopia, dysphagia, difficulty chewing due to bulbar muscle weakness weakness of the limbs and trunk	Myasthenia gravis	Anti-ACH "R"	Thymoma
2. Weakness, especially hip girdle weakness; ptosis; symptoms improve with exercise	LEMS	Anti–voltage gated Ca^{++} channel "R"	SCLCA
MUSCLE:			
1. Proximal muscle weakness, heliotrope skin rash, Gottron's sign on the MCP joints	Dermatomyositis	Unknown	Ovarian, NHL, lung, pancreatic, gastric; also Nasopharyngeal especially in SE Asians
2. Sudden-onset painful proximal weakness, elevated CK, and muscle biopsy with patchy necrosis.	Acute necrotizing myopathy	Unknown	Lung, breast, and GI

AB = Antibody; SCLCA = Small Cell Lung Cancer; LEMS = Lambert Eaton Myasthenic Syndrome; MCP = Metacarpal phalangeal; CK = Creatine Kinase; NHL = Non-Hodgkins Lymphoma; SE = Southeastern; GI = Gastrointestinal

teristic patterns. Early recognition may obviate the need for unnecessary testing and treatment and expedite appropriate management. Though hospitalists should enlist consultants for definitive management, their role in early recognition can be crucial.

Diagnosis

Establishing a diagnosis is especially difficult in patients with known malignancy and neurologic symptoms but undetectable characteristic antibodies in the serum that can confirm the diagnosis. However, absence of these antibodies does not exclude a paraneoplastic syndrome. In such instances, specific diagnostic tests such as neuroimaging studies, electromyography (EMG), electrophysiologic studies (EPS), positron emission tomography (PET) imaging, and cerebrospinal fluid (CSF) analysis may be of use in establishing a diagnosis.

- Neuroimaging studies such as magnetic resonance imaging (MRI) can detect signs of atrophy and thus assist in the diagnosis of limbic encephalitis and paraneoplastic cerebellar degeneration. However, more often than not, neuroimaging can be nonspecific.

- Whole-body PET scanning may be a helpful screening technique in detecting small occult tumors if there is a high index of suspicion for paraneoplastic syndrome.

- Presence of paraneoplastic antibodies in the CSF usually coincides with their presence in the serum. Nonetheless, examination of the CSF is especially helpful in garnering a diagnosis of PNNS in two other ways. In combination with MRI, it can reasonably exclude leptomeningeal carcinomatosis. Furthermore, by detecting inflammatory changes such as pleocytosis (30–40 white cells/mm^3), elevated IgG levels, slightly elevated protein levels (50–100 mg/dL), and oligoclonal bands in the CSF, it can confirm the presence of an inflammatory or immune-mediated neurologic disorder.

- Electrophysiologic studies are especially helpful with PNNS of the peripheral nervous system (such as LEMS and MG) and are associated with characteristic electrophysiologic findings. Though these findings may be seen even with neurologic syndromes not associated with a tumor, once a "syndrome" is established it may aid in focusing the search for neoplasm of specific organs (e.g., lung with LEMS).

Diagnosis of PNNS is made primarily on the basis of presentation of a clinically recognized neurologic syndrome, careful exclusion of other cancer-related disorders, and the use of appropriate diagnostic tests mentioned above. Given the challenges faced in diagnosing these syndromes, a set of guidelines were established by an international panel of neurologists to serve as a dependable diagnostic tool in the assessment of PNNS.[8]

Two broad categories were formed based on the finding of "classical" defined PNNS syndromes such as encephalomyelitis, limbic encephalitis, subacute cerebellar degeneration, opsoclonus-myoclonus, subacute sensory neuronopathy, chronic gastrointestinal pseudo-obstruction, LEMS, and dermatomyositis that are often seen in association with a tumor.

I) Definite syndromes[8]:

- Classical syndrome as described above in addition to a diagnosis of cancer within 5 years of the neurologic disorder.
- Nonclassical syndrome:
  A not-so-well-defined neurologic syndrome such as the ones described above, and there is complete resolution or improvement in symptoms with treatment of the cancer without concomitant treatment of the syndrome.
  OR
  Positive onconeural antibodies and development of cancer within 5 years of diagnosis of the neurologic disorder.
- Neurologic syndrome (classical or nonclassical) with "well-characterized" onconeural antibodies such as anti-Hu, CV2, Ri, Ma2, or amphiphysin and no cancer.

II) Possible syndromes[8]:

- Classical syndrome as defined above with high risk of underlying tumor.
- Neurologic syndrome with positive not-so-well-defined onconeural antibodies and no cancer.
- Nonclassical syndrome, no antibodies, and cancer diagnosis within 2 years of the neurologic disorder.

MANAGEMENT/TREATMENT

Valid and applicable evidence regarding treatment for most paraneoplastic neurologic syndromes is lacking. In patients with serious and progressive symptoms, biologically plausible and anecdotal reports may justify the use of two broad approaches for the treatment of PNNS, given the immunologic nature of the disorder.

1. Treating the underlying malignancy and thus removing the antigen source.

This is often not feasible, given the occult nature of the malignancy. In most cases, however, this is the only effective approach. In some instances, even eradication of the tumor is futile in reversing the neurologic disorder.

2. Suppression of the immune response (Table 74-2).

This treatment approach is based on the well-accepted concept that most paraneoplastic neurologic disorders are immune mediated. Since humoral and cell-mediated immunity may both play a role in the pathogenesis, suppressing both arms of the immune system has been incorporated into the treatment model. However, there is no established treatment protocol for most PNNS.

In paraneoplastic cerebellar degeneration and encephalomyelitis, which are T-cell mediated and are associated with anti-Yo and anti-Hu antibodies, respectively, tacrolimus and mycophenolate mofetil have been tried.

Plasma exchange or IV immune globulin (0.4 g/kg daily for 5 days) is beneficial in some conditions, such as MG and LEMS, in suppressing the immune response and ameliorating the neurologic status, at least temporarily.[9]

Use of 3,4-diaminopyridine (DAP), appears to be safe and effective in the treatment of LEMS based on many placebo-controlled studies and substantiated further by years of clinical experience.[10,11]

There are no established treatment protocols for most PNNS. In a majority of the cases, immunosuppression is not found to be helpful. However, if the neurologic symptoms are deteriorating, a combination of plasma exchange with intravenous

Table 74-2 PNNS That Often Respond to Treatment Strategies

Syndrome	Treatment
1. Eaton-Lambert myasthenia syndrome	– Immune-modulators: Plasmapheresis, IVIG, immune-suppressive agents (azathioprine, cyclosporine) – Release of ACH-enhancing treatment modalities: 3,4-Diaminopyridine, guanidine, and pyridostigmine.
2. Myasthenia gravis	– Immune modulators: Plasmapheresis – IVIG, glucocorticoids, immune-suppressive agents (azathioprine, cyclosporine) – Anticholinesterases – Thymectomy
3. Dermatomyositis	– Immune modulators: plasmapheresis, IVIG, glucocorticoids, immunosuppressive agents (azathioprine, methotrexate, cyclophosphamide)
4. Limbic encephalitis	– Immune modulators: IVIG, plasma exchange, glucocorticoids
5. Opsoclonus-myoclonus	– Immune modulators: Glucocorticoids, cyclophosphamide – Symptom control: Clonazepam and/or, valproate, thiamine
6. Stiff-man syndrome	– Immune modulators: IVIG, glucocorticoids – Symptom control: Diazepam, clonazepam, valproate
7. Acute necrotizing myopathy	Immunosuppression: Glucocorticoids, azathioprine

IVIG = Intravenous Immunoglobulin

immune globulin and immunosuppressants such as corticosteroids, cyclophosphamide, or tacrolimus should be initiated expeditiously. Though there remains an important question of whether immunosuppression stimulates tumor growth, so far there is no evidence reporting this.

Key Points

- The combination of an occult malignancy and disabling neurologic symptoms suggests immune-mediated eradication of tumor cells, and thus a more limited disease distribution, combined with autoimmune nervous system degeneration. Thus, PNNS may be the initial symptomatic presentation of cancer.

- Symptomatic paraneoplastic syndromes are rare, affecting approximately 0.01% of patients with cancer, but LEMS and MG occur in 3% of the patients with small cell lung cancer and approximately 15% of all patients with thymoma.

- Examination of the CSF is important in garnering a diagnosis of PNNS when combined with MRI, as it can reasonably exclude leptomeningeal carcinomatosis.

- Since humoral and cell-mediated immunity may both play a role in the pathogenesis, suppressing both arms of the immune system has been incorporated into the treatment model for PNNS, though there is no established treatment protocol.

- DAP (3,4-diaminopyridine) appears to be safe and effective in the treatment of LEMS based on many placebo-controlled studies and substantiated further by years of clinical experience.

SUGGESTED READING

Dalmau J, Gultekin HS, Posner JB. Paraneoplastic neurologic syndromes: pathogenesis and physiopathology. Brain Pathol 1999; (2):275–284.

Darnell RB, Posner JB. Paraneoplastic syndromes affecting the nervous system. N Engl J Med 2003; 349:1543–1554.

Graus F, Delattre JY, Antoine JC, et al. Recommended diagnostic criteria for paraneoplastic neurological syndromes. J Neurol Neurosurg Psychiatry 2004; 75(8):1135–1140.

Sanders DB, Massey JM, Sanders LL, et al. Edwards LJ. A randomized trial of 3,4-diaminopyridine in Lambert-Eaton myasthenic syndrome. Neurology 2000; 54(3):603–607.

Section
Ten

Hematology

75 Transfusion Medicine
    Debora Bruno, Jay H. Herman

76 Anemia
    Tyler Kang, Alan Lichtin

77 Sickle Cell Crises
    James R. Eckman, Allan F. Platt Jr.

78 Hemorrhagic and Thrombotic Disorders
    Jamie Siegel

CHAPTER SEVENTY-FIVE

Transfusion Medicine

Debora Bruno, MD, and Jay H. Herman, MD

BACKGROUND

Anemia is defined by decreased red blood cell (RBC) mass. Red blood cells have a life span of 100–120 days, and approximately 1% of the red cell mass is destroyed daily by macrophages located in the spleen, liver, and bone marrow. The bone marrow responds to this turnover with the production of reticulocytes released in the peripheral blood. Whenever this equilibrium is disrupted by either increased destruction of RBCs (hemolysis), loss (bleeding), or decreased production (bone marrow disease, i.e., aplastic anemia, leukemia) anemia develops. Most references consider hemoglobin levels of 14 g/dL and 12 g/dL, respectively, for men and women, as the lower normal values.[1] Anemia is covered in more detail in Chapter 76.

When diagnosing the underlying cause of a patient's anemia, two diagnostic approaches are usually used. The kinetic approach is summarized in Figure 75-1. One can also diagnose the etiology of anemia by measuring the RBC size through evaluation of the peripheral blood smear and assessment of the mean corpuscular volume (MCV) of red cells by automated cell counter devices. The normal MCV values are 80–100 fentoliters (fL). Anemias can then be classified in normocytic (normal MCV), microcytic (MCV <80 fL), and macrocytic (MVC >100 fL) (Box 75-1).

TRANSFUSION OF RED BLOOD CELLS—INDICATIONS

More important than hemoglobin levels as parameters for transfusion of RBCs is the assessment of the severity of symptoms related to the development of anemia. Symptoms result from a combination of how severe the anemia is and how fast it has developed, and, most importantly, the patient's cardiopulmonary reserve. For example, while a patient with active coronary artery disease might develop angina with a hemoglobin level of 9 g/dL and gastrointestinal bleeding, another patient might be asymptomatic with a hemoglobin level of 6 g/dL, due to iron deficiency anemia that has developed over months. When it comes to the indication for transfusion of RBCs, a rule of thumb remains assessment of each individual patient and the concomitant clinical scenario (Figure 75-2).

For several years, the "trigger" numbers for transfusion of RBCs in critically ill patients had been 10/30 (i.e., transfuse to keep hemoglobin levels above 10 g/dL and hematocrit above 30%). In 1999, Hébert et al.[2] in the Canadian Critical Care Trials Group reported the results of a prospective trial in which 838 patients were randomly assigned to either a liberal strategy of transfusion, in which hemoglobin threshold for transfusion was 10 g/dL (420 patients), or a restrictive strategy in which hemoglobin values were maintained at levels >7 g/dL (418 patients). Although differences in the mortality rate at 30 days did not reach statistical significance, the overall rate of in-hospital mortality was significantly lower in the restrictive-strategy group than in the liberal-strategy group (22.2 % vs. 28.1 %, P = 0.05). Very importantly, a subgroup analysis showed that among patients who were less severely ill (APACHE score, ≤20) and among those who were <55 years old, the patients assigned to the restrictive strategy of transfusion were half as likely to die within 30 days as those assigned to the liberal strategy. Patients who had clinically significant cardiac disease did not benefit from a restrictive transfusion strategy, which translated into no differences in mortality for this subgroup.

Liberal transfusion practices have been associated with pulmonary complications, increased hospital stays, and also increased rates of nosocomial infections. Taylor et al.[3] demonstrated that transfusion of packed RBCs is correlated with the occurrence of nosocomial infections, and there is a dose-response pattern (i.e., for each unit of packed RBCs transfused, the odds of developing nosocomial infection were increased by a factor of 1.5 in this particular study). The authors attribute these results to a possible immune modulation caused by the transfusion of allogeneic RBCs.

Complications of Transfusion of Red Blood Cells: Transfusion Reactions

Among the complications related to transfusion of RBCs, immune-mediated reactions play an important role. Physicians must be proficient in identifying manifestations and acting promptly to support the patients who develop those reactions (Table 75-1).

Figure 75-1 • Kinetic approach to the etiology of anemia.

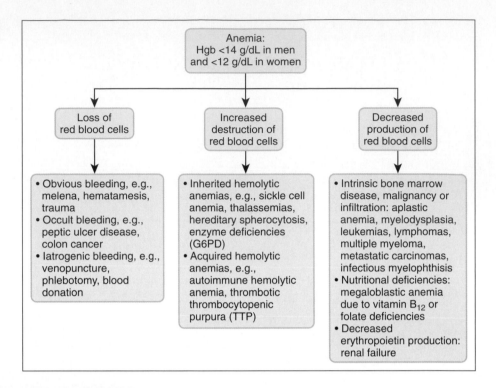

Box 75-1 Morphologic Approach to the Etiology of Anemia

Microcytic Anemias (MCV <80 fL):

- Iron deficiency
- Thalassemia
- Sideroblastic anemia
- Chronic disease/inflammation (commonly normocytic)
- Lead intoxication

Normocytic Anemias (MCV 80–100 fL):

- Renal insufficiency
- Chronic disease/inflammation (can be microcytic, hypochromic)
- Hemorrhagic (when iron deficiency has not yet developed)
- Hemolysis
- Aplastic anemia
- Bone marrow infiltration

Macrocytic Anemias (MCV >100 fL):

- Vitamin B$_{12}$ deficiency (pernicious anemia, malabsorption, dietary deficiency)
- Folate deficiency (dietary deficiency, increased requirements, alcoholism)
- Myelodysplasia
- Drug-induced disorders of DNA synthesis (e.g., methotrexate, zidovudine)
- Liver disease
- Hypothyroidism
- Reticulocytosis

MCV = mean corpuscular volume

Acute Hemolytic Transfusion Reactions (AHTRs)

AHTRs almost always result from clerical or procedural errors. They happen following the activation of complement by an inherited IgM anti-A or anti-B antibody when ABO incompatible blood is transfused. This leads to massive intravascular hemolysis. Symptoms and signs of AHTRs include fever and chills, pain at the infusion site, back/flank pain, hypotension, hemoglobinemia (pink plasma supernatant), and hemoglobinuria (dark urine). When it happens in the operating room, the patient might become hemodynamically unstable, and increased bleeding and oozing from surgical wounds and venopuncture sites might also be noted. It is imperative to stop the transfusion at the first sign of reaction. Usually, all the typical symptoms might not be present, and the first manifestation might be fever only. The bag of infused red cells should not be discarded, but sent to the blood bank for retyping. Intravenous access and fluids should be immediately started and the patient's blood samples obtained for a direct antiglobulin (Coombs') test, blood typing and cross-matches, and measurement of plasma hemoglobin concentration. A urine sample should be assessed for hemoglobinuria. The most serious complications of AHTRs include disseminated intravascular coagulation (DIC), shock, and acute renal failure from acute tubular necrosis.

Delayed Hemolytic Transfusion Reactions (DHTRs)

In contrast to AHTRs, these are secondary to the anamnestic production of antibodies (usually of the IgG class) to RBC antigens to which the patient has been previously exposed (i.e., pregnancy, previous transfusion) and that were not initially detected in typing screening methods due to initially low titers. They can also happen after a primary immune response takes place, leading to

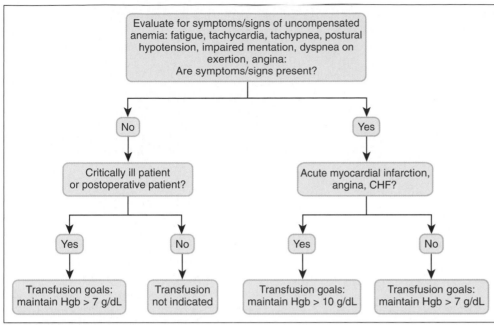

Figure 75-2 • Red cell transfusion algorithm. Each unit of packed red cells should increase the HgB levels by approximately 1.0 g/dL in a 70-kg patient.

Hgb = hemoglobin; MI = myocardial infarction; CHF = congestive heart failure

MI—myocardial infarcion

the development of a new antibody while the transfused red cells are still circulating. DHTRs are manifested by extravascular hemolysis and subsequent fall in hemoglobin, usually 5–10 days following the index transfusion. Often not clinically apparent, clues for the diagnosis include a newly positive direct Coombs' test or the detection of new antibodies in the patient's serum when another transfusion is requested to correct the anemia caused by the delayed hemolysis. The most important therapeutic approach is to avoid the offending RBC antigen and transfuse only antigen-negative units.

Febrile Non-Hemolytic Transfusion Reactions (FNHTRs)

Fever is probably the most common type of reaction related to the administration of blood products. Because fever may be the first manifestation of an acute hemolytic reaction to transfusion, the approach to the patient with a febrile reaction is the same as to an AHTR, until acute hemolysis has been ruled out. Febrile reactions often derive from the effects of cytokines such as IL-6, IL-8, and TNF-α, produced by donor leukocytes that were stored with the blood product, and that activate during storage and elaborate cytokines. The practice of storing blood products only after leukoreduction has proven to decrease the incidence of febrile reactions due to this mechanism. Another mechanism is antileukocyte agglutinins in the patient that react with donor leukocytes transfused with the product. Leukocyte reduction has been proven to decrease these reactions as well. However, FNHTRs have not been completely eliminated, even with "universal" leukocyte reduction.

Anaphylactic Transfusion Reactions (ATRs)

ATRs were classically described in patients who are IgA deficient and have developed anti-IgA antibodies after they receive plasma-containing blood products (fresh frozen plasma, platelets, RBCs

and intravenous immunoglobulin) containing IgA. Other anaphylaxis stimulants may cause these rare reactions in recipients who are not IgA deficient. The manifestations include dyspnea, angioedema, hypoxia, and hypotension. Those symptoms typically manifest within minutes after the transfusion is started. The transfusion should be immediately interrupted, and the reaction should be treated like any anaphylaxis, with the use of epinephrine, fluids, antihistamines, and steroids in the acute setting. Further reactions may be avoided for IgA-deficient patients by the selection of donors who are also IgA deficient. Washing of red cells or platelets to remove plasma contamination may not be sufficiently efficient for removal of the offending protein in order to prevent anaphylaxis.

Allergic (Urticarial) Transfusion Reactions

Urticarial transfusion reactions occur due to the presence in the blood product of proteins or allergens against which the recipient has IgE antibodies. The IgE triggers the release of histamine by mast cells and basophils, and the patient develops pruritus and sometimes hives. The transfusion can be interrupted and antihistamines administered. After there is reassurance that vital signs remain stable and there is no manifestation of symptom progression, safe restarting of the transfusion has been reported. Antihistamines might be given 30 minutes prior to future transfusions to prevent recurrence of symptoms.

Transfusion-Related Acute Lung Injury (TRALI)

TRALI has recently become a leading cause of reported transfusion-related fatalities reported to the Food and Drug Administration (FDA).[4] Currently, the most commonly accepted theory for the pathogenesis of TRALI is the "two-hit" insult; first an under-

Table 75-1 Transfusion Reactions

Transfusion Reaction	Common Signs	Common Symptoms	Onset	Treatment/Prevention
Acute hemolytic transfusion reactions (AHTRs)	Fever, tachycardia, hypotension, hemoglobinuria, hemoglobinemia, DIC	Chills, back and/or flank pain, dyspnea, nausea, vomiting, lightheadness	Within 24 hours of transfusion	• Stop transfusion • Maintain IV access and establish fluid resuscitation for maintenance of adequate urinary output • Other supportive care
Delayed hemolytic transfusion reactions (DHTRs)	Anemia, jaundice, fever Laboratory findings of hemolysis, positive DAT, and presence of a new red cell antibody	Chills, dyspnea—usually asymptomatic	At least 24 hours after transfusion, most commonly within 5–10 days	• Avoid future transfusions with red cells containing the offending antigen
Febrile non-hemolytic transfusion reactions (FNHTRs)	Fever (at least 1°C), tachycardia, blood pressure elevation	Chills, rigors, headache, sometimes dyspnea	Usually during transfusion or just after; resolves within 2–3 hours	• Stop transfusion • Rule out hemolytic reaction • Antipyretics • Leukocyte reduction may decrease incidence and prevent recurrence
Anaphylactic transfusion reactions	Hypotension, tachycardia, angioedema, stridor, bronchospasm, tachypnea, hypoxia	Dyspnea, chest tightness, urticaria, nausea, vomiting	Minutes after the transfusion is started	• Stop transfusion • Maintain IV access • Secure airway and provide oxygen • Antihistaminics, corticosteroids and epinephrine • In the case of IgA-deficient patients, provide blood from IgA deficient donors • Washed blood may offer some help
Allergic (not anaphylactic) transfusion reactions	Hives, erythema, flushing, stridor or wheezing if "anaphylactoid" reaction, but no hypotension or angioedema	Pruritus, dyspnea	Within minutes after transfusion started	• Stop transfusion • Antihistaminics and/or steroids
Transfusion-Related acute lung injury (TRALI)	Hypoxemia, cyanosis, tachypnea, fever, hypotension, pulmonary infiltrates without fluid overload (BNP <100)	Dyspnea	Usually develops 1 or 2 hours after the onset of transfusion (up to 6 hours) with resolution within 96 hours in most cases	• Stop transfusion • Implicated donor(s) will be investigated • Oxygen and mechanical ventilation if needed • Avoid diuretics • No role for corticosteroids
Acute hypotensive transfusion reactions	Profound hypotension (systolic pressure down to 70s and 60s) without other significant signs; flushing	Lightheadness, dizziness and anxiety	Within minutes after transfusion starts; quickly resolves after transfusion is discontinued	• Stop transfusion • Do not rechallenge patient with the same unit • IV fluids and vasopressors as needed • Hold ACE inhibitors for at least 24 hours prior to next transfusion • Avoid bedside leukoreduction filters
Post-transfusion purpura (PTP)	Petechiae, bleeding from mucosal sites, development of severe thrombocytopenia	Bleeding from mucosal sites	• Usually 5–7 days after RBC transfusion • Recovery in 7–48 days	• Intravenous immunoglobulin • High-dose corticosteroids • Plasma exchange • Platelet transfusions are of little or no value
Bacterial contamination	Rigors, high fevers, hypotension/shock	Chills, nausea and vomiting	Symptoms and signs usually develop during the transfusion	• Stop transfusion • Cultures from the transfused bags can be sent by blood bank • Blood cultures from the patient • Aggressive resuscitation • Broad-spectrum antibiotic coverage until implicated bacteria is isolated
Transfusion-associated circulatory overload (TACO)	Hypoxemia, tachypnea, systolic hypertension, pulmonary edema (BNP >100)	Dyspnea, headache, chest tightness	At end of transfusion or immediately after	• Elevate the head of the bed • Provide oxygen • Administer diuretics

DIC—disseminated intravascular coagulation; DAT—direct antiglobulin test; BNP—B-natriuretic peptide; ACE—angiotensin converting enzyme; RBC—red blood cell

lying stressful situation for the recipient allows neutrophils to be primed and adhere to the pulmonary endothelial bed (trauma, sepsis, massive transfusion, cardiac bypass surgery); and second, the transfusion of blood products containing donor antibodies against neutrophil antigens (NA2, NB1, NB2, 5b) and human leukocyte antigens (HLA) class I and II activates those primed neutrophils, and sometimes also monocytes and endothelial cells of the recipient. This combination leads to increased capillary permeability and noncardiogenic pulmonary edema. TRALI manifests as sudden onset of cough, fever, and hypoxia, usually starting within 1–2 hours after the onset of transfusion (up to 6 hours). Most patients require oxygen supplementation and sometimes intubation. There is a characteristically quick recovery, with resolution of symptoms usually within 96 hours. Diagnostic tools include presence of nonelevated B-natriuretic peptide (BNP) levels, tracheal-bronchial fluid/ serum protein ratio greater than 0.75, and transient leukopenia (seen immediately after symptoms develop, but evanescent).[5] Once a suspicion of TRALI is made, antibodies against neutrophils and HLA are tested in the serum of the putative donor, and, if confirmed, the donor is contacted and advised not to donate in the future.

Acute Hypotensive Transfusion Reactions

Hypotensive reactions are characterized by the early and abrupt onset of hypotension, often severe, with a drop of the systolic blood pressure down to the 70s or 60s, without many other signs or symptoms. Most symptoms patients experience are due to the sudden drop in blood pressure, including lightheadedness, dizziness, and anxiety. Another typical characteristic of this type of reaction is the fact that once the transfusion is stopped, the hypotension quickly resolves. These reactions are most likely due to the vasoactive effects of bradykinin and other peptides such as its active metabolite des-Arg^9-bradykinin. Increasing numbers of this type of reaction were seen in the1980s and early 1990s, coinciding with the more widespread use of angiotensin-converting enzyme (ACE) inhibitors. Bradykinin is generated by activated factor XII (commonly present in plasma in the nonactivated form) and metabolized in its majority by ACE. Factor XII can be activated by contact with a number of negatively charged surfaces, including dialysis membranes and leukoreduction filters. The isolated development of hypotension in patients being transfused should raise the suspicion of such a reaction. The transfusion must be stopped immediately, and the patient should not be rechallenged with that same unit. In case the patient is taking ACE inhibitors, the drug should be discontinued, and at least 24 hours should elapse before the next transfusion is attempted.

Post-Transfusion Purpura

This complication is seen most often in human platelet antigen 1a (HPA-1a)-negative multiparous women who, 5–10 days following transfusion from an antigen-positive donor, develop significant thrombocytopenia and have antibodies against the platelet antigen. This epidemiology is explained by previous immune sensitization during pregnancies from babies who inherited the offending platelet antigen from their fathers. For reasons not completely understood, recall of this alloimmunization triggers an autoreactive process, and the recipient's own antigen-negative platelets are destroyed as well. Intravenous immunoglobulin administration has been used with success in the treatment of this alloimmune/autoimmune disorder.

Transfusion-Transmitted Infectious Diseases

Though probably the complication of blood transfusion currently most feared by the recipients, one can actually say that ever since the emergence of AIDS in the 1980s, blood has never been safer. From more restrictive acceptance criteria of blood donors to the use of pathogen reduction methods and screening for virus using polymerase chain reaction (PCR) assays, great effort and cost have been mobilized in order to prevent the transfusion of infectious agents. As a result, the risk of HIV-transfusion transmitted infection now can only be estimated through mathematical modeling (1 in 2 million transfusions.[6] Similar numbers are projected for hepatitis C infection. However, constantly emerging infections for which transmission routes are not clear are always a concern. Over the last decade, outbreaks of variant Creutzfeldt-Jacob disease, West Nile virus infection, and severe acute respiratory syndrome (SARS) have led to more restrictive changes in the criteria of acceptance of blood donors and the use of more screening methods in analyzing donated blood. Unfortunately, the stricter the criteria for triage of blood donors become, the smaller becomes the donor pool to maintain the blood supply.

Bacterial contamination, on the other hand, is a much more common and sometimes fatal infectious complication of platelet transfusion. The prevalence of bacterial contamination is extremely low for red cells but 1 in 3,000 for platelets because platelets are stored at room temperature, and there is an increased risk for bacterial overgrowth from asymptomatic donor bacteremia or retention of skin plugs from venopuncture. Transfusion of platelet concentrates accounts for 85% of fatal septic reactions.

The organism most commonly implicated in bacterial contamination of red cells is *Yersinia enterocolitica* because it grows under refrigerated conditions, while both gram-negatives and skin flora have been implicated for platelets.[7] Changes to the antisepsis of the donor's skin at the time of collection and the practice of diverting the first 15 mL of collected blood for typing and infectious disease screening have been used, with the hope of reducing the bacterial load in skin fragments trapped in the phlebotomy needle. Currently, all platelet products in the U.S. are screened for bacterial contamination before transfusion.

Transfusion-Associated Circulatory Overload (TACO)

TACO is a rather common complication of transfusion of blood components, and it can be seen in up to 1 in 100 transfusions, especially in elderly patients and those with compromised cardiac function. A transfusion rate of approximately 2.0 mL/kg/hr is suggested to avoid this complication, which means that for an average-sized adult, one unit of packed red cells should be transfused over 2 hours, approximately. Elderly patients and those with impaired cardiac function can be safely transfused at a rate of

1 ml/kg/hr. One should also avoid transfusing more than 2 units of PRBCs within 24 hours, if the patient is not actively bleeding. Diuretics can be used in between units to avoid significant intravascular expansion.

RISKS OF NOT TRANSFUSING PATIENTS WITH ANEMIA

There is little published information on the risks of not transfusing patients with significant anemia. Observational studies suggest that moderate degrees of anemia are well tolerated in low-risk patients[8] and that a liberal transfusion practice might be deleterious even for critically ill patients.[2] Carson et al.[9] published a retrospective cohort study of 2,083 patients who declined RBC transfusions for religious reasons and underwent surgery. A total of 300 patients had a postoperative Hgb equal or less then 8 g/dL, and their mean age was 57 years. After adjusting for age, cardiovascular disease, and Acute Physiology and Chronic Health Evaluation (APACHE) II score, the authors concluded that the odds of death in patients with a postoperative Hgb level of < or = 8 g/dL increased 2.5 times for each gram decrease in Hgb level, which translated into 30-day inhospital mortalities of 0%, 9%, 30%, and 64%, respectively, for postoperative hemoglobin levels of 7.1–8.0 g/dL, 5.1–7.0 g/dL, 3.1–5.0 g/dL, and ≤3.0 g/dL. Thus, Hgb < 7.1 g/dL was associated with increased mortality.

COMPATIBILITY TESTING

Using a contemporary sample, a recipient/patient must have his or her blood typed for ABO and Rh type and screened for the existence of alloantibodies using a set of reagent red cells that carry most of the common antigen specificities. A standard, uncomplicated type and screen can often be completed within 30 minutes of receipt.[10] If alloantibodies are identified, ABO-compatible units lacking that specific antigen have to be selected in advance for possible use, and full cross matching using the patient's serum and a sample of the donor unit is required. This may often delay blood availability, since the testing takes longer, and specific antigen-negative units might not be available in that blood bank and have to be ordered. If the antibody screen is negative, then cross matching can be performed in a few minutes, using methods that ensure only ABO compatibility. Type and screen testing has to be repeated every 3 days to allow for detection of new alloantibodies the recipient might have developed after that period of time.

ALTERNATIVES TO ALLOGENEIC BLOOD TRANSFUSION

Recombinant Erythropoietin (EPO)

EPO poses an alternative to transfusion in cases of chronic anemia not associated with symptoms that require immediate intervention. This recombinant glycoprotein contains an identical amino acid sequence to that of endogenous erythropoietin and is currently indicated in the treatment of anemias in which relative endogenous EPO deficiency plays a role (i.e., renal insufficiency, malignancy, and HIV-infected patients undergoing treatment with zidovudine) (Figure 75-3).

The use of EPO is indicated for Hgb concentrations <10 g/dL, but it remains uncertain when the concentration is between 10 g/dL and 12 g/dL.[12] Recent research indicates EPO use maybe be associated with increased mortality. There seems to be no justification for the use of EPO as a preventive measure (i.e., hemoglobin levels >12 g/dL), except in the setting of autologous blood transfusion before major surgery. EPO is contraindicated in patients with uncontrolled hypertension.

Recommended starting doses of EPO for chronic renal insufficiency patients and zidovudine-treated HIV patients are 50–100 units/kg three times a week. Doses can be escalated up to 300 units/kg if patients fail to respond. Patients with malignancy who are being treated with chemotherapy can benefit from starting doses of 40,000 units once weekly, with dose escalation if necessary. It is essential to perform iron studies in patients receiving EPO, since a "functional" state of iron deficiency can be easily established by the increasing demands in erythropoiesis associated with the use of this drug.[13] Supplemental iron therapy is indicated for patients with transferrin saturation <20% and/or serum ferritin levels <100 ng/mL (Figure 75-4).

Darbepoetin, a new erythrocyte growth factor, binds to the same receptor as EPO. However, due to the presence of eight additional sialic acid residues and thus higher carbohydrate content, it has a longer serum half-life (2–3 times longer).[14]

Autologous Blood Donation

After the advent of HIV, the interest in preoperative autologous blood donation mushroomed. Patients feel safer having their own blood in storage in case of bleeding during surgical procedures. Good candidates for autologous blood donation include patients in good health, with no active cardiopulmonary disease, and with Hgb levels >11 g/dL. EPO together with iron replacement has proven effective at incrementing the amount of units collected per donor. The number of units obtained preoperatively is based on the number of units that would be cross matched before surgery if allogeneic blood were being used. Drawbacks to autologous donation[15] include the fact that half of autologous units obtained are never transfused, and autologous units can also be contaminated by bacteria and cause fatal septic reactions; clerical errors that lead to administration of ABO-incompatible units can still happen, and finally, it costs more than allogeneic blood donation.

Acute Normovolemic Hemodilution

This procedure also allows blood conservation during surgical procedures. It consists of removing the patient's RBCs just before the procedure and replacing the volume with crystalloid solutions, causing hemodilution. The bleeding that follows is mainly that of a diluted blood. Limited or moderate hemodilution leads to a decrease in hematocrit to 28%.[16] Later on, all blood that was removed and collected in bags containing anticoagulant is reinfused.

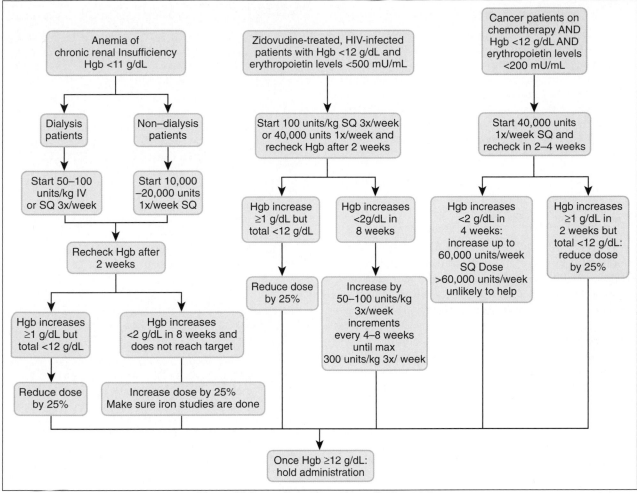

Figure 75-3 • Use of Recombinant Erythropoietin.

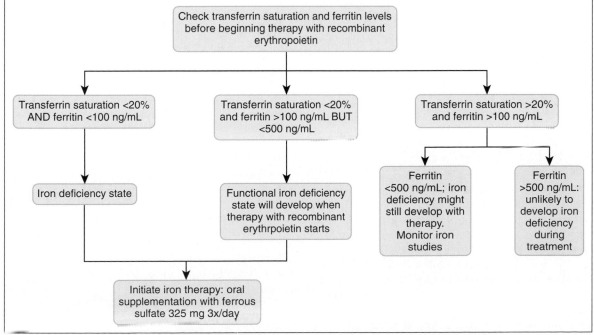

Figure 75-4 • Evaluation of iron studies prior to initiation of recombinant erythropoietin.

Cell Salvage

Recovery of red cells from the surgical site is possible using a collection system that includes a cardiotomy reservoir, a suction line, and an anticoagulant.[17] Indications for the use of cell salvage are many, including valve replacement surgeries, major spine orthopedic procedures, thoracoabdominal aortic aneurysm repair, and, very importantly, patients who refuse allogeneic blood transfusion due to religious beliefs and those patients who have developed red cell alloantibodies that are especially difficult to honor.

Red Blood Cell Substitutes

Research in the field of blood substitutes intensified in the early 1990s due to concerns regarding the transmission of infectious diseases through allogeneic blood transfusion. Currently, different types of modified hemoglobins are being tested in clinical trials, including a polyhemoglobin which is prepared based on the use of agents to cross-link hemoglobin intermolecularlly, as well as conjugated hemoglobin to polymers.[18,19] One of the challenges in the development of these artificial oxygen carriers comes from the fact that single tetrameric (not conjugated, not polymerized) hemoglobin molecules in these solutions have the potential to enter the interstitial space, bind nitric oxide, and cause symptomatic vasoconstriction.

Another problem is that plain oxygen carriers do not contain red cell enzymes such as catalase and superoxide dismutase that prevent tissue injury associated with reperfusion. Cross-linking of trace amounts of catalase and superoxide dismutase to polymerized hemoglobin has been attempted, resulting in decreased production of oxygen radicals by ischemic tissues.

Construction of artificial RBCs using membranes made of lipid containing polyethylene glycol (PEG) and biodegradable polymers such as polylactide and polyglycolides is also under investigation, but a number of regulatory hurdles must be overcome before such products can be effectively used in clinical practice. When this becomes a reality, issues such as dependence on voluntary blood donors for maintenance of blood supply, transmission of infectious diseases, and need for antigenic compatibility testing may all be solved.

EVALUATION OF EFFECTIVENESS OF RED BLOOD CELL TRANSFUSION

A dose of 1 unit of compatible red blood cells in an average-sized adult who is not bleeding or hemolyzing is supposed to increase Hgb levels by approximately 1.0 g/dL.[20] There is really not much evidence that supports the practice of measuring Hgb levels only 24 hours after transfusion, to allow for equilibration of Hgb concentration. This issue was addressed in a small study by Wiesen et al.,[20] who in 39 nonactively bleeding adult patients documented post-transfusion Hgb levels in the 15-minute, 1-hour, 2-hour, and 24- hour post-transfusion periods. The mean Hgb concentration increased by 2 g/dL, and no significant differences were noted among the 15-minute, 1-hour, 2-hour, and 24-hour Hgb values.

Key Points

- Assessment of each individual patient and the concomitant clinical scenario determines the indication for transfusion of RBCs.

- If patients do not have clinically significant cardiac disease, transfusion in the ICU should be restricted to maintaining Hgb and Htc to 7 g/dL and 21%, respectively, especially among patients who are less severely ill (APACHE score, ≤20) and <55 years old, as this is associated with reduced mortality.

- Transfusion of packed RBCs is correlated with increased occurrence of nosocomial infections in a dose–response pattern.

- Febrile non-hemolytic transfusion reactions (FNHTRs) are probably the most common type of reactions related to the administration of blood products.

- Transfusion-related acute lung injury (TRALI) has been the leading cause of reported transfusion-related fatalities reported to the FDA for the past few years.

- Bacterial contamination occurs about 1 in 3,000 for platelet transfusion because platelets are stored at room temperature, yielding an increased risk for bacterial overgrowth. Transfusion of platelet concentrates accounts for 85% of fatal septic reactions.

- Type and screen testing has to be repeated every 3 days to allow for detection of new alloantibodies the recipient might have developed after that period of time.

- Mean Hgb concentration increases by about 2 g/dL after transfusion, and no significant differences are noted among the 15-minute, 1-hour, 2-hour, and 24-hour Hgb values.

SUGGESTED READING

Hebert PC, Wells G, Blajchman MA, et al. A multicenter, randomized, controlled trial of transfusion requirements in critical care: transfusion requirements in critical care investigators, Canadian Critical Care Trials Group, N Engl J Med 1999; 340:409–417.

Taylor RW, Manganaro L, O'Brien J, et al. Impact of allogeneic packed red blood cell transfusion on nosocomial infection rates in the critically ill patient. Crit Care Med 2002; 30:2249–2254.

Looney MR. TRALI: Transfusion-Related Acute Lung Injury—a review. Chest 2004; 126:249–258.

Goodnough LT, Brecher ME, Kanter MH, AuBuchon JP. Transfusion medicine: first of two parts (blood transfusion). N Engl J Med 1999; 340:438–447.

Carson JL, Noveck H, et al. Mortality and morbidity in patients with very low postoperative Hb levels who decline blood transfusion. Transfusion 2002; 42:812–818.

Ford PA, Mastoris J. Strategies to optimize the use of erythropoietin and iron therapy in oncology patients. Transfusion 2004; 44:S15–S25.

Goodnough LT, et al. Transfusion medicine: second of two parts (blood conservation). N Engl J Med 1999; 340:525–533.

Shander A, Rijhwani T. Acute normovolemic hemodilution. Transfusion 2004; 44:S26–S34.

Vincent JL, Piagnerelli M. Transfusion in the intensive care unit. Crit Care Med 2006; 34(Suppl 5):S96–101.

CHAPTER SEVENTY-SIX

Anemia

Tyler Kang, MD, and Alan Lichtin, MD

BACKGROUND

Anemia is defined as a reduction in the red blood cell (RBC) mass as measured by either the hematocrit or the hemoglobin concentration. The hematocrit is typically three times larger than the hemoglobin level. Acquired anemia is not a disease per se, but rather a sign or symptom of an underlying disease, and thus every patient with anemia deserves careful evaluation to determine the cause.

The RBC mass is maintained in humans as the result of a continuous production of differentiated erythrocytes, generated by erythroid progenitors, and stimulated by the hormone erythropoietin. Iron and nutrients, such as vitamin B_{12} and folate, are necessary for RBC production, and energy sources are required to maintain the RBC membrane for RBCs to survive an average of 120 days.[1]

ASSESSMENT

Clinical Presentation

Many of the manifestations associated with an anemia are determined by the etiology of the underlying disease that is producing the anemia. If severe enough, all anemias result in symptoms of tissue hypoxia (i.e., the consequence of a low oxygen-carrying capacity of the blood). Therefore, several signs and symptoms are common to all anemias. Weakness, headache, feeling "cold," and exertional dyspnea are common nonspecific symptoms that may be mild if the anemia develops slowly.[2,3] Some patients complain of a pounding audible sensation with each heartbeat as cardiac output increases to compensate for the anemia. The presence of physical signs, such as pallor and tachycardia, can be severe but depend on the patient's previous cardiovascular status. Stress to the cardiovascular system may occur with mild anemia in patients with preexisting cardiovascular disease. However, even a healthy person begins to have cardiovascular stress at hemoglobin levels of less than 10 g/dL, as a result of the increased cardiac output required to compensate for the reduced oxygen-carrying capacity of blood.

Specific anemias will also present with other findings secondary to the underlying etiology. Pernicious anemia from B_{12} deficiency may present with neuropathy; immune-mediated hemolytic anemia may present with dark urine; sickle cell anemia may cause pain crises or avascular necrosis; iron deficiency may produce glossitis, cheilosis, abdominal pain with gastrointestinal bleed, and pica.

Differential Diagnosis

RBCs are produced and destroyed on a continuous basis. Anemia results when this equilibrium cannot be maintained because of (1) acute or chronic blood loss, (2) failure of production, or (3) increased destruction resulting in a shortening of the RBC life span. Box 76-1 provides an extensive listing of various etiologies for anemia separated by the presence or absence of a normal bone marrow response as measured by reticulocyte production.

Diagnosis

Preferred Studies

The first step in assessing a patient with anemia is always to exclude acute blood loss by history and physical examination, including stool guaiac for occult blood loss. Further analyses include a complete blood cell count (CBC) with red cell indices, including a calculation of the mean corpuscular volume (MCV); a review of the peripheral blood smear (PBS); and a corrected reticulocyte count. The reticulocyte count is the test most often forgotten by hospitalists when confronted by an anemic patient, so its importance must be stressed.

An important initial step in assessing anemia involves an examination of the PBS, the most cost-effective hematologic test. The RBC indices should never be substituted for an examination of the PBS, because the statistical averaging that occurs with an automated CBC loses valuable information about small populations of RBCs. An examination of the PBS reveals more information about specific RBC morphology, dimorphic populations, inclusion bodies, and accompanying white blood cell (WBC) morphology, all of which may not be available from an automated CBC.[4]

The corrected reticulocyte count serves to divide anemias into two major categories: (1) hyperproliferative anemias resulting from the loss or destruction of RBCs, with an associated increased bone marrow activity; and (2) hypoproliferative anemias, resulting from decreased bone marrow production.

Box 76-1 Differential Diagnosis of Anemia Based Upon Marrow Response

- **Anemias with increased reticulocyte count (marrow attempting to compensate by hyperproliferation or erythroid hyperplasia)**
  - Compensated acute blood loss occurring before depletion of iron stores
  - Hemolytic anemia
  - Thalassemia
  - Immune and autoimmune disorders
  - Drugs
    - α-Methyldopa (Aldomet)
    - Penicillins
    - Quinidine
    - Cephalosporins
  - Membrane defects
    - Hereditary spherocytosis/elliptocytosis
    - Paroxysmal nocturnal hemoglobinuria
  - Congenital enzymopathies
    - Glucose-6-phosphate dehydrogenase (G6PD) deficiency
    - Pyruvate kinase deficiency
    - Others
  - Hemoglobinopathies
    - Sickle cell anemia
    - Hemoglobin C disease
    - Others
  - Mechanical hemolysis
    - Heart valves
    - Disseminated intravascular coagulation
    - Thrombotic thrombocytopenic purpura
  - Infections
    - Malaria
    - Babesiosis
- **Anemias with decreased reticulocyte count (hypoproliferative marrow response)**
  - Macrocytic anemias (MCV >100 fl)
    - Pernicious anemia (vitamin B_{12} deficiency)
    - Folate deficiency
    - Alcoholism
    - Malabsorption
    - Liver disease
    - Myelodysplasia
  - Normochromic, normocytic (MCV >80 fl <100 fl)
    - Aplastic anemia
    - Myelophthisic disorders
    - Leukemias
    - Lymphomas
    - Multiple myeloma
    - Myelofibrosis
    - Myelodysplasia
    - Granulomatous diseases
    - Lipid storage diseases
    - Anemia of chronic disease (abnormal iron reutilization)
    - Chronic renal failure
    - Endocrine diseases (hypotestosteronism and hypothyroidism)
    - Hepatic failure
  - Hypochromic microcytic (MCV <80 fl)
    - Iron deficiency
    - Sideroblastic anemia
    - Lead intoxication
    - Thalassemia (usually demonstrates erythroid hyperplasia)
    - Anemia of chronic disease (severe)

Adapted from: Tefferi A. Anemia in adults: a contemporary approach to diagnosis. Mayo Clin Proc 2003; 78:1274.

Alternative Options

Results from the initial tests help determine whether more invasive or expensive testing is required, such as bone marrow aspiration, biopsy, and immunohistochemistry. Depending on the type of anemia suspected, further confirmatory laboratory tests may be helpful.

Hemolytic anemias are disorders characterized by an indirect hyperbilirubinemia, reticulocytosis, marrow erythroid hyperplasia, hemoglobinemia, and hemoglobinuria as well as decreased haptoglobin levels, especially in intravascular hemolysis.[5] Specific antibody testing (Coombs' test) is useful to diagnose immune-mediated processes. Hereditary disorders causing hemolysis such as hemoglobinopathies and sickle cell anemia can be diagnosed with hemoglobin electrophoresis.

Hypoproliferative anemias can be classified by RBC morphology and size.

- Macrocytic: Vitamin B_{12} and folate assays easily diagnose these nutritional deficiencies that cause macrocytic anemia; Schilling's test has recently fallen out of favor because of lack of reagents to perform the test. Anti-intrinsic factor and antiparietal cell antibodies can further delineate the cause of B_{12} deficiency (pernicious anemia). Intermediate metabolites dependent upon vitamin B_{12} or folic acid include methylmalonic acid (MMA) and homocysteine. One may see an elevated MMA level well before the serum B_{12} level falls. PBS would show hypersegmented neutrophils, pleomorphic RBCs, and dyserythropoiesis.[6]
- Normochromic normocytic: Anemia of chronic disease is characterized by low serum iron, low total iron-binding capacity (transferrin), low iron saturation, and normal or high ferritin level.[7] PBS and marrow examination can determine whether leukemia, lymphoma, or myelophthisic disorders are occurring.
- Hypochromic microcytic: Iron deficiency is characterized by low ferritin level and can be further characterized by increased total iron binding capacity, decreased total iron level, and low percent transferrin saturation.[8] Ferritin is the only test needed for initial screening for iron deficiency anemia

Figure 76-1 provides an algorithm for diagnosing the various etiologies for anemia. In the initial evaluation of a patient hospitalized with anemia, the hospitalist should order diagnostic testing (e.g., iron, B_{12}, folate) if possible prior to ordering blood transfusion. If the patient is hemodynamically compromised (angina, high output heart failure, edema), then transfusion may be mandatory,[9-11] but laboratory testing usually can be performed.

Prognosis

During Hospitalization

Acute anemia that requires hospitalization usually responds quickly to therapy, and the immediate outcome is usually favorable. It may take 2–4 weeks of replacement with iron, B_{12}, or folate to see significant rises in hemoglobin if the anemia is based on deficiency of these nutrients.[12,13] Chronic diseases that present with severe anemia will usually respond to temporizing measures such as transfusion, but the long-term prognosis will depend on the treatment of the underlying disorder. Occasionally, the process of hospitalization can be an important cause of added morbidity for hospitalized patients. Hospitalists should attempt to reduce the number of blood tests performed and limit phlebotomies to minimize the anemia associated with hospitalization.[13a]

Postdischarge

Anemia, as an acquired form, is usually the manifestation of an underlying disease. Therefore, the long-term outcome depends on the resolution of the underlying disorder. The acuteness of the underlying disease will also determine the chronicity of the anemia. For example, chronic diseases such as liver failure, renal failure, and rheumatologic or malignant diseases will have protracted courses of associated anemia. Patients with renal failure

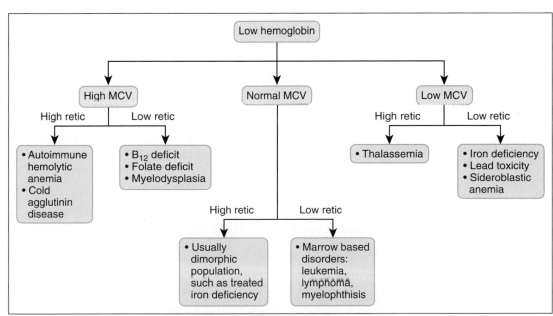

Figure 76-1 • Diagnostic Algorithm for Anemia.

who have low endogenous erythropoietin levels respond well to exogenous administration of erythropoietin.

Hereditary anemias such as sickle cell anemia and hemoglobinopathies will be chronic, and outcome depends on individual clinical factors.

MANAGEMENT

Treatment

Hemolytic Anemia

The treatment of choice for warm antibody immune-mediated hemolytic anemia is corticosteroids. Splenectomy is effective in about half of patients for whom corticosteroids fail. In cold agglutinin disease, cold avoidance is the best treatment option. Occasionally, plasmapheresis or rituximab therapy may be helpful.[14] Transfusion of RBCs is rarely indicated and usually complicated by the difficulty of typing and crossing the patient for compatible blood. Cases of drug-induced immune hemolysis are treated by removal of the inciting drug.

Sickle Cell Anemia

The therapy of sickle cell anemia and crisis is covered in detail in Chapter 77. The basic approach includes hydration and analgesia, with early treatment of infections and judicious use of transfusions.[15] Indications for transfusion include acute chest syndrome with hypoxia, symptomatic episodes of acute anemia, surgery with general anesthesia, or severe symptomatic chronic anemia. Transfusions may be useful in complicated obstetric problems, refractory leg ulcers, acute severe priapism, and refractory and protracted painful episodes. Straight transfusion, when the patient is given additional units of blood without removal of sickle blood, is best used when the hemoglobin concentration is lower than 8 or 9 g/dL. Exchange transfusion is better when the hemoglobin concentration is high, thus reducing the complications from increased viscosity. Iron overload with hemochromatosis due to repeated transfusions is a serious concern and should mitigate willingness to transfuse these patients.

Macrocytic Anemia

Therapy for vitamin B_{12} deficiency consists of monthly intramuscular injection of 100 to 1,000 mcg of B_{12}. It is important not to mistake folate deficiency with vitamin B_{12} deficiency, as folate cannot correct the neurologic deficits of B_{12} deficiency. In fact, replacing folic acid in a B_{12}-deficient patient will precipitate further neurologic decline.[16] If folate deficiency is diagnosed, folate replacement is mandated. If folate deficiency occurs secondary to malabsorption, correcting the cause of the malabsorption must take place (e.g., gluten-free diet in celiac disease.)

Normochromic Normocytic

Treatment of the underlying disease remains the only effective therapy for anemia of chronic disease. In renal failure, anemia is due to a deficiency of erythropoietin, the injection of which, along with iron, is usually sufficient to correct the anemia.[17]

Hypochromic Microcytic

In iron deficiency, treatment with iron salts such as ferrous sulfate, gluconate, or fumarate can replete stores in 2–6 months.[12] Notable reticulocytosis starts at about 7 days. Ferrous sulfate contains 65 mg of elemental iron per tablet while ferrous gluconate has 28 to 36 mg iron/tablet. One preparation is not more effective than the other. The recommended daily dose for the treatment of iron deficiency in adults is in the range of 150–200 mg/day of elemental iron. Thus, 195 mg of elemental iron would be delivered with prescribing 325 mg of ferrous sulfate orally three times daily between meals. However, this may provoke gastrointestinal side effects (nausea, vomiting, constipation), which are seen in 20% or more of patients. Using ferrous gluconate instead and having patients slowly increase from one tablet per day up to three may avoid this.

Treatment of thalassemia involves the transfusion of RBCs in severely affected children to reduce their own endogenous bone marrow activity and thus avoid bony hypertrophy and extramedullary hematopoiesis.[18] In adults, transfusion is beneficial but can lead to severe iron overload and organ damage from the hemochromatosis (e.g., heart failure). Deferoxamine is useful in these cases to chelate the excess iron and remove it from the body, but it must be given intravenously. Deferasirox (Exjade) is an effective oral alternative. Those with thalassemia minor or trait rarely require transfusion.

Alternative Options

Transfusion with RBCs to correct anemia may be the best option, but it is only a temporizing measure. In the event of acute blood loss sufficient to cause clinical detriment to the patient (i.e., end-organ damage), prompt repletion of RBC mass with transfusions is necessary to ensure adequate oxygenation of tissues.[9–11] However, correction of the underlying etiology of anemia is the ultimate goal. If GI bleeding is the cause of the anemia, identifying the source and treating it is the goal.

DISCHARGE/FOLLOW-UP PLANS

Patient Instruction

Once patients' acute clinical symptoms have been treated, either with temporizing transfusions or with treatments aimed at the underlying disease, they may be discharged with further outpatient follow-up. Patients should be instructed to monitor their own symptoms and watch for signs of relapse (e.g., in cases of sickle cell disease to monitor pain crisis, or in cases of acute bleeding to watch for signs of recurrence of blood loss). In the case of hemolytic anemia, it is important to instruct the patient to watch out for signs of hemoglobinuria manifested by dark urine or jaundice. Patients with chronic conditions are usually well educated about their signs and symptoms.

Outpatient Physician Communication

The hospitalist should maintain open lines of communication with the primary care clinician in order to have prompt follow-up with an early return visit and to check on any pending laboratory data which may still be unavailable at time of discharge. Follow-up on hereditary anemias such as thalassemia or sickle cell anemia is important in the education of patients with regard to potentially affected family members and offspring; family planning with geneticists may be crucial.[19]

Key Points

- Review of the peripheral blood smear and a corrected reticulocyte count are important tests in the initial evaluation of anemia.

- Ferritin is the single best screening test for iron deficiency anemia.

- It is important not to mistake folate deficiency with vitamin B_{12} deficiency, as folate cannot correct the neurologic deficits of B_{12} deficiency. In fact, replacing folic acid in a B_{12}-deficient patient will precipitate further neurologic decline.

- The treatment of choice for warm antibody immune-mediated hemolytic anemia is corticosteroids. Splenectomy is effective in about half of patients for whom corticosteroids fail.

SUGGESTED READING

Allison AC. Turnovers of erythrocytes and plasma proteins in mammals. Nature 1960; 188:37.

Weiskopf RB, Viele MK, Feiner J, et al. Human cardiovascular and metabolic response to acute, severe isovolemic anemia. JAMA 1998; 279:217.

Tefferi, A. Anemia in adults: a contemporary approach to diagnosis. Mayo Clin Proc 2003; 78:1274.

Weiss G, Goodnough LT. Anemia of chronic disease. N Engl J Med 2005; 352:1011.

Thavendiranathan P, Bagai A, Ebidia A, et al. Do blood tests cause anemia in hospitalized patients? The effect of diagnostic phlebotomy on hemoglobin and hematocrit levels. JGIM 2005; 20:520–24.

Petz LD. Treatment of autoimmune hemolytic anemias. Curr Opin Hematol 2001; 8:411.

Dhar M, Bellevue R, Carmel R. Pernicious anemia with neuropsychiatric dysfunction in a patient with sickle cell anemia treated with folate supplementation. N Engl J Med 2003; 348:2204.

CHAPTER SEVENTY-SEVEN

Sickle Cell Crises

James R. Eckman, MD, and Allan F. Platt, Jr, MS, PA-C

BACKGROUND

Sickle cell crisis can occur in individuals with inherited sickle hemoglobin disorders including phenotypes SS, SC, S beta 0 thalassemia, S beta + thalassemia, SD-Los Angeles, SE, SF, SG-Philadelphia, and SO-Arab. Patients with these disorders can have chronic hemolytic anemia, increased susceptibility to infections, end-organ damage, and intermittent ischemic episodes causing both acute and chronic pain. Sickle cell anemia (Hb SS), the most common sickle cell disease variant, results when an individual inherits a substitution of valine for the normal glutamic acid in the sixth position of the beta chain (sickle hemoglobin) from both parents. Sickle hemoglobin polymerizes, elongating and deforming the red cell into a rigid "sickle" shape when oxygen is released.[1-3]

Sickle cell disease is most common in descendents of individuals who resided in areas of the world where malaria is endemic. People who inherit one sickle gene (sickle cell trait) gain some protection from malaria, yielding evolutionary pressure to sustain it in the gene pool. In the United States, sickle cell disease is present in 1 in 400 African Americans. Sickle hemoglobin is found in Africans, Arabs, Turks, Greeks, Hispanic populations, Italians, and Asiatic Indians. There are four distinct sickle haplotypes, three originating in Africa and one of Arab-India origin.[1] Eight percent of American blacks are carriers of the sickle gene and make <50% sickle hemoglobin. The carrier state is usually asymptomatic, but hematuria and complications including splenic sequestration and sudden death can occur with severe hypoxia, dehydration, and elevated temperature.[4,5]

The clinical manifestations of sickle cell disease are thought to result from increased blood viscosity, changes in red blood cell deformability, fragility, and adherence to vascular walls. Markers of increased platelet activation are also prevalent in sickle cell patients. Clinically relevant deoxygenation, red cell dehydration, reduced pH, and elevated temperature all can provoke red cell sickling that causes increased blood viscosity and capillary plugging, producing vascular occlusion, hemorrhages, tissue infarction, and death.[1-3] Red cell survival is reduced from the normal of 120 days to about 15 days. The hemolytic anemia causes a high reticulocyte count, increased indirect bilirubin, and lactic dehydrogenase levels. Hemolysis, inflammation, and hyposplenism cause chronic elevation of the white blood cell and platelet counts.

The complex alterations in laboratory values make knowing the individual patient's baseline laboratory values critical for knowing what is "normal" for him or her. There are no characteristic "normal" laboratory values found in steady-state sickle cell disease. Baseline values of hemoglobin, hematocrit, reticulocyte count, lactic dehydrogenase, bilirubin, and pulse oximetry value for an individual patient should ideally be available for comparison during acute complications.

ASSESSMENT

Clinical Presentation

Prevalence and Presenting Signs and Symptoms

Pain is the most common presenting symptom. It is caused by bone and muscle ischemia, necrosis, or infarction, or the inflammatory response secondary to blood flow obstruction and sludging. Severity of pain has been reported to range from mild transient attacks of 5 minutes to excruciating pain requiring hospitalization for days to weeks. Cumulative ischemic tissue damage, bone infarction, and fibrosis can lead to chronic pain. The frequency of pain crisis varies with each individual and depends to some extent on his or her hemoglobin phenotype, physical condition, intercurrent illness, and psychological or social stress. The number of episodes per year correlates with the clinical severity of disease and early death in patients with sickle cell anemia over the age of 20.[6] A large study more than 15 years ago documented that about 39% of patients with sickle cell anemia had no episodes of pain, and 1% had more than six episodes per year. The 5% of patients with 3–10 episodes per year had one third of all episodes.[20]

Damage can occur to any organ in the body, including the brain, lungs, liver, spleen, kidneys, bones, muscles, and retina. **The single best question in evaluating a pain episode is: "Is this pain typical for your routine pain crisis?"** This helps differentiate routine sickle cell pain events from other complications that cause pain. Other signs and symptoms indicate a complication. Focal pain may also suggest complications common to sickle cell patients, such as splenic sequestration, premature gallstones, bone infarction, osteomyelitis, or avascular necrosis. Although numerous factors (dehydration, infection, stress, weather conditions, alcohol consumption) can trigger a pain crisis, no identifiable cause is apparent in the majority of cases.

Episodes can affect any area of the body, with the back, chest, extremities, and abdomen being most common. The pain severity can range from trivial to excruciating. About half of pain episodes are accompanied by vital sign abnormalities such as fever, tachypnea, or hypertension, or other symptoms such as nausea, vomiting, or focal swelling and tenderness. A detailed history and physical examination are important to identify correctable precipitating factors such as infection, dehydration, increased anemia, acidosis from any cause, emotional stress, extreme temperature exposure, or ingestion of other substances such as alcohol or other recreational drugs.

Fever is sepsis until proven otherwise. Bacterial infection is one of the main causes of morbidity and mortality in patients with sickle cell disease.[7] Splenic function is markedly decreased or absent in sickle cell anemia, leaving the individual at great risk for infection within encapsulated organisms such as *S. pneumoniae, H. influenza*, salmonella, meningococcus, and others.[7] Serious infections such as meningitis, pneumonia, sepsis, and osteomyelitis must be aggressively excluded and treated early and empirically to prevent morbidity and mortality.

Abdominal swelling and pain, combined with a falling hemoglobin level and increasing reticulocyte count, may signal a sequestration crisis. Splenic sequestration is a common cause of death in adults with sickle cell disease.[7] During splenic sequestration episodes, sickle cells are trapped in the spleen, causing left upper quadrant pain, enlargement of the spleen, and rapid fall in the hemoglobin level. Patients with hemoglobin SC and S beta thalassemia are at higher risk for splenic sequestration events as adults. Hepatic sequestration may also occur, causing right upper quadrant pain, a rapidly enlarging liver, and a falling hemoglobin level with high reticulocyte count.[9]

A falling hemoglobin and a low reticulocyte count point to failure of erythropoiesis by the bone marrow. Aplastic crisis can occur when parvovirus B19 infection stops new red blood production.[10] Infection, nutritional deficiency, relative erythropoietin deficiency, and surgery can also cause falling hemoglobin, with a decreased reticulocyte count, weakness, pallor, dyspnea, and dizziness. Treatment for aplastic crisis includes careful sequential monitoring and blood transfusions to support the hemoglobin level.

Chest pain can be the first sign of acute chest syndrome (ACS), which is an important cause of morbidity and mortality in sickle cell disease. The etiology of ACS includes obstruction of pulmonary vessels by sickled cells with infarction, pneumonia from viral and typical or atypical bacterial infection, and fat embolism from bone marrow necrosis.[11] Patients present with chest pain, a new infiltrate on chest radiograph, and fever; but they typically have negative blood cultures. Large prospective trials document ACS as the most frequently reported cause of death in adults with sickle disease, and it is a risk factor for early mortality.

The Cooperative Study of Sickle Cell Disease prospectively followed 3,751 patients enrolled from birth to the age of 66 for ACS, and documented 1,722 ACS episodes in 939 patients.[11] Adults were often febrile and complained of shortness of breath, chills, and severe pain. Severe hypoxia occurred in 18% of adults and could not be predicted by examination or laboratory findings. The death rate was four times higher in adults than in children.[11] Bronchoscopy with bronchial alveolar lavage may be diagnostic and therapeutic in cases of ACS. Patients should be treated with transfusions and antibiotics that cover community-acquired and atypical bacterial infections. ACS may be prevented by incentive spirometry in patients with chest and upper back pain.[12]

New onset of an unusual headache or neurologic signs can indicate a stroke, subarachnoid hemorrhage, or meningitis. Headaches in sickle cell anemia patients may be caused by any of the common etiologies or may be early symptoms of several life-threatening disorders such as meningitis, subarachnoid hemorrhage, or osteomyelitis of the jaw or skull. All sickle cell patients with a new, severe, or unusual headache should be evaluated with a CT scan, MRA, and LP.[14]

Priapism is common in males. Painful erections are difficult to treat and prevent. Prolonged or recurrent priapism can lead to impotence. Priapism can be precipitated by infection, sexual activity, and normal nocturnal erections.[15,16] Urologic consultation should be obtained.

Acute dysfunction in multiple organs can be fatal. Evidence of hepatic, renal, pulmonary failure; coagulopathy; or rhabdomyalysis can all indicate multiorgan system failure. The syndrome may develop in patients who previously exhibited relatively mild disease with little evidence of chronic organ damage and may be recurrent. High baseline hemoglobin levels may represent a predisposing factor.[17] Patients with acute multiorgan failure syndrome present with unusually severe pain. Deterioration often occurs on the third to fourth hospital day as the acute pain is improving. The onset of organ failure is associated with fever, a falling hemoglobin level, and decreased platelet count. Other findings include nonfocal encephalopathy, laboratory evidence of liver dysfunction, renal failure, and rhabdomyolysis. This potentially severe, life-threatening complication of pain episodes appears to be reversed with prompt, aggressive transfusion or exchange transfusion.

Right upper quadrant pain and increased jaundice suggests symptomatic gallstones. Over 50–70% of adult patients with sickle disease have pigment gallstones. Biliary complications include common duct stones, biliary sludge, cholelithiasis, and cholestasis. Ultrasound is a sensitive test for gallstones. HIDA scan may document cholecystitis.

Common syndromes are delineated in Table 77-1.

Differential Diagnosis

Pain Episode

The diagnosis of sickle cell pain episode (crisis) is clinical and must be based on history alone. Significant changes in physical findings or laboratory values suggest precipitating or concomitant complications. Localized or atypical pain suggests a complication other than simple pain episode.

Fever over 38°C, chills, white blood cell (WBC) count over 20,000 with a left shift, local swelling, or erythema suggest infection or some other inflammatory complication. Other considerations are acute chest syndrome, urinary tract infection, bacteremia, or multiorgan system failure.

Chest Pain

The complication to consider immediately is acute chest syndrome. This is characterized by chest pain, fever, hypoxia, and a new infiltrate on chest x-ray (CXR). Chest pain from rib and sternal infarction is also common. Other considerations are pneumonia, pulmonary embolus, myocardial infarction, pericarditis, pulmonary hypertension, pneumothorax, Gastroesophageal reflux

Table 77-1 Common Inpatient Problems

Signs and Symptoms	Diagnostic Tests and Differential	Treatment Options
Chills and fever,	Sepsis, pneumonia, osteomyelitis—CBC, WBC differential, (check for elevated bands and total WBC count), blood cultures	Empirically treat with antibiotics until cultures results are known
Headache	Stroke, aneurysm, meningitis—CT scan, MRI-MRA, LP	Treat etiology
Chest pain, dyspnea, cough	Chest syndrome, pneumonia—CXR, ABG, cultures	Treat empirically with antibiotics and transfusion
Abdominal pain and swelling	Splenic or hepatic sequestration, gallstones— Ultrasound or CT, CBC and chemistry profile	Transfusion for sequestration. Surgery for symptomatic gallstones
New weakness, parenthesis, difficulty talking	Stroke—CT or MRI-MRA	Transfuse acutely and chronic transfusion program for prevention
Pain in extremities, low-back "typical crisis pain"	Pain crisis—look for precipitating causes such as infection, dehydration, acidosis; CBC, retic count, chemistry profile and UA	Hydration with oral or IV water. Good pain management
Weakness, lethargy, pallor	Aplastic crisis; CBC with reticulocyte count	Transfusion support until bone marrow responds
Acute decline after routine pain crisis—multiple organ failure	Multiorgan system failure—evidenced by renal, hepatic, failure, ARDS, DIC,	Exchange transfusion can be life saving
Increasing jaundice	Increased hemolysis, hepatitis, or bile duct obstruction—CBC, retic count, chemistry profile, hepatitis screen. Abdominal ultrasound	Treat etiology
Increasing inpatient stays	Consider inadequate pain management, infection, increased anemia. Assess psychosocial aspects	Provide good pain management Consider hydroxyurea therapy to prevent pain. Case management
Focal bone pain	Consider bone infarction or osteomyelitis. If hip or shoulder pain, consider avascular necrosis (AVN)—CBC, and x-ray (or MRI) the area	For bone infarction and AVN, treat with long-acting NSAIDs, and decreased weight bearing.
Depression	Worry about death, pain, disability	Consider adding antidepressants, psychological and spiritual support

disease (GERD), referred pain from cholecystitis, cholelithiasis, or splenic infarction.

Abdominal Pain

Diffuse abdominal pain may occur during an uncomplicated pain episode. Bowel sounds are normal or increased, and rebound is absent. Severe or localized pain, decreased bowel sounds, increase in liver or spleen size, nausea, vomiting, or diarrhea suggest complications like splenic or hepatic sequestration, gallstones, or an acute abdomen from other causes. Sickle cell patients can have a urinary tract infection, perforated ulcer, ectopic pregnancy, appendicitis, pelvic inflammatory disease, or any other abdominal pathology seen in the general medical population.

Headache

Consider subarachnoid bleeding from aneurysms, cranial bone infarction, and meningitis if the headache is unusual or severe. Other causes of headache are similar to those seen in the general medical population.

Bone or Joint Pain

Localized bone or joint pain especially with swelling, erythema, or warmth suggests osteomyelitis, bone infarction, septic arthritis, or gout. Acute, monoarticular arthritis can accompany pain crisis, but this is a diagnosis of exclusion. Avascular necrosis (AVN) of the hips and shoulders should be considered when hip

and shoulder pain is recurrent or persistent. This complication is more common in patients with hemoglobin SC and hemoglobin S beta thalassemia.

Increasing Anemia

A falling hematocrit and falling or normal reticulocyte count suggest aplastic crisis, a lack of nutrients such as folic acid, or reduced erythropoietin from renal complications. Worsening anemia with a rising reticulocyte count suggests bleeding, sequestration crisis in the liver or spleen, or increased hemolysis.

Diagnosis

Preferred Studies

Hemoglobinopathies, including the many variants of sickle cell disease, are diagnosed using hemoglobin electrophoresis, isoelectric focusing (IEF), or high-performance liquid chromatography. The complete blood cell (CBC) count generally reveals anemia with elevated reticulocyte count; WBC and platelet counts are also increased. Hemolysis causes increased indirect bilirubin and LDH on the chemistry panel. X-rays may demonstrate marrow expansion in the spine.

Uncomplicated pain episodes cause no consistent changes in the patient's laboratory findings. The patient's history must be relied on for diagnosis of uncomplicated pain episodes. As noted above, an excellent question to ask the patient is: "Is this pain typical for your pain crisis?" If the pain is atypical, a search for other causes should be pursued. Headache, chest pain, focal bone pain, and abdominal pain should prompt a search for secondary causes and complications. Pain intensity should be assessed and recorded as a vital sign using a visual analog scale, or similar tool, at the beginning of treatment, and at set intervals throughout the hospital stay to document the response to treatment. Pulse oximetry values should be compared to the patient's base line SaO_2.

Minimum laboratory evaluation for symptoms should include a CBC with a WBC differential, platelet count, reticulocyte count, pulse oximetry, and urinalysis. A chemistry profile including electrolytes, blood urea nitrogen, creatinine, aspartate aminotransferase (AST), alanine aminotransferase (ALT), bilirubin is indicated and should be repeated every 2–3 days if the pain is unusually severe. The CBC and reticulocyte count should be monitored daily or every other day for prolonged stays.

Additional Evaluation

Urine culture should be done if urinalysis or urinary tract infection is suggested by history or physical examination. Blood cultures should be obtained if the patient is febrile or has a WBC over 20,000 or left shift. Other tests or procedures include: amylase if abdominal pain is present; electrocardiogram (ECG) for chest pain, palpitations, or congestive heart failure; arterial blood gases for unusually low O_2 saturation on pulse oximetry, dyspnea, chest syndrome, or suspected hypoxia. Do a CXR if the patient has a productive cough, dyspnea, chest pain, or cough with fever, WBC over 20,000 or left shift, or unusually low O_2 saturation on pulse oximetry.

Areas with localized pain or swelling should be x-rayed. If osteomyelitis is suspected, a bone scan or MRI should be done. Suspected AVN of the hips or shoulders should be evaluated by plain films and if negative followed by MRI if pain persists. An abdominal ultrasound is sensitive and specific if gallstones are suspected.

Prognosis

During Hospitalization

Twenty years of experience from the Georgia Comprehensive Sickle Cell Center at Grady Hospital in Atlanta have shown that 80% of patients presenting for emergency pain crisis resolve with 8 hours of prompt, aggressive pain and fluid management. For those requiring hospitalization, inpatient stays average 5.5 days, and 4 days if pain management is the only issue. The prognosis for uncomplicated pain crisis is excellent.[20] Other complications will require more prolonged stays.

Postdischarge

Life expectancy is increasing with good medical management. In the 1970s, life expectancy for sickle cell anemia was about 20 years. By 1994, data from the natural history study documented a mean survival of 44 years for those with Hb SS, and 64 for those with Hb SC. Median survival of individuals of all ages with sickle cell disease based on genotype and sex are[6]: 42 years for males with Hb SS, 48 years for females for HbSS, 60 years for males with Hb SC, and 68 years for females with Hb SC. Increased frequency of pain episodes predicts a shorter survival.[20]

Elevated blood levels of brain natriuretic peptide (BNP), greater than 160 pg/mL, predict a five-fold increased risk of death and a 78% percent chance of having pulmonary hypertension identified by echocardiogram. Chronically elevated lactate dehydrogenase (LDH) levels also are predictive of a poor prognosis and require aggressive treatment.[20a,20b]

Fortunately, life expectancy may be further increased by advances in treatment—such as hydroxyurea, the new pneumococcal vaccine Prevnar, stroke prevention with transcranial Doppler (TCD) screening of children for stroke prevention and prophylactic chronic transfusion program with a goal HbS of <30% of total hemoglobin, and potential cure with bone marrow transplants.[21]

MANAGEMENT

Treatment

General treatment measures include IV hydration with hypotonic fluids (D_5W or D_5, $^1/_2$ NS) to drive water into the red cells, pain medications, and oxygen if the patient is dyspneic or hypoxic. Pulse oximetry should be monitored as a vital sign but may be less reliable with severe anemia, irregular pulse, nail polish, and cold hands. Low oxygen saturation in symptomatic patients must be investigated with arterial blood gases, CXRs, and pulmonary testing.[22,23]

Pain Management

Pain should be assessed and recorded using a visual analog scale on a regular schedule. During the initial treatment period until the patient is definitely improving, pain medication should be given on a fixed or continuous basis not a p.r.n. (as needed) schedule. This will maintain a steady serum drug level, improving control of pain, minimizing complications, and decreasing anxiety. Patient-controlled analgesia (PCA) pumps delivering constant low-dose infusion of morphine with patient-controlled demand doses provide excellent treatment for patients with severe pain. All patients on opiates should be treated with stool softeners and laxatives to prevent constipation or fecal impaction.

The synthetic agonist-antagonist agents such as nalbuphine (Nubain) and buprenorphine (Buprenex) are alternative choices in relatively opiate-naïve patients, but can precipitate withdrawal symptoms similar to naloxone in patients with physical dependency. These agents also have an analgesic ceiling and should not be increased beyond recommended doses. See Box 77-1 for more details.

Evidence-based pain management guidelines were published by the American Pain Society in 1999, the Georgia Comprehensive Sickle Cell Center in 2000, the Sickle Cell Disease Care Consortium in 2002, the State of Pennsylvania in 2002, and the NIH in 2002. These are all available for order or viewing online at www.SCInfo.org. These guidelines offer clinicians excellent treatment options in the inpatient and outpatient setting.[24–26]

Sequestration Syndromes

Treatment consists of careful observation and aggressive blood transfusions.[8] Emergent splenectomy is occasionally required. In hepatic sequestration, treatment consists of aggressive simple transfusion or red cell exchange transfusion.

Box 77-1 Pain Management

Medications

Parenteral NSAID

- Ketorlac (Toradol) for adults >50 kg

- 15 to 30 mg IV q 6 hours for 5 days maximum.

- In adults <50 kg, give 15 mg IV as a loading dose and then 15 mg IV q 6 hours. The lower dose should be used in individuals over 65 years old and those with renal insufficiency. At present, 120 mg is the maximum total daily dose.

- Oral NSAID of choice should supplement any treatment plan for adults not using Ketorolac.

Parenteral Narcotics

- Morphine sulfate 0.1–0.2 mg/kg IV (up to 15 mg) q 3 hours.

- Nalbuphine HCl (Nubain), 0.3 mg/kg up to 20 mg IV q 3–4 hours.

  Total daily dose of nalbuphine should be limited to 160 mg. Do not use in patients who may be physically dependent on narcotics because withdrawal may be precipitated. Do not use with agonist narcotics because nalbuphine may block their analgesic action.

Additional Medications

- Add hydroxyzine HCl (Vistaril) 25 mg q 6 hours or diphenhydramine (Benadryl) 25–50 mg q 6 hours with morphine to prevent pruritus

- (Phenergan) 12.5 mg IM q 3 hours if allergy to hydroxyzine HCl exists or for individuals that have vomiting with narcotics.

Patient Controlled Analgesia (PCA)*

- Morphine PCA is the preferred therapy, although some centers use hydromorphone for PCA.

- Morphine concentration of 5 mg/mL for adults because they generally need relatively high doses to control the pain.

- Loading doses of morphine up to 0.05 mg/kg q 15 minutes times 4 may be given based on need.

- Demand doses of 0.018–0.04 mg/kg/dose with a 5–15 minute lockout are a usual range for patients with sickle cell disease.

- Continuous infusion doses, if necessary, may be given at night or around the clock. The usual dose ranges are between 0.01 and 0.04 mg/kg/hr.

Take Home Medications

- As a rule, the patient should be managed with a limited supply of oral analgesics consistent with the parenteral treatment protocol used in initial treatment. A 48-hour supply should be sufficient.

- Patients that have been on narcotics for more than a week may need a tapering schedule of narcotic analgesics to prevent physical withdrawal after abrupt stopping of narcotics.

*Please see discussion of PCA use in Chapter 94.

Gallstones

Symptomatic gallstones should probably be removed electively. Laparoscopic cholecystectomy has been found to be safe and cost effective in individuals with sickle cell disease.[18,19]

Role of Transfusion

Transfusion of packed red cells or exchange transfusion is indicated for TIA, stroke, acute chest syndrome, multiorgan system failure, or sequestration of red cells in the spleen or liver.[27-34] Box 77-2 presents a list of the indications. Several recent studies have shown that chronic transfusions can prevent serious sickle cell events, including central nervous system ischemia, ACS, pain crises, growth failure, and splenic dysfunction. The treatment goals for transfusion are to relieve symptoms and to treat or prevent complications. Because of the risks of iron overload, exposure to hepatitis, HIV, and other infectious agents, alloimmunization, induction of hyperviscosity, and limits on the resource, transfusion therapy should be used judiciously. However, red-cell pheresis can prevent the iron overload; and use

Box 77-2 Transfusion Indications

Definite Indications for Transfusion:

- Acute neurologic event

- Splenic sequestration

- Severe pneumonia or pulmonary infarction

- Severe anemia with cardiac decompensation

- Acute arterial hypoxia

- Aplastic crisis with severe anemia

- Hyperhemolytic crisis with enlarging liver/spleen

- Ophthalmological surgery

- Multiorgan system failure

Relative Indications:

- Symptomatic anemia

- Hepatic sequestration

- Leg ulcers refractory to conservative therapy

- Priapism resistant to acute treatment or recurrent

- Severe or prolonged pain episodes

- Frequent pain episodes

- Chronic respiratory insufficiency

- High-dose intravascular contrast studies

- Surgery with general anesthesia

- Pregnancy

Usually Not Indicated:

- Stable chronic anemia

- Pain episodes without absolute or relative indications

- Minor surgery under local or short general anesthesia

- Uncomplicated infections

- Chronic bone disease or organ failure without other indications

of phenotypic matching for E, C, Kell for all patients and extended phenotypic red-cell matching (matched for Kell, E, C, Kidd [Jkb], and Duffy [Fya]) for those with alloantibodies limits transfusion reactions.

Simple transfusion is indicated for severe anemia, aplastic crisis, hyperhemolytic crisis, symptomatic anemia during pregnancy, and in chronic transfusion programs. Exchange transfusions should be performed in patients with acute neurologic events, severe ACS, acute multiorgan failure, acute arterial hypoxia, ophthalmologic surgery, and, high-dose intravascular contrast studies. This can be accomplished either manually or by apheresis. The volume of packed cells to be given must be based on the hematocrit of the packed cells, the red cell mass of the patient, and the desired percentage of Hb A. The general goal of the following approaches is to establish <30% Hb S in the circulation with a hemoglobin of 10 g/dL. Hemoglobin levels of greater than 12 g/dL with >30% S may be associated with increased whole blood viscosity and complications.

With a relative indication for chronic transfusion, packed red cells should be given to raise the hemoglobin to Hb 10 g/dL and then once a week until the percent hemoglobin S is less than 50%. After the percent S is <50%, the hemoglobin can be increased to Hb of 12 g/dL. The patient should then be transfused every 3–4 weeks to keep the hemoglobin between 10 and 12 g/dL, and the percent S <30%.[27–34]

Iron overload occurs after 20–30 transfusions or with ferritin levels over 2,000 ng/mL. Iron chelation therapy should be administered with parenteral deferoxamine or the new oral chelating agent deferasirox (Exjade).[34a]

Preoperative Care

Anesthesia and surgery *are* associated with an increased incidence of morbidity and mortality in patients with sickle syndromes. Recent multicenter data found perioperative complications in 22% of sickle cell patients undergoing elective surgery. Optimal surgical outcome requires careful preoperative, intraoperative, and postoperative management by a team consisting of a surgeon, anesthesiologist, and hematologist. Potential sickle cell–related complications include ACS, pain episodes, hyperhemolytic crisis, relative aplastic crisis, alloimmunization with delayed transfusion reactions, and infections.

Sickle cell patients should have simple transfusions to raise their hemoglobin to 10 g/dL before surgery.[30] These simple transfusions were found to be safer than, and as effective in, preventing postoperative complications as exchange or aggressive transfusions to decrease the hemoglobin S level below 30%.[30] Postoperative complications such as ACS, fever, and alloimmunization with delayed transfusion reactions are common, still occurring in up to 30% of patients.[30]

Alloimmunization can be minimized by giving antigen matched blood for C, E, and Kell in all patients, and blood matched for K, C, E, S, Fy, and Jk antigens in those with alloantibodies.[31,33] All patients should receive adequate hydration; they should reduce body exposure to the cold before and during surgery, and they should receive incentive spirometry after surgery.

The patient with hemoglobin SS or SC with hemoglobin levels of >10 g/dL requires special consideration. Hyperviscosity is a clear contraindication to raising the hemoglobin level above 11 g/dL until the percentage of Hb S is <30%. Therefore, exchange transfusion or repeated simple transfusion over several weeks is required if the patient is undergoing surgery where the clinician feels it is necessary to provide cells containing hemoglobin A.[33]

Psychological Support

Hospitalized sickle cell patients are at risk for depression. Chronic pain and the day-to-day stresses associated with the illness may contribute to feelings of helplessness, a feeling of not being in control, and fear of death.[35–37] Major depression or mood disorders may increase pain and significantly interfere with daily functioning. Medical treatment for depression and the help of a trained mental health professional, along with establishment of a support system of family, friends, community members, chaplain, medical and mental health personnel, have been found to aid individuals in coping with both depression and sickle cell.

Occupational or physical therapy may help with pain and mood management. Pharmacologic treatment with specific serotonin reuptake inhibitors (SSRIs) tends to have the fewest side effects and can be very helpful in alleviating depressive symptoms. Tricyclic antidepressants may be especially helpful in patients with chronic pain syndromes.

PREVENTION

Pain events may be prevented by patients keeping well hydrated, avoiding temperature extremes, preventing infections, and by maintaining a healthy lifestyle. Diversions such as hobbies, work, games, and other recreation should be encouraged to distract from pain perception. Sickle cell patients should be under the care of a physician knowledgeable about sickle cell disease and experienced in the management of complications, preferably in a sickle cell center.

First Preventive Medication—Hydroxyurea

The chemotherapeutic agent hydroxyurea appears to work by stimulating production of fetal hemoglobin within red blood cells. Patients begin with low daily doses of 500 mg and are monitored every 2 weeks with complete blood counts for evidence of bone marrow suppression. The dose is increased until the maximum tolerated dose is obtained or a level of 35 mg/kg is reached. Adult patients on hydroxyurea have 50% fewer pain episodes, 50% fewer blood transfusions, and 50% less need for hospitalization.[38] Studies in children have shown efficacy and short-term safety, but the long-term effects are unknown.[39] Adult patients taking hydroxyurea for frequent painful sickle cell episodes have reduced mortality after 9 years of follow-up.[40] All Hb SS patients with frequent pain events or complications should be considered for therapy.

Cures with Bone Marrow and Stem Cell Transplants

Sickle cell disease can be cured by HLA-matched bone marrow transplantation. This therapy is now accepted treatment in symptomatic SS and S beta 0 thalassemia children under 16 with stroke, ACS, AVN, or frequent pain episodes. However, most patients lack a genotypically identical family donor.[41] Of the initial 50 patients transplanted, 2 died of graft-versus-host disease, and 4 patients have had return of sickle cell disease. The overall survival rate for HLA-identical sibling-donor stem-cell transplantation is 93%, and event-free survival is 82%.[41]

Emerging New Treatments

Preventive therapy is now under investigation to prevent red cell dehydration, to increase protective hemoglobin F, to decrease red cell adhesion, to increase nitric oxide, and to decrease the activation of the clotting system. New treatments for pulmonary hypertension include sildenafil and arginine.[42,43] The goal of correcting all these factors may lead to synergistic combination therapy that will be very effective.[1]

DISCHARGE/FOLLOW-UP PLANS

Patient Education

The best way to avoid problems is to prevent them from happening. The mnemonic FARMS helps patients to remember the basic principles for prevention:

F—for fluids and fever: Drink plenty of water, usually eight glasses a day for adults and more in heat or when exercising. Fever is an emergency and may indicate significant infection. If you get a fever, see your health care provider right away, and do not mask it with acetaminophen or NSAIDs.

A—for air: Make sure you do not get into problems with not enough oxygen like an unpressurized airplane, untreated asthma, or from smoking.

R—for rest: Get plenty of sleep, do not over do it, and take plenty of breaks when your body feels tired.

M—for prevention medications: Daily penicillin for children under six or hydroxyurea for pain prevention is recommended. The vitamin folic acid is needed to make new red blood cells

S—for situations to avoid: Try to avoid getting too hot or cold; avoid smoking, alcohol or illegal drugs. Exercise and work outdoors with the proper clothing for the season; drink plenty of water, and take frequent rest and water breaks. Carry a water bottle with you to keep drinking. Avoid swimming pools that are too cold or hot tubs that are too hot. Avoid emotional stress by pacing projects and work. Avoid situations that you know are upsetting. Join a support group, church, or faith-based group that offers spiritual and emotional support.

Outpatient–Physician Communication

A summary note of the hospitalization should be sent to the patient's clinician, including the final diagnosis, significant laboratory and x-ray findings, medications used, and follow-up questions. All sickle cell patients should be under the care of a hematologist or primary care physician knowledgeable about sickle cell disease. Follow-up should be arranged within 2 weeks after hospital discharge. This should be sooner if specific complications need evaluation. A listing of sickle cell clinic resources is available at www.SCInfo.org.

Key Points

- Pain is the most common presenting symptom. The single best question in evaluating a pain episode is: "Is this pain typical for your routine pain crisis?"

- Fever is sepsis until proven otherwise.

- Abdominal swelling and pain, combined with a falling hemoglobin level and increasing reticulocyte count, may be a sequestration crisis.

- New onset of an unusual headache or neurologic signs can indicate a stroke, subarachnoid hemorrhage, or meningitis.

- Uncomplicated pain episodes cause no consistent changes in a patient's laboratory findings.

- Simple transfusion is indicated for severe anemia, aplastic crisis, hyperhemolytic crisis, symptomatic anemia during pregnancy, and in chronic transfusion programs.

- Exchange transfusions should be performed in patients with acute neurologic events, severe ACS, acute multiorgan failure, acute arterial hypoxia, ophthalmologic surgery, and high-dose radiologic contrast studies.

- The goal of transfusion is to establish less than 30% Hb S in the circulation with a hemoglobin of 10 g/dL. Hemoglobin levels of greater than 12 g/dL with >30% S may be associated with increased whole blood viscosity and complications.

SUGGESTED READING

Stuart M, Nagel R. Sickle cell disease. Lancet 2004; 364:1323–1360.

Manci EA, Culberson DE, Yang YM, et al. Investigators of the Cooperative Study of Sickle Cell Disease. Causes of death in sickle cell disease: an autopsy study. Brit J Haematol 2003; 123:359–365.

Vichinsky EP, Neumayr LD, Earles AN, et al. Causes and outcomes of the acute chest syndrome in sickle cell disease. National Acute Chest Syndrome Study Group. N Engl J Med 2000; 342:1855–1865.

Management of Sickle Cell Disease, NIH Publication No. 02–2117.Revised May28, 2002 (Forth Edition). National Institutes of Health, National Heart, Lung, and Blood Institute. Available online at http://www.nhlbi.nih.gov/health/prof/blood/sickle/

Ohene-Frempong K. Indications for red cell transfusion in sickle cell disease. Semin Hematol 2001; 38(Suppl 1):5–13.

Eckman JR. Techniques for blood administration in sickle cell patients. Semin Hematol 2001; 38(Suppl 1):23–29.

Kwiatkowski JL, Cohen AR. Iron chelation therapy in sickle-cell disease and other transfusion-dependent anemias. Hematol Oncol Clin North Am 2004;18:1355–1377.

Machado RF, Anthi A, Steinberg MH, et al for MSH Investigators. N-terminal pro-brain natriuretic peptide levels and risk of death in sickle cell disease. JAMA 2006; 296:310–318

Lactate dehydrogenase as a biomarker of hemolysis-associated nitric oxide resistance, priapism, leg ulceration, pulmonary hypertension, and death in patients with sickle cell disease. Blood 2006; 107:2279–2285.

CHAPTER SEVENTY-EIGHT

Hemorrhagic and Thrombotic Disorders

Jamie Siegel, MD

BACKGROUND

Bleeding and thrombotic disorders comprise both rare (hemophilia) and common conditions (e.g., warfarin toxicity) that can complicate common medical conditions. They can be life threatening, and hospitalists need to be familiar with their management while consulting a hematologist for the more unusual afflictions. Table 78-1 lists the disorders reviewed in this chapter.

Inherited hemorrhagic disorders

HEMOPHILIA A OR B

Presentation

Hemophilia A (factor VIII deficiency) and hemophilia B (factor IX deficiency) are X-linked inherited disorders that occur once in approximately 5,000 male births. Hemophilia A is more common than hemophilia B. Of those born with hemophilia, 25% have no family history and are considered to result from spontaneous mutations.

Hemophilia A and B have the same clinical presentation. They are categorized into severe, moderate, or mild by the measured factor level and clinical presentation. Severe disease occurs when the factor level is <1%, moderate at 1–5%, and mild at >5% to <40%. Bleeding manifestations correlate with the level of deficiency. Those with severe hemophilia A or B will likely present in the first 1–2 years of life with spontaneous bleeding. In those with moderate disease, the presentation may occur later. Patients with mild hemophilia may not have a bleeding complication until they are adults, and it may only occur after trauma or surgery.

Because hemophilia A and B are X-linked disorders, they manifest predominantly in men. Women carriers have one X chromosome with the hemophilia mutation and one X chromosome without; their average factor VIII or IX level will be 50% of normal, but it may vary into the moderate range.

It is essential to understand that when a patient with hemophilia presents with a bleeding episode the only manifestation may be pain; the physical examination may be normal.[1] Life-threatening presentations include intracranial, oropharyngeal, and retroperitoneal hemorrhage.

A patient or his hemophilia treatment provider should inform you whether there is presence or history of an "inhibitor"—a specific antibody, or alloantibody, that inhibits proper functioning of the factor VIII or IX molecule.

Diagnosis

The patient or provider will often know the specific factor deficiency, the level of deficiency, and the presence or absence of an inhibitor. If the patient is unsure whether his deficiency is factor VIII or IX, then laboratory diagnosis is essential to determine the proper replacement therapy.

Ultrasound or CT scanning of the painful area may be ordered to evaluate the extent of bleeding. However, treatment of the suspected hemorrhage is necessary before the patient is sent for imaging. In addition, all invasive diagnostic testing must be preceded by replacement of the deficient factor product.[1]

Prognosis

Prognosis of a life-threatening bleed is determined by the ability to immediately administer adequate replacement therapy. For patients without an inhibitor, replacement and maintenance of a normal level of factor VIII or IX are imperative to control bleeding. In those patients with a specific factor inhibitor, bleeding may be more difficult to control and the prognosis worse, though currently available treatments can provide excellent hemostatic control even in this group of patients.

The prognosis for men with hemophilia in the past was determined by level of factor deficiency and site of bleeding episode. Before replacement therapies were available, death often occurred at a young age from bleeding episodes. Once factor concentrate became available, the prognosis from bleeding episodes improved. However, by 1985, 74% of patients who received the newly developed factor concentrate, derived from large pools of donated plasma, became infected with HIV. In addition, all who had been treated with clotting factor concentrates before 1985

Table 78-1 Disorders Causing Bleeding and Thrombosis

Hemorrhagic Disorders	Thrombotic Disorders
Inherited	Inherited
Hemophilia A, B, and C	Protein C
Von Willebrand disease	Protein S
Inherited platelet function defects	Antithrombin
	Factor V Leiden
Acquired	
Warfarin, associated bleeding	Acquired
Liver failure	Antiphospholipid antibody syndrome
	Heparin-induced thrombocytopenia (HIT)

were also exposed to hepatitis C virus (HCV); 85% of those patients are currently chronic carriers of HCV.[2]

Management

Immediate replacement with the proper factor VIII or IX concentrate is essential if there is an active bleed. A patient who presents with a head injury, with or without symptoms, must also be treated immediately. Patients with bleeding into limbs and joints should also be treated with rest, immobilization, ice, compression, and elevation (mnemonic of RICE).

The initial treatment of hematuria is bedrest and increased fluid intake. If the bleeding does not resolve, replacement with factor concentrate to achieve a level of at least 30% is administered for 2–3 days. Antifibrinolytic agents (such as aminocaproic acid, Amicar), while useful for dental procedures, are contraindicated in management of hematuria because of the risk of thrombus formation with subsequent obstruction in the ureters. Radiologic evaluation of the kidneys is indicated with the first episode of hematuria.

Clotting Factor Replacement Therapy

For those with severe and moderate hemophilia A and B, replacement of the specific deficient clotting protein is usually required. Patients with mild and moderate hemophilia A may have response, defined by an increase in their factor VIII level, to the synthetic agent desmopressin acetate (DDAVP). Factor concentrate may still be necessary to obtain a level considered adequate for hemostasis for certain situations. For hemarthrosis, a level of 30% is adequate, but replacement up to a level of 100% is required for head injury, oropharyngeal or retroperitoneal bleed, or surgery.

Factor VIII or IX replacement therapy is available in a concentrated form that requires reconstitution with saline before intravenous administration. This allows for self-treatment or "home therapy." The concentrated forms of factors VIII and IX are either plasma derived or made by recombinant technology. Treatments used in the past such as cryoprecipitate (for factor VIII deficiency) or fresh frozen plasma (for factor VIII or IX deficiency) are now considered substandard approaches.

If a patient has never been exposed to treatment, then the recommended choice of replacement product is to use a recombinantly engineered product rather than a plasma-derived product.[1] While the plasma-derived products undergo multiple

viral inactivation steps, there is continued concern about emerging pathogens entering the blood supply.[2]

Dosing of factor VIII and IX concentrate is based on the patient's weight. The plasma volume of an adult is approximately 40 mL/kg. The one international unit (IU) measurement, as recorded by the coagulation laboratory, was assigned based on that amount of clotting activity found in 1 mL of fresh, normal-pooled (many donors) plasma. Therefore, every milliliter of plasma carries 1 unit of each of the clotting factors. To replace a specific factor to a 100% level in the plasma volume, 1 unit of factor per milliliter of plasma needs to be replaced. Therefore, to achieve a factor VIII level of 100% in an adult, one would infuse 40 units/kg of body weight. Because factor IX distributes into both intra- and extravascular space, the dosing for factor IX needs to be doubled to achieve the same replacement level in the plasma volume. Factor VIII is expected to have a half-life of 8–12 hours whereas factor IX has a half-life of 18–24 hours.

Treatment for patients who develop alloantibodies to factor VIII, called inhibitors, require "bypassing products," which will result in thrombin generation and fibrin clot formation. The bypassing factors now available include anti-inhibitor coagulant complex (Feiba VH) and Novo VII. Feiba VH supplies multiple activated and nonactivated clotting factors, including factors II, VII, IX, and X. Novo VII is covered in more detail below.

Novo VII (Recombinant Factor VIIa)

Recombinant activated factor VII (rVIIa) was developed as a specific bypassing agent in the treatment of hemophilia with inhibitors.[3] Recombinant factor VIIa, when complexed with tissue factor, activates the clotting cascade, resulting in clot formation. The expectation is that this thrombus formation only occurs locally at the site of injury where tissue factor is released and complexed with the activated factor VII. Thus, it theoretically limits the extent of thrombosis.

Approved present uses of rVIIa include treatment of bleeding episodes and surgical procedures for patients with hemophilia A and B and inhibitors. It was also approved recently for use in patients with inherited factor VII deficiency. The dosing is determined by the underlying diagnosis and indication.

Recombinant VIIa may be the only available treatment for patients with rare bleeding disorders such as factor XI deficiency who have developed a specific factor inhibitor and those with Glanzmann's thrombasthenia (see below) before or after they have acquired alloantibodies to platelet transfusion. In addition, recombinant VIIa may be needed in situations where there is a specific coagulation factor inhibitor that may have developed in patients with rare inherited factor deficiency disorders or underlying disorders that have been associated with the development of an acquired factor V, VIII, or von Willebrand factor inhibitor. These are all uses that have not been FDA approved but may be appropriate with hematologic consultation.

Recombinant factor VIIa has been increasingly used for other "off-label" indications: those for which the efficacy and safety have not been adequately evaluated. The predicted low risk of thrombosis has now been challenged as extensive thrombosis has been reported. An FDA Adverse Event Reporting System review has concluded that both arterial thrombosis and venous thrombosis result from Novo VII and are associated with serious morbidity and mortality.[4]

Follow-up Plans

Ensure that necessary factor concentrate is available by communicating with the appropriate Hemophilia Treatment Center staff before discharge. Laboratory testing is usually not indicated prior to hospital discharge unless factor levels associated with treatment dosing are needed.

HEMOPHILIA C

Clinical Presentation

Factor XI deficiency, sometimes referred to as hemophilia C, is an uncommon bleeding disorder in the general population; however, the incidence may be as high as 8% in patients of Jewish heritage.[5] The typical clinical presentation is unexpected bleeding during or after an invasive procedure or more often as an unexpected prolonged activated partial thromboplastin time (aPTT) test ordered in preparation for invasive procedure.[6]

A person with factor XI deficiency does not bleed spontaneously, regardless of the factor level. This is in contrast to hemophilia A or B, in which levels of <1% are associated with spontaneous bleeding. Bleeding can occur rarely with circumcision but more often occurs later in life with menarche, dental procedures, or when a patient has elective surgery. The bleeding is neither predictable nor consistent.

Diagnosis

The diagnosis requires laboratory confirmation of a decreased factor XI level as a cause of a prolonged aPTT.

Prognosis

In those patients who have severe factor XI deficiency, there is a 33% risk of developing an alloantibody after exposure to plasma.

Management

Prophylactic treatment with fresh frozen plasma is the present standard of care before invasive procedures or surgery. There are no approved factor XI concentrates available in the United States. These products are available in Europe but have been associated with an increased risk of thrombosis.

Plasma therapy is dosed according to patient's weight. Often, the goal factor XI level is 50% and is achieved by initiating the plasma therapy at least 24 hours before a major procedure. Infusion of lesser volumes of plasma is often given the same day a minor procedure is performed. Factor XI has a half-life of 40–80 hours. Antifibrinolytic agents (e.g., aminocaproic acid) have been used successfully for dental procedures.

Follow-up plans should be reviewed with a hematologist or hemophilia treatment center staff.

VON WILLEBRAND DISEASE

Presentation

Von Willebrand disease is considered to be the most common inherited bleeding disorder and is estimated to occur in 1% of the population. An autosomally transmitted disorder with variable penetrance, it results in decreased or abnormal production of the von Willebrand protein, which is essential for primary hemostasis supporting platelet adhesion. In addition, it functions to stabilize and carry the factor VIII molecule.

Von Willebrand disease is classified into three types based on whether there is a qualitative or quantitative defect. Type I von Willebrand disease is a mild/moderate quantitative defect; the von Willebrand protein is normal but produced in deficient amounts. Type III von Willebrand disease is a severe quantitative defect and results in unmeasurable levels of the von Willebrand protein. Type II von Willebrand disease includes a heterogeneous group all with a qualitatively abnormal von Willebrand protein. This manifests as decreased functional ability to support platelet adhesion or a decreased capacity to stabilize and carry the factor VIII molecule.

The disorder is characterized by excessive bruising and bleeding, but the clinical presentation can be unpredictable and variable. Von Willebrand disease can manifest first in a young woman when she begins menstruation and is best identified by the pediatrician or gynecologist. Often, oral contraceptives are prescribed for the symptomatic manifestation while appropriate diagnosis and alternative treatment options may not be considered with the first bleeding episode, and the diagnosis is missed.[7,8]

Diagnosis

In the past, the aPTT assay system was sensitive to the mild decrease in the factor VIII level seen with von Willebrand disease and would be prolonged. Now, routine laboratory testing, particularly the aPTT, may be normal. The bleeding time test may be normal as well.

Diagnosis requires testing levels of the von Willebrand factor antigen (vWF:Ag), ristocetin cofactor activity (vWF:RCoF), and the factor VIII coagulant activity (FVIII). These tests are ordered to classify the subtype of von Willebrand disease as well as to measure the level of protein available. The von Willebrand antigen assay is a direct measure of the available protein. The ristocetin cofactor activity is an *in vitro* system that measures the functional ability of the von Willebrand protein to promote platelet adhesion. It is thought to have the best correlation with clinical symptoms.

Other laboratory testing in the diagnosis of von Willebrand disease includes multimer analysis, an immunoelectrophoretic procedure that separates the von Willebrand proteins by size and evaluates the amount of the large- and intermediate-sized proteins. These are disproportionately decreased in some of the type

II variants. Molecular diagnostic studies will likely become an essential component of the testing panel.

Prognosis

Patients with Von Willebrand disease can live full lives with no effect on their prognosis unless the patient has unexpected and severe bleeding or has developed an infectious complication secondary to blood product usage.

Management

DDAVP, or desmopressin acetate, a vasopressin analog, was found to increase the von Willebrand levels as well as factor VIII levels. "DDAVP testing" is performed in a controlled setting because a patient's individual response to DDAVP is reproducible and can therefore predict efficacy for future management. The documented level of response to DDAVP subsequently guides its use in clinical situations. For example, in the event of a life-threatening bleed, a decision should be made whether the response to DDAVP is adequate or if replacement with a von Willebrand factor concentrate is indicated.

The presently available von Willebrand factor concentrate, Humate P, is dosed by ristocetin cofactor units according to body weight in kilograms. Guidelines for dosing are available with each vial of medication.

The intravenous dose of DDAVP is 0.3 mcg/kg (maximum of 30 mcg) diluted in 50 mL of normal saline. The infusion should be administered no more rapidly than 30 minutes to prevent blood pressure fluctuations or severe facial flushing and headache. DDAVP can also be administered intranasally via Stimate Nasal Spray and is given in a dose of 150 mcg in each nostril. Only one dose is used if the patient weighs <50 kg. Contraindications to the use of DDAVP include uncontrolled hypertension, underlying coronary artery disease or other vascular disease, and seizure disorder.

Antifibrinolytic agents such as aminocaproic acid (Amicar) are very useful in patients with von Willebrand disease when undergoing surgical procedures that involve mucosal surfaces. Often, a patient can receive one or two doses of DDAVP followed by 3–10 days of aminocaproic acid and have adequate hemostasis. The dosing of aminocaproic acid can go as high as 24 g in a day, but often 2 g every 6 hours is adequate for hemostasis and is not associated with the gastrointestinal side effects seen at higher doses. Aminocaproic acid is also an effective agent for control of excessive menstrual bleeding.

Laboratory testing before discharge is not indicated unless it is necessary to establish the diagnosis. Follow-up with a hemophilia treatment center or the patient's hematologist should be recommended to the patient.

INHERITED PLATELET FUNCTION DEFECTS

Presentation

Inherited platelet function defects are a recognized cause of milder bleeding disorders, mostly symptomatic with mucosal bleeding, and now also considered a common cause of unexplained menorrhagia in women. Platelet function defects are a group of disorders that include abnormalities of the platelet membrane, storage granules, signaling pathways, and enzyme defects.[9] Glanzmann's thrombasthenia and Bernard-Soulier syndrome are the better known, but much less common, platelet abnormalities. These latter two disorders are autosomal recessive disorders of the platelet membrane; they present earlier in life and have significant bleeding and bruising symptoms. Bernard-Soulier is also characterized by thrombocytopenia and giant platelets.

Diagnosis

The diagnosis of a platelet function defect requires testing in a special hemostasis laboratory performed on a fresh specimen drawn by special technique and requires up to 4 hours to complete. The bleeding time test is no longer considered useful in the diagnosis or exclusion of this disorder but is still used to document a laboratory response to DDAVP testing. Definitive diagnosis of Glanzmann's thrombasthenia and Bernard-Soulier syndrome can be made by testing for the glycoprotein membrane complexes, IIb/IIIa and Ib-V-IX, respectively.

Prognosis

Patients with Glanzmann's thrombasthenia and Bernard-Soulier have more severe bleeding, resulting in poorer outcomes.

Management

The administration of DDAVP will decrease clinical bleeding in some patients with inherited platelet disorders. DDAVP is not effective in all patients, particularly Glanzmann's thrombasthenia and Bernard-Soilier. Platelet transfusion may be needed to prevent or control bleeding. Alternatively, use of an antifibrinolytic agent may be tried first to control menorrhagia or the mucosal bleeding associated with dental procedures.

If the patient has received platelet transfusion in the past and requires treatment again, evaluation for alloantibodies to platelets should be performed. In those patients with severe platelet function abnormalities in whom there is a significant risk of development of platelet alloimmunization, the recombinant factor VIIa bypassing product, Novo VII, appears to be effective.

Acquired Hemorrhagic Disorders

WARFARIN-ASSOCIATED BLEEDING

Warfarin (Coumadin) overdose and associated bleeding can result in significant morbidity and mortality and, increasingly, malpractice litigation. However, evidence-based guidelines endorsed by the American College of Chest Physicians, the seventh and most recent edition published in 2004,[10] facilitate management of this iatrogenic complication.

Table 78-2 Management of Warfarin Toxicity

INR Level	Recommended Action When __No__ Bleeding
<5	Withhold next dose of warfarin.
≥5.0 but ≤9.0	Stop warfarin for two doses or withhold for one dose, and give a dose of vitamin K (1–2.5 mg orally). Restart warfarin at a lower dose once in appropriate range.
≥9.0	Vitamin K 5–10 mg orally and withhold warfarin.
>20	Warfarin is withheld; vitamin K 10 mg given IV slow infusion*; Replacement of coagulation factors (FFP, prothrombin complex concentrate)
	Recommended Action When Bleeding Present
Above baseline	Warfarin is withheld; vitamin K 10 mg given IV slow infusion*; Replacement of coagulation factors (FFP, prothrombin complex concentrate, recombinant factor VIIa)
	Recommended Action with Life-Threatening Bleeding
Above baseline	Administration of prothrombin complex concentrate† or recombinant factor VIIa Vitamin K 10 mg slow IV infusion* and stop warfarin.

FFP—fresh frozen plasma given as 2–3 units initially.

*Slow infusion over 20–60 minutes.

†30 units/kg.

Warfarin is a vitamin K antagonist and results in the production of ineffective procoagulant proteins II, VII, IX, and X. It also interferes with the production of the natural anticoagulant proteins, proteins C and S.

Presentation

Patients present with bleeding manifestations or with an elevated international normalized ratio (INR) without associated bleeding. Prognosis is determined by the bleeding manifestations and the ability to reverse the coagulopathy.

Management

First, one must evaluate the risk of the bleeding episode or the elevated INR. If there is no bleeding, then reduction of the INR alone is indicated. If there is associated bleeding, then immediate hemostasis is needed. Life-threatening bleeding requires immediate replacement of the depressed vitamin K–dependent factors. This can be accomplished with fresh frozen plasma or with prothrombin complex concentrates. Prothrombin complex concentrates (PCCs), originally developed as a concentrated source of factor IX for patients with hemophilia B, also contain factors II, VII, and X. Correction of the effects of warfarin on the vitamin K–dependent factors is also accomplished with replacement of vitamin K. However, the reversal accomplished with vitamin K is delayed by the time necessary to produce the normally carboxylated vitamin K–dependent factors.

Management of warfarin overdose is determined by both the level of the INR and the presence of clinical bleeding. Guidelines for management of elevated INRs and bleeding associated with warfarin are delineated in Table 78-2.[10] Of note, vitamin K is more effective and predictable in its action if given orally versus subcutaneously. The effect of vitamin K should be apparent in 24–48 hours. Warfarin-associated intracerebral hemorrhage is covered in Chapter 91.

Patients suffering warfarin toxicity require close outpatient follow-up, preferably in a clinic with monitoring expertise, as patients experiencing an INR >6 are at increased risk for future hemorrhage.

HEMOSTATIC ABNORMALITIES ASSOCIATED WITH LIVER FAILURE

Presentation

Patients with liver disease will often present with gastrointestinal bleeding secondary to gastritis, gastric ulceration, or often variceal bleeding. This bleeding is thought to be exacerbated by the coagulopathy associated with liver dysfunction. Patients with liver disease are also considered to be at risk for excessive bleeding with dental or other invasive procedures.[11–13]

All of the coagulation proteins, except factor VIII, are synthesized solely by the hepatocyte. In progressive liver disease, factors II, V, VII, and X will decrease first. These are also the factors of the extrinsic and common coagulation pathways and are measured by the PT and the PT/aPTT, respectively. This may explain why the PT will prolong before the aPTT in progressive liver disease. Functional fibrinogen levels will also decrease with progressive impairment of hepatic synthetic function, either as a result of decreased or abnormal production of the fibrinogen protein.

Diagnosis of liver disease as the cause of the presenting coagulopathy requires evaluation of liver function, including albumin. The PT may be the best marker of liver impairment, may be the first sign of disease, and has been shown to be an important prognostic marker for survival. However the PT is not helpful (unless it is severely abnormal) in predicting bleeding for those patients who need liver biopsy or a surgical procedure.[11]

Thrombotic complications are also associated with chronic liver disease. This is related to decreased levels of the natural anticoagulants that are also produced by the hepatocyte, Protein C, protein S, antithrombin, tissue factor pathway inhibitor, and plasminogen. In addition, increased levels of the von Willebrand protein seen with hepatic disease may be associated with a pro-thrombotic state.[13]

Diagnosis

The diagnosis of hemostatic abnormalities associated with liver disease begins with PT and aPTT tests. There are discrepancies in the PT reagents that cause variation in their reflection of specific factor-level deficiencies on the prothrombin time. This variance in factor sensitivity is not corrected for by the INR. Thus, the INR should be used with caution to interpret the coagulation abnor-malities seen with liver disease,[11] though it is a component of the MELD score (see Chapter 56). In addition, the PT and aPTT coag-ulation tests are poor markers of level of disease and risk of bleed-ing. Elevated PT does portend a worse prognosis in acute viral, toxic, or alcoholic hepatitis.

Management

The use of fresh frozen plasma should be limited to bleeding episodes or in preparation for invasive procedures. The dose of fresh frozen plasma is based on the patient's plasma volume. The usual recommendation is 10–15 mL/kg of body weight to achieve factor levels of 25–30%. Cryoprecipitate may be needed in a patient with a fibrinogen level of less than 100 units. Novo 7 has been used in patients with liver failure and life-threatening bleeding unresponsive to these therapeutic approaches, but this is off-label use.

Thrombotic Disorders

Testing for inherited causes of thrombophilia has become com-monplace, despite the lack of studies examining the application of this information to the individual patient. The perceived need to discover why a patient had a thrombosis, to "have an answer," seems to override the established lack of usefulness of widespread and extensive testing. Nevertheless, the less common inherited deficiencies of protein C, protein S, and antithrombin do confer a greater risk of recurrent thrombosis. Identification of an asymptomatic carrier of one of these three disorders may alter management decisions for that patient. The more common factor V Leiden and prothrombin gene 20210 mutations do increase the risk of thrombosis when evaluated in population analyses. However, their influence on medical decisions for an individual patient has not been established.[14]

Environmental risk factors, immobilization, surgery, malig-nancy, pregnancy, puerperium, exogenous hormones, and travel all play an important role in thrombosis and risk of recurrent thrombosis—it is multifactorial in etiology. This needs to be considered when therapeutic decisions are made

for thrombosis prophylaxis, either for a transient stimulus such as surgery or for the long-term prevention of spontaneous events.[15]

INHERITED PROTEINS C AND S AND ANTITHROMBIN DEFICIENCY

Presentation

The inherited disorders, protein C, protein S, and antithrombin deficiency, are relatively rare abnormalities but are associated with an increased risk of thrombosis over a person's lifetime.

Diagnosis

These disorders are best evaluated in the steady state, not in the setting of an acute medical problem. The laboratory levels can be falsely low if measured during an acute thrombotic event because of consumption of plasma coagulation proteins during the episode. Protein C and protein S are also vitamin K dependent; therefore, measurement of the levels when the patient is on war-farin may result in decreased levels, potentially resulting in a patient being assigned a diagnosis incorrectly. Acquired protein S deficiency occurs with the hormonal milieu created by oral con-traceptive agents and pregnancy. In addition, a low protein S has been associated with liver disease, nephrotic syndrome, and HIV disease.

Management

Management of these disorders consists of treatment of the acute thrombosis, decisions regarding long-term management, and optimal protection during pregnancy and the puerperium. Labo-ratory testing to be performed in the hospital before discharge is not recommended. Follow-up plans should be made with a hematologist.

MUTATIONS: FACTOR V LEIDEN, PROTHROMBIN GENE 20210, AND METHYLENETETRAHYDROFOLATE REDUCTASE (MTHFR, C677T HOMOZYGOUS, OR C677T/A1298C COMPOUND HETEROZYGOUS)

Presentation

Factor V Leiden, the most common cause of inherited throm-bophilia (40–50% of cases), results from a single point muta-tion causing one amino acid substitution in the factor V molecule. This results in a factor V coagulation protein that is more resistant to inactivation by activated protein C as compared to the native or "wildtype" factor V protein. The prothrombin gene 20210 mutation is also associated with a single nucleotide substitution and is associated with an elevated prothrombin level. The MTHFR mutations have been associated with elevated homocysteine levels, which in turn is associated with arterial and venous thrombosis. These two sets of mutations, the C677T homozygous and the C677T/A1298C compound heterozygous, have the weakest direct association with thrombosis.

Diagnosis

Molecular diagnostic testing will identify these genetic mutations. The activated protein C resistance (APC) testing for the functional abnormality created by the factor V Leiden mutation is available but less commonly ordered.

Prognosis

The risk of thrombosis is best understood when looking at women with and without the factor V Leiden mutation exposed to oral contraceptive pills (OCPs). The baseline incidence of a thrombotic event for a woman with neither factor V Leiden or use of OCPs would be 8 per 100,000, women/years. If a woman without the gene mutation uses OCPs, her risk of a thrombotic event increases to 30 per 100,000, or four-fold over baseline. In women who have the factor V Leiden mutation and who do not use OCPs, the risk of thrombosis is 57 per 100,000 women/years, or a seven-fold increase over baseline. Combining the risk factors results in an incidence of 285 thrombotic events per 100,000 women/years, or a 36-fold increase over baseline. Based on these statistics, patients are told that they have a seven-fold increased risk, or a 36-fold increased risk.[16] What is not explained is that at a rate of 285/100,000 women/years the chance of occurrence of an event still remains low, at a rate of 0.3% per year for women with the factor V Leiden gene mutation who use oral contraceptive agents.

Management

Testing asymptomatic family members is not indicated. If the testing is performed, it should be performed by the patient's personal physician or after consultation with a hematologist. As with patients suffering deficiencies of protein C, S, or antithrombin, prophylactic therapy for asymptomatic disease is not indicted. For patients suffering a first deep venous thrombosis (DVT), extended warfarin therapy is indicated, but benefit beyond 1 year is not indicated. Eventually, the risk of major induced hemorrhages probably exceeds the number of clinically significant thrombotic events. There does not appear to be an increase in overall mortality among patients with these mutations.

ACQUIRED THROMBOTIC DISORDERS

Antiphospholipid antibody syndrome and heparin-induced thrombocytopenia are two acquired thrombotic disorders resulting from the development of a pathologic antibody. Both disorders are characterized by venous and arterial thrombosis, which can be acute and severe in presentation. Both are associated with antibody identification in the laboratory that is difficult to perform and interpret.

ANTIPHOSPHOLIPID ANTIBODY SYNDROME

Presentation

A patient with the antiphospholipid antibody (APA) syndrome will often first present with a symptomatic thrombosis, venous or arterial. The thrombotic event may be more severe or extensive than those associated with other precipitating thrombophilic risk factors; however, the severity of the presentation does not predict or preclude antiphospholipid antibody syndrome as a cause. The events may also occur in more unusual sites such as the mesenteric system or intracranially, but again this is neither sensitive nor specific to the disorder. What is clearly associated with the APA syndrome is a higher rate of recurrence when anticoagulation is interrupted or discontinued.

Antiphospholipid antibodies are a heterogeneous group of autoantibodies that interact with phospholipid dependent proteins in the laboratory testing system.[17] Originally, this syndrome was referred to as "the lupus anticoagulant," and prolonged aPTT erroneously came to be considered the only manifestation of this disorder. Later, a clot-based phospholipids-dependent coagulation test was established as a second sensitive system to detect this group of antibodies. The term "anticardiolipin antibody syndrome" came about because this immunologic test system developed by rheumatologists was also used to identify patients who fit into the overall syndrome.

The clinical syndrome includes venous thrombosis, arterial thrombosis, complications of pregnancy including spontaneous abortion, and intrauterine growth restriction. In addition, patients with APA syndrome may have valvular heart disease, thrombocytopenia, nephropathy, neurologic manifestations, and livedo reticularis.

Diagnosis

The Sapporo diagnostic classification system for antiphospholipid syndrome, updated in 2005, separates clinical and laboratory criteria and requires that at least one criterion from each set be met. The clinical criteria include either one objectively confirmed episode of vascular thrombosis or pregnancy morbidity—as defined by unexplained death beyond the 10th week of gestation, premature birth of normal neonate before the 34th week because of preeclampsia, placental insufficiency, or three or more unexplained consecutive spontaneous abortions before the 10th week. The laboratory criteria require evidence of a lupus anticoagulant, anticardiolipin antibody (IgM or IgG) in medium or high titer, or antibody (IgM or IgG) to the β2 glycoprotein I identified on two or more occasions at least 12 weeks apart.[17]

Management

The initial treatment is the same as with any patient with an acute thrombosis. Long-term therapy with warfarin is recommended, either to achieve an INR of 2–3 or to achieve an INR of greater than 3. Although it has been suggested in retrospective studies that this latter "high-intensity" warfarin is needed, this has not been verified in prospective randomized trials.[18] The current recommendation for a first episode of venous thrombosis is to maintain an INR of 2.0–3.0. Optimal duration of anticoagulation is unknown, but recommendations for indefinite anticoagulation are suggested because of the high incidence of recurrent thrombosis if the anticoagulation is discontinued once there is verification of persistence of the APA abnormality. Laboratory testing should be performed before anticoagulation is initiated as it may be the only opportunity to perform the clot-based assays for diagnosis. The serologic assays can be ordered any time to confirm the diagnosis. Follow-up plans must be made for warfarin management.

HEPARIN-INDUCED THROMBOCYTOPENIA AND THROMBOSIS (HIT AND HITT)

Presentation

Heparin-induced thrombocytopenia is an antibody-mediated disorder responding to the neoantigen formed when there is platelet activation with release of platelet factor 4. The creation of the heparin/platelet factor 4 (PF4) complex triggers an antibody response within 5–10 days of exposure to heparin. The risk of developing this disorder is related to the form of heparin used and the clinical situation associated with the use of heparin. The risk of developing thrombosis was originally reported to be as high as 25–50%, with a subsequent risk of developing a fatal thrombosis of 50%.

The recognition of a "rapid-onset" HIT pattern has been explained by re-exposure of a patient to heparin within 100 days of last exposure. The antibody is present, and with administration of heparin it rapidly interacts to create PF4/heparin/IgG immune complexes.

The patient presentation will be with thrombocytopenia (HIT) or with an acute thrombotic event (HITT), arterial or venous. Venous and arterial thrombosis, venous limb gangrene, and digital ischemia may all result. The thrombotic event, despite its presentation with thrombocytopenia, can be extensive and ongoing. However, there may only be subtle swelling of an extremity.

Diagnosis

The diagnosis is first considered on clinical grounds. Often, there is an unexplained fall in the platelet count of ≥50%. Laboratory testing for the disorder and radiographic confirmation of a thrombotic event will follow.

Patients on heparin who experience a decrease in the platelet count should be evaluated for signs of vascular occlusion. Some physicians even consider performing duplex ultrasound, ventilation/perfusion scan, or spiral computed tomography (CT) scan in order to detect subclinical thrombosis, given the prognosis and urgency of treatment. Conversely, if there is clinical suspicion for vascular compromise in a patient receiving heparin, then a platelet count should be ordered as part of the evaluation.

Alternative causes of thrombocytopenia can be considered, but the interventions required for a possible diagnosis of heparin-associated thrombocytopenia must be immediately initiated. In a patient who is postoperative and thrombocytopenic, all medications should be reviewed and evaluation for infection, sepsis, and other causes of disseminated intravascular coagulation investi-gated. Thrombosis unrelated to heparin occurs in the postoperative setting, but consideration that heparin is the culprit is part of proper management.

Final diagnosis of HIT or HITT can be made with certainty when a positive heparin antibody is found. A diagnosis of HIT or HITT is made presumptively when (1) the clinical scenario is consistent, (2) no other cause is identified, and (3) the platelet count recovers with removal of heparin exposure. A scoring system for clinical evaluation has been introduced.[19] Evaluation with the enzyme-linked immunosorbent assay (ELISA) for the heparin/PF4 antibody remains an important negative laboratory confirmation.[20]

Prognosis

The prognosis of this disorder continues to improve with current therapeutic and management guidelines. However, if not identified and managed appropriately, HIT/HITT remains a life- and limb-threatening disorder.

Management

Initial management requires immediate discontinuation of heparin in all forms, including heparin-coated catheters and heparin flushes. Clinical evaluation for thrombosis, such as digital ischemia or swelling in any of the extremities, needs to be performed with appropriate imaging studies. Assessment of the potential risk of bleeding must then be determined before an anticoagulant is started.

If anticoagulation therapy is appropriate, then the next choice to be made is between the two direct thrombin inhibitors, Lepirudin and Argatroban. If not already assessed, renal and hepatic function must be evaluated before initiating the pharmacologic treatment of a potential or evident thrombosis. These are the only two drugs approved for treatment of HIT and HITT and are renally or hepatically cleared, respectively. Bivalirudin, a third direct thrombin inhibitor, has been approved for anticoagulation in those patients who need percutaneous coronary intervention.

Argatroban: The initial infusion rate of 2 mcg/kg/min has been recommended in the package insert. The elimination of the drug is via the hepatobiliary system with a half-life of 40–50 minutes. If there is severe hepatic disease, then the drug should not be used; otherwise, significant dose reduction is necessary. The direct thrombin activity of this drug prolongs the prothrombin time, which makes monitoring the coumadin with INR problematic. A higher INR needs to be reached before discontinuation of the drug. Instructions for this modification have been made by the company and are in the package insert.[21]

Lepirudin: The initial infusion rate of 0.15 mg/kg/hr is recommended when the patient has normal renal clearance. An initial bolus of 0.4 mg/kg may be given. The target aPTT would be 1.5–2.5 times the patient's baseline. However, the present rate of bleeding with this drug has been reported to be as high as 17.6%. A lower target aPTT range of 1.5–2.0 times the baseline is considered to have similar efficacy and less bleeding,[21] and starting at a rate of 0.1 mg/kg/hr may be more prudent.[22]

In view of the initial laboratory presentation of HIT, thrombocytopenia, the inclination is to administer platelet transfusions to prevent bleeding. This disorder is not associated with bleeding, and there have been reports of worsening thrombosis when platelets have been infused. Therefore, platelet transfusions should not be used unless there is life-threatening bleeding thought to be caused by the platelet deficiency.

Administration of warfarin needs to be delayed until the platelet count has recovered to at least 100,000. In addition, sufficient overlap between the parenteral anticoagulation and warfarin should be for a minimum of 5 days and for a target therapeutic INR for at least 2 days before discontinuation of the direct thrombin inhibitor. Heparin-induced thrombocytopenia is a severe, ongoing thrombotic process with associated consumption of protein C. If warfarin is initiated before the thrombotic process has been effectively controlled, then venous gangrene and skin necrosis may result; the rapid decrease in the protein C with the administration of warfarin results in a relative hypercoagulable balance.

- Antiphospholipid antibody syndrome and heparin-induced thrombocytopenia result from the development of a pathologic antibody associated with unpredictable venous and arterial thrombosis. Antibody identification in the laboratory is difficult to perform and interpret.

- A diagnosis of HIT is made presumptively when (1) the clinical scenario is consistent, (2) no other cause is identified, and (3) the platelet count recovers with removal of heparin exposure.

Key Points

- When a patient with hemophilia presents with a bleeding episode, the only manifestation may be pain, and the physical examination may be normal.

- Hematology consultation and follow-up should be sought for management of patients with hemophilia.

- Antifibrinolytic agents such as aminocaproic acid are very useful in patients with von Willebrand disease when undergoing surgical procedures that involve mucosal surfaces.

- There does not appear to be an increase in overall mortality among patients with mutations causing thrombotic disorders of factor V Leiden or deficiency of protein C or S or Antithrombin.

SUGGESTED READING

Ludlam CA, Powderly WG, Bozzette S, et al. Clinical perspectives of emerging pathogens in bleeding disorders. Lancet 2006; 367:252–261.

Roberts HR, Monroe DM, White GC. The use of recombinant factor VIIa in the treatment of bleeding disorders. Blood 2004; 104:3858–3864.

Ansell J, Hirsh J, Poller L, et al. The pharmacology and management of the vitamin K antagonists. Chest 2004; 126:204S–233S.

Reverter JC. Abnormal hemostasis tests and bleeding in chronic liver disease: are they related? Yes. J Thromb Haemost 2006; 4:717–720.

Mannucci PM. Abnormal hemostasis tests and bleeding in chronic liver disease: are they related? No. J Thromb Haemost 2006; 4:721–723.

Christiansen SC, Cannegieter SC, Koster T, et al. Thrombophilia, clinical factors, and recurrent venous thrombotic events. JAMA 2005; 293:2352–2361.

Lim W, Crowther MA, Eikelboom JW. Management of antiphospholipid antibody syndrome. JAMA 2006; 295:1050–1057.

Warkentin TE, Greinacher A. Heparin-induced thrombocytopenia: recognition, treatment, and prevention. Chest 2004; 126:311S–337S.

Section
Eleven

Rheumatology, Immunology, and Dermatology

79 Acute Arthritis in the Hospitalized Patient
Brian F. Mandell

80 Systemic Vasculitis
Alexandra Villa-Forte, Brian F. Mandell

81 Allergic Reactions and Angioedema
Neil Winawer, Mandakolathur Murali

82 Dermatology in Hospitalized Patients
Calvin McCall, Murtaza Cassoobhoy, Lesley Miller

CHAPTER SEVENTY-NINE

Acute Arthritis in the Hospitalized Patient

Brian F. Mandell, MD, PhD, FACR

BACKGROUND

Acute inflammatory arthritis involving one or several joints in the hospitalized or emergency room patient is usually due to crystal-induced disease (e.g., gout). However, the possibility of septic arthritis with its associated morbidity and mortality mandates an accurate and expeditious diagnostic evaluation. Acute polyarticular arthritis suggests the presence of a systemic inflammatory disease; infection with a virus, particularly hepatitis B or C; or a serum sickness reaction. Bacterial infection and crystalline disease can also be polyarticular.

ASSESSMENT

Clinical Presentation

Patients with acute inflammatory arthritis who are able to describe their symptoms will generally note the presence of pain with the joint at rest. The pain worsens significantly with active or passive motion of the involved joint. Constitutional features may or may not be present in crystal-induced[1] or septic arthritis.[2] A history of prior episodes of acute arthritis should be elicited; prior arthritis is quite common in patients with postoperative flares of gouty arthritis.[3] The pattern of arthritis may provide a diagnostic clue to the etiology of the patient's problem that warranted admission. Prodromal illnesses should be defined. Recent diarrhea, conjunctivitis, or uveitis could be manifestations of reactive arthritis. Prior hepatitis or intermittent fever warrants exclusion of an underlying inflammatory or infectious process. Peripheral neurologic symptoms or findings suggest vasculitis.

A focused physical examination (Box 79-1) should document the presence (pain with passive motion of the affected joint, capsule tenderness, effusion) and location of inflammatory arthritis, detect the number of affected joints (particularly important yet difficult in patients unable to give a reliable history), identify the presence of enthesitis or tendonitis (common in reactive arthritis or spondylitis), and detect stigmata of systemic processes or allergic reactions (rash; nail fold, retinal, or conjunctival infarcts; tophi; neuropathy). Tophi should be sought overlying peripheral joints, on the ulnar aspect of the forearms, in olecranon bursae, and in external ear tissue. In the setting of indwelling intravenous catheters and possible bacteremia, fibrocartilage joints (sternoclavicular, sacroiliac) and the spine should be carefully examined as potential sites of metastatic infection. If polyarticular disease is documented, a complete examination should be done looking for evidence of a generalized inflammatory process.

Fever may be absent in patients with documented bacterial arthritis and is present in a significant portion of hospitalized patients with acute crystal induced arthritis.[1] Evaluation of fever in the intubated or unresponsive patient should include a careful joint examination, especially since unrecognized crystalline arthritis can cause postoperative fever. Rigors are uncommon in both infectious and crystal-induced arthritis.

Differential Diagnosis

The differential diagnosis in the hospitalized patient with acute arthritis always includes crystalline and septic arthritis. Attacks of gout or pseudo-gout following surgery or medical hospitalization are common, and they are likely due to acute fluxes in the serum urate (or calcium) levels in response to hydration, dehydration, circulating cytokine elevation, and medication institution or withdrawal. In one report, attacks of gout occurred at a mean of 4.2 days following surgical admission.[3] In hospitalized patients, gout seems to present in a polyarticular pattern at a higher frequency than in outpatients. Older and post-transplant patients may have polyarticular involvement with the first attack of gout, but most gouty patients with polyarticular involvement will have a history of prior attacks.

Rarely, crystalline and septic arthritis may coexist, usually in the patient with chronic gouty arthritis, who then develops a localized joint infection. Whether this occurs because the crystal deposition of gout had damaged the joint structures or affected the function of vascular endothelial cells in synovium to permit bacterial seeding is unknown. No clinical or laboratory parameter reliably permits the recognition of co-infection and gout.

Patients with acute polyarticular arthritis are less likely to have a bacterial infection, but both streptococcal (pneumococcus in particular) and staphylococcal polyarticular arthritis are well described and should be excluded with joint fluid cultures. Disseminated neisserial infections may cause migratory oligo- or polyarticular joint pains prior to settling in one or a few joints[6], one third of patients may have an associated tenosynovitis. Patients with disseminated gonococcal (GC) infection may also have

---

Box 79-1 Physical Examination Findings in Acute Arthritis

Pain with passive motion of the affected joint

Capsule tenderness

Joint effusion

Enthesitis or tendonitis (common in reactive arthritis or spondylitis)

Stigmata of systemic processes or allergic reactions

- Rash

- Infarcts—nail fold, retinal or conjunctival

- Tophi (overlying peripheral joints, ulnar aspect of the forearms, olecranon bursae, external ear tissue)

- Neuropathy

Fibrocartilage joint (sternoclavicular, sacroiliac) and spine involvement

- Potential sites of metastatic infection

Box 79-2 Diagnostic Studies in Acute Arthritis

Arthrocentesis—Mandatory

- Polarized microscopic examination

- Bacterial culture of the fluid (blood culture vials maybe ideal)

- Synovial fluid cell count and differential

- Gram stain

Imaging Studies

- MRI for suspected sternoclavicular joint infection

- Ultrasound of hip or shoulder to confirm synovial effusion

Laboratory Tests

- Urine sediment to assess renal involvement

- Microbiologic cultures

  - GC cultures of pharynx, rectum, and cervix (vaginal in postmenopausal women) or urethral (men)

  - *Mycobacterium marinum* in patients with a history of water exposure (aquariums, fishing)

- Acute phase reactants, ANA, RF, and other autoimmune serologies

  - Usually not helpful in the initial diagnostic evaluation of acute monoarticular arthritis.

- C-reactive protein (CRP)

  - Useful in following the response to therapy in septic arthritis.

- Synovial fluid glucose, protein, and LDH have **no** diagnostic value.

  - Synovial biopsy for unexplained chronic inflammatory monoarticular arthritis.

- CBC

  - Not helpful in determining the cause of acute arthritis unless accompanied by a striking increase in bands or eosinophils

- Serum urate level

  - **Not** a useful diagnostic test in the evaluation of acute arthritis

---

sparsely distributed purpura or hemorrhagic pustules on the extremities.

Other causes of acute arthritis developing in the hospitalized patient are less common, and without extremely suggestive features from the history or examination, crystal disease and infection should be initially excluded prior to pursuing these diagnoses. When there are features suggestive of an underlying disorder (i.e., abdominal pain, heme-positive stool), specific diagnoses (inflammatory bowel disorder [IBD], gut ischemia due to vasculitis) can be explored in conjunction with excluding joint infection. Potential drug or serum sickness reactions should be considered if multiple joints are involved.

PROGNOSIS

Acute monoarticular or oligoarticular (<4 joints) arthritis is most frequently due to gout, less commonly due to pseudogout. However, up to 20% of hospitalized patients with acute mono- or oligoarticular arthritis may have a joint infection. The mortality associated with septic arthritis is approximately 12%, and joint-related morbidity is significantly higher.[5] Thus, infection must be considered and excluded in all cases of acute mono- or oligoarticular arthritis. Special concern must be exercised for staphylococcal septic arthritis in patients with an apparent "monoarticular flare" in a chronic polyarticular disease such as rheumatoid arthritis. A delay in appropriate therapy is associated with poor functional joint outcome.

DIAGNOSIS

Preferred Diagnostic Studies

The diagnostic test of choice in acute arthritis is arthrocentesis with polarized microscopic examination and routine bacterial culture of the fluid (Box 79-2). Synovial fluid cell count and differential are useful because they will establish whether the fluid is inflammatory, but will not reliably distinguish between infec-

tion and crystal-induced arthritis. Both etiologies generally have >85% neutrophils in the synovial fluid. Although the mean synovial white count in septic arthritis is higher than in gout, there is significant overlap; 26% of patients with documented septic arthritis may have initial synovial white cell counts <20,000/mm^3.[8] The fluid leukocytosis will decrease with response to therapy. Gram stain is insensitive for the detection of joint fluid bacteria (~50%), but is useful to guide initial antibiotic choice if positive.[11] Optimal diagnostic decision-making requires arthrocentesis from all patients with acute monoarticular arthritis. In patients with acute oligoarticular or polyarticular arthritis, ideally at least two joints should be aspirated for diagnosis if crystals are not observed in the first joint fluid. If crystals are identified in the synovial fluid, an effort should be made to distinguish gout (urate crystals) from pseudogout (calcium pyrophosphate crystals). Fluid should be saved without anticoagulant for later examination by a more experienced observer if necessary. If infection remains a clinical likelihood, all joints should be aspirated as part of the initial therapy for (possible) bacterial arthritis. Fluid should be promptly sent to the laboratory for routine bacterial culture. Some authors have suggested that the sensitivity of synovial fluid bacterial culture can be increased by using blood culture vials as transportation vehicles. Fluid culture remains the gold standard for diagnosis of infectious arthritis.

Imaging rarely plays a role in the diagnosis of acute arthritis. One exception is a suspected infection of the sternoclavicular joint.[4] Since this joint abuts the mediastinum and may be associated with abscess formation and mediastinitis not detectable by examination, MRI or CT imaging is indicated. Intravenous drug users seem particularly predisposed to get an infection of this joint. Ultrasound may be useful in confirming the presence of a synovial effusion of deep-seated joints such as the hip or shoulder since acute effusions may not be detected in these joints by routine physical examination.

Alternative Studies in Patients with Arthritis

Patients with a generalized inflammatory process should have microscopy of fresh urine sediment to assess for the presence of renal involvement. If disseminated gonococcemia (GC) is a reasonable possibility, pharyngeal, rectal, and cervical (vaginal in postmenopausal women) or urethral (men) cultures should be obtained in addition to routine blood cultures. GC is infrequently cultured from blood or from joint fluid and skin lesions, perhaps because many of these inflammatory manifestations are due to immune complex deposition. Culture of joint fluid for fungus or mycobacteria is not necessary in the initial evaluation of acute arthritis, unless the clinical scenario warrants specific consideration of these infections. Acute phase reactants, antinuclear antibodies (ANA), rheumatoid factor (RF), and other autoimmune serologies have little if any role in the initial diagnostic evaluation of acute monoarticular arthritis. The ANA may be useful in patients with oligo- or polyarticular arthritis if there is a specific concern for the possibility of systemic lupus erythematosus (SLE). It is unlikely that SLE or RA will initially present with acute monoarthritis. The C-reactive protein (CRP), although not helpful with diagnosis, can be useful in following the response to therapy in septic arthritis. If a documented infection is slow to respond clinically, with a CRP that is not decreasing, the possibility of an occult abscess or adjacent osteomyelitis should be considered. Measurement of synovial fluid glucose, protein, and lactate dehydrogenase (LDH) has no diagnostic value. The utility of fluid polymerase chain reaction (PCR) and lactate studies is dependent upon the clinical scenario as well as local laboratory expertise and standardization; these are not presently routine tests. Fluid anaerobic cultures can be obtained in the clinical setting where there is a likely anaerobic source for infection. In patients with a history of water exposure (aquariums, fishing), infection with *Mycobacterium marinum* should be considered, and the microbiology laboratory notified of this possibility so appropriate incubation conditions can be established. This infection has a predilection to affect the tendon sheaths of the distal extremities, as well as joints.[9] Rarely, synovial biopsy is a necessary test in the pursuit of a diagnosis, usually with unexplained chronic inflammatory monoarticular arthritis. Complete blood cell count may

be helpful; however, leukocytosis may occur in arthritis of any cause and is common in hospitalized patients, particularly postoperatively. Thus, the presence or absence of an elevated white count, unless accompanied by a striking increase in bands or eosinophils, is not overly helpful in determining the cause of acute arthritis. Leukopenia can occur in the setting of arthritis with SLE or overwhelming infection, but not with the primary systemic vasculitic syndromes. The serum urate level is not a useful diagnostic test in the evaluation of acute arthritis. It may be in the normal or low normal range with acute gout,[7] and is frequently elevated in patients without gouty arthritis who may have pseudogout or septic arthritis. Wide fluctuations in the serum urate level occur in patients who have ingested significant amounts of alcohol, have been fasting, or have received certain medications or rapid volume repletion.

MANAGEMENT

Treatment

Initial (Box 79-3)

If the synovial fluid is inflammatory with >85% neutrophils, no crystals are observed, and there is no obvious explanation for the acute mono- or oligoarticular arthritis, the patient should usually be treated empirically for septic (bacterial) arthritis until the cultures return. Treatment, as with most closed space infections, should include adequate drainage and intravenous antibiotics. Drainage can be percutaneous if feasible. If the joint is difficult to aspirate due to location (i.e., hip) or because of thick fluid, then early arthroscopic drainage and lavage should be strongly considered. Arthrotomy is another option, although recovery of joint function may be longer when this approach to drainage is necessary. There are no adequate prospective randomized trials comparing these drainage procedures. Studies that suggested a better outcome with percutaneous drainage were retrospective. They were not randomized, and the results are not conclusive. Nonetheless, prompt percutaneous drainage when feasible is a reasonable initial approach. It should be repeated as often as necessary to keep the joint decompressed. If the affected joint had been previously damaged by arthritis or the patient is significantly immunosuppressed, an early invasive drainage procedure should be considered; but there are no data to support this clinical approach. If, for any reason, a septic joint cannot be adequately aspirated, surgical drainage is appropriate. GC infection with arthritis may be the exception to this approach.

There is no indication for intra-articular antibiotics. The joint can be initially immobilized for pain control, but passive and then active range-of-motion exercises should be initiated as soon as feasible in order to facilitate return of normal joint function. Nonsteroidal anti-inflammatory drugs may facilitate therapy and hasten functional improvement, but should be avoided until there is a confirmed diagnosis since at times the response to antibiotics may play a role in the diagnostic decision-making process (particularly with GC infection where cultures are often negative and in patients who had received antibiotics prior to joint fluid culture). Choice of initial empiric antibiotic therapy should be dictated by the suspected organism and the local antibiotic sensitivity profile. Staphylococcus (MRSA) should generally be considered a possibility. In otherwise healthy, sexually active patients, GC should be considered, even in the absence of any pelvic symptoms in women. Gram-negative infections should be considered in patients with underlying illnesses such as diabetes, cancer, urinary tract disorders, immunosuppression, or a history of recent hospitalization or antibiotic use.[5–10] Dosing should be based on the assumption that bacteremia is present.

If crystals are identified in the synovial fluid, the initial anti-inflammatory therapy of the acute arthritis is identical, but the long-term management may be different. Septic and crystalline arthritis can coexist, but this is fortunately uncommon.[13] Thus, unless there is a compelling reason to suspect infection, it is reasonable to treat only for crystal induced arthritis if crystals are definitely identified. It is reasonable in the hospitalized patient to send the fluid for culture even when crystals are seen, although there are no data to quantify the "yield" of this strategy. Acute gout (or pseudogout) will respond to once-daily moderate doses of corticosteroids (approximately 40 mg daily of prednisone equivalent). Sufficient dose and duration are necessary to avoid recurrence of the arthritis, which has been described as "rebound." Controlled dosing studies do not exist. Once the acute attack has resolved, the steroids should be tapered over another 7–10 days. Glucose control issues with the use of steroids can generally be easily managed in the hospitalized patient, but the increased risk of postoperative infection associated with hyperglycemia should be considered. Intra-articular steroid is effective, but in the hospitalized patient, this should be avoided until cultures return negative.

Alternative Treatments

Alternative anti-inflammatory approaches to crystalline arthritis include adrenocorticotrophic hormone (ACTH), high doses of nonsteroidal anti-inflammatory drugs (NSAIDs), or colchicine. Oral colchicine given hourly until "relief or development of diarrhea" is rarely utilized, since the gastrointestinal (GI) side effects are almost invariable and generally occur before relief is provided. The choice between steroids and NSAIDs is generally made based upon the relative potential for side effects in the individual patient. Any NSAID is likely effective, but should be utilized in high anti-inflammatory doses for a similar duration. With either corticosteroids or NSAIDs,[13] significant pain relief may begin within 6 hours. The issues of gastric toxicity/protection and comorbidities (renal insufficiency, bleeding potential) must be considered when choosing a therapy. Intravenous colchicine (1–3 mg total dose) is effective and has value in selected patients, but it is fraught with potential life-threatening toxicity if dosed incorrectly. Thus, many clinicians avoid administering colchicine by the intravenous route.

Subsequent

Frequent aspiration should be continued until infection is excluded, as long as the fluid is reaccumulating. Occasionally, crystals are not seen in the first fluid analysis. Crystals should be looked for, and cultures repeated at each aspiration. Synovial fluid cell counts can be followed; with successful therapy, the neutrophil count falls by approximately 50% daily. If the cell count is rising, cultures remain positive, or the fluid thickens, an arthroscopic or open drainage procedure is warranted in the setting of culture documented or strongly suspected septic arthritis. If the fluid is culture negative and remains inflammatory without a

diagnosis after approximately 3 days, mycobacterial and fungal infection can be considered.

PREVENTION

It is worthwhile to consider adding prophylactic therapy against a future attack of gout for several months after an attack. If the patient has potential for fluctuations in serum urate levels, he or she may be especially at risk for further attacks. In the absence of renal insufficiency or liver dysfunction, oral colchicine 0.6 daily to bid can be a useful prophylactic therapy.[14] Diarrhea is the most common adverse effect of low-dose colchicine. In the setting of renal insufficiency, or occasionally due to drug interactions (statins, macrolide antibiotics), a reversible axonal neuropathy/myopathy can develop. The initiation of hypouricemic therapy should be avoided in the setting of an acute gout attack, since sudden drops in serum urate level can provoke another attack.[14]

DISCHARGE/FOLLOW-UP

The patient with septic arthritis should generally receive parenteral antibiotics for approximately 4–6 weeks of total therapy. Plans should be made to institute physical therapy to ensure preservation of joint function. NSAID therapy for several weeks during physical therapy is a reasonable adjunctive therapy, if there are no contraindications. Radiographs to exclude periarticular osteomyelitis should be considered predischarge, since a longer course of antibiotic therapy may be prescribed. Plans should be confirmed for follow-up joint evaluation and intravenous catheter removal.

Outpatient Communication

For the patient with gout, hypouricemic therapy can be considered in the future. Because of this possible (future) specific intervention for gout, it is important to notify the patient or primary care provider whether urate crystals were or were not documented. Even more important is to alert the patient if calcium crystals were seen, and NOT urate crystals; otherwise, hypouricemic therapy may be mistakenly administered as treatment for presumed gout by the patient's outpatient physician.

Box 79-3 Treatment of Acute Arthritis

- **Crystal-Induced Arthritis (gout or pseudogout)**
  - Prednisone 40 mg q daily
    - Taper over 7–10 days after acute attack has resolved.
  - NSAID
  - Colchicine
- **Bacterial Arthritis**
  - Adequate aspiration or drainage
  - Antibiotics

Key Points

- Acute inflammatory arthritis in the hospitalized patient is usually due to crystal-induced disease, but this should not be assumed without evaluation.

- Attacks of gout or pseudogout following surgery or medical hospitalization are common, occurring at a mean of 4.2 days following surgical admission.

- Acute polyarticular arthritis suggests the presence of a systemic inflammatory disease.

- Fever may be absent in patients with documented bacterial arthritis and is present in a significant portion of hospitalized patients with acute crystal-induced arthritis.

- Up to 20% of hospitalized patients with acute mono- or oligoarticular arthritis may have a joint infection, and this must be considered and excluded in all cases of acute mono- or oligoarticular arthritis.

- Although the mean synovial white count in septic arthritis is higher than in gout, there is significant overlap; 26% of patients with documented septic arthritis may have initial synovial white cell counts <20,000/mm^3.

- Acute phase reactants, ANA, RF, and other "autoimmune" serologies have little if any role in the initial diagnostic evaluation of acute monoarticular arthritis.

- The serum urate level is not a useful diagnostic test in the evaluation of acute arthritis.

- Prompt percutaneous drainage, when feasible, is a reasonable initial approach; but if a septic joint cannot be adequately aspirated, surgical drainage is appropriate; GC infection with arthritis may be the exception.

SUGGESTED READING

Bieber JD, Terkeltaub RA. Gout: on the brink of novel therapeutic options for an ancient disease. Arthritis Rheum 2004; 50(8):2400–2414.

Pioro MH, Mandell BF. Septic arthritis. Rheum Dis Clin North Am 1997; 23(2):239–258.

Craig MH, Poole GV, Hauser CJ. Postsurgical gout. Am Surgeon 1995; 61:56–59.

Garcia-De La Torre I. Advances in the management of septic arthritis. Rheum Dis Clin North Am 2003; 29:61–75.

Ho G, DeNuccio M. Gout and pseudogout in hospitalized patients. Arch Intern Med 1993; 153:2787–2790.

Craig MH, Poole GV, Hauser CJ. Postsurgical gout. Am Surgeon 1995; 61:56–59.

Bardin T. Gonococcal arthritis. Best Pract Res Clin Rheum 2003; 17:201–208.

Schumacher HP, Boice JA, Daikh DI, et al. Randomised double blind trial of etoricoxib and indomethacin in treatment of acute gouty arthritis. BMJ 2002; 324:1488–1492.

Garcia-De La Torre I. Advances in the management of septic arthritis. Rheumatic Dis Clin North Am 2003; 29:61–75.

Coutlakis PJ, Roberts WN, Wise CM. Another look at synovial fluid leukocytosis and infection. J Clin Rheumatol 2002; 8:67–71.

CHAPTER EIGHTY

Systemic Vasculitis

Alexandra Villa-Forte, MD, MPH, and Brian F. Mandell MD, PhD

BACKGROUND

The vasculitides are a group of rare regional or systemic inflammatory disorders characterized by the variable presence of blood vessel wall inflammation, resulting in vessel occlusion, hemorrhage, or aneurysm formation. Blood vessels of different sizes, types, and location can be differentially affected. The vasculitides are classified as primary when there is no known cause or secondary when occurring as a consequence of another primary disorder such as infection, rheumatologic disease, malignancy, or drug allergy.[1] The primary vasculitides can be classified according to vessel size (Table 80-1) and the presence and distribution of parenchymal inflammation.[2] Therapeutic decisions are based on the specific diagnosis and the distribution, extent, and severity of disease.

ASSESSMENT

Clinical Presentation

Presenting Signs and Symptoms

Clinical presentation varies greatly amongst the different vasculitic syndromes. The presentation depends on the size, location, and type of blood vessels involved, as well as the degree of associated parenchymal inflammation. Some vasculitides (polyarteritis nodosa, Takayasu's arteritis) affect only blood vessels, while Wegener's granulomatosis (WG) may predominantly have tissue inflammation with minimal vasculitis. The systemic component of a vasculitic syndrome can be confined to one organ (e.g., skin, nerve, or kidney) or can affect multiple tissues. As a result, the clinical presentation may be as a multisystem illness or a limited clinical presentation with ischemic symptoms related to one or a few organs.

Patients may present with classical patterns of specific vasculitic syndromes, such as the triad of unremitting sinusitis, lung nodules, and glomerulonephritis seen in some patients with WG. Nonspecific symptoms such as fever, weight loss, malaise, myalgia, and arthralgia commonly occur with systemic presentations, but are not always present. Unexplained or atypical ischemia, or the concomitant or sequential involvement of certain organ systems should raise the suspicion for a vasculitic syndrome: kidneys (glomerulonephritis), skin (palpable purpura), neuropathy (mononeuritis multiplex), and lungs (infiltrates,

nodules, or hemorrhage). Leukopenia, thrombocytopenia, and striking adenopathy are not typical features of the primary vasculitic syndromes.

Differential Diagnosis

The most important concept when initially assessing a patient suspected of having a vasculitis is to recognize that the same symptoms and signs may also occur as a consequence of other disease processes that may mimic vasculitis. Thus, it is of utmost importance to distinguish a vasculitic process from its mimics (Box 80-1). Some of the diseases in the differential diagnosis of the primary vasculitides may be associated with a secondary vasculitis, and it is important to identify these clinical situations since therapeutic management can be quite different (e.g., polyarteritis nodosa or microscopic polyangiitis due to chronic hepatitis B or C).

The differential diagnosis of a pulmonary-renal syndrome includes several processes besides primary vasculitis, such as anti-glomerular basement membrane (GBM) disease, Systemic Lupus Erythematosus (SLE), and bacterial pneumonia with glomerulonephritis. Lung infiltrates can result from active vasculitis, infections, hypersensitivity, or drug toxicity (e.g., pneumonitis from cyclophosphamide or methotrexate). Hematuria may reflect active glomerulonephritis, damage from previous active vasculitis (glomerular injury), or hemorrhagic cystitis caused by cyclophosphamide. Persistent unexplained hematuria without cellular casts in the urinary sediment of a patient previously treated with cyclophosphamide should be investigated with cystoscopy to exclude bladder malignancy.[12]

Diagnosis

Use of clinical acumen is the primary method of diagnosing vasculitis, supported by biopsy or angiography when indicated and feasible. Patient history and physical examination will usually provide the initial clinical clues to the presence of vasculitis. Unexplained ischemia, chronic parenchymal inflammation, or constitutional features of inflammation should prompt consideration of possible vasculitis. Vasculitis should be specifically suspected in the presence of a systemic illness associated with peripheral neuropathy, glomerulonephritis, lung hemorrhage or recurrent infiltrates, palpable purpura, or when a constellation of symptoms/findings suggests a specific vasculitic syndrome.

Table 80-1 CLASSIFICATION—By Size of Predominantly Involved Blood Vessel

Large-sized vessel	Giant cell (temporal) arteritis
	Takayasu arteritis
Medium-sized vessel	Polyarteritis nodosa
	Kawasaki's disease
Small-sized vessel	Wegener's granulomatosis
	Churg-Strauss syndrome
	Microscopic polyangiitis
	Henoch-Schönlein purpura
	Essential cryoglobulinemic vasculitis
	Cutaneous leukocytoclastic angiitis

Box 80-1 Potential Clinical Mimics of Vasculitis

- Buerger's disease
- Atherosclerosis (cholesterol emboli)
- Thrombotic thrombocytopenic purpura
- Hypercoagulable syndromes (antiphospholipid syndrome)
- Vasospasm
- Amyloidosis
- Angiocentric malignancies

Certain patterns of clinical manifestations may lead directly to the suspicion of a specific vasculitic syndrome such as giant cell arteritis, WG, Churg-Strauss syndrome, or Takayasu's arteritis. If the diagnosis of vasculitis is suspected, consultation with an expert (e.g., rheumatologist) is reasonable.

Preferred Studies

There is no screening or confirmatory laboratory test for the diagnosis of vasculitis. A high index of suspicion for a vasculitic syndrome should arise from history and physical examination and can be subsequently supported by certain laboratory tests, once infection and other reasonable diagnoses are excluded. Most patients with a systemic vasculitis will have an elevated erythrocyte sedimentation rate (ESR) and C-reactive protein (CRP); but active vasculitis may occur without raised ESR or CRP. An elevated ESR >100 mm/hr does not specifically suggest vasculitis. Other common but nonspecific laboratory abnormalities include anemia of chronic disease, leukocytosis, and thrombocytosis. Eosinophilia at high levels supports the diagnosis of Churg-Strauss syndrome in the appropriate clinical setting.[3] Laboratory abnormalities may reflect specific organ involvement. Documentation of cellular casts is critical in the diagnosis of glomerulonephritis, and a freshly spun urine sediment should be examined by an experienced physician in every patient with an undiagnosed multisystem disorder or suspected vasculitis.

The role of antineutrophil cytoplasmic antibodies (ANCAs) in the diagnosis and assessment of disease activity is controversial. A positive ANCA is very common in patients with active generalized WG or microscopic polyangiitis, but is not equivalent to a confirmed case of vasculitis. About 80–90% of all ANCAs found in WG exhibit a cytoplasmic pattern (cANCA) by indirect immunofluorescence (IIF) and are directed against proteinase 3 (PR3). This specific antibody is infrequently found in other vasculitic or inflammatory disorders. Most other ANCAs in WG are directed against myeloperoxidase (anti-MPO) and are characterized by a perinuclear pattern (pANCA) by IIF. The ANCA specificity is identified by enzyme-linked immunoabsorbent assay (ELISA). Anti-MPO ANCAs have lower specificity for the different primary vasculitides. They can be found in patients with microscopic polyangiitis (MPA), Churg-Strauss syndrome, idiopathic rapidly progressive glomerulonephritis, and WG, as well as in nonvasculitic conditions (e.g., systemic lupus erythematosus [SLE], inflammatory bowel disease, endocarditis and drug-induced vasculitis).[4–7] The sensitivity of PR3-ANCA in WG depends on disease severity and activity and varies from 55–75% in patients with mild, limited, active disease to >90% in patients with active generalized disease.[8]

In WG, the combined use of IIF and ELISA for antigen identification results in diagnostic specificity of up to 98%.[9] Thus, in the setting of a high clinical suspicion for WG associated with the presence of PR3-ANCA, once infection is reasonably excluded, the diagnosis of WG can be provisionally made and therapy initiated without histopathologic confirmation. However, if the patient's response to therapy is unexpected in any way, tissue sampling should be aggressively pursued.

Although biopsy has been the definitive diagnostic test for vasculitis, when typical features of a specific vasculitic disorder are present and infection excluded, the diagnosis can be made and treatment initiated without biopsy confirmation. However, if the clinical suspicion for a specific disorder is not extremely high, or if the clinical picture is not totally "typical," a tissue confirmation should always be pursued. Thus, the "need" for biopsy may vary with the experience (estimated pretest likelihood) of the clinician. While considered the gold standard diagnostic test for the vasculitides, biopsy may not confirm the diagnosis. Involvement of the blood vessel may be segmental, and the characteristic findings may be missed by pathologic examination, even in the presence of disease.

Another important point to consider when making a decision regarding biopsy is the yield of the specific test. Biopsy of asymptomatic sites ("blind" biopsy) has a very low yield and should be avoided.[10] This includes biopsy of asymptomatic and/or electrodiagnostically normal sural nerves. The decision regarding biopsy site should include consideration of the likelihood of getting a disease specific diagnosis; if WG is suspected, renal biopsy is not likely to distinguish glomerulonephritis of WG from MPA or rapidly progressive glomerulonephritis (RPGN). Immunofluorescence will, however, distinguish WG from SLE or hepatitis C–associated glomerulonephritis. When a biopsy is planned, an adequate amount of tissue (needle biopsy usually not sufficient) should be obtained from a clinically involved area. Another limitation of tissue diagnosis is the location of the vessel involved. Large and some medium-sized vessels may not be available to biopsy and diagnosis. Takayasu's arteritis and polyarteritis nodosa (PAN) are often not confirmed by histopathology. The diagnosis of these and other vasculitides frequently relies on angiographic abnormalities. Characteristic angiographic abnormalities include stenosis or occlusion, irregular vessel walls, poststenotic dilatation and aneurysm formation. None of these findings is totally sensitive or specific for vasculitis.

The approach to a patient with suspected vasculitis begins with establishing the presence of vasculitis and then determining if the vasculitis is primary or secondary. Once a patient has been diagnosed with a primary vasculitis, the next step is to attempt to classify the specific vasculitic syndrome since treatment and prognosis differ among the different vasculitides. Classification is not always possible on the first encounter with the patient. It is important to remember that the specific criteria proposed by the American College of Rheumatology for each major vasculitic syndrome were not intended for initial diagnosis of early disease, but were designed for the purpose of classifying patients with well-defined disease for clinical trials.[11] The third step of the process is to determine the organ involvement, severity, and extent of the disease, all of which influence treatment decisions.

Prognosis

The combination of severity of the vasculitis, pattern of organ involvement, extent of organ damage, and occurrence of opportunistic infections determine prognosis. Patients with alveolar hemorrhage can rapidly deteriorate, requiring mechanical ventilation, yet we frequently see severely ill patients in the intensive care setting who subsequently respond to immunosuppressive therapy and achieve nearly complete recovery. The apparent severity of disease does not necessarily determine how the patient will respond to therapy, and lack of immediate clinical response may not indicate therapy failure. Glomerulonephritis in particular may take longer than other organ manifestations to respond to treatment, and patients may require temporary dialysis. On the other hand, a rising creatinine level during adequate immunosuppressive treatment and overall improvement does not mean there should necessarily be an increase in the intensity of treatment. Unnecessary augmentation of immunosuppression in an effort to abate renal deterioration due to severe prior damage may lead to infection, morbidity, and even death.

MANAGEMENT

Treatment

Patients with undiagnosed severe multisystem or ischemic disease qualify for admission to the hospital for diagnostic evaluation. When assessing a patient with known vasculitis, there are several possibilities that may lead to the patient's admission to the hospital. Patients may be admitted because of active vasculitis, treatment toxicity, infection, or disease-associated morbidity (e.g., complications from chronic renal insufficiency, DVT). It is essential to identify the specific problem(s) and to recognize that a combination of problems can simultaneously occur in the same patient. In the immunosuppressed febrile patient or the patient with pulmonary infiltrates, infection must be aggressively excluded prior to, or concurrent with, intensification of immunosuppression.

Immunosuppressive therapies have significantly decreased the mortality of the primary vasculitides. Since many deaths occur soon after presentation, there is a need for prompt diagnosis and institution of appropriate treatment. The systemic vasculitides vary greatly, and although immunosuppressive agents are always used to treat all of them, they are not all treated identically. Each primary vasculitic syndrome has unique clinical features and may present with different degrees of severity. Some require immediate aggressive treatment, while others may respond to less intense therapy. Giant cell arteritis (GCA) is treated with glucocorticoid monotherapy, while WG requires dual therapy with steroids and a second immunosuppressive agent. There is no adequate evidence to support the use of other immunosuppressive medications in GCA, with or in place of steroids.[13] In contrast, there are data showing that steroids alone are insufficient to sustain remission in WG.[14] Glucocorticoids may be used alone as initial therapy for selected patients with PAN, although severe presentations may warrant treatment with high doses of steroids and cyclophosphamide.[15,16]

Excluding infection and objectively defining disease activity are mandatory in the assessment of the patient admitted to the hospital with a previous diagnosis of vasculitis. Other important disease definitions that affect treatment decisions include severity of disease, the presence of an associated complicating disease process, and individual patient factors that need to be considered (e.g., history of medication toxicity, contraindications to certain medications, presence of previous organ damage, age). Patients with WG and perhaps other vasculitides are prone to develop thromboembolic disease. Occult pulmonary embolism and atherosclerosis may cause diagnostic confusion.

As a general rule, most primary vasculitides are initially treated with glucocorticoids, and some will require a combination of this and a second immunosuppressant from the outset of treatment. Aggressive therapy with high doses of steroids and a second immunosuppressant such as cyclophosphamide is usually indicated in the presence of life-threatening or major organ function–threatening clinical manifestations. In selected patients, such as those with leukocytoclastic vasculitis confined to the skin, steroids may be given as single treatment or not at all.[17] On the other hand, some vasculitides such as WG require combination therapy with steroids and a second immunosuppressant to induce and maintain remission. Glucocorticoids are most commonly started at a dose of 1 mg/kg/day and cyclophosphamide at 2 mg/kg/day given all at once in the morning with large amounts of fluids to avoid hemorrhagic cystitis. Some clinicians use high-steroid "pulse" doses in severe disease. Drug-induced leukopenia is not necessary to achieve disease remission and should be avoided since it increases the risk of concomitant severe infection.[18] Complete blood counts should be obtained regularly to permit adjustment of the dose of cyclophosphamide and prevent leukopenia. Although the question of whether to use daily oral cyclophosphamide or monthly intravenous therapy still is a subject of debate, most experts in the field favor the former since there is not sufficient evidence of superior results with monthly therapy, and it is easier to maintain control over the leukocyte count by adjusting the dose of daily oral cyclophosphamide.[19] Selected patients with less severe disease may be treated with steroids alone or in the case of milder WG, with GC and methotrexate, usually at a starting dose of 15 mg/week.[20] Intracellular folic acid depletion caused by the methotrexate may increase toxicity, and folic (1 mg/day) or folinic acid (5 mg/week) should be given. For patients with contraindications for the use of methotrexate (e.g., serum creatinine greater than 2.0 or liver disease), azathioprine can be used in combination with steroids, at a dose of 100–200 mg/day, adjusted to avoid leukopenia (Table 80-2).[21] Azathioprine causes febrile reactions, which can mimic systemic infection, in ~7% of patients.[21]

Table 80-2 Drug Toxicity

Glucocorticoids	Methotrexate
Osteoporosis	Bone marrow suppression
Osteonecrosis	Mucositis, nausea, vomiting, diarrhea
Diabetes	Malaise, fatigue, fever, dizziness
Cataracts, glaucoma	Acute or chronic hepatotoxicity
Sleep disturbance	Pneumonitis
Anxiety/psychosis	
Myopathy	
Acne	
Increased risk of infection	

Cyclophosphamide	Azathioprine
Bone marrow suppression	Bone marrow suppression
Nausea, vomiting	Nausea, vomiting, diarrhea
Hemorrhagic cystitis	Fever
Myeloproliferative diseases	Hypersensitivity reaction
Bladder cancer	Hepatotoxicity
Pneumonitis	Skin rashes
Alopecia, skin rashes	Increased risk of infection
Neutropenia	Pancreatitis
Increased risk of infection	

A major challenge when making treatment decisions in patients with established disease is accurately assessing disease activity in several types of vasculitis (e.g., Takayasu's arteritis).[22] Objective parameters such as the ESR are not always reliable; clinical features similar to those of active vasculitis occur with other conditions, and new ischemic symptoms can result from fibrous or thrombotic occlusive disease.

All patients taking combination immunosuppressive therapy should be given prophylactic therapy against *Pneumocystis jiroveci*. The most commonly used regimen is sulfamethoxazole/trimethoprim (a double-strength tablet, once daily on alternate days); other options for those with sulfa allergy include dapsone daily or monthly inhaled pentamidine. Since long-term use of steroids is associated with the development of osteoporosis, calcium and vitamin D should be given to all patients taking them. A bisphosphonate should be considered in patients with anticipated chronic steroid use. Influenza and pneumococcal vaccination should be up to date in all patients, prior to initiating immunosuppressive therapy if at all possible. Baseline PPD to assess for latent tuberculosis infection should be placed prior to long-term corticosteroid therapy.

DISCHARGE/FOLLOW-UP PLANS

At the time of discharge planning, the patient should be following the initial therapeutic plan to avoid any delay with consequent morbidity and mortality. Predischarge PPD status should be recorded. Careful outpatient follow-up plans with a clinician skilled in the use of immunosuppressants should be confirmed. Ideally, the therapy should be monitored and reevaluated no later

than 2 weeks after discharge. Response to treatment should be assessed, and adjustment of medication doses according to laboratory test results should not be delayed. Potential white cell nadir from cyclophosphamide (10–14 days) should be calculated and a plan should be made to check the white cell count at that time, with plans confirmed that a clinician will receive and review the results. The discharge summary should include biopsy reports and detailed radiograph reports, particularly chest films/CT scans and angiograms. Doses of immunosuppressants should be recorded. Neurologic examination, description of pulses, bruits, and four-extremity blood pressures (in patients with larger vessel disease) should be recorded.

Newly diagnosed patients need to be educated about their vasculitic syndrome, especially on how to take the medications, how to avoid toxicity, and how to recognize clinical symptoms and signs that should trigger an immediate phone call to their doctor or a visit to the emergency room (e.g., new cough, fever, or hemoptysis). The patient should also be made aware of the importance of regularly scheduled blood testing to monitor response to therapy and drug toxicity in the outpatient setting.

Key Points

- Unexplained ischemia, chronic parenchymal inflammation, or constitutional features of inflammation should prompt consideration of possible vasculitis.

- Vasculitis is not necessarily the final diagnosis; drug allergy, infection, and malignancy must be excluded.

- The antineutrophil cytoplasmic antibody test (ANCA) is not a screening test for vasculitis. In the appropriate setting, a positive ANCA can strongly support the clinical diagnosis of Wegeners granulomatosis, microscopic polyangiitis, or drug-induced vasculitis.

- Examination of fresh urine sediment should be performed in all patients with unexplained multisystem disease or suspected vasculitis; glomerulonephritis is usually asymptomatic.

- Aggressive therapy with high doses of steroids and a second immunosuppressant such as cyclophosphamide, azathioprine, or methotrexate is usually indicated in the presence of life-threatening or major organ function–threatening clinical manifestations, and in generalized WG.

- Patients taking intense combination immunosuppressive therapy should be given prophylactic therapy against *Pneumocystis jiroveci*.

SUGGESTED READING

Luqmani RA, Robinson H. Introduction to, and classification of, the systemic vasculitides. Best Pract Res Clin Rheumatol 2001; 15:187–212.

Hoffman GS, Kerr GS, Leavitt RY, et al. Wegener granulomatosis: an analysis of 158 patients. Ann Intern Med 1992; 116:488–498.

Jayne D, Rasmussen N, Andrassy K, et al. A randomized trial of maintenance therapy for vasculitis associated with antineutrophil cytoplasmic autoantibodies. N Engl J Med 2003; 349:36–44.

Langford CA. Management of systemic vasculitis. Best Pract Res Clin Rheum 2001; 15:281–297.

Kerr GS, Hallahan CW, Giordano J et al. Takayasu's arteritis. Ann Intern Med 1994; 120:919–929.

Gonzalez-Gay M, Garcia-Porrua C, Pujol RM. Clinical approach to cutaneous vasculitis. Curr Opin Rheum 2005; 17:56–61.

CHAPTER EIGHTY-ONE

Allergic Reactions and Angioedema

Neil Winawer, MD, and Mandakolathur Murali, MD

BACKGROUND

A hypersensitivity reaction occurs when the immune system produces an inflammatory response to an offending allergen. Allergic reactions represent a specific class of hypersensitivity reaction mediated by IgE antibody in response to agents such as insect venoms, food, beta-lactam antibiotics, and latex products. These reactions manifest clinically as a spectrum, ranging from mild (e.g., urticaria) to life threatening (anaphylaxis). Anaphylactic reactions, requiring epinephrine, account for approximately 1 in every 2,000 ambulance trips, and result in as many as 1,000 fatalities per year. This estimate is conservative given the variable presentation of the disorder, underreporting, and the lack of a consensus definition distinguishing severe allergic reactions from anaphylaxis.[1,2]

Anaphylaxis can also occur in the inpatient setting and complicates as many as 1 in 2,700 hospital admissions.[3] Many of these reactions, however, are non–IgE mediated and are referred to as "anaphylactoid." These include reactions to radiocontrast dye, angiotension-converting enzyme (ACE) inhibitors, opiates, and NSAIDS. Since anaphylactoid reactions are clinically indistinguishable from anaphylaxis, they are often grouped together under the general term *anaphylaxis.*

Definition and Classification

When a patient suffers an acute adverse event from to a drug or agent he or she is often labeled as being "allergic." This terminology can be misleading to patients and physicians, as true or classic allergic reactions are strictly defined by the immune system's production of IgE antibody. Other types of immunologic reactions (e.g., hemolytic anemia related to penicillin) occur via different mechanisms (Table 81-1). Some hypersensitivity reactions are difficult to classify given the lack of evidence supporting a predominant immunologic mechanism. These include cutaneous drug reactions such as maculopapular rashes, fixed drug eruptions, exfoliative dermatitis, Stevens-Johnson syndrome (SJS), and toxic epidermal necrolysis (TEN).[4,5]

Nonimmunologic mechanisms account for the largest percentage of adverse drug reactions.[6] While the majority of these events are classified as side effects (e.g., gastritis secondary to NSAIDS) or toxicities (e.g., increased liver enzymes secondary to statins), mast cells can also be activated by other mechanisms such as activation of neurokinin and complement receptors, producing a clinical picture identical to that of immediate hypersensitivity reactions. Since mast cells are the culprit in most cases of anaphylaxis (whether immune or nonimmune), it is crucial to understand their role in the inflammatory response.

Pathophysiology

When IgE antibody is formed in response to a specific allergen, it binds to high-affinity receptors, called Fc epsilon Type I, located on mast cells and basophils. Upon reexposure to that agent, cross-linking of cell-bound IgE antibody occurs, resulting in Fc epsilon receptor aggregation and activation, leading to the release of inflammatory mediators from mast cells (Fig. 81-1). It is these mediators (e.g., histamine, prostaglandins, tryptase, leukotrienes, etc.) that directly contribute to the allergic response by causing smooth muscle contraction, bronchoconstriction, vasodilation, increased vascular permeability, and edema. In addition to an IgE mast cell response, allergic reactions also are mediated by a subset of CD4+ T-cells called T-helper type 2 (TH2) cells, which preferentially produce interleukin 4, 5, and 13. Mast cell and basophil-bound IgE contribute to the early (or immediate) phase of allergic response; interleukin 5 recruits and activates eosinophils, contributing to the late (or chronic) phase of allergic inflammation. CD4+ TH2 cells also produce chemokines such as RANTES, eotaxin, and MIP-1alpha that escalate the cellular components of the late phase allergic response.

ASSESSMENT

Clinical Presentation

Prevalence and Presenting Signs and Symptoms

The clinical manifestations of allergic reactions are varied and depend on several factors. These include the amount of antigen, its route of administration, and the end organ response to vasoactive mediators. Most allergic reactions involve the skin, resulting in pruritus. This is often associated with a transient wheal and flare (urticaria). If the reaction is more severe and a larger number of mast cells (located in the deep dermis) are recruited, patients may develop angioedema (Fig. 81-2). Nonallergic cutaneous drug eruptions may have a variety of clinical presentations ranging from mild inflammation (e.g., maculopapular rash) to

Table 81-1 Immunologic and Nonimmunologic Reactions

A Hypersensitivity Reaction Is Defined as an Immune-Mediated Response to an Agent in a Sensitized Patient. An Allergic Reaction Is a Hypersensitivity Reaction Specifically Mediated by IgE.[17] Examples of Various Reactions Include:

Immune

Type	Example
Type I reaction—IgE mediated	Anaphylaxis from peanuts
Type II reaction—cytotoxic	Hemolytic anemia from penicillin
Type III reaction immune complex	Serum sickness from antithymocyte Globulin
Type IV reaction—delayed, cell-mediated	Contact dermatitis from poison ivy
Fas/Fas ligand-induced apoptosis	SJS, TEN
Other poorly defined mechanisms	Drug-induced lupus-like syndromes anticonvulsant hypersensitivity

Nonimmune

Side effects	Hyperkalemia from trimethoprim/sulfamethoxazole
Drug toxicity	Dysrhythmia from digoxin
Drug-drug interaction	Increased Coumadin level secondary to antibiotics
Pseudoallergic	Anaphylactoid reaction from radiocontrast

IgE = Immunoglobulin E; SJS = Stevens-Johnson Syndrome; TEN = Toxic Epidermal Necrolysis.

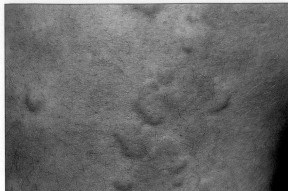

Figure 81-2 • Urticaria in close up, showing characteristic weals, surrounded by an erythematous flare. From: Forbes CD, Jackson WF. Color Atlas and Text of Clinical Medicine, 3rd Edition St. Louis, Missouri, 2003.

full dermal involvement causing vesicles, bullae, and even denuded skin (e.g., SJS, TEN).

Signs and symptoms of anaphylactic reactions usually begin within 5 minutes of exposure to the offending agent and include flushing, pruritus, urticaria, angioedema, shortness of breath, wheezing, chest tightness, nausea, vomiting, cramping abdominal pain, diarrhea, and lightheadedness. Systemic mast cell degranulation may also cause severe peripheral vasodilatation, hypotension, and subsequent cardiovascular collapse. Further, swelling of the larynx, tongue, epiglottis, or oropharynx may cause complete obstruction, leading to asphyxiation. Often, these events are preceded by hoarseness, a key clinical clue of laryngeal edema. Anaphylaxis also may affect the lower airways, causing bronchospasm, wheezing, and pulmonary edema. Progression of these findings results in severe hypoxemia, which can precipitate altered mental status and seizures.

Aside from anaphylaxis, there are other types of hypersensitivity reactions that are severe and warrant hospitalization. Stevens-Johnson syndrome (SJS) and toxic epidermal necrolysis (TEN) are bullous and necrolytic reactions to drugs or infections and can be life threatening. SJS is the most severe form of erythema multiforme and involves blistering lesions with epidermal loss occurring over less than 10% of the patient's body surface area. Patients often develop painful erosions of the oral mucosa and lip (90%), as well as conjunctivitis (85%). TEN is characterized by fever and epidermal loss of 30% or more of body surface area.[7] Mucosal erosions are also a prominent feature of TEN, often making it difficult to clinically distinguish from SJS.

Differential Diagnosis

The diagnosis of anaphylaxis is a clinical one based upon the patient's history and clinical presentation. Diagnostic testing is rarely indicated. However, in some clinical situations such as perioperative anaphylaxis, unexplained syncope, or recurrent anaphylaxis, determination of serum total and beta tryptase can confirm an anaphylactic event as they remain elevated for 4–8 hours.

There are several disease processes that can mimic the clinical features of anaphylaxis. For example, vasovagal reactions, cardiac arrhythmias, bronchoconstriction, and hypoglycemia can be partly associated with hypotension, pallor, diaphoresis,

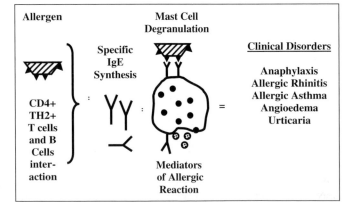

Figure 81-1 • Pathophysiology of a Type I hypersensitivity reaction. An allergic reaction refers to the immune system's production of IgE antibody in response to an offending antigen (allergen). The antibody binds to high-affinity IgE receptors on mast cells and basophils, resulting in sensitization to that antigen. Subsequent exposure to the allergen results in cross linking of mast cell and basophil bound IgE antibodies, triggering the release of inflammatory mediators (principally histamine) that cause vasodilatation and increased vascular permeability.

shortness of breath, and wheezing. However, cutaneous findings such as pruritus and urticaria are absent in these conditions.

Hereditary angioedema is a rare autosomal dominant disease that is characterized by a low or nonfunctioning C1 esterase inhibitor (C1 INH). Patients present with bouts of angioedema involving the larynx, face, lips, abdomen, genitalia, and extremities. Patients will often note prior bouts of angioedema and will relate a family history of these episodes. While hereditary angioedema is an uncommon disorder, it remains crucial for the clinician to distinguish between this entity and anaphylaxis, given the significant differences in treatment. In hereditary angioedema the complement cascade produces vasoactive kinin proteins; mast cells are not activated. Therefore, treatment with antihistamines, steroids, and epinephrine does not alter the disease process. Acute episodes are managed with supportive care and the administration of heat-vaporized C1 esterase inhibitor concentrate.[8] If the clinical picture remains uncertain, a serum total tryptase level can help to determine if the process was mast cell mediated. Additionally, obtaining a C4 level is a cost-effective screening test as a normal result effectively rules out hereditary angioedema (Fig. 81-3).

Systemic mastocytosis is another rare disorder that is characterized by an overabundance of mast cells in the gastrointestinal tract, liver, spleen, bone marrow, and skin. Patients typically present with symptoms of pruritus, flushing, and/or abdominal pain. Characteristic findings include hepatomegaly, splenomegaly, lymphadenopathy, anemia, and/or coagulopathy. Some patients may display the classic skin findings of urticaria pigmentosa. If mastocytosis is suspected, serum total and beta tryptase levels are useful diagnostic tests. A total tryptase level over 20 ng/mL with an increase in the alpha subunit is suggestive of the diagnosis. The beta subunit is usually normal (in contrast to anaphylaxis wherein the beta tryptase is elevated). A bone marrow biopsy and flow cytometry of marrow cells that are positive for CD25+, CD2+, c-kit, or CD117+ cells are diagnostic.

Many types of nonallergic hypersensitivity reactions can occur in the skin. The most common of these is a drug-induced exanthem that results in lesions that are macular, papular, or morbilliform in appearance. Hypersensitivity vasculitis has many causes and is typically characterized by palpable purpura (See Chapter 80). Another common clinical feature is urticarial vasculitis. In this entity, the individual hives last greater than 48 hours, often show pigmentary changes, and resolve with some scaling. Photosensitivity reactions may produce an eczematous rash in sun-exposed areas, and a fixed drug eruption is characterized by a solitary well-demarcated erythematous lesion. More severe eruptions that involve exfoliation, desquamation, and blistering can mimic SJS and TEN. These include exfoliative dermatitis, pemphigus vulgaris, bullous pemphigoid, and exanthematous pustulosis. Additionally, thermal burns, phototoxic eruptions, and pressure blisters can sometimes histologically resemble SJS or TEN. Skin biopsy and immunofluorescence studies often help to distinguish these vesiculobullous skin disorders.

MANAGEMENT

Treatment

The initial evaluation of allergic reactions is based on the underlying severity of the presentation. If the patient is experiencing shortness of breath or airway swelling, he or she should be treated as a medical emergency. If the patient is en route to the hospital or if intravenous access is not immediately available then an injection of epinephrine (0.3 ml of 1:1000) should be given directly into the muscle of the anterolateral thigh.[9] If the patient is hemodynamically unstable aggressive crystalloid fluid resuscitation should be instituted. Intravenous H_1 receptor antagonists (e.g., diphenhydramine) and H_2 receptor antagonists (e.g., ranitidine) should be given, as activation of histamine receptors in the splanchnic vascular bed represents a capacitance compartment, which contributes to hypotension. Patients recalcitrant to initial therapy should receive intravenous administration of aqueous epinephrine at a dose of 0.1–0.3 mL in 10 mL normal saline over several minutes (1:33,000 to 1:100,000 dilution). If patients are refractory to treatment secondary to long-standing beta-blocker therapy, they can be administered glucagon (1 mg in 1 L of D5W ↑ at 5 to 15 mL/min), given the drug's positive inotropic and chronotropic effects (mediated via cyclic AMP, not beta receptors). If at any point the patient is unable to maintain a patent airway, he or she should be intubated immediately.

If the patient is hemodynamically stable but is experiencing wheezing or shortness of breath, then supplemental oxygen should be initiated along with aerosolized beta-agonists (albuterol 2.5 mg in normal saline diluted to a total of 3 mL) every 20 minutes for the first hour, followed by repeat doses every 1–4 hours as needed. Antihistamines (e.g., diphenhydramine 25–50 mg) should be started and given as needed every 4–6 hours. Systemic glucocorticoids, (e.g., methylprednisolone 1–2 mg/kg per 24 hr) while not acutely affecting symptoms, may aid in the treatment of prolonged reactions.

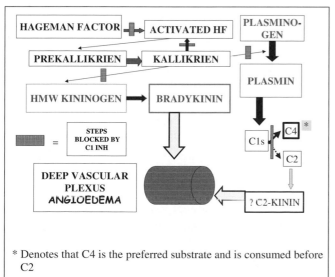

* Denotes that C4 is the preferred substrate and is consumed before C2

Figure 81-3 • Pathophysiology of Hereditary Angioedema. In an acute attack (due to absent or nonfunctional C1 esterase inhibitor) activated C1 allows the complement cascade to go unopposed, producing the vasoactive peptides, C2 kinin and bradykinin. In this reaction, the complement proteins, C2 and C4 are consumed. Hence, during an acute episode, these levels will be low. In between attacks, the value of C2 is normal, but C4 is always low as there is always a low level of activated C1 that cleaves C4 (C4 is the preferred substrate). Thus, a normal C4 level rules out the disease, while C2 levels reflect the activity of the disease.

Patients with predominantly cutaneous findings should be treated according to the appearance of their skin lesions. Urticaria and angioedema should generally be treated with antihistamines. Treatment with H_2 receptor antagonists and/or tricyclics (e.g., Doxepin) may provide additional benefit, given their blocking effects on histamine receptors. Patients with more severe eruptions such SJS or TEN should have a multifactorial approach focusing on electrolyte repletion, maintaining fluid balance, pain control, and preventing secondary infection. The use of adhesive tapes should be avoided and all nonessential medications discontinued. Recognizing the clinical findings of SJS/TEN is essential, as prompt withdrawal of the offending drug has been shown to significantly reduce mortality by as much as 30% per day.[10] When the etiology of the reaction is unknown, all nonessential medications should be stopped. The administration of corticosteroids in SJS/TEN is controversial and may be of benefit if started early in the disease process. The administration of intravenous immunoglobulin in patients with TEN has demonstrated benefit in one small uncontrolled study that has yet to be duplicated.[11]

PREVENTION

While the most effective method of preventing allergic reactions is avoidance, sometimes this is not always feasible. This is particularly the case in patients with a history of radiocontrast allergy who need to undergo further radiologic testing. Patients with a history of mild allergic reactions to radiocontrast (e.g., urticaria) can be pre-dosed with 50 mg of oral prednisone at different intervals the day of the procedure (13, 7, and 1 hour before) along with 50 mg of diphenhydramine parentally 1 hour prior to the procedure. Patients with more severe anaphylactoid reactions can additionally be given 300 mg of cimetidine orally along with 25 mg of oral ephedrine.[12] The use of low-osmolality radiocontrast also helps to minimize the likelihood of an allergic reaction.[13] It is advisable to hold any β-blockers for 6–12 hours prior to the study, provided there is no contraindication.

Often patients give a history of allergic reactions to commonly prescribed drugs such as antibiotics. In these circumstances, it is important to accurately gauge the likelihood of future reactions to similar agents. Most patients who report a non–life-threatening allergy to penicillin do not produce IgE antibodies to penicillin (80–90%). Among the remaining 10–20% of patients with a potential for cross reactivity to cephalosporins only 2–8% had an allergic reaction when challenged with cephalosporins (first-generation cephalosporins may pose a greater risk than second- and third-generation cephalosporins). However, as many as 50% of patients with a prior history of anaphylaxis to penicillin will produce IgE antibodies against penicillin. Given the lethal nature of the reaction and high risk of cross reactivity, patients with a history of penicillin anaphylaxis should be skin tested to major and minor determinants of penicillin. If skin tests are negative, the patient can receive a cephalosporin at no greater risk than the general population. If skin tests are positive, recommendations may include: (1) administering an alternative antibiotic, (2) cautious graded challenge with appropriate monitoring, recognizing that there may be a 2% chance of inducing an anaphylactic reaction, or (3) desensitization to the required cephalosporin.[14]

Patients may also relate a history of sulfur allergy. This typically refers to a class of drugs known as sulfonamides (e.g., sul-famethoxazole, sulfonylureas, thiazide diuretics, loop diuretics, carbonic anhydrase inhibitors, celecoxib, etc.). Most patients with a hypersensitivity reaction to one sulfur drug are typically advised not to receive others of the same class. The evidence, however, indicates that patients with a history of sulfonamide antibiotic allergy have at least an equally high risk of developing an allergic reaction to penicillin as compared to a sulfonamide nonantibiotic.[15] This suggests that a general predisposition to allergic reactions among certain patients might be at work, as opposed to a specific cross-reactivity with the sulfa moiety. Therefore, any drug treatment decisions in patients with a prior medication allergy should be based on the underlying need for the particular drug, as well as the severity of the patient's hypersensitivity.

Patients who develop angioedema from an ACE inhibitor should be taken off the drug to prevent future attacks. Since the reaction is a class effect and not dose dependent, patients should not be rechallenged with another ACE inhibitor or treated at a lower dose. It is also important to note that only 60% of these reactions occur within the first week of taking the drug, and that reactions can occur years after being on the agent.[16] An area of controversy surrounds whether or not these patients can be safely treated with angiotension receptor blockers (ARBs). While there have been a few case reports of ARB-induced angioedema in patients with a history of ACE-inhibitor angioedema, it is relatively uncommon. Decisions regarding whether these patients should receive an ARB need to be individualized. If the patient has a strong indication for an ARB (e.g., diabetic nephropathy, heart failure) and the episode of angioedema was non–life threatening, then the drug should be instituted with caution and close monitoring.

DISCHARGE/FOLLOW-UP PLANS

Patient Education

Upon discharge those patients with mild persistent allergic symptoms should receive a brief outpatient taper of corticosteroids and antihistamines as needed. Many patients, however, will have complete resolution of their symptoms. In these individuals, emphasis should focus on prevention of future allergic reactions. This entails providing information and fully educating patients about their disease process. Prior to discharge, patients should be able to verbalize understanding of potential triggers as well as recognize those substances which may cross-react and produce similar reactions. Patients experiencing anaphylactic reactions should be given medical alert bracelets and be provided with instructions on how to self-administer an injection of epinephrine (EpiPen) in the event of a repeat episode. Patients should be referred to an allergist for skin-prick testing and desensitization therapy if indicated.

Outpatient Physician Communication

The patient's primary care physician must be informed of all adverse reactions occurring in the hospital. All such reactions should be documented clearly in both the inpatient and outpatient medical record. This is particularly important as it pertains to drug reactions so that patients do not unknowingly receive the same medication in the future.

Key Points

- Since anaphylactoid reactions are clinically indistinguishable from anaphylaxis, they are often grouped together under the general term **anaphylaxis**.

- The diagnosis of anaphylaxis is a clinical one, based upon the patient's history and clinical presentation. Diagnostic testing is rarely indicated.

- In some clinical situations such as perioperative anaphylaxis, unexplained syncope, or recurrent anaphylaxis, determination of serum total and beta tryptase can confirm an anaphylactic event, as they remain elevated for 4–8 hours.

- Development of angioedema from ACE inhibitors is a class effect and not dose dependent. Only 60% of these reactions occur within the first week of taking the drug, while reactions can occur years after being on the agent.

- Recognizing the clinical findings of SJS/TEN is essential, as prompt withdrawal of the offending drug has been shown to significantly reduce mortality by as much as 30% per day.

- In patients with a history of radiocontrast allergy who need to undergo further radiologic testing, preventive treatment includes: steroids, H_1 and H_2 blockers, use of low-osmolality radiocontrast, and holding of any β-blockers for 6–12 hours prior to the study, provided there is no contraindication.

SUGGESTED READING

Sampson HA, Munoz-Furlong A, Bock SA, et al. Symposium on the definition and management of anaphylaxis: summary report. J Allergy Clin Immunol 2005; 115:584–591.

Neugut AI, Ghatak AT, Miller RL. Anaphylaxis in the United States: an investigation into its epidemiology. Arch Intern Med 2001; 161:15–21.

Laporte JR, deLatorre FJ, Gadgil DA, et al. An epidemiologic study of severe anaphylactic and anaphylactoid reactions among hospital patients: methods and overall risks. The International Collaborative Study of Severe Anaphylaxis. Epidemiology 1998; 9:141–146.

Garcia-Doval I, LeCleach L, Bocquet H, et al. Toxic epidermal necrolysis and Stevens Johnson syndrome: does early withdrawal of causative drugs decrease the risk of death? Arch Dermatology 2000; 136:323–327.

Wolff K. Treatment of toxic epidermal necrolysis. Arch Dermatology 2003; 139:85–86.

Strom BL, Schinnar R, Apter AJ, et al. Absence of cross-reactivity between sulfonamide antibiotics and nonsulfonamide antibiotics. N Engl J Med 2003; 349:1628–1635.

CHAPTER EIGHTY-TWO

Dermatology in Hospitalized Patients

Calvin McCall, MD, Murtaza Cassoobhoy, MD, and Lesley Miller, MD

INTRODUCTION

Skin eruptions are an extremely common manifestation of disease. Hospitalists will encounter patients who are admitted under their care with a primary dermatologic process (e.g., severe drug eruption) or as part of a systemic disease process. This chapter is organized based on that framework. The first section reviews some common skin diseases that a hospitalist should be able to identify and manage. The second section focuses on approaches to patients who present with fever or vasculitis and have a rash as part of their multiorgan disease involvement. Consultation with a dermatologist should be considered for patients with a rash when the full differential diagnosis is in question and a biopsy may aid in the diagnosis. A dermatologist should also be consulted to assist in the treatment of serious dermatologic diseases such as toxic epidermal necrolysis.

ADVERSE CUTANEOUS DRUG REACTIONS

Background

The most common adverse event caused by medical treatment for hospitalized patients is due to complications of drug therapy (19%).[1] Adverse cutaneous drug reactions (ACDRs) occur in 2.2% of all hospitalized patients.[2] Most of these reactions are mild, but a few of them can be severe and life threatening. It is important for a hospitalist to not only recognize that a drug may be causing the reaction, but also to be able to distinguish which type of reaction it is. Features that are a red flag for a life-threatening drug reaction are listed in Box 82-1.

There are many different types of ACDRs, and this section will review the common ones (exanthem, urticaria) and those that are life threatening (anaphylaxis, blistering drug eruptions). The hospitalist should consider an ACDR in the differential diagnosis of any new eruption in a hospitalized patient. At the same time, it is important to exclude infection, particularly a viral exanthem that may look very similar to an exanthematous reactions caused by drugs. A complete review of the patient's medications should be performed, including their temporal relationship to the onset of the eruption. The patient or family members should be asked about a history of similar reactions to any agents, including prescription and over-the-counter drugs. In most cases, the drug should be immediately stopped if it is suspected of causing an eruption.

EXANTHEMATOUS REACTIONS

Assessment

Clinical Presentation

These are the most common type of ACDR and can be caused by any drug. Penicillins, sulfonamides, carbamazepine, allopurinol, nonsteroidal anti-inflammatory drugs and isoniazid are some of the medications that frequently (1–5%) cause exanthematous reactions. For the first exposure to the drug, the reaction can occur up to 3 weeks after starting the medication. In the case of penicillin, can occur for 2 weeks after it is stopped. This is one of the few eruptions that can be truly maculopapular. The rash is red and pruritic, but not painful, and symmetrically involves the trunk and extremities, commonly sparing the face (Fig. 82-1).

Differential Diagnosis

Viral exanthems appear very similar to drug exanthems, but frequently begin on the face. Secondary syphilis, atypical pityriasis rosea, and widespread contact dermatitis should be considered.

Diagnosis

This is a clinical diagnosis that can be confirmed by skin biopsy, though biopsy will not assist in identifying the offending agent.

Prognosis

The majority of exanthematous reactions resolve after discontinuation of the drug and treatment. However, the rash may worsen for a few days after stopping the drug. The patient should be closely monitored for more serious reactions, such as toxic epidermal necrolysis (TEN), hypersensitivity syndrome, and serum sickness, which can all begin with an exanthematous eruption.

Box 82-1 Features of a Life-Threatening Drug Reaction

Clinical Findings

Cutaneous

- Confluent erythema
- Facial edema or central facial involvement
- Skin pain
- Palpable purpura
- Skin necrosis
- Blisters or epidermal detachment
- Positive Nikolsky's sign*
- Mucous-membrane erosions
- Urticaria
- Swelling of tongue

General

- High fever (temperature >40°C)
- Enlarged lymph nodes
- Arthralgias or arthritis
- Shortness of breath, wheezing, hypotension

Laboratory Results

- Eosinophil count >1000/mm^3
- Lymphocytosis with atypical lymphocytes
- Abnormal results on liver-function tests

Roujeau JC, Stern RS. Severe Adverse Cutaneous Reactions to Drugs. (N Engl J Med 1994; 331:1272–1285).

*The outer layer of the epidermis separates readily from the basal layer with lateral pressure.

Management

Treatment

The offending drug must be discontinued. Oral antihistamines can help alleviate itching. Steroids may be used if the itching is not controlled with antihistamines and there are no contraindications to steroid use.

Discharge/Follow up Plans

The patient should be counseled to notify any future medical provider about his or her drug allergy, and a medical alert bracelet should be considered. The discharge summary should clearly review the nature of the reaction and the offending drug.

URTICARIA (HIVES)/ANGIOEDEMA/ANAPHYLAXIS

Assessment

Clinical Presentation

These are the second-most common types of drug reaction and are covered in detail in Chapter 81, Allergic Reactions and Angioedema. They can be considered as a spectrum of the same dis-

order mediated either by IgE-, complement-, or kinin-metabolism induced pathways. Urticaria is distinguished by superficial wheals that are transient for hours and pruritic (Fig. 82-2).

Angioedema involves the deep dermal and subcutaneous tissues involving the face, especially the lips and tongue. Patients with angioedema need to be closely monitored for respiratory compromise due to severe tongue or laryngeal swelling while being treated. Anaphylaxis is the most severe and life threatening of these disorders, and is characterized by respiratory distress due to laryngeal edema and hypotension due to vascular collapse. Antibiotics (especially the penicillins), anesthetics, and radiocontrast agents are the most common causes of serious anaphylactic reactions. Angiotensin-converting enzyme (ACE) inhibitors are a common cause of angioedema (0.1–0.7%) due to bradykinin inhibition. Angioedema can occur at any time during their use and prohibits future use of ACE inhibitors. Angiotensin-receptor antagonists are not known to affect bradykinin metabolism, but must be used cautiously in these patients, as they appear to have a higher recurrence of angioedema.[3]

Differential Diagnosis

Foods, insect bites, and contact allergens commonly cause urticaria. The allergen may not be identified in many people. Urticaria that does not blanch is suggestive of vasculitis as an etiology.

Diagnosis

The diagnosis is straightforward, based on the appearance of the eruption. A detailed history of exposures is necessary to help elucidate the cause.

Management

Treatment

The treatment of urticaria and mild angioedema begins with stopping the offending drug and using antihistamines. H$_1$ blockers should be used initially, and H$_2$ blockers can be added if symptoms are not controlled. The treatment for severe angioedema and anaphylaxis is more critical. Airway patency must be closely monitored. In addition to intravenous antihistamines, intravenous fluid resuscitation, epinephrine (0.3–0.5 mL of 1 : 1000 dilution subcutaneously, repeat in 15–20 minutes if needed) and steroids, either intravenous (hydrocortisone 100 mg every 6 hours) or oral (prednisone 60 mg initially), need to be immediately administered.

Discharge/Follow-up Plans

The patient should be counseled to notify any future medical provider about his or her drug allergy and a medical alert bracelet should be considered. If steroids need to be given, they should be tapered over 2 weeks. The discharge summary should clearly discuss the nature of the reaction and the offending drug.

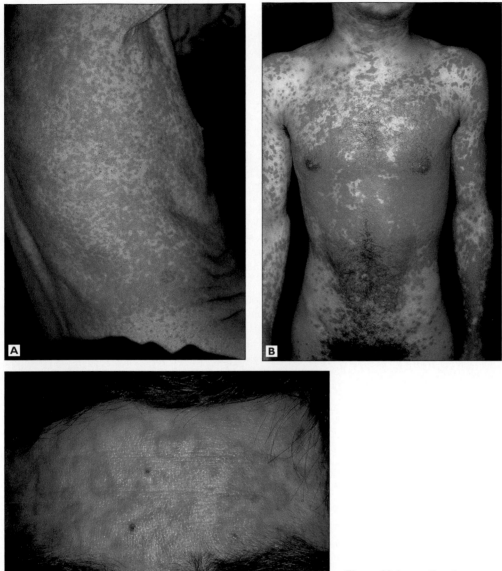

Figure 82-1 • Exanthematous drug eruption. From dermtext.com Figure 23-1.

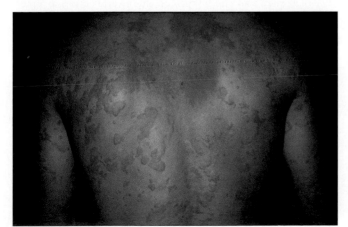

Figure 82-2 • Urticaria secondary to penicillin. From: dermtext.com Figure 23.2.

BLISTERING DRUG ERUPTIONS

Assessment

Clinical Presentation

Steven Johnson syndrome (SJS) and toxic epidermal necrolysis (TEN) are severe blistering diseases that usually are drug induced. They both can start out with a similar pattern of erythema and skin tenderness and then can evolve to diffuse bullae and eventually epidermal detachment and necrosis (Fig. 82-3). SJS is less severe, while patients with TEN appear toxic and have a much higher mortality rate. Associated findings with both disorders include fever, severe pain, and multiorgan involvement. Acute renal failure from acute tubular necrosis and epithelial erosions in the respiratory and gastrointestinal tract can occur.

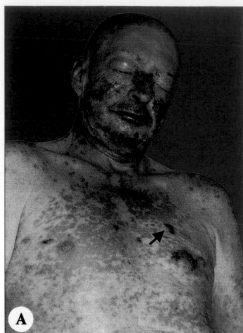

Figure 82-3 • SJS vs. SJS-TEN overlap. From: dermtext.com Figure 22.6.

Differential Diagnosis

Erythema multiforme was initially felt to be related to SJS, but it is now considered a distinct syndrome secondary to herpes simplex infection. Staphylococcal scalded skin syndrome, autoimmune bullous diseases, and graft-versus-host disease can present similar to TEN.

Diagnosis

Skin biopsy with frozen section can confirm the diagnosis of TEN and distinguish it from the other bullous diseases.

Prognosis

The mortality rate in SJS is 5%, but in TEN it can be as high as 30% among the elderly.

The recurrence can be even more severe than the initial episode if the patient is re-exposed to the offending drug.

Management

Treatment

Treatment includes immediately stopping the offending drug. If more than 10% of the body surface area is involved or the course is rapidly worsening, the patient should be transferred to a burn unit. Aggressive intravenous fluid and electrolyte replacement is needed. Corticosteroid use is controversial but may be helpful in the early stages. High-dose intravenous immunoglobulins can stop progression of TEN if started early in the course. Antibiotics should only be used if superimposed bacterial infection or sepsis is suspected.

Discharge/Follow-up Plans

The patient should be counseled to notify any future medical provider about his or her drug allergy, and a medical alert bracelet should be worn at all times. The discharge summary should clearly discuss the nature of the reaction and the offending drug.

DERMATOLOGIC MIMICS OF CELLULITIS

BACKGROUND

Cellulitis is one of the most common soft tissue infections in patients, often leading to hospital admission for further evaluation and treatment. The assessment and management of cellulitis are covered in detail in Chapter 36, Skin and Soft Tissue Infections. This section will review the dermatologic diseases that can present similar to cellulitis and how they can be distinguished. Usually, the hospitalist will consider these etiologies after the patient fails to respond to empirical antibiotic therapy, but there can be clues early in the presentation that may alert the hospitalist to other possibilities.

Cellulitis usually presents as an acute (few days) of a red, hot, edematous plaque that is well demarcated and extremely tender. The plaque can progress and form bullae. A portal of entry such as a break in the skin may be present. Risk factors include chronic skin disorders such as eczema or ulcers and fungal infections, especially *tinea pedis*. Fever is almost always present, and, depending on the severity, sepsis may occur.

Chronic Venous Insufficiency

Patients with chronic venous insufficiency (CVI) have a history of longstanding, intermittent edema that worsens with standing and resolves after leg elevation. However, patients with CVI can have an acute worsening of the edema after unusually prolonged standing or physical activity that can lead to more pain, redness, and warmth than they have experienced. Other skin diseases superimposed on CVI may also mimic cellulites, such as ulcers, stasis dermatitis, or lipodermatosclerosis (Fig. 82-4). Lipodermatosclerosis is an indurated, erythematous plaque on the lower third of the leg that can be painful acutely and causes a "piano leg" appearance with edema above and below the affected area.

If both lower extremities are involved, CVI should be considered as a possible etiology, as bilateral cellulitis is rare. Absence of fever further supports the unlikelihood of cellulitis. The diagnosis is made clinically, based on longstanding edema in the both lower legs that improves with elevation.

Bedrest, elevation of the legs, and compression therapy can result in marked improvement over 24 hours, and antibiotics are not necessary. If a patient has ulcers due to CVI or the findings are significantly worse in one leg, superimposed cellulitis may be present, and empiric antibiotics should be considered.

Contact Dermatitis

Contact dermatitis is an inflammatory reaction in the skin due to a foreign substance. Patients with leg ulcers and venous

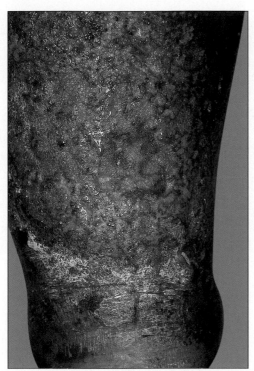

Figure 82-4 ● Stasis dermatitis. From: dermtext.com Figure 14.4.

insufficiency are at higher risk to develop contact dermatitis of the lower legs. However, this reaction can occur anywhere on the body. The patient should be asked about any recent exposures to possible offending agents such as detergents, solvents, metals, and plants. Acutely, the eruption can look very similar to cellulites, presenting as a well-demarcated erythematous plaque. However, it not as painful as expected with cellulitis and more pruritic. The patterns of skin involvement can also help, especially any linear or sharply angulated areas that point to an "outside job." Skin biopsy and patch testing can be used to confirm the diagnosis.

Treatment with topical corticosteroids is usually sufficient, but systemic steroids may be needed for severe cases. These should be tapered over a 2-week period to prevent a relapse.

Deep Venous Thrombosis

Deep venous thrombosis (DVT) typically presents as unilateral leg pain, swelling, erythema, and warmth that can easily be mistaken for cellulitis. Fever and leukocytosis can be present in both conditions. Use of a clinical decision rule can aid in determining the clinical probability of DVT. However, history and physical may not be clearly diagnostic for distinguishing the two conditions, and evaluation with D-dimer and ultrasound should be performed if DVT is suspected. The assessment and management of DVT are reviewed in detail in Chapter 26.

Carcinoma Erysipelatoides

Carcinoma erysipelatoides is caused by metastatic spread of malignant cells to cutaneous lymph vessels. It most commonly occurs in breast cancer. The clinical appearance can be confused with cellulitis because it presents as an erythematous plaque. If fever and leukocytosis are not present and the involved area is on the breast, carcinoma erysipelatoides should be considered. Mammography and tissue biopsy can confirm the diagnosis. Treatment is dependent on the underlying malignancy.

SKIN INFECTIONS

COMMUNITY-ACQUIRED METHICILLIN-RESISTANT *STAPHYLOCOCCUS AUREUS*

Background

Hospitalists are quite familiar with nosocomial methicillin-resistant *Staphylococcus aureus* (MRSA) that has been increasing in prevalence since its emergence 40 years ago. Acquisition of MRSA is typically associated with health care institutions (hospitals and long-term care facilities) and patients who have prolonged hospitalizations, past antimicrobial use, indwelling catheters, or hemodialysis. Infections due to MRSA present a considerable challenge to hospitalists since their presence increases mortality and length of hospital stay. Since the 1990s, novel strains of MRSA have been isolated from patients who have had no recent associations with hospitals. These infections have been termed community-acquired MRSA (CA-MRSA).

The prevalence of CA-MRSA has been steadily increasing, and patients are relatively young, healthy, and without risk factors for MRSA. Because of this increased prevalence, it is important for the hospitalist to be aware of this emerging infection and to recognize, treat, and isolate patients who may harbor this infection, even though they have been admitted for a different problem. MRSA is more prevalent than methicillin sensitive S. aureus in some communities.

Assessment

Clinical Presentation

Most patients from whom CA-MRSA is isolated present with skin or soft tissue infections. Frequently, the patient states that he or she has a "spider bite" and may not have noted any break or open wound in the involved area. The continuum of skin findings ranges from mild folliculitis to abscesses or furuncles (deeper seated abscess) to carbuncles (interconnecting abscesses). The skin around the lesions can be red, warm, and tender as well (Fig. 82-5). There may be a single lesion or multiple lesions, and the extremities and trunk are commonly involved. Occasionally, the patient may have bacteremia with CA-MRSA.

Differential Diagnosis

The most common organisms that can cause similar skin infections include methicillin-sensitive *Staphylococcus aureus* and group A streptococcus. A ruptured epidermoid cyst may be mistaken for an abscess, but usually the patient recalls having prior episodes of swelling in the affected area.

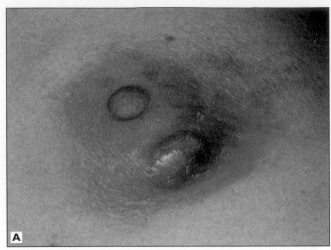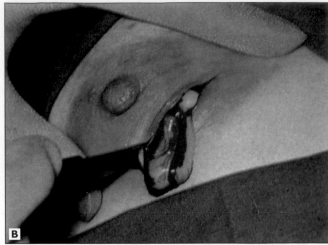

Figure 82-5 • Staphylococcal abscess. From: Forbes and Jackson: Colour Atlas and Text of Clinical Medicine Figure 1.80, 1.81.

Diagnosis

The Centers for Disease Control and Prevention (CDC) has established criteria to distinguish CA-MRSA from HA-MRSA isolates. According to these criteria, CA-MRSA is diagnosed when a culture is obtained in the outpatient setting or within 48 hours after admission to the hospital. The patient must not have experienced any of the following during the year before infection: hospitalization; admission to a nursing home, skilled nursing facility, or hospice; dialysis; or surgery. In addition, the patient must be without permanent indwelling catheters or medical devices that pass through the skin into the body.

Management

Treatment

Incision and drainage is the first-line treatment for any fluctuant skin infections. It alone may be sufficient for an isolated lesion that is adequately drained. However, if there are multiple lesions, concurrent cellulites, or incision and drainage is inadequate, antibiotics should be started. Antibiotic selection can be guided by local susceptibility patterns and sensitivity of the isolate once available. If the skin and/or soft tissue infection is the reason for admission, the patient should be started on intravenous vancomycin. If the skin infections are mild and not the primary reason for admission, oral antibiotics may be used. Trimethoprim-sulfamethoxazole, clindamycin, minocycline, and linezolid have been used successfully, though resistance to clindamycin is on the rise. Our approach is to start with trimethoprim-sulfamethoxazole for 7–10 days if CA-MRSA is suspected. If the response is inadequate, the antibiotics are changed depending on the susceptibility pattern of the isolate, or rifampin is added to the regimen. Rifampin should not be used as monotherapy, as resistance can rapidly develop. Linezolid and daptomycin are reserved for severely ill patients with HA-MRSA. Any patient hospitalized with MRSA should be placed in contact isolation to prevent further spread.

CANDIDIASIS IN THE HOSPITALIZED PATIENT

Background

Mucosal and cutaneous candidal infectious have a variety of presentations, and they are quite common in hospitalized patients. While these infections are rarely the reason for admission to the hospital, they often present comorbid to a patient's underlying medical problems, and they sometimes develop as a direct result of a patient's hospitalization. A brief discussion of the most commonly encountered superficial candidal infections in hospitalized patients, oral and cutaneous candidiasis follows.

Assessment

Clinical Presentation

Presenting Signs and Symptoms

The most common presentation of oral candidiasis is pseudomembranous candidiasis, or thrush, which presents as white, cheesy patches on the tongue, buccal mucosa, palate, and oropharynx. These patches scrape off with a tongue blade and may reveal friable underlying tissue. Predisposing factors include diabetes mellitus, antimicrobial therapy, corticosteroids (including inhaled, systemic and topical), denture use, and immunosuppression, including HIV and malignancy.[4]

Cutaneous candidiasis most frequently presents as intertrigo. The surfaces most often involved are the inguinal, perineal, inframammary, and finger web spaces, where occlusion, heat, and moisture lead to overgrowth of yeast. Hospitalized patients are at increased risk for developing intertrigo. Other risk factors include diabetes mellitus, systemic antibiotic therapy, and obesity. "Diaper dermatitis" is an important entity to consider in incontinent hospitalized patients, as urine ammonia combined with the above factors creates an ideal environment for candida infection.[4]

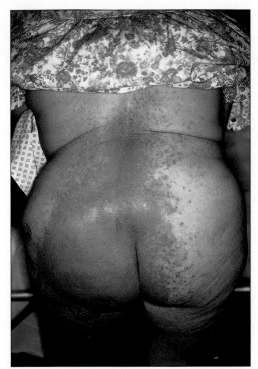

Figure 82-6 • Cutaneous candidiasis in a hospitalized, diabetic patient. From: dermtext.com Figure 77.19.

Intertrigo lesions present as macerated erythematous plaques with peripheral scale and often satellite papules or pustules (Fig. 82-6).

Differential Diagnosis

Oral candidiasis can be confused with leukoplakia, which presents with white plaques that do not scrape off as candidal plaques do. Intertrigo can appear similarly to contact or atopic dermatitis.

Diagnosis

Oral and cutaneous candidiasis may be diagnosed by performing a potassium hydroxide preparation of a scraping from a lesion. Microscopic examination should reveal pseudohyphae.

Prognosis

The prognosis for candidal infections is good, and most outbreaks respond well to standard treatment, as long as risk factors are well controlled.

Management

Treatment

Initial

The first aim of treatment for candidiasis is to control underlying risk factors like diabetes and immunosuppression. Antifungal regimens for oral candidiasis include topical therapy with Clotrimazole troches five times a day for 2 weeks, or Nystatin pastilles, one to two pastilles five times a day for 2 weeks, and systemic therapy

with oral fluconazole 200 mg to start, then 100 mg daily for 13 days. For cutaneous candidiasis, in addition to controlling the above risk factors, treatment should start with controlling local factors such as moisture, heat, and occlusion. Drying agents like acetic acid solution, zinc oxide paste, and Burow's solution may help decrease moisture. Polyene and azole topical antifungal preparations are the mainstay of treatment. Cutaneous candidal infections should respond to a 14-day course of these agents applied twice daily. In cases accompanied by severe inflammation, a short (1-week) course of a midpotency topical corticosteroid may be necessary in addition to antifungal therapy.

Subsequent

Oral agents may be required in addition to topical therapy for resistant or recurrent infections. Fluconazole is most commonly used, at a dose of 100 mg daily for 1-2 weeks. Fluconazole-resistant infections may respond to itraconazole or ketoconazole 200 mg daily for 5–7 days. Both fluconazole and itraconazole have significant medication interactions that are important to be aware of in the hospitalized patient.

Prevention

Controlling local factors such as moisture, heat, and occlusion will help prevent cutaneous candidal infections, as will achieving optimal control of diabetes mellitus, when present.

Discharge/Follow-up Plans

Patients should be discharged with instructions to complete the prescribed course of antifungal therapy started in the hospital. Follow-up with a dermatologist may be necessary if the patient fails to respond to the full course of treatment. Patients should be educated about the importance of controlling risk factors including diabetes mellitus and local factors such as moisture and occlusion.

HIV-RELATED DERMATOSES

Background

Cutaneous disease frequently accompanies HIV infection and AIDS. Rashes and other skin disease may be the presenting complaint of a patient with HIV/AIDS or may be an incidental finding. The hospitalist should be familiar with the most common of these skin diseases and should know how to initiate treatment and when to refer to a dermatologist. Patients with HIV/AIDS often present with characteristic infections, severe manifestations of common skin diseases, common rashes with uncommon presentations, or extreme worsening of existing skin disease. In fact, the severe presentation of a common rash, like seborrheic dermatitis or herpes simplex, may be the primary clue to HIV diagnosis. Several of the most common cutaneous diseases associated with HIV/AIDS and their diagnosis and treatment are outlined below.

Seborrheic Dermatitis

Seborrheic dermatitis is the most common dermatosis associated with HIV infection, occurring in up to 85% of patients with

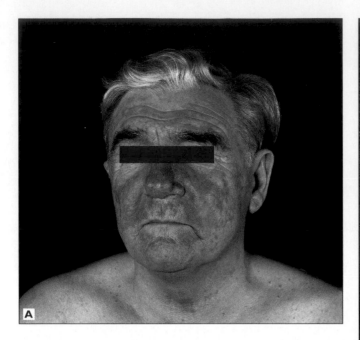
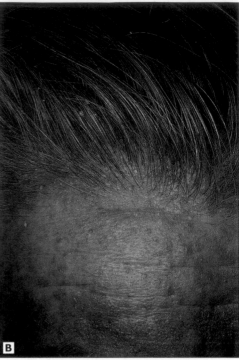

Figure 82-7 • Seborrheic dermatitis. From: dermtext.com Figure 14.2.

HIV[5,6]. Though classified as an inflammatory disorder, it has been associated with *Pityrosporum* yeast infection. The condition is characterized by discrete, erythematous, scaling, greasy plaques located most commonly on the scalp, eyebrows, eyelids, nasolabial folds, and ears (Fig. 82-7). It less commonly involves the central back and chest, as well as the axillae and groin. These lesions are usually asymptomatic but may be pruritic. As with other inflammatory conditions, the diagnosis is usually made clinically. In severe cases, marked erythema and scale on the face may be confused with psoriasis or fungal infection, which may be ruled out with a potassium hydroxide preparation. Seborrheic dermatitis is not only more severe, but often more resistant to treatment in patients with AIDS. The goal in treating seborrheic dermatitis is control rather than cure, as it is a chronic, recurrent disease. The lesions are treated with low-potency topical corticosteroids and imidazole antifungal agents (ketoconazole 2% shampoo or cream). A brief course of a systemic imidazole like itraconazole may be necessary. Alternative treatments for scalp involvement include shampoos containing tar, selenium sulfide, or pyrithione zinc. Although the use of mid-potency corticosteroids is generally avoided on the face, a short course (not exceeding 7 days) of these agents may be necessary to treat a severe eruption.

Herpes Zoster

The incidence of herpes zoster decreases with decline in immune function, and this infection affects approximately 25% of patients with HIV.[5] The eruption is usually preceded by 2–3 days by pain and paresthesia in the affected dermatome. The most commonly affected dermatomes are thoracic, followed by lumbar and trigeminal. The eruption consists initially of grouped erythema-tous macules and papules, which develop into vesicles on an erythematous base in a dermatomal distribution. Vesicles can become ulcerative, necrotic, or even verrucous. Most commonly, 1 or 2 dermatomes are affected, but it is not unusual to see an adjacent third dermatome involved. Lesions are unilateral, and with the exception of a few scattered vesicles, they do not cross the midline. It is important to look for involvement of the nose tip, as this is an indicator of potential ocular involvement necessitating ophthalmology consultation (Fig. 82-8).

In immunocompromised patients, herpes zoster may become disseminated, with scattered, widespread vesicles erupting outside of a dermatomal distribution. Atypical presentations of zoster include paresthesias without cutaneous eruption or motor nerve involvement. Common complications include secondary infection and post-herpetic neuralgia. Diagnosis is based on a typical history and physical examination findings, although VZV (varicella zoster virus) culture, direct fluorescent antibody stain, and biopsy with special stains may be performed in cases with atypical presentations.

Treatment with antiviral therapy shortens the duration of illness, decreases severity of pain, and possibly decreases the incidence of postherpetic neuralgia. In immunocompromised patients, antiviral therapy limits cutaneous dissemination and visceral involvement. These results are more likely if treatment is initiated in the first 48 hours after the onset of the rash. Immunocompromised patients should be prescribed valacyclovir 1 g PO TID for 7 days or until lesions are healed. Famciclovir 500 mg PO TID for 7 days is an alternative, but the previous standard of Acyclovir 800 mg PO five times a day for 7–10 days is problematic from a compliance standpoint. If the eruption is severe or spreads on oral therapy, intravenous acyclovir 10 mg/kg IV every 8 hours for 7–14 days should be initiated. Patients who do not respond

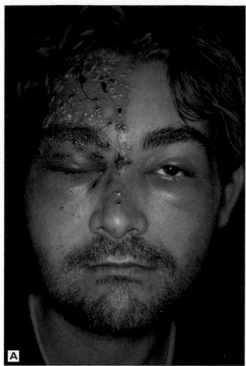
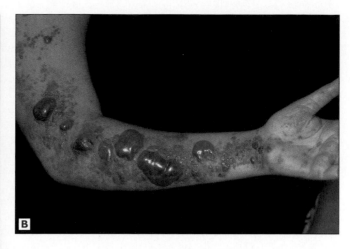

Figure 82-8 • Herpes zoster. From: dermtext.com Figure 80.12.

to IV acyclovir may require treatment with intravenous foscarnet.

Patients with disseminated zoster should be placed on respiratory isolation. The use of adjunctive systemic corticosteroid therapy has been advocated, but studies reveal that only otherwise healthy patients over the age of 50 benefit from the addition of steroids to acyclovir therapy. Amitriptyline reduces both acute and chronic pain associated with herpes zoster. Non-opiate or opiate analgesics are often necessary for pain control, and if pruritus is prominent, a systemic antihistamine is also indicated.

Prurigo Nodularis

The inciting factor in this eruption is pruritus, which is a common symptom in HIV disease. Lichenified, dome-shaped, firm nodules develop as a result of chronic scratching. Lesions are often hyperpigmented but may be erythematous or skin colored. They are multiple and are often excoriated. As lesions are caused by scratching, they are only located in areas within the patient's reach, but are most common on the back, legs, and arms. The central back is often spared, as this area is hard to reach (Fig. 82-9). Getting a history of chronic pruritus preceding the eruption is helpful for the diagnosis, but as lesions may be confused with tumors, especially in an immunocompromised patient, skin biopsy may be necessary to confirm the diagnosis. Patients should also undergo evaluation for a correctable cause of pruritus, which may include folliculitis. Patients are sometimes treated empirically for staphylococcal folliculitis. Treatment consists of patient education and high-potency topical corticosteroids applied BID under occlusive dressings. Nighttime amitriptyline can be a useful adjunctive therapy.

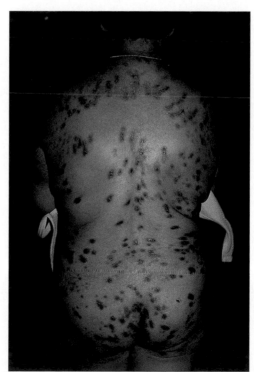

Figure 82-9 • Prurigo nodularis. From: dermtext.com Figure 7.7

Kaposi's Sarcoma

Kaposi's sarcoma (KS) is an AIDS-defining skin malignancy of the capillary endothelium, and it affects 15% of people with AIDS.[6] It is associated with human herpes virus 8. The incidence of KS has significantly declined in recent years with advances in therapy for HIV infection. Lesions begin as erythematous macules or papules and later develop into oval-shaped, violaceous, or red/brown plaques or nodules in patients with light skin, and dark brown or black lesions in patients with dark skin (Fig. 82-10). KS lesions occur on the trunk, extremities, face, and oral mucosa, most commonly on the tip of the nose and hard palate.[6]

These lesions are usually asymptomatic. Visceral lesions may also occur, affecting the lungs, gastrointestinal (GI) tract, and lymph nodes. Differential diagnosis includes bacillary angiomatosis, and the diagnosis of KS must be confirmed by biopsy.

In many cases, lesions have an indolent course and do not require treatment, although patients may elect to have treatment to alleviate symptoms if present or for cosmetic reasons. Treatment for individual lesions consists of cryotherapy with liquid nitrogen. Alternatives included intralesional vinblastine chemotherapy, interferon alpha, or radiation therapy. Systemic therapy may be needed for extensive internal involvement with KS. Improvement of CD4 cell counts with HAART can lead to resolution of KS lesions. Recurrences of the neoplasm are common with all forms of therapy.

Herpes Simplex

Herpes simplex (HSV) infections are quite common in HIV-infected patients. In fact, chronic ulcerating HSV infection that lasts for more than 1 month is an AIDS-defining illness.[7] The appearance of lesions is often preceded by a prodrome of burning or tingling at the eruption site. Lesions start out as grouped vesicles on an erythematous base that later ulcerate. Lesions may occur in the oral, anal, and genital regions; and they must be differentiated from those caused by cytomegalovirus (CMV), syphilis, chancroid and granuloma inguinale (Fig. 82-11). In immunocompromised patients, HSV is often complicated by severe, persistent, deep ulcers and disseminated infection with visceral involvement. Any ulcerative lesion should be evaluated by Tzanck smear to look for multinucleated giant cells. Viral culture, PCR, or biopsy can also help differentiate HSV from other infections. Immunocompromised patients with HSV often require both longer courses of treatment and chronic suppressive therapy. Treatment for HSV is with oral acyclovir, 400 mg five times a day for 14–21 days or until lesions heal and then 400 mg BID indefinitely to prevent recurrences. Alternatives include famciclovir 500 mg BID for 7 days, followed by 500 mg BID for suppression or valacyclovir 500 mg BID for 5–10 days followed by 500 mg BID for suppression. As with herpes zoster, herpes simplex can disseminate, requiring treatment with systemic antiviral agents (acyclovir 5 mg/kg IV every 8 hours for 7 days).

Eosinophilic Folliculitis

Eosinophilic folliculitis (Ofugi disease) is a rare skin condition that is seen in the United States primarily in patients with AIDS. The etiology is thought to be infectious, although no causative organism has been identified. It presents as erythematous papules,

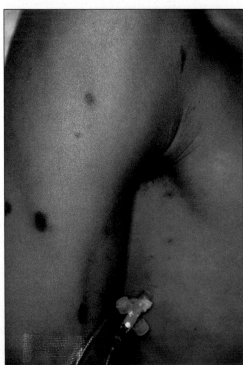

Figure 82-10 • Kaposi's sarcoma in a patient with AIDS. From: dermtext.com Figure 115.18.

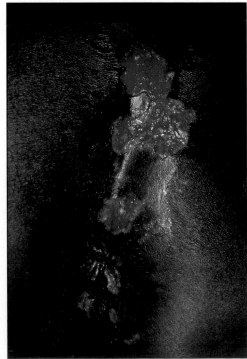

Figure 82-11 • Chronic herpes simplex in a patient with HIV infection. From: dermtext.com Figure 78.4.

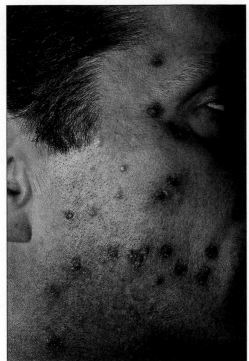

Figure 82-12 • Eosinophilic folliculitis. From: dermtext.com
Figure 78.8.

sterile pustules, and nodules on the face, trunk, and extremities (Fig. 82-12). In patients with dark skin, the lesions may be skin colored or hyperpigmented. The lesions are nonscaling and extremely pruritic. Associated laboratory findings include eosinophilia, leukocytosis, and elevated IgE levels. Differential diagnosis includes infective folliculitis, acne, and pustular drug eruption. Culture of pustule contents and/or biopsy may be necessary to distinguish between these entities.[6] Eosinophilic folliculitis is very difficult to manage, and the disease often persists despite treatment. Treatment options include topical corticosteroids, dapsone, metronidazole, isotretinoin, or ultraviolet B phototherapy.

RASH AND FEVER

Background

The approach to the hospitalized patient with a fever and rash can be very challenging because of the vast number of potential etiologies. Infectious diseases, inflammatory diseases, and malignancies all may produce fever and rash. Some patients with fever and rash require no therapy, while others require immediate intervention (e.g., meningococcemia or Rocky Mountain spotted fever), including some level of isolation. The hospitalist must fully assess all patients with fever and rash, develop a differential diagnosis, and institute an appropriate management plan. The history and physical examination are the most important tools in determining the etiology of a fever and rash; ancillary studies are of limited value.

Box 82-2 Components of the History and Physical

- **Time and circumstance surrounding the onset of the rash**
  - Date and time the patient or hospital staff first noticed the eruption

    It is very important to determine if the rash began before admission and if the patient underwent procedures immediately preceding the onset of the rash
  - Changes in the severity of the rash since its onset
  - Changes in the characteristics of the rash including the direction of spread
    - Some rashes begin on the face and chest progressing centrifugally; others begin distally and spread centripetally
  - Interventions or circumstances that have modified the rash
- **Past medical history**
  - Complete medication history
    - Especially medications recently started
    - Prescription medications, over-the-counter medications, borrowed medications, and recreational drugs
    - Medications administered in the hospital, including those administered during tests and procedures
  - Chronic infections, immune status, connective tissue diseases, malignant diseases, and any known drug allergies
- **Review of systems**
  - Upper respiratory or gastrointestinal complaints may suggest a viral infection
  - Arthralgias—seen in cutaneous vasculitis, disseminated gonococcal infection, erythema infectiosum (parvovirus B-19), erythema marginatum, hepatitis, Lyme disease, Reiter's disease, rheumatoid arthritis, Still's disease, and systemic lupus erythematosus
- **Recent exposures**
  - Changes in diet, recent travel, especially foreign travel, recent immunizations, sexual contacts, exposure to ill persons, excessive sun exposure, and exposures to wild or domestic animals

---

Assessment

Clinical Presentation

The history and physical should focus on specific issues relevant to making the diagnosis and treatment. These are detailed in Box 82-2.

The physical examination should be complete with an emphasis on cutaneous structures, including the scalp, hair, and nails.
- General examination with emphasis on examination of:
  - Major joints and neck
  - Neurologic status
  - Lymphatics, liver, and spleen
  - Mucous membranes
- Skin examination:
  - Determine the type of primary lesions present
  - Determine the configuration of the primary lesions

Table 82-1 Fever with Erythema

Localized erythema:	Generalized erythema:
Acute febrile neutropenic dermatosis (Sweet's syndrome)	Drug allergy
Dermatomyositis	HIV seroconversion reaction
Erysipelas	Kawasaki's disease
Erythema infectiosum	Mononucleosis
Familial Mediterranean fever	Necrolytic migratory erythema
Kawasaki's disease	Pustular psoriasis
Leptospirosis	Respiratory syncytial virus infection
Lyme disease	Scarlet fever
Sarcoidosis	Staphylococcal scalded skin syndrome
	Staphylococcal toxic shock syndrome
	Still's disease

Box 82-3 Fever with Vesicles or Bullae

Acute febrile neutropenic dermatosis (Sweet's syndrome)

Coxsackievirus infection

Echovirus infection

Erysipelas

Erythema multiforme

Graft vs. host disease

Herpes simplex

Herpes zoster

Miliaria

Mycoplasma infection

Pyoderma gangrenosum

Rickettsialpox

Staphylococcal scalded skin syndrome

Stevens-Johnson syndrome

Vaccinia

Varicella

Vibrio vulnificus infections

Box 82-4 Fever with Other Cutaneous Manifestations

Furuncles—Furunculosis due to *S. aureus*, MRSA, CA-MRSA

Nodules—acne fulminans, erythema nodosum, Lofgren's syndrome, erythema induratum

Target lesions—erythema multiforme, Stevens-Johnson syndrome

Ulcerations—HSV or CMV in immunocompromised, pyoderma gangrenosum

82-2 because they so often coexist. They may be variable in size and color. Petechiae, purpura, and ecchymoses refer to extravasated blood; and these lesions do not blanch with pressure. Vesicles, bullae, and special lesion types are also included in the tables. The distribution of lesions may provide a primary clue to the diagnosis. Lesions of the palms and soles are more common in: atypical measles, drug reactions, erythema multiforme, hand-foot-mouth disease, Kawasaki disease, Rocky Mountain spotted fever, secondary syphilis, and toxic shock syndrome. Mucous membranes are often involved in herpes simplex, mononucleosis (petechia), Kawasaki disease, scarlet fever, toxic shock syndrome (strawberry tongue), rubeola (Koplik's spots), and rubella (Forchheimer spots).

Diagnosis

Skin biopsy upon recommendation of a dermatologist may be needed to determine the correct etiology. Depending on the differential diagnosis considered, tissue may be sent for routine hematoxylin and eosin staining; special stains for bacteria, fungi, spirochetes, and acid-fast bacilli; immunohistochemical staining; immunofluorescence studies; and culture for bacteria, fungi, acid-fast organisms, and viruses. A dermatology consultant should guide this testing. With the exception of facilities capable of performing rush processing, biopsy results will usually require more than 72 hours, and cultures longer. Therefore, the clinician will need to rely on clinical observation, and in rare cases, direct microscopy (e.g., potassium hydroxide preparation, Tzanck preparation, crush preparation). Biopsies and cultures may be most helpful by confirming the diagnosis in a patient with a rash and fever. Acute and convalescent serologic studies should also be considered in the case of suspected viral infections.

- Randomly scattered
- Grouped as in herpes simplex or herpes zoster
- Determine the distribution of the lesions
  - Localized
  - Generalized
  - Mucous membrane involvement

Differential Diagnosis

Due to the large number of potential etiologies, it is necessary to develop a logical method for reaching a differential diagnosis for the patient with a fever and rash. One such method is to group the differential diagnoses according to the type of primary lesion. It is important to realize that rashes evolve, and more than one type of lesion may be present at the time of the examination. In Boxes 82-1, 82-2, 82-3, 82-4 and Tables 82-1 through 82-4, erythema refers to confluent redness of the skin that blanches with pressure. Macules (flat) and papules (raised) are grouped in Table

Table 82-2 Fever with Cutaneous Macules and/or Papules

Bartonella infection	Miliaria
Brucellosis	Mononucleosis
Colorado tick fever	Mycobacterial infection
Cytomegalovirus infection	*Mycoplasma* infection
Dengue	*Pseudomonas* infection
Drug allergy	Rat bite fever
Erythema chronicum migrans	Relapsing fever
Erythema infectiosum	Rickettsialpox
Exanthem subitum (roseola infantum, sixth disease)	Rocky Mountain spotted fever
Fungal infections, disseminated	Rubeola, rubella, atypical measles
Candida spp.	*Salmonella* infection
Cryptococus neoformans	Sarcoidosis
Histoplasma capsulatum	Scarlet fever
Blastomyces dermatitidis	Secondary syphilis
Coccidioides immitis	Staphylococcal infection
Fusarium spp.	Systemic lupus erythematosus
Gonococcemia	Toxic shock syndrome
Gram-negative bacteremia	Toxoplasmosis
Hepatitis B	Tularemia
Herpes simplex	Typhus
Herpes zoster	Varicella
Human herpes virus 6 infection	Viral exanthems
HIV	Enterovirus
Leptospirosis	Adenovirus
Listeriosis	Echovirus
Lyme disease	Coxackievirus
Meningococcemia	Rotavirus

Table 82-3 Fever with Cutaneous Petechiae, Purpura, or Ecchymoses

Bacteremia	Rocky Mountain spotted fever
Brazilian purpuric fever	Rubeola, rubella, atypical measles
Brucellosis	Scarlet fever
Colorado tick fever	Toxic shock syndrome
Corynebacterium infection	Typhus
Dengue	Vasculitis
Drug allergy	Infections (e.g., hepatitis B)
Gonococcemia	Autoimmune diseases
Hemorrhagic fevers, viral	Neoplasms, lymphomas and leukemias
Malaria	Viral exanthems
Meningococcemia	Adenovirus
Mononucleosis	Echovirus
Rat bite fever	Coxsackievirus
Relapsing fever	Wegener's granulomatosus
Respiratory syncytial virus infection	Yellow fever

Prognosis

Some patients with fever and rash will require no therapy and will recover uneventfully. In others, the prognosis is directly related to the clinician's success determining the etiology and initiating appropriate therapy promptly. Drug eruptions may persist indefinitely if the offending agent is not recognized and discontinued. In the case of meningococcemia or Rocky Mountain spotted fever, the prognosis is good if the patient is diagnosed and treated early, but the prognosis is very poor otherwise.

Table 82-4 Selected Diseases that Present with Rash and Fever

Disease	Major skin findings	Diagnostic tests	Therapy	Isolation
Meningococcemia	Erythematous macules evolving to petechiae and purpura	Culture of blood, CSF, or skin (treatment must be initiated prior to result)	Cefotaxime 2 g IV q 4 hr or Ceftriaxone 2 g IV q 12 hr	Airborne
RMSF	Erythematous macules initially, petechiae and purpura may appear late	Indirect immunofluorescence assay	Doxycycline 100 mg twice daily; second line is chloramphenicol 50–100 mg/kg/day IV	None
CA-MRSA	Furuncles	Culture and sensitivity	TMP/SMX twice daily or clindamycin 300 mg twice daily and rifampin 600 mg/day	Enhanced contact
Zoster	Dermatomal erythema and vesicles	Viral culture, direct immunofluorescence	Immunocompetent: acyclovir 800 mg orally 5 times daily	Airborne
SJS/TEN	Tender cutaneous erythema with blisters and erosions, mucosal lesions common	Biopsy (consider frozen section)	Identification and removal of offending agent, supportive care, consider burn unit admission	None

TMP/SMX—trimethoprim/sulfamethoxazole 160 mg/800 mg; SJS/TEN—Stevens Johnson syndrome/toxic opidermal necrolysis; CA-MRSA—community-acquired methicillin resistant *S. aureus*; RMSF—rocky mountain spotted fever; CSF—cerebrospinal fluid

Management

Treatment

Therapy for the patient with a fever and rash may involve isolation, topical therapies, systemic therapies, and transfer to specialized units. Infectious etiologies present the most critical need for correct diagnosis and management. Any patient suspected of having meningococcemia must be isolated, and appropriate antibiotics should be started immediately. Rapid antibiotic therapy is also imperative for patients having symptoms of Rocky Mountain spotted fever. For uncomplicated viral exanthems, macular and/or papular drug eruptions, and similar eruptions, soothing topical lotions (e.g., calamine) and antihistamines orally may be helpful. For more symptomatic eruptions and those suspected of progressing to a life-threatening state, systemic immunosuppressive agents may be needed. In the case of severe drug eruptions (SJS, TEN), transfer of the patient to a burn unit may be life saving.

Discharge/Follow-up Plans

Patients with persistent eruptions at the time of discharge should be given a follow-up appointment with a dermatologist and a sufficient amount of medication to use until that appointment.

BLISTERING DISEASES

Background

The hospitalist will encounter patients with blisters under three circumstances: (1) admissions to the hospital from the Emergency Department because of a new or existing blistering disease; (2) patients with known blistering admitted for an additional, possibly unrelated, medical problem; and (3) on rare occasions, hospitalized patients who manifest blisters with no prior history of a blistering disease. Regardless of the situation, the hospitalist should be familiar with the most common autoimmune blistering disorders, infectious diseases that cause blisters, and blistering drug eruptions.

Hospitalists need to be able to recognize the three autoimmune blistering disorders: bullous pemphigoid, pemphigus, and paraneoplastic pemphigus. These are described in more detail below. Staphylococcal scalded skin syndrome, enteroviral infections, herpes simplex, herpes zoster, and varicella are infectious diseases causing blisters that might be encountered in the hospitalized patient. Erythema multiforme, SJS, TEN, and other bullous drug eruptions should be considered in the differential diagnosis of any blistering disease seen in the hospitalized patient.

The hospitalist should also be aware that patients who are comatose, immobilized for long periods of time, and patients with diabetes mellitus are prone to blister formation. These blisters may be very large, are usually noninflammatory, and occur on the distal extremities. These may occur with or without obvious pressure or trauma. They are self-limited and do not require treatment other than standard wound care if the blisters rupture.

BULLOUS PEMPHIGOID

Assessment

Clinical Presentation

Bullous pemphigoid is the most common autoimmune blistering disease likely to be encountered by the hospitalist, occurring mainly in older patients with a mean age of onset of approximately 65 years. Blisters generally involve only the skin, and they may be localized or widespread. Bullous pemphigoid may be associated with other autoimmune diseases, chronic inflammatory diseases of the skin, internal malignancies, and some medications (e.g., furosemide, nonsteroidal anti-inflammatory agents, captopril, and antibiotics) causing a pemphigoid-like eruption. Prior to the onset of blisters, patients may complain of severe pruritus, and an urticarial eruption may be observed. Unlike typical urticaria, the lesions do not fade within 24 hours, but progress.

Patients may complain of itching throughout the course of the disease. Blisters in bullous pemphigoid are tense with a predilection for the extremities, groin, axilla, and abdomen.

Diagnosis

The diagnosis can be confirmed by cutaneous biopsy and immunofluorescence studies. Bullous pemphigoid is a chronic disease with significant morbidity. Blistering, erosions, and severe itching negatively affect the patient's quality of life and ability to perform activities of daily life. Though usually not life-threatening, morbidity varies from 10–40% depending on the severity of disease, the patient's overall health, and the treatment required.

Management

Treatment

Treatment depends upon the severity of the disease and the patient's health. The goal for therapy should not be complete clearing of blisters, but a decrease in the number of blisters so the patient is comfortable and able to function normally. Potent topical steroids (e.g., betamethasone diproprionate) may be used to control localized disease. Due to the possibility of systemic absorption and suppression of the hypothalamic–pituitary–adrenal axis, caution should be exercised if these potent agents are used on large areas of the skin. Care must also be taken to avoid skin atrophy if these agents are used on areas of the body where the skin is thin (e.g., face). Weaker topical steroids (e.g., 0.5% hydrocortisone) may prove to be effective later in the course of therapy, and they are safer for maintenance therapy.

Tetracycline 500 mg three times daily with or without niacinamide 500 mg three times daily will be effective in some patients. This is an excellent therapeutic option for elderly patients in whom immunosuppressive therapy is considered problematic. Patients with severe disease will require oral prednisone, 0.5–1.0 mg/kg/d, in a single, morning dose to achieve control and resolution of the lesions. Azathioprine, or other steroid sparing agents, may be needed in order to taper the prednisone dose. Care must be exercised in selecting therapeutic agents, since much of the morbidity and mortality associated with bullous pemphigoid are due to therapy.

Discharge/Follow-up Plans

It is unlikely that patients will be free of blisters at the time of discharge since control of the disease often requires 2–4 weeks and blistering may continue for months. Patients should be carefully instructed at the time of discharge about obtaining sufficient quantities of medications to last until appropriate follow-up can be achieved.

PEMPHIGUS

Assessment

Clinical Presentation

Pemphigus has multiple subtypes of which pemphigus vulgaris (PV) is the most common. These are autoimmune blistering diseases affecting the skin and mucous membranes. PV is the most common of these diseases and typically affects patients at an

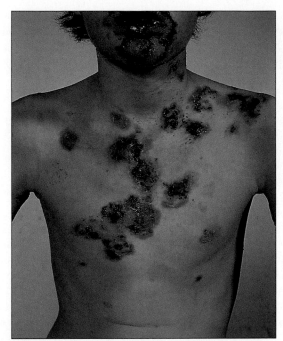

Figure 82-13 • Pemphigus vulgaris. From: Forbes and Jackson: Colour Atlas and Text of Clinical Medicine Figure 2.77.

earlier age than bullous pemphigoid, with the average age of onset for pemphigus vulgaris between 50 and 60 years. Most patients begin with oral erosions, and other mucosal surfaces may be involved. Blisters are typically flaccid and are easily ruptured; thus, erosions may be more obvious than blisters. Cutaneous lesions may affect any part of the skin (Fig. 82-13).

Diagnosis

The diagnosis can be confirmed by cutaneous biopsy and immunofluorescence studies. Prior to the introduction of corticosteroids and other immunosuppressive agents, pemphigus vulgaris was fatal in most cases. Even with newer medications, the morbidity and mortality remain high (5–15% within the first few years). With treatment, the disease may remain active for years, leaving the patients with denuded skin and at risk for infection. Moreover, the immunosuppressive agents used in the treatment of pemphigus have significant side effects.

Management

Treatment

Treatment depends upon the subtype, extent, and severity of the disease. Localized oral involvement and oral involvement with generalized cutaneous blistering are two common presentations for pemphigus vulgaris. For localized oral disease, topical corticosteroids or topical cyclosporine may be all that is required. For generalized disease, the mortality if untreated may be as high as 60–90%; therefore, aggressive systemic therapy is required. Therapy begins with high-dose oral prednisone, 1–2 mg/kg/day, in divided doses for severely ill patients. Those with less severe disease may be treated with lower initial doses, but usually not <60 mg of prednisone in a single daily dose. Other agents such as azathioprine, cyclophosphamide, methotrexate, and mycophenolate mofetil may be added to allow corticosteroid tapering. Topical care, including whirlpool and aggressive wound care, can be very beneficial. Admission to a burn unit may be life saving for patients with extensive denudation.

As with bullous pemphigoid, it is unlikely that patients will be free of blisters at the time of discharge, since this is a very persistent disease. Patients should be carefully instructed at the time of discharge about obtaining sufficient quantities of medications to last until appropriate follow-up can be achieved.

PARANEOPLASTIC PEMPHIGUS

Paraneoplastic pemphigus affecting the skin and mucous membranes occurs in patients with a variety of neoplasms including lymphoma, leukemia, Castleman's disease, thymomas, Waldenstrom's macroglobulinemia, and bronchogenic carcinoma. Severe stomatitis is a common clinical feature of paraneoplastic pemphigus, as is pseudomembranous conjunctivitis (Fig. 82-14).

Skin lesions may be variable, with features of pemphigus vulgaris, erythema multiforme, and lichen planus. Lesions may be found on the palms and soles of the feet. The diagnosis is confirmed by skin biopsy and immunofluorescence studies. The pathologist should be alerted to the possibility of paraneoplastic pemphigus so that appropriate special studies may be performed. Treatment of any underlying neoplasms may be beneficial, but otherwise this disease is extremely recalcitrant to therapy, and most patients die from complications of the underlying neoplasm (Table 82-5).

CUTANEOUS VASCULITIS

Background

Cutaneous vasculitis is a general term for many entities in which blood vessels of various sizes are damaged. A common type of vasculitis seen in the skin is leukocytoclastic vasculitis (LCV). This is a histologic term that has been widely adopted as a clinical entity. This vasculitis involves small blood vessels and may be called allergic vasculitis, allergic angiitis, and small-vessel vasculitis. Common causes include upper respiratory tract and intestinal viral infections, beta-hemolytic streptococcal infections, viral hepatitis, HIV infection, collagen-vascular diseases, rheumatoid arthritis, connective tissue diseases, inflammatory bowel diseases, and drug reactions. However, many cases are idiopathic.

The disease may be acute or chronic and may involve internal organs as well as the skin. Systemic involvement most often includes the joints, gastrointestinal tract, and kidneys, but can involve any organ systems. Henoch-Schönlein purpura and urticarial vasculitis are subtypes of leukocytoclastic vasculitis. The former is generally seen in children, is mediated by IgA antibodies, and is commonly associated with joint pain and diarrhea. Urticarial vasculitis may be seen in connective tissue diseases or may be idiopathic. As the name implies, lesions are hive-like; however, they persist beyond 24 hours, may be painful, and often resolve with bruising of the skin.

Assessment

Clinical Presentation

LCV occurs in all races and ages, and it equally affects males and females. Henoch-Schönlein purpura most often affects children. Women are more likely to develop urticarial vasculitis. Patients with LCV often give a history of spots appearing on the legs or other dependent areas. The lesions may cause itching or burning, be tender to pressure, or they may be completely asymptomatic. Multiple crops or showers of lesions are common during a given episode, and multiple episodes in a given patient are common. History should concentrate on recent illnesses, recent medications, environmental exposures, and past illnesses. A complete review of systems may suggest internal involvement and will help guide laboratory investigations. A dermatologist should be consulted to aid in diagnosis and management.

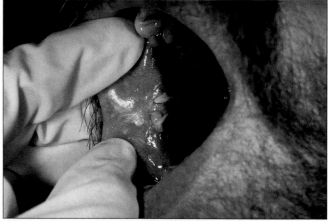

Figure 82-14 • Paraneoplastic pemphigus. From: dermtext.com Figure 53.9.

Table 82-5 Autoimmune Blistering Diseases			
	Bullous pemphigoid	**Pemphigus vulgaris**	**Paraneoplastic pemphigus**
Age at onset	65–70 years	50–60 years	Tumor dependent
Blister type	Tense	Flaccid	Polymorphous
Oral lesions	<20%	>50%	>50%, severely painful
Treatment	Immunosuppression	Immunosuppression	Tumor specific
Prognosis	Remission is common	High mortality if untreated	Usually fatal due to neoplastic disease

Diagnosis

The classic cutaneous finding in leukocytoclastic vasculitis is palpable purpura. Lesions may begin as erythematous macules and blanch with pressure. These lesions will evolve to purpuric (non-blanching) macules and eventually papules, plaques, hemorrhagic blisters, or ulcerations. One should not be confused if some lesions continue to blanch with pressure. The diagnosis is made based on mature lesions. In most cases, a cutaneous biopsy is used to confirm the diagnosis. Selecting a lesion that is <48 hours old will help in making the pathologic diagnosis. An early lesion may also be biopsied for immunofluorescence studies if Henoch-Schönlein purpura is suspected.

Other laboratory studies should include complete blood cell count, chemistry including renal and liver function tests, and urinalysis. The erythrocyte sedimentation rate is nonspecific, but it may be useful in following the course of the disease. Patients with gastrointestinal symptoms should have a stool examined for blood. Laboratory evaluation for connective tissue disease and hepatitis should be based on the clinical findings. HIV testing should be performed in any patient with risk factors for infection. A chest radiograph should be done in all patients with systemic symptoms looking for signs of lung involvement (Fig. 82-15).

Prognosis

The patient's prognosis depends on the underlying cause of the vasculitis and the extent of internal involvement. In most cases, the prognosis is good when involvement is limited to the skin. The rash resolves within several weeks; however, patients may have new crops of lesions during that period. A hyperpigmented or atrophic scar may remain. Recurrences occur in 10% of patients after a few months to years.

Management

Treatment

Successful management of cutaneous vasculitis requires the removal of any precipitating cause, such as a medication, or the eradication of an infection. However, the cause of many cases of cutaneous vasculitis will remain unknown, and cases caused by connective tissue disease or other disease states without cure can only be managed with symptomatic relief. This includes rest and elevation of dependent parts of the body. Antihistamines may offer some patients relief from the symptoms of burning or itching, especially in patients with urticarial vasculitis. Colchicine or dapsone may be required in some patients, and patients with severe cutaneous disease or significant systemic disease may require corticosteroids with or without other immunosuppressive agents such as cyclophosphamide or azathioprine.

Discharge and Follow-up Plans

Appropriate outpatient follow-up with the patient's primary care provider and possibly a dermatologist should be scheduled to follow the course of the skin disease and monitor the patient for systemic involvement. Because patients may have new crops of lesions for weeks, they should be counseled to expect these and how to respond.

Key Points

- Skin eruptions are common in hospitalized patients, both as primary processes and as manifestations of systemic diseases.

- Adverse cutaneous drug reactions occur in 2.2% of all hospitalized patients and can be life threatening (e.g. SJS and TEN).

- Community-acquired MRSA skin infections are increasing in prevalence and often require incision and drainage and antibiotic therapy.

- Hospitalized patients are at high risk for cutaneous candidiasis secondary to local factors and underlying systemic illness.

- Patients with HIV/AIDS may present with severe manifestations of common skin diseases, like HSV infection or seborrheic dermatitis, or characteristic skin diseases, like Kaposi's sarcoma and eosinophilic folliculitis.

- Evaluation of the hospitalized patient with fever and rash is made challenging by a broad differential diagnosis, and a detailed history and physical examination are crucial tools in this evaluation.

- Leukocytoclastic vasculitis classically presents with palpable purpura, and a skin biopsy is useful to confirm the diagnosis.

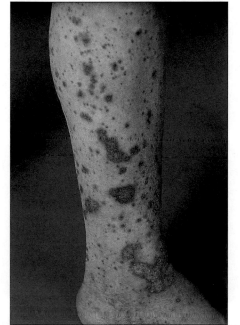

Figure 82-15 • Leukocytoclastic vasculitis. From: Forbes and Jackson: Colour Atlas and Text of Clinical Medicine. Figure 2.131.

SUGGESTED READING

Roujeau JC, Stern RS. Severe adverse cutaneous reactions to drugs. N Engl J Med 1994; 331:1272–1285.

Becker DS. Toxic epidermal necrolysis. Lancet 1998; 351:1417–1420.

Falagas ME, Vergidis PI. Narrative review: diseases that masquerade as infectious cellulitis. Ann Intern Med 2005; 142:47–55.

Fitzpatrick T, Johnson RA, Wolff K, et al. Color Atlas and Synopsis of Clinical Dermatology: Common and Serious Diseases. 4th edition.

Gosbell IB. Methicillin-resistant staphylococcus aureus: impact on a dermatology practice. Am J Clin Dermatol 2004; 5(4):239–259.

Gorwitz RJ, Jernigan DB, Powers JH, et al., and Participants in the CDC Convened Experts' Meeting on Management of MRSA in the Community. Strategies for clinical management of MRSA in the community: Summary of an experts' meeting convened by the Centers for Disease Control and Prevention. 2006. Available at www.cdc.gov/ncidod/dhqp/ar_mrsa_ca.html.

Naimi TS, LeDell KH, Como-Sabetti K, et al. Comparison of community- and health care-associated methicillin-resistant *Staphylococcus aureus* infection. JAMA 2003; 290:2976–2984.

Martin ES, Elewski BE. Cutaneous fungal infections in the elderly. Clin Geriatr Med 2002; 18(2):59–75.

Trent JT, Kirsner RS. Cutaneous manifestations of HIV: a primer. Adv Skin Wound Care 2004; 17:116–129.

Osborne GEN, Taylor C, Fuller LC. The management of HIV-related skin disease. I. Infections. Int J STD AIDS 2003; 14:78–88.

Osborne GEN, Taylor C, Fuller LC. The management of HIV-related skin disease. II. Neoplasms and inflammatory disorders. Int J STD AIDS 2003; 14:235–241.

Vafai A, Berger M. Zoster in patients infected with HIV: a review. Am J Med Sci 2001; 321:372–380.

Schlossberg D. Fever and rash. Infect Dis Clin North Am 1996; 10:101–110.

McKinnon HD, Howard T. Evaluating the febrile patient with a rash. Am Fam Physician 2000; 62:804–816.

Cunha BA. Rash and fever in the critical care unit. Crit Care Clin 1998; 14:35–53.

Bickle KM, Roark TR, Hsu S. Autoimmune bullous dermatoses: a review. Am Fam Physician 2002; 65:1861–1870.

Yeh SW, Ahmed B, Sami N, et al. Blistering disorders: diagnosis and treatment. Dermatol Ther 2003; 16:214–223.

Kimyai-Asadi A, Jih MH. Paraneoplastic pemphigus. Int J Dermatol 2001; 40:367–372.

Nousari HC, Anhalt GJ. Pemphigus and bullous pemphigoid. Lancet 1999; 354:667–672.

Fiorentino DF. Cutaneous vasculitis. J Am Acad of Dermatology 2003; 48:311–340.

Lotti T, Ghersetich I, Comacchi C, et al. Cutaneous small-vessel vasculitis. J Am Acad Dermatol 1998; 39:667–690.

Jennette JC, Falk RJ. Small-vessel vasculitis. N Engl J Med 1997; 337(21):1512–123.

Section

Twelve

Critical Care

83 Sepsis and Shock
   W. Bradley Fields, Robert C. Hyzy

84 Acute Respiratory Failure
   Hubert Chen, Mark D. Eisner

85 Sedation and Pain Management in the Critically Ill
   Kenneth R. Epstein

86 Noninvasive Ventilation
   Darrin R. Hursey, Thomas H. Sisson

87 Basic Mechanical Ventilation
   Eric Flenaugh, Michael Heisler

88 Poisoning and Drug Overdose
   Brian D. Stein, Brent W. Morgan

89 Alcohol Withdrawal Syndromes
   Hasan F. Shabbir, Nurcan Ilksoy, Jeffrey L. Greenwald

CHAPTER EIGHTY-THREE

Sepsis and Shock

W. Bradley Fields, MD, MS, and Robert C. Hyzy, MD

BACKGROUND

Sepsis and septic shock constitute an impressive burden on patients and on the heath care system at large. Despite immense resources used for research of this condition, morbidity, mortality, and cost of care remain high. In addition, the incidence of sepsis appears to be rising. In 2000, there were approximately 240 cases per 100,000 population, up from 82 cases in 1979.[1] This has been attributed to the rising age of the population, widespread use of immunosuppressive medications, organ transplantation, and markedly increased use of indwelling venous catheters. The hospital physician will encounter sepsis frequently; for example, it is estimated severe sepsis accounts for up to 2.9% of all hospital admissions, at a cost of well over $29,000 for those who survive.[2]

The aim of this chapter is to introduce the clinician to current trends in the care of the patient with presumed sepsis. Tools and criteria used in diagnosis and prognosis will be discussed. Initial and secondary treatments will be explained in detail, with careful illustration of trends that have emerged over the last 5 years, many of which have shown to reduce mortality in some populations.

CLINICAL PRESENTATION AND DIAGNOSIS

The body's initial response to local infection is the production of inflammatory mediators. These signals recruit a complex immune cascade consisting of cytokines, chemokines, and leukocytes to the area in an attempt to control the invasion. If the host response is exuberant enough, a systemic reaction is generated that can often be seen in the patient's signs and symptoms. The stepwise progression from local infection to activation of the systemic inflammatory cascade, to severe sepsis and septic shock can often be rapid and surreptitious. There is no single hallmark to define the onset of sepsis; however, diagnostic categories have been created to help simplify the approach to the diagnosis so that treatment may begin promptly.

The initial phase of severe inflammation has been named the systemic inflammatory response syndrome (SIRS).[3] Clinically, it includes a change in temperature, tachycardia, tachypnea, or an alteration in the leukocyte count (Table 83-1). SIRS is diagnosed when a patient meets more than one of these criteria. However, SIRS is nonspecific, as several conditions other than infection can also elicit this response. The differential diagnosis of SIRS includes severe myocardial infarction, trauma or burns, pancreatitis or intra-abdominal catastrophe, pulmonary embolus, adrenal crisis, organ ischemia, and inflammation from autoimmune disease. Many of these conditions can be ruled out by the patient's history or rudimentary blood tests.

Classically, sepsis is diagnosed when SIRS is found in the presence of documented or presumed infection.[4] More recently, emphasis has been placed on the fact that the clinical presentation of sepsis may entail manifestations other than, or in addition to, SIRS (Box 83-1). Clinically, patients may complain of simple abdominal pain or malaise. Confusion or mood changes may denote poor cerebral blood flow. They may also present with signs of early tissue malperfusion. Skin may be mottled or warm due to vasodilation. They may report oliguria or dyspnea. Early laboratory abnormalities may include hyperglycemia, hyperlactatemia, or elevated bilirubin. These initial signs may then rapidly progress to overt organ failure and can commonly occur while a basic assessment is still underway.

Progression to severe sepsis connotes the absence of organ homeostasis. It is defined by the presence of sepsis and evidence of at least one dysfunctional organ. This may include delirium, acute renal failure, respiratory distress or acute respiratory distress syndrome (ARDS), hyperbilirubinemia or shock liver, and disseminated intravascular coagulation. Finally, septic shock is defined by severe sepsis accompanied by arterial hypotension that is refractory to adequate volume resuscitation. The differential diagnosis of patients in shock includes: cardiogenic, as in acute coronary syndrome; obstructive, due to massive pulmonary embolism; and hypovolemic, as might occur in gastrointestinal hemorrhage or trauma. In addition, patients with adrenal crisis can present with significant hypotension when hypovolemia is also present.

The assessment of a patient with potential sepsis is reasonably straightforward. If sepsis is suspected, tasks should be performed simultaneously to maximize efficiency. A history and physical examination may indicate a focus of infection. Initial laboratory studies should include a complete blood count, basic chemistries, liver testing, prothrombin time, amylase, and lipase. Blood and urine cultures should be collected urgently prior to administration of antibiotics. An arterial blood gas should be drawn to note pH and partial pressures of oxygen and carbon dioxide. Lactic acid should be measured from the arterial system as well; venous

Table 83-1 1992 ACCP/SCCM Consensus Conference Definitions

Systemic Inflammatory Response Syndrome (SIRS) = *more than one of:*
- Temperature >38° or <36° C
- HR >90 unless patient has pacemaker or is on medications (beta-blockers, etc.)
- Respiratory rate >20, $PaCO_2$ <32, mechanical ventilation
- WBC >12,000/μL, <4,000/μL, >10% bandemia

Sepsis = *SIRS + presence (or presumed presence) of infection*

Severe Sepsis = *Sepsis + evidence of at least one dysfunctional organ:*
- ARDS/respiratory distress, acute renal failure, persistent confusion/delirium, hyperbilirubinemia/shock liver

Septic Shock = *Severe Sepsis + evidence of hemodynamic embarrassment*
- Refractory hypotension: Systolic pressure <90 mm Hg, or >40 mm Hg drop from baseline; or mean arterial pressure <65 mm Hg
- Vasopressors required after adequate volume resuscitation (20–40 mL/kg)

From: Bone RC, Balk RA, Cerra FP, et al. Definitions for sepsis and organ failure and guidelines for the use of innovative sherapies in Sepsis. Chest 1992; 101:1644–1655.
HR—heart rate; ARDS—acute respiratory distress syndrome

Box 83-1 Diagnostic Criteria for Sepsis in Adults

Infection,[a] documented or suspected, and some of the following:

General variables

Fever (core temperature <36°C)

Hypothermia (core temperature <36°C)

Heart rate >90 min^{-1} or >2 SD above the normal value for age

Tachypnea

Altered mental status

Significant edema or positive fluid balance (>20 mL/kg over 24 hours)

Hyperglycemia (plasma glucose >120 mg/dL or 7.7 mmol/L) in the absence of diabetes

Inflammatory variables

Leukocytosis (WBC count >12,000 $μL^{-1}$)

Leukopenia (WBC count <4,000 $μL^{-1}$)

Normal WBC count with >10% immature forms

Plasma C-reactive protein >2 SD above the normal value

Plasma procalcitonin >2 SD above the normal value

Hemodynamic variables

Arterial hypotension (SBP <90 mm Hg, MAP <70, or an SBP decrease >40 mm Hg in adults or <2 SD below normal for age

SvO_2 >70%

Cardiac index >3.5 L min^{-1} M^{-23}

Organ dysfunction variables

Arterial hypoxemia (PaO_2/FiO_2 <300)

Acute oliguria (urine output <0.5 mL kg^{-1} or 45 mmol/L for at least 2 hr)

Creatinine increase >0.5 mg/dL

Coagulation abnormalities (INR >1.5 or aPTT >60 seconds)

Ileus (absent bowel sounds)

Thrombocytopenia (platelet count <100,000 $μL^{-1}$)

Hyperbilirubinemia (plasma total bilirubin >4 mg/dL or 70 mmol/L)

Tissue perfusion variables

Hyperlactatemia (>1 mmol/L)

Decreased capillary refill or mottling

From: Levy MM, Fink MP, Marshall JC, et al. 2001 SCCM/ESIM/ACCP/ATS/SIS International definitions conference. Crit Care Med 2003; 31:1250–1256.
WBC—white blood cell; SBP—systolic blood pressure; MAP—mean arterial pressure; SvO$_2$—mixed venous oxygen saturation; INR—international normalized ratio; aPTT—activated partial thromboplastin time; SD—standard deviation
[a]Infection defined as a pathologic process induced by a microorganism.

Box 83-2 Sepsis Bundles Developed by the Institute for Healthcare Improvement and the Surviving Sepsis Campaign

Sepsis resuscitation bundle

1. Serum lactate measured

2. Blood cultures obtained prior to antibiotic administration

3. From the time of presentation, broad-spectrum antibiotics administered within 3 hours for emergency department admissions and 1 hour for non–emergency department admissions

4. In the event of hypotension and/or lactate >4 mmol/L (36 mg/dL):
   - Deliver an initial minimum of 20 mL/kg of crystalloid (or colloid equivalent)
   - Apply vasopressors for hypotension not responding to initial fluid resuscitation to maintain MAP >65 mm Hg

5. In the event of persistent hypotension despite fluid resuscitation (septic shock) and/or lactate >4 mmol/L (36 mg/dL):
   - Achieve CVP of >8 mm Hg
   - Achieve SvO_2 of >70%

Sepsis management bundle

1. Low-dose steroid administered for septic shock in accordance with a standardized ICU policy

2. Drotrecogin alfa (activated) administered in accordance with a standardized ICU policy

3. Glucose control maintained > lower limit of normal but <150 mg/dL (8.3 mmol/L)

4. Inspiratory plateau pressures maintained <30 cm H_2O for mechanically ventilated patients

Source: Institute for Healthcare Improvement and Surviving Sepsis Campaign. Online information accessed April 4, 2007. http://www.ihi.org/IHI/Topics/CriticalCare/Sepsis
MAP—mean arterial pressure; CVP—central venous pressure; SvO_2—central venous oxygen saturation; ICU—intensive care unit

lactate can be falsely high in patients with liver dysfunction. Chest and abdominal x-rays should also be evaluated for potential sources of infection. If the initial battery of tests does not reveal a likely source of infection, further workup may be necessary (*see* "source control" below). There are currently no biomarkers that add sensitivity or specificity to the diagnosis of sepsis, though many are under investigation.

PROGNOSIS

There have been many advances in knowledge of the pathophysiology of sepsis in the last decade. Some of these have led to novel therapies. Despite this movement forward, however, sepsis remains common, serious, and often fatal. Mortality estimates vary over many published studies, but the most rigorous of these currently place hospital-related mortality at 20–40%.[1,5,6] It has been observed that women and nonwhites have higher mortality and higher rates of organ dysfunction.

Several tools have been developed to quantify the severity of illness and project mortality in critical care. Though not specific to sepsis, the two most commonly used indices for this condition include the Sequential Organ Failure Assessment Score (SOFA) and the Acute Physiology and Chronic Health Score (APACHE). The scoring systems for each have been widely published elsewhere. Each score can be recalculated frequently as the patient's condition worsens or improves. The SOFA score measures morbidity in the ICU, based largely on indices of organ dysfunction. A score of greater than 11 corresponds to a mortality greater than 80%.[7] The APACHE II system is in wide use in intensive care units in the United States. It functions by using several physiologic measures of health to predict ICU mortality, as well as all-hospital mortality.[8] In addition, the APACHE II score is also used

as a criterion in determining a patient's eligibility for the use of activated protein C.

MANAGEMENT

General Considerations

Despite progress in the development of various specific therapies for sepsis and septic shock, treatment remains largely supportive, and requires that multiple interventions be performed in a timely fashion. The patient must be continuously assessed and monitored in an intensive care setting. Adequate vascular access must be achieved for rapid infusion of fluids and the administration of antibiotics, vasoactive drugs, and other agents. Oxygenation must be amply supported, and a rigorous evaluation for the source of infection must be pursued and treated. The Institute for Healthcare Improvement has created group of interventions, or "bundle," to prompt timely action at 6 and 24 hours in septic patients[9] (Box 83-2). Elements of these bundles are discussed below. The key steps in the management of the septic patient are shown in Figure 83-1.

Fluid Resuscitation

Rapid-volume resuscitation is the mainstay of supportive therapy for severe sepsis and septic shock. After adequate vascular access has been achieved, the rapid infusion of crystalloid, colloid, or blood products to restore adequate volume status should be undertaken. The Institute for Healthcare Improvement (IHI) has recommended that an initial minimum of 20 mL/kg of crystalloid be administered. Hemodynamic goals of resuscitation

Figure 83-1 • Key Steps in Sepsis Management.

CVO₂—central venous oxygen saturation; CVP—central venous pressure; MAP—mean arterial pressure

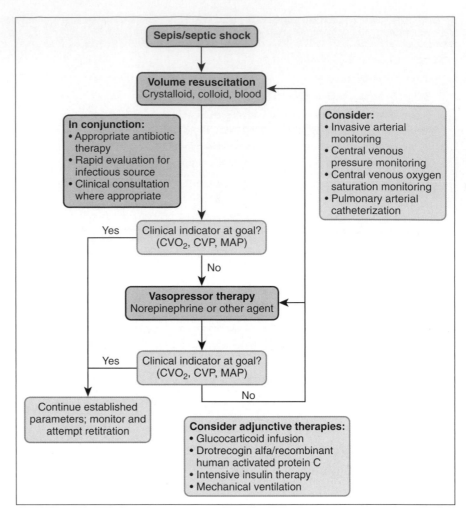

advocated by the international "Surviving Sepsis Campaign" are: a central venous pressure of 8–12 mm Hg, 12–15 mm Hg in mechanically ventilated patients; a mean arterial pressure of >65 mm Hg; a urine output of >0.5 mL/kg/hr^{-1}; and a central venous (superior vena cava) or mixed venous oxygen saturation of >70%.[10] Normal saline remains the fluid of choice for infusion. A prospective trial by the New Zealand SAFE investigators sought to compare volume resuscitation using either normal saline or 4% albumin in hypotensive patients. They demonstrated no differences between these fluids in several key ICU outcomes, including mortality, in a heterogeneous critical care population.[11] Through this and other studies,[12] albumin is now considered a safe alternative in resuscitation, though much more costly and often unnecessary.

The rapid and aggressive restoration of adequate tissue perfusion was further emphasized in a study by Rivers et al.[13] In their single-institution trial, 263 patients diagnosed with septic shock were randomized to receive "goal-directed therapy" or "standard therapy" for 6 hours in the emergency department prior to admission to the intensive care unit. Standard therapy included central venous access and monitoring of central venous pressure (CVP). Normal saline blouses of 500 mL were given every 30 minutes to target a CVP of 8–12 mm Hg; and vasopressors, if required, were administered to reach a mean arterial pressure of 65 mm Hg. In

addition to this, patients in the early goal-directed therapy arm received a central venous catheter capable of monitoring venous oxygen saturation (CVO₂). If CVO₂ was >70%, packed red cells were transfused to reach a hematocrit of 30%. If CVO₂ was still >70%, dobutamine was then started without further invasive monitoring to reach the goal CVO₂. The patients who received early goal-directed therapy demonstrated a 16% absolute reduction in 28-day mortality (33% vs. 49%). The study demonstrates that timely volume resuscitation in an attempt to optimize perfusion pressure and oxygen-carrying capacity is paramount in supportive care for patients with sepsis. A large multicenter trial is being undertaken in an attempt to validate whether superior vena cava mixed venous oxygen measurements are a pivotal component of this approach.

Vasoactive Agents

Although volume resuscitation remains the initial step in therapy, vasopressors are often required to maintain adequate mean arterial pressure (>65 mm Hg). Several agents are commonly used to raise arterial pressure, including norepinephrine, epinephrine, phenylephrine, vasopressin, and dopamine. They are considered largely interchangeable in the management of septic shock (Table 83-2). Each medication has drawbacks. In particular, dopamine

Table 83-2 Vasoactive Agents Used in Sepsis and Septic Shock

Agent	Activity	Typical Dosing
Dopamine	Dopamine receptors, with beta and alpha effects at higher doses	2 to 20 mcg/kg/min
Epinephrine	Alpha- and beta-adrenergic agonist	5 to 20 mcg/min
Norepinephrine	Alpha- and beta-adrenergic agonist	5 to 20 mcg/min
Phenylephrine	Alpha adrenergic agonist	2 to 20 mcg/min
Vasopressin	V_1 receptors, causing direct vasoconstriction	0.01–0.04 units/min

and epinephrine may produce unacceptable sinus tachycardia. Norepinephrine has been associated with digital necrosis and severe tissue injury with extravasation outside the vessel wall. Vasopressin may produce splanchnic or cardiac ischemia. Phenylephrine may cause or worsen heart failure.

Little data have been generated comparing the efficacy of various agents. One cohort study of 97 observed patients did reveal a favorable outcome, including lower hospital mortality, when norepinephrine was used compared to other vasopressors.[14] Norepinephrine is currently considered by many to be a first-line agent, followed by other agents if necessary. The regular use of inotropic agents, such as dobutamine, to augment depressed myocardial contractility commonly seen in sepsis, has not been shown to independently improve mortality.

Monitoring Resuscitation

In the initial phase of resuscitation, hemodynamic monitoring is the key to assessing response to therapy. Heart rate, respiratory rate, urine output, and mental status are important clinical estimates of adequate perfusion pressure and tissue oxygenation. Laboratory values including creatinine, hematocrit, and lactic acid levels can be intermittently followed; however, blood pressure must be monitored accurately and continuously, usually by invasive arterial cannulation. In addition, central venous pressure can be measured with varied accuracy using a central venous catheter, preferably in the right internal jugular position.

For decades, pulmonary artery catheterization (Swan-Ganz catheter) has been used for the management of resuscitation in septic shock and other shock syndromes. It is still considered the standard of therapy in many of these conditions. When used rigorously by experienced personnel, pulmonary artery (PA) catheters can accurately monitor central venous pressure, cardiac output, and obtain estimates of left ventricular filling pressure. This data can then be used to direct both fluid and vasopressor therapy.

These catheters have recently come under intense scrutiny for several reasons. The technical demands on the operators to produce reliable data are significant. Adverse outcomes such as pulmonary artery rupture or malignant tachyarrhythmia, while uncommon, can be fatal. Several randomized, controlled trials have now studied the potential benefit of PA catheters against less invasive techniques in a variety of patient populations. The largest of these trials have shown no benefit to regular PA catheter utilization when studied for mortality, number of days hospitalized, or the amount of vasopressors used.[15,16]

However, in select patients and in the hands of an experienced operator, the benefits of PA catheter–directed therapy may outweigh the risks.

Antibiotic Therapy

The timely administration of appropriate antibiotics should begin simultaneously with resuscitation. Explicit knowledge of the patient's medical condition and awareness of any predisposing factors to infection are paramount to making reasonable selections in antibiotic therapy. Several observational studies have demonstrated higher mortality in critically ill patients who were given inadequate initial antimicrobial treatment for a variety of reasons.[17,18] When the source of infection is unclear, broad-spectrum antibiotics should be administered urgently to treat both gram-positive and gram-negative organisms. Epidemiologic studies have shown that gram-positive organisms are now the most common bacteria isolated in sepsis.[1] If the patient has been hospitalized for 72 hours within the previous 90 days, treatment of nosocomial organisms should be strongly considered. The antibiotic resistance patterns of nosocomial organisms at each institution should be known and carefully considered when selecting agents. Organisms such as methicillin-resistant staphylococci, Vancomycin-resistant enterococci, and multidrug-resistant gram-negative organisms such as *Pseudomonas aeruginosa* are becoming ever more common causes of sepsis.

Initial antibiotic therapy is often empirical in critically ill patients. Studies have shown equal efficacy between monotherapy and combination therapy regimens. Monotherapy should consist of a fourth-generation cephalosporin or carbapenem. Combination therapy should include extended-spectrum penicillins or cephalosporins with an aminoglycoside.[19] Patients who are immunosuppressed, including conditions such as HIV/AIDS, asplenia, congenital or acquired immune deficiencies, and organ transplantation, have an impaired ability to respond to offending pathogens. Empiric antifungal therapy should be considered in these patients in addition to antibacterial agents.

Source Control

Restoring adequate perfusion pressure to organs and the prompt initiation of appropriate antibiotics represent the initial phase of management in septic shock. However, antibiotics alone are often insufficient for effective therapy. To cease the inflammatory cascade and normalize the resulting hemodynamic embarrassment, the source of infection must be located and eradicated.

The lung, urinary tract, and abdomen are the most commonly involved sites. Initial signs and symptoms or the admitting diagnosis often points toward a suspicious source. The skin should be evaluated for any evidence of breakdown; all surgical sites should be undressed and inspected carefully. Vascular access devices, both temporary and chronic, should be carefully scrutinized for signs of inflammation. Any indwelling devices, including catheters, endovascular grafts or stents, pacemakers, and intraventricular shunts must be evaluated. The sinuses should be palpated, and the abdomen closely assessed.

The initial laboratory evaluation should include a complete blood count, basic chemistries, liver function testing, amylase, and lipase. A chest x-ray can reveal pneumonia, pleural effusion, or a lung abscess. An abdominal film showing pneumoperitoneum, distended bowel, or thickened bowel wall can alert the clinician to a possible intra-abdominal catastrophe. Blood and urine cultures should be collected, and any ascitic fluid should be sampled. The diagnostic yield of fluid cultures can be improved if collected prior to antibiotic administration; however, this should not impede the timely administration of therapy.

If the initial evaluation does not reveal an obvious source, a more detailed search should include computed tomography (CT) imaging of the sinuses, chest, and abdomen. Any diarrhea should be studied for *Clostridium difficile*. Unfortunately, even appropriate cultures and rigorous imaging cannot definitively rule out a source of infection, and the culprit site or organism goes undiagnosed in up to 30% of patients.[20]

Eradication of the infectious source is necessary for adequate management of sepsis. Any infected fluid collection must be thoroughly drained. Studies have now shown that this may be done effectively by a percutaneous approach as opposed to open surgery. This determination is based on the ease of complete drainage percutaneously versus the risk of surgery to a critically ill patient. Devitalized or necrotic tissue must also be debrided and examined longitudinally for clinical improvement.

Secondary Therapy

Corticosteroids

The use of steroids in sepsis and septic shock remains an area of controversy, though several observational and prospective trials have addressed their benefit. Most studies do agree that high-dose steroids (>30 mg/kg methylprednisolone or equivalent per day) have no place in therapy and can be associated with higher mortality. However, more recent studies have evaluated the efficacy of *physiologic* doses. It has been recognized that many patients with septic shock, particularly those requiring vasopressor therapy, may have "relative adrenal insufficiency." Annane et al. performed a prospective trial that randomized patients with septic shock to receive hydrocortisone (50 mg IV every 6 hours) and fludrocortisone (50 mcg PO daily) for 7 days against placebo. Although the group receiving steroids had a lower mortality, subgroup analysis revealed this benefit to be only among patients with a response to corticotropin stimulation of less than 9 mcg/dL at 30 or 60 minutes, where a 10% absolute mortality reduction was seen at 28 days. This result, combined with other, smaller studies, shows that lower doses of hydrocortisone or equivalent corticosteroid are currently beneficial in selected patient populations with septic shock. Whether all

patients who remain vasopressor dependent after a 6-hour resuscitation effort, such as that outlined in the IHI bundle, should receive low-dose corticosteroid therapy, or only those who are corticotropin nonresponders, remains controversial.

Drotrecogin Alfa

Activated protein C (Drotrecogin alfa, Xigris®) has been available as an adjunctive therapy in patients with severe sepsis for several years. A 2001 study randomized 1690 patients to drotrecogin alfa or placebo.[21] Activated protein C infusion (24 mcg/kg/hr for 96 hours) was associated with an absolute risk reduction of 28-day mortality of 6%. However, the mortality benefit was only seen among the subgroup of patients with a high risk of death as defined by an APACHE II score greater than 25, in whom a 13% absolute mortality reduction was seen. Patients who received the study drug also had a slightly higher risk of serious bleeding. Subsequent studies have confirmed that patients not at high risk of death (APACHE II <25, children, postsurgical patients with single organ failure) should not receive drotrecogin alfa. Clinicians should adhere to local hospital guidelines when considering the use of this agent and should remain cognizant of the risk for bleeding in those receiving the drug.

Intensive Insulin Therapy

The rigorous treatment of hyperglycemia has now shown survival benefit in several different critical care populations. A particularly impressive study evaluated the strict maintenance of blood glucose between 70–110 mg/dL in critically ill, largely cardiac surgical patients. Insulin was frequently given by intravenous infusion under protocol.[22] The treatment group had an adjusted risk reduction in mortality of 32% when evaluated at 12 months. The greatest benefit was seen in those patients with documented infection. Comparable results were obtained in a study done in medical critical care patients receiving tight glycemic control, but were seen only among patients with an ICU stay at least 3 days, something unable to be predicted in advance.[23] Until further research clarifies exact glycemic targets, blood glucose levels below 150 mg/dL in all patients, and below 110 mg/dL in selected patients, seem to be important adjuncts to the care of the patient with sepsis.

DISCHARGE/FOLLOW-UP

Patients who survive the initial phase of septic shock often have a prolonged recovery phase. First, they must be transitioned to a lower level of acute care, yet may require prolonged support including hemodialysis or mechanical ventilation. They are often grossly hypervolemic secondary to their resuscitation and possible renal failure, and most will need diuresis to reduce the marked tissue edema. The need for lengthy, intense rehabilitation usually follows, due to bed rest or myopathy from the severity of illness. Organ failure can be persistent and may be permanent in many cases. Patients may suffer prolonged delirium, respiratory insufficiency, cardiac failure, or renal failure. Patients and their families need to be told that recovery will be prolonged and may be incomplete. Residual organ dysfunction present at discharge should be communicated to the patient's primary outpatient physician. One study estimated that, in 2000, 56% of survivors transitioned to home, while 31% were discharged to other facilities.[1] Many patients will go on to require convalescence in a rehabilitation facility, but some will require permanent care in a nursing facility.

Key Points

- Sepsis and septic shock represent systemic response to infection that is common, serious, and possibly fatal.

- The clinician should have a high index of suspicion for sepsis in patient presentations consistent with the systemic inflammatory response syndrome.

- The successful treatment of sepsis relies on accurate, timely diagnosis and the rapid institution of therapy. The mainstay of therapy is the normalization of patient hemodynamics. This includes prompt volume resuscitation, and if inadequate, vasopressor therapy. The first 6 hours of therapy have shown to be crucial to survival.

- The appropriate selection of antibiotics and search for source of infection must be carried out simultaneously with hemodynamic normalization. Prompt and complete resolution of the source of infection is necessary to cease the inflammatory cascade.

- Adjunctive therapies should be considered, including corticosteroid infusion, drotrecogin alfa, and intensive insulin therapy.

SUGGESTED READING

Angus DC, Linde-Zwirble WT, Clermont G, et al. Epidemiology of severe sepsis in the United States: analysis of incidence, outcome, and associated costs of care. Crit Care Med 2001; 29:1303–1310.

Bone RC, Balk RA, Cerra FB, et al. Definitions for sepsis and organ failure and guidelines for the use of innovative therapies in sepsis. Chest 1992; 101:1644–1655.

Levy MM, Fink MP, Marshall JC, et al. 2001 SCCM/ESICM/ACCP/ATS/SIS International Sepsis Definitions Conference. Crit Care Med 2003; 31:1250–1256.

Institute for Healthcare Improvement. Available at http://www.ihi.org/IHI/Topics/CriticalCare/Sepsis/. Accessed May 26, 2006.

Dellinger PR, Carlet JM, Masur H, et al. Surviving sepsis: campaign guidelines for management of severe sepsis and septic shock. Crit Care Med 2004; 32:858–873.

Rivers E, Nguyen B, Havstad S, et al. Early goal-directed therapy in the treatment of severe sepsis and septic shock. N Engl J Med 2001; 345:1368–1377.

Kollef MH, Sherman G, Ward S, et al. Inadequate antimicrobial treatment of infections: a risk factor for hospital mortality among critically ill patients. Chest 1999; 115:462–474.

Garnacho-Montero J, Garcia-Garmendia JL, Barrero-Amodovar A, et al. Impact of adequate empirical antibiotic therapy on the outcome of patients admitted to the intensive care unit with sepsis. Crit Care Med 2003; 31:2742–2751.

Bochud PY, Bonten M, Marchetti O, et al. Antimicrobial therapy for patients with severe sepsis and septic shock: an evidence-based review. Crit Care Med 2004; 32:S495–S512.

Van den Berghe G, Wilmer A, Hermans G, et al. Intensive insulin therapy in the medical ICU. N Engl J Med 2006; 354:449–461.

CHAPTER EIGHTY-FOUR

Acute Respiratory Failure

Hubert Chen, MD, MPH, and Mark D. Eisner, MD, MPH

BACKGROUND

Acute respiratory failure is one of the most feared complications of the hospitalized patient. Respiratory failure occurs when oxygenation or ventilation becomes sufficiently impaired to threaten the function of vital organs. Such patients can decompensate quickly, requiring that the physician make a number of important decisions within a brief period of time. It is therefore essential that the hospitalist be familiar with the different types of respiratory failure and be comfortable with the management of these patients.

In general, respiratory failure can be divided into two major categories: *hypoxemic respiratory failure* and *hypercapneic respiratory failure*. It is critical to distinguish these types of respiratory failure early, so that the proper treatment can be initiated. Once oxygenation and ventilation have been restored, a more thorough search for the underlying cause of respiratory failure can be pursued. This chapter focuses on differentiating the various causes of acute respiratory failure and provides a general approach to treating these patients.

ASSESSMENT

Clinical Presentation

Incidence

Acute respiratory failure is both a common reason for hospitalization, as well as a frequent complication among hospitalized patients. The annual incidence of acute respiratory failure in the United States has been estimated to be as high as 137 hospitalizations per 100,000 residents, increasing exponentially with each decade of life.[1] In one multicenter study,[2] approximately 32% of all ICU admissions met a diagnosis of acute respiratory failure, defined as a Pa_{O2}/F_{iO2} of <200 mmHg and the need for respiratory support. An additional 24% of patients developed respiratory failure while in the ICU, the most prominent risk factors being infection, neurologic failure, and older age. Studies of acute respiratory distress syndrome (ARDS), a specific type of hypoxemic respiratory failure characterized by diffuse pulmonary infiltrates in the absence of elevated left arterial pressures, have reported an annual incidence between 14–28 cases per 100,000 residents.[3–5]

Presenting Signs and Symptoms

Acute respiratory failure can present in various ways, ranging from overt respiratory distress to nonspecific changes in mental status. Typically, patients will present with respiratory distress. Although the definition of respiratory distress is subjective, it can be easily recognized by a trained clinician. Tachypnea is usually present, as both hypoxemia and hypercapnia are potent respiratory stimulants. In certain circumstances, however, respiratory drive may be depressed, such as in the case of opiate overdose. Depth and pattern of breathing are often affected as well. Use of accessory muscles, retractions, or the presence of a paradoxical breathing pattern (inward movement of the abdomen during inspiration) indicate diaphragmatic fatigue and the need for additional ventilatory support.

Respiratory distress may not be apparent in all patients with acute respiratory failure. In elderly patients, the first sign of hypoxemia may be agitation, confusion, or decreased responsiveness. Stoic or noncommunicative patients may present with increased respiratory rate, cyanosis, or low oxygen saturation. For patients already on supplemental oxygen, a progressive increase in oxygen requirement may be the only indication of impending respiratory failure. In extreme cases, patients may present completely obtunded, as seen in hypercapneic patients with "CO_2 narcosis."

Physical examination, although often nonspecific, will sometimes give clues to the underlying cause of respiratory failure. For example, elevated neck veins, fine pulmonary rales, and peripheral edema suggest left-sided heart failure. Diffuse wheezing and prolonged expiratory phase usually indicate bronchospasm or obstructive airway disease. Certain signs, such as purse-lipped breathing, are more specific to a particular condition like emphysema. The finding of diaphoresis in the setting of respiratory distress should alert the physician to the high probability of impending respiratory arrest.

Clinicians should focus their examination on findings which indicate a focal abnormality. The presence of stridor, for instance, suggests upper airway obstruction as seen in patients with thyroid cancer, postintubation subglottic stenosis, or angioedema. A unilateral decrease in breath sounds and dullness to percussion could represent lobar pneumonia or a large pleural effusion. Hyperresonance and asymmetric chest elevation are concerning for pneumothorax. The absence of findings can also be useful in ruling out certain conditions. In patients with respi-

Table 84-1 Common Causes of Respiratory Failure

Failure to oxygenate	Failure to ventilate
1. Low inspired partial pressure of oxygen High altitude	1. Central nervous system abnormality Brainstem lesion—*stroke, tumor* Spinal cord lesion—*trauma, poliomyelitis, amyotrophic lateral sclerosis* Drug-induced—*sedatives, opiates, alcohol*
2. Diffusion impairment Destruction of alveolar surface area—*emphysema* Obliteration of air-blood interface—*pulmonary fibrosis, pulmonary vascular disease*	2. Neuromuscular disorder Peripheral neuropathy—*Guillain-Barré syndrome* Neuromuscular junction disorder—*myasthenia gravis, botulism* Muscle disorder—*polymyositis, muscular dystrophy*
3. Ventilation-perfusion mismatch Low $\dot{V}/\dot{Q}$ ratio—*obstructive airway disease, atelectasis* High $\dot{V}/\dot{Q}$ ratio—*pulmonary embolism*	3. Chest wall, diaphragm, and pleural disorders Extrathoracic—*flail chest, kyphoscoliosis, massive ascites, morbid obesity* Intrathoracic—*pneumothorax, pulmonary effusion*
4. Right-to-left shunt Intrapulmonary—*pulmonary edema, alveolar hemorrhage, pneumonia, ARDS* Intracardiac*—*patent foramen ovale, atrial or ventricular septal defect*	4. Upper airway obstruction External—*goiter, thyroid cancer, bulky adenopathy* Internal—*foreign body, laryngospasm, subglottic stenosis, angioedema*
5. Alveolar hypoventilation *(see failure to ventilate)*	5. Lower airway obstruction Obstructive airway disease—*asthma, COPD, bronchiolitis*
	6. Dead space ventilation Airway—*bronchiectasis, cystic fibrosis* Alveolar—*bullous emphysema*

*not considered primary respiratory failure

---

ratory distress and an unremarkable chest exam, nonparenchymal conditions such pulmonary embolism must be considered.

Differential Diagnosis

Acute respiratory failure can be divided into *hypoxemic respiratory failure* and *hypercapneic respiratory failure.* While the lungs are the primary site for gas exchange, normal respiration relies on the integrated function of multiple organ systems (including the nervous system, musculoskeletal system, and cardiovascular system). Respiratory failure may result from impairment of any of these essential components. In framing the differential diagnosis of acute respiratory failure, it is important to approach the problem both in terms of basic physiologic principles, as well as using a systems-based approach.

There are five main physiologic causes of hypoxemia (Table 84-1, left column). The first two mechanisms, low inspired partial pressure of oxygen and diffusion impairment, rarely cause acute respiratory failure in the hospital setting. The majority of patients with *hypoxemic respiratory failure* have some degree of ventilation-perfusion ($\dot{V}/\dot{Q}$) mismatch or right-to-left intrapulmonary shunt. $\dot{V}/\dot{Q}$ mismatch usually refers to any condition that produces an imbalance between ventilation and perfusion within alveolar units. $\dot{V}/\dot{Q}$ mismatch is commonly due to impaired ventilation, as occurs in patients with obstructive airway disease or significant atelectasis. $\dot{V}/\dot{Q}$ mismatch, however, may also result from impaired perfusion (while ventilation is preserved), as in the case of pulmonary embolism.

Shunt can be viewed as an extreme case of $\dot{V}/\dot{Q}$ mismatch, in which alveolar units are being perfused, but not ventilated. Intrapulmonary shunt is typically caused by an alveolar-filling process, such as pneumonia, pulmonary edema, or alveolar hemorrhage. The prototypic example of hypoxemic respiratory failure due to shunt is ARDS, which may result from pneumonia, aspiration, sepsis, or trauma. ARDS represents a common pathway in which lung injury results in diffuse alveolar damage, increased vascular permeability, and filling of the alveoli with a protein-rich edema fluid. Other types of right-to-left shunt also exist, such as intracardiac shunt, but are not considered primary respiratory failure.

The other major class of respiratory failure is *hypercapneic respiratory failure.* In this condition, hypoxemia occurs secondary to alveolar hypoventilation. Causes of hypoventilatory failure are best categorized by the component of the respiratory system affected (*see* Table 84-1, right column). For example, respiratory drive may be suppressed at the level of the central nervous system, as in patients who have received excess sedation. Hypoventilation can also occur as a result of neuromuscular weakness (e.g., myasthenia gravis) or due to an anatomic restriction (e.g., kyphoscoliosis, morbid obesity). More commonly, alveolar hypoventilation results from obstruction of the lower airways, such as during an asthma or COPD exacerbation.

Finally, it is important to keep in mind that a number of nonpulmonary disorders can also be associated with respiratory distress. Systemic illnesses, such as septic shock and pancreatitis are well known to induce lung injury and ARDS. Conditions associated with profound metabolic acidosis, particularly diabetic ketoacidosis, substantially increase ventilatory demand and work of breathing. Hyperventilation due to fever, pain, and anxiety can sometimes mimic respiratory distress, but may also be present in patients with true respiratory failure, making it difficult for the clinician to distinguish cause from effect.

Diagnosis

Primary Studies

The initial evaluation of most patients with acute respiratory distress should include the following:

Pulse oximetry. A quick determination of oxygen saturation can be easily obtained by pulse oximetry. Although useful in identifying hypoxemia, pulse oximetry does not provide any information regarding ventilation. For example, a person may have impaired oxygen transfer (e.g., pneumonia) yet still have a normal oxygen saturation due to compensatory hyperventilation. Furthermore, pulse oximetry may not always accurately reflect arterial oxygen tension. In patients with profound hypoxemia, estimates of oxygen saturation by pulse oximetry are notoriously poor. In the presence of abnormal hemoglobins, such as in carbon monoxide poisoning or methemoglobinemia, pulse oximetry can also be misleading.

Arterial blood gas (ABG). ABG analysis allows the clinician to simultaneously assess both oxygenation and ventilation. If oxygenation is impaired, calculating the alveolar-arterial (A-a) gradient can help distinguish hypoxemia due to hypoventilation from other causes of hypoxemia. The A-a gradient can be estimated by subtracting measured arterial P_{O2} (P_{aO2}) from the alveolar P_{O2} (P_{AO2}), calculated using the alveolar gas equation:

$$P_{AO2} = F_{iO2}(P_B - P_{H2O}) - \frac{P_{ACO2}}{R}$$

where F_{iO2} is the fraction of inspired oxygen concentration, P_B is barometric pressure (760 mm Hg at sea level), P_{H2O} is water vapor pressure (47 mm Hg), P_{ACO2} is approximated using arterial P_{CO2}, and R is the respiratory quotient (usually 0.8). An increased A–a gradient suggests that the hypoxemia observed cannot be accounted for solely by hypoventilation. Aside from assessing arterial gas concentrations, an ABG can also be sent for co-oximetry if the presence of carboxyhemoglobin or methemoglobinemia is suspected.

Chest radiograph. While the ABG helps to identify physiologic abnormalities, the chest radiograph is used to evaluate for presence of any parenchymal abnormalities. Although frequently nonspecific in appearance, certain patterns on chest radiograph can be suggestive of specific pathology. For example, bihilar alveolar infiltrates and Kerley B lines indicate heart failure, whereas focal consolidation is more consistent with pneumonia. The chest radiograph can also be helpful in ruling out the presence of extrapulmonary disease, such as a pneumothorax or large pleural effusion. The absence of any significant chest radiograph findings should lead the clinician to consider non-parenchymal processes such as obstructive airway disease or a pulmonary vascular process.

12-lead electrocardiogram (ECG). Cardiac causes of acute respiratory distress, such as arrhythmia, myocardial ischemia, and heart failure, are common in the hospital setting. Therefore, it is always essential that an ECG be obtained as part of the evaluation of any patient with undiagnosed respiratory distress.

Secondary Options

Once the patient has been stabilized, a more comprehensive workup for the underlying cause of respiratory failure can be pursued. Choice of further testing depends on clinical suspicion.

Thoracic imaging. In cases where the chest radiograph is nonspecific, computed tomography (CT) of the chest may yield additional information. CT angiography, in particular, has been shown to have adequate sensitivity and specificity for the detection of clinically significant pulmonary emboli.[6,7] Even when negative for pulmonary embolism, CT angiography can provide other clues to the diagnosis. Pulmonary $\dot{V}/\dot{Q}$ scanning is another option when pulmonary embolism is suspected, but is frequently indeterminate in the presence of other ventilatory defects.[8] Echocardiogram may also be useful, especially when evaluating for congestive heart failure, cardiac ischemia, pulmonary hypertension, valvular pathology, or pericardial tamponade.

Specific laboratory tests. Testing for B-type natriuretic peptide (BNP) is now available at most hospital laboratories. Plasma levels of BNP can help to distinguish heart failure from other types of respiratory failure. In patients with acute dyspnea, a low BNP level (<50 pg/mL) has been demonstrated to have a negative predictive value of 96%.[9] Likewise, D-dimer testing can be useful in ruling out pulmonary embolism, particularly when highly sensitive assays such as the ELISA are used. In the setting of a low pretest probability, a low D-dimer has a negative predictive value of 99%[10] (*see* Chapter 27, Pulmonary Embolism). D-dimers, however, are often elevated in hospitalized patients for other reasons, thereby limiting the clinical utility of this test.[11]

Pulmonary function testing. Spirometry is difficult to obtain in patients with respiratory distress and thus rarely performed. One scenario in which bedside spirometry can be diagnostic is in the setting of upper airway obstruction. Blunting of the inspiratory limb of the flow-volume loop, when present, supports a diagnosis of an extrathoracic obstruction. If neuromuscular weakness is suspected as the cause of respiratory failure, measurements of maximal inspiratory and expiratory pressures can also be useful. For patients who remain intubated, inspiratory force and vital capacity provide similar information.

Bronchoscopy. Traditionally, bronchoscopy has played a limited role in the diagnosis of acute respiratory failure. Indications for bronchoscopy usually include ruling out specific pathology such as central airway obstruction, occult pulmonary hemorrhage, or infection. In cases of suspected ventilator-associated pneumonia, distal airway sampling via bronchoscopy has been shown to help guide antibiotic therapy, as well as improve ICU outcomes[12] (*see* Chapter 34, Nosocomial pneumonia).

Preferred Approach

Causes of acute respiratory failure are wide and varied; therefore, it is best to have a systematic approach to the diagnosis. Figure 84-1 depicts a conceptual algorithm for approaching patients with acute respiratory failure. After first assessing the immediate need for intubation, an ABG, ECG, and chest radiograph should be ordered. As these studies are underway, the clinician ought to have an opportunity to perform a focused history and physical examination.

As discussed, an ABG is essential in quantifying the severity of hypoxemia and determining whether hypercapnia is present. By calculating the A–a gradient, one can determine whether the observed hypoxemia can be explained primarily on the basis of alveolar hypoventilation. Hypoxemia with a normal A–a gradient should lead the clinician to consider the differential diagnosis for hypercapneic respiratory failure. On the other hand, if an

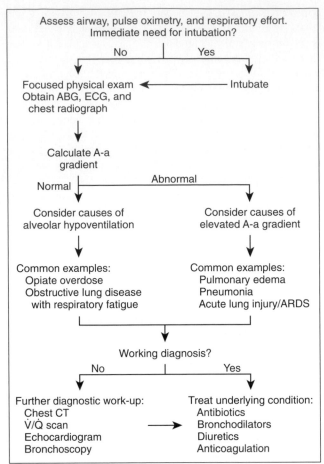

Figure 84-1 • Conceptual approach to acute respiratory failure.

increased A–a gradient is found, then one ought to evaluate for conditions in which $\dot{V}/\dot{Q}$ mismatch or shunting occur. Response to 100% oxygen can be used to determine whether right-to-left shunt is present. Unlike $\dot{V}/\dot{Q}$ mismatch, hypoxemia due to shunt does not respond completely to increases in inspired oxygen. When present, intrapulmonary shunt is typically associated with an alveolar-filling process detectable by chest radiograph. If there are no radiographic findings to account for intrapulmonary shunt, then a work-up for pulmonary embolism or intracardiac shunt ought to be pursued.

Prognosis

During Hospitalization

The hospital course of patients with acute respiratory failure depends largely on the nature of the underlying condition. Patients with hypercapneic respiratory failure due to drug overdose tend to recover without major sequelae, while those with ARDS have mortality rates as high as 60%.[13] Studies of acute respiratory failure (including all types) have shown overall mortality rates ranging from about 30–40%.[1–3] One multicenter study of critically ill patients with acute respiratory failure showed that length of stay was longer, and ICU mortality rate was more than twice that of patients without respiratory failure.[2] Independent risk factors for death include age, multiorgan system failure,

malignancy, HIV, chronic renal failure, liver cirrhosis, and sepsis.[1,2]

In particular, much research has been focused on outcomes of patients with ARDS.[13] In this population, it has been found that the majority of deaths are attributable to sepsis or multiorgan dysfunction rather than a primary respiratory cause. Risk factors for death in ARDS are similar to those for acute respiratory failure. Notably, however, it has been found that indexes of oxygenation and ventilation are not good predictors of outcome. Although mortality remains high, recent evidence suggests that the mortality rate for ARDS may be decreasing.[13]

Postdischarge

Extended survival is common among patients with acute respiratory failure who survive to discharge.[14] Although nearly half of survivors have evidence of impaired functional capacity several years later, only a fraction of this impairment can be directly attributed to the sequelae of respiratory failure.[14] Among ARDS survivors, evidence shows that lung function generally returns to near normal levels but plateaus quickly thereafter.[15] Residual impairments in lung function and quality of life continue to be detected even several months after hospitalization.[16,17]

MANAGEMENT

Treatment

Initial Management

Initial management for patients with acute respiratory failure should always address airway patency, oxygenation, and ventilation, in the stated order.

Airway management. Patency of the airway is crucial. If obstruction of the upper airway is present, any other intervention will prove futile until airflow is restored. Ability to protect the airway should also be assessed. Presence of a decreased gag or cough reflex may be an indication that a patient cannot adequately manage his or her own secretions. Attempts at securing the airway should begin with the least invasive approach. In patients with altered level of consciousness, obstruction is commonly due to occlusion by the tongue. In many cases, the airway can be opened by repositioning of the head and applying a jaw thrust maneuver. Simple appliances such as a plastic oral pharyngeal airway or nasopharyngeal tube can be inserted to temporarily stent the airway open (Fig. 84-2). If a foreign body or thick secretions are present, direct laryngoscopy may be required for removal of the object or for suctioning. In patients who are unconscious or unable to maintain an airway, oral or nasal endotracheal intubation is often necessary. In certain situations, endotracheal intubation may not be feasible, in which case an emergency cricothyrotomy should be performed.

Supplemental oxygen. Restoration of normoxia is critical, as irreversible brain damage occurs after only minutes without oxygen. Hypercarbia and acidosis, on the other hand, are better tolerated by the body unless extreme or prolonged. In general, the immediate goal should be to establish an oxygen saturation of >90% or P_{aO2} of >60 mm Hg. Delivery of oxygen is usually started at F_{iO2} of 100%, then titrated to maintain adequate oxygenation. Although high levels of inspired oxygen can result in worsening of hypercapnea in certain patients (e.g., COPD), oxygen therapy should not be withheld if significant hypoxemia exists.

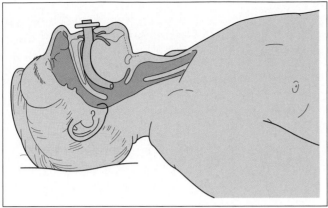

Figure 84-2 • Use of an oral pharyngeal airway device to prevent upper airway occlusion by the tongue.

Box 84-1 Indications for endotracheal intubation
1. Airway patency
Upper airway obstruction
Altered level of consciousness
2. Pulmonary toilet
Inability to clear secretions
3. Oxygenation
Refractory hypoxemia despite supplemental oxygen
4. Ventilation
Severe respiratory acidosis
Apnea
5. Work of breathing
Extreme respiratory distress
Respiratory muscle fatigue

In the spontaneously breathing patient, oxygen can be delivered by nasal cannula or facemask. Fraction of inspired oxygen delivered by nasal cannula depends on minute ventilation and the entrainment of room air, and thus cannot be reliably determined in patients with respiratory distress. Facemasks, by providing a higher flow rate, allow oxygen to be titrated more carefully. If necessary, a "Venturi" mask can be used to deliver specified concentrations of oxygen while ensuring adequate airflow to the patient. More recently, high-flow oxygen blenders (≥ 80 L/min) have been developed that can deliver high-flow humidified oxygen at predetermined concentrations via nasal cannula. If normal oxygenation cannot be achieved with the use of supplemental oxygen, then positive-pressure ventilation may be required.

Noninvasive positive-pressure ventilation (NIPPV). The increased availability of NIPPV has proven to be useful in certain patient populations. NIPPV is particularly effective in treating patients with acute hypercapneic respiratory failure. Studies in patients with COPD have demonstrated NIPPV to be effective in reducing the rate of intubation, length of stay, and mortality.[18] Similar trials of NIPPV for acute hypoxemic (nonhypercapneic) respiratory failure have shown mixed results, depending on the population in question.[19] NIPPV is best reserved for those in whom the cause of respiratory failure can be reversed over several hours. For example, in patients with hypoxemia due to cardiogenic pulmonary edema, the application of NIPPV has been shown to improve outcomes.[20] In cases such as ARDS, where prolonged respiratory support is required for recovery, intubation and mechanical ventilation should be considered (*see* Chapter 86, Noninvasive ventilation).

Endotracheal intubation. Prediction rules for when or whether to intubate have not been well studied. While certain parameters have been suggested as guidelines (Box 84-1), often the entire clinical picture needs to be taken into account. As mentioned, airway protection and hypoxemia are both common indications for intubation when other noninvasive modalities have failed. The presence of hypercarbia alone, however, is not always a reliable indicator (as P_{aCO2} is often elevated in patients with chronic hypoventilation). On the other hand, serial ABGs demonstrating an acute increase in P_{aCO2} and a drop in pH is much more suggestive of impending respiratory failure, as this indicates that ventilation is no longer sufficient to meet metabolic demand.

Degree of respiratory distress, work of breathing, and change in mental status also need to be taken into account. The decision of when to consider a trial of NIPPV versus immediate intubation remains subject to debate. NIPPV is felt to be most beneficial in patients with early respiratory failure and a pH of greater than 7.1.[21] Patients who are severely acidemic should probably be intubated immediately.

Subsequent Management

Once airway, oxygenation, and ventilation have been addressed, subsequent treatment should be aimed at the underlying cause of respiratory failure. The early initiation of empiric board-spectrum antibiotics is recommended for all patients at high risk for pneumonia. In patients with evidence of obstructive airway disease, use of inhaled bronchodilators and systemic corticosteroids is indicated. If volume overload is suspected, then intravenous diuretics should be administered. Specific treatments for the different causes of respiratory failure are discussed in their respective chapters.

Patients with acute respiratory failure often require prolonged mechanical ventilation, particularly those with ARDS. Much research has been focused on possible treatments for ARDS; however, the only strategy to demonstrate a clear survival benefit is the use of low tidal volume ventilation. In a large, multicenter trial performed by the ARDS Network, mortality was reduced by 22% in patients treated with low tidal ventilation (6 mL/kg of predicted body weight) versus those ventilated at traditional tidal volumes (12 mL/kg).[22] Surprisingly, this benefit was observed, despite the fact that hypoxemia was somewhat worse in the group receiving lower tidal volumes. These findings suggest that low tidal ventilation may work by minimizing ventilator-associated lung injury rather than by the correction of hypoxemia. Consequently, this low tidal volume approach, also referred to as "protective lung strategy," should be adopted in all patients with acute lung injury or ARDS (for detailed protocol, see ARDS Network website at http://www.ardsnet.org/lowvtrefcard.pdf).

PREVENTION

Prevention measures should focus on reducing the risk of pneumonia, aspiration, pulmonary embolism, and other common causes of respiratory failure. Measures used to prevent pulmonary complications in hospitalized patients include use of incentive spirometry, frequent ambulation, aspiration precautions, prophylaxis for deep venous thrombosis, and avoidance of CNS depressants whenever possible. In addition, high-risk patients who have not been previously immunized against pneumococcus should be vaccinated prior to discharge.

DISCHARGE/FOLLOW-UP PLANS

Respiratory failure is often an indicator of advanced medical illness; therefore, the primary care provider should be contacted at least at the time of admission and at discharge.[23] In the case of patients who are gravely ill, efforts should be made to invite the primary provider to important family meetings. Oftentimes, the primary provider will have an established relationship with the patient, which may facilitate discussions regarding withdrawal of care or placement in hospice if necessary.

Survivors of acute respiratory failure frequently develop muscle wasting and weakness, requiring discharge to a subacute care unit for rehabilitation.[17] On rare occasion, patients may even need to be discharged to a chronic ventilator facility. Such patients may transition through the care of several physicians before finally returning home. In such circumstances, coordinating the transfer of care with the primary provider is absolutely essential.[24] Once the patient has recovered, the primary provider may wish to readdress the patient's desire for medical intervention should he or she develop respiratory failure again in the future.

Key Points

- The annual incidence of acute respiratory failure increases exponentially with each decade of life.

- In elderly patients, the first sign of hypoxemia may be agitation, confusion, or decreased responsiveness.

- The initial evaluation of patients with acute respiratory distress should include: airway assessment, pulse oximetry, ABG, CXR, and ECG.

- An ABG is important for determining whether the primary cause of respiratory failure is impaired oxygenation (hypoxemic respiratory failure) or failure to ventilate (hypercapneic respiratory failure).

- Non-invasive ventilation in patients with hypercapneic respiratory failure due to obstructive airway disease and in patients with acute cardiogenic pulmonary edema may prevent the need for intubation.

- A protective lung strategy utilizing a low tidal volume approach should be adopted for patients with acute lung injury or ARDS that require intubation and prolonged mechanical ventilation.

SUGGESTED READING

Vincent JL, Akca S, De Mendonca A, et al. The epidemiology of acute respiratory failure in critically ill patients. Chest 2002; 121(5):1602–1609.

Hayashino Y, Goto M, Noguchi Y, et al. Ventilation-perfusion scanning and helical CT in suspected pulmonary embolism: meta-analysis of diagnostic performance. Radiology 2005; 234(3):740–748.

Maisel AS, Krishnaswamy P, Nowak RM, et al. Rapid measurement of B-type natriuretic peptide in the emergency diagnosis of heart failure. N Engl J Med 2002; 347(3):161–167.

Crowther MA, Cook DJ, Griffith LE, et al. Neither baseline tests of molecular hypercoagulability nor D-dimer levels predict deep venous thrombosis in critically ill medical-surgical patients. Intensive Care Med 2005; 31(1):48–55.

Ware LB, Matthay MA. The acute respiratory distress syndrome. N Engl J Med 2000; 342(18):1334–1349.

Garland A, Dawson NV, Altmann I, et al. Outcomes up to 5 years after severe, acute respiratory failure. Chest 2004; 126(6):1897–1904.

Herridge MS, Cheung AM, Tansey CM, et al. One-year outcomes in survivors of the acute respiratory distress syndrome. N Engl J Med 2003; 348(8):683–693.

Liesching T, Kwok H, Hill NS. Acute applications of noninvasive positive pressure ventilation. Chest 2003; 124(2):699–713.

CHAPTER EIGHTY-FIVE

Sedation and Pain Management in the Critically Ill

Kenneth R. Epstein, MD, MBA, FACP

BACKGROUND

In the intensive care unit (ICU), critically ill patients frequently experience pain and anxiety, which medical staff should attempt to alleviate. Among the many causes of pain and anxiety in the ICU are the underlying disease process, the performance of diagnostic and therapeutic procedures, the use of mechanical ventilation, loss of control or autonomy, uncertainty regarding prognosis, and physical isolation from familiar surroundings and loved ones.[1] Although all critically ill patients experience pain and anxiety, the need for sedation and analgesia is particularly important for patients who are mechanically ventilated or delirious.

In addition to its clinical importance, effective treatment of pain and anxiety correlates directly with resource utilization and length of stay in the ICU. Both under- and over-treatment can prolong length of stay. Under-treatment can worsen autonomic nervous system function and other physiologic parameters, while over-treatment can worsen delirium and prolong time to extubation. In addition to causing extreme discomfort, unrelieved pain can result in inadequate sleep, may worsen delirium, and is a common cause of agitation. Pain evokes a stress response, resulting in tachycardia, increased myocardial oxygen consumption, hypercoagulability, immunosuppression, and persistent catabolism.[2] Effective treatment of pain and anxiety can decrease these autonomic nervous system responses, decrease myocardial work, and improve oxygen consumption.

Pain intensity or need for analgesia is not affected by gender, age, or personality adjustment.[3] In one study of patients' perception of pain and pain management in a critical care unit, 64% were often in moderate to severe pain while in the ICU. Pain intensity correlated with waiting for an analgesic, expectation of less pain, and longer stay in the ICU.[4] In another study of ICU patients, 74% rated their pain as moderate to severe, despite the fact that 95% of house staff and 81% of nurses reported that the patients were receiving adequate pain control.[5]

ASSESSMENT AND DIAGNOSIS

Assessment of Pain in the ICU

Various scales exist for assessment of pain in the patient who is cognitively intact and able to communicate either verbally or nonverbally. These scales include the verbal rating scale, visual analog scale, and numeric rating scale (e.g., 0–10, where 0 is no pain and 10 is the worst pain ever experienced). However, critically ill patients are often not able to communicate due to delirium, encephalopathy, pharmacologic sedation, or neuromuscular blockade. In these patients, the clinician must use behavioral or physiologic assessment to estimate the patient's pain. For example, the Behavioral Pain Scale allows medical staff to assess pain-related behaviors such as grimacing, other facial expressions, agitation, and posturing and to measure it in a standardized fashion (Table 85-1).[5a] Physiologic measures such as heart rate, blood pressure, and respiratory rate also can correlate directly with the level of patient agitation. Assessing and treating patients' pain and agitation not only provides comfort, but improves outcomes with decreased duration of mechanical ventilation and nosocomial infections.[5b]

Patients may be in pain from the endotracheal tube, the various intravenous lines, and the procedures being done on the patient. However, it is also imperative to rule out other causes of pain. The level of sedation should be light enough to allow the clinician to perform a thorough physical examination, in order to rule out abdominal or other tenderness, examine the skin for integrity, and look for any other medical causes of pain.

Assessment of Sedation

Common indications for sedation are listed in Table 85-2.[6] The presence of anxiety or agitation is often the primary reason to sedate a critically ill patient. However, once anxiety or agitation is detected, the first step should be to rule out any underlying physiologic abnormality. Examples include hypoxia, hypoglycemia, hypotension, pain, and alcohol or other drug withdrawal.[2] Sedation should only be used after pain and reversible physiologic causes have been treated. Since pain and discomfort are main causes of agitation, they should be treated with analgesics before sedatives are administered.

Once the decision to sedate a patient is made, ongoing monitoring is critical. The Society of Critical Care Medicine practice guidelines recommend frequent use of sedation scales that are both valid and reliable.[2] They also recommend the use of protocol-driven sedation plans. In a study on implementing a sedation and delirium monitoring program for nurses in the ICU, the biggest barriers to implementation were physician buy-in and time.[7]

Table 85-1 Behavioral Pain Scale

Behavioral Pain Scale	Description	Score
Facial expression	Relaxed	1
	Partially tightened (e.g., brow lowering)	2
	Fully tightened (e.g., eyelid closing)	3
	Grimacing	4
Upper limbs	No movement	1
	Partially bent	2
	Fully bent with finger flexion	3
	Permanently retracted	4
Compliance with ventilation	Tolerating movement	1
	Coughing but tolerating ventilation for most of the time	2
	Fighting ventilator	3
	Unable to control ventilation	4

From: Payen JF, Bru O, Bosson JL, et al. Assessing pain in critically ill sedated patients by using a behavioral pain scale. Crit Care Med 2001; 29:2258–2263.

Table 85-2 Indications for Sedation

Indication	Comments
Analgesia	Adequate analgesia is the first priority when choosing a sedating agent.
Anxiety and agitation	Due to inability to communicate, continuous noise, continuous lighting, excessive sensory stimulation, sleep deprivation, as well as pain
Dyspnea	The sensation of dyspnea can cause severe anxiety.
Delirium	Can worsen agitation
To facilitate nursing and other care	Is only an indication if the agitation is creating a risk situation for the patient
To prevent pulling out lines or self-extubation	Goal is sedation at lowest level possible
To decrease excess oxygen consumption	Primarily by decreasing anxiety and agitation
To achieve amnesia	Only an indication if neuromuscular blocking agents are used

From: Gehlbach BK, Kress JP. Sedation in the intensive care unit. Curr Opin Crit Care 2002; 8:290–298.

Table 85-3 Sedation Scales

A. Riker Sedation-Agitation Scale

Score	Description
7	Dangerous agitation
6	Very agitated
5	Agitated
4	Calm and cooperative
3	Sedated
2	Very sedated
1	Unarousable

From: Riker RR, Picard JT, Fraser GL. Prospective evaluation of the Sedation-Agitation Scale for adult critically ill patients. Crit Care Med 1999; 27:1325–1329.

B. Motor Activity Assessment Scale (MAAS)

Score	Description
6	Dangerously agitated
5	Agitated
4	Restless and cooperative
3	Calm and cooperative
2	Responsive to touch or name
1	Responsive only to noxious stimuli
0	Unresponsive

From: Riker RR, Picard JT, Fraser GL. Prospective evaluation of the Sedation-Agitation Scale for adult critically ill patients. Crit Care Med 1999; 27:1325–1329.

C. Ramsay Scale

Score	Description
6	Asleep—No response to light glabellar tap or loud auditory stimulus
5	Asleep—A sluggish response to light glabellar tap or loud auditory stimulus
4	Asleep—A brisk response to light glabellar tap or loud auditory stimulus
3	Awake—Patient responds to commands only
2	Awake—Patient cooperative, oriented, and tranquil
1	Awake—Patient anxious and agitated or restless or both

From: Ramsay MA, Savege TM, Simpson BR, et al. Controlled sedation with alphaxalone-alphadalone. Brit Med J 1974; 2(920):656–659.

D. Richmond Agitation-Sedation Scale

Score	Description
−5	Unarousable
−4	Deep sedation
−3	Moderate sedation
−2	Light sedation
−1	Drowsy
0	Alert and calm
+1	Restless
+2	Agitated
+3	Very agitated
+4	Combative

From: Sessler CN, Gosnell MS, Grap MJ et al. The Richmond Agitation-Sedation Scale. Amer J Respir Crit Care Med 2002; 166:1338–1344.

Note: All scales are reported as the single number, measured at some uniform time interval.

Use of a sedation protocol has been shown to reduce both mean ventilator time and length of stay in the ICU.[8]

Several sedation scales have been shown to be valid and reliable in assessing the degree of a patient's sedation acutely and over time. These include the Ramsay Scale (RS), Sedation-Agitation Scale (SAS), Glasgow Coma Scale (GCS), Motor Activity Assessment Scale (MAAS), and the Richmond Agitation-Sedation Scale (RASS). The various scales and their components are shown in Table 85-3. The scales are all used by recording, at standard intervals, the digit that corresponds to the patient's level of sedation and agitation. These assessment tools (*see* Table 85-3) are used to maintain the desired level of sedation as staff varies by shift in the ICU and as goals change. The desired level of sedation should be explicitly identified by the physician managing the patient, and then nursing staff can adjust treatments according to protocol to achieve this level.

Each scale has advantages and disadvantages. The GCS is most often used in the assessment of brain-injured and comatose patients. The Ramsay Scale is probably the most commonly used scale at present, but probably because it is older and simple to use. However, the Ramsay Scale and the MAAS only allow the clinician to rate the patient from awake to unresponsive. The Riker Scale adds the ability to also measure and record the degree of agitation. The RASS may be the most useful, because it allows the clinician to rate degrees of sedation (−1 to −4) and degrees of agitation (+1 to +4) on the same scale, using a negative to positive number format, and it provides an assessment of mental function beyond level of consciousness.

The Bispectral Index System (BIS)

All of the standard sedation scales discussed above require subjective measurement, though the RASS has been shown to be valid and reliable in research studies. Nonetheless, there is potential for variation in the score, based on individual interpretation of the patient's level of sedation. Interest in developing quantitative and physiologic measurements of sedation led to the Bispectral Index. The BIS uses specially designed electroencephalographic (EEG) electrodes that connect either to a standalone monitor or to a module integrated into the existing bedside monitors.[9] A computerized algorithm then reviews the EEG data and produces a numeric value between 0 (isoelectric EEG) and 100 (maximum value of awakeness). The BIS is affected by muscle movement, although newer versions attempt to control for the degree of electromyographic (EMG) activity, which can falsely elevate the score. It is also affected by the degree of underlying neurologic illness, such as encephalopathy, as well as other physiologic states. Research so far has not supported any consistent advantages to using the BIS over the currently validated sedation scales, and its potential role in routinely monitoring sedated patients remains to be determined. However, the BIS may have some clinical utility for patients in deep levels of sedation. The BIS can continue to monitor depth of sedation from the point of unresponsiveness down to complete EEG suppression. There can be a wide range of BIS levels in patients with minimum sedation scores. For similar reasons, the BIS may have utility in paralyzed ICU patients.

Assessment of Delirium

Given the links between pain, agitation, and delirium, understanding how to assess the delirious ICU patient is critical to overall management. Due to the multiorgan system illness that patients suffer in the critical care setting, the prevalence of delirium is high. In one study, 81.7% of mechanically ventilated medical ICU patients had delirium, which lasted on average 2.1 days. Patients with dementia have a much higher risk of delirium in the ICU.[10] Given its profound negative impact on outcomes, identification and treatment of delirium are important. After

adjusting for multiple demographic and clinical variables, the presence of delirium was associated with 39% higher ICU costs, 31% higher total hospital costs,[11] longer length of stay in the ICU, and higher mortality.[12,13]

Delirium can be functionally defined as an acutely changing or fluctuating mental status, inattention, disorganized thinking, and an altered level of consciousness that may or may not be accompanied by agitation.[2] The tool that has been most studied, and found to be valid and reproducible, is the Confusion Assessment Method for the Intensive Care Unit (CAM-ICU). This instrument assesses both observed behaviors and nonverbal responses to simple questions as well as visual and auditory recognition tasks. When CAM-ICU was compared to the reference standard of a delirium expert who used the DSM-4 criteria, the scale showed excellent reliability and validity when used by nurses and physicians.[14,15] As with pain, delirium should be identified and underlying reversible etiologies identified and treated instead of simply sedating patients to obliterate symptoms.

MANAGEMENT

Treatment

Treatment for pain, agitation, and delirium must be individualized and titrated to the patient's response. As discussed above, sedation should only be used for the treatment or prevention of anxiety, agitation, and as an adjunct in the treatment of pain. Analgesics and sedatives should not be routinely used as "chemical restraints" in the absence of these clear indications.

Many pharmacokinetic and pharmacodynamic differences exist among both analgesic and sedative agents. A thorough discussion of this topic is beyond the scope of this chapter, and is covered in Chapter 94. However, certain general principles are worth noting. In critically ill patients, there is a wide variation in organ function and hemodynamics that creates significant interindividual variation. An "appropriate dose" of a medication pharmacologically may be toxic in one patient and provide minimal analgesia or sedation in another. Hepatic metabolism and renal excretion are often altered in the critically ill patient, resulting in serum half-lives that may vary considerably from expectation. Additionally, oral doses of medications are often administered via a nasogastric or other enteral feeding tube. Conversion of a tablet or capsule into a form suitable for administration through a tube can considerably alter a medication's properties, rendering it less effective or more toxic.[16] Enteral absorption is also unpredictable. Therefore, dosing of medications must be individualized to the patient, and the use of a standardized sedation scale to assess effect is recommended.

Analgesic Agents

Opioids

Opioids are the mainstay of treatment of pain in the ICU. This class of medications also produces some sedation and anxiolysis, but the effect is less predictable and less titratable. Short-term, however, there may sometimes be a role for analgesia-based sedation, where an opioid analgesic is administered initially titrated to comfort, and a sedative is added only if

Table 85-4 Properties of Opioids

Name	Onset of Action	Duration of Action	Metabolism/Excretion	Comments
Morphine	5–10 min	Up to 4 hr	Hepatic metabolism Renal excretion	Half-life may be significantly prolonged in patients with hepatic or renal disease
Hydromorphone	5 min	Up to 4 hr, often much less	Hepatic metabolism Renal excretion	Shorter duration of action than morphine due to lack of active metabolites
Meperidine	3–5 min	1–4 hr	Hepatic metabolism with active metabolites	Primary metabolite is normeperidine, which is a CNS stimulant and may cause seizures
Fentanyl	1 min	0.5–1 hr	Hepatic metabolism to inactive product Not renally excreted.	Good choice for renal failure Best for rapid treatment of pain Long-term use, morphine, or hydromorphone are preferable
Remifentanil	<1 min	5–10 min	Metabolism independent of hepatic and renal function[18] Renal excretion	Rapid metabolism requires slow taper to avoid withdrawal syndrome[17,18]

necessary.[17] Due to the pharmacologic variability in effect in the critically ill discussed above, there are no minimum or maximum doses. The dose must be individualized, based on the patient's renal and hepatic function, and most importantly, on the clinical effect.

Due to their effect on the mu-2 receptors, opioids can cause respiratory depression with decreased respiratory rate. Chronically, patients develop tolerance to the respiratory depressant effect, but acutely this is a concern in the spontaneously breathing or partially ventilated patient. They also can cause a decreased response to hypoxia, which makes them useful agents for patients with subjective feelings of dyspnea. When administering opiates, health care providers should remember their side effect of decreased GI motility with constipation and institute preventive treatment (e.g., a stimulant such as senna) at the time of administration.

Table 85-4 reviews the pharmacologic properties of the opioids that are commonly used in the critical care setting. Hypotension can occur with all opioids, particularly in hypovolemic or hemodynamically unstable patients. Hypotension can, however, occur in stable, euvolemic patients due to sympatholysis, vagally mediated bradycardia, and histamine release (particularly in morphine, meperidine, and codeine).[2] In the hemodynamically unstable patient, as well as in those with renal insufficiency, hydromorphone or fentanyl causes less hypotension, and are therefore recommended. Some patients will report an allergy to morphine, but in many cases this is not a true allergy. Due to histamine release in the mast cells, morphine may result in pruritus and allergic-type reactions. If it is necessary to use morphine, the pruritus can be treated with antihistamines. Hydromorphone has some distinct advantages in that it does not cause the histamine effect of morphine. Meperidine, an agent with a potentially toxic metabolite, can cause seizures and should not be routinely used

in the ICU setting (see Table 85-4). It offers no real advantages over the other agents, and many hospitals have removed it from their formularies.

Fentanyl is a good choice for patients with renal failure. It is hepatically metabolized to an inactive product, and there is no renal metabolism. Remifentanil has the most rapid onset of action, and it is quickly degraded to inactive metabolites. It is therefore very easy to titrate remifentanil to clinical effect. Because of the short and predictable half-life, higher doses can be used, making it an effective agent for analgesia while decreasing the need for concomitant sedatives.[17] In a study comparing remifentanil with fentanyl for analgesia in the ICU, both were equally efficacious,[17] but the remifentanil group required less frequent and lower doses of propofol to achieve sedation than did the fentanyl group.

Nonsteroidal Anti-inflammatory Drugs (NSAIDs)

Although NSAIDs have some theoretical benefit in reducing opioid requirements, they actually have a much higher risk-to-benefit ratio, due to their potential to cause side effects including gastrointestinal bleeding, other bleeding due to platelet inhibition, and development of worsening renal function. Therefore, the benefit of NSAIDs in reducing the need for opioids in the critically ill patient is unclear, and this has not been adequately studied.

Acetaminophen

Acetaminophen is a useful oral analgesic for mild-to-moderate pain. However, excessive doses must be avoided due to the risk of hepatoxicity. In selected patients who can take oral medication and have mild discomfort, acetaminophen has a role.

Table 85-5 Properties of Benzodiazepines

Name	Onset of Action	Duration of Action	Metabolism/Excretion	Comments
Midazolam	0.5–5 min	2 hr	Hepatically metabolized Renally excreted	Half-life may be significantly prolonged in patients with hepatic or renal disease.
Lorazepam	5 min	Up to 6 hr	Renal excretion	Due to longer duration of action, need to watch for evidence of drug accumulation, especially in those with renal failure.
Diazepam	1–3 min	Single dose: 30–60 min	Hepatic metabolism with active metabolites	With prolonged administration, duration of action can be many hours to days.
Chlordiazepoxide	Variable	Variable and prolonged	Hepatic metabolism with multiple active metabolites	Clinical effect variable, based on hepatic disease and age.

Agents for Sedation

Benzodiazepines

The mechanism of action of benzodiazepines is through the potentiation of GABA receptor complex-mediated inhibition of the CNS. In addition to anxiolysis, benzodiazepines are potent amnestic agents, and in high doses they are hypnotic. They all have anticonvulsant properties. Like opioids, benzodiazepines can cause dose-dependent CNS-mediated respiratory depression. This effect, however, is less potent than that of opioids. Benzodiazepines tend to decrease tidal volume, whereas opioids exert their respiratory effect by lowering respiratory rate.[6] Benzodiazepines also have a synergistic effect with opioids in producing sedation.

Lipid soluble, they are distributed into peripheral tissues and accumulate with prolonged infusion. The drug may be released back in to the bloodstream, resulting in extended sedation even though the infusion has stopped. Table 85-5 reviews some of the key pharmacologic properties of the benzodiazepines, but pharmacokinetics and pharmacodynamics may be quite different in the critically ill. For instance, increasing evidence indicates that midazolam may not be a short-acting agent in critically ill patients, especially those over 50 years of age.[16] This drug, however, remains a very useful drug for short-term use in critically ill patients without significant hepatic or renal disease. The pharmacokinetics of lorazepam are less affected by age or critical illness than are those of midazolam, so it is preferable for long-term sedation in the ICU. However, due to its longer duration of action, clinicians need to watch for evidence of drug accumulation. Both lorazepam and midazolam are more water soluble and have shorter durations of action than diazepam, so they are preferable in the critical care setting.

Propofol (Diprivan)

Propofol is also a GABA agonist,[18] but it may act at a different site than benzodiazepines, and its exact mechanism of action is unclear. A very short-acting intravenous anesthetic agent, it has become popular for continuous sedation of patients undergoing mechanical ventilation. As with all sedatives, however, the clini-

cal effect is variable in the critically ill, so dosing needs to be titrated to effect.

It has a rapid onset (1–5 min) and short duration of action (2–8 min). It is therefore more effective as a continuous infusion than as a bolus injection. Even with prolonged infusion, the duration of action remains relatively short (less than an hour) if it is discontinued within 24–48 hours, making it a very useful drug for quick weaning from mechanical ventilation. Propofol metabolism and excretion are not affected by hepatic or renal dysfunction, but concern about significant myopathy with prolonged infusions beyond 48 hours exists.

It is not known how effective propofol is as an analgesic. Propofol use should therefore be accompanied by the use of an opioid if the patient is expected to be in pain, or if painful procedures are planned. Concurrent opioid administration may increase the amnestic and hypnotic effects of propofol.[16] Propofol has more potent cardiovascular effects than do benzodiazepines. It can cause hypotension, especially if the patient is hypovolemic. It can also cause myocardial depression, which is useful in patients with ischemic heart disease, but can be problematic in patients with left ventricular dysfunction.

Propofol is very highly lipid soluble, and it is prepared in a lipid emulsion. Bacteria and fungi can grow in the emulsion, so strict aseptic technique must be used. The clinician must monitor triglyceride levels and discontinue the medication if levels increase. Also, since the lipid provides caloric input, it may be necessary to adjust the lipids in parenteral nutrition formulas. In one study of 159 ICU patients receiving propofol, 18% developed elevated triglycerides. Pancreatitis developed in 10% of those patients who developed hypertriglyceridemia.[19] The risk of developing hypertriglyceridemia was increased in patients who were older, had longer ICU stays, and who had longer duration of therapy with propofol.

Etomidate

Etomidate is a short-acting induction anesthetic. It has a rapid onset of action and a short half-life. This medication is particularly useful in patients with cardiovascular dysfunction and instability. Its primary use in the critically ill is for short-term use, such as in emergent intubation. Continuous sedation with etomidate can result in adrenal depression and increased mortality,[20] so it is not recommended for continuous infusion or long-term use.

Dexmedetomidine (Precedex)

This centrally acting α_2 agonist has been approved for sedation of intubated and mechanically ventilated patients in the ICU, but is restricted to 24 hours or less.[20a] In addition to its sedating effect associated with minimal depression of respiratory drive, it has analgesic properties due to binding on receptors in the spinal cord. Most experience has been in surgical patients undergoing cardiac and vascular procedures, and careful administration with slow loading is necessary to avoid side effects. Hypotension can occur in up to 30% of patients and nausea in 10% or more. Other adverse side effects include atrial fibrillation and bradycardia. More experience is needed before routine use in medical ICU patients.

Barbiturates

Barbiturates have much longer serum half-lives than the other agents, so they are not routinely used for sedation in critically ill patients. The exception is in patients with acute head injury, where they are very effective sedatives due to their ability to decrease cerebral blood flow and metabolic oxygen consumption.[16] The barbiturate used most often in this setting is pentobarbital.

Butyrophenones (Haloperidol)

The mechanism of action of this class of drugs is that of dopamine antagonist. Compared to older neuroleptic agents such as chlorpromazine, haloperidol is less sedating, has less anticholinergic side effects, and causes less hypotension. Haloperidol has a long half-life and can be given as intermittent intravenous injections. The clinician can start with a loading dose of 2 mg, followed by repeat doses (doubling the previous dose as necessary) every 15–20 minutes until agitation is decreased. Haloperidol prolongs Q-T interval, and may increase the risk of torsades de pointes. It is therefore important to monitor for electrocardiographic changes. It also can induce extrapyramidal symptoms, although intravenous doses may not have as high a risk as oral doses.[2]

Daily Interruption of Sedation

Continuous infusion of sedatives provides a more uniform degree of sedation than does intermittent bolus administration. However, a potential disadvantage to continuous infusion is the inability to assess any improvement in mental status. For this reason and others, the continuous infusion of IV sedation has been associated with prolongation of mechanical ventilation, prolonged length of intensive care stay, and extended hospitalization.[21] Prolongation of mechanical ventilation has been associated with increased risk of ventilator-associated pneumonia, barotrauma, airway complications, and unanticipated extubation with resultant oxygen desaturation.[22]

Daily interruption of sedative infusion to awaken the patient allows the clinician to perform a more accurate assessment of the patient's neurologic and mental status, allowing daily reassessment of the dose necessary for sedation. As the patient improves, lower doses of sedatives can be used on subsequent days. Daily awakening also allows a more accurate physical examination and earlier detection of problems such as increased abdominal tenderness.

In one study, interrupting sedative infusions daily (long enough for the patient to awaken) shortened the median duration of mechanical ventilation from 7.3 days to 4.9 days, and the median length of stay in the intensive care unit from 9.9 days to 6.4 days.[23] Kress et al. also found that this protocol reduced the total dose of benzodiazepines administered by almost half, but did not alter the total dose of propofol used.[23] Another study found that daily interruption decreased the incidence of complications, including ventilator-associated pneumonia, bacteremia, barotrauma, and venous thromboembolism. The overall rate of complications was 2.8% for the daily interruption group versus 6.2% for the control group (P = 0.04).[24] An exception to the practice of daily interruption includes patients requiring neuromuscular paralysis who should not be awakened until the paralytic agent has worn off.

Preferred Choice of Sedative

The ideal sedative would have a rapid onset of action with rapid recovery, have low risk of drug accumulation, be easy to titrate, exhibit no tachyphylaxis or withdrawal symptoms, cause no hemodynamic instability, and be inexpensive.[6] No single drug currently meets all these criteria. Each class of drugs, and individual drugs within the classes, offers certain benefits and disadvantages, and may be preferred in a specific clinical situation.

For instance, if one of the goals of pharmacologic management of pain and anxiety in the critical care setting is amnesia of the period of critical illness, then benzodiazepines produce the most consistent effect. The amnestic effects of propofol and opioids are more dose dependent.[16] Conversely, propofol may produce a greater percentage of hours of sedation at the desired level (Grade 2–5 on Ramsay scale) compared with midazolam.[25,26] Also, propofol may lead to a more rapid recovery after interrupting sedation and a more predictable recovery to total consciousness.[27] Although propofol is more expensive than midazolam, it has been reported to be more cost effective due to shorter ICU stays.[25,28] For patients receiving more than 48 hours of ventilation, continuous propofol sedation may result in fewer ventilator days than intermittent lorazepam boluses.[29]

No matter what agent is chosen, it is essential to dose at sufficient levels to achieve effective sedation. Attempting to minimize the amount of sedative initially may result in increased anxiety and agitation, which may worsen cardiac and pulmonary instability.[6] One way to achieve sedation goals, while minimizing adverse effects, is to use combinations of drugs in a synergistic manner rather than using excessive doses of one drug. For example, combining an opioid analgesic with a sedative, both at moderate doses, is preferable to a very high dose of the sedative alone with no analgesic. Evidence suggests that the choice of sedative may be less important than its proper dosing and titration to optimize effect and minimize complications.[2,30]

Both analgesics and sedatives can increase the risk of delirium. In one study comparing lorazepam, midazolam, fentanyl, morphine, and propofol for the risk of delirium, use of lorazepam was an independent risk factor for daily transition to delirium.[31] In

Table 85-6 Society of Critical Care Medicine 2002 Clinical Practice Guidelines Recommendations on Use of Sedatives and Analgesics

Analgesia:	If hemodynamically stable: Morphine 2–5 mg IV push q 5–15 min
	If hemodynamically unstable: Fentanyl 25–100 mcg IV push q 5–15 min; or
	hydromorphone 0.25–0.75 mg IV push q 5–15 min
	Repeat until pain controlled, then give as scheduled dose plus PRN
Sedation:	Acute agitation: Midazolam 2–5 mg IV push q 5–15 min until acute event controlled
	Ongoing sedation: Lorazepam 1–4 mg IV push q 10–20 min until at goal, then q 2–6 hours scheduled plus PRN; or
	propofol—Start at 5 mcg/kg/min, titrate q 5 min until at goal
	If >3 days of propofol, then convert to lorazepam
Delirium:	Haloperidol 2–10 mg IV push q 20–30 min, then 25% of loading dose q 6 hr

From: Jacobi J, Fraser GL, Coursin DB, et al. Clinical practice guidelines for the sustained use of sedatives and analgesics in the critically ill adult. Crit Care Med 2002; 30:119–141.

patients receiving a cumulative dose of more than 20 mg in 24 hours, there was a 100% probability of delirium. As noted above, the medication that has been most extensively studied for the treatment of delirium in the critical care setting has been haloperidol. As with opioids and sedative agents, the dose of haloperidol to achieve adequate treatment of agitation due to delirium must be individualized, starting low and titrating up to the most effective dose. There has recently been discussion regarding the use of some of the newer agents for management of agitation, such as olanzapine and ziprasidone, but there have been no systematic studies in the ICU setting comparing these agents to older agents. Risperidone may also have a place as a treatment option, but it is only available orally.

Table 85-6 presents the most recent Society of Critical Care Medicine consensus practice guidelines on the choice of analgesics, sedatives, and antidelirium medications.[2] These are the most widely accepted standard recommendations.

PREVENTION

All pain and anxiety cannot be prevented in the critical care setting. In the noncommunicating patient, assessment may be difficult, so it is imperative to treat early on the assumption that anxiety and pain are present. If the patient is undergoing procedures that are usually uncomfortable or painful, it is best to assume that the patient will feel pain and treat accordingly; it is always preferable and more effective to prevent pain than to treat existing pain. Therefore, when ongoing patient discomfort is expected, analgesics should be administered on a continuous or scheduled basis, rather than "as needed" only. Additional bolus doses can be administered as required. An awareness of physiologic and behavioral signs of discomfort allows treatment to be started early, and unnecessary suffering can be prevented.

The goal in the management of delirium in the critically ill patient should also be focused on prevention and early detection. A large degree of delirium may be due to critical illness as well as physiologic and metabolic abnormalities, and it is therefore not preventable. However, methods to prevent or minimize delirium include frequent efforts to orient the patient to time and place and frequent explanations to the patient as to what is occurring, both in terms of illness and procedures. Even if a patient is somewhat sedated, it is best to continually provide these explanations as a means to minimize confusion and delirium.

Key Points

- Hospital staff commonly underestimate the amount of pain experienced by patients in the ICU. In the past, up to three fourths of ICU patients rate their pain as moderate to severe, despite the fact that up to 80% or more of nurses and physicians believe that patients are receiving adequate pain control.

- In addition to causing extreme discomfort, unrelieved pain can result in inadequate sleep, may worsen delirium, and is a common cause of agitation.

- Both under- and over-treatment of pain and anxiety can prolong length of stay. Under-treatment can worsen autonomic nervous system function and other physiologic parameters, while over-treatment can worsen delirium and prolong time to extubation.

- Assessing and treating patients' pain and agitation not only provide comfort, but improve outcomes with decreased duration of mechanical ventilation and fewer nosocomial infections.

- Sedation should only be used for agitatio after pain and reversible physiological causes have been treated.

- Tools such as the Richmond Agitation-Sedation Scale (RASS) should be used to assess the level of sedation and direct dosing of medications.

- Delirium should be evaluated using an instrument such as the Confusion Assessment Method for the Intensive Care Unit (CAM-ICU) and treated when diagnosed.

SUGGESTED READING

Jacobi J, Fraser GL, Coursin DB, et al. Clinical practice guidelines for the sustained use of sedatives and analgesics in the critically ill adult. Crit Care Med 2002; 30:119–141.

Chanques G, Jaber S, Barbotte E, et al. Impact of systematic evaluation of pain and agitation in an intensive care unit. Crit Care Med 2006; 34:1691–1698.

Pun BT, Gordon SM, Peterson JF, et al. Large-scale implementation of sedation and delirium monitoring in the intensive care unit: a report from two medical centers. Crit Care Med 2005; 33:1199–1205.

Brattebo G, Hofoss D, Flaatten H, et al. Effect of a scoring system and protocol for sedation on duration of patients' need for ventilator support in a surgical intensive care unit. BMJ 2002; 324(7350):1386–1389.

Ely EW, Shintani A, Truman B, et al. Delirium as a predictor of mortality in mechanically ventilated patients in the intensive care unit. JAMA 2004; 291:1753–1762.

Ely EW, Inouye SK, Bernard GR, et al. Delirium in mechanically ventilated patients: validity and reliability of the confusion assessment method for the intensive care unit (CAM-ICU). JAMA 2001; 286:2703–2710.

Pandharipande P, Ely EW. Narcotic-based sedation regimens for critically ill mechanically ventilated patients. Crit Care 2005; 9:247–248.

Schweickert WD, Gehlbach BK, Pohlman AS, et al. Daily interruption of sedative infusions and complications of critical illness in mechanically ventilated patients. Crit Care Med 2004; 32:1272–1276.

Carson SS, Kress JP, Rodgers JE, et al. A randomized trial of intermittent lorazepam versus propofol with daily interruption in mechanically ventilated patients. Crit Care Med 2006; 34:1326–1332.

Ely EW, Truman B, Shintani A, et al. Monitoring sedation status over time in ICU patients: reliability and validity of the Richmond Agitation-Sedation Scale (RASS). JAMA 2003; 289:2983–2991.

Pandharipande P, Shintani A, Peterson J, et al. Lorazepam is an independent risk factor for transitioning to delirium in intensive care unit patients. Anesthesiology 2006; 104:21–26.

Turkmen A, Altan A, Turgut N, et al. The correlation between the Richmond agitation-sedation scale and bispectral index during dexmedetomidine sedation. Eur J Anaesthesiol 2006; 23:300–304.

CHAPTER EIGHTY-SIX

Noninvasive Ventilation

Darrin R. Hursey, MD, and Thomas H. Sisson, MD

BACKGROUND

Noninvasive ventilation (NIV) refers to the delivery of mechanical ventilatory support to the lungs using an interface that does not require endotracheal intubation or tracheostomy. The earliest application of this technique began over 150 years ago with the development of tank-like body ventilators that supported respiration by generating negative pressure around a patient's thorax. These "iron lungs" gained widespread use during the polio epidemics of the 1900s. In the 1980s, noninvasive positive pressure ventilation gained popularity with the advent of the nasal mask that allowed the delivery of continuous positive airway pressure (CPAP) for treatment of obstructive sleep apnea.

More recently, because of the complications associated with endotracheal intubation, there has been an increasing interest in the use of noninvasive ventilation to treat both acute and chronic respiratory failure. Recent studies have explored the use of NIV in three separate clinical settings: 1) to avert the need for endotracheal intubation in the setting of acute respiratory failure, 2) to facilitate early weaning from invasive ventilation, and 3) to support patients with chronic respiratory failure in whom invasive ventilation is not desired.

RATIONALE

NIV is an attractive treatment modality because it offers many of the benefits of invasive ventilation while avoiding many of its complications.[1] In a patient with hypercapneic respiratory failure, the administration of positive-pressure ventilation can augment tidal volume and thereby increase minute ventilation. Successful augmentation of an individual patient's minute ventilation will reduce arterial CO_2 and, at the same time, improve arterial oxygenation. In addition, NIV allows the application of positive end-expiratory pressure (PEEP). This intervention can offset the intrinsic PEEP that frequently complicates an exacerbation of obstructive lung disease. The successful counterbalance of intrinsic PEEP results in a decrease in the patient's work of breathing. The application of positive pressure at end-exhalation can also recruit collapsed or underventilated alveoli, which in turn ameliorates ventilation/perfusion mismatching and helps correct hypoxemia.

RISKS

Invasive ventilation offers many of the same benefits associated with NIV but is associated with significant risk.[2] The placement of an endotracheal tube can result in trauma, including fractured teeth or laryngeal injury. Tracheomalacia or tracheal stenosis can also result from prolonged tube placement. The major risk associated with invasive ventilation, however, is that of infection. By bypassing the natural airway defense mechanisms, endotracheal intubation is associated with a significant rate of pneumonia and sinusitis. Although NIV is not without risk, the complications tend to be less severe.[2] One major problem is skin necrosis from prolonged mask-related pressure on the bridge of the nose. Careful application of the straps to avoid excess pressure and the use of Duoderm or other products on the skin can help minimize the risk. Less common complications include pneumothorax and conjunctivitis. The administration of positive-pressure ventilation can also cause gastric distention, particularly in the setting of diseases that reduce lung compliance (e.g., acute respiratory distress syndrome [ARDS], pneumonia). Gastric distention can precipitate emesis and increase the risk of aspiration, which has been reported to occur in up to 5% of patients treated with NIV.[3] Ultimately, the most serious risk of NIV is its tendency to inappropriately delay endotracheal intubation in patients who require invasive support. Careful patient selection and close monitoring, detailed later in this chapter, can help minimize the various complications.

MODES OF ADMINISTRATION

NIV can be administered as either a continuous positive pressure or with different levels of inspiratory and expiratory support. CPAP provides the same pressure during both inspiration and expiration. The expiratory positive airway pressure (EPAP) against which the patient must exhale can help recruit collapsed or underventilated alveoli and thereby improve oxygenation. It can also decrease the work of breathing by increasing FRC and decreasing the effort needed for a patient to initiate inspiration. Furthermore, CPAP has been shown to reduce both left ventricular preload and afterload, which makes this an attractive modality for the treatment of pulmonary edema. CPAP is typically delivered by small, portable devices designed for this mode, but standard critical care ventilators can also be employed for this purpose.

Bilevel support delivers different, independently set inspiratory positive airway pressures (IPAP) and expiratory positive airway pressures (EPAP). The ventilator senses the patient's inspiratory effort and provides the set IPAP response. This augments inspiration, resulting in an increase in tidal volume and minute ventilation that, in turn, reverses hypercarbia. The applied respiratory pressure can also help reverse hypoxemia by reducing $\dot{V}/\dot{Q}$ mismatch and enhancing alveolar ventilation. As with CPAP, bilevel pressure support can be delivered by portable devices or by standard critical care ventilators.

Proportional assist ventilation (PAV) is a mode in which volume and pressure are generated in proportion to patient effort. Therefore, the patient is in control of the entire respiratory cycle, and as a result patient–ventilator synchrony improves. Ultimately, this translates into improved patient tolerance of NIV. This is a relatively new mode of ventilation that is not yet available in the United States.

Volume-limited ventilation differs from CPAP and bilevel pressure support in that a set volume of gas is delivered by the ventilator rather than a set pressure. This mode of ventilation typically requires the use of a critical care ventilator in order to optimize the delivery of a fixed tidal volume. Volume-limited ventilation can be delivered either in an assist control (A/C) mode or as intermittent mandatory ventilation (IMV). With both modes, a tidal volume and a respiratory rate are chosen. The two modes differ only when the patient is breathing above the set respiratory rate. With A/C, the ventilator delivers a full tidal volume with every patient breath. In IMV, no support is provided by the ventilator for the breaths that occur at a frequency above the backup rate. To date, there have been no studies that have demonstrated an advantage of volume-controlled versus pressure-controlled NIV in the treatment of acute respiratory failure. Therefore, the choice of modality should be determined by the institutional experience with each approach as well as patient response.[1]

INTERFACES

One of the most important considerations when initiating NIV is the choice of interface (the connection between the patient and ventilator). A significant percentage of patients cannot tolerate NIV, and most frequently the interface is responsible. Careful selection and proper application can help lessen the likelihood of patient intolerance and decrease the chances of NIV failure.[4]

The nasal mask was the first interface developed, and it remains the most commonly used device. It consists of a triangular- or cone-shaped clear plastic mask that fits over the bridge of the nose. It is held in place by a number of straps, which vary in the number and configuration, depending on the manufacturer. Nasal masks have the advantage of being smaller, inducing less claustrophobia, and allowing easier secretion clearance. However, they can be problematic in the patient who is a "mouth breather" because air escaping through the mouth limits the resultant tidal volume. They are also prone to causing pressure sores over the bridge of the nose (Fig. 86-1). The oronasal interface is a full face mask that covers the mouth and nose. This device is useful in patients in whom excessive mouth leaking

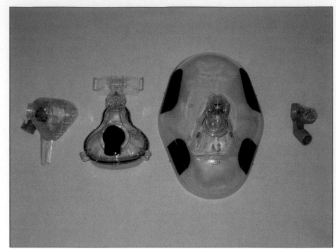

Figure 86-1 • Common interfaces used in the application of noninvasive ventilation. From left to right: nasal mask, oronasal mask, full face mask, and nasal pillows.

cannot be controlled. In one study, this interface was more efficacious in lowering $PaCO_2$ than nasal masks. Thus, in the setting of acute respiratory failure, this approach may be superior. On the other hand, full face masks are associated with several disadvantages. They are more likely to cause claustrophobia; they interfere with speech, eating, and expectoration; and they can potentially lead to aspiration. There is also a concern about potential for asphyxiation in the event of ventilator failure.

Another potential interface is the nasal pillows that insert directly into the nostrils and eliminate pressure on the bridge of the nose (*see* Fig. 86-1). They are useful in patients who cannot tolerate nasal or oronasal masks. Mouthpieces held in place with lip seals are yet another alternative for patients who cannot tolerate the other interfaces. These devices are used much less frequently than nasal or full face masks, but they are a viable alternative when the more commonly used approaches fail.

EVALUATION OF PATIENTS FOR NIV

If NIV is to be effective, it must be employed in the proper setting. Patient selection is critical in order to maximize the likelihood of success. Patients who are in acute respiratory distress and are at risk for requiring intubation could potentially benefit from this therapy. Such patients will typically have subjective and objective evidence of respiratory distress, including dyspnea, tachypnea, accessory muscle use, and tachycardia. Laboratory evidence of respiratory failure, including acute CO_2 retention and hypoxia, should also be present. Patients should also have an appropriate clinical condition (Box 86-1), such as an acute COPD exacerbation, cardiogenic pulmonary edema, or community-acquired pneumonia. Furthermore, they should not meet exclusion criteria (Box 86-2). Criteria that absolutely contraindicate the institution of NIV include the presence of cardiac or respiratory arrest, significant facial trauma, and upper airway obstruction. Other conditions that should be considered as contraindications to the use of NIV include the presence of nonrespiratory organ dysfunction (e.g., hemodynamic instability, CNS dysfunction, and upper gastrointestinal (GI) bleeding), an inability to handle secretions, and an increased risk of aspiration.[4] When choosing to implement NIV, clinical judgment is crucial: if

---

Box 86-1 Acute Respiratory Conditions Appropriate for NIV

COPD with respiratory acidosis (pH 7.25–7.35)

Cardiogenic pulmonary edema

Community-acquired pneumonia (particularly in setting of COPD)

Hypoxic respiratory failure from other causes

Hypercapnic respiratory failure secondary to neuromuscular disease, obesity hypoventilation syndrome, or chest wall deformity

Weaning from endotracheal intubation

Respiratory failure in "Do Not Intubate" patients

COPD—chronic obstructive pulmonary disease

Box 86-2 Contraindications to NIV*

Cardiac or respiratory arrest

Nonrespiratory organ failure, including severe encephalopathy (GCS <10), severe upper GI bleeding, hemodynamic instability, and unstable cardiac arrhythmia

Facial surgery, trauma, or deformity

Upper airway obstruction

Inability to cooperate or protect the airway

Inability to clear respiratory secretions

High risk for aspiration

*See Fig. 86-2.
GCS—Glasgow coma scale

Box 86-3 Predicting Response to NIV

Predictors of success

    High $PaCO_2$ and low A-a gradient

    pH between 7.25 and 7.35

    Improvement in pH, $PaCO_2$, and respiratory rate within an hour of initiating NIV

    Good level of consciousness

Predictors of failure

    High APACHE score

    Copious secretions

    Edentulous patient

    Poor nutritional status

    Altered level of consciousness

$PaCO_2$—arterial partial pressure of carbon dioxide; APACHE—acute physiology, age, chronic health evaluation

---

Box 86-4 Monitoring the Patient during NIV

Subjective assessment of patient comfort, level of consciousness, accessory muscle usage, coordination with ventilator

Heart rate, respiratory rate, blood pressure, continuous pulse oximetry.

Arterial blood gas analysis at 1–2 hours and then as needed to evaluate improvement in ventilation and oxygenation

---

individual patients with impending respiratory failure fit any of the exclusion criteria, endotracheal intubation should be performed immediately.

Predicting response to NIV has proven difficult. A recent guideline on NIV[5] has evaluated the available evidence, and the recommendations are listed in Box 86-3. Patients with a good level of consciousness, less severe physiologic derangements at baseline, and clinical improvement within 1 hour of starting therapy have the greatest likelihood of a favorable outcome. Conversely, patients with more severe derangements, higher APACHE score, more copious secretions, or an altered level of consciousness are more likely to fail this approach.[1]

EVIDENCE OF EFFICACY

Chronic Obstructive Lung Disease

NIV has been most thoroughly studied in patients with acute exacerbations of chronic obstructive pulmonary disease (COPD). There have been multiple randomized controlled trials examining the effectiveness of NIV in this setting. A recent meta-analysis of 15 randomized controlled studies showed that NIV, when added to standard medical therapy, reduced the rates of endotracheal intubation, length of hospitalization, and inhospital mortality rates.[6] It is important to note that only patients with severe COPD exacerbations (pH <7.30 or expected hospital mortality rate

>10%) realized this benefit. Patients admitted with less severe exacerbations had no improvement in these parameters with the addition of noninvasive support. This underscores the importance of patient selection; the patient should be ill enough that he or she would benefit from NIV, but not so ill that immediate endotracheal intubation is required.

Based upon these results, NIV should be strongly considered in addition to standard medical therapy for patients admitted with severe exacerbations of COPD. At the present time, there are no studies that support the use of a particular type of ventilator or interface when treating patients admitted with a COPD exacerbation. Although low levels of CPAP appear to be beneficial in this setting, there has not yet been a randomized control trial comparing the modalities, so this mode cannot be recommended over bilevel support. Otherwise, initial therapy should be based upon availability of equipment and provider preference. Response to therapy should be closely monitored (Box 86-4), and the equipment and mode should be adjusted accordingly.

Cardiogenic Pulmonary Edema

CPAP has been shown to improve both oxygenation and respiratory rate, and to decrease the need for endotracheal intubation in patients hospitalized with cardiogenic pulmonary edema.[7] However, the decreased rate of intubation, perhaps because of inadequate study size, has not translated into an improved mortality. Fewer studies have examined the effect of bilevel ventilation in patients with acute pulmonary edema. In a recent multicenter trial, the addition of bilevel support to standard medical therapy helped improve dyspnea, respiratory rate, and the ratio of PaO_2 to FiO_2.[7] However, mortality rate, length of stay, and intubation rate were not affected. With subgroup analysis, the authors found that, in those patients who were hypercapneic ($PaCO_2$ >45 mm Hg) on presentation, the intubation rate was decreased with the addition of NIV (6% vs. 29%). Previous studies had found an increased rate of myocardial infarction in patients undergoing bilevel ventilation, but this was not observed in this recent trial.

Based upon the current literature, either CPAP or bilevel noninvasive ventilation should be considered in patients who present with cardiogenic pulmonary edema and who have not quickly responded to standard medical therapy. This recommendation is particularly salient in those individuals who demonstrate hypercapnea. In ischemic patients, bilevel ventilation should be used with caution. Otherwise, both CPAP and bilevel support appear to be effective treatment modalities; and until further data are available, the initial choice should be guided by availability, provider preference, and patient comfort.

Community-Acquired Pneumonia

The role for NIV in patients admitted with community-acquired pneumonia has also been investigated. A recent prospective, randomized study[8] demonstrated that the addition of NIV to standard medical therapy for patients admitted with community-acquired pneumonia and acute respiratory failure (respiratory rate >35, PaO_2/FiO_2 <250, and/or $PaCO_2$ >50 mm Hg) reduced respiratory rate, the need for endotracheal intubation (21% in the study group vs. 50% in the control group), and ICU length of stay (1.8 +/− 0.7 days vs. 6 +/− 1.8 days). In a subgroup analysis, only the patients with underlying COPD, all of whom were hypercapneic, had a reduction in their requirement for mechanical ventilation when treated with NIV. In addition, the patients with COPD treated with NIV also had an improvement in their 2-month survival (88.9% vs. 37.5%).

Based on these results, the use of NIV should be strongly considered in patients with community-acquired pneumonia and acute hypoxemic or hypercarbic respiratory insufficiency, as long as contraindications do not exist. Prior to initiating this therapy, one must consider whether the use of an interface for noninvasive ventilation will interfere with secretion clearance and/or the performance of aggressive pulmonary toilet.

Hypoxemic Respiratory Failure

Multiple studies have investigated the efficacy of NIV in acute hypoxemic respiratory failure. As mentioned in the previous section, current evidence supports the use of bilevel noninvasive ventilation in patients with hypoxemic respiratory failure secondary to community-acquired pneumonia. The role of noninvasive ventilation in the general setting of acute hypoxemic respiratory failure has been further explored in a recent meta-analysis of eight randomized controlled trials.[9] Four of the eight trials independently found NIV to significantly reduce the rate of intubation, whereas the other studies revealed no difference. The combined results of all eight investigations favored the use of NIV with respect to reducing the risk of endotracheal intubation (23% absolute risk reduction). The meta-analysis also found noninva-

sive ventilation to improve ICU length of stay (absolute reduction of 2 days) and decrease ICU mortality (17% absolute risk reduction), compared to standard treatment. Because of the significant heterogeneity in the trial results, the authors were hesitant to endorse the routine use of NIV in hypoxemic respiratory failure. The variable outcomes were likely due to differences in the patient populations of each study. Certain etiologies appear to respond better than others, including hypoxemic respiratory failure in the immunosuppressed patient and in the post lung resection patient. Other studies corroborate the benefit of noninvasive ventilation in the immunocompromised individual (e.g., AIDS with *Pneumocystis* pneumonia[3] and solid organ transplant recipients[10]). In patients with acute lung injury or ARDS, the data are inconclusive, but considering the typically protracted nature of these disorders, NIV is unlikely to play a significant role.

Asthma

Only a few randomized controlled studies have examined the use of NIV in acute exacerbations of asthma. A recent blinded study randomized 30 patients to receive either bilevel pressure ventilation or subtherapeutic (sham) ventilation for 3 hours in addition to standard bronchodilator therapy.[11] The investigators found that the addition of NIV resulted in a >50% improvement in FEV_1 for 80% of the patients. In contrast, only 20% of the patients in the control group had a >50% improvement in their FEV_1. With the improvement in FEV_1, the treatment patients also had a reduced rate of hospitalization. Although these results are encouraging, further investigations are required to confirm this benefit before noninvasive ventilation becomes standard treatment for severe asthma exacerbations.

WEANING FROM INVASIVE VENTILATION

Several studies have examined the use of NIV to facilitate the weaning of patients from invasive mechanical ventilation. One trial explored the utility of noninvasive ventilation in patients who failed a T-piece trial after 48 hours of endotracheal intubation.[12] Patients who received NIV had a faster weaning time (10.2±6.8 days vs. 16.6±11.8 days) and a shorter ICU length of stay (15.1±5.4 days vs. 24.0±13.7 days). Presumably by lessening endotracheal intubation time, NIV also decreased the incidence of nosocomial pneumonia and improved 60-day survival. A subsequent study confirms the benefits of NIV in shortening the duration of invasive ventilation in those patients who have encouraging weaning parameters but fail a 2-hour spontaneous breathing trial.[13] One limitation of these studies is the fact that the majority of the recruited patients were intubated for an exacerbation of COPD. Using this modality to expedite the weaning of patients on invasive ventilation for other causes of acute respiratory failure cannot be recommended based on the available literature.

An important distinction must be drawn between the use of NIV in patients who have failed to wean from invasive ventilation and its use in patients with post-extubation respiratory distress. A recent study compared NIV to standard medical therapy, including reintubation, in patients who had been intubated for greater than 48 hours and experienced respiratory distress within 48 hours of extubation.[14] The study was stopped early because there was no difference in reintubation rate, and there was a significant increase in the mortality rate (25% vs. 14%) in the NIV group. This mortality difference likely resulted from a delay in reintubation in the patients managed with noninvasive ventilation. This, in turn, predisposed the patients to the development of adverse events, including cardiac ischemia or aspiration. Therefore, NIV should not be used in this clinical setting.

DO NOT INTUBATE ADVANCED DIRECTIVES

There have been several reports examining the use of NIV in patients who refuse endotracheal intubation. In a recent prospective cohort trial, 114 patients with acute respiratory failure and a do not intubate order were treated with NIV.[15] Of these, 49 survived to discharge (43%). This demonstrates that NIV can be used to treat respiratory failure in patients for whom invasive ventilation is indicated but refused. In terminally ill patients for whom more invasive therapy is not desired, NIV also has the potential to limit symptoms while allowing the patient to maintain their autonomy and interaction with their family. In this circumstance, the use of NIV must be explained as a form of life-support, and the ability of this modality to limit symptoms must be weighed against potential complications and the possible prolongation of suffering.

INITIATING THERAPY AND MONITORING RESPONSE

Once a patient has been deemed to be a candidate for NIV, therapy should be initiated as soon as possible (a protocol is presented in Fig. 86-2). One must first decide where to administer NIV. Studies have demonstrated that NIV can be safely initiated in the emergency department[16] or on general wards.[17] After initiation, expert opinion recommends high-level monitoring by both nursing and respiratory therapy, and the management team should have the capability of responding quickly to deterioration.[1] If these criteria can be met on the general ward or in the emergency department, patient care can be continued in these settings. If not available, NIV can be initiated outside the ICU, but subsequent transfer to a unit with close monitoring should occur promptly. Furthermore, if NIV is administered outside of an ICU setting and no improvement with this modality occurs within 60–120 minutes, prompt transfer to the ICU is recommended because endotracheal intubation will likely be required. Discussing the process of NIV with the individual patient, including the goals of treatment and the potential side effects, is critically important for a successful outcome. Selection of ventilator and interface should be based on operator familiarity. Gently applying the selected interface and initially having the patient hold it in place can improve comfort and compliance. In addition, cautious adminis-

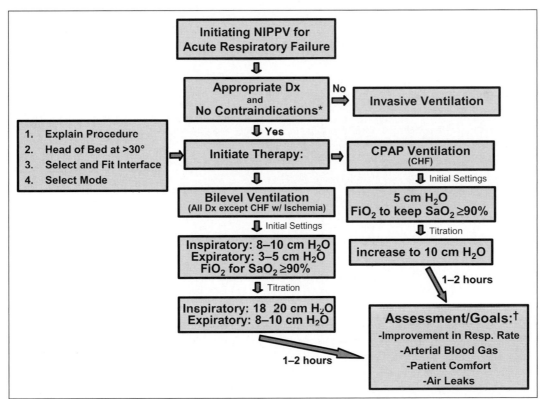

Figure 86-2 • Protocol for initiating noninvasive ventilation

NIV = noninvasive ventilation.
Dx = diagnosis
CHF = congestive heart failure
FiO$_2$ = Fraction of inspired oxygen
SaO$_2$ = arterial oxygen saturation
CPAP = continuous positive airway pressure

*See Box 86-1 and 86-2
†See Box 86-4

tration of sedatives/anxiolytics can help patients adapt to the noninvasive support. For the initiation of therapy, a bilevel mode with an inspiratory pressure of 8–10 cm H_2O and an expiratory pressure of 3–5 cm H_2O has been used in many of the experimental trials (for cardiogenic pulmonary edema, one should consider CPAP).

Appropriate monitoring (see Box 86-4) of the patient's response to NIV is critical. The patient's comfort level, level of consciousness, respiratory rate, and heart rate should be monitored closely. It may be necessary to adjust straps or change interface type if there are excessive air leaks or if the patient is too uncomfortable. After 1–2 hours, a repeat arterial blood gas should be obtained to document improvement in $PaCO_2$ and PaO_2. Those patients who will benefit from NIV should demonstrate improvements in their respiratory rate, heart rate, and arterial blood gas during this initial 1–2 hour period. A lack of improvement or deterioration in any of these parameters should prompt a serious consideration of endotracheal intubation.

Treatment with NIV can continue as long as the patient's condition improves. One of the benefits of NIV is the ability to temporarily discontinue support in order to provide medication, allow the patient to eat, participate in physical therapy, etc. These interruptions should be limited during the first 24 hours of therapy. However, after this time, as long as the patient continues to improve, these breaks can be extended so that the patient spends progressively less time with ventilatory support. These breaks should initially be limited to the daytime hours, and the patient should continue to receive NIV during the night. By continuing to extend the amount of time spent off the ventilator, the patient can be efficiently weaned off of NIV altogether.[5]

Key Points

- Noninvasive ventilation allows for delivery of mechanical ventilatory support to the lungs using an interface that does not require endotracheal intubation or tracheostomy. It offers many of the benefits of invasive ventilation while avoiding many of the potential complications.

- There are a variety of interface and ventilatory mode options available, allowing therapy to be tailored to the individual patient and clinical presentation.

- Noninvasive ventilation can be beneficial in patients with COPD, cardiogenic pulmonary edema, community-acquired pneumonia, select causes of hypoxemic respiratory failure, and as a means of weaning from invasive mechanical ventilation.

- Noninvasive ventilation can be safely initiated in the emergency department or on the general wards, provided that high-level monitoring from nursing staff and respiratory therapy is available.

- Close monitoring is essential in order to assess for signs of clinical decompensation, requiring endotracheal intubation and transfer to the intensive care unit.

SUGGESTED READING

Mehta S, Hill N. Noninvasive ventilation. Am J Respir Crit Care Med 2001; 163:540–577.

Acton R, et al. Noninvasive ventilation. J Trauma 2002; 53:593–601.

International Consensus Conferences in Intensive Care Medicine. Noninvasive positive pressure ventilation in acute respiratory failure. Am J Respir Crit Care Med 2001; 63:283–291.

British Thoracic Society Standards of Care Committee. Non-invasive ventilation in acute respiratory failure. Thorax 2002; 57:192–211.

Nava S, et al. Noninvasive mechanical ventilation in the weaning of patients with respiratory failure due to chronic obstructive pulmonary disease. Ann Intern Med 1998; 128:721–728.

CHAPTER EIGHTY-SEVEN

Basic Mechanical Ventilation

Eric Flenaugh, MD, and Michael Heisler, MD, MPH

BACKGROUND

Hospitalists provide a significant percentage of care in intensive care units (ICU) across the United States; up to 80% of hospitalists care for patients in the ICU.[1] There were approximately 14,000 hospitalists in the United States in 2005, with a projected increase to greater than 20,000 by 2010.[2] At the same time, intensivists care for only one third of patients in the ICU, and a severe shortage of these physicians will occur by 2007 and worsen until 2030 as the United States population ages and the demand for critical care services increases.[3] The role of hospitalists in the ICU will therefore continue to increase, requiring knowledge and skills in the care of patients on ventilators.

INDICATIONS FOR MECHANICAL VENTILATION

The indications for mechanical ventilation are acute respiratory failure (66% of patients), coma (15%), acute exacerbations of chronic obstructive pulmonary disease (13%), and neuromuscular disorders (5%). Acute respiratory distress syndrome, heart failure, pneumonia, sepsis, complications from surgery, and trauma account for the majority of etiologies among patients presenting with acute respiratory failure.[4]

A more thorough discussion of the causes of respiratory failure can be found in Chapter 84, but can be classified as follows:

1. Failure of gas exchange—the inability to provide adequate oxygenation or ventilation, resulting in hypoxia or hypercarbia, respectively.
2. Failure to support respiration—including impairment of the central respiratory drive center (drugs or central nervous system [CNS] injury) or the peripheral neuromuscular support system (e.g., myasthenia gravis).
3. Failure of protective mechanisms—impaired ability to maintain airway protection (aspiration risks, vocal cord injury) or loss of other protective mechanisms (excessive secretions, impaired cough).

The objectives of mechanical ventilation are therefore to decrease the work of breathing and reverse life-threatening hypoxemia or acute progressive respiratory acidosis.

INITIATING MECHANICAL VENTILATION

There are six variables that must be addressed when initiating mechanical ventilation: mode, fraction of inspired oxygen (FiO_2), tidal volume, rate, peak flow, and positive end-expiratory pressure. Table 87-1 summarizes basic guidelines for initiating mechanical ventilation.

MODE

Volume-Cycled versus Flow-Cycled versus Pressure-Cycled Ventilation

The mode, or cycling, of mechanical ventilation is classified according to the manner in which the inspiratory phase is terminated—by volume, flow, or pressure. In *volume cycled ventilation*, the most common form, each breath is cycled based on a predetermined tidal volume set by the physician. The ventilator delivers the necessary pressure to achieve this preset volume, and the patient receives a designated minute ventilation (total tidal volume per minute). In *flow cycled ventilation*, the inspiratory phase of the breath cycle is initiated when the patient spontaneously triggers air flow and terminated when the flow of air decreases to a preset level. At this point, the expiratory phase begins and lasts until another inspiratory phase is triggered. In *pressure controlled ventilation*, the physician sets an upper pressure limit. During each inspiration, the ventilator terminates the inspiratory phase when this pressure is achieved. Thus, changes in the compliance of lung parenchyma and resistance of airways determine the variable tidal volume delivered. The different modes of ventilation are summarized in Table 87-3.

Volume-Cycled Ventilation

There are three basic modes of volume-cycled ventilation: controlled mechanical ventilation (CMV), assist controlled ventilation (ACV), and synchronized intermittent mandatory ventilation (SIMV). These vary based on how the inspiratory phase is initiated.

Table 87-1 Recommended Initial Ventilator Settings for Special Circumstances

	COPD	ARDS	Shock	Preserved Lung Function (e.g., Surgery, overdose)
Mode	ACV	ACV/PCV*	ACV	ACV
FiO$_2$	.40–.60	1.0	.30–.50	.30–.50
Tidal volume cc/kg	4*–6 *Limit auto PEEP	4–6	5–7	5–7
Minute volume liters/minute	3–6 Permissive hypercapnea may be required	7–10 Permissive hypercapnea may be required	7–10 Adjust to treat academia	4–6
Peak flow liters/minute	70–90	60	60–70	60–80
PEEP cm H$_2$O	5–8* Adjust to approximate but not exceed intrinsic PEEP	5–20 Adjust to achieve SaO$_2$ >90%	0 to 5 Limit increased intrathoracic pressures to avoid hypotension	0 to 5

Abbreviations:

COPD—chronic obstructive pulmonary disease; ARDS—acute respiratory distress syndrome; P$_{Plateau}$—plateau pressure; ACV—assist control ventilation; PCV—pressure cycled ventilation

*If P$_{Plateau}$ >30 cm H$_2$O despite 4 cc/kg tidal volume

Controlled Mechanical Ventilation (CMV)

In this mode of ventilation, the physician attempts to control completely the patient's respiration by setting a tidal volume and rate with the intent of limiting spontaneous respiratory efforts. The ventilator forces inspiration regardless of any intrinsic efforts by the patient. CMV is indicated in patients with depressed or no respiratory drive (intoxication, traumatic brain, or spinal cord injury) or when super-physiologic ventilatory requirements are necessary.

Assist Control Ventilation (ACV)

Assist control ventilation is similar to CMV except that it allows the patient to initiate inspiration and breathe at an equal or higher rate than that set by the physician. The ventilator has either a pressure or flow sensor that, when triggered, allows the patient to initiate breaths potentially exceeding the preset rate. The ventilator delivers a set tidal volume whether inspiration is initiated by the patient ("assisted breath") or by the ventilator if the patient does not inspire in a timely manner. The patient receives the predetermined tidal volume for each breath, even those above the preset rate. The ventilator provides up to two thirds of the work of breathing when the peak flow and sensitivity are adjusted to allow synchrony with the ventilator, even if the patient is triggering all of the breaths.

Synchronized Intermittent Mandatory Ventilation (SIMV)

In SIMV mode, the physician sets a tidal volume and rate, and the ventilator delivers a breath based on these settings. Using a trigger sensor (pressure or flow), the ventilator can synchronize the intermittent ventilator breaths with the patient's inspiratory effort (i.e., synchronized IMV or SIMV). Patient effort is required to trigger the sensor increasing the work of breathing. Additionally, the patient is able to breathe spontaneously through the ventilator tubing generating tidal volumes dependent entirely on the patient's effort (unassisted breaths) or supported with pressure

support ventilation (see below). Ventilator synchronization with the patient's respiratory effort avoids delivering a mandatory "preset" breath at the same time the patient generates a spontaneous breath and thus avoids breath stacking and excessive tidal volume, which can cause barotrauma. In comparison to ACV, the work of breathing in SIMV can be significantly higher in patients requiring high levels of ventilator support. This should be taken into consideration when selecting the initial ventilator settings (see Table 87-1).

Flow-Cycled Ventilation

Spontaneous or Pressure Support Ventilation (PSV)

This mode has no predetermined minimum minute ventilation (i.e., rate or tidal volume is not set). Patients are allowed to breathe spontaneously and must generate their own tidal volume. The clinician must ensure the patient has an intact respiratory drive prior to initiating this mode. The tidal volume generated is dependent upon the patient's respiratory muscle effort, airway mechanics, compliance of the respiratory system, and a support pressure determined by the clinician. The patient generates an inspiratory flow to initiate the breath cycle, and the ventilator provides pressure to support the patient in generating a tidal volume until the flow decreases to a preset value. Then the inspiratory phase is terminated, and the patient is allowed to exhale. The physician can augment the amount of tidal volume by adjusting the amount of "pressure support" and base it upon the amount of assistance required by the patient. Values may range from 5 to 25 cm H$_2$O.

Pressure-Cycled Ventilation

The goal of pressure-cycled ventilation is to limit excessive and potentially harmful effects of positive pressure ventilation that arise from the generation of elevated peak alveolar pressures. This is accomplished when the physician predetermines and sets a "target- pressure" that the ventilator will not exceed. The ventilator will provide an inspiratory flow to generate tidal volume until the target pressure is reached, at which point flow will cease and the expiratory phase begins. This mode, when the appropriate target pressure is selected, allows an optimal distention of the alveoli while using prolonged inspiratory times or high levels of $PEEP_E$ to improved oxygenation. Indications for the use of PCV include[5]:

1. Patients with ARDS requiring FiO_2 concentration >60%
2. $PEEP_E$ >12–14 cm H_2O to maintain SaO_2 >90%.
3. Patients with peak inspiratory pressures measuring >45 cm H_2O.
4. Patients with plateau pressures >30–35 cm H_2O.

FiO₂

As opposed to supplemental oxygen provided through nasal cannula or facemasks, oxygen concentrations are more accurate when delivered through an endotracheal tube in a closed system. As discussed in Chapter 84, oxygen should be delivered in concentrations that will maintain a SaO_2 >90% or a PaO_2 >60 torr. As the patient's requirement decreases, evidenced by a rising PaO_2/FiO_2 ratio, the FiO_2 can be decreased. The SPO_2 obtained via pulse oximetry correlates with SaO_2 within +/− 2%, assuming a normal pulse oximetry waveform.

Maintaining super-physiologic concentrations of oxygen, also called hyperoxia, injures the alveolar and capillary endothelium, resulting in increased permeability and loss of compliance and gas exchange surface area.[6,7] Oxygen toxicity may develop within the first 24–72 hours when the FiO_2 exceeds 80%. Even at levels as low as 60%, airway erythema, vascular congestion, and alveolar epithelial injury may occur. The risk of injury declines as FiO_2 concentration decreases to <50%. Thus, clinicians should aim for an FiO_2 <50% within the first 72 hours of mechanical ventilation whenever possible, while aiming for oxyhemoglobin saturation >90%.[8]

Tidal Volume

When selecting both tidal volume and rate, the clinician should consider minute ventilation goals (rate × volume), work of breathing, and the deleterious effects of over-distention of the alveolar unit. Traditional values for tidal volume were determined using the calculation of 10–15 cc/kg of ideal body weight. However, studies demonstrated that these volumes could result in over-distention of the alveoli with secondary pressure and volume-related injury.[9] Recent studies by the ARDSNet Group showed improved outcomes when tidal volumes of 5–7 cc/kg ideal body weight were used to treat patients with acute lung injury (ALI) and especially acute respiratory distress syndrome (ARDS), as long as adjustments are made to maintain the plateau pressure (peak alveolar pressure) <30 cm H_2O.[10]

Rate

Once the tidal volume is determined, the physician can then determine the rate based on the patient's minute ventilation requirements and respiratory drive. For example, a normal person's minute ventilation ranges 4–6 L/min to maintain a PCO_2 35–43 torr. However, in a person with acidemia, the minute ventilatory requirements may double, requiring 8 to 12 liters per minute. In this situation, a patient with a tidal volume of 0.5 L would require a rate of 16–24 breaths per minute to meet the requirements. Likewise, a patient with a minute ventilation of 4–6 L/min and alkalemia may require a rate of 6–10 breaths/min. Adjustments may also be made based on the desired amount of unloading of the respiratory muscles. For example, a patient with severe acidemia may require a minute ventilation in excess of 3–4 times normal, and voluntary respiratory muscle use required to meet this demand generates additional CO_2 and lactic acid. This, in turn, increases minute ventilation demand. Matching or even exceeding the patient's spontaneous respiratory rate by 3–5 breaths/min reduces patient effort, and thus muscle oxygen consumption and CO_2 production.

Peak Flow

Peak flow is the rate (liters per minute) at which the preset tidal volume is delivered. Patients in respiratory distress can generate inspiratory flow rates up to 600 L/min in response to the sensation of air hunger. Flow rates below patient demands can increase the work of breathing as the patient tries to pull air faster than the ventilator is providing. It also adds to patient discomfort. Flow rates above optimal levels may also create discomfort as the air jet stimulates the cough reflex. However, studies indicate that low peak flows creating air hunger are several times more uncomfortable than flows above the optimal level.[9] Optimal levels are determined at the bedside while simultaneously monitoring the patient's respiratory efforts and the ventilator's pressure and flow waveforms. A patient breathing with a peak flow rate that is too low will generate low or negative pressure levels that are evident on the waveform tracings, throughout the inspiratory phase of the breath cycle. On examination, the patient may have nasal flaring, tracheal retraction, or paradoxical abdominal breathing during the inspiratory phase. In most patients, optimal flow can be achieved with rates between 70–100 L/min.

Extrinsic Positive End-Expiratory Pressure (PEEP₍)

$PEEP_E$ is the lowest level of airway pressure that the ventilator allows the patient to reach at the end of the expiratory phase (i.e., at the point when expiratory flow of air reaches 0 L/min). This is different from pressure support (discussed above) that assists in generating tidal volume during the inspiratory phase of the respiratory cycle. If the $PEEP_E$ is set at 7 cm H_2O, then the airway pressure will not fall below this level at the end of expiration. $PEEP_E$ assists in achieving the goals of mechanical ventilation by performing one of two functions:

1. In patients with impaired alveolar distention from edema or inflammation, $PEEP_E$ improves oxygenation by recruiting collapsed alveoli, redistributing lung fluid, and preventing surfactant breakdown.
2. In patients with a large amount of autoPEEP or intrinsic PEEP ($PEEP_I$), such as COPD or asthma patients, there is an increased pressure gradient between the alveolus and the atmospheric pressure. In order for the patient to generate flow into the already distended alveolus, the diaphragm and respiratory muscles must generate enough negative pressure to overcome the level of auto PEEP. However, if extrinsic PEEP is applied at a level just below the level of $PEEP_I$, then the gradient is decreased, requiring less work to generate flow into the alveolus. On the contrary, if the level of $PEEP_E$ exceeds the level

of $PEEP_I$, then severe and potentially life-threatening air trapping may result.[12] The level of $PEEP_I$ can be determined by asking the respiratory therapist to briefly and gently occlude the expiratory valve at the end of the expiratory cycle, allowing the $PEEP_I$ to equilibrate throughout the ventilator circuit, and measuring the pressure.[13,14]

$PEEP_E$ also decreases shunting of venous blood by increasing gas exchange surface area. When selecting the level of $PEEP_E$, the clinician's goal is to optimize the SaO_2 and decrease the FiO_2 requirements while attempting to limit additional injury to the patient caused by over-distention of areas of healthy lung or impairing hemodynamics by diminishing venous return to the heart (see below). This requires close patient monitoring of both the acute responses to changes in the level of $PEEP_E$, as well as attention to trends in hemodynamics and oxygen saturation levels. Likewise, as the patient's condition improves and the FiO_2 is decreased to acceptable levels (<50%), gradual reductions of $PEEP_E$ are required to limit a rapid collapse of recruited alveoli and subsequent hypoxemia secondary to shunting.[11]

Table 87-1 summarizes recommended ventilator settings for special circumstances.

MONITORING AND COMPLICATIONS

The most common complications of mechanical ventilation can be categorized in to three major categories:

1. Positive Pressure Effects

Increased intrathoracic pressures pose a risk to both the pulmonary parenchyma and the cardiopulmonary circulation. Monitoring the plateau pressures as one makes adjustments to the ventilator settings may avoid lung injury by avoiding pressures of 30 cm H_2O or more, which cause prolonged over-distention of the alveolar unit. Elevated plateau pressures along with the shearing forces from the dynamics of deflating and inflating of alveoli can cause ventilator-associated lung injury (VALI), pneumomediastimun, or pneumothorax. Furthermore, elevated intrathoracic pressure may impair venous return and depress cardiac output, especially in the setting of high levels of PEEP, breath stacking (autoPEEP), and low intravascular volume status.[5,9]

2. Endotracheal Tube–Related Complications

The presence of an endotracheal tube during mechanical ventilation increases the risk of ventilator-associated pneumonia (VAP)[15] and direct injury to the large airways. Oropharyngeal secretions may collect around the cuff of the endotracheal tube in patients with inadequate oral suctioning and hygiene, posing a risk for micro-aspiration and the development of nosocomial pneumonia (see Chapter 34). The incidence of VAP has been reported to be 3% per day during the first 5 days of mechanical ventilation, 2% per day for days 5–10, and 1% per day of mechanical ventilation thereafter, significantly increasing ICU length of stay and mortality rates.[16] Prolonged presence of the endotracheal tube or high cuff pressure can result in local injury to the larynx and trachea that may cause vocal cord injury, fistula, tracheomalacia, and postintubation stenosis (Figs. 87-1 and 87-2). A recent meta-analysis of randomized studies comparing early tracheostomy (within the first 7 days of mechanical ventilation)

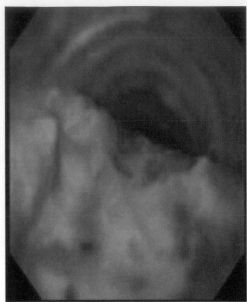

Figure 87-1 • Tracheal Wall Injury: Bronchoscopic picture of tracheal erosion and granulational tissue from prolonged intubation.

and late tracheostomy (after 14–16 days of mechanical ventilation) showed that early tracheostomy can significantly decrease the length of mechanical ventilation as well as the length of ICU stay, and there is no significant decrease in incidence of VAP or mortality. However, the risks of these complications are significantly decreased by early liberation from the ventilator.[17]

3. Acid-Base Disturbances

Monitoring arterial blood gases, pulse-oximetry, and end tidal CO_2 concentrations and individualizing the goals of long-term and acute therapy is essential in preventing severe acid-base complications. For example, a patient with chronic hypercarbia from chronic obstructive pulmonary disease (COPD) may have a compensatory metabolic alkalosis. If the ventilator settings are adjusted to correct the patient's PCO_2 to a normal range, then his or her kidneys may excrete the excess bicarbonate stores. Once mechanical ventilation is no longer required to correct the underlying pulmonary insufficiency, the patient may develop profound acidemia from an unbuffered respiratory acidosis. Thus, the physician should adjust the ventilator settings (i.e., the minute ventilation) and allow hypercarbia for patients with COPD who chronically retain CO_2, aiming for a mild respiratory acidosis to preserve the signal to the kidneys to retain bicarbonate for buffering baseline acidemia.

DISCONTINUING MECHANICAL VENTILATION

Because prolonged mechanical ventilation increases the risk of developing many of the complications listed above, physicians should be aggressive in their efforts to liberate the patient from mechanical ventilation. However, since patients who require reintubation have significantly higher VAP and mortality rates,[16] physicians should employ a systematic approach, using defined criteria for assessing the likelihood of successful extubation, to prevent premature extubation. The assessments for discontinuing mechanical ventilation should begin immediately following its

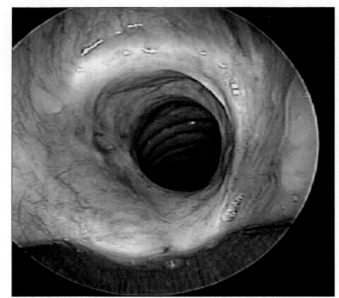

Figure 87-2 • Tracheal Stenosis: Bronchoscopic picture of tracheal narrowing from prolonged intubation.

Table 87-2 Assessment Criteria for Discontinuation of Mechanical Ventilation

Criteria	Parameters
Vital signs	T <38°C, HR <110–120 bpm, RR <30 bpm, minimal to no pressor requirements
Examination	Reversal of underlying condition, cough, alert
Oxygenation	PaO_2 >60 torr and FiO_2 ≤.40, PEEP <8, PaO_2/FiO_2 >150
Metabolic	pH >7.25, normal electrolytes (K, PO_4, mg), gb >8–10

Adapted from: Vallerdu I, Calaf N, Subirana M, et al. Clinical characteristics, respiratory functional parameters, and outcome of a two-hour T-piece trial in patients weaning from mechanical ventilation. Am J Respir Crit Care Med 1998; 158:1855–1862; and MacIntyre NR. Evidence-based guidelines for weaning and discontinuing ventilatory support: a collective task force facilitated by the American College of Chest Physicians; the American Association for Respiratory Care; and the American College of Critical Care Medicine. Chest 2001; 120S:375–396; and Kollef MH, Shapiro SD, Silver P, et al. A randomized, controlled trial of protocol-directed versus physician-directed weaning from mechanical ventilation. Crit Care Med 1997; 25:567–574; and Meade M, Guyatt G, Cook D, et al. Predicting success in weaning from mechanical ventilation. Chest 2001; 120:300–424.

initiation and continue regularly until ventilatory support is discontinued.

Assessment for reversal of the underlying cause of the respiratory failure should be the first step in determining candidacy for discontinuing mechanical ventilation (Table 87-2) prior to changing to a weaning mode of ventilation. For example, an intubated patient with septic shock requiring vasoactive agents is unlikely to maintain prolonged extubation if his or her hemodynamic instability requires continued use of high doses of pressors. Likewise, patients with respiratory failure secondary to oxygenation or ventilatory failure should demonstrate improvements in the PaO_2/FiO_2 ratio and PEEP requirements or improved pH/PCO_2 measurements and minute ventilation requirements, respectively. Respiratory drive and the ability to protect the airway (reflexes vs. tracheostomy) should be present. If the initial assessment indicates the patient is a candidate for discontinuation from mechanical ventilation, a weaning trial should be initiated.

Spontaneous Breathing Trial (SBT) versus SIMV Weaning

SIMV Weaning

In the past, the SIMV mode was felt to be a bridge between ACV and spontaneous mode, and was commonly used as a weaning mode. The use of SIMV mode for ventilator weaning was subsequently shown to increase the time to extubation by an average of 2.3 days over the use of spontaneous breathing trials for weaning.[18]

Spontaneous Breathing Trials

A SBT can be performed by allowing the patient to breathe spontaneously with either a pressure support of 5–8 cm H_2O or continuous positive airway pressure (CPAP) of 5 cm H_2O for a period 30–120 minutes, or with the endotracheal tube disconnected from the ventilator and connected to a flow of supplemental oxygen (T-piece trial).

Two large controlled studies of successful discontinuation of mechanical ventilation indicated that disease reversal, hemody-

namic stability, and weaning parameters were best assessed during a SBT.[18,19] Table 87-3 defines predictive parameters with high likelihood ratios for successful extubation in patients receiving ventilatory support and for those during a SBT.

Summary of the Weaning Process

1. Assess weaning candidacy (Table 87-2).
2. Change to a spontaneous mode of mechanical ventilation and assess the parameters in Table 87-3.
3. If criteria are met, start SBT by placing patient on a T-piece trial or CPAP of 5–8 cm H_2O for 5–10 minutes. Observe patient at bedside while assessing SBT parameters (Table 87-3).
4. If criteria are met, leave patient on SBT for 30–120 minutes with continued assessment of SBT criteria, vital signs, pulse oximetry, and patient tolerance of breathing challenge. Arterial blood gas testing may be useful for patients with limited reserve or marginal tolerance of the SBT.
5. If the patient tolerates the SBT, liberation from mechanical ventilation should be performed. If the SBT is not tolerated, then continued therapy with reassessment and correction of those factors limiting extubation should occur.

There is no required length of time for monitoring the patient in an ICU setting post extubation. However, the risk of complications such as laryngeal edema, stridor, and reintubation is highest in the first 24 hours.

CONCLUSION

Approximately 1.5 million nonsurgical patients are placed on ventilators each year in the United States.[20] These patients consume a significant percentage of ICU-related health care resources and are a major determinant of ICU length of stay, morbidity, and mortality. The clinical outcome of patients on ventilators is clearly improved when they are managed by physicians who routinely practice in the critical care setting. In the United States, this role will increasingly be filled by hospitalists.

Table 87-3 Predictors of Successful Extubation

ASSESSMENTS MADE DURING MECHANICAL VENTILATION			ASSESSMENTS MADE DURING SBT		
Criteria	Parameters	Assessment	Criteria	Parameters	Assessment
Minute ventilation	≤10 L/min	Respiratory muscle demand	Respiratory rate	<35 bpm	Respiratory muscle demand
Peak flow during cough	≥160 L/min	Ability to clear secretions	Tidal Volume/vital capacity	V_T/V_C <.40	Respiratory muscle strength (likelihood to fatigue if >.40)
Required suctioning for secretions	>q2hr requirement	Risk of airway compromise	Rapid shallow breathing index (frequency/tidal volume)	f/V_T <105	Inspiratory muscle weakness
Cuff leak (average of 3 consecutive breaths)	≥110 mL	Presence of laryngeal edema	Maximum inspiratory pressure	≤30 cm H_2O	Inspiratory muscle strength

COMPARISON OF VENTILATOR MODES

	Physician Interactions	Patient Interactions	Advantages	Limitations
Volume Cycled				
CMV	Physician presets rate and tidal volume.	Patient has no influence on the $\dot{V}_E$	Accurately establishes $\dot{V}_E$	Patient discomfort Limited ability to assess patient effort.
ACV	Physician presets rate and tidal volume for a minimum $\dot{V}_E$	Patient may influence $\dot{V}_E$ by spontaneously over-breathing the set rate but receives preset tidal volume.	Patient establishes $\dot{V}_E$ with decreased work of breathing compared to other modes. Useful as an initial mode of ventilation.	Respiratory alkalosis. Risk of auto PEEP and barotrauma.
SIMV	Physician presets rate and tidal volume.	Patient may influence $\dot{V}_E$ by spontaneously over-breathing the set rate but generates own tidal volume. May require addition of PSV.	Ventilator synchrony over ACV. Less risk of barotraumas compared to ACV.	Increased work of breathing. May delay ventilator weaning.
Flow Cycled				
PSV	Physician presets a level of positive pressure.	Rate, tidal volume, and flow are determined by the patient. Preset level of positive pressure assists patient in generating a tidal volume when a breath is initiated.	Effective as a weaning mode Respiratory muscle reconditioning is enhanced. Reduces sedation requirements	Requires spontaneous respiratory effort. Not useful as initial mode for patients requiring respiratory muscle unloading.

Abbreviations:
$\dot{V}_E$—minute ventilation; CMV—controlled mechanical ventilation; ACV—assist control ventilation; SIMV—synchronized intermittent mandatory ventilation; f/V_T—respiratory rate (frequency)/tidal volume; V_T—tidal volume; V_C—vital capacity PSV—pressure support ventilation

Table 87-3 Predictors of Successful Extubation—Cont'd

COMPARISON OF VENTILATOR MODES

	Physician Interactions	Patient Interactions	Advantages	Limitations
Pressure Cycled				
PCV	Physician presets a targeted maximum airway pressure, rate, and an inspiratory-time to expiratory-time ratio.	Tidal volume is dependent upon the compliance of the respiratory system. Patient may influence VE by spontaneously over-breathing the set rate.	Improves physician's control of peak alveolar pressures. Improves oxygenation.	Patient discomfort. Increased intrathoracic pressures may decrease cardiac output.

Adapted from: Esteban A, Frutos F, Tobin MJ, et al. A comparison of four methods of weaning patients from mechanical ventilation: the Spanish Lung Failure Collaborative Group. N Engl J Med 1995; 332:345–350; *and* Ely EW, Baker AM, Dunagan DP, et al. Effect on the duration of mechanical ventilation of identifying patients capable of breathing spontaneously. N Engl J Med 1996; 335:1864–1869; *and* Esteban A, Alia I, Gordo F et al. Extubation outcome after spontaneous breathing trials with T-tube or pressure support ventilation: the Spanish Lung Failure Collaborative Group. Am J Respir Crit Care Med 1997; 156:459–465; *and* Vallerdu I, Calaf N, Subirana M, et al. Clinical characteristics, respiratory functional parameters, and outcome of a two-hour T-piece trial in patients weaning from mechanical ventilation. Am J Respir Crit Care Med 1998; 158:1855–1862; *and* MacIntyre NR. Evidence-based guidelines for weaning and discontinuing ventilatory support: a collective task force facilitated by the American College of Chest Physicians; the American Association for Respiratory Care; and the American College of Critical Care Medicine. Chest 2001; 120S:375–396; *and* Kollef MH, Shapiro SD, Silver P, et al. A randomized, controlled trial of protocol-directed versus physician-directed weaning from mechanical ventilation. Crit Care Med 1997; 25:567–574; *and* Bach J, Saporto L. Criteria for extubation and tracheostomy tube removal for patients with ventilatory failure. Chest 1996; 110:1566–1571; *and* Capdevila XJ, Perrigault PF, Perey PJ, et al. Occlusion pressure and its ratio to maximum inspiratory pressure are useful predictors for successful extubation following T-piece weaning trial. Chest 1995; 108:482–489; *and* Meade M, Guyatt G, Cook D, et al. Predicting success in weaning from mechanical ventilation. Chest 2001; 120:300–424.

Key Points

- Oxygen toxicity may develop within the first 24–72 hours when the FiO_2 exceeds 80%. Clinicians should aim for a FiO_2 <50% within the first 72 hours of mechanical ventilation whenever possible, while aiming for oxyhemoglobin saturation >90%.

- Tidal volumes of 5 to 7 cc/kg ideal body weight improve outcomes when used to treat patients with ALI and especially ARDS, as long as adjustments are made to maintain the plateau pressure (peak alveolar pressure) <30 cm H_2O.

- Flow rates below the patient demands increase the work of breathing, and add to patient discomfort. Low peak flows creating air hunger are several times more uncomfortable than flows above the optimal level.

- When selecting the level of $PEEP_E$, the goal is to optimize the SaO_2 and decrease the FiO_2 requirements while attempting to limit additional injury to the patient caused by overdistention of areas of healthy lung or impairing hemodynamics by diminishing venous return to the heart.

- Monitoring the plateau pressures as one makes adjustments to the ventilator settings may avoid lung injury by avoiding pressures of 30 cm H_2O or more, which cause prolonged overdistention of the alveolar unit.

- Early tracheostomy (within the first 7 days of mechanical ventilation) compared to late tracheostomy (after 14–16 days of mechanical ventilation) can significantly decrease the length of mechanical ventilation as well as the length of ICU stay, but there is no significant decrease in incidence of VAP or mortality.

- Adjust the ventilator settings (i.e., the minute ventilation) to allow hypercarbia for patients with COPD who chronically retain CO_2, aiming for a mild respiratory acidosis to preserve the signal to the kidneys to retain bicarbonate for buffering baseline acidemia.

- Employ a systematic approach, using defined criteria for assessing the likelihood of successful extubation, to prevent premature extubation. The assessments for discontinuing mechanical ventilation should begin immediately following its initiation and continue regularly until ventilatory support is discontinued.

- Spontaneous breathing trials are preferred for weaning, as the use of SIMV mode for ventilator weaning appears to increase the time to extubation.

SUGGESTED READING

Tobin MJ. Advances in mechanical ventilation. N Engl J Med 2001; 344(26):1986–1996.

The Acute Respiratory Distress Syndrome Network. Ventilation with lower tidal volumes as compared with traditional tidal volumes for acute lung injury and the acute respiratory distress syndrome. N Engl J Med 2000; 342:1303–1308.

MacIntyre NR. Evidence-based guidelines for weaning and discontinuing ventilatory support: a collective task force facilitated by the American College of Chest Physicians; the American Association for Respiratory Care; and the American College of Critical Care Medicine. Chest 2001; 120S:375–396.

Meade M, Guyatt G, Cook D, et al. Predicting success in weaning from mechanical ventilation. Chest 2001; 120:300–424.

Chastre J, Fagon JY. Ventilator-associated pneumonia. Am J Respir Crit Care Med 2002; 165(7):867–903.

Griffiths J, Vicki BS, Morgan L, et al. Systematic review and meta-analysis of studies of the timing of tracheostomy in adult patients undergoing artificial ventilation. BMJ 2005; 330(7502): 1243–1247.

Kelley MA, Angus D, Chalfin D, et al. The critical care crisis in the United States. Chest 2004; 125:1514–1517.

CHAPTER EIGHTY-EIGHT

Poisonings and Drug Overdose

Brian D. Stein, MD, and Brent W. Morgan, MD

INTRODUCTION

Patients with drug overdoses and poisonings are commonplace on the floors of any hospital, including countless cases of iatrogenic exposures as well. Annually, there are slightly over 2 million reported cases of toxic exposures to United States poison control centers.[1] The true number is undoubtedly higher and estimated at approximately 5 million. Of these exposures, children make up the majority of the cases. Adults, however, make up 90% of the case fatalities. Of these fatalities, roughly 80% are intentional exposures and are secondary to drug abuse or suicide.[1] Of all reported poisonings in 2003, approximately 75% were managed outside of health care facilities. Of those seen at health care facilities, nearly 50% were admitted to the hospital.[1] The most common adult exposures were analgesics, sedative hypnotics, cleansing substances, antidepressants, bites/envenomations, alcohols, and cardiovascular drugs, respectively.[1] This chapter will review the approach to the poisoned patient and specific treatments for poisoning or overdoses commonly encountered in the hospital.

Adults with toxic exposures represent a diverse population who may present in a variety of ways, including seizures, respiratory arrest, altered mental status, cardiac arrhythmias, gastrointestinal (GI) complaints, hypotension, and metabolic acidosis. The initial approach to the poisoned patient should focus on resuscitation and stabilization, history and physical examination, GI tract decontamination, appropriate use of laboratory tests, administration of specific antidotes, and the utilization of enhanced elimination techniques for selected toxins. The United States system of Poison Control Centers tracks the epidemiology of poisoning and serves as a reservoir of information that can be helpful in managing these challenging cases.

History and physical examination: While extremely important, the history of the overdosed patient can be unobtainable or unreliable. Essential details in the history include the substance, time of exposure, route, intent of the exposure, and onset of symptoms as well as any other pertinent past medical or psychiatric history. Specific attention should be paid to the patient's vital signs, level of consciousness, pupillary examination, temperature, and neurologic examination. Bear in mind, patients may not have any signs or symptoms if a substance with delayed toxicity has been ingested (Table 88-1).

Diagnostic tests: Laboratory and radiologic studies should be guided by the history and physical examination. All patients admitted with toxic exposures should have a comprehensive metabolic panel performed that includes transaminases to assess for renal and hepatotoxicity as well as an anion gap acidosis. Rapid urine drug screens are generally not necessary in intentional ingestions but can be useful if an accurate history is unobtainable. Obtaining serum levels of salicylate and acetaminophen should be considered in all cases of intentional overdose, due to their availability and frequent involvement in ingestions; checking an acetaminophen level is a mandatory part of the evaluation.

TREATMENT: GASTROINTESTINAL DECONTAMINATION

Potential options for GI decontamination include gastric lavage, single-dose activated charcoal, multidose activated charcoal, and whole bowel irrigation (WBI) with polyethylene glycol. The clinician should always consider the risk-to-benefit ratio before performing GI decontamination, since most cases involving mild to moderate poisoning do well without GI decontamination.

Once considered a main stay in the treatment of the poisoned patient the use of gastric lavage is no longer routinely recommended.[2] The potential benefit diminishes as time from the initial ingestion passes. The procedure can be associated with complications including laryngospasm, perforation of the GI tract, and aspiration pneumonia. The clinician could consider the use of gastric lavage in cases involving a recent potentially lethal toxic ingestion, especially if the substance is not bound to activated charcoal. Activated charcoal administration and WBI also have known risks to the patient, and should not be performed in a patient with an unprotected airway.

Single-dose activated charcoal is widely used for GI decontamination in the poisoned patient, despite the lack of evidence that it improves clinical outcome.[3] Studies indicate that its potentially greatest benefit occurs if administered within 1 hour of ingestion. Activated charcoal can cause complications, especially if aspirated into the lungs.

In animal and human volunteer studies, multidose charcoal has been shown to enhance the elimination of several drugs.[4] However, no controlled studies have been performed that show a reduction in morbidity or mortality. The proposed mechanisms of

Table 88-1 Classification of Agents That Can Produce Delayed Toxicity

Pharmaceuticals	Biologicals	Pharmaceutical Dosage forms	Chemicals
Acetaminophen	Coral snakes	Concretions	Acetonitrile
Astemizole	Cyanogenic compounds	Drug packets	HFl
Aspirin	Mushrooms	Enteric-coated	Methanol
Iron		Sustained release	Organophosphates
Lomotil			
Methadone			
Thyroid hormone			
Tricyclic antidepressants			
Valpromide			

Adapted from: Bosse GM, Matyunas NJ, Delayed toxidromes. J Emerg Med, 17(4):679–90, 1999 Jul–Aug.

Table 88-2 Potential Antidotes in the Treatment of the Poisoned Patient

Drug or Toxin	Antidotes
Acetaminophen	N-Acetylcysteine
Black widow spider, venomous snakes, and scorpions	Species-specific antivenin
Digoxin	Digoxin-specific antibodies
Carbon monoxide	Normobaric and hyperbaric oxygen
Lead	DMSA or BAL and EDTA
Inorganic arsenic	DMSA
Mercury	DMSA
Thallium	Prussian blue
Beta-blockers	Glucagon
Calcium channel blockers	Calcium, glucagon
Hydroflouric acid	Insulin and dextrose
INH and other hydrazines	Calcium, magnesium
Insulin and other hypoglycemic agents	Pyridoxine
Sulfonylurea	Glucose
Valproic acid	Octreotide
Cyanide	Carnitine
Iron	Amyl nitrite, sodium nitrite, thiusulfate Hydroxocobalamin (not available in United States) Deferoxime
Opiates	Naloxone
Benzodiazepines	Flumazenil
Ethylene glycol and methanol	Fomepizole
Methemoglobinemia	Methylene blue
Coumarins	Vitamin K
Heparin	Protamine
Tricyclic antidepressants	Sodium bicarbonate
Anticholinergies	Physostigmine
Organophosphates and carbmates	Atropine
Organophosphates	Pralidoxime

The reader is referred to a more detailed text for indications and dosage. The above antidotes have not all been approved by the Food and Drug Administration at the time of publication.

DMSA—dimercaptosuccinic acid; BAL—British anti-Lewisite (dimercaprol); EDTA—ethylenediaminetetraacetic acid

action of multidose charcoal include the binding of residual drug in the GI tract and enhancing elimination via interrupting the enteroenteric and enterohepatic circulation. Multidose charcoal can be considered as an option in the management of carbamazepine, dapsone, phenobarbital, quinine, and theophylline ingestions. Side effects attributed to multidose charcoal include bowel obstruction in addition to aspiration.

WBI has a limited role in the management of the poisoned patient.[5] No controlled trials have been performed, so evidence of benefit is derived from volunteer studies, animal studies, and case reports. Potential uses of WBI include ingestions of: iron and other toxic metal that are not bound by charcoal, sustained-release or enteric-coated medications, and packets of illicit drugs. In adults, WBI is best administered via a nasogastric tube at a rate of 1,500 to 2,000 mL/hr. Once instituted, WBI should be continued until rectal effluent is clear. In cases when radiologic studies confirm the presence of toxins in the GI tract, WBI should be continued until subsequent follow-up studies are negative.

Following determination of the need for GI decontamination and application in appropriate cases, the clinician should administer an appropriate antidote after consultation with the local Poison Control (Table 88-2). Overdoses and poisonings that hospitalists may commonly encounter are reviewed in more detail below.

ACETAMINOPHEN

Background

Acetaminophen accounts for more overdoses and overdose-related fatalities each year in the United States than any other medicinal agent. In adults, the ingestion of 150 mg/kg or 7.5–10 g (the equivalent of 15–20 extra-strength tablets) has the potential to produce liver damage; however, 4–6 g may be enough to produce damage in those with heavy alcohol use or preexisting hepatic disease.[6] Most patients who ingest doses in excess of 350 mg/kg develop severe liver toxicity (defined as a peak aspartate aminotransferase or alanine aminotransferase levels greater than 1,000 international unit/L) unless treated.[7] Acetaminophen is commonly ingested in overdoses involving multiple medications and should be part of screening in all intentional overdoses.

Assessment

Clinical presentation: Signs and symptoms from acetaminophen toxicity may be subtle and nonspecific, ranging from asymptomatic to fulminant hepatic failure. There are four classic phases of toxicity, and patients may present in any of the four phases, depending on the time of ingestion and the formulation (immediate vs. sustained release). Phase 1 occurs in the first 24 hours and commonly involves anorexia, malaise, pallor, diaphoresis, and nausea and vomiting. Phase 2 occurs from 24–48 hours after an untreated overdose. It includes liver function test abnormalities and right upper quadrant pain. Signs and symptoms of Phase 2 may occur even in light of improving symptoms of phase 1. Phase 3 occurs at 48–96 hours after ingestion and involves symptoms of severe hepatotoxicity, including encephalopathy, coagulopathy, and hypoglycemia. If a patient survives phase 3, he or she enters phase 4, which is a recovery period and is usually complete by day 7.

Differential Diagnosis: Differential diagnosis is broad and includes any toxic, infectious, environmental, or metabolic cause of hepatocellular injury.

Diagnosis: Diagnosis is made by history and a postingestion serum acetaminophen level above the toxic range on the Rummack-Mathew nomogram (Fig. 88-1). Serum levels obtained prior to 4 hours after ingestion are not interpretable secondary to ongoing drug absorption and distribution. The Rummack-Mathew nomogram is only applicable in cases involving a single acute ingestion. If a patient has ingested extended-release preparations of acetaminophen, the serum level may peak later.

Algorithm: Treatment is indicated for patients with a postingestion acetaminophen level above the "possible hepatic toxicity" line on the Rummack-Mathew nomogram (see Figure 88-1), and for patients with an unknown time of ingestion and a serum acetaminophen level of greater then 10 mcg/mL, with single ingestions of greater than 150 mg/kg, with any evidence of hepatotoxicity and a history of acetaminophen overdose, and for patients with repeated excessive acetaminophen ingestion and a serum level greater than 10 mcg/mL or transaminase elevation. Patients who present more than 24 hours after an acute ingestion and have either detectable serum acetaminophen or transaminase elevation require treatment.

Prognosis: N-acetylcysteine (NAC) is believed to be 100% effective when administered within the first 8–10 hours.[3] Among patients who develop fulminant hepatic failure and do not receive liver transplants, acetaminophen-induced fulminant hepatic failure has the highest survival rate; this raises the threshold for transplantation. Prolongation of the prothrombin time (PT) is an important prognostic factor, and fresh frozen plasma should not be given routinely unless there is evidence of bleeding. Administration of vitamin K with subsequent decline in PT or international normalized ratio (INR) suggests viable liver tissue, while lack of response is a poor prognostic factor. Metabolic acidosis, hypoglycemia, and renal failure are all poor prognostic signs.

Management

Treatment: NAC should be administered to patients falling above the treatment line on the modified Rumack-Matthew nomogram or those at increased risk. NAC is administered as a 140 mg/kg oral loading dose and then 70 mg/kg every 4 hours for 17 doses.[8,9] Patients with intractable nausea and vomiting or other conditions precluding oral administration should be given IV NAC. Intravenous NAC is preferred in cases of fulminant hepatic failure. Of note, the adverse reaction rate is considerably higher with IV NAC than oral treatment.[8] Acetadote® (IV NAC) was approved in 2004 by the Food and Drug Administration (FDA), and the full treatment dose of 300 mg/kg can be administered in a 24-hour period. After the an initial IV dose of 150 mg/kg IV over 15 minutes, then 12.5 mg/kg/hour for 4 hours is given, and finally 6.25 mg/kg/hour for the next 16 hours. This treatment should be initiated within 8 hours of the overdose and immediately if time of ingestion is uncertain. It may be continued if liver enzymes continue to rise. Cimetidine has not proven to be of any benefit.

Patients with fulminant liver failure should be identified and transferred to a center with expertise in the management of liver failure and capability to perform liver transplantation (see

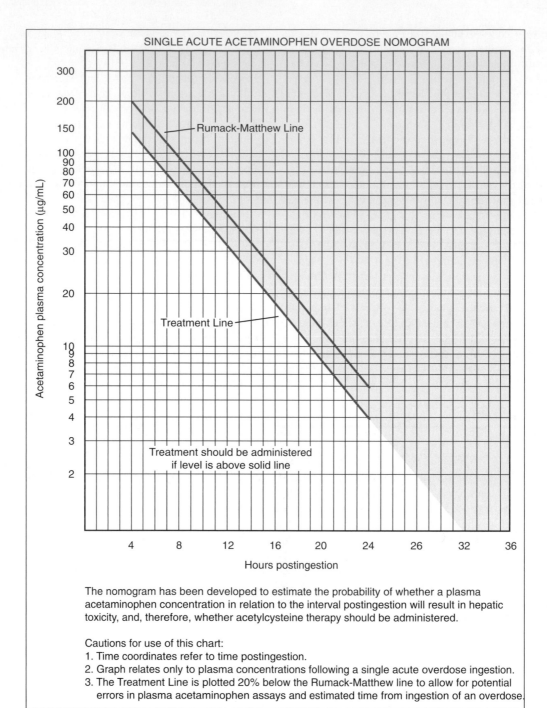

Figure 88-1 • Rummack-Mathew nomogram. From: Ford MD, et al., eds. Clinical Toxicology, 1st ed. St. Louis, MO: W.B. Saunders; 2001.

Chapters 55 and 56). One set of criteria for transplantation includes either an arterial pH <7.30 or grade III–IV encephalopathy, a prothrombin time >100, or a serum Cr >3.4.[9]

Disposition: Disposition will be guided by other medical or psychiatric needs once treatment is complete. For patients in whom no acetaminophen is detectable and no elevation in serum transaminases has developed 36 hours or more post ingestion, there is little risk of hepatotoxicity, and these patients can be safely discharged.

SALICYLATES

Background

Salicylates are present in a variety of prescription and over-the-counter medications. While aspirin is implicated in most cases of salicylate toxicity, ingestion of topical liniments, bismuth subsalicylate, and salicylic acid (used in wart removal) can also result in toxicity. The incidence of salicylate toxicity has decreased, but due to continued widespread use of salicylates it remains an important problem. Patients with chronic salicylate toxicity have a higher mortality than acute ingestions, as chronic ingestions can increase the half-life to >20 hours.

Assessment

Clinical Presentation

Tinnitus, vertigo, nausea, vomiting, and diarrhea are features present in early salicylate intoxication. Tinnitus may be present even at levels within the therapeutic range. More severe intoxication may result in a respiratory alkalosis or mixed metabolic acidosis and respiratory alkalosis. Altered mental status, coma, noncardiogenic pulmonary edema, and even death may occur in severe intoxication. The classic respiratory alkalosis may be absent if a CNS depressant has been coingested.

Differential Diagnosis

Salicylate toxicity should be considered in any patient presenting with an anion gap metabolic acidosis (see Chapter 53). It is often mistaken for altered mental status from sepsis, meningitis, or dementia in elderly patients on chronic salicylate therapy.

Preferred Studies

The therapeutic range for serum salicylates is 10–30 mg/dL. The level correlates poorly to signs and symptoms of toxicity, but symptoms generally occur at a level above 40 mg/dL. A level greater than 100 mg/dL in an acute ingestion is an indication for dialysis, while a level of 60 mg/dL in a symptomatic patient with chronic ingestion may also indicate a need for dialysis. The level should be repeated at 2-hour intervals until two consecutive levels show a decrease from the peak level. Bear in mind, levels may peak later in delayed-release or enteric-coated aspirin preparations. Plasma potassium, glucose, and creatinine should be monitored closely. An arterial blood gas should be obtained along with a lactate level in the presence of acidosis. A chest radiograph should be performed to evaluate for salicylate induced noncardiogenic pulmonary edema, as this may complicate rehydration and may also indicate a need for dialysis.

Prediction Rule

Toxicity may occur with acute ingestions of 150 mg/kg. Chronic ingestions of greater than 100 mg/kg day may also cause toxicity. Mortality from chronic salicylate toxicity has been estimated as high as 25% versus 1% for acute toxicity.[12]

Management

Treatment

Gastric lavage may be considered if within an hour of an acute ingestion. Activated charcoal is also indicated acutely and may be repeated. Urinary alkalization is the mainstay of treatment with a goal urine pH of 7.5–8.0 and a serum pH of 7.45–7.5. Sodium bicarbonate should be administered early and not withheld because of respiratory alkalosis. Arterial blood gases may need to be checked every 2 hours to keep pH <7.6 and above 7.45.

The distribution of salicylates is pH dependent. The primary respiratory alkalosis caused by salicylates actually helps keep salicylates out of the tissue compartment by maintaining the molecule in an ionized form. With a drop in pH from acidosis,

salicylic acid shifts to a unionized state and can readily cross the blood–brain barrier, resulting in greater toxicity. In cases of salicylism requiring intubation, clinicians should strive to avoid a drop in the pH once they place a patient on mechanical ventilation and hyperventilate patients to maintain alkalemia.

Aggressive hydration and electrolyte correction may be necessary to manage dehydration and hypokalemia. Indications for hemodialysis depend on the serum salicylate value or associated symptoms (Box 88-1). Serial salicylate levels should be performed at 2-hour intervals until a downward trend is noted in two serial measurements.

Discharge/Follow-up

Patients with acute, single ingestions of non–enteric-coated salicylates of <150 mg/kg who remain asymptomatic and have 6-hour postingestion levels within the nontoxic range and a repeat level that indicates downward trend can be safely discharged.

Patients with intentional ingestions meeting the above criteria can be safely transferred to a psychiatric service.

OPIOIDS

Background

The surge in prescribed opiate medications and a rising incidence of heroin abuse in the United States have made opioid intoxication commonplace in emergency departments and hospital wards across the nation. Most heroin-related fatalities are also accompanied by significant blood levels of alcohol or benzodiazepines.

Assessment

Clinical Presentation

Opioid toxicity produces a classic syndrome characterized by depressed level of consciousness, respiratory depression, and miosis. Studies have used a Glasgow Coma Scale score of less than 12 and a respiratory rate less than 12 to define respiratory depression and depressed level of consciousness.[13] Additional toxicities may include hypotension, noncardiogenic pulmonary edema, aspiration pneumonitis, ileus, nausea, vomiting, and pruritus.

Differential Diagnosis

Other causes of depressed mental status and miosis should be considered. These include hypoxia, CNS infection, head trauma,

---

Box 88-1 Hemodialysis Indications in Salicylate Toxicity

Serum levels >100 mg/dL in acute ingestion

Serum levels >60 mg/dL in chronic intoxication

Pulmonary edema

Renal failure

Congestive heart failure

Altered mental status and acidemia

hypoglycemia, central α_2 receptor agonists, organophosphates or carbamates, phenothiazines, phencyclidine, sedative-hypnotic drugs, and pontine hemorrhage.

Diagnosis

The diagnosis of opioid toxicity is often made clinically as described above. A rapid response to naloxone supports the diagnosis of opioid intoxication, but is not diagnostic. Toxicologic screens are not generally helpful in the management of patients with opioid toxicity, as screening results are often unavailable until after significant patient management must occur. Screens are helpful in identifying patients with poly-substance use and helping confirm the diagnosis. Of note, opioid screens lack sensitivity and many may not detect some of the synthetic and semi-synthetic opioids, including hydrocodone, oxycodone, methadone, and propoxyphene. In addition, fentanyl and its derivatives are not detectable on routine screens. Serum quantitative levels are of no clinical benefit.

Algorithms

The patient with a suspected overdose should first be stabilized with supportive measures. Naloxone should be administered in the appropriate setting. Of note, chronic users of opioids should first be given a small dose of naloxone (e.g., 0.4 mg), as it may precipitate severe withdrawal symptoms, instead of the standard 2-mg dose. Patients should undergo toxicologic screening to identify other drugs or medications concurrently being taken. All patients with opiate toxicity from oral overdose should have an acetaminophen level drawn, as a large percentage of oral opiates are coupled with acetaminophen.

Prognosis

As long as a hypoxic insult has not occurred, full recovery is expected once medical stabilization has occurred.

During Hospitalization

Patients admitted with opioid intoxication or chronic opioid use should be monitored for signs of withdrawal that include pupillary dilatation, lacrimation, rhinorrhea, piloerection, yawning, sneezing, nausea, vomiting, and diarrhea. These symptoms can be managed with long-acting opioid medications, such as methadone. Clonidine also may be used to decrease withdrawal symptoms.

Management

Treatment

Preferred Treatment: Treatment of opiate toxicity initially involves supportive measures. Airway protection and hemodynamic stabilization should be obtained prior to initiating additional therapy. IV naloxone is the drug of choice in opioid overdose but may be administered via IM and SQ routes if an IV line is not available. It also can be administered via endotracheal tube in an intubated patient. The initial recommended IV dose is 0.4 mg. If no clinical response is seen, additional 1–2 mg doses can be administered at 3–5 minute intervals up to a total of 10 mg. Greater than 10 mg may be necessary to reverse the effects of semi-synthetic oral opiates.[14] Naloxone's onset of action occurs within minutes and lasts 45–90 minutes. Repeat boluses

may be needed to maintain its effects, as the half-life of most opiates far exceeds that of naloxone. Infusion may be used at 0.4–0.8 mg/hr if necessary. In acute ingestions, gastric decontamination may be indicated.

Alternative

Nalmefene is another opioid antagonist with a 4- to 10-hour duration of action. It has been avoided, largely due to the risk of inducing an extended period of withdrawal.

Discharge/Follow-up Plans

Disposition, observation guidelines, and indications for admission of opioid-toxic patients are controversial. Situations that warrant extended observation or admission include recurrence of respiratory depression, development of noncardiogenic pulmonary edema, or ingestion of long-acting opioids or opioids with anticipated delayed absorption. In cases of intentional overdoses, the patient should have psychiatric evaluation prior to discharge. Patients with opioid abuse should be referred to appropriate treatment programs at time of discharge.

TOXIC ALCOHOLS

Background

Ethylene glycol and methanol ingestion remain important causes of toxic alcohol poisoning that may result in significant morbidity and mortality if misdiagnosed or left untreated. Ethylene glycol is present in antifreeze and industrial solvents while methanol is a component of many paint removers, de-icing solutions, and varnishes. Ingestion of either ethylene glycol or methanol in minute amounts can result in death or other permanent sequelae. Both alcohols are converted to toxic metabolites by alcohol dehydrogenase, which is the target of pharmacologic therapy. Both are commonly coingested with alcohol, which can delay toxicity.

Assessment

Clinical Presentation

Classically, ethylene glycol toxicity presents as a continuum of symptoms. Initial symptoms are similar to ethanol toxicity and include inebriation, ataxia, and nausea and vomiting but may progress to coma or cerebral edema. Symptoms can occur as early as 30 minutes to 2 hours post ingestion. Variable levels of anion gap metabolic acidosis may be present. Hypocalcemia may be present as well. If untreated, symptoms may progress to cardiovascular dysfunction and cardiogenic or noncardiogenic pulmonary edema. Later presentation includes flank pain and acute renal failure. Cranial neuropathies may be seen up to weeks after ingestion has occurred.

Methanol toxicity may present in a similar fashion to ethanol toxicity as well. Patients will often present alert, however, having passed through the initial period of inebriation. Headache, dizziness, and nausea and vomiting are common presenting symptoms. Visual complaints ranging from blurred vision to complete blindness may be present secondary to retinal and optic nerve injury. Variable degrees of anion gap metabolic acidosis may be present.

Table 88-3 Anion Gap Acidosis

Pneumonic	Substance	Substance responsible for Anion Gap
C	Carbun monoxide	Lactic acid and
	Cyanide	Ketoacids
A	AKA	Ketoacids
	Azides	Lactic acid
T	Toluene	Hippuric acid
M	Methanol	Formic acid
	Metaformin	Lactic acid
U	Uremia	Phosphoric and sulfuric acid metabolites
D	DKA	Ketoacids
P	Phenformin	Lactic acid
	Paraldehyde	
I	Iron	Lactic acid
	INH	
	Ibuprofen	Propionic acid
L	Lactate	Lactic Aacid
E	Ethylene glycol	Glycolic and oxalic acid
S	Salicylates	Salicylic acid

AKA—alcoholic ketoacidosis; DKA—diabetic ketoacidosis; INH—isoniazid

Differential Diagnosis

The differential diagnosis for ethylene glycol or methanol poisoning includes any condition that may cause an anion gap metabolic acidosis (Table 88-3).

Diagnosis

Diagnosis is made by clinical history and laboratory evaluation. The presence of a metabolic acidosis with a large anion gap and an osmolar gap in conjunction with altered mental status is suggestive of methanol or ethylene glycol poisoning. Serum ethylene glycol or methanol levels may be measured directly by gas chromatography. Levels do not always correlate with toxicity, as much of the parent compound may already have been metabolized. In ethylene glycol poisoning, 50% of patients will have calcium oxalate crystals in their urine on admission to the hospital.[15] Hypocalcemia is also prevalent in ethylene glycol toxicity.

Preferred Studies

Recommended studies include serum electrolytes, blood urea nitrogen (BUN), creatinine, glucose, serum osmolality, arterial blood gas analysis, and lactate level. Specific methanol and ethylene glycol levels are recommended but are not always readily available. Serum salicylates, acetaminophen, and routine serum toxicologic screening is also recommended. Both an ECG (to assess for QT prolongation) and a chest radiograph (for suspected aspiration or pulmonary edema) are recommended. Ionized calcium and urinalysis for calcium oxalate crystals are recommended in ethylene glycol toxicity.

Prognosis

If left untreated, ingestion of as little as 100 mL of ethylene glycol or methanol may prove fatal. Toxicity from both typically resolves completely after medical treatment. Patients with ethylene glycol toxicity may require dialysis for several months secondary to renal toxicity; however, this typically resolves as well. Ocular toxicity with methanol ingestion may be permanent. Clinical symptoms and mortality correlate more closely with degree of metabolic acidosis than measured methanol or ethylene glycol levels.

Management

Treatment

Treatment for both ethylene glycol and methanol toxicity includes supportive care, administration of alcohol dehydrogenase inhibitors such as fomepizole or ethanol, administration of sodium bicarbonate for acidosis, and hemodialysis for removal of the toxic alcohol and correction of severe metabolic derangements. Indications for treatment with fomepizole or ethanol include a plasma methanol or ethylene glycol concentration of >20 mg/dL; a history of ingestion with an osmol gap >10 mosm/L; or strong suspicion of ingestion in conjunction with any combination of arterial pH <7.3, serum bicarbonate <20 meq/L, an osmol gap >10 mosm/L; or the presence of calcium oxalate crystals in the urine.[16,17] Fomepizole is the antidote of choice for toxic alcohol ingestion, with a loading dose of 15 mg/kg and maintenance dosing of 10 mg/kg every 12 hours for four doses, and then 15 mg/kg every 12 hours thereafter. It is dialyzable, and dosing should be adjusted with hemodialysis. Ethanol may be administered if fomepizole is unavailable; however, its use is not FDA approved, and intensive care unit (ICU) monitoring is recommended. Ethanol is also less ideal in poly-substance ingestions and in patients with altered mental status. Both fomepizole and ethanol can be discontinued once serum levels of the toxic alcohol are <20 mg/dL.

Traditionally, serum concentrations of 50 mg/dL of ethylene glycol or methanol were indications for hemodialysis; however, this cutoff has been questioned with the advent of treatment with fomepizole. Other indications for dialysis are the inability to maintain a serum pH >7.30 with bicarbonate therapy, renal failure in ethylene glycol ingestion, and visual impairment in the setting of methanol ingestion. Dialysis may be discontinued once the serum levels are below the toxic range and metabolic acidosis corrected.

Folic acid may be of some therapeutic benefit in methanol toxicity; however, its use is off label. Additionally, pyridoxine and thiamine administration may be of some benefit in ethylene glycol toxicity, though there is no clinical evidence that their administration is beneficial in nutritionally replete patients.

Discharge

Patients may be discharged with routine follow-up once the underlying metabolic abnormalities have been corrected. It is recommended that serum osmolality and toxic alcohol level be measured again 12 hours after dialysis, as redistribution may occur, resulting in an increased level. Residual end-organ damage will dictate outpatient follow-up.

SYMPATHOMIMETICS

Background

Sympathomimetics are drugs whose properties mimic those of a stimulated sympathetic nervous system. Two of the most commonly abused sympathomimetics are cocaine and amphetamines. Amphetamines are a relatively large class of agents and include methamphetamine, MDMA (ecstasy), pseudoephedrine and phenylpropanolamine. The Drug Abuse Warning Network (DAWN) estimates that cocaine and amphetamines use accounts for more than 160,000 emergency department visits in the United States each year.[18]

Assessment

Clinical Presentation

Cocaine and amphetamines cause a sympathomimetic response including tachycardia, hypertension, agitation, hyperthermia, diaphoresis, and mydriasis. Other findings can include rhabdomyolysis; cardiac ischemia from coronary vasospasm or increased myocardial demand in the setting of coronary artery disease; dysrhythmias; seizures; and, because of excessive hypertension, intracranial hemorrhage or aortic dissection. After the effects of the drug have worn off, patients may have prolonged somnolence and lethargy because of preceding profound sleep deprivation while they were using the drug.

Differential Diagnosis

The differential diagnosis of cocaine and amphetamine toxicity includes hypoglycemia, thyrotoxicosis, pheochromocytoma, mania, psychosis, sedative hypnotic and ethanol drug withdrawal, serotonin syndrome, and use of the following substances: phencyclidine, methylxanthines, and monoamine oxidase inhibitors.

Diagnosis

The diagnosis is made on historical and clinical grounds. Urine drug screen can be confirmatory.

Preferred Studies

Symptomatic patients typically require serum electrolytes, liver transaminases, complete blood count, electrocardiogram, chest x-ray, cardiac enzymes, and evaluation for rhabdomyolysis. A cranial CT should be obtained in patients with altered mental status or seizures, and in those patients with suspected intracranial bleed or infarction.

Prognosis

The majority of patients presenting with acute toxicity from cocaine and amphetamine usually recover without permanent sequelae. Approximately 6% of patients with cocaine-associated chest pain sustain a myocardial infarction.[19] Continued use of cocaine or amphetamines after discharge can result in neurologic and cardiac sequelae as well as disruption of patients' social lives with loss of jobs, marriages, and friends.

Management

Treatment

Gastrointestinal decontamination should be considered in patients with oral exposures. There is no specific antidote. Management is mainly supportive, with attention directed to the clinical effects and intravenous hydration. Cocaine and amphetamines cause an increase in endogenous catecholamines, and aggressive use of benzodiazepines is frequently warranted to enhance central nervous system inhibitory pathways. Hyperthermia is associated with increased mortality. Cooling measures should be instituted emergently in the hyperthermic patient.

Hypertension that is unresponsive to benzodiazepines can be treated with nitroglycerin, nitroprusside, or phentolamine. Tachycardia should be treated with benzodiazepines, intravenous hydration, and cooling if needed.[19] Because of the concern for unopposed α receptor stimulation, beta-blockers should be avoided in the treatment of hypertension and tachycardia.[21] They can worsen the hypertension.

Myocardial ischemia can be treated with aspirin, nitrates, benzodiazepines, and phentolamine. Cardiac catheterization should be used in appropriate cases.[20] Thrombolytic therapy should be used with caution if at all, as it may have a higher risk-to-benefit ratio in drug-induced coronary syndromes.[22]

Discharge

Patients can be discharged when the vitals signs and mental status have normalized, the patient appears free of the effects of medications, and no serious pathology has been found. Both methamphetamines and cocaine are highly addictive, and patients admitted for side effects from sympathomimetic abuse should be enrolled in drug treatment programs at the time of discharge.

CARBON MONOXIDE

Background

Carbon monoxide (CO) is an odorless, colorless, and tasteless gas produced during the incomplete combustion of carbon-based compounds and via hepatic metabolism of the solvent methylene chloride. Carbon monoxide poisoning is a leading cause of poisoning death worldwide. In the United States alone, there are an estimated 2,000 to 3,000 deaths from accidental and intentional carbon monoxide exposure each year.[23] Carbon monoxide impairs the oxygen-carrying capacity of hemoglobin as its main mechanism of toxicity.

Assessment

Clinical Presentation

Carbon monoxide poisoning causes clinical effects by producing tissue hypoxia. The central nervous system and cardiovascular system appear most vulnerable. Clinical symptoms of mild poisoning can be difficult to diagnosis, as they mimic those of a viral illness and include headache, nausea, vomiting, malaise, and fatigue.

Severe cases of poisoning can present with neurologic symptoms that can include impaired cognition, altered mental status, coma, and seizures. Other symptoms can include syncope, ventricular dysrhythmias, tachycardia, and tachypnea followed by bradycardia, bradypnea, and death.

Differential Diagnosis

The differential diagnosis includes viral syndromes, gastroenteritis, myocardial infarction, stroke, asphyxia, drug overdoses that can produce coma with or without metabolic acidosis, and myxedema coma.

Diagnosis

Diagnosis is made by clinical history and laboratory confirmation. Once the diagnosis is confirmed, the clinician should consider the possibility of other-undiagnosed victims who have not presented for evaluation or have yet to be found.

Preferred Studies

Patients with mild exposure can be managed in the emergency department with carboxyhemoglobin levels from either arterial or venous blood and a pregnancy test in women of childbearing age. Patients with more severe poisoning typically also require an electrocardiogram, chest x-ray, an arterial blood gas, serum chemistries, complete blood count, cardiac enzymes, and urinalysis. Patients with persistent neurologic findings may require a computed tomography (CT) or magnetic resonance imaging (MRI) of the brain. Neuropsychologic testing may help in the identification of subtle deficits.

Prognosis

Patients who sustain a myocardial injury from carbon monoxide poisoning have an increased risk of mortality.[24] Neurologic effects are relatively common after severe carbon monoxide poisoning. The neurologic effects can appear initially or several days after exposure and may resolve in several months or result in permanent sequelae.

Management

Treatment

The treatment of carbon monoxide poisoning includes supportive care and the administration of oxygen. Carbon monoxide binds to hemoglobin at an affinity 200–250 times that of

oxygen.[25] The half-life of carbon monoxide can be considerably shortened by increasing the dose of oxygen administration. For example, 100% oxygen via a nonrebreather mask and hyperbaric oxygen diminish the half-life of carbon monoxide to roughly 1.5 hours and 0.5 hours, respectively, compared to 4.5 hours for room air. All suspected carbon monoxide–poisoned patients should receive 100% oxygen via a non-rebreather mask until the diagnosis is confirmed with laboratory testing. Once the diagnosis is confirmed, oxygen therapy should continue until the patient is asymptomatic or the carbon monoxide level is normal.

The use of hyperbaric oxygen for the treatment of carbon monoxide poisoning is still controversial.[26] However, it should be strongly considered in carbon monoxide–poisoned patients who had a loss of consciousness, any neurologic signs or symptoms, cardiac complications, a level of >25%, and in pregnant patients. Consult with your local Poison Control or hyperbaric physician in these instances.

Discharge

Patients without evidence of neurologic impairment or cardiac injury can be discharged after oxygen therapy. They should be cautioned about the potential for delayed neurologic sequelae and should have follow-up arranged. The degree of neurologic impairment or cardiac injury will dictate follow-up in patients with severe poisoning.

Key Points

- All patients presenting to the hospital with an intentional overdose should undergo measurement of serum acetaminophen levels.

- The use of gastric lavage is no longer routinely recommended, as its potential benefit is limited and it can be associated with laryngospasm, perforation of the gastrointestinal tract, and aspiration pneumonia.

- Activated charcoal administration and WBI should not be performed in a patient with an unprotected airway.

- NAC is believed to be 100% effective when administered within the first 8–10 hours after acetaminophen overdose.

- Beta-blockers should be avoided in treating cocaine and amphetamine toxicity.

- Potential indications for hyperbaric oxygen in the treatment of carbon monoxide poisoning: loss of consciousness, pregnancy, neurologic signs or symptoms, cardiac ischemia, and a COHb level of >25%.

SUGGESTED READING

Watson WA, Litovitz TL, Klein-Schwartz W, et al. 2003 annual report of the American Association of Poison Control Centers Toxic Exposure Surveillance System. Am J Emerg Med 2004; 22:335–404.

Vale JA, Kulig K. American Academy of Clinical Toxicology. European Association of Poisons Centres and Clinical Toxicologists. Position paper: gastric lavage. J Toxicol Clin Toxicol 2004; 42:933–943.

Position statement and practice guidelines on the use of multi-dose activated charcoal in the treatment of acute poisoning. American Academy of Clinical Toxicology; European Association of Poisons Centres and Clinical Toxicologists. J Toxicol Clin Toxicol 1999; 37:731–751.

Position paper: whole bowel irrigation. J Toxicol Clin Toxicol 2004; 42:843–854.

Barceloux DG, Bond GR, Krenzelok EP, et al. American Academy of Clinical Toxicology Ad Hoc Committee on the Treatment Guidelines for Methanol Poisoning. Related Articles, American Academy of Clinical Toxicology practice guidelines on the treatment of methanol poisoning. J Toxicol Clin Toxicol 2002; 40:415–446.

Drug Abuse Warning Network, 2003: Interim National Estimates of Drug-Related EmergencyDepartment Visits: U.S. Department of Health and Human Services Substance Abuse and Mental Health Services Administration. Available at http://DAWNinfo.samhsa.gov. Toxicology in ECC. Circulation 2005; 112;126–132.

Henry CR, Satran D, Lindgren B, et al. Myocardial injury and long-term mortality following moderate to severe carbon monoxide poisoning. JAMA 2006; 295(4):398–402.

Juurlink DN, Buckley NA, Stanbrook MB, et al. Hyperbaric oxygen for carbon monoxide poisoning.[update of Cochrane Database Syst Rev. 2000;(2):CD002041; PMID: 10796853]. Cochrane Database Syst Rev (1):CD002041, 2005.

CHAPTER EIGHTY-NINE

Alcohol Withdrawal Syndromes

Hasan F. Shabbir, MD, Nurcan Ilksoy, MD, and Jeffrey L. Greenwald, MD

BACKGROUND

Alcoholism continues to be a major health problem in the United States, with approximately 8 million people meeting criteria for alcohol dependence. About half a million of these individuals suffer from severe withdrawal symptoms.[1,2]

Alcohol-related issues are thus also common among hospitalized patients. It is estimated that 12.5–30% of inpatients have ongoing alcohol abuse or dependence issues.[3] In 2002–2003, more than 4 million hospitalizations had alcohol abuse or dependence-related problems as the primary or secondary discharge diagnosis.[4] Hospitalists must be able to recognize those patients at risk for withdrawal and initiate the appropriate therapy to prevent complications of alcohol withdrawal syndrome (AWS), some of which are potentially fatal.

Pathophysiology

The exact mechanism of alcohol's depressant effect on the central nervous system (CNS) is not completely understood. Alcohol appears to inhibit dopamine and central adrenergic receptors and has an action similar to gamma-aminobutyric acid (GABA)—an inhibitory neurotransmitter. With chronic exposure, the brain compensates to offset the inhibitory effect of alcohol on neuronal excitability, impulse conduction, and transmitter release. Abrupt cessation or reduction of ethanol consumption can result in brain hyperexcitability. This effect manifests clinically with a spectrum of symptoms from anxiety, tremors, and agitation to hallucinosis, seizures, and delirium. Tremors result from excess noradrenergic activity, and hallucinosis may be caused by excess dopamine.[3] Seizures and delirium tremens are thought to occur from this hyperexcitability in some patients with long-term alcohol-related neuronal changes.[1] Although the exact pathophysiology is not well understood, risk factors for each manifestation of AWS have been identified and are reviewed in the Clinical Presentation section below.

Definition of Alcohol Withdrawal (DSM-IV)[6]

To meet the definition of alcohol withdrawal, an individual must meet the following criteria:

A. Cessation of (or reduction in) alcohol use that has been heavy and prolonged.

B. Two (or more) of the following, developing within several hours to a few days after Criterion A:

1) autonomic hyperactivity (e.g., sweating or pulse rate greater than 100)
2) increased hand tremor
3) insomnia
4) nausea or vomiting
5) transient visual, tactile, or auditory hallucinations or illusions
6) psychomotor agitation
7) anxiety
8) grand mal seizures

C. The symptoms in Criterion B cause clinically significant distress or impairment in social, occupational, or other important areas of functioning.

D. The symptoms are not due to a general medical condition and are not better accounted for by another mental disorder.

CLINICAL PRESENTATION

Alcohol withdrawal syndrome may be a progressive condition requiring hospitalization.

Alcohol withdrawal symptoms appear in susceptible individuals as the blood alcohol level falls below a certain threshold. This threshold varies between individuals and is dependent upon a number of factors, but primarily the long-term alcohol consumption history. In some patients, only a reduction in ethanol intake, rather than actual cessation may precipitate the withdrawal. The presence and severity of withdrawal depend, in part, on the amount and the duration of alcohol consumption.

In the following section, the four major types of AWS are discussed: minor withdrawal (including autonomic hyperactivity, anxiety and tremors), alcoholic hallucinosis, withdrawal seizures, and delirium tremens. There can be significant overlap between some of these stages.[5,7] Each type of withdrawal will be discussed in detail below.

Minor Alcohol Withdrawal

Minor withdrawal commonly includes anxiety and tremors Pharmacotherapy is warranted for hospitalized patients with minor withdrawal.

Minor AWS symptoms can occur within 6–12 hours after cessation of drinking, even while the patient has a measurable blood alcohol level. As it is characterized by a state of autonomic hyperactivity, symptoms may include anxiety, tremulousness, insomnia, hypertension, tachycardia, nausea, vomiting, or diarrhea. Of note, the hemodynamic symptoms of "minor" AWS may be severe with difficult to control hypertension and tachyarrhythmias. Myalgias may also be seen.

Not all patients will exhibit all elements of minor withdrawal; however, these symptoms, particularly in the hospitalized individual, may be slow to resolve, with resolution taking as long as 2 weeks.[5,7,8]

Binge drinkers rarely develop significant withdrawal unless the binge was prolonged or was in addition to a history of significant continuous consumption. Other factors predictive for alcohol withdrawal include concomitant medical/surgical illness, higher breath/blood alcohol levels, older age, time since the last drink, and a history of (1) detoxifications, (2) delirium tremens, (3) AWS seizures, and (4) longer duration of alcohol dependence.[9] Minor withdrawal in the hospitalized patient should be recognized and treated promptly (see "Pharmacotherapies" below).

Alcoholic Hallucinosis

Hallucinations associated with alcohol withdrawal occur early in the course of the process and are accompanied by an otherwise intact sensorium.

Approximately 10–25% of hospitalized patients with chronic alcohol use experience hallucinations. These hallucinations usually occur relatively early in the course of withdrawal (during the first 24–48 hours).[7,10] They are generally visual hallucinations, but auditory hallucinations, and less commonly tactile or olfactory hallucinations, may also occur. Formication is a classic tactile hallucination characterized by a sensation of bugs crawling on the skin. It is important to understand that what differentiates these hallucinations from those that may accompany delirium tremens is that outside of the hallucinosis, the patient's sensorium is intact.[8,10] This symptom of alcohol withdrawal is not predictive of subsequent progression to delirium tremens.

Major Alcohol Withdrawal: Seizures and Delirium Tremens

Seizures

Generalized tonic-clonic seizures may occur early in the withdrawal timeline and may not be preceded by any other warning signs. Risk factors include prolonged history of alcohol consumption and history of withdrawal seizures.

Withdrawal seizures may occur in 5–33% of chronic alcohol abusers. Greater than 90% of seizures happen within 8–48 hours of the individual's last drink, with peak activity between 12–24 hours. They are usually generalized tonic-clonic, self-limited seizures, and are rarely focal in nature, unless there is underlying neuropathology. Fewer than 3% result in status epilepticus. These events classically are single, though approximately a quarter of patients will have more than one. Recurrent seizure activity occurs within 6 hours of the initial seizure in 85% of patients who have recurrences.[11] Like tremulousness, withdrawal seizures may occur before the blood alcohol level becomes undetectable.

Of note, seizures may not necessarily be preceded by any other manifestation of alcohol withdrawal. That is, alcohol withdrawal seizures may occur without preceding minor withdrawal symptoms or signs.

Withdrawal seizures are more common in patients who have a history of multiple episodes of withdrawals or detoxifications, a phenomenon known as "kindling." This controversial phenomenon is explained by cumulative long-term changes in brain excitability.[5,10,12] Additionally, patients with histories of withdrawal seizures appear to be at higher risk for developing them again during future withdrawal episodes. Other predictors include a long history of alcohol consumption (e.g., >10 years) and a history of alcohol-related hospitalizations.[9] Concurrent abuse of certain drugs may also be a predictor of alcohol withdrawal seizures.[9]

Rathlev et al. found that patients who present having had a single withdrawal seizure were less likely to have a recurrent seizure if the blood alcohol level at the time of presentation was >100 mg/dL.[11] Age, history of seizures, and quantity of alcohol consumed failed to identify patients at risk for recurrent seizures.[13]

Causes other than alcohol withdrawal should be considered if (1) seizures are focal in nature, (2) if there is no definite history of recent abstinence from drinking, (3) if there is status epilepticus, or (4) if the patient has a history of fever or trauma.[14]

Delirium Tremens

Delirium tremens (DTs) is a potentially fatal condition, often requiring ICU care. Features include marked autonomic hyperactivity, hallucinations, and agitation, with confusion. Proven risk factors include time since last alcohol consumption and comorbid medical conditions.

DTs is seen in 5–8% of patients hospitalized with alcohol withdrawal.[10,16] It is characterized by profound autonomic hyperactivity including fever, tachycardia, hypertension, diaphoresis, and by the development of agitation, confusion, disorientation, and hallucinations. DTs occur in some chronic alcohol abusers from 2–14 days (usually 3–5 days) after abstaining from alcohol.[10,15]

One must use caution when interpreting time courses for alcohol withdrawal. While there is some variability in the time course,[10] the real variability may be in when the patient actually consumed alcohol last prior to being admitted. For example, DTs may occur on day 1 of hospitalization if the patient actually stopped consuming alcohol 3 days prior to admission.

Disorientation and global confusion must be present for the diagnosis of DTs. Furthermore, the hallucinations are prominent and well formed. While patients with tremors and hallucinosis are colloquially referred to as being in "the DTs," this is not correct unless a global delirium is also present.

DTs is the most serious complication of alcohol withdrawal. Mortality from DTs has been reported as high as 20%; however, with current evidence-based medical therapy, mortality has declined to 5% in the hospital setting. In 90% of cases, DTs resolves within 4 days. In hospitalized patients, with concurrent medical procedures and illnesses, it may last as long as 2 weeks.[8,10]

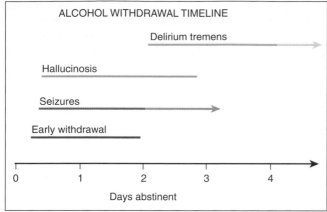

ALCOHOL WITHDRAWAL TIMELINE

Delirium tremens

Hallucinosis

Seizures

Early withdrawal

0   1   2   3   4

Days abstinent

Figure 89-1 • Alcohol withdrawal timeline.

Box 89-1 Differential Diagnosis of Alcohol Withdrawal

Other intoxicants
(e.g., amphetamines, LSD, and cocaine)

α-Blocker withdrawal

Anxiety disorder

Pheochromocytoma

Psychosis/paranoia

Epilepsy

Head trauma

Meningoencephalitis

Hypoglycemia

Thyrotoxicosis

Delirium
(e.g., due to sepsis, electrolyte abnormality, acid-base disorder, etc.)

Risk factors for developing DTs include presence of concurrent medical illness, daily heavy and prolonged alcohol consumption, history of previous delirium tremens or withdrawal seizures, and age >30.[12,16] Neither the duration of consumption nor any particular laboratory value have been consistently identified to portend increased risk in the literature. Smaller studies have suggested that earlier age at onset of alcohol consumption, longer duration of dependence, the presence of electrolyte and liver function abnormalities, and prior DTs are predictive of increased risk of recurrence.[9]

Ferguson et al.[16] identified only two factors that were positive predictors of DTs in their inpatient study: the presence of a concurrent medical illness (adjusted odds ratio = 5.1) and a greater number of days since last drink (adjusted odds ratio = 1.3). When applying the predictive model created by combining these two factors to the group studied, the area under the Receiver Operator Curve was 0.76. They went on to dichotomize the number of days since last drink to create a scale using fewer than 2 days versus 2 or more. With this model, of the patients with no risk factors, 9% developed the DTs. One or two risk factors were associated with 25% and 54% of patients developing the DTs, respectively. Quantity and duration of consumption were not analyzed in this study; however, prior withdrawal events, age, several laboratory values (albumin, potassium, sodium, BUN, AST), and physiologic parameters, including respiratory rate and systolic blood pressure, failed to demonstrate any independent predictive value[16] (Fig. 89-1).

ASSESSMENT

Differential Diagnosis

Although the history and physical examination are usually sufficient to establish the diagnosis of AWS, clinicians must keep in mind that other conditions may present with similar symptoms.

Both severe hypoglycemia and thyroid storm may mimic alcohol withdrawal with heightened autonomic activity. Several other alcohol-related disorders may present with seizures or mental status changes. These include Wernicke's encephalopathy, hepatic encephalopathy, and head trauma with or without subdural hematoma.[5]

Other substances of abuse (amphetamine, cocaine) can result in signs of increased sympathetic activity and altered mental status as well. Withdrawal from sedative-hypnotics such as benzodiazepines may cause signs and symptoms similar to those seen in AWS (Box 89-1). To determine the presence of AWS, especially because many of the complications of withdrawal can begin early on after alcohol cessation, it is mandatory to perform a thorough initial evaluation.

The Initial Evaluation

A number of key issues in the initial history, physical, and laboratory examinations are vital to manage alcohol withdrawal properly. The history must include a (1) consumption history (including quantity and frequency), (2) detoxification history, (3) history of seizures, and (4) history of delirium tremens. History obtained from family members or friends may be helpful to corroborate or append the patient's information. Determining time of last drink and assessing the presence of auditory, visual, and tactile hallucinations, are parts of the complete alcohol-withdrawal history. Concurrent conditions must be identified, as AWS may exacerbate these conditions or complicate their management.

A complete psychosocial history helps gauge the amount of substance abuse, elucidates some of the underlying factors involved in the abuse, and clarifies the level of social support resources available to the patient.

During physical examination, identifying evidence of chronic liver disease is important, as it may affect medication choices. Evaluation of the patient's hemodynamic, neurologic, and mental status is critical to determine the patient's stage of withdrawal.

Routine laboratory tests, including electrolytes, glucose, complete blood counts, coagulation profiles, and liver function tests, are useful in general management but do not specifically help predict or manage AWS. An alcohol level may help identify if the symptoms at hand are attributable to alcohol withdrawal, though this evaluation is inexact. Toxicologic testing may be considered, as co-consumption of other illicit substances is common,[13] and may confound the diagnosis as symptoms of both ingestion and withdrawal of other substances are similar to those of alcohol withdrawal.

TREATMENT

Treatment Setting

Most patients in alcohol withdrawal do not need hospitalization unless there is a comorbid condition requiring it, or signs and symptoms are severe. Marked autonomic symptoms despite initial treatment warrant consideration of an ICU stay.

Only 10–20% of all patients suffering from alcohol withdrawal need hospitalization. Severe withdrawal symptoms, difficulty tolerating oral medications, and poor social support are indicators of poor outcomes in the outpatient setting.[1] Heavy alcohol consumption, history of seizures, history of delirium tremens, and multiple detoxifications should also direct the care providers to consider a hospital admission. Intensive care admission should be considered for patients with marked agitation, hypertension (SBP > 180), or tachycardia (HR > 130), which are not promptly responding to initial benzodiazepine administration.

Pharmacotherapies

Vitamins, Nutrition, and Volume Replacement

The basics of supportive treatment include the administration of vitamins, especially thiamine, and administration of adequate nutrition and volume replacement. If a dextrose-containing infusion is planned, intravenous or intramuscular thiamine should be given to avoid the Wernicke-Korsakoff's syndrome.[17] Though conventionally given before glucose is administered, the data for this recommendation are limited, and other authors have advocated no need for concern about the order of medications as long as parenteral thiamine is given in close proximity to the glucose infusion.[18] Oral thiamine may follow if the patient is able to take oral medications. Supplementation of potassium, magnesium, and phosphate are also often necessary in this patient population.

Benzodiazepines

Benzodiazepines form the cornerstone of AWS management due to their efficacy as anticonvulsants and sedatives along with low overall cost. No single benzodiazepine has proven to be superior to another in randomized trials, but expert opinion suggests long-acting benzodiazepines such as diazepam and chlordiazepoxide are generally preferred.

According to a meta-analysis by the American Society of Addiction Medicine, benzodiazepines, as a class, successfully reduce AWS symptoms and decrease the risk of the development of seizures (absolute risk reduction of 7.7 cases/100 patients) and delirium (absolute risk reduction of 4.9 cases/100 patients).[17] The largest study in that meta-analysis demonstrated only one case of seizure and one case of delirium out of 103 patients receiving chlordiazepoxide as compared with nine cases of seizures and eight cases of delirium out of 130 patients receiving placebos [RR = 0.14 (95% CI 0.2–1.09, P = 0.046 for seizures; RR = 0.16 (95% CI 0.02–1.24, p = 0.08)].[19]

For inpatients with concurrent medical illnesses who are considered high risk for the development of AWS, a prophylactic initial dose of benzodiazepine should be considered, irrespective of the current presence of withdrawal symptoms to decrease the likelihood of them developing. Thereafter, two basic methods of benzodiazepine administration may be used: fixed dose or symptom triggered.

The "fixed dose" method administers benzodiazepines on a schedule (not as needed), typically with a 3- to 5-day taper. The dose is decreased by 20% each day.[20] Additional doses are given as needed in between scheduled doses.

"Symptom triggered" methods utilize protocols for assessing the amount of alcohol withdrawal present and direct nursing staff to administer benzodiazepines. The Clinical Institute Withdrawal Assessment Scale for Alcohol, Revised (CIWA-Ar) scale is a well-validated eight-question scale (Table 89-1) that assesses the severity of alcohol withdrawal. One must use this and similar scales cautiously with inpatients, as medical illnesses themselves may produce some of the symptoms and signs (vomiting, diaphoresis, anxiety, etc.) that are scored. Refer to Table 89-2 for samples of scheduled taper and symptom-triggered protocols.

Randomized trials have shown the two approaches to be equally efficacious and safe, but symptom-triggered methods result in less medication requirement, less sedation, and fewer days of therapy.[21,22] The symptom-triggered method does require a significant level of nurse training, and some experts maintain that it is suited only for dedicated detoxification or substance withdrawal units[5,21] or hospitals with experience in managing AWS.

The choice of which benzodiazepine is to be used should be based on half-life, onset of action, route of administration, and presence or absence of significant liver disease. These factors are summarized in Table 89-3, which includes the most common benzodiazepines utilized in alcohol withdrawal. Short-acting benzodiazepines should be avoided, except in patients with significant hepatic dysfunction or in the elderly, in whom oversedation may be of significant concern due to decreased medication metabolism. Diazepam, chlordiazepoxide, and clorazepate offer long half-lives, which are preferable whether the symptoms are mild or advanced, since self-tapering occurs. Diazepam's immediate onset of parenteral action allows usage every 5 minutes as needed, making it a good choice for the critically ill uncontrolled patient with seizures or DTs. Significant doses of chlordiazepoxide (900 mg) and diazepam (500 mg) have been required in the management of patients with DTs.[23] It should be noted that only lorazepam has an intramuscular route available.[24]

Finally, it should be noted that rarely a patient will not respond to benzodiazepines at all, even when given in very high doses. Phenobarbital and propofol may become necessary in these cases of benzodiazepine-resistant delirium tremens.

Other Drugs

Phenobarbital and propofol have been used for the treatment of AWS for cases refractory to benzodiazepines. Neuroleptics should only be considered adjunctive therapy as insufficient evidence is present for using them as monotherapy for AWS.

Phenobarbital is effective in cases refractory to benzodiazepines, as its sedative effects are synergistic with benzodiazepines. It has been used successfully in cases with uncontrolled agitation, delirium, hypertension, and tachycardia, despite high-

Table 89-1 CIWA-Ar Scale for Alcohol Withdrawal

Clinical Institute Withdrawal Assessment Scale for Alcohol, Revised CIWA-Ar

Nausea and vomiting—Ask "Do you feel sick to your stomach? Have you vomited?" Observation:
0 No nausea or vomiting
1
2
3
4 Intermittent nausea with dry heaves
5
6
7 Constant nausea, frequent dry heaves, and vomiting

Paroxysmal sweats—Observation:
0 No sweats visible
1 Barely perceptible sweating, palms moist
2
3
4 Beads of sweat obvious on forehead
5
6
7 Drenching sweats

Agitation—Observation:
0 Normal activity
1 Somewhat more than normal activity
2
3
4 Moderately fidgety and restless
5
6
7 Paces back and forth during most of the interview or constantly thrashes about

Headache, fullness in head—Ask "Does your head feel different? Does it feel like there is a band around your head?" Do not rate for dizziness or lightheadedness. Otherwise, rate severity:
0 Not present
1 Very mild
2 Mild
3 Moderate
4 Moderately severe
5 Severe
6 Very severe
7 Extremely severe

Anxiety—Ask "Do you feel nervous?" Observation:
0 No anxiety, at ease
1 Mildly anxious
2
3
4 Moderately anxious, or guarded, so anxiety is inferred
5
6
7 Equivalent to acute panic states as Seen in severe delirium or acute Schizophrenic reactions

Tremor—Arms extended and fingers spread apart. Observation:
0 No tremor
1 Not visible, but can be felt fingertip to fingertip
2
3
4 Moderate, with patient's arms extended
5
6
7 Severe, even with arms not extended

Visual disturbances—Ask "Does the light appear too bright? Is the color different? Does it hurt your eyes? Are you seeing anything that is disturbing to you? Are you seeing things you know are not there?" Observation:
0 Not present
1 Very mild sensitivity
2 Mild sensitivity
3 Moderate sensitivity
4 Moderately severe hallucinations
5 Severe hallucinations
6 Extremely severe hallucinations
7 Continuous hallucinations

Tactile disturbances—Ask "Have you any itching, pins and needles sensations, any burning, any numbness, or do you feel bugs crawling on or under your skin?" Observation:
0 None
1 Very mild itching, pins and needles, burning or numbness
2 Mild itching, pins and needles, burning or numbness
3 Moderate itching, pins and needles, burning or numbness
4 Moderately severe hallucinations
5 Severe hallucinations
6 Extremely severe hallucinations
7 Continuous hallucinations

Auditory disturbances—Ask "Are you aware of sounds around you? Are they harsh? Do they frighten you? Are you hearing anything that is disturbing to you? Are you hearing things you know are not there?" Observation:
0 Not present
1 Very mild harshness or ability to frighten
2 Mild harshness or ability to frighten
3 Moderate harshness or ability to frighten
4 Moderately severe hallucinations
5 Severe hallucinations
6 Extremely severe hallucinations
7 Continuous hallucinations

Orientation and clouding of sensorium—Ask "What day is this? Where are you? Who am I?"
0 Oriented and do serial additions
1 Cannot do serial additions
2 Disoriented for date by no more than 2 calendar days
3 Disoriented for date by more than 2 calendar days
4 Disoriented for place and/or person

The score is a simple sum of each item score (maximum score = 67).

Adapted from: Sullivan, JT, Sykora, K, Schneiderman, J, et al. Assessment of alcohol withdrawal: the revised clinical institute withdrawal assessment for alcohol scale (CIWA-Ar). Br J Addict 1987; 84:1353. This scale is not copyrighted and may be used freely.

Table 89-2 Sample Scheduled Taper and Symptom Triggered Regimens for the Treatment of Alcohol Withdrawal

Fixed Dose Regimen	Symptom Triggered Regimen
Standing dose: 　Chlordiazepoxide 50 mg PO QID for 4 doses then 　Chlordiazepoxide 25 mg PO QID for 8 doses PRN CIWA-Ar ≥8: 　Chlordiazepoxide 25–100 mg PO every 2 hours	Initial dose*: 　Chlordiazepoxide 50 mg PO once PRN CIWA-Ar ≥8: 　Chlordiazepoxide 25–100 mg PO every 2 hours
Standing dose: 　Diazepam 20 mg PO QID for 4 doses then 　Diazepam 10 mg PO QID for 8 doses PRN CIWA-Ar ≥8: 　Diazepam 10–20 mg PO every 2 hours	Initial dose*: 　Diazepam 20 mg PO once PRN CIWA-Ar ≥8: 　Diazepam 10–20 mg PO every 2 hours
Standing dose[†]: 　Lorazepam 4 mg PO QID for 4 doses then 　Lorazepam 2 mg PO QID for 4 doses PRN CIWA-Ar ≥8: 　Lorazepam 1–4 mg PO every 2 hours	Initial dose*: 　Lorazepam 4 mg PO once PRN CIWA-Ar ≥8: 　Lorazepam 1–4 mg PO every 2 hours

*For inpatients with concurrent acute illness, at least one standing dose is recommended. For patients not meeting this criterion, this dose may be omitted.

[†]Lorazepam and similar shorter acting benzodiazepines should be reserved for elderly patients or patients with significant hepatic dysfunction.

Modified from: Saitz R, Mayo-Smith MF, Roberts MS, et al. Individualized treatments for alcohol withdrawal: a randomized double-blind controlled trial. JAMA 1994; 272(7):519–523.

Table 89-3 Pharmacokinetics of Selected Benzodiazepines

Drug	Half-Life	Onset of Action	Route of Administration	Dose Equivalence
Diazepam (Valium)	20–50 hr	IV- immediate PO-?	PO, IV	10 mg
Chlordiazepoxide (Librium)	6–25 hr	IV-? PO-?	PO, IV	50 mg
Clorazepate (Tranxene)	48–96 hr	1–2 hr	PO	15 mg
Lorazepam (Ativan)	10–15 hr	IV-5–20 min IM-20–30 min PO-?	PO, IV, IM	2 mg
Oxazepam (Serax)	6–8 hr	?	PO	30 mg

Source: Lexi-Comp. Lexi-Comp Online Drug Information. Available at www.lexi.com. Accessed 1/6/05.

dose benzodiazepines.[19] Its use should be limited to the intensive care unit (ICU), as intubation may become necessary. Typical dosing is 130–260 mg every 15 minutes as needed.

Propofol is reported to be effective for refractory alcohol withdrawal delirium in a number of case series.[25] Dosing requires intubation, and a bolus of 1 mg/kg followed by titration to control symptoms formulates typical therapy. Patients treated with propofol for delirium tremens often require the medicine for a number of days before weaning is possible.[25]

Haloperidol may be used as an adjunctive medication in the combative or belligerent withdrawing patient. The intramuscular dosing capability allows for emergency administration in case intravenous access is lost. Typical dosing is 1–5 mg intravenously every 10 minutes as needed, or 2–10 mg intramuscularly every 20 minutes as needed, with 24 hour dosing limited to 30–40 mg. Its side effects include lowering the seizure threshold and prolongation of the QTc interval, which may limit the usefulness of this drug.

Anticonvulsants have been studied in alcohol withdrawal, including phenytoin and carbamazepine. Their utility has been inconsistent, and they have been untested in DTs so these drugs are not recommended as monotherapy for alcohol withdrawal.[1,9,17] If there is a primary seizure investigation underway, it is reasonable to initiate a course of phenytoin therapy until other causes of seizures are excluded; however, the routine use of phenytoin to treat or prevent known alcohol withdrawal seizures is not recommended[9] (see Management of Alcohol Withdrawal Seizures below).

β-blockers are an important drug in elderly patients and patients with known coronary artery disease who present with alcohol withdrawal. Much of the 5–10% mortality rate from delirium tremens is from associated cardiac complications. In addition, β-blockers may reduce alcohol craving when given with benzodiazepines.[5] As a negative chronotropic and anti-hypertensive agent, it has the risk of masking some autonomic symptoms of alcohol withdrawal. With no anticonvulsant effect, β-blockers should only be utilized in an adjunctive manner in the management of AWS.

Clonidine is not an effective agent for alcohol withdrawal, and it has the danger of masking autonomic symptoms that may lead to inadequate therapy. Moreover, it has no anticonvulsant properties.[1] Its use is therefore not recommended.

Alcohol Withdrawal Seizure Prophylaxis

An initial single dose of a benzodiazepine (e.g., diazepam 10–20 mg orally) is recommended for patients hospitalized with a significant, concurrent medical illness who have a history of withdrawal seizures, repeated detoxifications, or substantial daily alcohol consumption with recent cessation, regardless of autonomic activity and symptoms at presentation, unless there is a clear contraindication.[26]

Management of Alcohol Withdrawal Seizures

The management of an alcohol withdrawal seizure is relatively uncomplicated, as it is usually self-limiting and unlikely to recur, particularly after benzodiazepines are administered. Patients presenting with or who develop a withdrawal seizure should receive at least one dose of a benzodiazepine. In a study by D'Onofrio, only 3% of patients receiving an initial dose of 2 mg of intravenous lorazepam developed a recurrent seizure within 6 hours, compared with 24% of those who did not.[26] The routine use of phenytoin to treat withdrawal seizures is discouraged, unless the patient is known to have an underlying seizure disorder or the presenting seizures are atypical for alcohol withdrawal.[9]

Management of Delirium Tremens

Treatment of DTs requires intensive monitoring and should, generally, occur in an intensive care setting. Airway, hemodynamic, acid-base, electrolyte, and vascular access issues require close monitoring while high dose parenteral benzodiazepines are used. Choosing which benzodiazepine to use and deciding the method of administration (intravenous bolus vs. intravenous infusion) depends upon vascular access, coexisting compounds within the drug formulation, and whether the patient is intubated or not. As soon as possible, patients should be transitioned to oral benzodiazepines. Adjunctive phenobarbital or propofol is typically utilized when high-dose benzodiazepines are insufficient.

An example of an initial benzodiazepine regimen for the treatment of DTs was presented by Mayo-Smith, et al.[23] in their evidence-based practice guideline. It suggests diazepam 5 mg intravenously initially. If that is not effective, it may be repeated in 5–10 minutes. Thereafter, doubling the dose is recommended, and again the new higher dose is repeated in 5–10 minutes. This pattern of doubling the dose and then repeating in 5–10 minutes should continue until satisfactory sedation is achieved, with close monitoring for over-sedation. Intermittent rebolusing may be required hourly to maintain light sedation and hemodynamic stability.[23] Diazepam is phlebitic, and its use in patients without central venous access should be very limited. Lorazepam is a satisfactory alternative.

Continuous benzodiazepine infusions may be chosen in patients who are intubated, those without central venous access requiring increasing doses of benzodiazepine boluses, and in patients with DTs being managed by nursing staff trained to *rapidly* titrate benzodiazepines to achieve light sedation. Lorazepam and midazolam are common benzodiazepine intravenous infusions. Lorazepam's onset of action is slower, and therefore the risk of oversedation is somewhat higher. Of note, the intravenous preparation of lorazepam contains propylene glycol, and toxicity associated with this vehicle may be significant in patients requiring substantial doses. Midazolam has a short half-life, is hepatically metabolized, and has an *active* metabolite that is excreted by the kidneys. Therefore, in patients with normal hepatic and renal function, the risk of relapsing DTs is present when midazolam is rapidly decreased or discontinued.

As stated above, intravenous phenobarbital and propofol may be needed for DTs refractory to high-dose benzodiazepines. Intubation and mechanical ventilation are required to safely administer propofol.

DISCHARGE PLANNING

Once the patient with AWS regains baseline mental status and near normal hemodynamic parameters, medical stability for discharge has been achieved, assuming concurrent medical issues have also resolved.

Please refer to Chapter 16 for details on transition from treatment of alcohol withdrawal to treatment of alcohol abuse and dependence. It is critical to provide the patient with alcohol withdrawal aftercare with a primary care physician; substance abuse counselors and support organizations like Alcoholics Anonymous may also assist during the transition to recovery period. The patient should clearly hear the inpatient caregiver's professional opinion that follow-up of the alcohol-related issues is very important.

SUMMARY

Alcohol withdrawal is a common medical condition with significant morbidity and mortality. Close attention should be paid to risk factors for the various manifestations of alcohol withdrawal, which include hyperautonomic symptoms like tremor, hypertension, and tachycardia, as well as hallucinosis, seizures, and delirium tremens. A careful evaluation must be conducted to assure exclusion of mimicking diseases and other substances.

Patients with significant alcohol consumption histories who are admitted with active medical or surgical issues, and those with histories of withdrawal seizures or DTs should have prophylactic benzodiazepine administration upon initial admission, regardless of their CIWA-Ar score or symptomatology upon presentation. After initial alcohol withdrawal prophylaxis is delivered, we recommend CIWA-Ar protocol-driven symptom triggered benzodiazepine therapy for most cases of AWS in all inpatient settings with the capacity and training to do so. This protocol has proven to be effective in AWS management, and it reduces length of stay and total benzodiazepine requirements.

Expert opinion suggests long-acting benzodiazepines should be used as first-line therapies, except in patients with significantly reduced hepatic metabolism, such as the elderly and patients with advanced cirrhosis. When agitation is very severe, intravenous or intramuscular haloperidol is an effective adjunctive therapy, but benzodiazepines must be continued. DTs refractory to high-dose benzodiazepines in the ICU should be treated with phenobarbital or propofol.

A patient may be safely discharged when hemodynamic parameters and mental status normalize. Professional medical and substance abuse follow-up is required to assure proper treatment for alcohol abuse or dependence.

Key Points

- AWS are common and potentially fatal if not properly recognized and treated. A history should include details of consumption and prior manifestations of AWS. Mimicking syndromes should be ruled out, and the presence of other substances must be investigated.

- One-time benzodiazepine administration for alcohol withdrawal seizure prophylaxis is warranted for nearly all hospitalized patients with alcohol dependence, regardless of symptoms.

- Long-acting benzodiazepines are the mainstay for the treatment of AWS unless there is reduced hepatic metabolism. Beta-blockers and haloperidol are useful adjunctive medications in many patients.

- Both fixed-dose and symptom-triggered approaches to benzodiazepine treatment of alcohol withdrawal are efficacious and safe, but the symptom-triggered methods result in less medication administration, less sedation, and fewer days of therapy. The symptom-triggered method does require a significant level of nurse training and patient monitoring.

- The presence of disorientation and global confusion, (not simply hallucinosis alone) are necessary to make the diagnosis of delirium tremens, the most morbid of the alcohol withdrawal syndromes.

- Phenobarbital and propofol have been successfully used in cases of DTs in cases refractory to benzodiazepines.

- Substance abuse follow-up should be arranged upon discharge from the hospital.

SUGGESTED READING

Kosten TR, O'Connor PG. Management of drug and alcohol withdrawal. N Engl J Med 2003; 348:1786.

Kozak LJ, Hall MJ, Owings, MF. National Hospital Discharge Survey: 2000 Annual Summary with Detailed Diagnosis and Procedure Data. Vital Health Stat 2002; 153(13):1–194.

Moore RD, Bone LR, Geller G, et al. Prevalence, detection, and treatment of alcoholism in hospitalized patients. JAMA 1989; 261(3):403–407.

HCUP. National and regional estimates on hospital use for all patients from the HCUP Nationwide Inpatient Sample (NIS). Available at www.hcup.ahrq.gov/hcupnet.asp. Accessed 8/5/05.

Alcohol withdrawal. In: First M, ed. Diagnostic and Statistical Manual—Text Revision. 4th ed., Washington, DC: American Psychiatric Association, 2000; 216.

Chang PH, Steinberg MB. Alcohol withdrawal. Med Clin North Am 2001; 85(5):1191–1212.

Rathlev NK, Ulrich A, Fish SS, et al. Clinical characteristics as predictors of recurrent alcohol-related seizures. Acad Emerg Med 2000; 7(8):886–891.

American Society of Addiction Medicine. American Society of Addiction Medicine's Working Group on Pharmacological Management of Alcohol Withdrawal. Pharmacological Management of Alcohol Withdrawal. A Meta-analysis and Evidence-Based Practice Guideline. JAMA 1997; 278(2):144–151.

Reoux JP, Miller K. Routine hospital alcohol detoxification practice compared to symptom triggered management with an objective withdrawal scale (CIWA-Ar). Am J Addict 2000; 9:135–144.

Mayo-Smith MF, Beecher LH, Fischer TL, et al. Management of alcohol withdrawal delirium: an evidence-based practice guideline. Arch Int Med 2004; 164(13):1405–1412.

Section

Thirteen

Neurology

90 Ischemic Stroke
Geno J. Merli, Rodney Bell

91 Intracerebral Hemorrhage
Geno J. Merli, Robert Rosenwasser, Mark V. Williams

92 Coma
Chong-Sang Kim, Alpesh N. Amin

93 Altered Mental Status: Delirium
Michael D. Wang, Solomon Liao, Alpesh N. Amin

94 Pain Management of the Hospitalized Patient
David J. Axelrod

95 Palliative Care in the Hospital
Stephanie Grossman, S. Melissa Mahoney

CHAPTER NINETY

Ischemic Stroke

Geno J. Merli, MD, FACP, and Rodney Bell, MD

BACKGROUND

Management of acute ischemic stroke is a multidisciplinary, time sensitive, team process involving prehospital emergency medical technicians, emergency medicine physicians, neurologists, neurosurgeons, neurointensivists, radiologists, nurses, and hospitalists. The evaluation of a patient with suspected acute ischemic stroke should be performed immediately. This assessment is most often expeditiously performed in the emergency department in order to select patients eligible for thrombolytic therapy who are less than 3 hours from the onset of symptoms. More often than not, patients have exceeded the time interval, and the hospitalist is called to admit the patient. The history and physical examination will direct the development of a differential diagnosis of the etiology and subsequent appropriate management.

At many hospitals, the hospitalist admits all patients presenting with a "brain attack," and a neurologist provides consultative services. Thus, hospitalists need to have a thorough understanding of the assessment and management of patients suffering a stroke. This chapter discusses the management of acute ischemic stroke from the initial presentation through acute phase of care in the hospital setting and discharge.

ASSESSMENT

Clinical Presentation

Prevalence

The incidence of stroke has continued to increase since the mid 1960s, with up to 700,000 new cases reported in the United States each year.[1] There are two main stroke categories of etiologic importance: (1) ischemic stroke, accounting for about 83% of cases, and (2) hemorrhage stroke.[2] Ischemic strokes are attributable to arterial thrombosis (20%), embolism (25%), small vessel disease (25%), and cryptogenic causes (30%). Hemorrhagic strokes are further subcategorized as intraparenchymal (60%) or subarachnoid hemorrhage (40%).[3] Management of hemorrhagic strokes is covered in detail in Chapter 91.

Presenting Signs and Symptoms

Stroke patients usually present with a history of sudden or rapid onset of focal neurologic symptoms, which may be gradually progressive or waxing and waning. Tables 90-1 and 90-2 define the symptoms and signs associated with the ischemia and infarction of different central nervous system regions.[4]

Diagnosis

First, detailing the patient's risk factors for cardiac and cerebrovascular disease will assist in guiding further testing and future management. In addition, the following history should be elicited: medications, recent head or neck trauma, current alcohol use, illicit drug use, hormone replacement therapy or oral contraception, family or personal history of thrombotic events, history of miscarriages, and migraine headaches.

The physical examination should focus on the neurologic and vascular systems, including blood pressure in both arms, heart rate and rhythm, cardiac auscultation, palpation and auscultation of peripheral pulses, deep tendon reflexes, motor and sensory assessment, and mental status. A standardized approach using the National Institute of Health (NIH) Stroke Scale (see Appendix 1 at the back of the book) facilitates comparison of the neurologic examination over time, even among different examiners. With this information, the hospitalist should localize the ischemic event to either the posterior or anterior circulation as well as cortical versus subcortical areas.

Laboratory testing should include: urine drug screen, complete blood count (CBC) with differential, platelets, electrolytes, blood urea nitrogen (BUN), creatinine, prothrombin time, activated partial thromboplastin time (APTT), electrocardiogram, and chest X-ray (Table 90-3).[4]

Upon completion of the above, a noncontrast computed tomography (CT) of the head is performed—the imaging study of choice to distinguish between primary hemorrhagic and ischemic stroke. Hemorrhagic findings show up quickly after onset as an area of hyperdensity versus ischemic stroke, which initially does not have any findings but eventually will progress to an area of hypodensity in 6–12 hours. An area of hypodensity in the region consistent with neurologic findings signifies that ischemia has been present for over 6 hours, and the patient may not be a candidate for thrombolytic therapy. CT scan is relatively insensitive in detecting acute and small cortical or subcortical infarctions, especially in the posterior fossa.

Table 90-1 Anterior versus Posterior Circulation: Symptoms and Signs of Cerebral Ischemia

Anterior	Posterior

Motor dysfunction of contralateral extremities or face or both
  Clumsiness
  Weakness
  Paralysis
	Motor dysfunction of ipsilateral face and/or contralateral
	    extremities
	  Clumsiness
	Weakness

Loss of vision in ipsilateral eye	Paralysis
Homonymous hemianopia	Loss of vision of 1 or both homonymous visual fields
Aphasia (dominant hemisphere)	Sensory deficit of ipsilateral face and/or contralateral extremities
Dysarthria	Numbness or loss of sensation

Sensory deficit of contralateral extremities or face (or both)
  Numbness or loss of sensation
  Paresthesias
	Paresthesias
	Typical, but nondiagnostic in isolation
	  Ataxia
	  Vertigo
	  Diplopia
	  Dysphagia
	  Dysarthria

From: Flemming KD, Brown RD, Petty GW, et al. Evaluation and management of transient ischemic attack and minor cerebral infarction. Mayo Clinic Proceedings 2004;79:1071–1086 with permission.

Table 90-2 Cortical versus Subcortical Symptoms and Signs of Cerebral Ischemia

Cortical	Subcortical
Aphasia	Face, arm, leg more equally affected
Visual field defect	Classic lacunar syndromes
Hemi-neglect	Pure motor
Cortical sensory loss	Pure sensory

Abulia	Ataxic hemiparesis
	  Clumsy-hand dysarthria
	  Sensorimotor stroke

Adapted from: Flemming KD, Brown RD, Petty GW, et al. Evaluation and management of transient ischemic attack and minor cerebral infarction. Mayo Clinic Proceedings 2004; 79:1071–1086 with permission.

Differential Diagnosis

The goal of the initial diagnostic evaluation is to confirm that the patient's signs and symptoms are due to ischemic stroke and not another systemic or neurologic illness. The risks of thrombolytic therapy for stroke mandate certainty of diagnosis, and thus hospitalists need to recognize the common patterns of neurologic abnormalities seen in patients with ischemic stroke. Importantly, up to a third of patients presenting with acute onset of focal neurologic deficits may **not** have a stroke. Other conditions that can mimic acute stroke include hypoglycemia, seizures, syncope, toxic or metabolic disorders, brain tumors, or subdural hematoma. Commonly, though not always, associated with global rather than focal neurologic symptoms, they can be readily identified by diagnostic testing (Table 90-4).[5]

One study at an urban teaching hospital enrolled more than 300 consecutive patients presenting with a possible stroke. A consensus panel of stroke experts who reviewed the clinical details, imaging studies, and "other relevant investigations" determined a final diagnosis of stroke in 69% of patients. Specific independent clinical variables appeared to predict the final diagnosis. Having an exact time of onset, definite focal symptoms, presence of neurologic signs (especially if they could be lateralized to the left or right side of the brain, and abnormal vascular findings suggested a stroke. Patients with a stroke mimic tended to have cognitive impairment and abnormal signs in other systems.

Having completed the above initial evaluation, the next management step is to determine the etiology for stroke and intervene with the appropriate assessment and treatment. The evaluation of stroke can be differentiated, based on the various causes: embolic (atrial fibrillation, patent foramen ovale (PFO) and atrial septal aneurysm (ASA), extracranial vessel, intracranial vessel), small vessel disease (lacunar), and coagulation disorders.

Embolic Stroke Diagnostic Studies

Approximately 25% of cerebral infarctions are due to cardioembolic etiologies. These percentages do not change with age, but the source of embolism does. Atrial fibrillation is present in 1% of the population, but this arrhythmia is found in 10% of patients over the age of 75 years. Risk factors such as prior stroke or transient ischemic attack (TIA), history of hypertension, heart failure, advanced age, diabetes, coronary artery disease, left atrial thrombus, spontaneous echo contrast (SEC), and left ventricular dysfunction associated with atrial fibrillation increase the risk of stroke as high as 10–12% per year.[6]

The association between PFO and cerebral infarction has been controversial, due to varying results from epidemiologic studies. A population-based echocardiographic study reported the prevalence of PFO to be 25% in the general population.[7] Risk factors believed to increase the probability that PFO is associated with cerebral infarction include size, shunting characteristics (right to left) as defined by the number of bubbles crossing per cardiac cycle, associated ASA, known deep vein thrombosis (DVT), and cortical stroke.[8] Transthoracic echocardiography (TTE) is noninvasive and provides an estimate of left ventricular function and the presence of left ventricular thrombus. Transesophageal echocardiography (TEE) is superior for the detection of aortic atheromatous disease or dissection, left atrial thrombosis, and PFO.[9] The complication rate with TEE is less than 0.02% with experienced operators.[9]

Table 90-3 Immediate Testing: Acute Stroke

All Patients	Selected Patients Based on Clinical Findings
CT scan of brain (without contrast)	Hepatic panel
Electrocardiogram	Toxicologic screen
Blood glucose	Blood alcohol
Serum electrolytes	Pregnancy test
Creatinine/BUN	Arterial blood gas (hypoxia suspected)
Complete blood count with differential	EEG
Platelets	Troponins
PT and a PTT	Lumbar puncture (if subarachnoid hemorrhage is suspected and CT is negative for blood)
Urine drug screen	Drug levels for specific medications

CT—computed tomography; BUN—blood urea nitrogen; EEG—electroencephalogram; PT—prothrombin time; aPTT—activated partial thromboplastin time

Table 90-4 Mimics of Transient Ischemia or Cerebral Infarction

Transient Ischemia	Cerebral Infarction
Seizure	Seizure
Migraine equivalent (variant)	Systemic infection
Metabolic derangement, e.g., hypoglycemia	Brain tumor Subdural or ICH
Multiple sclerosis	HSV encephalitis Dementia

ICH—intracranial hemorrhage; HSV—herpes simplex virus

Table 90-5 Classification of Lacunar Strokes

Syndrome	Localization
Pure motor hemiparesis	Posterior internal capsule, corona radiate
Pure sensory stroke	Thalamus
Ataxia hemiparesis	Pons: posterior internal capsule, corona radiata
Clumsy-hand dysarthria	Pons
Sensory-motor stroke	Posterior internal capsule and thalamus

Adapted from: Petty GW, Brown RD Jr, Whisnant JP, et al. Ischemic stroke subtypes: a population based study of incidence and risk factors. Stroke 1999; 30:2513 2516.

Atrial Fibrillation

Patients presenting with acute stroke and atrial fibrillation are managed as those with atrial fibrillation alone. An evaluation for the cause of atrial fibrillation should be completed concomitantly with controlling the heart rate.

Patent Foramen Ovale/Atrial Septal Aneurysm (PFO/ASA)

The management of PFO/ASA is controversial. In a prospective multicenter observational study, 581 patients aged 18–55 years with cryptogenic ischemic stroke were given aspirin.[8] After 4 years, the recurrent stroke risk was 2.3% among persons with PFO alone, 15.2% with PFO and ASA, 4.2% without PFO/ASA. This study suggests that some patients with stroke and PFO are at high risk and require treatment other than antiplatelet therapy. Options included warfarin, closure of the PFO with an endovascular device, or open heart surgery with PFO repair. Studies of both device closure and surgery suggest a recurrent stroke risk of 3–4% per year.[12]

Extracranial Vessel Sources

Approximately 15–20% of strokes are secondary to large extracranial vessel disease, which includes the extracranial portion of the carotid artery, the vertebral artery, and the aorta.[13] The probability of extracranial vessel disease due to atherosclerosis increases with risk factors such as hypertension, hyperlipi-demia, diabetes, and smoking. A number of tests can be used to assess carotid, vertebral, and aortic vessels (Table 90-6).

Color flow duplex carotid ultrasound is operator dependent. Magnetic resonance angiography (MRA), computed tomographic angiography (CTA), or conventional angiography may be superior for pathologies such as fibromuscular dysplasia, arteritis, or dissection. Computed tomographic angiography should be avoided in patients with renal failure or dye allergy. The main limitations of MRA are cost and availability. Conventional arteriography is considered the gold standard for assessment of the cerebral vessels. However, it is an invasive procedure for assessing the degree of internal carotid artery (ICA) stenosis, though it is better for detecting plaque morphology, evidence of dissection, and fibromuscular dysplasia than standard MRA.[17] The risk of cerebral infarction, TIA, or hematoma formation during the procedure is 0.5–1% in addition to renal failure and contrast allergy. Currently, transesophageal echocardiography is superior to MRA of the aortic arch for detection and quantification of aortic plaque.

Large Vessel Intracranial Sources

Epidemiology studies have shown that 5–8% of strokes are due to large vessel intracranial disease.[18] The pretest probability increases among women; Asian, African, or Hispanic Americans; diabetic patients, patients with cortical symptoms, or recurrent stereotypical TIAs in a single vascular territory; and in patients with posterior circulation events. Intracranial disease may be due

Table 90-6 Tests for Evaluation of Stroke Etiology

Test		Sensitivity	Specificity
Transcranial Doppler ultrasound	**Extracranial Vessel**[14] Internal carotid artery (ICA) stenosis >70%	87–95%	86–97%
	Intracranial Vessel[15] Detecting stenosis >50%	89–98%	87–96%
CT angiography	**Extracranial Vessel** Detecting stenosis >70% Detecting carotid occlusion	74–100% 100%	83–100%
	Intracranial Vessel Detecting 30–64% stenosis, Detecting 70–99% stenosis Occluded segments.	61% 78% 100%	
MRA	**Extracranial Vessel**[16] Detection of extracranial internal carotid stenosis greater than 70% Occlusion	83–95% 98–100%	89–94% 98–100%
	Intracranial Vessel Detecting stenosis >50%	85–88%	96–97%

to atherosclerosis, dissection, vasculitis, noninflammatory vasculopathy, moya moya disease, and vasospasm.

Evaluation options include transcranial Doppler ultrasound, CT angiography, MRA, and conventional angiography. Table 90-6 lists the sensitivity and specificity of the various tests. Transcranial Doppler ultrasound noninvasively assesses the proximal intracranial internal carotid artery, the M-1 segment of the middle cerebral artery, the A-1 segment of the anterior cerebral artery, the vertebral arteries, and the proximal aspect of the basilar artery.[19] Computed tomographic angiography is limited by the need for contrast. Magnetic resonance imaging can image the brain, and MR angiography can evaluate the vessels.[20] Conventional arteriography is superior to noninvasive studies for evaluating arteries distal to the circle of Willis, such as those involved in vasculitis. It is also superior for detecting arteriovenous malformations or dural arteriovenous fistulas that may present with transient neurologic deficits and for defining plaque and vessel pathology.

Small Vessel Disease (Lacunar Stroke)

Lacunar infarctions account for up to 20% of all cerebral ischemic events. Lacunar infarctions are associated microscopically with microatheroma, lipohyalinosis, and fibrinoid necrosis. They are the result of occlusion of a penetrating end artery. Lacunes predominate in the basal ganglia, thalamus, centrum semiovale, brainstem, and internal capsule. Lacunar syndromes can also occur with emboli, either from the carotids or atrial fibrillation. Typical lacunar syndromes and locations are presented in Table 90-5.

Antiplatelet agents and aggressive risk factor modification are the recommended approach to managing this stroke entity. Extracranial carotid artery assessment is recommended in patients with lacunar infarcts in the anterior circulation.

Coagulation Disorders

Coagulation disorders account for 1–4.8% of all strokes.[4] The following abnormalities have been associated with arterial cerebral infarctions: sickle cell disease, polycythemia vera, essential thrombocythemia, heparin induced thrombocytopenia, disseminated intravascular coagulation, thrombocytosis, protein C or S deficiency (acquired or congenital), antithrombin III deficiency, antiphospholipid antibody syndrome, lupus anticoagulant, and hyperhomocysteinemia. Assessing patients for the above diagnosis should begin by completing a CBC with differential, aPTT, INR, and platelet count.

Prognosis

With a 5-year mortality of >50%, stroke is a deadly disease that ranks with serious cancers such as hepatic carcinoma and invasive bladder cancer. A 2003 analysis of the Perth Community Stroke Study database showed that 60% of stroke patients die within 5 years and 80% within 10 years.[35,36] The risk of death among 1 year survivors remains fairly consistent at 10% per year, and the annual case fatality rate is 5% per year.[37]

MANAGEMENT

Treatment

The initial approach to a patient diagnosed with a stroke hinges on whether or not the patient is a candidate for thrombolytic therapy. Restoring blood flow through thrombolytic therapy (either intravenous or intra-arterial) is the ideal goal in stroke treatment, but this must be accomplished within 3 hours of symptom onset. This decision should be made in consultation with a neurologist. Appendix 2 at the back of the book provides an example of a checklist for eligibility criteria for thrombolytic therapy. Additionally, thrombolytic therapy should be administered as part of a well-structured protocol, as this results in risk similar to, or less than, the original treatment study. Of note, multiple studies demonstrate that deviation from the protocol yields unacceptable outcomes.[38] If your institution lacks such a protocol, then therapy should follow the approach described below.

For patients who are not eligible for thrombolytic therapy, treatment focuses on:[27]

- Antiplatelet therapy
- Ensuring adequate oxygenation and perfusion
- Monitoring heart rhythm and blood pressure
- Controlling temperature and glucose
- Treating underlying infections and other medical conditions
- Preventing medical complications such as DVT, malnutrition, and pressure sores
- Secondary prevention

The role of the hospitalist in the management of patients with stroke is to manage the concomitant medical problems and prevent poststroke complications which increase the morbidity and mortality of this already deadly disease.

Antiplatelet or Anticoagulation Therapy

If there are no contraindications, antiplatelet therapy with aspirin, 160–300 mg daily, should be started within 48 hours of onset of presumed ischemic stroke. Aspirin reduces the risk of early recurrent ischemic stroke without a major risk of early hemorrhagic complications and improves long-term outcome. Anticoagulants such as heparin or low molecular weight heparin (LMWH) appear to offer no benefit over aspirin, except in specific situations. Anticoagulation may be of benefit among patients with large vessel atherosclerotic disease and those deemed to be suffering ongoing thromboembolic stroke, and those with emboli from a cardiac source such as valvular disease or a mechanical heart valve. It does not appear to render any acute benefit among patients with atrial fibrillation or acute stroke of uncertain etiology.

Maintaining Oxygenation and Perfusion

Patients with acute stroke should have pulse oximetry monitoring with a target oxygen saturation of >95% to prevent hypoxemia and potential worsening of the neurologic injury. Elective endotracheal intubation should be reserved for patients with a threatened airway or decreased level of consciousness or brainstem stroke with impaired oropharyngeal motility and loss of protective reflexes. Keeping the patient completely recumbent increases cerebral blood flow but should not be sustained beyond 24 hours, and patients must be able to protect their airway.

Cardiac Arrhythmias

The most common arrhythmia observed in acute stroke is atrial fibrillation. Electrocardiographic changes secondary to stroke include ST segment depression, QT interval prolongation, inverted T waves, and prominent U waves.[21,22] Reportedly, patients sustaining right hemispheric infarction have a high risk of arrhythmias secondary to disturbances in sympathetic and parasympathetic nervous system function.[23] Myocardial infarction has also been reported as a complication following acute ischemic stroke.[24] Thus, patients with acute ischemic stroke should be placed in a monitored setting to detect life-threatening arrhythmias or atrial fibrillation

Blood Pressure

Arterial hypertension is common following stroke, but physicians should limit their impulse to treat it. Elevation of blood pressure following acute stroke can result from the stress of stroke (possibly a response to increase brain perfusion), pain, preexisting hypertension, a physiologic response to hypoxia, or increased intracranial pressure. Reducing blood pressure within the first 24 hours may actually worsen the outcome. In general, the blood pressure of patients suffering an acute ischemic stroke should be allowed to be higher than normal to optimize perfusion of the peri-infarct area. Additionally, treatment with antihypertensive agents may result in excessive reduction in cerebral blood flow as autoregulation is lost in the ischemic areas.

The current consensus on hypertensive management is to use medications when the systolic blood pressure is >220 mm Hg and diastolic >120 mm Hg,[26] or if the patient is suffering from hypertensive encephalopathy, aortic dissection, acute renal failure, acute pulmonary edema, or acute myocardial infarction. Chapter 32 thoroughly reviews management of blood pressure in hypertensive emergencies and urgencies. Otherwise, the blood pressure should **not** be treated acutely and antihypertensive therapy withheld for up to 10 days in patients with acute ischemic stroke.

Blood Glucose Control

Hypoglycemia can cause focal neurologic signs that mimic stroke as well as contributing to possible brain injury. Rapid reversal of hypoglycemia is critical. Hyperglycemia is also an important management issue following acute stroke. Many patients with diabetes mellitus have vascular disease and an increased risk for stroke. These patients will frequently have significant hyperglycemia post stroke, and elevated glucose is associated with poorer outcomes. Management of elevated blood glucose should be similar to that for treatment of other acutely ill patients who have hyperglycemia. Target blood sugar levels should be <180 mg/dL.[27]

Fever

Fever is common in the first 48 hours after acute ischemic stroke and not frequently associated with infection. Increased temperature in the setting of acute ischemic stroke has been associated with poor neurologic outcome, possibly due to increased metabolic demands, enhanced release of neurotransmitters, and increased free radical production. A recent meta-analysis suggested that fever after stroke onset is associated with a marked increase in morbidity and mortality.[28] Any source of fever should be evaluated for an etiology and aggressively managed with oral antipyretic or cooling devices.

Deep Vein Thrombosis Prophylaxis

The first 14 days following acute stroke is the greatest risk period for developing deep vein thrombosis and/or pulmonary embolism. The reported incidence of deep vein thrombosis during the first 2 weeks varies from 27–75%, depending on the endpoint assessment methodology.[29–31] Autopsy studies in patients 1 month post stroke have revealed pulmonary embolism as the principal cause of death in 13–16% of cases.[32,33]

In order to prevent this complication, prophylaxis with mechanical and/or pharmacologic agents must be provided for this patient population. In patients with ischemic stroke who do not receive thrombolytic therapy and anticoagulation, the use of unfractionated heparin (5,000 units, SC, q 8hr) or low molecular weight heparin (enoxaparin 40 mg, SC, q 24hr) is the recommended prophylaxis for preventing deep vein thrombosis.[34] This level of anticoagulation can be given along with aspirin. Sequential compression devices should be used if there is a contraindication to anticoagulation.

Nutrition and Mobilization

Early evaluation by a dietician and physical therapist may be essential. A dietician can help assess the patient's nutritional status and recommend supplements to treat or prevent malnutrition (see Chapter 4). Speech therapy assessment may be needed to assess swallowing function for dysphagia so that patients do not aspirate. Physical therapy can help mobilize the patient and prevent pressure sores. Occupational therapy assessment may be needed for patients suffering major hemiparesis for assistance with splints and adaptation to their new deficit to optimize their functioning. Standardized orders for admission of patients with stroke should include the option for early consultation with nutrition, and speech, physical, and occupational therapy.

PREVENTION

Atrial Fibrillation–Associated Stoke

Patients with atrial fibrillation and stroke should be started on warfarin after 48 hours. The target INR is 2–3. Some patients may be selected for cardioversion or TEE-guided cardioversion. In this group, warfarin is maintained for 3–4 weeks. Prior to cardioversion, the INR should ideally be 2.5 or higher. Following cardioversion and restoration of normal sinus rhythm, the warfarin is maintained for 3–4 weeks, again with a goal INR of 2–3.

The recent Atrial Fibrillation Follow-up Investigation of Rhythm Management (AFFIRM) demonstrated that rate control plus anticoagulation in patients with atrial fibrillation is an acceptable primary therapy and produces a similar composite outcome (death, disabling stroke, major bleeding, cardiac arrest) as rhythm control plus anticoagulation.[10] Although high rates of anticoagulation were used in both arms, most strokes occurred in patients who were not taking warfarin or had an INR <2.0. The results of AFFIRM suggest that both restoration of sinus rhythm and atrial fibrillation rate control with concomitant chronic anticoagulation have similar morbidity and mortality rates.

Patients with persistent or paroxysmal atrial fibrillation are at high risk of stroke if they have any of the following features: primary ischemic stroke, TIA, systemic embolism, age >75, moderately or severely impaired left ventricular systolic function and/or congestive heart failure, hypertension, or diabetes. They should receive anticoagulation with warfarin to a target INR of 2–3.

The CHADS$_2$ Index was derived from risk factors identified in the Atrial Fibrillation Investigators (AFI) and Stroke Prevention in Atrial Fibrillation (SPAF) trials. In this model, the CHADS$_2$ score is calculated by assigning one point each for the presence of CHF (C), history of hypertension (H), age >75 years (A), or diabetes (D), and adding two points for history of stroke or TIA (S$_2$),

Table 90-7 CHADS$_2$ Index

Score	Stroke Rate/100 pt yrs	Adjusted Stroke Rate (95% CI)
0	1.2	1.9 (1.2–3.0)
1	2.8	2.8 (2.0–3.8)
2	3.6	4.0 (3.1–5.1)
3	6.4	5.9 (4.6–7.3)
4	8.0	8.5 (6.3–11.1)
5	7.7	12.5 (8.2–17.5)
6	44.0	18.5 (10.5–27.9)

Adapted from: Gage BF, Waterman AD, Shannon W, et al. Validation of clinical classification schemes for predicting stroke: results from the National Registry of Atrial Fibrillation. J Am Med Assoc 2001; 285:2864–2870.

C = Congestive Heart Failure; H = Hypertension; A = Age >75; D = Diabetes; S$_2$ = Stroke or Transient Ischemic Attack

producing the acronym CHADS$_2$.[11] The CHADS$_2$ index was validated in a chart review of 1,733 patients with atrial fibrillation and found to be highly predictive of stroke (Table 90-7).

Lipid Lowering

All patients suffering a stroke should undergo lipid profile testing. Treatment with a statin should be considered, as aggressive lowering of cholesterol has been shown to reduce the risk of subsequent stroke. The statin can be started in the hospital with eventual goal of LDL <100.

DISCHARGE/FOLLOW-UP PLANS

Close follow-up with both the patient's primary care provider (PCP) and neurology consultant should be arranged within a week of discharge. The PCP will need to coordinate any home health services, including physical therapy.

Patient Education

Having a stroke is a traumatic event for a patient. Given the potential cognitive impact, family members or friends should be enlisted to assist with care. Patients will need assistance with quitting smoking if they abused tobacco prior to the stroke. Additionally, they will need to adjust their diet to optimally control their blood pressure, lipids, and blood glucose. Patients should be counseled to be compliant with new medications such as statins and/or aspirin. If they will be taking warfarin as an outpatient, they will need to have close follow-up for INR testing and dosage adjustment. Discharge counseling should focus on the importance of follow-up with a PCP and their neurologist.

Outpatient Physician Communication

The PCP should be made aware of all new treatments such as aspirin and statins. Additionally, the PCP should be alerted to the need to restart antihypertensive medications and control any hyperglycemia. The hospitalist should ensure close follow-up of patients taking warfarin, ideally in an anticoagulation clinic skilled in its management.

Key Points

- Patients with stroke should be rapidly evaluated to determine if they are appropriate candidates for thrombolytic therapy.

- Consider mimics of stroke in your initial evaluation, recognizing that as many as one third of patients presenting with acute onset of focal neurologic deficits do **not** have a stroke.

- Administer aspirin, but avoid full anticoagulation with heparin unless there is a specific indication.

- Prevent common complications such as hypoxia, hyperglycemia, and fever, which increase morbidity and mortality.

- Administer DVT prophylaxis.

- Initiate secondary prevention treatments prior to hospital discharge.

SUGGESTED READING

American Heart Association. Heart Disease and Stroke Statistics www.americanheart.org

American Stroke Association. What are the types of stroke? www.strokeassociation.org

Flemming KD, Brown RD, Petty GW, et al. Evaluation and management of transient ischemic attack and minor cerebral infarction. Mayo Clin Proc 2004; 79(8):1071–1086.

Hand PJ, Kwan J, Lindley RI, et al. Distinguishing between stroke and mimic at the bedside: the brain attack study. Stroke 2006; 37:769–775.

Peterson GE, Brickner ME, Reimold SC. Transesophageal echocardiography: clinical indications and applications. Circulation 2003; 107:2398–2402.

Berge E, Abdelnoor M, Nakstad PH, Sandset PM. Low molecular-weight heparin versus aspirin in patients with acute ischemic stroke and atrial fibrillation: a double-blind randomized study. HAEST Study Group. Lancet 2000; 355(9211):1205–1210.

AFFIRM Investigators. A comparison of rate control and rhythm control in patients with atrial fibrillation. N Engl J Med 2002; 347:1825–1833.

Nederkourn PJ, van der Graaf Y, Hunick MG. Duplex ultrasound and magnetic resonance angiography compared with digital subtraction angiography in carotid artery stenosis: a systematic review. Stroke 2003; 34:1324–1332.

Adams HP, Adams RJ, Del Zoppo GJ, et al. Guidelines for the early management of patients with ischemic stroke: 2005 guidelines update a scientific statement from the Stroke Council of the American Heart Association/American Stroke Association. Stroke 2005; 36:916.

Hajat C, Hajat S, Sharma P. Effects of poststroke pyrexia on stroke outcome: a meta analysis of studies in patients. Stroke 2000; 31:410–414.

Hillbom M, Erila T, Sotaniemi K, et al. Enoxaparin vs heparin for prevention of DVT in acute ischemic stroke: a randomized, double blind study. Acta Neurol Scand 2002; 106:84–92.

Albers GW, Amarenco P, Easton JD, et al. Antithrombotic and thrombolytic therapy for ischemic stroke. Chest 2004; 126:483S–512S.

Bravata DM, Ho SY, Brass LM, et al. Long term mortality in cerebrovascular disease. Stroke 2003; 34:699–704.

CHAPTER NINETY-ONE

Intracerebral Hemorrhage

Geno J. Merli, MD, FACP; Robert Rosenwasser, MD, FACS; and Mark V. Williams, MD, FACP

BACKGROUND

Intracranial hemorrhage (ICH), whether intracerebral or subarachnoid, can be a devastating event for patients. The estimated lifetime costs of intracerebral hemorrhage, which includes patient care and lost productivity, are about $125,000 per person year with an aggregate cost of $6 billion per year in the United States.[5] If we compare it to the estimated lifetime costs of subarachnoid hemorrhage ($5.6 billion) and ischemic stroke ($29 billion), it is clear that ICH places a significant economic burden on society.[6,7] Comprising both intracerebral hemorrhage and subarachnoid hemorrhage, this chapter reviews the clinical presentation of intracerebral hemorrhage, diagnosis, and treatment.

With the decreasing availability of neurologists and neurosurgeons in the hospital, especially at night and on weekends, hospitalists increasingly are being asked to admit these patients to the hospital. While background knowledge of ICH is essential, hospitalists must still insist on appropriate involvement of a neurologist or neurosurgeon in the care of these potentially complicated cases.

ASSESSMENT

Clinical Presentation

Prevalence

Intracerebral hemorrhage has an estimated prevalence of 37,000 cases per year in the United States.[1] It is twice as prevalent as subarachnoid hemorrhage and accounts for approximately 10% of all strokes.[1] The most recent population-based studies using computerized tomographic (CT) verification estimated that the overall incidence of ICH is between 12 and 15 cases per 100,000 population.[2] The worldwide incidence ranges from 10–20 cases per 100,000 population.[1] ICH is more common in men than women, those older than 55 years, and ethnic groups such as Blacks and Japanese.[1,3] The National Health and Nutrition Examination Survey Epidemiologic Follow-up Study reported the incidence among blacks in the United States was 50 per 100,000, which is twice the incidence among whites.[4] The incidence in the Japanese population was 55 per 100,000, quite similar to the black population.[3]

Intracranial saccular aneurysms, the primary cause of subarachnoid hemorrhage (SAH), are fairly common—present in about 5% of people. However, actual SAH is far rarer, afflicting less than 0.02% of the population for about 30,000 cases per year in North America.

Presenting Signs and Symptoms

The clinical manifestations of intracerebral hemorrhage relate to its location, extent of the bleed, and the presence of intraventricular hemorrhage. About half of spontaneous intracerebral hemorrhages originate in the basal ganglia, a third in the cerebral hemispheres, and a sixth in the brainstem or cerebellum[19] (Fig. 91-1). Rapid onset of a focal neurologic deficit occurs frequently with associated headache of variable intensity, reduced level of consciousness, and nausea and vomiting. The neurologic signs may not follow a typical distribution as in a large artery stroke. Seizures occur in approximately 10% of all patients, with intracerebral hemorrhage and in approximately 50% of patients with lobar hemorrhage.[14] Almost all seizures occur at the onset of bleeding or within the first 24 hours of the event and are not predictive of the development of future seizure recurrence.[20,21] Over 90% of patients will have hypertension exceeding 160/100 mm Hg, regardless of any previous history of high blood pressure.[22] Dysautonomia in the form of central fever, hyperventilation, hyperglycemia, and tachycardia or bradycardia is also common.[19]

Subarachnoid hemorrhage most commonly occurs due to rupture of a saccular aneurysm with rapid onset of symptoms. Classically presenting with the "worst headache of my life" in 97% of patients, they also may have nausea, vomiting (about 50%), brief loss of consciousness, or a seizure. Of note, up to 20% of patients with the complaint of the worst headache of their life will have a subarachnoid hemorrhage. Onset of meningismus may be delayed several hours. The well-described "sentinel headache" occurs in from 10–50% of patients, and typically precedes a major hemorrhage by 1–3 weeks.[4a]

Differential Diagnosis

The causes of ICH are divided into primary and secondary etiologies. Primary hemorrhage is unrelated to underlying congenital or acquired central nervous system lesions or abnormalities. Table 91-1 documents the most common causes of primary and secondary intracerebral hemorrhage.[5]

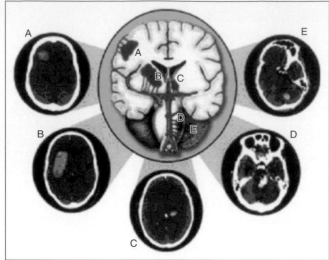

Figure 91-1 • Hemorrhage Sites. A. Deep White Matter, B. Basal Ganglia, C. Thalamus, D. Pons, E. Cerebellum. Center Image from Qureshi AI, Tuhrim S, Broderick JP, Batjer HH, Hondo H, Hanley DF. Spontaneous intracerebral hemorrhage. N Engl J Med 2001;344:1450–1460. Other images from Manno EM, Atkinson JLD, Fulgham JR, Wijdicks EF. Emerging medical and surgical management strategies in the evaluation and treatment of intracerebral hemorrhage. Mayo Clin Proc 2005;80:420–433.

Table 91-1 Etiologies of Intracerebral Hemorrhage

Primary	Secondary
Hypertension	Vascular malformations
Cerebral amyloid angiopathy	Arteriovenous malformations
Anticoagulant/fibrinolytic	Dural arteriovenous fistula
Antiplatelet agents	Cavernous malformations
Drug Use	Aneurysm
Amphetamines	Saccular
Cocaine	Mycotic
Phenylpropanolamine	Fusiform
Other illicit drugs	Tumors
Other bleeding diathesis	Primary brain tumors
	Secondary metastasis
	Hemorrhagic transformation of cerebral infarct
	Venous infarction with hemorrhage secondary to cerebral vein thrombosis
	Moyamoya disease

Emerging medical and surgical management strategies in the evaluation and treatment of intracerebral hemorrhage. Adapted from: Manno EM, Atkinson JLD, Fulgham JR, et al. Mayo Clinic Pro 2005; 80(3):420–433.

Chronic hypertension accounts for approximately 75% of all cases of primary ICH.[11,12] The remaining 25% is a result of cerebral amyloid angiopathy, anticoagulant/fibrinolytic/antiplatelet use, drugs (amphetamines, cocaine, phenylpropanolamine, etc.), or bleeding diathesis. Cerebral amyloid angiopathy is the deposition of congophilic amyloid-B protein in the cerebral and leptomeningeal vessels. Cerebral amyloid angiopathy is found in 50% of patients over the age of 80 years.[13] This pathologic process is estimated to account for more than 20% of all ICH in patients older than 70 years.[14] The National Institute of Neurological Disorders and Stroke (NINDS) trial rated the overall risk of ICH after tissue plasminogen activator use in ischemic stroke to be 6.4%.[15] Risk factors for this high rate were age greater than 70 years, serum glucose level greater than 300 mg/dL, National Institute of Health Stroke Scale score higher than 20, and early ischemic changes noted on computerized tomography.[16]

The long-term use of warfarin increases the risk of ICH tenfold.[17] Intracerebral hemorrhage secondary to sudden elevation in blood pressure, multifocal cerebral vessel spasm, or drug-induced vasculitis can result from the use of cocaine, amphetamine, or phenylpropanolamine.[18]

Underlying vascular abnormalities such as arteriovenous malformations, cerebral aneurysm, or cavernous angiomas are an important cause of secondary ICH. These vascular abnormalities occur in a younger population. ICH can also occur when bleeding occurs into primary or metastatic brain lesions.

Risk factors for SAH include cigarette smoking, hypertension, alcohol, family history, and phenylpropanolamine. Additionally, exercise or exertion appears to be a trigger for SAH.

Diagnosis

Even with nonspecific clinical findings, CT without contrast of the head will provide immediate information that will distinguish between cerebral infarction and intracerebral hemorrhage. The CT scan also defines the size, location, and the presence of intraventricular, subarachnoid, or subdural blood.

The location of the bleed frequently identifies possible underlying etiologies for the event. Hemorrhages that originate in the deep subcortical structures (putamen, caudate, thalamus, pons, cerebellum, or periventricular deep white matter), particularly in patients with a history of hypertension, result from rupture of the deep perforating arteries. Single or multiple hemorrhages in elderly persons that extend to the cortical surface are most likely attributable to amyloid angiopathy.[23,24]

Magnetic resonance imaging (MRI) is as sensitive as CT for detecting ICH during the acute bleed.[5] It can be useful as a follow-up study for dating hemorrhages or identifying small vascular lesions that may have been missed with a noncontrast head CT. Use of MRI is limited in early detection of ICH by the time required to obtain imaging and by the limited ability to monitor a patient while in the scanner.[1]

Evidence is contradictory regarding the value of cerebral angiography in intracerebral hemorrhage. One study reported low yield from cerebral angiography in identifying an underlying lesion in patients older than 45 years who had a history of hypertension and had hemorrhages in deep subcortical structures.[25] On the other hand, cerebral angiography revealed underlying lesions in 84% of patients in another study. These lesions appeared to have some structural abnormality detected in previous neuroimaging.[26] The findings on CT that should prompt cerebral angiography include the presence of subarachnoid or intraventricular blood, an abnormal calcification or prominent draining vein, or blood that extends to the perisylvian or interhemispheric fissure.[26] Young patients with no clear source of hemorrhage should also have angiography.

Diagnosis of SAH also relies on noncontrast head CT, with greatest accuracy on the initial day of the event (sensitivity >90%) and steadily declining thereafter. If the head CT reveals no evidence of hemorrhage, a lumbar puncture must be performed.

While red blood cells and xanthochromia are the classic findings, spectrophotometry to detect the blood breakdown products (e.g., bilirubin) appears to be more accurate. After making the diagnosis of SAH, cerebral angiography should be pursued. Alternatives include CT angiography and magnetic resonance angiography (MRA), but both of these noninvasive tests are primarily used for screening and planning, as they do not have the desired resolution. Of note, from 15–20% of patients with SAH will not have an etiology identified on initial angiography and should have this repeated in 4 days to 2 weeks.

Prognosis

The 30-day mortality and morbidity associated with ICH ranges between 30% and 40% in hospital-based studies and up 52% in community-based trials.[8] The 1-year mortality following ICH is approximately 50%, with half of all deaths occurring in the first 48 hours after onset of symptoms. The subsequent annual mortality is 8% per year for 5 years, with almost 50% of the deaths attributable to the original hemorrhage, myocardial infarction, sudden death, pneumonia, or extracranial hemorrhage.[9]

Among survivors, only 21–38% of patients are functionally independent at 6 months.[10] About 1 in 10 patients suffering an SAH die before reaching the hospital, and only a third recover to baseline after treatment. Strokes (hypodense lesions on CT) from vasospasm following the acute event afflict about half of survivors.

A scoring system for prognosticating the 30-day mortality used the following prediction: large ICH volume, coma, older age, intraventricular hemorrhage, and infratentorial location[27] (Table 91-2). The mortality after the first 30 days is the result of secondary complications from comorbid conditions.

Patients suffering ICH in the setting of anticoagulation with warfarin have a worse prognosis, with more than half dying within 30 days of onset.[27a] The degree of INR prolongation correlates with outcomes; up to two thirds of patients with INR >3 will not survive. Additionally, neurologic status on presentation predicts mortality, with up to 96% of patients unconscious on admission dying.

MANAGEMENT

Treatment

Beyond any definitive neurosurgical intervention, treatment should focus on supportive measures to mitigate subsequent damage from the hemorrhage. Efforts should focus on careful management of the airway and oxygenation; fluids, electrolytes, and glucose; blood pressure; seizures; coagulation status and hemostasis; venous thromboembolism prophylaxis; and management of intracranial pressure. Patients with a subarachnoid hemorrhage should receive Nimodpine[27b] and be carefully evaluated for the presence of vasospasm and treated accordingly.[27c]

Airway Management and Oxygenation
Rapid neurologic decline and depressed consciousness can result in hypoxemia or hypercapnia, causing cerebral vasodilatation and high intracranial pressure. Recognition of this risk should direct care to airway protection and maintenance of adequate

Table 91-2 The Intracerebral Hemorrhage Score

Glasgow Coma Scale Score	Points
3–4	2
5–12	1
13–15	0
Intracerebral Hemorrhage Volume (mL)	
>30 mL	1
<30 mL	0
Intraventricular Hemorrhage	
Yes	1
No	0
Age (years)	
>80	1
<80	0
Infratentorial Origin	
Yes	1
No	0
30 Day Mortality for Total Points	
5 +	100%
4	97%
3	72%
2	26%
1	13%
0	0%

The ICH Score: a simple, reliable grading scale for intracerebral hemorrhage
Adapted from: Hemphill JC 3rd, et al. Stroke 2001; 32:891–897.

oxygenation. If the patient has significant alteration in mental status and inability to protect the airway, rapid-sequence intubation should be performed, ideally by someone expert in this technique to minimize any increase in intracranial pressure.

Intravenous Fluids, Electrolytes, Glucose
The goal of fluid management in intracerebral hemorrhage is to achieve euvolemia and maintain intravascular volume in order optimize cerebral perfusion. Dextrose solutions should be avoided, since hyperglycemia is detrimental to damaged brain tissue. When present, hyperglycemia should be corrected slowly because a rapid decrease in the serum glucose level may worsen cerebral edema because of the concomitant decrease in serum osmolality.[28] Electrolyte, phosphorus, and magnesium abnormalities must be corrected. In diabetics, all oral agents should be discontinued and patients placed on insulin infusion to maintain blood glucose levels to less than 140 mg/dL. Once the patient has stabilized from the acute event, oral therapy may be reinstituted if needed.

Blood Pressure
Hypertension within the first 6 hours of ICH should be aggressively managed to optimize cerebral perfusion pressure. The goal is to maintain cerebral perfusion pressure while also preventing expansion of the hemorrhage. (See below for management in SAH.) Gentle lowering of the mean arterial pressure (MAP) appears to ensure adequate cerebral blood flow as local cerebral autoregulation appears to remain functional. The American Stroke Association guidelines recommend that the MAP be maintained at or below 130 mm Hg for patients with ICH.[1] In patients who have had craniotomy, mean arterial pressure

Table 91-3 Antihypertensive Medications in Patient with Acute Intracerebral Hemorrhage

Drug	Type	Dose	Contraindications
Labetalol	α_a, β_1, and β_2 Receptor antagonist	10–80 mg bolus, every 10 min, up to 300 mg 0.5 mg–2 mg/min infusion	Bradycardia Bronchospasm, heart failure
Metoprolol			
Nicardipine	Calcium channel blocker	5–15 mg/hr infusion	Severe aortic stenosis, myocardial ischemia
Enalapril	ACE inhibitor	0.625 mg bolus, 1.25 mg–5 mg every 6 hr	Variable blood pressure response Sudden hypotension In high rennin states

ACE—angiotensin converting enzyme

Table 91-4 Management of the Anticoagulated Patient with Intracerebral Hemorrhage

Drug	Management	
Warfarin	Vitamin K	10 mg IV slow infusion over 20 minutes (10 mg in 50 mL 0.9% saline)
	Fresh frozen plasma	
	Profilnine	INR <4, 25 units/kg, IV, 2–3 minutes INR >4, 50 units/kg, IV, 2–3 minutes
Unfractionated heparin	Protamine 1 mg for every 100 units, unfractionated heparin	
Low molecular weight heparin	Protamine 1 mg for every 1 mg of enoxaparin dose	
Aspirin	Platelet transfusion	
Clopidogrel	Platelet transfusion	

INR = Intermational Normalization Ratio

should be maintained at or below 100 mm Hg.[19] Systolic blood pressures of 160 mm Hg or greater are associated with hematoma enlargement.

Table 91-3 reviews available medication options. The common finding of increase in blood pressure may persist for a few days following the initial event and is attributable to persistent headache, increased circulating brainstem-mediated release of catecholamines secondary to increased intracranial pressure, or withdrawal of antihypertensive medications. Blood pressure is best controlled by the use of labetalol, metoprolol, nicardipine, or angiotensin-converting enzyme inhibitors. These agents have the advantage of not affecting intracranial pressure. Sodium nitroprusside and intravenous or topical nitrates should be avoided, since they cause cerebral vasodilatation and increased intracranial pressure.

Seizures

Seizure activity increases cerebral blood flow and intracranial pressure that can result in neuronal injury and destabilization of a patient with an acute intracerebral hemorrhage.[1] The 30-day risk of clinically evident seizures after ICH is approximately 8%.[29] Most seizures occur at the time of ICH or shortly thereafter, with lobar location of bleeding an independent predictor of early seizure activity. Acute seizures at the time of presentation should be treated with lorazepam followed by phenytoin or fosphenytoin, valproic acid, or phenobarbital. The role of seizure prophylaxis for patients suffering ICH remains controversial. The American Heart Association guidelines recommend seizure prophylaxis for

up to 1 month, after which time therapy can be discontinued in the absence of seizure activity.[1]

Anticoagulated Patients (Table 91-4)

Patients on warfarin anticoagulation are at increased risk for intracerebral hemorrhage, and approximately 15% of cases of ICH are associated with warfarin therapy. Moreover, these patient have a higher risk of progressive bleeding and clinical deterioration.[30] Rapid correction of the INR is critical to reducing the risk of continued intracerebral bleeding. The effects of warfarin can be reversed with fresh frozen plasma, prothrombin-complex concentrates, and vitamin K. Caution should be exercised in using fresh frozen plasma since the volume (15 mL/kg) from rapid administration might compromise patients with poor cardiac reserve. The use of vitamin K orally, subcutaneously, or intravenously should be reserved for the patient in whom long-term reversal of warfarin is contemplated. Our approach is to use the prothrombin-complex along with 5 mg of vitamin K subcutaneously to reverse the warfarin effect.[31] Of note, oral vitamin K is more predictably effective than subcutaneous administration but may not be possible in the patient with altered mental status. The use of recombinant activated factor VII concentrate, which potentiates the clotting process, is not approved for the previously mentioned patient population, and we do not advocate its for patients with warfarin-associated intracerebral hemorrhage. Nonetheless, preliminary research is intriguing. For patients receiving unfractionated heparin or low molecular weight heparin, protamine sulfate will reverse the effect of these agents. The management of intracerebral hemorrhage in patients taking aspirin or clopidogrel should take into consideration the time of the last dose of these agents. An afflicted patient having taken these antiplatelet agents within 7 days of the event should receive platelet transfusion.

Hemostatic Therapy: Preventing Hematoma Expansion

One of the key factors in acute intracerebral hemorrhage is expansion of the hematoma and its damage to neural tissue. A prospective study showed that early hematoma growth occurred in 26% of patients within 1 hour after the initial CT scan and in another 12% within 20 hours.[32] Another study reported hematoma expansion occurring in 20% of patients within 3 hours from onset of the intracerebral hemorrhage, but it rarely occurred after the first 24 hours.[33] Risk factors for the expansion of intracerebral hemorrhage include poorly controlled diabetes and systolic blood pressures greater than 200 mm Hg on hospital admission.

Recombinant activated factor VII may diminish or stop hematoma expansion after acute intracerebral hemorrhage. It is a powerful initiator of hemostasis and is currently approved for treatment of bleeding in patients with hemophilia who are resistant to factor VIII replacement therapy. Using this concept, a randomized, double-blind, placebo-controlled study of 399 patients was completed using doses of 40 mcg/kg, 80 mcg/kg, and 160 micrograms per kilogram versus placebo.[34] All patient were treated within 4 hours of the diagnosis of intracerebral hemorrhage. The mean increase was 29% in placebo versus 16%, 14%, and 11% in the escalating doses of recombinant activated factor VII, respectively (P value 0.011). This outcome was associated with a 38% reduction in mortality and significantly improved functional capacity at 90 days. A side effect of the stimulation of the clotting process was a 5% increases in arterial thromboembolic adverse events.

Deep Vein Thrombosis and Pulmonary Embolism Prophylaxis

The incidence of deep vein thrombosis and pulmonary embolism in intracerebral hemorrhage has not been defined. Using the 7th American College of Chest Physicians consensus conference, intracerebral hemorrhage patients would be considered high risk for deep vein thrombosis and pulmonary embolism but at increased risk for bleeding. Therefore, mechanical devices alone are the best clinical option during the first week following acute hemorrhage. A recently completed randomized, prospective trial comparing elastic stockings versus elastic stockings plus intermittent pneumatic compression sleeves[35] demonstrated significant benefit to use of the combination therapy, with a 4.7% rate of thrombotic events compared to 15.9% among patients prescribed only elastic stockings. Once the patient becomes more mobile and not able to wear the intermittent pneumatic compression devices consistently, then consider treatment with unfractionated heparin (5,000 units, SC, q8 or 12hr) or low molecular weight heparin (enoxaparin 40 mg, SC, q24hr or dalteparin 5,000 units, SC, q24hr) if the risk of hemorrhage is acceptable.

Treatment of Elevated Intracranial Pressure

Emergency management of increased intracranial pressure (ICP) in a patient with acute intracerebral hemorrhage requires involvement of a neurosurgeon or a neuro-intensivist. Options to lower ICP include elevation of the head to 30 degrees, 20% mannitol (0.25–1 g/kg) infusion, and hyperventilating the patient to a pCO2 of 28–32 mm Hg. These are temporizing measures until either a ventriculostomy or intracerebral bolt is placed for monitoring and fluid drainage. Corticosteroids are not recommended for intracerebral hemorrhage patients, since randomized controlled trial found no benefit and a greater risk for medical complication in the steroid group.[36]

Subarachnoid Hemorrhage and Vasospasm

All patients with SAH should be initially managed in an intensive care unit (ICU), ideally with assistance from a neuro-intensivist and neurosurgeon. Treatment focuses initially on optimizing blood pressure and correcting metabolic derangements, as noted above. Narcotics provided for pain relief will also help reduce blood pressure fluctuations and risk of rebleeding. Blood pressure control is dependent on balancing cerebral perfusion and risking rebleeding. Nimodipine administration improves outcomes through reduction in neurologic deficits and mortality from vasospasm. Statins also appear to reduce vasospasm. Transcranial Doppler ultrasound is used to monitor the degree of vasospasm. Once the aneurysm is definitively treated with neurosurgical clipping or interventional radiology placing coils in the aneurysm, then efforts aim to increase intravascular volume and pressure.

Surgical Intervention

The surgical management of intracranial hematoma varies, depending on the size of the hemorrhage, timing, location, and concomitant symptoms. A number of clinical trials indicate there is no benefit from early surgical intervention to evacuate intracerebral hemorrhages.[37–39] Most recently the international Surgical Trial in Intracerebral Haemorrhage (STICH) randomized 1,033 patients with intracerebral hemorrhage for either early surgical evacuation or medical management.[40] Of note, patients were randomized by an "uncertainty principle" based on whether the surgeon was uncertain about the best possible treatment. The trial revealed no benefit from early surgical intervention. Another meta-analysis of surgical versus medical management also did not demonstrate a benefit from surgery.[41] However, most neurosurgeons concur that urgent surgical intervention is indicated in patients with infratentorial hematomas 3 cm or larger in diameter or smaller with brainstem compression, because of the rapid deterioration to coma and brainstem herniation.[42,43]

Timing of surgery in patients with SAH is influenced by the severity of the bleed. Patients without neurologic deficits do well with early surgery, while those with large bleeds and deficits on presentation have significant edema, initially making a delay in surgery for 10–14 days desirable. However, early surgery allows aggressive therapy of resultant vasospasm. Use of endovascular coils is altering the approach.

DISCHARGE/FOLLOW-UP PLANS

Many of these patients will require rehabilitation, and all need close neurologic follow-up. Patients suffering a SAH remain at higher risk of recurrence, despite successful treatment by a neurosurgeon or radiologist. Thus, careful coordination of follow-up plans and treatment needs to occur prior to discharge. All patients should have appointments with their outpatient physicians arranged, and family or friends should be made aware of this to help ensure compliance.

Patient Education

Patients who smoke need aggressive counseling and help to quit. Blood pressure control is paramount, as modest reductions markedly reduce the recurrence of ICH. Additionally, among patients who suffered a SAH, it may be reasonable to screen first-degree relatives for cerebral aneurysms.

CONCLUSIONS

Intracerebral hemorrhage will remain an important medical issue as the population ages in this country. The focus for the hospitalist as part of the care team is to assist in the accurate diagnosis and most importantly to medically manage the patient following his or her initial cerebral insult. Controlling blood pressure, tight blood sugar management, seizure prevention, deep vein thrombosis prophylaxis, and maintaining intravascular volume remain the mainstays for hospitalist care of the patient with intracerebral hemorrhage.

Key Points

- Almost all seizures in patients with intracerebral hemorrhage occur at the onset of bleeding or within the first 24 hours of the event and are not predictive of the development of future seizure recurrence.

- Noncontrast CT is the diagnostic test of choice, but lumbar puncture should be performed in all patients suspected of subarachnoid hemorrhage who have a negative CT.

- Patients with a SAH should receive nimodipine and be carefully evaluated for the presence of vasospasm.

- Anticoagulated patients with an elevated INR require rapid correction of the INR to reduce the risk of continued intracerebral bleeding.

- Controlling blood pressure, tight blood sugar management, seizure prevention, deep vein thrombosis prophylaxis, and maintaining intravascular volume remain the mainstays for hospitalist care of the patient with intracerebral hemorrhage.

- Labetalol, and not nitroprusside, should be used to control high blood pressure.

SUGGESTED READING

Manno EM, Atkinson JLD, Fulgham JR, et al. Emerging medical and surgical management strategies in the evaluation and treatment of intracerebral hemorrhage. Mayo Clin Proc 2005; 80(3): 420–433.

Vermeer SE, Algra A, Franke CL, et al. Long-term prognosis after recovery from primary intracerebral hemorrhage. Neurology 2002; 59:205–209.

Qureshi AI, Tuhrim S, Broderick JP, et al. Medical progress: spontaneous intracerebral hemorrhage. N Engl J Med 2001; 344:1450–1460.

Mayer S, Rincon F. Treatment of intracerebral haemorrhage. Lancet Neurol 2005; 4:662–672.

Rinkel GJ, Feigin,VL, Algra A, et al. Calcium antagonists for aneurysmal subarachnoid haemorrhage. Cochrane Database Syst Rev 2005.

Wijdicks EF, Kallmes DF, Manno EM, et al. Subarachnoid hemorrhage: neurointensive care and aneurysm repair. Mayo Clin Proc 2005; 80:550–559.

Mayer SA, Brun NC, Begtrup K, et al. Recombinant activated factor VII for acute intracerebral hemorrhage. N Engl J Med 2005; 352:777–785.

Lacut K, Bressollette L, Le Gal G, et al. VICTORIAh (Venous Intermittent Compression and Thrombosis Occurrence Related to Intra-cerebral Acute hemorrhage) Investigators. Prevention of venous thrombosis in patients with acute intracerebral hemorrhage. Neurology 2005; 65(6):865–869.

Mendelow AD, Gregson BA, Fernandes HM, et al. STICH Investigators. Early surgery versus initial conservative treatment in patients with spontaneous supratentorial intracerebral haematomas in the International Surgical Trial in Intracerebral Haemorrhage (STICH): a randomized trial. Lancet 2005; 365:387–397.

Fernandes HM, Gregson B, Siddique S, et al. Surgery in intracerebral hemorrhage the uncertainty continues. Stroke 2000; 31:2511–2516.

CHAPTER NINETY-TWO

Coma

Chong-Sang Kim, MD, and Alpesh N. Amin, MD, MBA

BACKGROUND

Arousal and awareness of the self and the environment comprise consciousness. Varying stages of loss of consciousness (minimally conscious state, vegetative state, and coma) will be reviewed in this chapter. Coma, defined as an unarousable state of unresponsiveness with eyes closed, is an utter lack of consciousness. Rarely lasting longer than 2–4 weeks, coma may result from traumatic and nontraumatic brain injury.[1] The vegetative state (VS) is characterized by complete unawareness of the self and the environment with preserved arousal, sleep-wake cycles, and varying degrees of brainstem and hypothalamic autonomic function. VS may be persistent or transitory. VS evolves from coma, or may progress from degenerative and metabolic brain disorder or result from severe developmental brain malformation.[2,3] In the minimally conscious state (MCS), the patient shows depressed consciousness and inconsistent but reproducible behavior appropriate to the environmental cue. MCS follows coma or VS.[3,4]

Locked-in syndrome is differentiated from coma, VS, and MCS. Locked-in syndrome is a state of preserved arousal and awareness with anarthria (loss of the motor ability that enables speech) and complete paralysis, except for minimal eye movements. Brainstem stroke is the most common underlying cause; however, Landry-Guillain-Barré syndrome, myasthenia gravis, botulism, medication, or poisoning with neuromuscular paralyzing agents may present with a similar clinical picture.[1,4]

The Glasgow Coma Scale (GCS) measures the patient's response in motor function, speech, and eye opening[5] (Table 92-1). In following the course and predicting short-term outcome of coma, GCS, despite certain limitations,[6] compares very favorably with the more extensive Acute Physiology and Chronic Health Evaluation (APACHE) II and III.[7–9]

ASSESSMENT

Clinical Presentation

Prevalence

Traumatic brain injury (TBI) is a major cause of coma in the United States and abroad with an estimated average incidence of 150/100,000/year and a fatality rate of between 22 and 30/100,000/year in the United States. Young people between age 15 and 24 constitute the largest group of TBI-related coma, and males outnumber females by a factor of 2 or more.[6]

Nontraumatic coma may be due to hypoxia-ischemia, metabolic/toxic causes, sepsis, or intracranial structural lesion, including stroke. A quarter to one third of coma was drug-induced among teens and adults in reports of nontraumatic coma that included drug-induced etiology.[9,10] A study of nontraumatic coma, excluding the drug-induced etiology, found that hypoxic-ischemic cause was present in 31% and cerebral infarction or intracerebral hemorrhage in 36%.[11]

Presenting Signs and Symptoms

In the hospital setting, coma of either type may be present at admission or develop during hospitalization. The coma may result from worsening or complication of the patient's existing illnesses or from other causes such as cardiorespiratory arrest, cerebral infarction, intracranial hemorrhage, brainstem stroke, anaphylactic shock, septic shock, acute renal failure, status epilepticus, or medication or as a complication of anesthesia.[12]

Diagnosis

Following a rapid initial assessment and stabilization of respiration/oxygenation and circulation, the first order of diagnostic task should focus on the search for an underlying cause that needs to be addressed expeditiously in order to restore consciousness and/or minimize brain injury. (See Figure 92-1.)

History obtained by careful review of available patient records or interviews with family, friends, and/or medical personnel, frequently yields important diagnostic information. As a general rule, history is often helpful in establishing a cause, whereas physical signs point to the anatomical localization, depth of coma, or presence of increased intracranial pressure. Evaluation should include and document:

1. Breathing pattern
2. Lid and corneal reflex (symmetry or absence)
3. Eye movements on oculocephalic and oculovestibular reflex test
4. Pupil size/symmetry, pupillary light reflex
5. Fundoscopic eye examination

Table 92-1 Glasgow Coma Scale

Best Motor Response	
Obeys	M6
Localizes (to pain)	5
Withdraws (from pain)	4
Abnormal flexion	3
Extensor response	2
Nil	1
Verbal Response	
Oriented	V5
Confused	4
Inappropriate words	3
Incomprehensible sounds	2
Nil	1
Eye Opening	
Spontaneous	E4
To speech	3
To pain	2
Nil	1

6. Tonic neck reflex (when cervical spine fracture is not present)
7. Spontaneous or pain-induced upper and lower limb extensor or upper limb flexor posturing

Presence or absence of the pupillary light reflex correlates respectively with metabolic or structural coma.[1] In anoxic-ischemic coma, periodic stereotypical eye/eyelid movements, slow opening and closing of eyes, or rhythmic eyelid flutter with or without focal or generalized myoclonus accompany electroencephalographic periodic burst suppression discharges with a poor prognosis. In this situation, GCS is spuriously higher, or closer to normal, than the actual depth of coma.[13] Of note, extensor posturing may be present also in a metabolic or toxic coma.[14,15]

Some measures are simultaneously diagnostic and therapeutic, such as blood chemistry/toxicology followed by intravenous infusion of electrolytes, fluid, glucose, and pharmaceutical interventions such as flumazenil or naloxone.[16]

CT or MRI of the head is invaluable in most cases of coma of undetermined cause. For example, one might find epidural or subdural hematoma, mass, or brainstem pathology. In post-traumatic coma, special precaution is necessary before embarking on imaging studies due to the possibility of cervical spine fracture. Until absence of cervical spine fracture/injury has been confirmed, the C-spine should remain stabilized in the setting of trauma-related altered mental status. Spinal fluid examination is appropriate and indicated for suspected intracranial infection in the absence of contraindications to lumbar puncture, such as uncorrected coagulopathy or increased intracranial pressure due to a mass lesion.

Electroencephalography (EEG) provides insight into brain function in a manner not always available from clinical examination or structural imaging, and can be very helpful in diagnosing some cases of coma. EEG aids in diagnosis and treatment of status epilepticus and nonconvulsive status epilepticus. EEG also may help direct attention to a certain metabolic or infectious cause; for example triphasic delta waves in hepatic or renal encephalopathy; burst suppression pattern in posthypoxemic encephalopathy, heavy sedative medication, or prion disorder; and focal temporal rhythmic slow waves in herpes encephalitis.[17] If seizure is suspected as the etiology for coma, then obtaining evaluation with an EEG becomes critical, as status epilepticus requires urgent therapy to suppress the seizure activity.

Prognosis

TBI inducing a coma of GCS = 3 (no eye opening, and no verbal nor motor response), the lowest possible score, carries a mortality of approximately 80% and 8–10% functional survival.[18] Prognosis favors youth in coma from TBI.[18,19] Age is not a prognostic factor in nontraumatic coma.[20,21] A study of 188 patients older than 10 years with nontraumatic coma and initial GCS grade of 3–5, showed that 15% of the patients were awake at the end of 2 weeks and 85% dead or in persistent coma. For the group with GCS of 6–8, 53% were awake after 2 weeks while 47% were dead or in persistent coma. Hypoxic-ischemic coma had the worst 2-week outcome of 79% dead or comatose. Drug-induced coma had the most favorable outcome of 73% conscious at 2 weeks. Coma due to other causes was intermediate. Incorporation of the cause of coma into the GCS may improve its utility as a 2-week prognostic tool of coma outcome.[20]

A prospective study of 500 patients with nontraumatic, non–drug-induced coma lasting longer than 6 hours, found that all but one of those with absence of two of the following reflexes died on the first day: pupillary light, corneal, or oculocephalic/oculovestibular.[21] Based on the results of this study, a likelihood ratio nomogram using positive and negative predictive values of various physical signs of coma at 24 hours can provide a prognostic value[22] (see Table 92-2 and Fig. 92-2). For both traumatic and nontraumatic coma excluding drug-induced coma, GCS is also a fairly reliable prognostic tool for short-term survival[8,9] and, in TBI, the long-term functional recovery as measured by Glasgow Coma Outcome Scale (GCOS)[23] (Table 92-3). However, more recent research involving >20,000 patients raised questions of whether GCS is capable of discrimination of individual clinical prognostication and outcome prediction among patients suffering TBI.[24]

MRI, functional MRI, positron emission tomography (PET),[25] EEG, various evoked potential studies,[26] and CSF markers of brain injury[27] may complement but not supplant careful serial clinical assessment for prognostication. Abnormal brain-evoked responses in coma help in prediction of early poor outcome. Although helpful, the absence or presence of evoked responses or event-related brain potentials does not consistently predict degree of recovery of cognitive function having limited electrophysiological correlation with the complex and dynamic process of human cognitive process.[26]

An analysis of 596 patients with nontraumatic coma of GCS 9 or less for at least 6 hours demonstrated that those patients with high risk for poor outcome had a 2-month mortality rate of 93%. Implementation of a "Do Not Resuscitate" (DNR) order on the fourth day of coma for high-risk patients resulted in an incremental cost savings of $140,000 in 1998 dollars per quality-adjusted life-year without affecting the outcome.[11] The very poor prognosis of nontraumatic coma with low GCS and the cost may temper the enthusiasm of overly aggressive treatment efforts.

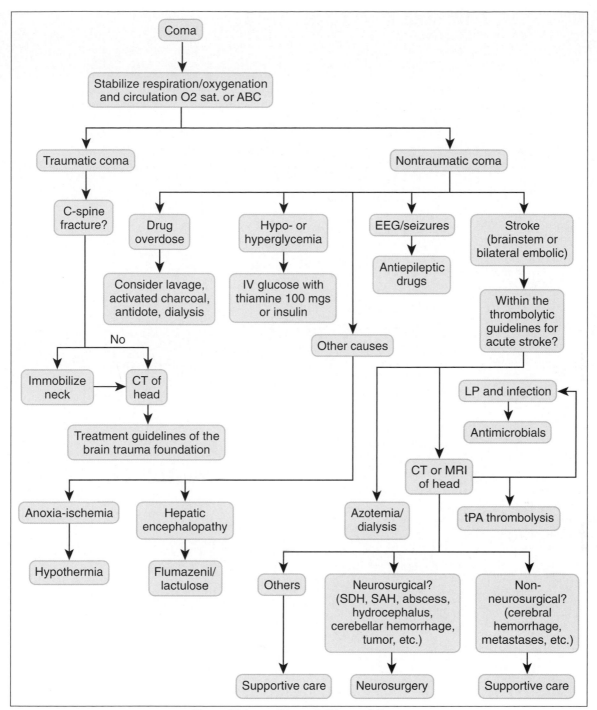

Figure 92-1 • Diagnostic Scheme of Coma.

Table 92-2 Data from Levy et al. Prognosis in Nontraumatic Coma. Ann of Intern Med 1981; 94(3):293. About Patients with Nontraumatic Coma of >6 hours' Duration (Excluding Drug-Induced Coma), Showing the Relation between Physical Signs at 24 Hours and Their Long-Term Outcome

	Severe disability or worse	Moderate or good recovery	Sensitivity	Specificity	Positive predicted value	Negative predicted value	Likelihood ratio (positive test)	Likelihood ratio (negative test)
Verbal response								
Incomprehensible or none	187	45	0.96	0.26	0.81	0.67	1.30	0.16
Orientated, confused, or inappropriate	8	16						
Eye opening response								
To pain/none	270	42	0.89	0.48	0.87	0.53	1.69	0.24
Spontaneous/to noise	34	38						
Pupillary light reflex								
Absent	78	1	0.26	0.99	0.99	0.26	20.59	0.75
Present	225	79						
Corneal reflex								
Absent	90	0	0.32	1.00	1.00	0.29	20*	0.68
Present	190	77						
Spontaneous eye movements								
Roving dysconjugate other or none	210	19	0.69	0.77	0.92	0.40	2.94	0.40
Orienting or roving conjugate	94	62						
Oculocephalic responses								
Abnormal/absent	292	61	0.96	0.24	0.83	0.59	1.26	0.18
Normal	13	19						
Oculovestibular responses								
Abnormal	265	45	0.96	0.32	0.85	0.64	1.40	0.14
Normal	12	21						
Motor responses (best limb)								
Flexion, extension or none	206	15	0.68	0.81	0.93	0.40	3.66	0.40
Obeying, localizing or withdrawing	98	66						
Deep tendon reflexes								
Absent	67	4	0.24	0.95	0.94	0.26	4.67	0.80
Present	213	74						
Skeletal muscle tone								
Absent	120	4	0.44	0.89	0.94	0.30	3.98	0.63
Present	155	74						

*Not able to calculate exactly

From Overell J, Bone I, Fuller GN. An aid to predicting prognosis in patients with non-traumatic coma at one day. J Neurol, Neurosurg Psychiatry 2001; 71:i24.

MANAGEMENT

Treatment

Coma Due to Traumatic Brain Injury

The Brain Trauma Foundation (BTF) published Guidelines for Severe Traumatic Brain Injury (those with GCS below 9),[18] which recommend the following (Figure 92-1):

1. Initial maintenance of systolic blood pressure above 90 mm Hg
2. Maintenance of airway and arterial O_2 saturation of at least 90% in the field or PaO_2 of 60 mm Hg
3. Intracranial pressure monitoring for certain groups of patients, preferably from the ventricles (guided by a neurosurgeon or neurointensivist)
4. Maintenance of cerebral perfusion pressure of 70 mm Hg
5. Intermittent hyperventilation for increased intracranial pressure keeping $PaCO_2 \geq 30$ mm Hg
6. Intermittent use of mannitol at 0.25 g/kg to 1 g/kg to reduce increased intracranial pressure while maintaining euvolemia and serum osmolarity of less than 320 m/Osm/L
7. Use of pentobarbital if refractory (at 10 mg/kg over 30 minutes, 5 mg/kg each hour for 3 doses, then 1 mg/kg/hr) to mannitol
8. Prophylactic anticonvulsant or carbamazepine for the first 7 days
9. Corticosteroid should not be used for treatment of coma due to TBI.[18]

Adherence to the BTF Guidelines resulted in a nine-fold improvement in outcomes (GCOS 4 and 5) relative to the odds of poor outcome in a historical comparison.[28]

Nontraumatic coma

After restoration and stabilization of adequate respiratory function and circulation, therapy should aim at the underlying etiology of coma. It may include:

1. Normalization of metabolic aberration (e.g., electrolytes,[29] acidosis,[30] hypo-[31] or hyperglycemia,[32] hyperammonemia,[33–35] hypothyroidism,[36] hyperthyroidism,[37] B_{12} deficiency,[38] hypopituitarism with secondary adrenal insufficiency,[29] azotemia)
2. Consideration of removal of ingested toxins or drugs with gastric lavage, activated charcoal, and use of therapy with reversal agents such as flumazenil[16] or naloxone
3. Thrombolytic therapy with tPA for acute cerebral infarction presenting within a 3-hour time window from the onset of symptoms[39]
4. Anticonvulsants for convulsive or nonconvulsive status epilepticus[17]

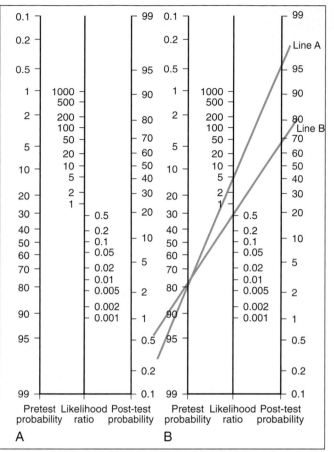

Figure 92-2 • Nomogram. The likelihood ratio (shown in bold type) is a useful way to use these probabilities clinically. The likelihood ratio of a positive test indicates the effect of the worse neurologic state while the likelihood ratio of a negative test indicates the effect of the better state on outcome.

Using Table 92-2 and the likelihood ratio nomogram, the effect of a negative or positive test can be appreciated. From the population of patients admitted in coma examined in one day, 79% have a poor outcome (305/385), so the pretest probability for a poor outcome is 79%. The likelihood ratio indicates the effect of the different elements of clinical examination. If, for example, their best motor response is flexion or worse (likelihood ratio of positive test is 3.66), then using a straight edge on the nomogram the post-test probability of a poor outcome is about 95% (Fig. 92-2B, line A). If, however, their best motor response is withdrawing or better (likelihood ratio of negative test is 0.4), the post-test probability of a poor outcome falls to about 60% (Fig. 92-2B, line B). As the signs are not independent of one another, the prognosis should be taken from the most informative sign rather than from combining the signs.

From Overell J, Bone I, Fuller GN. An aid to predicting prognosis in patients with non-traumatic coma at one day. J Neurol, Neurosurg Psychiatry 2001; 71:124; and Sackett, Straus, Richardson, et al. Evidence-Based Medicine. Toronto: Churchill Livingstone, 2000.

Table 92-3 Glasgow Coma Outcome Scale		
Good recovery	5	Regains normal life or to the previous level of function.
Moderate disability	4	Achieves independent activities in daily living but not the previous level of function.
Severe disability	3	Regains some cognitive function but depends on others for support.
Vegetative state	2	Awake but no sign of cognitive function.
No recovery	1	In coma till death.

5. Antimicrobial therapy for sepsis or meningitis/encephalitis
6. Neurosurgery consultation to assist with special measures and medications for subarachnoid or other intracranial hemorrhage, tumor, or abscess

Antiepileptic drugs (AEDs) in Convulsive or Nonconvulsive Status Epilepictus (SE)

Status epilepictus (SE) is defined as more than 30 minutes of continuous seizure activity or two or more sequential seizures without full recovery of consciousness between seizures.[40] Refractory SE (RSE) is defined as SE that fails to respond to first- and second-line AEDs.[41] RSE occurs in 9–31% of SE. Lorazepam is the preferred initial AED for SE. Diazepam may be substituted if lorazepam is not available. Phenytoin or fosphenytoin is the second AED in most situations.[42]

A systematic review of 28 published studies of RSE treated with midazolam, propofol, and pentobarbital noted 48% mortality. Continuous intravenous infusion of pentobarbital titrated to the suppression of the EEG background activity by use of intermittent EEG monitoring was associated with a lower frequency of breakthrough seizures and a higher incidence of hypotension. Midazolam and propofol were infused more often to titrate to suppress visible seizure activity rather than to suppress the EEG background activity in the published studies. A randomized, prospective, controlled study to compare efficacy of anticonvulsants for refractory status epilepticus is needed.[41]

Lorazepam is given 0.1 mg/kg at 2 mg/min initially to the maximum of 0.3 mg/kg. Lorazepam may be repeated every 2–3 hours at a lower dosage. Diazepam may be substituted as the initial AED at the dosage of 0.15 mg/kg and at the rate of 5 mg/min.[42] Phenytoin or fosphenytoin is the next AED in most hands at 20 mg/kg, with infusion rate of 50 mg/min. Although fosphenytoin may be given at a higher rate of infusion, our experience is that it can cause hypotension at the recommended infusion rate of 150 mg/min, especially in elderly patients. Maintenance dose is 1.5 mg/kg tid. Fosphenytoin has, if needed, the advantage of administration of intramuscular (IM) injection for maintenance.[42] If the patient has adequate IV access, phenytoin can be given and is much cheaper. Midazolam is administered at 0.2 mg/kg as the initial dose and maintained at 0.75 mcg-10 mcg/kg/min.[42] Propofol is given at 1–2 mg/kg and maintained at 2–15 mg/kg/hr. Both midazolam and propofol have a short half-life.[42] Pentobarbital is infused at 10–15 mg/kg as the initial dose and maintained at 0.5 mg/kg/hr.[42]

Intravenous valproate is emerging as an alternative AED for SE with fewer side effects. A retrospective study showed 77.1% control of seizure activity for 12 hours (27 out of 35 patients). The dosage used was 15 mg/kg over a time period of 30 minutes followed by an infusion rate of 1–2 mg/kg/hr over 12–24 hours.[43] If no agent controls RSE, general anesthesia may be warranted.[42]

Neuroprotective Agents in Anoxic-Ischemic Coma

Post anoxic-ischemic brain injury and its mitigation is the object of intense investigations, due to its prevalence and potential gravity. Human trials of neuroprotective agents have proved disappointing, including inhibitors of oxygen free radical generation, free radical scavengers, antagonists of excitatory amino acids, calcium channel blockers, nitric oxide synthase inhibitors, corticosteroids, monosialogangliosides, and growth factors.[44,45]

Hypothermia in Anoxic-Ischemic Coma

The International Liaison Committee on Resuscitation recommends that hypothermia of 32°C to 34°C be administered for 12 to 24 hours to adults with spontaneous circulation after cardiac arrest when the initial rhythm was ventricular fibrillation. The committee further states, "Such cooling may be beneficial for other rhythms or in-hospital cardiac arrest." Currently, there are insufficient data to recommend hypothermia for children who suffer cardiac arrest.[46] Sedation and neuromuscular blockade will prevent shivering and the resulting elevation of temperature.

Flumazenil in Drug-induced and Hepatic Coma

Despite anecdotal reports of successful use of flumazenil in intoxication with baclofen,[47] antihistamine,[48] gabapentin,[49] carisoprodol,[50] promethazine,[51] and alcohol,[52] no controlled study exists to attest to such efficacy except in benzodiazepine intoxication.[16]

A literature review of 12 randomized trials of 765 patients, found no significant effect on recovery or survival from hepatic encephalopathy but significant effect on short-term improvement of hepatic encephalopathy in some patients with chronic liver disease.[53,54] A meta-analysis of six double-blind randomized controlled trials including 641 patients concluded that flumazenil induces clinical and electroencephalographic improvement among patients with hepatic encephalopathy.[54]

For reversal of benzodiazepine-induced coma, 0.2 mg of flumazenil is infused intravenously over 30 seconds. After 30 seconds, another 0.3 mg of flumazenil may be given over 30 seconds. If the desired level of consciousness is not attained, 0.5 mg IV over 30 seconds at 1-minute intervals may be given to a cumulative dose of 3 mg. For resedation, a repeat 1 mg dose may be given at 20-minute intervals, not to exceed 3 mg at any given hour.

Naloxone in Opiate- and Other Drug-induced Coma

Anecdotal reports of efficacy of naloxone in ibuprofen,[55] valproate,[56] pentazocine,[57] and other drug overdose[58] exist in the literature. To reverse opiate overdose, naloxone is given 0.4–2 mg IV first and repeated every 2–3 minutes as needed, up to 10 mg of cumulative dose. If the patient is suspected of chronic narcotic abuse, the lower dose of 0.4 mg should be given to avoid severe narcotic withdrawal.

Vegetative State, Minimally Conscious State, and Brain Death

VS is classified as permanent after 3 months in a nontraumatic coma or after 12 months in traumatic coma.[59] MCS, especially after TBI, does not preclude ultimate moderate or good functional outcome with the passage of time and therapy.[3,60] Ethical, moral, religious, and legal issues of treatment remain controversial.[61] Least controversial may be the continuation of life support measures for a pregnant woman with a viable fetus until delivery when a surrogate decision-maker is in agreement.[62]

The concept and terminology of brain death are medically and legally accepted in the United States and abroad.[63] In the United States, the following requirements must be present:

1. *Prerequisites:* Proximate cause of the neurologic catastrophe is known and demonstrably irreversible and compatible with the clinical diagnosis of brain death, exclusion of confounding

conditions (no severe electrolyte, acid-base, or endocrine disturbance), no drug intoxication, and core temperature of 32°C or higher

2. *Evidence of coma:* No cerebral or motor response of cerebral origin to pain in all limbs and supraorbital pressure

3. *Absent brainstem reflexes:* No pupillary light reflex, no oculocephalic, oculovestibular reflex to 50 mL of cold water irrigation for 1 minute, no evidence of facial sensory and motor response (corneal reflex, jaw reflex, grimacing to deep pressure on nail bed, supraorbital ridge, or temporomandibular joint), and absence of gag and cough reflex

4. *Apnea:* Apnea during and after an adequate interval of no mechanical ventilation, typically for 8 minutes or longer, at the end of which $PaCO_2$ is at least 60 mm Hg or 20 mm Hg higher than the baseline normal $PaCO_2$[64]

In summary, traumatic and nontraumatic coma (excluding drug-induced) with the lowest GCS score carries mortality of 80%. In traumatic coma, adherence to the BTF Guidelines improves outcome. Hypothermia for anoxic-ischemic coma helps reduce the severity of brain injury. Flumazenil improves short-term outcome of hepatic coma. In nontraumatic coma, absence of corneal reflex and no withdrawal response to pain on the third day of coma foretell no recovery, vegetative state or severe disability. Controversy remains regarding the care of patients with vegetative or minimally conscious state.

Key Points

- Extensor posturing may be present in a metabolic or toxic coma and thus may be seen in a potentially reversible condition.

- Presence or absence of pupillary light reflex correlates respectively with metabolic or structural coma.

- Age is a prognostic factor in traumatic coma but not in nontraumatic coma.

- Adults suffering from coma due to cardiac arrest with spontaneous circulation after an initial rhythm of ventricular fibrillation benefit from hypothermia of 32–34°C if administered for 12 to 24 hours.

- Traumatic and nontraumatic coma (excluding drug-induced) with the lowest GCS score are associated with a mortality of 80%.

- Nontraumatic coma with absent corneal reflex and no withdrawal response to pain on the third day portends no recovery, vegetative state, or severe disability.

- EEG is essential in diagnosing and treating coma due to non-convulsive status epilepticus.

- Neuroimaging studies are essential in diagnosis and treatment of coma due to unknown cause or trauma

SUGGESTED READING

Plum F, Posner JB. The Diagnosis of Stupor and Coma. 3rd ed. New York: Oxford University Press, 1982.

Levy DE, Caronna JJ, Singer BH, et al. Predicting outcome from hypoxic-ischemic coma. JAMA 1985; 253(10):1420.

Practice parameters for determining brain death in adults (summary statement). The Quality Standards Subcommittee of the American Academy of Neurology. Neurology 1995; 45(5):1012–1014.

Practice parameters: assessment and management of patients in the persistent vegetative state (summary statement). The Quality Standards

Subcommittee of the American Academy of Neurology. Neurology 1995; 45(5):1015.

Practice Paraneters: prediction of outcome in comatose survivors after cardiopulmonary resuscitation (an evidence-based reviews). Neurology 2006; 67:203–210.

The Brain Trauma Foundation. The American Association of Neurological Surgeons. The Joint Section on Neurotrauma and Critical Care. Trauma Systems. J Neurotrauma 2000; 17(6):457. http://www2.braintrauma.org/guidelines/index.php.

Cooper PR, Goldfinos JG, eds. Head Injury. New York: McGraw-Hill, 2000.

Nolan JP, Morley PT, Vanden Hoek TL, et al. Therapeutic hypothermia after cardiac arrest: an advisory statement by the Advanced Life Support Task Force of the International Liaison Committee on Resuscitation. Circulation 2003; 108(1):118.

Goulenok C, Bernard B, Cadranel JF, et al. Flumazenil vs. placebo in hepatic encephalopathy in patients with cirrhosis: a meta-analysis. Aliment Pharmacol Ther 2002; 16(3):361.

Giacino W. The vegetative and minimally conscious states: current knowledge and remaining questions. J Head Trauma Rehabil 2005; 20(1):30.

Lowenstein DH. Treatment options for status epilepticus. Curr Opin Pharmacol 2005; 5(3):334.

Claassen J, Hirsch LJ, Mayer S, et al. Treatment of refractory status epilepticus with pentobarbital, propofol, or midazolam: a systematic review. Epilepsia 2002; 43(2):146.

Peters PE. Intravenous valproate as an innovative therapy in seizure emergency situations including status epilepticus: Experience in 102 adult patients. Seizure 2005; 14(3):164.

Overell J, Bone I, Fuller GN. An aid to predicting prognosis in patients with non-traumatic coma at one day. J Neurol Neurosurg Psychiatry 2001; 71(Suppl 1): i24–i25.

CHAPTER NINETY-THREE

Altered Mental Status: Delirium

Michael D. Wang, MD, Solomon Liao, MD, and Alpesh N. Amin, MD, MBA

BACKGROUND

Delirium in hospitalized patients remains largely under recognized. The implications for this under-recognition and the resultant under-treatment are: (1) prolongation of hospital stay, (2) increased complications, (3) unnecessary suffering by patients and their families, and (4) inappropriate disposition from the hospital. The heterogenous presentation of delirium contributes to this under-recognition. It can present with hypo- or hyperactive behavior or both. It can last a few hours or a few months. Additionally, the term "delirium" is not as commonly used or understood as hypertension and pneumonia, although it has specific descriptive criteria, well-described implications, and potential treatment. While the nomenclature for delirium is well defined, a host of alternative terms have been used—altered mental status, acute confusional state, metabolic encephalopathy, organic brain syndrome, ICU psychosis, sundowning. Though they appear to mean the same things, the lack of explicit and common criteria for these alternative terms render them less useful in the clinical setting.

Recognizing the delirious patient is critically important because of the possibility of serious underlying medical conditions that lead to this condition. An acute alteration of cognition may be considered the "fever" of the psychiatry examination. As opposed to patients with other confusional states, such as dementia, depression, and schizophrenia, delirium is the manifestation of an underlying acute medical problem and should be considered a medical emergency.

Delirium is the manifestation of a multifactorial assault on the vulnerable brain. The supply-demand model provides a conceptual framework for its pathophysiology. The more demands (or insults) on the brain, the less supply (cerebral reserve), the more likely this temporary cognitive dysfunction occurs. At the biochemical level, cerebral cholinergic deficiency is the leading theory, although abnormalities in lymphokines, serotonin, dopamine, cortisol, glutamate, and gamma-aminobutyric acid are also proposed.[2] An understanding of these frameworks is the basis for the evaluation and treatment of delirium.

ASSESSMENT

Clinical Presentation

Prevalence and Presenting Signs and Symptoms

Delirium is common in elderly hospitalized patients. Studies suggest that delirium is present in 10% of patients in the emergency department[3] and in 10–25% of older patient upon admission. Another 5–10% of patients develop delirium subsequently during the admission.[1] Delirium occurs on average in 37% of elderly postoperative patients. Occurrence is as high as 70–80% of ICU patients.[7] The fact that up to one in four medical patients and one in three surgical patients may have or develop delirium makes this a critical topic for the adult hospitalist.

History-taking should focus on gathering the information needed to make the diagnosis. Based on the Diagnostic and Statistical Manual of Mental Disorders (DSM-IV) criteria (Box 93-1), the hospitalist should look for: (1) an acute change in cognition; (2) a disturbance of consciousness; (3) a perceptual disturbance, associated with reduced ability to focus, sustain, or shift attention; and (4) an underlying medical cause. Because the patient's confusion precludes a reliable history from the patient, the clinician will need to gather information from collateral sources, such as family members, caregivers, or nursing staff. These informants who have been with the patient for hours to days will often report that the patient is acutely confused, disoriented, not the same person, out of it, more irritable, sleepy, or lethargic. A change in usual function or behavior is often noted. Clues to recent changes in behavior include a recent fall, new incontinence, poor appetite, or new noncompliance with the care plan. The patient may be noted even to mistake caregivers for other people, or unfamiliar objects for threatening ones. Identifying a fluctuation in the course of the patient's behavior and cognition provides further confirmation of the diagnosis of delirium.

While third-party informants will generally volunteer the above information, the physician needs to probe for further data on history. Family members or caregivers often do not recall or identify hallucinations and delusion unless specifically asked,

Table 93-1 Confusion Assessment Method

I and 2 Required, Plus Either 3 or 4	CAM	CAM-ICU
1. Acute onset, fluctuating course	Behavior fluctuation	Changes on RASS or GCS
2. Inattention	Easily distractible, difficulty keeping track	Attention screening Examination (visual recall of 5 pictures and A test of 10 letters)
3. Disorganized thinking	Rambling, irrelevant conversation, illogical flow of ideas	>50% of yes-no questions wrong, and inability to follow visual and verbal commands of holding up 2 fingers
4. Altered level of consciousness	Hyperalert to comatose	Hyperalert to comatose

Data from: Inouye SK, van Dyck CH, Alessi CA, et al. Clarifying confusion: The confusion assessment method. Ann Intern Med 1990; 113:941–948; and Ely W, Inouye SK, Bernard GR, et al. Delirium in Mechanically Ventilated patients. JAMA 2001; 286:2703–2710.
CAM—confusion assessment method; RASS—Richmond Agitation-Sedation Scale; GCS—Glasgow Coma Scale.
http://www.icudelirium.org/delirium/training-pages/CAM-ICU%20trainingman.2005.pdf

---

Box 93-1 DSM IV Criteria for Delirium

Criterion A: Impairment of ability to focus, sustain, or shift attention

Criterion B: Change in cognition or perception

Criterion C: Acute change over hours to days and fluctuation over the course of the day

Criterion D: Due to a general medical condition, substance intoxication or withdrawal, or other

---

though these findings are common in delirium and support the diagnosis. Determining the sequence of signs of delirium such as sundowning and the characteristics of the sleep-wake cycle disturbance is key to timing potential pharmacologic regimens. Review of the patient's medications should focus on recent changes as well as drugs for which levels can be checked. A thorough review of systems (e.g., fever, chest pain, headache), a good social history (e.g., alcohol consumption), and review of medications (looking for anticholinergics and sedatives) including compliance help the physician to identify the underlying medical cause.

On physical examination, the clinician should focus on testing the patient's sensorium and looking for the underlying medical cause. The patient may appear restless, fidgety, uncooperative or withdrawn, sedate, or depressed in affect. Although the patient may answer close-ended questions without apparent difficulty, the patient will require frequent redirection or repeat questioning to ascertain more complex details. These patients often fall asleep during the interview when not stimulated. They may have trouble recalling details of their history or trouble finding their words.

Cognitive testing should focus on attention. While the Mini-Mental State Examination (MMSE) is a screening test for Alzheimer's dementia, it includes elements useful to the diagnosis of delirium, such as tests of attention, spelling a word backwards (WORLD), and subtracting backward in decrements (serial 7's). Other tests of attention include serial 3's, counting from 20 to 1 backward, recounting the days of the week or months of the year backward. The most basic attention tests are the digit span and the A test. In the forward digit span, the patient is given a random set of numbers and asked immediately to repeat them. A normal person should be able to do a 7-digit span (the digits in a telephone number). A digit span below 5 is abnormal. Utilizing the A test can be useful, where the patient is asked to

indicate (with a raised hand or finger) when he hears the letter A, but not upon any other letter.

Differential Diagnosis

The differential diagnoses for delirium include dementia, mood disorders, schizophrenia, and other psychotic disorders. What separates delirium from these other conditions is its acute onset and the secondary nature (i.e., delirium reverses when the underlying cause is removed). While dementia, depression, and substance abuse are risk factors for the development of delirium, these disorders can be distinguished from delirium through careful history and physical examination. Dementia, for example, is of gradual onset over a time frame of months to years, without fluctuations and without attention deficits until its severe stages. Affective disorders may have overlapping symptoms, such as hallucinations and paranoid delusions, but have prominent mood features and do not have characteristic attention disturbances or fluctuations in cognition. Nevertheless, 40% of psychiatric referrals for depression in the hospital turn out to be a different diagnosis, often being delirium.

Diagnosis

Preferred Studies

As important a syndrome as delirium is, the literature suggests poor sensitivity of health care professionals for detection of delirium. Accurate detection has been documented by only 35% of emergency personnel,[3] 19% of inpatient nursing,[4] and 27% of inpatient medical physicians. Delirium by its nature fluctuates in its course, making single daily physician visits suboptimal for its detection and characterization. Patients' typically poor sleep patterns in the hospital confounds mental status assessment in the early morning; hospitalists' ability to round more than once during the day is an advantage in heightened detection of delirium. Gross assessment for level of alertness and orientation may mislead. One study suggested a good specificity at 95–100%, but only a poor 50% sensitivity for delirium using level of consciousness alone as an indicator. Orientation, on the other hand, showed a sensitivity of 88–90%, but a specificity of 55–80%.[6]

The Confusion Assessment Method, CAM (Table 93-1) is an easy-to-administer, validated tool, developed for both the inpatient ward and ICU settings. The sensitivity and specificity in the original study were 94–100% and 90–95%, respectively,

> **Box 93-2 Potential Causes of Delirium**[22]
>
> - Drugs and drug withdrawal
> - Eye and ear problems
> - Low oxygen states
> - Infection, indwelling bladder catheter
> - Retention (urine, stool, physical restraints)
> - Intracranial process (e.g., postictal state, trauma, subdural, stroke, infection)
> - Undernutrition and under-hydration
> - Metabolic derangements
> - Sleep deprivation

when compared to the gold standard of psychiatry consultation.[6] The CAM-ICU is adapted for intubated, critically ill patients and yielded sensitivities of 93–100% and specificities of 98–100%.[7] See Appendix 3.

Because delirium is a clinical diagnosis, no tests are definitive. An electric encephalogram may show diffuse slowing of brain waves, which will be interpreted by the neurologist as a "metabolic encephalopathy." Brain imaging, such as computed tomography (CT) and magnetic resonance imaging (MRI), are low yield in neurologically nonfocal patients. Lumbar punctures are rarely indicated, unless there is suspicion for a central nervous system (CNS) infection or inflammatory disorder.

Risk Factors and Causes

Delirium can be understood as an accumulation of substantial risk factors of the brain with additional insults triggering an episode of delirium. Elie et al.[3] performed a systematic review of risk factors with statistically significant odds ratios. This list included age, dementia, medical illness, male gender, depression, alcohol, abnormal sodium and potassium, dehydration, hearing impairment, visual impairment, and diminished activities of daily living. Undertreated pain appears to be a greater risk factor for delirium than opioid use.[17]

The diagnosis of delirium is linked by definition to an underlying medical problem, and therefore ascertaining the underlying causes becomes an essential part of the diagnostic workup. The list for putative causes of delirium is extensive and basically includes many medical problems and medications. Box 93-2 lists potential precipitating causes.[22] Common causes in the elderly patient are infections (pulmonary or urinary), medications, ischemia (cardiac more commonly than CNS), and metabolic abnormalities (including electrolytes). Medication culprits are most commonly drugs with anticholinergic activity and sedative properties (e.g., diphenhydramine [Benadryl]).

Prediction Rules

Prediction rules are available for diagnosing delirium in medical and surgical patients. Research suggests that interventions may be more helpful at preventing delirium than reducing the length or severity of delirium after its onset. Therefore, an important underappreciated helpful clinical approach is to identify high-risk patients and install aggressive preventive measures so as to avoid the development of delirium. Inouye et al.[6] developed and validated a model incorporating the predisposing baseline

vulnerability of a patient juxtaposed with precipitating insults.[9] In her model, baseline risk factors included visual impairment, severe illness, cognitive impairment, and blood urea nitrogen (BUN)/creatinine ratio of 18 or greater. Precipitants were use of physical restraints, malnutrition, use of bladder catheter, more than three medications added, and any iatrogenic event. The number of predisposing factors and precipitating factors correlated with risk for developing delirium. Utilizing just the precipitating factors, low risk (no factors present) predicted a risk of <5%. High risk (three or more precipitants) predicted a 35% risk. These concepts can also be applied to preoperative risk assessment. In the elective vascular surgery model developed by Marcantonio et al.,[11] age 70 or older, alcohol abuse, cognitive impairment, physical impairment, abnormal electrolytes, and aneurysm or thoracic surgery predicted risk similarly to Inouye's model. Three or more of these features predicted a 50% risk.

Prognosis

During Hospitalization

Delirium is a marker of higher mortality risk,[16] as it is associated with being seriously ill. Inhospital complications associated with delirium include increased length of stay, increased iatrogenic complications, functional decline, cognitive decline, and higher rate of long-term care placement in these frail and elderly patients. Traditionally, delirium is thought to be a reversible syndrome that reverses with correction of the underlying medical problems over a timeframe of days to weeks. However, the reality is that in 15–25% of cases, the underlying medical problem is not discovered in the hospital, and in many cases where the medical problem is resolved, the delirium is not immediately reversed.[1]

Post Discharge

Even when the underlying cause is reversed in the hospital, follow-up studies of patients show that many do not return back to their baseline mental status for months or even a year.[5] Patients who develop delirium in the hospital are much more likely to develop dementia and overall have greater functional decline and higher mortality rates. Persistent (beyond 1 month) hypoactive delirium in both hospital and nursing home patients with dementia is related to an even poorer prognosis that should prompt a consideration of referral to hospice.

Terminal delirium is common at the end of life and portends a prognosis of days. Delirium occurs in up to 80% of hospice patients during their last days of life.[15,22] This type of delirium is a common final pathway for dying patients and may serve to protect them from being aware of their pain and suffering.

MANAGEMENT

Treatment

Preferred

Nonpharmacologic interventions are preferred over pharmacologic ones. Treatment of delirium focuses on removing or minimizing the insults and precipitants, modifying the consequences of adverse behavior, and facilitating optimal rehabilitation. Interventions depend on the behavior. For those with the hypoactive form, routine repositioning, early mobilization, consultation with physical and occupational therapy, and higher vigilance for subtle medical problems can help reduce complications. For those with hyperactive form, the risks include falls, injuries from iatrogenic tethers (e.g., indwelling bladder catheters), and even physical injury to staff and patient. Low beds, minimizing iatrogenic devices (e.g., minimizing side-rails and physical restraints), increasing nursing continuity and attention (e.g., bed near nursing station, one-to-one nursing observation), and increased family presence may be helpful. A constant reorientation and a calm, soothing environment that avoids extremes of understimulation or overstimulation is the best setting of care.

Careful medication review is important, looking specifically to stop medications with anticholinergic and CNS-affecting properties, as well as for medications recently started or stopped. Antipsychotics are considered first-line pharmacotherapy (except in delirium tremens, where benzodiazepines are preferred) for adjuvant management of potentially dangerous behavior. Several antipsychotics have supportive data, and there are probably no differences in efficacy among them.[18] Initial drug doses of oral medications include haloperidol at 0.5–1 mg every 4–6 hours as needed, risperidone 0.25–0.5 mg twice daily, olanzapine 2.5–5 mg nightly, or quetiapine 25 mg three times daily. Routine low-dose antipsychotics can be given a few hours before anticipated sundowning. Administration of large doses of an as-needed antipsychotic or a sedative late at night or early morning can perpetuate the sleep-wake cycle disturbance. Physical restraints can worsen delirium and should be used only for a few hours on an agitated patient to buy time while medications take effect. For patients unable to swallow, the dissolvable olanzapine or risperidone formulations are options. A parenteral as-needed dose can be given as backup (e.g., haloperidol 0.5–1 mg IM or IV q 4–6 hr). Extrapyramidal symptoms are probably rare with the atypical antipsychotic agents, since patients with delirium already have a deficiency in cholinergic activity and because the antipsychotic doses used are generally low and for short term. The more concerning short-term adverse effects include sedation, orthostasis, QT interval prolongation, risk of neuroleptic malignant syndrome, and lowering of seizure threshold. Of note, cumulative data suggest an association with increased mortality in elderly patients with dementia on longer-term use of atypical antipsychotics.

Alternative Options

Except in the case of alcohol-related delirium, benzodiazepines should be only used after an antipsychotic is on board and additional sedation is necessary. Benzodiazepines can cause a "paradoxical response," because they disinhibit the frontal lobe. If a benzodiazepine is to be used, low doses of a short-acting one is preferable (e.g., lorazepam [Ativan], 0.5 mg).

For refractory delirium in end-stage patients that causes distress, palliative sedation is an ethically reasonable option. This sedation can be achieved with a midazolam infusion (intravenous or subcutaneous) or phenobarbital or pentobarbital given enterally (including rectal) or parenterally. For more information on palliative sedation, please see Chapter 95 on Palliative Care.

PREVENTION

Clinical trials support multifaceted interventions that can reduce delirium incidence. Interventions that appear to work for medical patients involve alterations of the care process to minimize psy-

choactive medications and optimize sleep, reduce sensory deprivation, and increase physical function, hydration, and cognitive orientation.[13,14] Catheters, tubes, telemetry, pulse oximeters, and pneumatic compression stockings should be minimized. Optimizing nursing continuity and education also maybe helpful. Marcantonio's 2001 study in the *Journal of the American Geriatric Society*[12] showed that routine preoperative geriatric medicine consultation may reduce the incidence of delirium in inherently high-risk hip fracture patients.

DISCHARGE/FOLLOW-UP PLANS

Patient/Family Education

Education of family members and the support system is paramount to ongoing cognitive and physical rehabilitation. Patients are at risk for ongoing cognitive impairment that can impede self-management expected of patients upon discharge. If the patient goes home, family members or caregivers should be instructed to be vigilant for medication compliance, new symptoms of illness, falls, and adequate nutrition and hydration. Home health care should be considered. However, since most patients with delirium are sent to a rehabilitative setting, families should be educated about the duration, reversibility, and prognosis of the delirium. Hospice should be offered for patients with terminal delirium or persistent delirium with poor prognosis.

Outpatient Physician Communication

If antipsychotics are initiated in the hospital, the reason should be clearly documented and communicated to the primary care physician, so that the drug can be reevaluated or stopped at 5–7 days after resolution of symptoms. Given the risk for persistent cognitive symptoms, careful cognitive follow-up and consideration for subspecialty referral (geriatrics, psychiatry, or neurology) are recommended.

Key Points

- Delirium is common, but underdetected in older hospitalized patients, occurring in 10–25% of medical patients, a third of surgical patients, and higher in ICU settings.

- Attention, a core feature of delirium, can be tested by digit span, serial 7's or 3's, spelling backward, and the A test.

- The differential diagnosis of delirium includes dementia, depression, schizophrenia, and other psychotic disorders.

- Treatment of delirium focuses on treating the underlying causes and minimizing the consequences of delirium behavior.

- In cases of necessity to prevent injurious behavior, chemical restraints are preferred over physical ones, and antipsychotics are preferred over benzodiazepines.

- Best preventive interventions have a multidisciplinary, comprehensive approach involving nursing, physical therapy, occupational therapy, and geriatrics-trained physicians.

SUGGESTED READING

Marcantonio ER, Flacker JM, Wright RJ, et al. Reducing delirium after hip fracture: a randomized trial. J Am Geriatr Soc 2001; 49:516–522.

Inouye SK, Bogardus ST Jr, Charpentier PA, et al. A multicomponent intervention to prevent delirium in hospitalized older patients. N Engl J Med 1999; 340:669–676.

Marcantonio ER, Simon SE, Bergmann MA, et al. Delirium symptoms in post-acute care: prevalent, persistent, and associated with poor functional recovery. J Am Geriatr Soc 2003; 51:4–9.

Lundstrom M, Edlund A, Karlsson S, et al. A multifactorial intervention program reduces the duration of delirium, length of hospitalization, and mortality in delirious patients. J Am Geriatr Soc 2005; 53:622–628.

Ely EW, Inouye SK, Bernard GR, et al. Delirium in mechanically ventilated patients: validity and reliability of the confusion assessment method for the intensive care unit (CAM-ICU). JAMA 2001; 286:2703–2710.

Weber JB, Coverdale JH, Kunik ME. Delirium: current trends in prevention and treatment. Intern Med J 2004; 34:115–121.

Mitchell SL, Kiely DK, Hamel MB, et al. Estimating prognosis for nursing home residents with advance dementia. JAMA 2004; 291:2734–2740.

Morrison RS, Magaziner J, Gilbert M, et al. Relationship between pain and opioid analgesics on the development of delirium following hip fracture. J Gerontol A Biol Med Sci 2003; 58:76–81.

CHAPTER NINETY-FOUR

Pain Management of the Hospitalized Patient

David J. Axelrod, MD, JD

BACKGROUND

Pain is a common finding and a major cause of suffering in the hospitalized patient. Pain, an unpleasant perceptual experience, occurs with actual or potential tissue damage.[1] With few reliable objective criteria to quantify it, one must listen to the patient to assess pain effectively and to evaluate response to therapy. For the hospitalist who is meeting a patient in a hospital setting without an established prior relationship, a patient in pain presents significant challenges.

Prior to 1960, there was only one textbook on pain and no pain journals or pain societies. Today, the assessment and treatment of pain receive increased attention. The Joint Commission (previously known as the Joint Commission on Accreditation of Healthcare Organization or JCAHO) recently mandated standards for pain management,[2] and the American Pain Society advocates using pain as "the fifth vital sign."[3] Treating pain not only relieves the suffering of patients, but it also improves health outcomes. Studies confirm that high levels of symptom distress are associated with a diminished quality of life, a decreased satisfaction with inpatient care,[2-4] delayed discharge, and an increased likelihood for increased level of care after discharge,[5] all of which result in higher health care expenditures.

ASSESSMENT

Clinical Presentation

Prevalence

Pain affects the majority of hospitalized patients, with studies indicating that 52–74% of patients on medical wards or medical surgical units experience pain.[6,7] Chronic pain is also quite prevalent, affecting 20% of Americans or about 30 million people.[8] It is therefore important to screen for pain at every hospital visit, particularly in postoperative patients, where the prevalence of pain is higher.

Presenting Signs and Symptoms

Although pain is a subjective experience, some physical signs indicate pain. These include facial grimacing, tachycardia, and hypertension. Although it is important to assess for signs of pain, these signs are not required for a diagnosis due to their poor sensitivity and specificity. Patients may experience severe pain without physical signs. One should attempt to objectively rate a patient's subjective pain, using one or more of the conventional pain measurement scales. Conducting a pain assessment at each visit helps to diagnose pain and to determine response to treatment.

The reporting of pain by patients using simple scales of intensity with a numeric rating provides vital information to evaluate response to analgesic therapy.[9] The visual analog scale (VAS) is used to give a subjective numerical value to the patient's rating of pain. The VAS rating should be charted along with vital signs. For more in-depth evaluation, a variety of measurements scales are used. The Wong-Baker FACES Pain Rating Scale (Fig. 94-1) enables one to quantify pain based on facial expression. A disease-specific measure such as the McGill Pain Assessment Questionnaire (MPQ) helps to determine functionality. The VAS and MPQ are the most commonly used self-rating instruments in clinical and research settings.[10]

Differential Diagnosis

Pain can be a symptom of many different illnesses. Pain can be categorized into four primary types: nociceptive, inflammatory, neuropathic, and functional[11] (Fig. 94-2) (Table 94-1). Nociceptive pain includes acute pain from trauma or surgery and some chronic pain such as arthritis and cancer pain. It is usually finite and localized and subsides with healing or removal of the noxious substance.[12] Nociceptive pain serves a protective function by alerting the body to the occurrence of tissue damage. Neuropathic pain is associated with disease or injury of the peripheral or central nervous system, and it manifests in medical conditions such as diabetic neuropathy, trigeminal neuralgia, postherpetic neuralgia, and spinal cord injury.[13] The patient with neuropathic pain will typically have both paresthesias and dysesthesias.[14] Inflammatory pain is a spontaneous and hypersensitive response to tissue damage and inflammation.[15] Functional pain results from an abnormal central processing of sensory input.[17] If there is a suspicion that a patient falsely claims to have pain, one should consider malingering, psychiatric illness, substance dependence, and addiction in the differential diagnosis. Of note, physicians should not leap to suspecting the patient is falsifying his or her complaints, but initially assume the pain is real. Correctly classifying the type of pain helps to tailor the most beneficial treatment and identify the underlying pathology. See Table 94-2.

Figure 94-1 • Wong-Baker FACES Pain Rating Scale.
From: Hockenberry MJ, Wilson D, Winkelstein ML.
Wong's Essentials of Pediatric Nursing, 7th ed. St. Louis:
Elsevier, 2005; 1259.

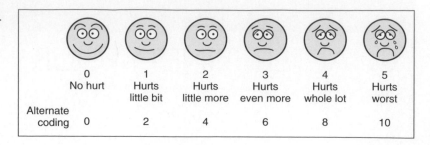

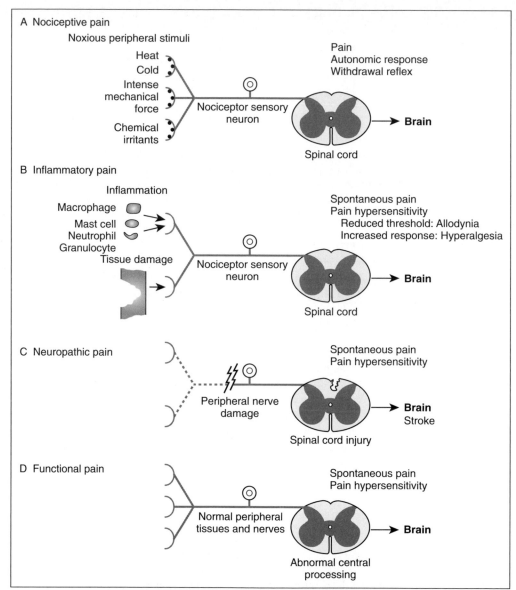

Figure 94-2 • The Four Primary Types of Pain. From: Woolf CJ. Pain: moving from symptom control toward mechanism-specific pharmacologic management. Ann Intern Med 2004; 140:442–451.

Diagnosis

The diagnosis of pain is a clinical one, based predominantly on patient history. Physical examination, pertinent labs, and certain studies provide some diagnostic value. As there usually are no objective signs to indicate the diagnosis of pain, and some patients may be unable to verbalize their pain, physicians must elicit this complaint. It is crucial to give credence to patient reports of pain. Unfortunately, complaints of pain are often dismissed or minimized by physicians and nurses.

A pain history includes the character of the pain, the intensity, the location, aggravating and alleviating factors, and

Table 94-1 Etiologies of Pain

Nociceptive Pain	Neuropathic Pain	Inflammatory Pain	Functional Pain
Arthropathies	AIDS neuropathy	Rheumatoid arthritis	Irritable bowel syndrome
Burns	Chemotherapy neuropathy	Surgery	Fibromyalgia
Infarction	Diabetic neuropathy	Trauma	Noncardiac chest pain
Inflammation	Postamputation		Tension-type headache
Myalgia	Multiple sclerosis		Abnormal response of nervous system
Myofascial pain	Spinal stenosis		
Polymyalgia rheumatica	Complex regional pain syndrome		
Sickle cell pain	Regional pain syndrome		
	Phantom limb pain		
	Postherpetic neuralgia		
	Trigeminal neuralgia		
	Parkinson's disease		
	Spinal cord injury		
	Post stroke pain		

Table 94-2 Pain Terms Plus Definitions from the Published IASP List of Pain Terms

Pain Term	Definition
Allodynia	Pain due to a stimulus that does not normally provoke pain
Causalgia	A syndrome of sustained burning pain, allodynia, and hyperpathia after a traumatic nerve lesion, often combined with vasomotor or pseudomotor dysfunction and later trophic changes
Central pain	Pain initiated or caused by a primary lesion of dysfunction in the central nervous system
Dysesthesia	An unpleasant abnormal sensation, whether spontaneous or evoked
Hyperalgesia	An increased response to a stimulus that is normally painful
Hyperpathia	A painful syndrome characterized by an abnormally painful reaction to a stimulus, especially a repetitive stimulus, as well as an increased threshold
Neuralgia	Pain in the distribution of a nerve or nerves
Neuropathic pain	Pain initiated or caused by a primary lesion or dysfunction in the nervous system
Noxious stimulus	A noxious stimulus is one that is damaging to nerves
Parasthesia	An abnormal sensation, whether spontaneous or evoked
Peripheral neuropathic pain	Pain initiated or caused by a primary lesion or dysfunction in the peripheral nervous system

From: Mersky H, Bogduk N, eds. Classification of Chronic Pain: Descriptions of Chronic Pain Syndromes and Definitions of Pain Terms. 2nd ed Seattle: IASP Press, 1994.

associated signs and symptoms. If a patient complains of pain, it is important to clarify the anatomical site of pain, the onset of pain, and any temporal relationships. A careful physical examination with palpation of the pertinent areas can help localize areas of pain.

For cognitively impaired patients who may not be able to give a history, observation for certain signs can be helpful. These include nonverbal cues and behaviors, vocalizations, facial expressions, and change in behavior.[18] If examination of a patient reveals localized areas of pain, further diagnostic studies such as x-ray, ultrasound, CT, or MRI may be indicated to rule out underlying pathology.

MANAGEMENT

The goal of treating pain is to alleviate symptoms and to give the patient an improved quality of life. Complete eradication of pain

may not always be a realistic or necessary goal of treatment. Treating pain involves several different modalities, including medical management, procedural interventions, and nonpharmacologic methods.

Medical management remains the mainstay in hospital treatment of pain. Analgesics fall into three main categories: nonopioids, opioids, and adjuvant medications. The world health organization (WHO) developed a three-step analgesic guide to the medical management of pain.[19] The ladder, although not validated, is a well-used instrument and a standard tool for treatment of any pain (Fig. 94-3).

For mild pain, treating with acetaminophen or a nonsteroidal anti-inflammatory (NSAID) is the first step. Acetaminophen is generally a safe medication but must be used cautiously in patients who have liver disease or drink excessive alcohol. The maximum dose of acetaminophen is 1 g per day. If pain is associated with inflammation, NSAIDs present a good option (Table

94-3). Their use is limited by a ceiling effect on pain treatment and by toxicities, especially gastrointestinal complications. Therefore, prescribers should implement preventive strategies, such as taking the medication with food and using H_2 blockers or proton pump inhibitors. At this time, use of COX-2 inhibitors should be reserved for situations when traditional NSAIDs are contraindicated. Ketorolac (Toradol) is the only NSAID available for parenteral use. Use of ketorolac should be limited to 5 days, but it is a good option to spare the use of opioids. Renal toxicities are also a concern with the use of NSAIDs. High doses of NSAIDs can cause acute renal failure, especially among elderly patients; for patients with underlying chronic renal insufficiency, NSAIDs should be avoided.

Historically, adjuvant pain medications were agents that had primary indications other than for pain but were often employed to augment pain treatments. Now, many of these medications are used primarily for analgesia. Good evidence supports use of some adjuvant medications as analgesics; for others, the evidence is evolving. The most common application of adjuvant pain medications is in pain syndromes that are difficult to manage with conventional analgesia.

Neuropathic pain, which is often unresponsive to typical analgesic medications, often responds to adjuvant medications. Medications used for neuropathic pain include antiepileptics, antiarrhythmics, corticosteroids, and antidepressants.[20] Gabapentin (Neurontin) is the adjuvant pain medication typically used first line for neuropathic pain. It should be started at a dose of 300 mg/day the first day, and titrated up to a maximum of 1,200 mg 3 times a day. Pregabalin (Lyrica) appears to inhibit release of excitatory neurotransmitters, including some involved in pain (substance P and glutamate) and purportedly requires less titration than gabapentin while demonstrating effectiveness within 1 week. Doses of 50 mg TID increased to 100 mg TID over 7 days result in sustained relief from neuropathic pain. Antidepressants, particularly tricyclics,[21] also have demonstrated efficacy with neuropathic pain.[22] Amitriptyline is started at 25 mg/day and increased by 25 mg a day to a maximum dose of 300 mg a day. Venlafaxine and duloxetine, SNRI antidepressants, are particularly effective for diabetic neuropathic pain.[23]

Scant evidence supports the use of benzodiazepines for treating pain. They may in fact exacerbate pain and have the potential to lead to cognitive impairment and physical and psychological dependence. There may be a role for treatment of acute muscle spasm and neuropathic pain with longer-acting benzodiazepines such as clonazepam.[24] In a preliminary case series, clonazepam has successfully treated cancer-related neuropathic pain.[25]

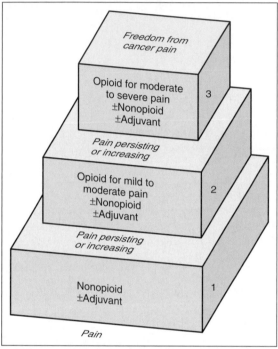

Figure 94-3 • WHO Analgesic Ladder. From: World Health Organization. Cancer Pain Relief and Palliative Care: Report of a WHO Expert Committee. Geneva, Switzerland: World Health Organization, 1990. Technical report series 804.

Table 94-3 Pharmacologic Dosing of Non-Opioid Medications			
Drug	**Usual Analgesic Dose**	**Dose Interval**	**Maximum Daily Dose**
Acetaminophen	500–1000 mg	4–6 hours	4000 mg
NSAIDs			
Aspirin	500–1000 mg	4–6 hours	4000 mg
Ibuprofen	400 mg	4–6 hours	2400 mg
Indomethacin	25 mg	8–12 hours	200 mg
Ketorolac	Age < 65: 30 mg IM/IV	6 hours	120 mg
	Age > 65: 15 mg IM/IV		60 mg (limit use to 5 days only)
Naproxen	500 mg initially then		1250 mg first day then
	250 mg or	6–8 hours	1000 mg
	500 mg	12 hours	
Meloxicam	7.5 mg daily	24 hours	15 mg per day

Opioids

Opioids are well established as effective and safe for treating both acute and chronic pain[26] of both nociceptive and neuropathic origins.[27] Opioids exert their pain-relief effects by binding to the μ opioid receptor. However, there is large individual variation in response to opioids.[28] Opioids, unlike NSAIDs, do not have a dose-related ceiling, and dose escalation is limited only by adverse effects.[29] The numerous administration options for opioids (oral, transmucosal, IV/IM, transdermal, rectal, intrathecal, intranasal, and subcutaneous infusion) provide considerable flexibility.[29]

When initiating opioid therapy, start treatment with short-acting opioids, and titrate the dose to achieve satisfactory analgesia without adverse effects. Respiratory depression can occur when excessive doses are given. However, respiratory depression rarely occurs in a patient who has pain, and concern for this complication should not prevent appropriate use of opioids.[30]

Morphine represents a common first choice, as it is the most studied and most used of the opioids. The initial dose is 5–15 milligrams orally or intravenously. However, in the elderly and in the opioid naïve, it may be reasonable to start with 1 milligram.

One can also use hydromorphone (Dilaudid), oxycodone, or fentanyl. Hydromorphone, a semisynthetic opioid agonist, shares a similar analgesic and side effect profile with morphine, but is 6–7 times more potent on a milligram basis.[31] Oxycodone provides equivalent analgesia and lipid solubility, but has a greater oral bioavailability compared to morphine and may cause fewer hallucinations and less itching.[32] Fentanyl, a lipid-soluble synthetic opioid, has the administration versatility of being available intravenously, orally as a lollipop, and transdermally. Methadone also can be used first line, particularly in patients who are at risk for addiction. Meperidine has toxic metabolites and may cause seizures, mood alterations, and confusion. There is no evidence that meperidine does not raise the pressure of the sphincter of Oddi and thus is not preferable to morphine for pancreatic or biliary pain. In general, use of meperidine should be avoided. Many hospitals are successfully removing meperidine from their formulary because of its side-effect profile, and hospitalists should aim to never use this medication in treatment of pain.

There is little difference between opioids with respect to speed of analgesic effect. Onset of action varies with the route of administration, with intravenous being fastest and appropriate for patients in severe pain. The WHO ladder recommends using strong opioids such as morphine, oxycodone, hydromorphone, or methadone, for severe pain that is not controlled with weak opioids.[33] Alternatives to using opioid agonists include tramadol, a weak opioid agonist; and buprenorphine, pentazocine, butorphanol, and nalbuphine, which are partial agonists.

Once the patient's pain has been stabilized with short-acting opioids, the dose should be converted to an equi-analgesic long-acting stable dose that will give steady blood levels of the medication (Table 94-4). Long-acting opioids are less "positively reinforcing" and thus are believed to present lower risk of addiction, although little data exist to confirm this.

When treating with opioids, it is important to manage side effects such as constipation, nausea, and pruritus. Prophylactic use of senna and stool softeners is a good strategy. Antihistamines can help with pruritus. Nausea should be treated with medications such as metoclopramide, as needed.

When using opioids, one must be cognizant of tolerance, dependence, and addiction.

Tolerance refers to the need for higher doses of a medication to achieve the desired effects. Chronic use of opioids will lead to tolerance of both the side effects (except constipation) and the analgesic properties. Tolerance and dependence are a predictable result of the use of opioids. For patients who do not have a history of addiction, the risk of addiction from being treated with opioids in the hospital is exceedingly low.[34] However, some previously addicted hospitalized patients may present with pain. Clinical experience shows that patients who have addiction and who are in acute or chronic pain can be treated effectively with opioids and with adjuvant medications.[35] Nevertheless, the physician must be alert for signs of a relapse and treat appropriately.

Different opioids have partial cross-tolerance, and therefore opioid rotation is often helpful. There are several reasons to rotate from one opioid to another opioid. These include lack of efficacy, intolerable side effects, change in patient's status, and practical considerations.[36,37] The first step in changing opioids is to calculate the total daily use of opioid. Referring to a table of equi-analgesic dosing (see Table 94-4), convert all opioids used to morphine equivalents. Simply add each one together in morphine equivalents to determine a total daily dose. The dosing and schedule of opioids should be individually tailored to the specific patient and circumstance. When changing the opioid in the case of intolerable side effects, it is recommended to reduce the calculated total dose by 33%.[36] If the reason for rotating opioids is for better pain control, then one can be more aggressive with the dosing and can increase the total opioid dose by 25–50%.[38]

Breakthrough Pain

Immediate-release opioids should be used only intermittently. The short-acting opioid provides a "rescue" for times of acute pain from end-of-dose failure, incident pain, or for breakthrough pain[36] that may develop during the course of treatment with long-acting opioids. In general, the doses for breakthrough pain should be 10–20% of the total daily opioid dose, or 25–30% of

Table 94-4 Opioid Equianalgesic Conversions of Selected Opioids (Milligrams)

Drug	IV/IM Dose	PO Dose	Starting Oral Dose
Morphine	10	30	30–60
Hydromorphone	1.5	7.5	4–8
Methadone	10	10	5–10
Oxycodone	—	20–30	5–30
Meperidine	75	300	
Codeine	130	200	30–60
Fentanyl	0.1	—	
Hydrocodone		30	5–10
Oxymorphone	1		
Levorphanol	2	4	

From: Inturrisi CE. Clinical pharmacology of opioids for pain. Clin J Pain 2002; 18:S3–S13; and Gammaitoni AR, Fine P, Alvarez N, et al. Clinical application of opioid equianalgesic data. Clin J Pain 2003; 19(5):286–297.

the single-standing dose.[36] Use of the same type of opioid for both long-acting and short-acting treatment simplifies titration of the medications.

Alternative Options

Alternatives for treatment of pain include using patient-controlled analgesia (PCA), multimodal pain treatment, topical analgesics, and nonpharmacologic treatment.

Patient-Controlled Analgesia

An effective option for patients in continuous pain is to implement PCA. PCA allows for individual titration of pain medication. This method is primarily used in patients who are unable to be treated effectively with oral medications and who will need treatment for greater than 24–36 hours. PCA permits the patient to self-administer doses of parenteral medication at frequent intervals. The rationale of the PCA is that it allows opioid analgesia to produce serum levels at or slightly more than the minimum effective analgesic concentration (MEAC), with small incremental doses that can be administered promptly when the levels fall below the MEAC.[39] Thus, the PCA should be used once the pain is under control to help maintain a steady level of medication to prevent and treat further pain. PCA prevents delay of treatment, as the patient does not need to wait for nursing. This allows the patient control over the subjective determination of his or her pain and also prevents overdosing of opioids by requiring the patient to actively administer the medication.

Most PCAs administer morphine and hydromorphone or fentanyl. The bolus dose to promote pain control should be great enough to reach the MEAC for the next 30–60 minutes without the need for additional doses. Young adults often require a bolus dose of morphine of 1.5–2 mg, while older adults without tolerance should start at 1 mg. The lockout interval is the minimum amount of time between dosing intervals. A lockout of 20 minutes is usually sufficient. Many doctors also specify a maximum number of doses in a 1-hour or 4-hour time span.

For many patients, PCA is a safe alternative to scheduled or as-needed dosing of opioid medication. In a recent meta-analysis, PCA in the postoperative setting compared with conventional opioid treatment was found to improve analgesia and decrease the risk of pulmonary complications. It also demonstrated that patients prefer PCA.[40] Under investigation is the use of a transdermal fentanyl PCA, which has been shown to provide equivalent pain control when compared to morphine.[41]

Topical medications can be helpful for localized pain. Lidocaine patch 5% is approved by the FDA for treating postherpetic neuralgia. Capsaicin cream is used for neuropathic pain and for osteoarthritis. Transdermal clonidine and topical EMLA (a mixture of lidocaine and prilocaine) are also used for localized pain.

Multimodal Analgesia

The multimodal approach to pain therapy involves treatment with a combination of different classes of analgesic modalities. This includes analgesic medications as well as regional analgesia, such as spinal and epidural anesthesia. Integration of multimodal and multidisciplinary care can enhance recovery and reduce hospital stay.[42] In situations where medical management has failed, it is helpful to consult a pain service to implement multimodal analgesia.

Nonmedical Treatment

Transcutaneous electrical nerve stimulator (TENS) has been used to treat both acute and chronic pain for many years. It creates a feeling of light touch and pressure by transmitting electrical currents across the surface of the skin. The theory is that it prevents firing of the C fibers that transmit pain from the dorsal horn of the spinal cord. TENS has been shown to be effective for use in mild pain. In one study, compared to naproxen, TENs provided superior pain control for mild rib fractures.[43] Other nonpharmacologic treatments of pain include biofeedback, massage therapy, acupuncture, cognitive therapy, and physical therapy.

DISCHARGE/FOLLOW-UP PLANS

Upon discharge, it is important to avoid abrupt cessation of an opioid, as withdrawal can occur. Instead, plan to taper the opioid slowly. Contact the outpatient physician to formulate a plan to either taper off opioids or to continue long-term treatment with opioids. Good communication with an outpatient physician is imperative for appropriate pain management.

Patient Education

At the time of discharge, the patient should understand the dosing of the medications he or she is being prescribed and should be made aware of side effects and toxicities. With NSAIDs and acetaminophen, the patient should understand that these medications have a ceiling dose above which toxicities can occur. They should be informed that NSAIDs should be taken with food and that acetaminophen should not be taken with alcohol. If the patient is discharged with opioids, the patient must be made aware that opioids need to be tapered slowly to prevent withdrawal. The patient should know the signs of opioid withdrawal, which include agitation and restlessness, diarrhea, tachycardia, nausea, and vomiting. They should also be aware of opioid side effects, such as constipation, drowsiness, and mental status changes, and instructed how to treat these side effects. The patient should be instructed not to drive or operate heavy machinery (including cars) when under the influence of opioids. The patient should also understand that complete eradication of pain is not always realistic. Ongoing assessment and treatment of patient should be continued with an outpatient physician.

Outpatient Physician Communication

The primary care physician should be contacted to discuss the treatment plan. In particular, the outpatient physician needs to know the dosing and the planned length of treatment, the tapering schedule, if appropriate, and other treatment plans. The amount of opioid medication prescribed should be enough to last until the appropriate outpatient follow-up, preferably within 1–2 weeks. At that time, the outpatient physician will assume the pain management for the patient. Close follow-up is imperative.

Key Points

- Pain is a common finding and a major cause of suffering in the hospitalized patient.

- Using simple scales of pain intensity, such as the visual analog scale, for patients' self-report of pain provides vital information to evaluate response to therapy.

- The goal of treating pain is to alleviate symptoms and give the patient an improved quality of life. Complete eradication of pain may not always be realistic or necessary.

- Medical management with nonopioids, opioids, and adjuvant medications is the mainstay in treatment of pain among hospitalized patients.

- Analgesic use should follow the guidelines set forth in the World Health Organization analgesic ladder, a well-used instrument which provides a standard for treatment of pain.

- The most common use of adjuvant pain medications is in the treatment of pain syndromes, such as neuropathic pain, that are difficult to manage with conventional analgesia.

- Opioids, unlike NSAIDs, do not have a dose-related ceiling, and dose escalation is limited only by adverse effects.

- Upon discharge, it is important to avoid abrupt cessation of an opioid, as withdrawal can occur. Plan to taper the opioid slowly, and arrange close follow-up with an outpatient physician.

SUGGESTED READING

Gammaitoni AR, Fine P, Alvarez N, et al. Clinical application of opioid equianalgesic data. Clin Journal Pain 2003; 19:286–297.

Inturrisi CE. Clinical pharmacology of opioids for pain. Clin J Pain 2002; 18:S3–S13.

Jensen TS, Gottrop H, Sindrup SH, et al. The clinical picture of neuropathic pain. Eur J Pharmacol 2001; 429:1–11.

Katz J, Melzack R. Measurement of pain. Surg Clin North Am 1999; 79(2):231–252.

Kris AE, Dodd MJ. Symptom experience of adult hospitalized medical-surgical patients. J Pain Symptom Manage 2004; 28:451–459.

Lehmann KA. Recent developments in patient-controlled analgesia. J Pain Symptom Manage 2005; 29(5S):S72–S89.

Woolf CJ. Pain: moving from symptom control toward mechanism-specific pharmacologic management. Ann Intern Med 2004; 140:441–451.

CHAPTER NINETY-FIVE

Palliative Care in the Hospital

Stephanie Grossman, MD, and S. Melissa Mahoney, MD

BACKGROUND

Palliative care is an interdisciplinary approach to relieve suffering and improve the quality of life for patients with a life-threatening or advanced chronic illness. This includes malignant as well as nonmalignant diseases. Symptom management and expertise at communicating with patients to identify goals of care are core skills of palliative care. Pain, anxiety, depression, anorexia, nausea, constipation, bowel obstruction, dyspnea, delirium, and dysphagia should all be assessed during a palliative care evaluation. (Specific management of these symptoms is addressed in other chapters of this book.) It is important to also recognize and treat "total pain," the combination of physical; emotional, psychic, or interpersonal; and spiritual or existential pain. Each type can exist and interact with the others, contributing to overall suffering. Assessment and treatment of each type of pain should be integrated with other appropriate medical treatments.

IMPLEMENTATION

Ideally, palliative care should be offered at the point of diagnosis, simultaneous with the offering or implementation of other treatment options. As the illness progresses, the proportion of palliative versus curative treatments tends to increase. Toward the last stages of palliative care, hospice can be considered on the continuum of care if the patient is determined to have a prognosis of less than 6 months. However, this "terminal phase," particularly in nonmalignant chronic illness, may last months to years and thus warrant palliative care but not hospice care. Curative options may no longer be available, or the degree of suffering involved with curative treatment exceeds the patient's preferences or goals of care.

This gradual shift compares with the traditional model of care that focuses exclusively on curing illness and prolonging life; hospice care is introduced when "nothing more can be done." In fact, the traditional model fails to adequately address the multitude of palliative treatment options that improve the quality of life and are available, even during the dying process so as to ensure that a patient does not suffer (Fig. 95-1).

PALLIATIVE CARE IN THE HOSPITAL

Palliative care is a particularly important skill in the hospital setting. Hospitalized patients are typically older with an acute illness overlapping complex medical issues, or an exacerbation of an underlying illness that requires hospitalization. Common conditions (Box 95-1) include but are not limited to strokes, dementia, heart failure (HF), chronic obstructive pulmonary disease (COPD), end-stage renal disease, or acquired immune deficiency syndrome (AIDS). These patients may also have an underlying malignancy for which they are receiving treatment. Very often, despite the introduction of the Patient Self-Determination Act of 1990, these patients do not have advanced directives or designated medical powers of attorney. The hospitalist may indeed be the first person to recognize that the burden of life-prolonging efforts exceeds the benefit, yet may have difficulty integrating prognostication with patient and/or family goals of care. Often, these difficult conversations take place with a patient's surrogate who has not previously had relevant communication with his or her loved one.

Prognostication

The ability to prognosticate illnesses accurately is helpful in the communication process with patients and their families. Patients with metastatic cancer or multiorgan system failure have a more predictable pattern of decline compared to those with organ specific entities such as CHF or COPD. At the same time, the ability of the hospitalist to glean the "big picture" of multiple insults is more important than the organ-specific prognostication by various specialists. Indeed, such fragmentation of care by specialists may also lead to conflicting messages to the patient and families. For example, while a patient's kidney failure may be resolving, and thus the nephrologist tells the family the patient is doing better, the concomitant combination of dementia, stroke, heart failure, and pneumonia indicates a poor prognosis.

The performance status of a patient prior to hospitalization can aid a clinician in determining a more accurate prediction of death over time. Several guidelines are available to help with prognostication. These include consensus guidelines developed by the

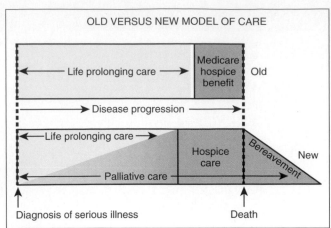

OLD VERSUS NEW MODEL OF CARE

Figure 95-1 • Palliative Care versus Traditional Model of Care (figure of contrasting models of care). From: Weissman, DE. MCW Pocket Cards. Communication Phrases Near the End of Life and The Family Goal-Setting Conference. MCW Research Foundation Inc., Milwaukee, Wisconsin, 2002.

Box 95-1 Common Conditions for Which Palliative Care is Helpful

- Cancer
- Stroke
- Dementia
- Heart failure
- COPD
- End-Stage renal disease
- AIDS

COPD = Chronic Obstructive Pulmonary Disease; AIDS = Acquired Immune Deficiency Syndrome

Box 95-2 Symptom Management in Palliative Care

- Pain
- Delirium
- Anxiety and/or depression
- Dyspnea
- Anorexia
- Nausea
- Dysphagia
- Constipation
- Bowel obstruction

National Hospice and Palliative Care Organization (NHPCO) that identify patients with noncancer diagnoses who are likely to have a life expectancy of 6 months of less if the illness were to run its normal course. The Karnofsky Performance Scale is more oriented toward hospitalization based on functional status. The Palliative Care Performance Scale is similar but also includes nutritional limitations and mental status deterioration and may be a better predictor of hospice length of stay.

Ultimately, prognostication can empower patients and/or surrogates in determining how they wish to live the remainder of their lives. This may tip the balance toward forgoing further attempts at potential but not certain curative therapy, and thus avoiding further suffering. It may also allow the patient and/or surrogate to determine location of death. In the U.S., 90% of patients wish to die at home. Unfortunately, 23% of deaths currently take place at home, 23% in nursing homes, and 49% in hospitals. Finally, appropriate provision of palliative care may coincidentally lead to less inappropriate utilization of resources.

Symptom Management

Particularly in the hospital, symptoms during the dying process can be distressing for both the patient and the family. As noted earlier, distressing symptoms (e.g., pain, anxiety, nausea, consti-

pation, dyspnea) should all be addressed during a palliative care assessment (Box 95-2).

Pain

Both patients and significant others strongly desire freedom from pain at the time of death, and fear of pain at the time of death terrifies many. However, clinicians may be hesitant to prescribe opioids at the time of death secondary to the fear of hastening death. According to the "rule of double effect," when a desirable effect is intended the risk of a foreseen, but unintended, undesirable effect is acceptable. Careful titration of opioids may prevent the need for application of this rule. However, in the case of a dying patient, the rule of double effect is acceptable to prevent unnecessary distress and suffering. Pain may be treated with opioids delivered through multiple routes, including oral and nonoral (e.g., subcutaneous, sublingual, intravenous). Management of pain is reviewed in detail in Chapter 94.

Dyspnea and the Death Rattle

Dyspnea can be alleviated with morphine or an analgesic equivalent. The "death rattle" is a gurgling or rattling sound sometimes made in the throat of a dying patient secondary to the inability to clear oral secretions. This can be treated, or even prevented, with anticholinergics, such as a scopolamine gel or patch; sublingual hyoscyamine; intravenous glycopyrrolate; a nebulizer solution consisting of atropine, morphine, and dexamethasone; or atropine and furosemide.

Anxiety and Delirium

Benzodiazepines such as lorazepam and alprazolam are effective for anxiety, but should be used cautiously as they may worsen delirium. Delirium can be managed with haloperidol, methotrimeprazine, or chlorpromazine.

Nausea

The most common causes of nausea affect the chemoreceptor trigger zone of the brain and include drugs and metabolic abnormalities. Neuroleptics such as haloperidol and serotonin 5HT3 receptor agonists such as ondansetron are effective treatments in these instances. The gastrointestinal tract is also a source of nausea: obstruction or poor gastric motility may respond to metoclopramide. The patient should also be assessed for constipation. Nausea as a result of increased intracranial pressure responds well to dexamethasone, while nausea secondary to vestibular disease may respond to meclizine, decongestants, or a transdermal scopolamine patch. Anxiety is also a cause of nausea and can be treated as noted above.

Constipation and Bowel Obstruction

Constipation may be caused by drugs (especially opioids), poor oral intake, dehydration, decreased intestinal mobility, and metabolic abnormalities such as hypercalcemia. Consistency of stool on rectal exam should guide treatment (i.e., use of a stool softener such as docusate, or use of a laxative such as senna, or bisacodyl or sorbitol). If constipation persists, a suppository or enema may be helpful, but if the impaction is in the proximal colon, magnesium citrate or sorbitol may be more effective.

If complete bowel obstruction is present and the patient is not a candidate for surgery, opioids should be escalated to control pain. Often, cramping and nausea are caused by increased secretions, and this can be managed by anticholinergic agents such as hyoscyamine or glycopyrrolate. Octreotide will also relieve secretions but is much more expensive.

COMMUNICATION

Communication is the cornerstone of palliative care (see Table 95-1 for helpful communication phrases by situation). Caring for hospitalized patients with chronic, life-threatening or terminal illness requires dialogue regarding goals of care and may involve such topics as artificial nutrition and hydration, advanced care planning, use of antibiotics for infection, extent of diagnostic testing, desire for rehospitalization after discharge, and use of artificial respiration. Once prognosis has been established, the next step toward setting any goal of care with patients and families involves open and effective communication which clarifies prognosis, elicits patient and family knowledge and preferences, and finally seeks to reconcile both.

Communication between practitioners and patients or families, whether it involves clarifying prognosis, breaking bad news or establishing goals of care, should always follow a few general guidelines. Practitioners should be familiar with the medical facts of the case by reviewing the chart, speaking with consultants, and conducting any necessary literature review. Adequate interruption-free time should be set aside for meeting with the patient to review the situation and discuss options. If possible, patients and families should be given lead time to allow all interested parties to be present. The meeting should take place in a comfortable, private setting with all parties seated, if possible. Discussion should begin with finding out how much is known by the patient and family. One way to ascertain this is to ask, "What is your understanding of your medical situation at this point?" If the patient and family lack understanding, it is important to clarify how much they would like to know by asking, "Would you like to know all of the details or more of a general overview?" In the context of palliative care, and especially in goal-setting, it can be helpful to ask how the current medical situation has affected changes in function (activity, sleep, eating, and mood). Once this information has been elicited from the patient and family, then

Table 95-1 Helpful Communication Phrases by Situation

1. Discussing artificial feeding/hydration
   a. "What do you know about artificial ways to provide food?"
   b. "All dying patients lose interest in the days and weeks leading up to death; this is the body's signal that death is coming."
   c. "I am recommending that the (tube feeding/hydration) be discontinued (or not started), as these will not improve his or her living; these treatments, if used, may only prolong his or her dying."
   d. "Your (relation) will not suffer; we will do everything necessary to improve comfort."
   e. "Your (relation) is dying from (disease); he or she is not dying from dehydration or starvation."

2. Responding to a patient or family who is angry
   a. "It sounds/appears as though you are angry."
   b. "You appear angry. Can you tell me what is upsetting you?"
   c. "I wish that things were different. How can we move forward? How can I help?"

3. Assessing the impact of illness on a patient's quality of life
   a. "How has your disease interfered with your daily activities, your family and friends?"
   b. "Have you been feeling worried or sad about your illness?"
   c. "What symptoms bother you the most? What concerns you the most?"
   d. "How have your religious beliefs been affected by your illness?"
   e. "Many people wonder about the meaning of all this—do you?"

4. Discussing advanced care planning
   a. "I'd like to talk with you about possible health care decisions in the future. This is something I do with all my patients, so I can be sure that I know and can follow your wishes. Have you ever completed an advance directive?"
   b. "What do you understand about your health situation?"
   c. "If you were unable to make your own medical decisions, who would you like to make them for you? Have you spoken to this person?"
   d. "When you think about dying, have you thought about what the end would be like or how you would like it to be?"
   e. "Have you discussed your wishes with your family?"

5. Death pronouncement
   a. "I wish there was more we could have done. I am very sorry for your loss. This must be very difficult for you; is there anyone I can call for you?"
   b. "In the days to weeks to come, please contact me if I can answer any questions about your (insert relation)'s illness."

From: Weissman DE. MCW Pocket Cards. Communication Phrases Near the End of Life and The Family Goal-Setting Conference. MCW Research Foundation Inc Milwaukee, Wisconsin, 2002.

new diagnostic or prognostic information should be presented in a straightforward but compassionate manner, avoiding medical jargon and checking in frequently with patients and families to ensure they understand the new information being presented. Practitioners should respond to emotion after the delivery of bad news. Allow a period of silence and acknowledge emotion with an empathic statement such as, "I can see this is very difficult for you." Once information is exchanged, a summary statement can be provided by the practitioner, allowing time and opportunity for final questions from the patient and family.

Many times, practitioners encounter patients and families who have views of illness that are different from their own. This may stem from cultural or religious differences. It is important to acknowledge such differences and explore them. One way to do so is to simply state, "I know different people have different ways of understanding illness . . . please help me understand how you see things." Understanding these differences can often facilitate efforts to resolve or avoid conflicts, set realistic goals, and allow all parties to be heard.

Once information has been exchanged regarding condition and prognosis, whether from specialists or hospitalists themselves, hospitalists are often faced with the challenging task of helping patients and families make decisions regarding future medical care. From a purely medical perspective, this involves the complicated task of weighing the benefits and burdens of each test, procedure, and care option. Often, when these discussions take place,

Table 95-2 Guidelines for Conducting an Effective Family Meeting

1. Preparation
   a. Review the chart—know all the medical facts, including diagnosis, prognosis and treatment options.
   b. Review/obtain family psychosocial issues; keep an open mind regarding reported conflicts.
   c. Identify medical decision-maker.
   d. Coordinate opinions among consulting physicians.
   e. Clarify your goals for the meeting (what do you hope to get accomplished?).
   f. Decide who you would like to attend the meeting—inform them of time and location.
   g. Check your own emotions.

2. Establish proper setting
   a. Private, comfortable
   b. Turn your pager off or to vibrate
   c. Have everyone seated—circle seating if possible

3. Introduction/goals/relationship
   a. Allow everyone to state his or her name and relationship to the patient.
   b. Verify medical decision-maker.
   c. State your goals for the meeting, and ask patient and family members to state their goals.
   d. Ask nonmedical questions about the patient to build relationship (*Can you tell me something about your father?*).

4. Family understanding of the medical condition
   a. *Tell me your understanding of the current medical condition.*
   b. Encourage all present to respond.
   c. For patients with chronic conditions, ask for a description of changes in function (activity, eating, sleep, mood) observed over the last weeks or months.

5. Medical summary
   a. Summarize the "big picture" in a few sentences. Use the word "dying" if appropriate.
   b. Respond to specific medical questions, if asked.

6. Silence/reactions
   a. Respond to emotional reactions.
   b. Be prepared for common questions (*How long? What do we do now? How can you be sure?*).

7. Prognostication
   a. If appropriate/necessary, provide prognostic information using ranges (days to weeks, weeks to months).
   b. Allow silence; respond to emotional reactions with empathy.

8. Decision-making (go to step 9 if no decisions need to be made)
   a. Review options, make recommendations, assess reactions.
   b. Decisional patient: *"What decision(s) are you considering?"*
   c. Nondecisional patient: *"What do you believe the patient would choose if he or she were able to communicate?"*
   d. If consensus is reached, summarize and confirm.
   e. If no consensus, mutually decide on specific time-limited goals.

9. Goal setting (go to 10 if goals were established in 8)
   a. Allow family/patient to state their goals (*Knowing that time is short, what is important in the time that is left?*).
   b. Review all current and planned interventions—make recommendations to continue or stop. If appropriate, discuss artificial hydration/feeding/DNR orders, etc. with clear recommendations.
   c. Summarize all the decisions made.

10. Document and discuss
    a. Write a note which includes who was present, what decisions were made, and the follow-up plan.
    b. Discuss with relevant team members.
    c. Check your emotions.

the focus turns away from the patient and toward the particular test, procedure, or care option. Especially when the prognosis is poor, these choices can be daunting for patients and families. They will often feel pressure to choose a more aggressive option over a less aggressive one just so they feel they are "doing everything." An alternative approach that palliative care offers is to first elicit from the patient and family a broad understanding of the patient's hopes and goals before developing a specific medical plan. Some key phrases which may help in this situation include the following: "Given what we now know about your medical condition, how can we help you live well? What fears or worries do you have about your illness or medical care? If you have to choose between living longer and quality of life, how would you approach this balance? What do you hope for your family? In what way do you feel you could make this time especially meaningful to you?" Once these broader goals are discussed, physicians, patients, and families often see what particular tests, procedures, and care options may contribute or detract from the previously set goals.

A key communication tool that hospitalists can help facilitate is the family meeting. In the busy hospital setting, it is invaluable to assemble all parties, including patient, family, physicians, nurses, social work, and chaplaincy to discuss a particular patient's care. This meeting can ensure all parties are receiving accurate information and can help patients and families in decision-making regarding all aspects of care. Guidelines for conducting an effective family meeting are listed in Table 95-2. Key aspects include proper preparation, establishing an appropriate setting, assessing patient and family knowledge of the medical condition, summarizing the medical facts, responding to emotion, establishing goals, and executing appropriate follow-up.

A GOOD DEATH

Determinants of a good death are only partly in the hands of a skilled clinician and are a highly individualized decision. Some patients may indeed desire sacrificing good pain management with the desire to be fully aware at the time of death. Others may feel that a good death is fighting to the very end. Social and religious components can be distinct from the medical care that can be provided. Again, this emphasizes the need for an interdisciplinary approach of palliative care that focuses on communication and management of uncomfortable symptoms.

CONCLUSION

Ideally, all physicians would be expert in providing palliative care. Unfortunately, most physicians have not received adequate training, and it is unrealistic to expect them to learn this on an as-needed basis. A palliative care team, often including a specially trained physician, nurse, social worker, and chaplain, provides a significant resource to improve the overall quality of care delivery to hospitalized patients. An extended team may include pain management specialists, a psychiatrist or psychologist, a member of the ethics committee, a clinical pharmacist, nutritionist, physical and occupational therapist, and a member of the administration. Palliative care is a rapidly growing specialty, and hospitalists will commonly find themselves in need of this expertise to relieve suffering and improve the quality of life for patients with a life-threatening or advanced chronic illness.

Key Points

- Palliative care is an interdisciplinary approach to relieve suffering and improve the quality of life for patients with a life-threatening or advanced chronic illness through intense symptom management and effective communication.

- Palliative care should be offered at the point of diagnosis of any life-threatening illness. As the illness progresses, the proportion of palliative versus curative treatments tends to increase, but both can be offered simultaneously.

- Regarding prognostication, the ability of the hospitalist to glean the "big picture" of multiple insults is more important than the organ-specific prognostication by various specialists. The latter can often be confusing to families.

- In the United States, 90% of patients wish to die at home. Unfortunately, 23% of deaths currently take place at home, 23% in nursing homes, and 49% in hospitals. Appropriate provision of palliative care may lead to less inappropriate utilization of resources.

- Fear of pain at the time of death terrifies many. Clinicians may be hesitant to prescribe opioids at the time of death secondary to the fear of hastening death. According to the "rule of double effect," when a desirable effect is intended, the risk of a foreseen, but unintended, undesirable effect is acceptable.

- Discussing goals of care with patients and families involves open and effective communication which clarifies prognosis, elicits patient and family knowledge and preferences, and finally seeks to reconcile both.

- Discussion of medical information should begin with finding out how much is known by the patient and family. One way to ascertain this is to ask, "What is your understanding of your medical situation at this point?"

- A key communication tool which hospitalists can help facilitate is the family meeting.

SUGGESTED READING

Billings JA. What is palliative care? J Palliative Med 1998; 1:73–81.

Block SD. Psychological considerations, growth, and transcendence at the end of life: the art of the possible. JAMA 2001; 285:2898–2905.

Block SD, Billings JA. Learning from the dying. N Engl J Med 2005; 353:1313–1315.

Meier DE. Palliative care in hospitals. J Hosp Med 2006; 1:21–28.

Pantilat S. Palliative care and hospitalists: a partnership for hope. J Hosp Med 2006; 1:5–6.

Quill TE, Townsend P. Bad news: delivery, dialogue, and dilemmas. Arch Intern Med 1991; 151:463–468.

Quill TE. Initiating end-of-life discussions with seriously ill patients; addressing the "elephant in the room." JAMA 2000; 284:2502–2507.

Steinhauser KE, Christakis NA, Clipp EC, et al. Factors considered important at the end of life by patients, family, physicians, and other care providers. JAMA 2000; 284:2476–2482.

Tulsky JA, Fischer GS, Rose MR, et al. Opening the black box: how do physicians communicate about advance directives. Ann Intern Med 1998; 129:441–449.

Ambuel B, Weissman DE. Fast Facts and Concepts #16. Moderating an end-of-life family conference. August, 2005. 2nd Edition. End-of-Life Palliative Education Resource Center www.eperc.mcw.edu.

Ambuel B. Fast Facts and Concepts #29. Responding to patient emotion. August 2005, 2nd edition. End-of-Life Physician Education Resource Center www.eperc.mcw.edu.

Weissman DE. MCW Pocket Cards. Communication Phrases Near the End of Life and The Family Goal-Setting Conference. MCW Research Foundation Inc., Milwaukee, Wisconsin 2002.

Section

Fourteen

Consultative Hospital Medicine

96 *The Hospitalist as Consultant*
David J. Rosenman, Geno J. Merli

97 *Anesthesia Effects and Complications*
A. Scott Keller, Christopher J. Jankowski

CHAPTER NINETY-SIX

The Hospitalist as Consultant

David J. Rosenman, MD, and Geno J. Merli, MD, FACP

BACKGROUND

Much has been written about the roles and responsibilities of the medical consultant. Rather than reiterate in detail the basic principles of medical consultation, we summarize them briefly and then discuss issues specifically related to the hospitalist as consultant. General principles for providing optimal medical consultation may be useful to any hospitalist but particularly to those who expect to serve formally as a consultant. This chapter summarizes several of the most common issues relevant to the consulting hospitalist and also some unique ones. Subsequent chapters address in more detail medical management in the preoperative and postoperative periods, the medical complications of pregnancy, and consultation for the psychiatric patient.

One physician should have primary responsibility for a patient's overall care. This physician, in referring a patient for consultation, typically requests diagnostic or therapeutic guidance but not assumption of the primary management of the patient's care. If you as a hospitalist are honored with such a consultation, respond in a timely fashion—at least within 24 hours, or preferably sooner. Given time pressures in hospitals today and the emphasis on shortening length of stay, consultations should be provided as quickly as possible and ideally on the same day as the request. Communication with the primary physician requesting consultation will clarify the urgency of the need to evaluate the patient and provide recommendations. Subsequent communication during the consultation needs to be clear and directed to the referring physician; discussion with the patient may follow but only with the prior consent of the requesting physician or service. Although continuation of the consultation is at the discretion of the referring service (e.g., in the case of a conflict of opinion), consultants retain the right to share their opinions with the patient as well as with the referring physician.[1] Goldman et al. outlined the "10 Commandments" for effective consultations (Box 96-1).[2] They provide simple and straightforward directions for success.

SCOPE OF THE CONSULTATION REPORT

Although internists may be accustomed to thorough and comprehensive evaluations, consultation reports serve a more focused purpose. The consultation report should begin by addressing the reason for consultation. Ideally, there should be a written order requesting the consult in the medical record. This is necessary, as Medicare will reimburse a consultation only when specific criteria are met, as noted in Box 96-2. An initial statement such as "Dr. (Referring Physician) requested consultation to evaluate this patient's (medical condition)" will aid billing and collection.

Issues unrelated to the reason for consultation should be organized by problem and communicated to the requesting physician so that appropriate recommendations can be made to address the problem(s). Preferably, additional items will be few in number and the discussion of each recommendation concise. Details related to particular therapies (doses, frequencies, durations, etc.) should be included. Generally, recommendations for therapy are more likely to be implemented than recommendations for further diagnostic studies.

Every consultation must begin with a clear understanding of what the requesting physician needs. Ideally, this is provided to the consultant with a written or oral case summary. If the reason for the consultation is not apparent, the consulting hospitalist is responsible for obtaining clarification. Excellent interprofessional communication is fundamental to providing high-quality consultative service.[3,4] In the ideal consultation, communication between all parties is clear, accurate, timely, respectful, to the point, and for the benefit of the patient. These qualities should characterize all communication throughout the process, including the initial request by the referring service, the consultation report, and any follow-up. Principles of clear and effective communication apply to the written document as well. Unless specifically requested, eschew lengthy evaluation and commentary regarding every chronic illness a patient may be suffering; focus on the specific request of the referring physician.

ASSESSING OPERATIVE RISK AND THE IMPLICATIONS OF "CLEARING" A PATIENT FOR SURGERY

Preoperative evaluation guidelines have proved to be successful for risk stratifying noncardiac surgery patients for adverse cardiac events and for directing specific interventions to high-risk groups to decrease morbidity and mortality. A common request by surgeons is for patients to be medically "cleared" for surgery. By most interpretations, the word "cleared" connotes a certainty

---

Box 96-1 Ten Commandments for Effective Consultation

1. Determine the question.
2. Establish urgency.
3. Look for yourself.
4. Be as brief as appropriate.
5. Be specific and concise.
6. Provide contingency plans.
7. Honor thy turf.
8. Teach with tact.
9. Remember that talk is cheap and effective.
10. Follow up.

From: Goldman L, Lee T, Rudd P. Ten commandments for effective consultations. Arch Intern Med 1983; 143:1753–1755.

Box 96-2 Medicare Criteria for Consultation Payment

- A physician whose opinion regarding evaluation/management of a specific problem is requested by another physician.

- A request for a consultation and the need for consultation are documented in the patient's medical record.

- The consultant prepares a written report of the findings, which is provided to the referring physician.

---

or guarantee (e.g., "absolved," "freed," "authorized," or "certified") that is inappropriate for perioperative cardiovascular risk stratification. Terms such as "cleared" and "okayed" must not be used to describe a patient's candidacy for anesthesia or surgery[12] because all patients are at some risk for perioperative cardiovascular complications. Instead, the consulting physician's goal is to identify patients who may have a risk that is higher than average and to recommend diagnostic or therapeutic interventions that may reduce that risk.[11] Perioperative cardiopulmonary complications are significant contributors to the morbidity and mortality of hospitalized patients, and thus deserve special attention. A validated assessment instrument or algorithm should be applied; if the resulting conclusion is that a patient's risk for a perioperative cardiovascular event is average or acceptable for the planned surgery, then this conclusion should be stated. Information about specific guidelines is provided in Chapter 102 ("Cardiovascular Preoperative Risk Assessment and Evaluation").

In addition to estimating a patient's risk, the consulting physician may help the surgical or anesthesia services by recommending perioperative prophylactic measures or providing additional information that may further reduce a patient's risk for complication. Acknowledging boundaries of professional expertise is important, however, and the medical consultant should refrain from making recommendations regarding the type of anesthesia.

PERIOPERATIVE MEDICATIONS

The consulting physician is expected to optimize a patient's medication regimen perioperatively. This includes the appropriate dosing of preoperative medications such as glucocorticoids, insulin, oral hypoglycemics, antihypertensives, and anticoagulants. After the procedure, the consulting physician provides not only the management recommendations for continuing the use of preoperative medication but also directs the postoperative addition of drugs, such as anticoagulants for venous thromboembolic prophylaxis (if not started preoperatively). Chapter 102 reviews in detail management of medications in the perioperative period.

IMPROVING COMPLIANCE WITH RECOMMENDATIONS

Several factors increase the likelihood that recommendations will be followed. A prompt response (within 24 hours) generally leads to compliance by the referring physician or service. A small number of recommendations (no more than five) is preferred. Crucial or critical recommendations should be identified and separated from routine recommendations. The consultation report should focus on central issues and make specific, relevant recommendations. The most effective consultations use definitive language. Recommendations for medications should specify drug dosage, frequency, route, and duration. Consultations that include frequent follow-up and documentation in the progress notes are usually followed more closely by the referring physician than are transient evaluations. Direct oral communication also helps. Therapeutic recommendations are more likely to be followed than diagnostic recommendations, and recommendations are generally observed more closely when illnesses are more severe.[11]

THE HOSPITALIST IN THE ROLE OF CONSULTANT

Hospitalists, by virtue of their site of practice, are not usually considered as consultants but instead as requestors of consultation services. Hospitalists, after all, help manage patient care from emergency department admissions to discharge. Thus, it may not be intuitive to request expert recommendations from such physicians, but with their broad range of expertise, hospitalists can offer recommendations on various medical problems.

The hospitalist often acts in an advisory capacity to the patient's primary physician. Examples include the orthopedic surgeon seeking guidance in management of anticoagulation for a patient with a prosthetic heart valve, a psychiatrist requesting recommendations for glycemic control in a patient with diabetes mellitus, or a gynecologic oncologist who wants advice about respiratory therapy for a patient with chronic obstructive pulmonary disease. Hospitalists who are trained in general medical fields and who work in a specific site of care are potential consultants for anything related to general medical or perioperative care in the hospital.

Even specialists trained in general medical care may request consultation from a hospitalist. While a general physician may also have specialty expertise, the converse does not always apply to specialists, and physicians in a number of specialties do not practice acute-care medicine.[5] The expertise of the hospitalist may also go beyond clinical medicine to include insight into more effective systems of health care delivery.[6] Sustained trends in inpatient care support the notion that hospitalists may be insightful consultants who improve patient care.[7] As hospitalists embrace an understanding of systems of care, they may be better prepared to recommend resources and services provided for patients by hospitals and related facilities.

CONSULTATION VERSUS COMANAGEMENT

The hospitalist may act as a consultant in one of two ways: as a "pure consultant" or as a "comanager" who works in tandem with the requesting service. The hospitalist acting as a pure consultant provides an assessment of the patient's condition and offers recommendations to the service or primary physician who provides the patient's care as described above.[8] The consulting hospitalist acting as a comanager assists the requesting physician or service by providing direct patient care within a scope that, ideally, is predetermined. The main difference between these two roles usually is that the comanaging hospitalist writes orders. In various settings, the comanagement model has been shown to benefit patient care.[9,10]

Curbside Consultation

"Curbside," or informal, consultation is a common request received by hospitalists because of their visibility and accessibility in the hospital. Having expertise in numerous medical issues, hospitalists are often sought for advice; however, requests for curbside consultation that are not clear or well defined should be deferred, or a formal consultation should be requested. Formal consultation affords the best care for the patient and reduces medicolegal liability.

Consultation for Nonsurgical versus Surgical Patients

As noted earlier, hospitalists may act as consultants in various settings, not all of which are perioperative. Subsequent chapters in this section discuss details relating to specific situations, including those pertaining to patients on obstetric and psychiatric services.

The bulk of this "Consultative Hospital Medicine" section, however, is devoted to perioperative assessment and care—a con-

siderable and growing segment of the hospitalist's typical workload. Box 96-3 summarizes the five core responsibilities of the hospitalist providing perioperative consultation. Appropriately completing these responsibilities provides the best possible management.

Key Points

- The general principles of medical consultation apply to consultation by hospitalists.

- The referring and consulting physicians should mutually agree on whether the hospitalist serves as a "pure consultant" or "comanager."

- Hospitalists may be asked to "risk stratify" patients preoperatively but should avoid using terminology such as "cleared" for surgery.

- Formal consultation with documentation in the medical record is preferred over "curbside" consultation, and should be accompanied by a formal order requesting consultation and the reason.

- Certain factors are thought to improve compliance with a consultant's recommendations.

SUGGESTED READING

Goldman L, Lee T, Rudd P. Ten commandments for effective consultations. Arch Intern Med 1983; 143:1753–1755.

Black C, Cheese IL. Hospitalists and consultant physicians in acute medicine. Clin Med 2002; 2:290–291.

Pham HH, Devers KJ, Kuo S, et al. Health care market trends and the evolution of hospitalist use and roles. J Gen Intern Med 2005; 20:101–107.

Huddleston JM, Long KH, Naessens JM, et al. Hospitalist-Orthopedic Team Trial Investigators. Medical and surgical comanagement after elective hip and knee arthroplasty: a randomized, controlled trial. Ann Intern Med 2004; 141:28–38.

Cohn SL. The role of the medical consultant. Med Clin North Am 2003; 87:1–6.

Box 96-3 Core Responsibilities of the Hospitalist Providing Perioperative Consultation

1. Identify the pertinent medical problems.
2. Integrate this information with the physiologic stresses of anesthesia and surgery.
3. Anticipate potential perioperative problems.
4. Assess the patient's risk and need for further interventions.
5. Communicate effectively with the surgeon and anesthesiologist.

CHAPTER NINETY-SEVEN

Anesthesia Effects and Complications

A. Scott Keller, MD, MS, and Christopher J. Jankowski, MD

INTRODUCTION

Hospitalists are uniquely positioned to work with anesthesiologists and surgeons in perioperative patient management. In particular, hospitalists can provide both preoperative assessment and postoperative care, with the goal of decreasing patient morbidity and mortality. Furthermore, by understanding the effects and possible complications of anesthesia, hospitalists will be better able to identify and optimize medical conditions that may be of concern perioperatively and can communicate these concerns to the anesthesiologist.

This chapter first provides a brief overview of anesthesia. Next, the major physiologic effects of general and regional anesthesia are covered. Finally, anesthesia-related complications likely to be encountered by the hospitalist are discussed. Recommendations are given to help prevent, recognize, and treat these complications.

OVERVIEW OF ANESTHESIA

Modern anesthetic techniques are extremely safe, with an estimated mortality of 1 per 250,000 cases.[1] The estimated incidence of complications related to anesthesia overdose, anesthesia reaction, and endotracheal tube misplacement was 0.72 per 1,000 surgical discharges in the United States in 2000.[2]

In broad terms, anesthesia can be divided into two types, general and regional.

- General anesthesia provides hypnosis, amnesia, analgesia, and muscle relaxation using intravenous and inhaled anesthetic agents. Some agents, such as the inhaled volatile anesthetics (sevoflurane, isoflurane, and desflurane), provide, to some degree, all four components of general anesthesia. Other agents provide only one or two components. For example, midazolam provides hypnosis and amnesia, but not analgesia or muscle relaxation. Likewise, opioids are profound analgesics, but do not provide the other components of general anesthesia.
- Regional anesthesia is the result of perineural injection of local anesthetics such as bupivacaine. Deposition of local anesthetics can occur centrally as in spinal (subarachnoid) and epidural blocks, collectively known as neuraxial anesthesia, or peripherally to individual nerves or plexi. The distribution of the resulting block corresponds to the distribution of the nerves bathed with local anesthetic. Regional anesthetics are often

supplemented with intravenous sedation. Regional techniques are also used to provide postoperative analgesia.

General and regional anesthesia are largely equivalent regarding morbidity and mortality. The decision regarding which technique to use is complex and depends on the location, extent, and anticipated duration of the proposed operation; the medical condition of the patient; and the skills and preferences of the anesthesia and surgical teams. This typically is a decision to be made by the anesthesiologist, not the consulting hospitalist, but the hospitalist can provide helpful information regarding medical risk assessment.

ANESTHESIA EFFECTS

While both general and regional anesthesia have the same goal of providing a safe and comfortable surgical experience for the patient, each has different physiologic effects and potential complications. Anesthetic agents can affect multiple organ systems,[3] although the effects are usually inconsequential in otherwise healthy patients. However, for patients with underlying disease states or in elderly patients who have diminished organ system reserve, anesthesia may have profound, if not deleterious, effects.[4]

This section discusses some of the major physiologic effects of general and regional anesthesia, while a detailed list of the effects and complications is provided in Tables 97-1 and 97-2. Although most of these effects occur intraoperatively and are treated by the anesthesiology team, some (such as prolonged sedation) are of concern postoperatively and may require intervention by the hospitalist.

Neurologic Effects

Most intravenous anesthetics augment the inhibitory γ-aminobutyric acid (GABA) neurotransmitter system, and inhaled anesthetics appear to inhibit synaptic transmission, especially in the reticular activating system. These agents, along with opioids, can lead to prolonged sedation. Local anesthetics (e.g., lidocaine and bupivacaine) block sodium ion channel conduction through nerve membranes. High doses may lead to systemic toxicity and cause tinnitus, a metallic taste, perioral numbness, muscle twitches (often of the eyes and lips), and seizures.[5] Ultimately, high doses may lead to depression of the central nervous, respi-

Table 97-1 Effects and Complications of General Anesthesia

Neurologic
Eye injury (corneal abrasion, ischemic optic neuropathy in prone patients)
Delirium
Intraoperative awareness
Prolonged sedation
Peripheral nerve damage from inappropriate patient positioning

Cardiovascular
Arrhythmias (usually tachyarrhythmias)
Coronary steal (predominantly isoflurane)
Decreased myocardial contractility
Decreased systemic vascular resistance
Hypertension
Hypotension
Intravascular volume depletion or overload
Myocardial ischemia

Pulmonary
Aspiration
Atelectasis
Attenuation of hypoxic pulmonary vasoconstriction
Bronchospasm
Cervical spine stress at C1-C2 during intubation
Decreased functional residual capacity
Decreased respiratory drive

Hypercarbia
Hypoxia
Impaired mucociliary clearance
Increased dead space
Laryngeal or subglottic edema
Laryngospasm
Management of the difficult airway
Negative-pressure pulmonary edema
Oropharyngeal injury from intubation
Tracheal stenosis
Vocal cord paralysis

Gastrointestinal
Ileus
Hepatic dysfunction
Postoperative nausea and vomiting

Renal
Decreased renal blood flow, glomerular filtration rate (GFR), and urine output
Urine retention from bladder atony

Hematologic
Deep vein thrombosis (primarily from surgical stimulation and immobilization)

Metabolic/Endocrine
Hyperkalemia worsened by succinylcholine

Table 97-2 Effects and Complications of Neuraxial Anesthesia

Neurologic
Accidental dural or subdural injection
Accidental total spinal anesthesia (apnea and hypotension)
Adhesive arachnoiditis
Backache
Delirium
Meningitis
Oversedation
Peripheral nerve damage from patient positioning
Post-dural headache
Spinal and epidural hematoma/abscess
Spinal cord ischemia/infarct
Systemic drug toxicity (epidural and peripheral blocks)

Cardiovascular
Arrhythmias (usually bradyarrhythmias)
Asystolic arrest (rare, but leading cause of death from spinal anesthesia)
Hypotension

Intravascular volume depletion or overload
Myocardial ischemia

Pulmonary
Decreased vital capacity
Decreased expiratory reserve volume
Decreased maximum expiratory and inspiratory airway pressures
Inhibition of phrenic nerve

Gastrointestinal
Ileus
Postoperative nausea and vomiting

Renal
Urine retention from detrusor blockade

Hematologic
Appropriate timing of anticoagulation
Deep vein thrombosis (primarily from surgical stimulation and immobilization), possibly lower risk than from general anesthesia

ratory, and cardiovascular systems.[5] Neuraxial anesthesia may cause self-limited transient neurologic symptoms in the sacral dermatomes, postdural puncture headache, or serious complications such as epidural hematoma and abscess. The effects of anesthesia and opioids may contribute to postoperative delirium, particularly in the elderly and those with preexisting cognitive deficits. Position-related peripheral nerve injuries from compression can occur unrelated to the actual anesthetic agent.

Cardiovascular Effects

The inhaled volatile anesthetics cause dose-dependent myocardial depression and decreased mean arterial pressure.[6] In addi-

tion, positive-pressure ventilation can decrease venous return (preload), reduce diastolic compliance, and increase right ventricular outflow impedance.[7] Neuraxial anesthetics block the sympathetic nervous system and cause arterial and venodilation along with decreased cardiac output. Neuraxial anesthetics can also cause bradycardia and rarely can induce asystole and cardiac arrest, while drug toxicity may lead to refractory arrhythmias.

Adverse hemodynamic effects, primarily transient hypertension and tachycardia, can occur with laryngoscopy, intubation, extubation, and emergence (awakening) from anesthesia. Conversely, induction (initiation) of anesthesia may cause hypotension as a result of vasodilation and myocardial depression, especially in patients who are volume depleted.

Aside from the effects of anesthesia, surgical stress produces a hypercoagulable and inflammatory state that may predispose patients to coronary plaque rupture and thrombus formation. In addition, the stress response to surgery is mediated by the hypothalamic-pituitary-adrenal axis, the renin-angiotensin system, and the sympathetic nervous system, and can cause significant hemodynamic changes.

Pulmonary Effects

General anesthesia can depress respiratory drive, decrease functional residual capacity (FRC), cause possible airway obstruction, impair mechanics of ventilation, and impair gas exchange.[7] Pulmonary gas exchange may be affected by atelectasis related to decreased FRC and due to the combined effects of neuromuscular blocking agents, patient positioning, and the inability to clear mucus secretions.[3] Of particular concern, airway reflexes are impaired during induction and emergence from general anesthesia, making patients more likely to aspirate.

Neuraxial anesthesia has only a minimal effect on tidal volume and respiratory rate, but it can decrease vital capacity and expiratory reserve volume. Also, maximum expiratory airway pressure, and, to a lesser extent, inspiratory pressure, are reduced.[8] This may limit a patient's ability to cough and may affect persons with chronic obstructive pulmonary disease (COPD), who depend on the muscles of expiration to overcome airway resistance.

Gastrointestinal Effects

Anesthesia can diminish gastric emptying, creating a risk for aspiration and postoperative nausea and vomiting (PONV). Causes of PONV include pain, hypotension and hypoperfusion of the medulla, volatile anesthetics, nitrous oxide, etomidate, and opioids, which stimulate the chemoreceptor trigger zone in the area postrema of the medulla.[9] All anesthetic agents affect bowel motility, but epidural anesthesia may allow quicker return of bowel function.[9,10] There have been rare reports of hepatotoxicity with anesthetic agents, primarily with the older agent halothane; the risk is increased with underlying liver disease.

POSTOPERATIVE COMPLICATIONS

Neurologic Complications

Oversedation

Description. Oversedation can result from prolonged effects of general anesthetic agents and from opioids given for postoperative analgesia. The major concerns are inability to protect the airway and respiratory depression, which may cause hypoxemia and hypercarbia.

Risk factors. Risk factors include advanced age, low body mass or poor nutritional status, and chronic hypercarbia. Also, liver disease or renal insufficiency may cause delayed drug metabolism and/or prolonged drug effects.

Treatment. First ensure there is an adequate airway and check vital signs, including oxygen saturation. Patients with severe res-

piratory depression may require intubation and mechanical ventilation. Next, discontinue any opioids or sedatives, and perform a neurologic assessment (cognitive status, cranial nerve function, and gross motor and sensory function). Observation without intervention is safe for patients who have no signs or symptoms of respiratory depression and who have normal vital signs and examination. However, all patients with prolonged sedation should be monitored with continuous pulse oximetry. Patients with respiratory depression may require an opioid antagonist such as naloxone. Unless respiratory depression is profound, give naloxone only in small, incremental doses of 40 mcg to prevent reversal of analgesia. Note that high doses of naloxone may precipitate nausea, vomiting, hypertension or hypotension, and cardiac arrest. Use opioid antagonists with caution in opioid-dependent persons, as they may lead to withdrawal symptoms.[12] Patients with sleep apnea may benefit from treatment with continuous positive airway pressure (CPAP).

Post-Dural Puncture Headache (PDPH)

Description. Post-dural puncture headaches (PDPH) occur in 31–75% of patients following accidental dural puncture during epidural anesthesia, and is caused by a persistent cerebrospinal fluid leak in the dura.[8] In contrast, PDPH occurs in only 0.02% to 3% of patients following spinal anesthesia due to the use of smaller needles.[8] These headaches are classically postural (improved when supine, worsened when upright). Associated symptoms can include diplopia, tinnitus, and diminished hearing.

Risk factors. Risk factors include young age, use of large-gauge needles, and pregnancy.

Treatment. Supine positioning will minimize symptoms, although it will not prevent PDPH. The mainstays of treatment are analgesics, hydration, and caffeine. If conservative measures are not effective, autologous lumbar epidural blood patch may be required. Patients should have routine neurologic assessments.

Epidural Hematoma

Description. Formation of a hematoma from bleeding in the epidural area following neuraxial anesthesia is rare, but may lead to spinal cord compression causing paraplegia or cauda equina syndrome.

Risk factors. Risk factors include anticoagulation, thienopyridine antiplatelet therapy (clopidogrel and ticlopidine), recent thrombolytic therapy, underlying coagulopathy, and traumatic needle placement.

Treatment. A review of reported cases showed the time from onset of neurologic deficit to complete paralysis was approximately 15 hours.[13] Therefore, immediately evaluate a patient with any symptoms suggestive of cord compression, and order appropriate imaging and neurology/neurosurgery consultation. Emergent decompressive laminectomy may be indicated. However, the best treatment is prevention, and there are consensus guidelines regarding anticoagulation in the setting of neuraxial anesthesia.[14] These recommendations can be found at the website for the American Society of Regional Anesthesia and Pain Medicine at http://www.asra.com/items_of_interest/consensus_statements/

(*see* Chapters 100 for more detail). Highlights of the recommendations include:

- *Minidose subcutaneous heparin for thromboprophylaxis.* There are no contraindications to the use of neuraxial blocks, although delaying the heparin injection until after the block may reduce the risk of neuraxial bleeding. Since heparin-induced thrombocytopenia may occur during heparin administration, patients receiving heparin for greater than 4 days should have a platelet count assessed prior to neuraxial block and catheter removal.

- *Preoperative low molecular weight heparin (LMWH) thromboprophylaxis.* Delay neuraxial block at least 10–12 hours after a dose of LWMH.

- *Postoperative LMWH thromboprophylaxis (single daily dosing).* Give first dose 6–8 hours following surgery with neuraxial block, and the second dose no sooner than 24 hours after the first dose. Indwelling neuraxial catheters may be safely maintained. However, the catheter should be removed a minimum of 10–12 hours after the last dose of LMWH. Subsequent dosing should occur a minimum of 2 hours after catheter removal. Thromboprophylaxis using a twice-daily dosing regimen of LMWH may be associated with increased risk of spinal hematoma; indwelling neuraxial catheters should be avoided in these patients.

- *Therapeutic LMWH (for example, enoxaparin 1 mg/kg twice daily).* Delay neuraxial block at least 24 hours after the LMWH dose.

- *Warfarin.* Stop 4–5 days prior to neuraxial block; the international normalized ratio (INR) should be within normal limits.

- *Thienopyridine antiplatelet therapy.* Stop clopidogrel 7 days prior to neuraxial block. Stop ticlopidine 14 days prior to block.

- *NSAIDs.* There does not appear to be a significant risk of spinal hematoma in persons taking NSAIDs who undergo neuraxial anesthesia.

Cardiovascular Complications

Myocardial Ischemia

Description. Coronary artery disease is a leading cause of perioperative morbidity and mortality. Myocardial ischemia may result from adverse hemodynamic effects including hypertension, hypotension, or tachycardia; or from acute coronary plaque rupture, coronary thrombosis, or coronary vasospasm. Patients with an area of critical coronary stenosis may develop ischemia in areas distal to the stenotic lesion as a result of intra- and postoperative hemodynamic changes. Patients with noncritical coronary stenosis may suffer an acute plaque rupture with subsequent coronary thrombosis due to the surgically induced hypercoagulable state or from tachycardia inducing increased sheer stress. One third of perioperative cardiac events occur in patients with noncritical lesions, but preoperative cardiac testing will not identify these patients.[15]

Risk factors. Approximately 30% of adults undergoing surgery each year in the United States have coronary artery disease or have risk factors for it.[16] Many of these patients are potentially at risk for perioperative myocardial ischemia and can be identified preoperatively based on traditional cardiac risk factors and through the use of guidelines such as the American College of Cardiology/American Heart Association 2002 Perioperative Car-

diovascular Evaluation for Noncardiac Surgery.[17] In addition, severe aortic stenosis is a risk factor for myocardial ischemia and infarction (independent of coronary disease)[18] and may cause hypotension and decreased cardiac output.

Preoperative Treatment. Identify risk factors preoperatively, and risk stratify patients accordingly. Some patients may require preoperative noninvasive cardiac testing, although such tests generally should not be performed unless the result is expected to change patient management.[19] Continue cardiac medications as indicated, especially beta-blockers and clonidine. Certain patients not previously on a beta-blocker may benefit from perioperative beta-blockade.[20,21] Evaluate persons with suspected aortic stenosis preoperatively to determine severity of disease and if further treatment should be considered prior to an elective surgery. Persons with heart failure should be at their optimal baseline fluid status. Current guidelines[17,22] recommend postponing elective surgery in persons with a systolic blood pressure greater than 180 mm Hg and a diastolic blood pressure greater than 110 mm Hg. Such elevations in blood pressure may increase the risk of perioperative hemodynamic instability, myocardial ischemia, and cardiac arrhythmias. However, these guidelines are based on studies with small sample sizes and outcomes other than myocardial infarction.[23] There is no clear evidence that deferring anesthesia and surgery in these patients will reduce perioperative risk, especially in patients with no target organ damage.[24] Except in cases of extreme hypertension or severe target organ damage, patients can undergo surgery with acute control of hypertension if it is important not to delay surgery.[25]

Postoperative Treatment. Myocardial infarction most commonly occurs within the first 48 hours following surgery. Continue cardiac medications as tolerated and optimize blood pressure, heart rate, and fluid balance. Control factors that can contribute to hypertension or tachycardia (including pain, anxiety, hypoxemia, hypothermia, anemia, volume depletion or overload, fever, urine retention, and constipation) to decrease the risk of myocardial ischemia. Be vigilant for possible withdrawal syndromes from alcohol and other drugs.

Intravascular Fluid Balance

Description. Intraoperative fluid therapy is a delicate balance of maintaining adequate ventricular preload while avoiding fluid overload. Intraoperative fluid is given to compensate for any preoperative deficit (nil per os [NPO] status, vomiting, diarrhea, fever), to meet ongoing maintenance requirements, to provide medications, to treat transient episodes of hypotension, and to compensate for intraoperative fluid losses. Intraoperative fluid losses include bleeding, fluid shifts ("third spacing"), and insensible losses[26]; replacement of these losses generally accounts for the bulk of fluid administration. Additional fluid administration may be required in the early postoperative period to treat ongoing third spacing, which is a cytokine-mediated process. Despite the significantly positive fluid balance of many patients, the total intraoperative fluid administration is generally appropriate to compensate for losses and to maintain organ perfusion, and these patients are intravascularly euvolemic. However, excess fluid administration will increase the amount of third-spaced fluid and can impair left ventricular function in patients with underlying heart failure. The resulting decreased cardiac output can affect pulmonary, gastrointestinal, and renal function and may impair wound healing.[27]

Risk factors. Elderly patients and those with known systolic or diastolic cardiac dysfunction, mitral stenosis, severe liver dysfunction/cirrhosis, or renal insufficiency are at risk for postoperative fluid over-load. Patients who have a net fluid retention of more than 67 mL/kg/day (about 5 L in a 70-kg person) within the initial 36 postoperative hours may be at risk for pulmonary edema.[28]

Treatment. Unless there is evidence of decompensated heart failure, it is usually best to avoid diuresis above the amount provided by the patient's baseline medications. In certain cases, patients may benefit from having their diuretics held in the immediate postoperative period. Otherwise, intravascular volume depletion can occur that may cause cerebral or coronary ischemia or precipitate renal insufficiency. Note that urine output is typically reduced in the first 12–24 hours after surgery because of stress-induced elevation in anti-diuretic hormone, and does not necessarily imply renal insufficiency.[29] Assuming normal cardiac and renal function, patients will begin to mobilize the third-spaced fluids around postoperative day 2 or 3, and urine output will significantly increase without the need for diuretics. However, elderly patients may take twice as long as younger patients to mobilize and excrete overexpanded extracellular volume.[30] Patients with decreased left ventricular function may develop intravascular fluid overload as a result of fluid mobilization. These patients should be diuresed while carefully monitoring blood pressure, blood urea nitrogen (BUN), creatinine, and urine output.

Pulmonary Complications

Aspiration

Description. General anesthesia and deep sedation impair airway reflexes, making patients more likely to aspirate oropharyngeal and gastric contents.

Risk Factors. Many conditions increase the risk for aspiration during general anesthesia, including recently ingested food, prior dysphagia/debility, gastroesophageal reflux, bowel obstruction, pregnancy, obesity, diabetic gastroparesis, acute hyperglycemia, and advanced age.[31] Postoperative vomiting is also a risk factor.

Treatment. Therapy is mainly supportive, so prevention is key. Patients should follow NPO guidelines. It may be helpful to premedicate those at increased risk with nonparticulate antacids, H_2-receptor antagonists, or proton pump inhibitors. In cases of witnessed aspiration, perform suctioning immediately and treat the resulting chemical pneumonitis with aggressive supportive therapy, including mechanical ventilation, if necessary.[32] Secondary bacterial infection may develop and should be treated with antibiotics. Use of corticosteroids is controversial, but most likely will not improve long-term outcome following aspiration.[32]

Hypoxia

Description. Postoperative hypoxia occurs frequently and may persist for up to 1 to 5 days. Upper abdominal surgery generally leads to longer and more severe hypoxia than nonabdominal and nonthoracic surgery.[32] Causes in the early postoperative period include depressed respiratory drive, decreased FRC, limited inspiration due to pain, bronchospasm, pharyngeal secretions, atelectasis, and pulmonary edema. Negative-pressure pulmonary edema secondary to inspiratory efforts against a closed glottis during laryngospasm is a rare cause of hypoxia. Obstructive sleep apnea increases the risk for respiratory depression. Numerous other conditions may lead to hypoxia, including coronary ischemia, heart failure, pulmonary embolism (PE); and nosocomial pneumonia. PE classically presents, usually after the second postoperative day, with acute-onset of dyspnea with hypoxia, tachypnea, and tachycardia. Nosocomial pneumonia typically manifests later in the postoperative period.

Risk factors. Smokers and patients who have decreased pulmonary function due to age effects, COPD, asthma, sleep apnea, and obesity are at increased risk for postoperative hypoxia. Severe COPD imparts a ten-fold increase in the incidence of bronchospasm, pulmonary complications, and death.[7] Sleep apnea may be unmasked, induced, or worsened by anesthetic and analgesic agents[33] and should be identified preoperatively.

Treatment. As with other postoperative complications, prevention is of utmost importance. Patients should stop smoking at least 8 weeks before surgery, if possible.[34] Patients with asthma should be at their baseline before elective surgery. Instruct all patients on postoperative pulmonary toilet, including incentive spirometry, deep breathing exercises, and coughing. Frequently assess volume status to monitor for fluid overload. Patients with sleep apnea should bring their CPAP to the hospital; exercise caution when giving these patients sedatives and opioids. Patients suspected of having sleep apnea may benefit from a formal sleep evaluation prior to elective surgery. Patients with known respiratory disease may require continuous pulse oximetry in the initial postoperative period.

Provide supplemental oxygen and ventilatory support as necessary to hypoxic patients, and perform a thorough diagnostic workup. Treat patients with bronchospasm, pulmonary edema, or nosocomial pneumonia appropriately, noting the differences in possible causes in the postoperative period. When treating patients with evidence of acute coronary syndrome or PE, always consult with the surgical team prior to starting anticoagulation to determine the risk-to-benefit ratio of treatment versus operative-site bleeding. Surgical patients receiving anticoagulation may benefit from protective measures such as pressure dressings and elastic wraps to minimize bleeding.

Gastrointestinal Complications

Postoperative Nausea and Vomiting

Description. PONV is common, is a major concern for patients, and can lead to prolonged hospital stays and increased morbidity.

Risk Factors. Females, persons prone to motion sickness, patients who have previously suffered from PONV, and nonsmokers are at risk.[35,36]

Treatment. Reduce PONV by minimizing opioids (while providing adequate analgesia), by avoiding sudden patient movements, by maintaining hydration, by avoiding noxious stimuli, and by practicing relaxation techniques. Start feedings with a clear liquid diet that is slowly advanced. Give antiemetics and anxiolytics as needed. Supplemental oxygen may improve the symptoms of PONV.[37] Other effective treatments include acupressure at the P6 point[38] (2–5 minutes of pressure every 2–4 hours on the forearm 5 cm above the wrist crease, between the palmaris longus and the flexor carpi radialis tendons) and intermittent inhalation of isopropyl alcohol (i.e., alcohol swabs or pads, three deep sniffs with the pad 1 inch from the nose, repeat as needed every 5 minutes for three doses).[39]

Ileus

Description. Ileus is a nonobstructive delay in coordinated movement of the gastrointestinal tract.[40] Clinical signs and symptoms include diminished bowel sounds, abdominal pain and distention, nausea, vomiting, and delayed passage of flatus and stool.

Risk factors. Risk factors include the type of surgery (particularly intra-abdominal procedures), general anesthesia, and analgesic medications (especially opioids). Excessive fluid administration can cause gut edema and may contribute to an ileus.[40] Patients who have untreated hypothyroidism or chronic constipation or who take laxatives on a regular basis may be at increased risk for developing an ileus. Electrolyte abnormalities (hypokalemia, hyponatremia, hypomagnesemia, and hypercalcemia), hyperglycemia, and calcium channel blockers may also contribute to development of an ileus.

Treatment. Adequate pain relief is important in treating a postoperative ileus, since sympathetic stimulation from pain leads to decreased bowel motility. Although opioids can cause or worsen an ileus, always strive for optimal pain control, possibly with nonopioid analgesics. Other interventions that may help improve an ileus include early enteral feedings, early ambulation, and a short hospital stay.[10,40] Laxative agents such as magnesium citrate may be of benefit, and sugarless chewing gum given three times daily seems to be effective in stimulating bowel motility.[41,42] Motility agents such as metoclopramide may help, but should be avoided if there is any concern for bowel obstruction. A nasogastric tube may worsen an ileus, but one can be placed if the patient has significant discomfort from nausea, vomiting, and abdominal distention.

CONCLUSIONS

Hospitalists are uniquely positioned to help prevent and treat perioperative medical complications. With a basic understanding of the complexities and effects of anesthesia, hospitalists can identify and treat conditions preoperatively that may be of concern to the anesthesiologist. Furthermore, such knowledge will help hospitalists anticipate, diagnose, and treat postoperative complications. Only with a team effort can we ensure that each patient arrives in the operating room fully prepared and medically optimized, and is appropriately managed after surgery. Although we cannot guarantee success, we can improve the patient's chances for a good outcome.

Key Points

- Modern anesthetic techniques are extremely safe, with an estimated mortality of 1 per 250,000 cases.

- General and regional anesthesia are largely equivalent regarding morbidity and mortality. The decision regarding which technique to use is complex and depends on the location, extent and anticipated duration of the proposed operation, the medical condition of the patient, and the skills and preferences of the anesthesia and surgical teams.

- Over sedation can result from prolonged effects of general anesthetic agents and from opioids potentially leading to respiratory depression and inability to protect the airway. All patients with prolonged sedation should be monitored with continuous pulse oximetry.

- General anesthesia and deep sedation impair airway reflexes and make patients more likely to aspirate oropharyngeal and gastric contents.

- Epidural hematoma following regional anesthesia is rare, but may lead to spinal cord compression causing paraplegia or cauda equina syndrome. Risk factors include anticoagulation, thienopyridine antiplatelet therapy (clopidogrel and ticlopidine), recent thrombolytic therapy, underlying coagulopathy, and traumatic needle placement.

- Myocardial infarction most commonly occurs within the first 48 hours following surgery, so hospitalists should control factors that can contribute to hypertension or tachycardia (including pain, anxiety, hypoxemia, hypothermia, anemia, volume depletion or overload, fever, urine retention, and constipation).

- Despite the significantly positive fluid balance of many patients, the amount of intraoperative fluid administration is generally appropriate to compensate for losses and to maintain organ perfusion. Be cautious with diuretics in the immediate postoperative period.

- Postoperative hypoxia occurs frequently and may persist for up to 4–5 days. Causes in the early postoperative period include depressed respiratory drive, decreased functional residual capacity, limited inspiration due to pain, bronchospasm, pharyngeal secretions, atelectasis, and pulmonary edema.

- PONV is common and is seen most often in females, in people prone to motion sickness, in those who have previously suffered from PONV, and in nonsmokers.

- Adequate pain relief is important in treating a postoperative ileus, since sympathetic stimulation from pain leads to decreased bowel motility. Although opioids can cause or worsen an ileus, always strive for optimal pain control, possibly with nonopioid analgesics.

SUGGESTED READING

Ben-David B, Rawa R. Complications of neuraxial blockade. Anesthesiol Clin North Am 2002; 20:669–693.

Luckey A, Livingston E, Taché Y. Mechanisms and treatment of postoperative ileus. Arch Surg 2003; 138:206–214.

Horlocker TT, Wedel DJ, Benzon H, et al. Regional anesthesia in the anticoagulated patient: defining the risks (the second ASRA consensus conference on neuraxial anesthesia and anticoagulation). Reg Anesth Pain Med 2003; 28(3):172–197.

Eagle KA, Berger PB, Calkins H, et al. Perioperative cardiovascular evaluation for noncardiac surgery: ACC/AHA 2002 Guideline Update. J Am Coll Cardiol 2002; 39:542–553.

Liu LL, Wiener-Kronish JP. Perioperative anesthesia issues in the elderly. Crit Care Clin 2003; 19:641–656.

Caruso LJ, Kirby RR. Fluids, electrolytes, blood, and blood substitutes. In: Clinical Anesthesia Practice, 2nd ed. Kirby RR, Gravenstein N, Lobato EB, Gravensteon JS, eds. WB Saunders Company: 2002; 770–789.

Rosenthal MH. Intraoperative fluid management: What and how much? Chest 1999; 115:106S–112S.

Jin F, Chung F. Minimizing perioperative adverse events in the elderly. Br J Anaesth 2001; 87:608–624.

Conde MV, Im SS. Overview of the management of postoperative pulmonary complications. In: Rose BD, ed. Waltham, MA: 2005.

Jain SS, Dhand R. Perioperative treatment of patients with obstructive sleep apnea. Curr Opin Pulm Med 2004; 10:482–488.

Apfel CC, Roewer N. Risk assessment of postoperative nausea and vomiting. Int Anesthesiol Clin 2003; 41(4):13–32.

Mythen MG. Postoperative gastrointestinal tract dysfunction. Anesth Analg 2005; 100:196–204.

Section

Fifteen

Preoperative Assessments and Preparation

98 Preoperative Evaluation and Testing
Mark Enzler, Bradly J. Narr

99 Perioperative Medication Management
Nathan O. Spell, Steven L. Cohn

100 Perioperative Anticoagulation: Prophylaxis for Venous Thromboembolism (VTE)
Jason Stein, Michael P. Phy, Amir K. Jaffer

101 Management of Long-term Warfarin for Surgery
Jason Stein, Michael P. Phy, Amir K. Jaffer

102 Cardiovascular Preoperative Risk Assessment and Evaluation
Steven L. Cohn, Dennis M. Manning

103 Pulmonary Preoperative Risk Assessment and Evaluation
Rendell W. Ashton, Ognjen Gajic, Gerald W. Smetana

104 Perioperative Management of Diabetic Patients
Maged Doss, Guillermo E. Umpierrez

105 Nutrition in the Perioperative Period
Lisa Kirkland

CHAPTER NINETY-EIGHT

Preoperative Evaluation and Testing

Mark Enzler, MD, and Bradly J. Narr, MD

BACKGROUND

The objective of preoperative assessment is to become familiar with the surgical illness, coexisting medical conditions, and patient risk factors that may increase the risk of anesthesia. The history and physical examination are used to define those patients who may benefit from further evaluation and diagnostic testing, with the ultimate goal of reducing perioperative morbidity and mortality. The American Society of Anesthesiologists (ASA) has approved a Practice Advisory for Preanesthetic Care, based on best available evidence and current practice.[1] In the setting of non-emergent surgeries, the patient interview and physical examination should be performed prior to the day of surgery for patients with high severity of disease or for patients with low severity of disease undergoing procedures with high surgical invasiveness.

History

Obtain pertinent information from review of the medical and anesthesia records, if available in a timely fashion, and then interview the patient. Review of pertinent medical and surgical consultations or direct discussion with the medical or surgical staff may add important information or substitute when the medical record is unavailable.

A complete preoperative health assessment includes:

A. **Current surgical illness.** The provider should have a basic understanding of the surgical illness, diagnostic studies or therapies that have been employed, and indications for the planned surgical procedure.

B. **Medical history.** Review the status of known medical problems, with an emphasis on cardiopulmonary disease because it accounts for the majority of serious complications. Also ask about airway, renal, neurologic, gastrointestinal, musculoskeletal, and genitourinary problems.

C. **Current medications.** Review and record the patient's prescription and nonprescription medications, including dosing and schedule. Continue all necessary medications prescribed for the patient up through the morning of surgery with a small sip of water. Some medications should be held or adjusted prior to surgery, such as anticoagulants, insulin, oral hypoglycemics, and antiplatelet agents (*see* Chapter 99). Additionally, prophylactic therapy to prevent cardiac ischemia, surgical site infection, venous thromboembolism, endocardi-

tis, relative adrenal insufficiency, and aspiration may be indicated (Chapters 99, 103, and 112, respectively). The ASA has published guidelines for preoperative fasting status: a 2-hour fast is recommended after ingestion of clear liquids; 4-hour fast following breast milk; 6-hour fast following infant formula, nonhuman milk, or light meal; and 8-hour fast following ingestion of fried or fatty foods, and meat.[2] These guidelines are intended for relatively healthy individuals without risk factors for delayed gastric emptying. Patients undergoing emergency surgery or patients with predisposing factors for delayed gastric emptying (diabetic patients, narcotic use, morbidly obese patients) should follow more traditional nil-by-mouth (NPO) guidelines.

D. **Allergies and intolerances to medications or other agents** should be documented, including reaction type. Although the prevalence of penicillin allergy in the general population is unknown, the incidence of self-reported penicillin allergy ranges from 1–10%, and the frequency of life-threatening immunoglobulin E (IgE)-mediated anaphylaxis is estimated at 0.01 to 0.05%.[3] Some severe penicillin (PCN) reactions are non–IgE-mediated, such as hemolytic anemia, thrombocytopenia, interstitial nephritis, serum sickness, drug fever, morbilliform eruptions, erythema multiforme minor (EM), Stevens-Johnson, or toxic epidermal necrolysis (TEN). Consider referring the patient with a history of allergy to penicillin or cephalosporin for a formal allergy consultation and consideration of penicillin skin testing if beta-lactam therapy is being considered.

E. **Tobacco, alcohol, and illicit drug history.** Smoking contributes to many perioperative complications, including pneumonia, respiratory failure, cardiovascular events, and impaired healing of bones and surgical wounds. Assess the amount of tobacco used, and advise as well as assist the patient to quit smoking preoperatively if time allows. Preoperative smoking cessation of 6–8 weeks has been shown to decrease overall complications, although the optimal duration of tobacco cessation preoperatively is unknown.[4,5] The patient should be counseled to stop smoking at least 12 hours before surgery, use nicotine gum instead of smoking the morning of surgery, be provided with nicotine replacement postoperatively, and to stay smoke free for at least 1 week after surgery.[6]

Alcohol dependence may increase anesthetic requirements and can be associated with alcohol withdrawal syndrome (*see* Chapter X) which may include seizures, hallucinosis, or delirium tremens. Screening for alcohol abuse can be accomplished using the CAGE Questionnaire[7,8] (Table 98-1). Table 98-2 summarizes the Diagnostic and Statistical Manual of Mental Disorders-IV (DSM-IV) definitions of alcohol abuse and dependence.[41] Monitor the alcohol-dependent patient postoperatively for signs of withdrawal. We employ the Clinical Institute Withdrawal Assessment for alcohol scale (CIWA-Ar) as a rapid assessment tool that objectively quantifies the severity of alcohol withdrawal in the hospitalized patient and triggers benzodiazepine dosing according to the severity of alcohol-withdrawal symptoms.[9] The CIWA is a validated, reproducible tool that can be used by nursing staff to monitor and treat patients for alcohol-withdrawal syndrome.

Excess preoperative opioid or benzodiazepine use may also increase the requirements for anesthesia or adequate postoperative analgesia. Monitor these patients for withdrawal, and offer chemical dependency counseling if indicated.

F. **Family Medical History** should be documented, including bleeding disorders, reactions to anesthesia, or malignant hyperthermia (MH). MH is a life-threatening hypermetabolic crisis in susceptible individuals that occurs after exposure to succinylcholine or inhalational anesthetics. The prevalence of MH is estimated to be 1 in 8,500. There is a strong genetic predisposition to MH, as it is inherited as an autosomal dominant trait. Thus, patients with siblings and children of MH-susceptible patients have a 50% risk for this disorder. Although baseline creative kinase (CK) determinations may be of no value in screening for MH, relatives of MH-susceptible patients with an elevated CK level without recent trauma or muscle disorder have greater than 80% chance of being susceptible—although a normal CK level does not rule out MH suscep-tibility. Inform the anesthesiologist of any family history of MH, anesthesia, or operative complications.

FOCUSED REVIEW OF ISSUES PERTINENT TO THE PLANNED PROCEDURE

Current Status of Pertinent Known Medical Problems

1. **Cardiovascular status.** The presence of major or intermediate cardiac clinical indicators prior to a high- or intermediate-risk surgery may warrant preoperative cardiac evaluation[10]

(*see* Chapter 102). Inform the anesthesia team of the presence of cardiac pacemakers or implantable defibrillators. Uncontrolled hypertension is associated with wider fluctuations of blood pressure (BP) during induction of anesthesia and may increase the risk for perioperative cardiac ischemic events. It is appropriate to defer anesthesia and surgery where possible in a patient with admission arterial pressures greater than 180 systolic or 110 diastolic, especially if there is evidence of target organ damage.[11] This recommendation is made on the basis of evidence of risk in medical patients rather than data on perioperative risk.[12,13] Identify signs or symptoms of peripheral vascular disease such as claudication, rest pain, nonhealing ulcers, or deep venous thrombosis, particularly in patients undergoing major surgery or joint replacement.

2. **Pulmonary status.** Asthma may be accompanied by mucous plugging and acute bronchospasm after the induction of anesthesia or endotracheal intubation. Four percent of men and 2% of women have obstructive sleep apnea (OSA), the overwhelming majority of whom remain undiagnosed. Heavy or persistent snoring, sudden awakenings accompanied by choking, apneas as observed by the bed partner, and excessive sleepiness during daytime may suggest OSA. Patients with OSA have an increased risk of other comorbidities, such as cardiovascular disease, hypertension, heart failure, and atrial fibrillation, and there have been numerous reports of perioperative complications with patients with OSA.[14,15] Patients with diagnosed OSA should bring their continuous positive airway pressure (CPAP) or bilevel positive airway pressure (BiPAP) machines to the hospital on the day of surgery to be

Table 98-1 CAGE Questionnaire: Screen for Alcohol Abuse/Dependence

1. Have you ever felt you ought to **C**ut down on your drinking?
2. Have people **A**nnoyed you by criticizing your drinking?
3. Have you ever felt bad or **G**uilty about your drinking?
4. Have you ever had a drink first thing in the morning to steady your nerves or get rid of a hangover (**E**ye opener)?

Key: One positive response suggests closer assessment; two or more positive responses: 85% sensitive and 90% specific for alcohol abuse.[7]

From: Ewing JA. The CAGE questionnaire. JAMA 1984; 252:1905–1907, with permission.

Table 98-2 Alcohol Use Disorders—DSM-IV Definitions

Alcohol Abuse (one or more)	Alcohol Dependence (3 or more)
Failure to fulfill work, school, or social obligations	Tolerance
Recurrent substance use in physically hazardous situations	Substance taken in larger quantity than intended
Recurrent legal problems	Withdrawal
Continued use despite alcohol-related social/interpersonal problems	Persistent desire to cut down or control use
	Time is spent obtaining, using, or recovering from the substance
	Social, occupational, or recreational tasks are sacrificed
	Use continues despite physical and psychological problems

DSM = Diagnostic and Statistical Manual of Mental Disorders-IV. Published by the American Psychiatric Association. APA. Diagnostic and statistical manual of mental disorders: DSM-IV (by the DSM-IV Task Force of the American Psychiatric Association). 4 ed. Washington, DC; 1994.

used in the immediate postoperative period, during transfer to the postanesthesia care unit (PACU) and whenever sleeping.

3. **Gastrointestinal prophylaxis** with acid-lowering therapy may decrease the risk of aspiration in obese patients, pregnant women, and in those with a hiatal hernia.

4. **Hematologic status**, including hemostasis and severe (symptomatic) anemia.

5. **Functional status.** Knowledge of the patient's maximum physical activity level—in terms of metabolic equivalents (METs) may help predict the overall outcome in the perioperative period (Table 98-3). Patients who are unable to perform activities involving more than four METs without becoming symptomatic of chest pain or shortness of breath are at increased perioperative risk.[16,17]

6. **History of cervical spine instability** should be documented.

7. **Infection.** Documentation of recent fever, hepatitis B or C, antibiotic use, or active infection (especially TB) is important. A recent upper respiratory infection may predispose patients to pulmonary complications, including bronchospasm and laryngospasm. Open wounds or skin infections, particularly in the area of the planned surgery, may increase the risk of surgical site infection. Patients with HIV infection should have recent (3 months) CD4 cell count and HIV viral load results. Many antiretrovirals have significant drug–drug interaction potential.[18] Methicillin-resistant *Staphylococcus aureus* (MRSA) or vancornycin resistant enterococcus (VRE) infection or carrier state should also be noted.

If significant symptomatic or unstable comorbidities are encountered, obtain appropriate studies and/or preoperative consultations as indicated.

PHYSICAL EXAMINATION

Perform a general examination with the focus guided by the preoperative history.

Vital signs to be documented include blood pressure (in both arms with an appropriately sized cuff, and supine and standing if hypovolemia is suspected), oral temperature if infection is suspected, pulse rate and regularity, respiratory rate and pattern, and height and weight to determine medication dosing and adequacy of postoperative urine output.

Skin: Observe for rash, open lesions, bruising, or jaundice. Examine the back/buttocks and pressure points in elderly, frail bedbound patients to assess for pressure-induced ulcerations.

Airway: With the patient seated, note the mouth opening, thyromental distance, neck movement, ability to prognath (move jaw forward), and presence of loose or broken teeth, dentures, range of cervical spine motion in flexion, extension, and rotation. Physical findings that may contribute to difficult intubation are summarized in Table 98-4.[19]

Pulmonary: Observe the pattern of breathing, and document breath sounds. Rhonchi represent large airway secretions and should clear with cough. Inspiratory crackles may indicate an alveolar process. Purulent secretions and cough may suggest viral or bacterial infection. Significant wheezing may suggest reactive airway disease. Distant breath sounds with prolonged expiratory phase may suggest chronic obstructive pulmonary disease (COPD); if symptoms are at baseline with good exercise tolerance, then there is no benefit to delaying surgery.

Cardiac examination should focus on the detection of heart failure and aortic stenosis. Note the presence of murmurs (systolic, diastolic, quality, grade, and location), S_3 or S_4. Peripheral edema, elevated jugular venous distension, or a third heart sound may suggest poorly compensated heart failure. The presence of severe aortic stenosis (AS) is associated with a high risk of perioperative morbidity and mortality. The finding of a systolic ejection murmur at the right upper sternal border that radiates to the neck suggests the presence of AS. Clues that the disease is at least moderate in severity are peaking of the murmur late in systole, palpable delay of the carotid upstroke, and a soft single S_2 sound. Patients with significant AS, particularly in the presence of any of the classic symptoms of angina, syncope, or dyspnea or patients undergoing coronary-artery bypass surgery or surgery on the aorta or other heart valves should be evaluated by a cardiologist prior to elective surgery.[20]

Abdomen. Note any distention, ascites, mass or organomegaly (liver, spleen, bladder, kidney), or changes consistent with portal hypertension or peritonitis.

Table 98-3 Estimated Energy Requirements for Various Activities	
1 MET	Can you care for yourself? Eat, dress, or use the toilet? Walk 1–2 blocks on level ground at 2–3mph Walk indoors Do light work around the house (dusting; washing dishes)
4 METS	Climb a flight of stairs or walk up a hill Walk on level ground at 4 mph (6.4 km/hr) Do heavy work around the house (scrubbing floors or lifting or moving heavy furniture) Run a short distance Participate in moderate recreational activities like golf, bowling, dancing, doubles tennis, or throwing a baseball or football
Greater than 10 METS	Participate in strenuous sports like swimming, singles tennis, football, basketball, or skiing

MET = metabolic equivalent; km = kilometer; hr = hour; mph = miles per hour.

Modified from: Eagle KA, Berger PB, Caklins H, et al. ACC/AHA guidelines update for perioperative cardiovascular evaluation for noncardiac surgery: executive summary: A report of the American College of Cardiology/American Heart Association Task Force on Practice Guideline (Committee to Update the 1996 Guidelines on Perioperative Cardiovascular Evaluation for Noncardiac Surgery). Circulation 2002; 105:1257–1267.

Table 98-4 Components of the Preoperative Airway Physical Examination

Airway Examination Component	Nonreassuring Findings
1. Length of upper incisors	Relatively long
2. Relation of maxillary and mandibular incisors during normal jaw closure	Prominent "overbite" (maxillary incisors anterior to mandibular incisors)
3. Relation of maxillary and mandibular incisors during voluntary protrusion	Patient cannot bring mandibular incisors anterior to maxillary incisors
4. Interincisor distance	Less than 3 cm
5. Visibility of uvula	Not visible when tongue is protruded with patient in sitting position (e.g. Mallampati class greater than II)
6. Shape of palate	Highly arched or very narrow
7. Compliance of mandibular space	Stiff, indurated, occupied by mass, or nonresilient
8. Thyromental distance	Less than three ordinary finger breadths
9. Length of neck	Short
10. Thickness of neck	Thick
11. Range of motion of head and neck	Patient cannot touch tip of chin to chest of cannot extend neck.

This table displays some findings of the airway physical examination that may suggest the presence of a difficult intubation. The decision to examine some or all of the airway components shown in this table depends on the clinical context and judgment of the practitioner. The table is not intended as a mandatory or exhaustive list of the components of an airway examination. The order of presentation in this table follow the "line of sight" that occurs during conventional oral laryngoscopy.

Adapted from: ASA. Practice guidelines for management of the difficult airway: an updated report by the American Society of Anesthesiologists Task Force on Management of the Difficult Airway Anesthesiology 2003; 98:1269–1277, with permission.

Vascular. Perform auscultation for abdominal, carotid, and femoral bruits. Assess the pulses in a patient with a claudication history or planned extremity surgery in patients with significant cardiovascular risk factors.

Musculoskeletal/Extremities. Assess for injuries, range of motion, position of limbs with fractures, muscle wasting, deformities, weakness, capillary refill, venous stasis changes, clubbing, and cyanosis.

Neurologic examination may be cursory in healthy patients or extensive in patients with coexisting neurologic disease. Perform formal testing of strength, sensation, and reflexes in patients who are to undergo procedures that may result in neurologic deficits. Assess the mental status, cognition, peripheral sensorimotor function, asterixis, movement disorders, focal neurologic deficit, hearing/vision impairment if indicated by the planned surgery or medical history.

Laboratory Studies

Traditionally, the goal of preoperative laboratory testing has been to detect conditions that may alter the risk of surgery, unsuspected abnormalities that can be modified, or to obtain baseline results that can be helpful in the perioperative period. *Routine testing* is defined as a test ordered in the absence of a specific clinical indication or purpose. "Preop status" is not considered a specific clinical indication or purpose. Numerous studies have called into question the need to obtain "routine" preoperative testing in healthy patients.[21–23] An *indicated test* is a test that is ordered for a specific clinical indication or purpose. Preoperative tests may be ordered, required, or performed on a selective basis for purposes of guiding or optimizing perioperative management. The indications for such testing should be documented and based on information obtained from medical records, patient interview, physical examination, and the type and invasiveness of the planned procedure.

Table 98-5 Types of Surgical Procedures Based on Degree of Invasiveness

Class A, Minimally invasive
- Little potential to disrupt normal physiology
- Rarely associated with morbidity related to the anesthetic
- Rarely require blood administration, invasive monitoring, or postoperative management in a critical care setting
- *Examples:* cataract extraction, diagnostic arthroscopy, postpartum tubal ligation

Class B, Moderately invasive
- Modest potential to disrupt normal physiology
- May require blood administration, invasive monitoring, or postoperative management in a critical care setting
- *Examples:* carotid endarterectomy, abdominal hysterectomy, laparoscopic cholecystectomy

Class C, Highly invasive
- Typically produce significant disruption of normal physiology
- Almost always require blood administration, invasive monitoring, and postoperative management in a critical care setting
- *Examples:* total hip replacement, open aortic aneurysm resection, aortic valve replacement, posterior fossa craniotomy of aneurysm

Modified from: Roizen MF, Fleisher LA. Anesthetic implications of concurrent disease. In: Miller RD, ed. Miller's Anesthesia. Vol 1. 6th ed. Philadelphia: Elsevier-Churchill Livingstone, 2005: 1017–1149, with permission.

The ASA has published an *Advisory* for preoperative testing based on common practice and best available evidence.[1] Table 98-5 represents a simplified strategy for using clinical judgment in ordering preoperative testing for surgical class B and C procedures.[24] A careful history and physical examination of the

Table 98-6 American Society of Anesthesiologists Physical Status Classification

Status	Disease State
ASA Class 1	Nonorganic, physiologic, biochemical, psychiatric disturbance
ASA Class 2	Mild-to-moderate systemic disturbance that may not may be related to the reason for surgery
ASA Class 3	Severe systemic disturbance that may or may not better reason for surgery
ASA Class 4	Severe systemic disturbance that is life threatening with or without surgery
ASA Class 5	Moribund patient who has little chance of survival but is submitted to surgery as a last resort (resuscitative effort)
ASA Class 6	Brain dead organ donor
Emergency Operation (E)	Any patient in whom an emergency operation is required

ASA = American Society of Anesthesiologists

Adapted from: ASA. New classification of physical status. Anesthesiology 1963; 24:111, with permission from the American Society for Anesthesiologists.

patient are required, with special attention to testing whenever indicators of disease entities listed in the tables are discovered.

Specific Laboratory Testing

Electrocardiogram. An electrocardiogram (ECG) is recommended for patients with known cardiac risk factors. The validity of performing an ECG on all patients over a certain age is not supported by controlled studies.[1] The preoperative ECG may be helpful to establish a baseline that allows both preoperative myocardial evaluation and comparison with postoperative tracings. The significance of preoperative ECG abnormalities is discussed in Chapter 103.

The American College of Cardiology (ACC)/American Heart Association (AHA) guidelines recommend based on available evidence that preoperative ECGs should be obtained with recent chest pain or ischemic equivalent in clinically intermediate- or high-risk surgical patients scheduled for an intermediate- or high-risk operative procedure. The weight of evidence favors obtaining preoperative ECG in asymptomatic persons with diabetes mellitus (DM), prior coronary revascularization, asymptomatic men >45 years old, or women >55 years old, with two or more atherosclerotic risk factors (hypertension, stroke, DM, renal insufficiency, or hypercholesterolemia), or prior hospital admission for cardiac causes. On the other hand, ECG is not useful as a routine test in asymptomatic subjects undergoing low-risk operative procedures.[12]

Chest roentgenography is indicated for patients with a history of cardiac or pulmonary disease or with recent respiratory symptoms. Extremes of age, smoking, stable COPD, stable cardiac disease, or resolved recent upper respiratory infection (URI) are not necessarily indications for chest radiography.[1]

Pulmonary function testing and/or arterial blood gases (ABGs) should be considered for patients with symptomatic lung disease (asthma, COPD, restrictive lung disease), those undergoing lung resection, or in patients in whom uncharacterized lung disease is suspected. Consider pulmonary consultation in the setting of symptomatic lung disease or anticipated lung surgery[25] (see Chapter 103).

Serum electrolytes including potassium are indicated in patients taking various medications (such as diuretics, angiotensin converting enzyme (ACE) inhibitors, angiotensin receptor blockers, digoxin, amphotericin B, corticosteroids, *cis*-platinum), with chronic kidney disease, diabetes, endocrine disorders, major dysrhythmias, congestive heart failure, ischemic heart disease, hepatic disease, recent bowel preparation, planned major vascular surgery (with aorta cross-clamp), or patients order than 60 years undergoing prolonged surgery with major blood loss. Significant hypokalemia should be corrected prior to surgery. Serum magnesium should be obtained in the setting of severe hypokalemia and replenished if indicated. Preoperative blood urea nitrogen (BUN) and serum creatinine are recommended in the setting of diabetes mellitus, moderate-to-severe hypertension, severe liver dysfunction, atherosclerotic vascular disease, use of nephrotoxic agents (aminoglycosides, intravenous contrast, ACE inhibitors) or prior to operations at risk of perioperative renal ischemia including aortic cross-clamping or cardiac bypass surgery. Screening for hypophosphatemia would be reasonable in the setting of alcohol abuse, severe sepsis or trauma, malnutrition, or refeeding of starved patients.

Blood glucose is indicated in the setting of known diabetes mellitus, chronic steroid use, intracranial procedures, cardiac surgery, elderly (>60 years) or obsess patients undergoing moderate to major surgery.

Hemoglobin. Randomized prospective studies in patients who are having elective surgery without significant blood loss did not show that a preoperative hemoglobin predicts any adverse outcome.[21,26] Routine preoperative hemoglobin determination is not supported unless triggered by specific patient factors such as known anemia, coagulopathy, hematologic disorders, or the likelihood of significant bleeding requiring transfusion. No randomized prospective studies involving patients with anticipated blood loss have defined a hemoglobin level as a risk factor for anesthesia and surgery. The preoperative hemoglobin has been shown to be a predictor of transfusion risk in procedures with significant blood loss.[27-31] Antibody type and screen are indicated prior to Class C surgical procedures with anticipated significant blood loss. The decision for perioperative transfusion should be based on preoperative hemoglobin concentration, anticipated blood loss, and cardiorespiratory status.

Complete blood count (hemoglobin, platelet and leukocyte count) is reasonable in the setting of hematologic disorder, planned vascular procedure and patients on chemotherapy or other medications with possible myelosuppression side effects.

Coagulation studies are reasonable with known or suspected bleeding disorders, anticoagulant therapy, renal or liver dysfunction, malnourishment, malabsorption syndromes, alcoholism, family history of bleeding disorders associated with prior operations or dental work, or major blood loss surgery.

Liver enzyme (aspartate aminotransferase, alkalie phosphatase, and on occasion bilirubin) testing may be indicated in the setting of medication use associated with liver toxicity (such as statins, methotrexate, hydralazine), history of hepatitis or excessive alcohol ingestion, malignancy with chemotherapy, morbid obesity, recent prolonged or severe hypotension or in patients and undergoing major upper abdominal surgery associated with hepatic ischemia risk.

Urinalysis (UA) is indicated with suspected genitourinary disease, prior to specific procedures (e.g., prosthesis implantation, urologic procedures), or when urinary tract symptoms are present.[1] If a urinary tract infection (UTI) is suspected, consider obtaining a urine culture since the UA may be insensitive for the detection of some UTIs.[32–35]

Pregnancy Testing. Since the history and physical examination may be insufficient for identification of early pregnancy, pregnancy testing may be *considered* for all female patients of childbearing age. Clinical characteristics to consider include a history or physical findings suggestive of current pregnancy or uncertain pregnancy history.[1,36,37]

Timing of laboratory testing. Absent a material change in the patient's medical condition or history, values for laboratory and other testing obtained within the 6 months prior to surgery are probably sufficient. Individual hospitals often have their own criteria and policies, though not evidence based, that may differ from these recommendations. This usually results in performance of tests that are not medically indicated.

After finishing the patient and laboratory assessments, one can determine the ASA Physical Status Classification (Table 98-6). This serves as a general categorization of patient sickness and is a predictor of perioperative mortality.[38,39]

SUMMARY

The history and results from the physical examination should dictate the selective ordering of laboratory testing to assist in optimally preparing the patient for undergoing anesthesia. Some disease processes that could affect the anesthetic plan have been outlined above. The Institute for Clinical Systems Improvement (ICSI) summarizes:

"Positive findings" are the results from the preoperative basic health assessment that suggest that further evaluation is needed in order to assess or optimize surgical/anesthesia risk and care. Examples include a current infection, the presence of chest pains, or a markedly elevated blood pressure.[40]

There may be other positive findings that, although not relevant to the planned procedure, may be relevant to the patient's general health. The evaluation of these findings should follow standard medical practice and is beyond the scope of this chapter. This type of finding would not necessarily need to delay the procedure.[40]

Key Points

- Evaluation of the patient should occur prior to the day of surgery if the procedure is other than minimally invasive or the patient is not absolutely healthy.

- The history and physical examination remain the primary methods of preoperative assessment, defining those who may benefit from further evaluation and diagnostic testing.

- History of the current condition should determine exercise tolerance, history of present illness and its treatments, and an understanding of the planned surgical procedure.

- Have patients quit smoking 6–8 weeks before surgery.

- Susceptibility to Malignant Hyperthermia is inherited as an autosomal dominant trait.

- Identify signs of obstructive sleep apnea, as this increases postoperative morbidity.

- No research supports "routine" preoperative testing in healthy patients. Laboratory tests, ECG, or CXR should only be performed if there is a specific clinical indication or purpose.

SUGGESTED READING

ASA. Practice advisory for preanesthesia evaluation: a report by the American Society of Anesthesiologists Task Force on Preanesthesia evaluation. Anesthesiology 2002; 96:485–496.

ASA. Practice guidelines for preoperative fasting and the use of pharmacologic agents to reduce the risk of pulmonary aspiration: application to healthy patients undergoing elective procedures (ASA Task Force on Preoperative Fasting). Anesthesiology 1999; 90:896–905.

Park MA, Li JT. Diagnosis and management of penicillin allergy. Mayo Clin Proc 2005; 80:405–410.

Findlay JY. Is there an optimal timing for smoking cessation? In: Fleisher LA, ed. Evidence-Based Practice of Anesthesiology. Philadelphia: Saunders, 2004; 57–61.

Prys-Roberts C. Should antihypertensive medications be continued through the perioperative period? In: Fleisher LA, ed. Evidence-Based Practice of Anesthesiology. Philadelphia: Saunders, 2004; 68–76.

Dzankic S, Pastor D, Gonzalez C, et al. The prevalence and predictive value of abnormal preoperative laboratory tests in elderly surgical patients. Anesth Analg 2001; 93:301–308.

denHerder C, Schmeck J, Appelboom DJK, et al. Risks of general anaesthesia in people with obstructive sleep apnea. Br Med J 2004; 329:955–959.

Mercado DL, Petty BG. Perioperative medication management. Med Clin North Am 2003; 87:41–57.

Geerts WH, Pineo GF, Heit JA, et al. Prevention of venous thromboembolism. The Seventh ACCP Conference on Antithrombotic and Thrombolytic Therapy. Chest 2004; 126(3suppl):338S–400.

Chobanian AV, Bakris GL, Black HR, et al. The Seventh report of the Joint National Committee on Prevention, Detection, Evaluation, and Treatment of High Blood Pressure: The JNC 7 Report. Hypertension 2003; 42:1206–1252.

CHAPTER NINETY-NINE

Perioperative Medication Management

Nathan O. Spell, MD, FACP, and Steven L. Cohn, MD, FACP

BACKGROUND

The medical consultant performs an important service by reviewing medications before surgery, considering how these may pose unique hazards or, conversely, enhance safety in the perioperative period. This chapter will discuss several medication categories, including steroids, immunosuppressive agents, antiplatelet and nonsteroidal anti-inflammatory drugs, and herbal medications. Cardiopulmonary, anticoagulant, and antidiabetic medications are discussed in their respective chapters. It should be noted that our recommendations are based on the available evidence, several review articles,[1–3] and clinical experience, since well-conducted studies and high-level evidence are often lacking.

The following principles generally apply to perioperative medication management:

- Fewer medications are better. The likelihood of drug–drug interaction rises exponentially with medication number. The surgical period introduces new medications, including sedative-hypnotics, anesthetics, analgesics, antibiotics, and others. Reducing the number of medications a patient takes before surgery will thereby reduce the chance of adverse drug interactions. For most medications, five half-lives will be an adequate time to discontinue before surgery to eliminate the risk of drug effects.
- In general, continue medications providing stability in chronic diseases. However, certain medications with known potential for adverse effects (including anticoagulants, drugs with antiplatelet effects, and hypoglycemic agents) may need to be modified or discontinued perioperatively. For each medication, there is a balance between the adverse effects that may occur if the medication is stopped and the chance of harm from continuation through surgery.
- When possible, avoid stopping medications associated with a withdrawal syndrome. Specifically, chronic use of benzodiazepines, narcotic analgesics, and centrally acting sympatholytics such as clonidine may predispose patients to significant physiologic stresses if these medications are abruptly discontinued.
- Consider the nature of the surgery and its associated risks. Duration of surgery, type of anesthesia, anticipated blood loss, risk of venous thromboembolism, and the patient's ability to take oral medications for an extended period are factors that can influence medication management decisions.

- Inquire about the patient's use of nonprescription substances, as these may have important physiologic actions. Herbal products, over-the-counter medications, caffeine, tobacco, alcohol, and illicit drugs may all affect the course of the patient through surgery and recovery.
- For medications continued through surgery, anticipate problems that these mediations are known to cause; use extra vigilance or preventive measures where appropriate. For instance, estrogens and selective estrogen-receptor modulators increase the risk for venous thromboembolism (VTE).[4,5] For a patient taking these medications, it may be appropriate to increase the intensity or duration of prophylactic measures.
- Use prophylactic medications for VTE, surgical site infection, endocarditis, perioperative ischemia, and aspiration as indicated by recommended guidelines. These medications are discussed in other chapters.

PATHOPHYSIOLOGY

In the immediate perioperative period, blood pressure and heart rate may vary substantially. During the early stages of both general endotracheal and spinal anesthesia, blood pressure typically falls as a result of vasodilatation. Endotracheal intubation and extubation and pain in the postanesthesia period activate the sympathetic nervous system with resultant increase in blood pressure and heart rate. Serum cortisol rises, peaking about the time of extubation or early recovery and returning to baseline levels the next day for uncomplicated surgeries.[6]

Preoperative intravascular volume depletion or surgical blood loss will exacerbate hypotension of surgery and challenge compensatory mechanisms to maintain arterial blood pressure and organ perfusion. These compensatory mechanisms include sympathetic nervous system activation, vasopressin release, and activation of the renin-angiotensin-aldosterone axis. Within organs such as the kidney, prostaglandin production helps to maintain perfusion via local vasodilatation.

Surgery may disrupt gastrointestinal motility, resulting in an "ileus." Among common causes are surgeries within the abdomen and pelvis, electrolyte disturbances, and the use of narcotic analgesics and anticholinergic drugs. Such gastrointestinal dysfunction impairs the patient's ability to take and absorb oral medications. Renal or hepatic dysfunction after surgery reduces the clearance of many medications, forcing discontinuation, reduction of dose, and/or close serum drug level monitoring.

Inadequate adrenal cortical function may complicate surgery and recovery.[7] Some patients experiencing hypotension or circulatory collapse in the surgical intensive care unit have adrenal insufficiency. When physicians recognize this situation, treatment with adrenocortical steroid hormones has been shown to improve outcomes.[8] Patients at increased risk for adrenal insufficiency include those currently taking or having received corticosteroid therapy within the past year or those with diseases affecting pituitary or adrenal function. Additional discussion of this point follows.

It is well recognized that chronic use of corticosteroids and other immunosuppressive drugs predisposes patients to infections. The significance of this effect during the postoperative period is not clear, as studies reach opposite conclusions.[9–11]

CLINICAL ASSESSMENT/EVALUATION

Preoperative medical consultants should take a thorough medication history, including prior adverse drug reactions and use of prescription and nonprescription drugs, herbal products and nutritional supplements, alcohol, and recreational drugs. Knowing the details of the patient's medical history can help the consultant anticipate potential for cardiac, hepatic, and renal dysfunction that may affect medication metabolism. Patients with impaired metabolism may need additional time to clear medications before surgery and cautious dosing afterward.

Corticosteroids

Patients with illnesses for which steroids are commonly used require a careful history of the steroid doses and duration within the previous year. These patients may be divided into three categories:

1. Patients assumed to have adrenal insufficiency who have taken the equivalent of more than 20 mg of prednisone a day for more than 3 weeks within the last year or have an obvious cushingoid appearance.[12]
2. Patients at risk for adrenal suppression based on corticosteroid use or because of their diseases (cancer involving both adrenal glands, pituitary tumors or infiltrative diseases, among others). Daily use of the equivalent of between 5 mg and 20 mg of prednisone has potential to suppress adrenal function.[13] Patients in this group may either be treated as if they have adrenal insufficiency or assessed for adrenal dysfunction with a cosyntropin stimulation test. In the most commonly recommended protocol, 250 mcg of cosyntropin is injected intravenously or intramuscularly, and serum cortisol is measured just before and 30 and 60 minutes after the injection. The normal response is for the cortisol level to rise to at least 19 mcg/dL.[7]
3. Patients assumed to have normal adrenal function who have used any dose of steroids for less than 3 weeks or use inhaled, intranasal, or topical corticosteroids.[12]

Medications with Antiplatelet Activity

If concerned about platelet dysfunction that would affect perioperative management, whether based on history of bleeding or use of antiplatelet agents, order a platelet function assay. Take into

account the indication for use of the drug and its beneficial effects versus the potential for adverse effects perioperatively.

RECOMMENDATIONS/MANAGEMENT

Table 99-1 summarizes recommendations for perioperative medication management. Cardiopulmonary, anticoagulant, and diabetic medications are discussed in Chapters 101–104.

Corticosteroids and Immunosuppressive Medications

Corticosteroid dosing for surgery should take into account the surgical stress and the degree of likely adrenal insufficiency of the patient.[14]

- For patients using only inhaled, intranasal, or topical steroids, simply observe for signs of adrenal insufficiency and treat if necessary.[12]
- For patients taking oral steroids and thought to require replacement therapy, those undergoing surgeries with minor amounts of stress (e.g., performed under local anesthesia) may take their usual morning oral dose.
- For moderate stress surgeries such as joint replacement, administer a total IV hydrocortisone dose the day of surgery ranging from 50–75 mg[12] in divided doses every 6–8 hours. Give the first dose of IV hydrocortisone at the time of induction of anesthesia.
- Major surgeries require total doses of up to 200 mg of IV hydrocortisone the first day.[7]

Duration of corticosteroid supplementation also depends upon the patient and the surgery.

- Patients undergoing minor- or moderate-stress surgeries who take daily oral corticosteroids may resume their usual daily dose the day after surgery if they are hemodynamically stable.
- The patient who does not require chronic corticosteroid therapy may have the perioperative supplementation rapidly tapered and discontinued over 1–2 days.
- A patient undergoing major surgery, in whom a more prolonged and complicated postoperative course is expected, should have the corticosteroid dose more gradually tapered as the medical condition allows.

Beyond corticosteroids, consultants have little data on which to base recommendations for perioperative management of other immunosuppressive agents.[15] These medications include inhibitors of T-lymphocyte function (azathioprine, cyclosporine, tacrolimus, sirolimus), antimetabolites (methotrexate, mercaptopurine), and specific inhibitors of tumor necrosis factor (etanercept, infliximab, and adalimumab), interleukin-1 (anakinra) and CD20 (rituximab). The experience reported is generally favorable, indicating no significant increase in risk attributable to these agents in ordinary perioperative use[11,16]; however, patients in one study undergoing liver transplantation experienced significantly more incidents of sepsis on sirolimus.[10] Overall, it does not appear necessary to discontinue these drugs perioperatively, as we await more definitive studies.

Antiplatelet Medications

Antiplatelet agents may increase the risk for bleeding with major surgeries. Aspirin, an irreversible cyclo-oxygenase inhibitor, is the best studied. Although preoperative aspirin use with coronary

Table 99-1 Summary of Perioperative Medication Management

Medication Class	Recommendation
Anticoagulants (heparins, warfarin)	Continue for minor surgery. Discontinue at appropriate interval before major surgery. Consider bridging anticoagulation for patients at high risk of interim thrombosis.
Antiplatelet drugs	Continue for minor surgery. Discontinue clopidogrel at least 5 days before surgery. If discontinuing aspirin, do so at least 5–7 days before surgery.
Cardiovascular	Continue most agents.
Medications	Initiate beta-blockers in patients at high risk of perioperative cardiac morbidity. Withhold diuretics on the morning of surgery, especially if signs of volume depletion. Caution with ACE inhibitors and ARBs as they may cause hypotension with induction of anesthesia.
Lipid lowering agents	Continue "statins." Discontinue other agents.
Pulmonary agents	Continue.
Gastrointestinal agents	Continue.
Diabetic agents	Withhold oral hypoglycemics on morning of surgery (longer for metformin?); restart when patient resumes eating. For type 1 diabetics, continue some form of insulin (long acting or intravenous) at all times. For type 2 diabetics, decrease dose of morning intermediate insulin.
Thyroid agents (hypo- and hyperthyroidism)	Continue thyroid replacement. Continue antithyroid medication and postpone surgery until hyperthyroidism is controlled.
Oral contraceptives, hormone replacement, and SERMs	May discontinue 3 weeks before surgery only in patients at high risk for perioperative venous thromboembolism, otherwise continue.
Corticosteroids	Continue chronic corticosteroids. Increase dosage to account for surgical stress.
Psychotropic agents	Continue SSRIs but consider holding several weeks before CNS surgery. Continue tricyclic antidepressants, benzodiazepines, lithium and antipsychotics. Usually discontinue MAOs 10–14 days before surgery.
Chronic opioids	Continue. Substitute equianalgesic or higher doses for surgical pain.
Rheumatologic agents	Continue methotrexate. Limited data on other DMARDs and anticytokines; probably safe to continue. Continue hypouricemic agents.
Neurologic agents	Continue antiseizure medications. Hold antiparkinsonian agents briefly. Continue agents for myasthenia gravis.
Herbal agents	Discontinue all agents.

ACE—angiotensin converting enzyme; ARB—angiotensin receptor blocker; SSRI—selective seratonin reuptake inhibitor; MAD—monoamine oxidae inhibitor; CNS—central nervous system; DMARD—disease modifying anti-rheumatic drug.

Adapted from: Cohn and Macpherson, Perioperative Medicine—Just the Facts, 2006.[2]

artery bypass graft (CABG) surgery has been associated with increased bleeding and reoperation in some studies,[17] it has also been shown to reduce mortality when given within 5 days preoperatively[18] or within 48 hours post-CABG.[19] In minor surgical procedures such as vitreoretinal surgery and transbronchial biopsy, bleeding rates are low and are not significantly affected by aspirin use.[20,21] It does not appear to be necessary to stop aspirin and other platelet inhibitors for most surgeries, especially if these drugs provide important cardiovascular protective effects for the individual patient. There is a suggestion of a rebound effect within 4 weeks of discontinuing aspirin therapy[22]; however, a patient with low risk for cardiovascular events may benefit by stopping aspirin 5–7 days before major surgery, thereby reducing postoperative bleeding complications.

Clopidogrel and ticlopidine also permanently inhibit platelet function via action on adenosine diphosphate. These drugs should be stopped at least 5 days before coronary artery bypass

surgery, as they were associated with increased bleeding and morbidity in multiple studies.[23,24] The combination of aspirin and clopidogrel increases risk of bleeding, and their perioperative use for noncardiac surgery after coronary artery stenting is discussed in Chapter 102. Much less information is available about perioperative bleeding effects for other antiplatelet agents.

Nonsteroidal anti-inflammatory drugs (NSAIDs) other than cyclo-oxygenase-2 (COX-2) inhibitors reversibly inhibit platelet function but have less effect than aspirin. While effective for postoperative analgesia, NSAIDs may transiently reduce renal function in surgical patients via inhibition of prostaglandin synthesis. This does not appear to be a clinically significant effect in patients with normal renal function,[25] but less is known about patients with impaired renal function or those concomitantly taking angiotensin-converting enzyme inhibitors (ACEIs) and diuretics. They are often stopped before surgery, the time varying with the half-life of the drug.

Most antihypertensive medications are continued through surgery. However, management of ACEIs and angiotensin II receptor blockers (ARBs) is somewhat controversial, due to variable hemodynamic effects reported in several perioperative studies. In a small, randomized study, Comfere et al.[26] found that stopping ACEIs or ARBs before surgery reduced the risk of hypotension soon after general anesthetic induction, but there was no significant effect overall on surgical complications. Pigott et al.[27] found no difference in hypotension on induction of anaesthesia or in the use of vasoconstrictors after cardiopulmonary bypass. Similarly, Hohne et al.[28] did not find a significant blood pressure change related to ACEI use in patients undergoing minor surgery under spinal anesthesia. The incidence of postoperative renal insufficiency may be increased in patients on chronic ACEI therapy.[29] In sum, whether or not to continue ACEI or ARB therapy through surgery remains a judgment call, based on the potential benefits to the patient of effective control of hypertension and heart failure weighed against increased risk of intraoperative hypotension and postoperative renal impairment.

Alternative Medications

The general public and patients undergoing surgery commonly use alternative medications, specifically herbal medications and nutritional supplements.[30] While there is little research relating outcomes to alternative medicine use before surgery, many herbal medications have effects on platelet aggregation, clotting, and liver and central nervous system function.[31,32] The position of the American Society of Anesthesiologists reflects the general consensus that herbal medications should be discontinued 2 weeks or more before surgery.

Key Points

- Preoperative medical consultants should take a thorough medication history, including prior adverse drug reactions and use of prescription and nonprescription drugs, herbal products and nutritional supplements, alcohol, and recreational drugs.

- Fewer medications are better. The likelihood of drug–drug interaction rises exponentially with medication number.

- In general, continue medications providing stability in chronic diseases.

- Avoid stopping medications associated with a withdrawal syndrome.

- For medications continued through surgery, anticipate problems these mediations are known to cause.

- Assume patients have adrenal insufficiency if they have taken the equivalent of >20 mg of prednisone a day for >3 weeks within the last year or have an obvious cushingoid appearance. These patients require corticosteroid replacement for surgery.

- It does not appear to be necessary to stop aspirin and other platelet inhibitors for most surgeries (except coronary artery bypass grafting where these increase the risk for reoperation and mortality due to bleeding), especially if these drugs provide important cardiovascular protective effects for the individual patient.

- The general consensus is to discontinue herbal medications at least 2 weeks before surgery.

SUGGESTED READING

Spell NO. Stopping and restarting medications in the perioperative period. Med Clin North Am 2001; 85(5):1117–1128.

Cohn SL. Perioperative medication management in PIER, 2005. (http://pier.acponline.org/physicians/diseases/d835/d835.html).

Cooper MS, Stewart PM. Corticosteroid insufficiency in acutely ill patients. N Engl J Med 2003; 348:727–734.

Rivers EP, Gaspari M, Saad GA, et al. Adrenal insufficiency in high-risk surgical ICU patients. Chest 2001; 119(3):889–896.

Lamberts SW, Bruining HA, de Jong FH. Corticosteroid therapy in severe illness. N Engl J Med 1997; 337(18):1285–1292.

Merritt JC, Bhatt DL. The efficacy and safety of perioperative antiplatelet therapy. J Thromb Thrombolysis 2002; 13(2):97–103.

Kaye AD, Kucera I, Sabar R. Perioperative anesthesia clinical considerations of alternative medicines. Anesthesiol Clin North Am 2004; 22(1):125–139.

CHAPTER ONE HUNDRED

Perioperative Anticoagulation: Prophylaxis for Venous Thromboembolism (VTE)

Jason Stein MD, Michael P. Phy DO, MSc, and Amir K. Jaffer MD

BACKGROUND

Prophylaxis for venous thromboembolism (VTE) in surgical patients is a critical risk reduction measure in perioperative care. VTE is common and associated with significant morbidity, mortality, and health care costs. Every year in the United States, an estimated 2 million patients develop deep vein thrombosis (DVT), with approximately 200,000 dying from pulmonary embolism (PE). Nearly half of these cases and deaths are attributable to surgical patients.[1] Among the more than 30 million patients undergoing surgery each year, a significant proportion is considered at risk for VTE.[2]

PE resulting from DVT may be the most common cause of preventable hospital death.

Without prophylaxis, the incidence of proximal DVT and clinical PE in many surgical patients is unacceptably high: up to 60% in the highest risk surgical category—for example, those undergoing arthroplasty of the hip or knee, or hip fracture surgery. Among these highest-risk surgical patients, up to 10% will develop clinically evident PE, and half of these events will be fatal.[1]

Multiple clinical trials using routine venography to study postoperative prevalence suggest that VTE is often silent. Since the first clinical manifestation may be fatal PE, primary prevention should be the goal. Moreover, universal screening for postoperative DVT is neither cost effective nor reliable. Detection is further complicated by the fact that most symptomatic postoperative DVTs occur after hospital discharge. The best strategy to prevent postoperative VTE and chronic sequelae like post-phlebitic syndrome is to recommend prophylaxis for almost all surgical patients.

In most surgical settings, evidence supports a variety of methods for prophylaxis. Despite demonstrated safety, efficacy, and ease of administration, however, appropriate prophylaxis is underused. Critical pathways, pocket guides, or policies of VTE prophylaxis have not improved rates of adherence to high-grade recommendations.[3,4] Encouragingly, educational programs promoting guidelines may *contribute* to improved prophylaxis of surgical patients.[4]

As with hospitalized medical patients, all surgical patients should undergo an early VTE risk assessment linked to a menu of appropriate VTE prophylaxis options. How these fundamental steps are blended into the clinical workflow depends on the dynamics of any given hospital system. Clinical judgment should weigh additional patient and procedure-specific factors when selecting an appropriate method of prophylaxis.

PATHOPHYSIOLOGY

The pathophysiologic changes of stasis, intimal injury, and hypercoagulability predispose surgical patients to the development of VTE.

Stasis occurs through several mechanisms. Venographic contrast studies show that the supine position on the operating room table impedes venous return. Additionally, the anatomical position of the extremities providing the best surgical access—particularly in orthopedic, gynecologic, and urologic surgeries—impairs adequate venous drainage during the procedure.[5–7] Furthermore, anesthesia causes peripheral venodilation, which results in increased venous capacitance and decreased venous return during the operative procedure.[8,9]

Intimal injury occurs through these same mechanisms. Anatomical positions and anesthesia itself—especially with prolonged distortion of the veins and tourniquet use—can damage delicate venous endothelium and create transendothelial tears exposing highly thrombogenic subendothelial collagen.[10]

Hypercoagulability in the surgical patient is thought to emerge in the perioperative period. Reduced levels of antithrombin III in the 3–5 days following hip and knee surgery increase the propensity for thrombus formation.[11] The endogenous fibrinolytic system may also be suppressed with prothrombotic ratios of tissue plasminogen activator to plasminogen activator inhibitor-1.[12–14]

PREOPERATIVE EVALUATION

Clinical Assessment

History

Preoperative risk assessment for VTE must consider procedure (Table 100-1) and patient-specific factors (Table 100-2). Both factors, combined with the method of prophylaxis, influence overall VTE risk. Incorporating a standardized risk assessment at the time of the preoperative evaluation or admission is critical. Though many standardized risk-assessment tools exist, few have been rigorously validated. We advocate use of the recommendations in the Seventh ACCP Conference on Antithrombotic and Thrombolytic Therapy.[2]

VTE risk ranges from patients at *low risk*, who may require no special VTE prophylaxis beyond early ambulation, to those patients at *very high risk*, who require combination modalities and who may require extended prophylaxis. It is also critical to identify those patients for whom anticoagulant prophylaxis should be used cautiously, with special timing, or replaced entirely. Such patient groups include certain intracranial neurosurgery patients, trauma patients with particular bleeding concerns, and cases involving either spinal puncture or epidural catheter for regional anesthesia or analgesia (Table 100-3 and the section on Special Considerations with LMWH's, respectively).

Physical Examination

The physical examination should identify patient-specific risk factors for VTE (Table 100-2) potentially not appreciated in the history. These include obesity, evidence of prolonged immobility, cardiac dysfunction, varicose veins, or presence of an indwelling central venous catheter.

Table 100-1 Surgery Related Risk Factors for DVT*

Surgery Group	DVT Prevalence (%)
General surgery	15–40
Major gynecologic surgery	15–40
Major urologic surgery	15–40
Neurosurgery	15–40
Hip or knee arthroplasty	40–60
Hip fracture surgery	40–60
Major trauma	40–80
Spinal cord injury	60–80

*Rates based on objective diagnostic testing for DVT in patients not receiving thromboprophylaxis.

Revised from: Geerts WH, Pineo GF, Heit JA, et al. Prevention of venous thromboembolism: the Seventh ACCP Conference on Antithrombotic and Thrombolytic Therapy. Chest 2004; 126:338S–400S.

Table 100-2 Patient-Related Risk Factors for VTE

Surgery	Inflammatory bowel disease
Trauma	Nephrotic syndrome
Immobility, paresis	Myeloproliferative disorders
Malignancy	Paroxysmal nocturnal hemoglobinuria
Cancer therapy	Obesity
Previous VTE	Smoking
Increasing age	Varicose veins
Pregnancy and postpartum period	Central venous catheterization
Estrogen OCPs or HRT	Inherited or acquired thrombophilia
Acute medical illness	Selective estrogen receptor modulators
Heart or respiratory failure	

VTE—venous thromboembolism; OCP—oral contraceptive pills; HRT—hormone replacement therapy

Revised from: Geerts WH, Pineo GF, Heit JA, et al. Prevention of venous thromboembolism: the Seventh ACCP Conference on Antithrombotic and Thrombolytic Therapy. Chest 2004; 126:338S–400S.

Table 100-3 Neurosurgery, Trauma, and Acute Spinal Cord Injury

Procedure Risk Group	Recommended Prophylaxis
Intracranial neurosurgery	IPC device, with or without GCS. LDUH or postoperative LMWH may be acceptable alternatives. High-risk patients: GCS and/or IPC device with LDUH or postoperative LMWH.
Trauma, with identifiable risk factor for thromboembolism	Prophylaxis with LMWH, as soon as considered safe; if delayed, or contraindicated because of bleeding concerns: initial use of GCS, or IPC device, or both. If prophylaxis is suboptimal, screening of high-risk patients (spinal cord injury, lower extremity or pelvic fracture, major head injury, or indwelling femoral line) with duplex ultrasound is recommended. IVC filter insertion as primary prophylaxis is **NOT** recommended. Continue prophylaxis until hospital discharge (including inpatient rehabilitation). In patients with major impaired mobility, continuation of prophylaxis with LMWH or Coumadin (goal INR 2.5; range, 2.0–3.0) is suggested.
Acute spinal cord injury	Prophylaxis with LMWH to commence once primary hemostasis is evident. GCS and IPC may be offered in combination with LMWH or LDUH as an alternative to LMWH. IPC and/or GCS is recommended when anticoagulant prophylaxis is contraindicated early after surgery. LDUH, GCS, or IPC as sole prophylaxis is **NOT** recommended. Use of IVC filter insertion as primary prophylaxis is **NOT** recommended for prophylaxis against PE. In the rehabilitation phase, we recommend continued LMWH therapy, or Coumadin (goal INR 2.5; range, 2.0–3.0) is suggested.

IPC—intermittent pneumatic compression; GCS—graduated compression stockings; LDUH—low dose unfractionated heparin; LMWH—low molecular weight heparin; IVC—inferior vena cava; INR—international normalized ratio

Revised from: Geerts WH, Pineo GF, Heit JA, et al. Prevention of venous thromboembolism: the Seventh ACCP Conference on Antithrombotic and Thrombolytic Therapy. Chest 2004; 126:338S–400S.

Laboratory and Other Testing

No screening or other diagnostic tests are routinely recommended in the preoperative evaluation unless the patient has signs and symptoms to suggest VTE. If these exist, the patient should be further evaluated using standardized and validated nomograms combined with diagnostic testing.

Management

Ideally, VTE prophylaxis should begin preoperatively. Selecting appropriate prophylaxis depends on an accurate VTE risk assessment that can be performed by identifying the risk group for the type of surgery (surgery-specific tables: Table 100-3, Neurosurgery, Trauma, and Acute Spinal Cord Injury; Table 100-4, General Surgery; Table 100-5, Gynecologic Surgery; Table 100-6, Urologic Surgery; Table 100-7, Major Orthopedic Surgery). Important perspective on VTE risk comes from understanding the relevant factors unique to the surgery and to the patient (Table 100-1 and Table 100-2). Efforts to create simplified, pre-printed

risk assessments have led many institutions to stratify all surgical patients to one of 4 VTE risk categories (Table 100-8).

It is important to appreciate the mechanism, risks, benefits, limitations, and potential complications associated with each VTE prophylaxis agent (Table 100-9). Aspirin alone is not recommended for VTE prophylaxis in *any* surgical group. Early ambulation, however, is recommended for *all* surgical patients.

POSTOPERATIVE EVALUATION

Clinical Assessment

Continually assess all postoperative patients for hemostasis, hemodynamic stability, and compliance with VTE prophylaxis regimen. Patients on unfractionated heparin (UFH) or low molecular weight heparin (LMWH) require a complete blood count with platelets to assess for bleeding or evolving heparin-associated or heparin-induced thrombocytopenia. Patients on warfarin require monitoring of the international normalized ratio (INR).

Table 100-4 General Surgery

Procedure Risk Group	Recommended Prophylaxis
Low risk (Minor procedure in patients <40 yr, with no additional risk factors)	Early ambulation
Moderate risk (Non-major surgery in patients 40 to 60 yr, or have additional risk factors, or major surgery in patients <40 yr, with no additional risk factors)	LDUH 5,000 units BID or LMWH ≤3,400 units once daily
Higher risk (Non-major surgery in patients >60 yr, or with additional risk factors; major surgery in patients >40 yr, or with additional risk factors)	LDUH 5,000 units TID or LMWH >3,400 units daily
Higher risk, with greater-than-usual risk for bleeding	Mechanical prophylaxis with fitted GCS or IPC device, at least initially until bleeding risk decreases

LDUH—low dose unfractionated heparin; BID—twice daily; TID—three times daily; LMWH—low molecular weight heparin; GCS—graduated compression stockings; IPC—intermittent pneumatic compression

Revised from: Geerts WH, Pineo GF, Heit JA, et al. Prevention of venous thromboembolism: the Seventh ACCP Conference on Antithrombotic and Thrombolytic Therapy. Chest 2004; 126:338S–400S.

Table 100-5 Gynecologic Surgery

Procedure Risk Group	Recommended Prophylaxis
Brief procedure of ≤30 min for benign disease	Early mobilization
Laparoscopic procedures with additional VTE risk factors	Use one or more of the following; LDUH, LMWH, IPC, or GCS
Major gynecologic surgery for benign disease; no additional risk factors	LDUH 5,000 units BID; alternatively, LMWH ≤3,400 units daily or IPC device started just before surgery and used continually while the patient is not ambulating
Extensive surgery for malignancy, and for patients with additional VTE risk factors	LDUH 5,000 units TID, or LMWH >3,400 units daily. Alternative considerations include IPC alone continued until hospital discharge, or a combination of LDUH or LMWH plus mechanical prophylaxis with GCS or IPC.

LDUH—low dose unfractionated heparin; VTE—venous thromboembolism; LMWH—low molecular weight heparin; BID—twice daily; TID—three times daily; IPC—intermittent pneumatic compression; GCS—graduated compression stockings

Revised from: Geerts WH, Pineo GF, Heit JA, et al. Prevention of venous thromboembolism: the Seventh ACCP Conference on Antithrombotic and Thrombolytic Therapy. Chest 2004; 126:338S–400S.

Table 100-6 Urologic Surgery

Procedure Risk Group	Recommended Prophylaxis
Transurethral surgery or other low-risk procedure	Prompt mobilization
Major open urologic procedure	LDUH 5,000 units BID or TID. Acceptable alternatives; IPC and/or GCS
Highest-risk patients with multiple risk factors	Combination of LDUH or LMWH with GCS and/or IPC
Patients actively bleeding or high risk for bleeding	GCS and/or IPC until bleeding risk decreases

LDUH—low dose unfractionated heparin; BID—twice daily; TID—three times daily; IPC—intermittent pneumatic compression; LMWH—low molecular weight heparin; GCS—graduated compression stockings

Revised from: Geerts WH, Pineo GF, Heit JA, et al. Prevention of venous thromboembolism: the Seventh ACCP Conference on Antithrombotic and Thrombolytic Therapy. Chest 2004; 126:338S–400S.

Table 100-7 Major Orthopedic Surgery

Procedure Risk Group	Recommended Prophylaxis
Elective total hip replacement (THR)	LMWH therapy (started 12 hr before surgery, or 12–24 hr after surgery; or half the usual high-risk dose 4–6 hr after surgery, followed by the usual high-risk dose the following day); or adjusted-dose Coumadin therapy (goal INR 2.5; range, 2.0–3.0), started preoperatively or the evening after surgery; or fondaparinux 2.5 mg started 6 to 8 h after surgery Sole therapy with LDUH, aspirin, dextran, GCS, or IPC device is **NOT** recommended
Elective knee arthroplasty (TKA)	LMWH, fondaparinux, or adjusted-dose Coumadin (goal INR 2.5; range, 2.0–3.0) Sole therapy with LDUH, aspirin, or venous foot pump is **NOT** recommended Alternative: optimal use of IPC device
Hip fracture surgery (HFS)	LDUH 5,000 units TID, LMWH, fondaparinux, or adjusted-dose Coumadin (goal INR 2.5; range, 2.0–3.0) Sole therapy with aspirin is **NOT** recommended. Mechanical prophylaxis if anticoagulant prophylaxis is contraindicated because of high risk of bleeding
Duration of prophylaxis THR, TKA, or HFS	LMWH, fondaparinux 2.5 mg daily, or adjusted-dose Coumadin (goal INR 2.5; range, 2.0–3.0) for at least 10 days
THR or HFS	Can be given extended prophylaxis up to 28–35 days after surgery; LMWH, fondaparinux, or Coumadin

LMWH—low molecular weight heparin; INR—international normalized ratio; LDUH—low dose unfractionated heparin; GCS—graduated compression stockings; IPC—intermittent pneumatic compression; TID—three times daily

Revised from: Geerts WH, Pineo GF, Heit JA, et al. Prevention of venous thromboembolism: the Seventh ACCP Conference on Antithrombotic and Thrombolytic Therapy. Chest 2004; 126:338S–400S.

Management

Delay the initial postoperative anticoagulation dose for all patients until hemostasis is confirmed. This may require communication with the surgeon or the surgical team. In patients at high risk for bleeding, delay the initial postoperative anticoagulation dose until 12–24 after surgery *and* after hemostasis is confirmed.

Continue mechanical prophylaxis whenever anticoagulation is contraindicated. Except in **orthopedic** patients, discontinue pharmacologic prophylaxis when the patient is ambulating normally. Consider extended-duration prophylaxis with LMWH after gynecologic and general surgical procedures for cancer. Duration of VTE prophylaxis depends on the surgery and ongoing additional risk factors since certain types of patient-related risks and surgeries confer high risk for VTE, even after discharge from the hospital.

DISCHARGE RECOMMENDATIONS

Patient Education

The patient and responsible caregivers should receive (a) encouragement to achieve ambulation as soon as possible, (b) instructions on administering any ongoing pharmacologic prophylaxis regimens, and (c) education relating to signs of new VTE and how to report them in the post-discharge period.

Follow-up Management

At the time of discharge or at outpatient follow-up, routine screening with duplex ultrasonography is not recommended for asymptomatic patients who have received one of the recommended prophylaxis regimens.

Table 100-8 Venous Thromboembolism Risk Category and Risk Without Prophylaxis

Low Risk: Minor surgery in patients <40 years, with no additional risk factors
  Risk of calf DVT: 2%
  Risk of proximal DVT: 0.4%
  Risk of clinical PE: 0.2%

Moderate Risk: Minor surgery in patients with additional risk factor, or surgery in patients 40–60 years with no additional risk factor,
  Risk of calf DVT: 10–20%
  Risk of proximal DVT: 2–4%
  Risk of clinical PE: 1–2%

High Risk: Surgery in patients >60 years, or age 40–60 years with additional risk factors (prior VTE, cancer, molecular hypercoagulability)
  Risk of calf DVT: 20–40%
  Risk of proximal DVT: 4–8%
  Risk of clinical PE: 2–4%

Highest Risk: Surgery in patients with multiple risk factors (>40 years, cancer, prior VTE)

Hip or knee arthroplasty, or hip fracture surgery, or major trauma, or spinal cord injury
  Risk of calf DVT: 40–80%
  Risk of proximal DVT: 10–20%
  Risk of clinical PE: 4–10%

DVT—deep vein thrombosis; VTE—venous thromboembolism

Revised from: Geerts WH, Pineo GF, Heit JA, et al. Prevention of venous thromboembolism: the Seventh ACCP Conference on Antithrombotic and Thrombolytic Therapy. Chest 2004; 126:338S–400S.

Table 100-9 VTE Prophylaxis Agents

Agent and Mechanism	Considerations
GCS Decrease venous stasis in legs	No risk for bleeding, as effective as LDUH in moderate-risk general surgery patients, can be combined with pharmacologic agent
IPC Enhance blood flow in deep veins of legs and reduces levels of PAI-1 thereby enhancing endogenous fibrinolytic activity	No risk for bleeding, as effective as LDUH in high-risk general surgery patients, can be combined with pharmacologic agent Comfort can affect compliance, contraindicated if patient immobilized >72 hours without any form of prophylaxis, recent DVT, leg ulcers, severe PVD
LDUH Binds to antithrombin, potentiating its inhibition of thrombin and activated factor X.	Well studied, no monitoring needed, inexpensive, rapid onset of action, reversible, no difference in major hemorrhage, increased risk of HIT (especially in orthopedic patients)
LMWH Same mechanism as LDUH	No monitoring needed, more expensive than LDUH, rapid onset of action, rates of major hemorrhage comparable to LDUH, can be dosed once daily, less likely than LDUH to produce HIT and thrombosis
Coumadin Inhibits vitamin K–dependent activation of cofactors II, VII, IX, and X with dose adjusted to target INR 2–3 Fondaparinux Catalyzes factor Xa inactivation by AIII without inhibiting thrombin	Oral administration, reversible, effective with dosing beginning day of surgery—or day after, increased risk of DVT if used alone for prophylaxis,[16] conveniently continued into the outpatient setting, requires at least 3 days before therapeutic and required frequent monitoring until dose stable More study required. Promising characteristics: Fondaparinux—SQ route with no risk for HIT or thrombosis but most expensive option, questionable reversibility, may cause more bleeding[17]

VTE—venous thromboembolism; GCS—graduated compression stockings; IPC—intermittent pneumatic compression; PAI-1—plasminogen activator inhibitor-1; LDUH—low dose unfractionated heparin; LMWH—low molecular weight heparin; PVD—peripheral vascular disease; HIT—heparin induced thrombocytopenia.

Revised from: Geerts WH, Pineo GF, Heit JA, et al. Prevention of venous thromboembolism: The 7th ACCP Conference on Antithrombotic and Thrombolytic Therapy. Chest 2004; 126:338S–400S.

SPECIAL CONSIDERATIONS WITH LMWH

The American Society of Regional Anesthesia (ASRA) has developed a consensus statement regarding "Anesthetic Management of the Patient Receiving Low Molecular Weight Heparin (LMWH)." This report highlights the concern that symptomatic epidural hematomas can develop when a spinal or epidural catheter is inserted or removed in the patient who is anticoagulated with a LMWH.

The guideline recommends caution when antiplatelet or oral anticoagulant medications are administered in combination with LMWH, as they may increase the risk of spinal hematoma. Also, if spinal anesthesia is administered, a traumatic needle or catheter placement (evidence of blood during needle or catheter placement) necessitates delaying the initiation of LMWH therapy in this setting for 24 hours postoperatively.

If LMWH is used in the **preoperative** setting, the co-administration of antiplatelet or oral anticoagulant medication is contraindicated. Also, do not perform a lumbar puncture for at least 12 hours after the last thromboprophylaxis dose of LMWH and for at least 24 hours if treatment doses of LMWH have been used

If LMWH is used in the **postoperative** setting, the management is based on total daily dose, timing of the first postoperative dose, and the dosing schedule. In **single daily dosing,** administer the first postoperative LMWH dose 6–8 hours after completion of surgery, and give the second postoperative dose no sooner than 24 hours after the first dose. Indwelling neuraxial catheters may be safely maintained, but wait a minimum of 10–12 hours after the last dose of LMWH before removing the catheter. Do not administer subsequent LMWH dosing for a minimum of 2 hours after catheter removal. In **twice daily dosing,** administer the first dose of LMWH no earlier than 24 hours postoperatively. Remove indwelling catheters prior to initiation of LMWH thromboprophylaxis. If a continuous technique is selected, the epidural catheter may be left indwelling overnight and removed the following day, with the first dose of LMWH administered at least 2 hours after catheter removal. For further information regarding neuraxial anesthesia and anticoagulation, see the Second Consensus Conference on Neuraxial Anesthesia and Anticoagulation, April 25–28 at http://www.asra.com/.[15]

Key Points

- Venous thromboembolic events after surgery are common and particularly morbid; VTE prophylaxis is underutilized.

- Preoperative risk assessment of VTE is based on surgery-specific and patient-specific risk factors.

- Preoperative screening for VTE is not recommended in patients without signs or symptoms to suggest increased risk for VTE.

- Choice of prophylactic method and timing of initiation in the postoperative setting require good communication with the surgical team.

- Consider longer duration of prophylactic therapy in patients undergoing orthopedic procedures or gynecologic/general surgeries for cancer.

SUGGESTED READING

Geerts WH, Pineo GF, Heit JA, et al. Prevention of venous thromboembolism. The Seventh ACCP Conference on Antithrombotic and Thrombolytic Therapy. Chest 2004; 126:3385–4005.

CHAPTER ONE HUNDRED AND ONE

Management of Long-term Warfarin for Surgery

Jason Stein, MD, Michael P. Phy, DO, MSc, and Amir K. Jaffer, MD

BACKGROUND

Approximately 2 million patients take warfarin to prevent arterial or venous thromboembolism (VTE), and approximately 250,000 are assessed for bridging therapy every year in North America. Concern for bleeding complications due to surgery or procedures often requires dose reduction or discontinuation of the drug altogether. However, in most cases, the removal of anticoagulation places patients at increased risk for thromboembolic events. Although warfarin can be continued without dose alteration in certain minor procedures (Box 101-1), most surgeries require discontinuation of warfarin and possibly additional bridging therapy. For these patients, many clinicians use either unfractionated heparin (UFH) or low-molecular-weight heparin (LMWH) as an anticoagulation "bridge" before and after surgery.

PREOPERATIVE HISTORY

"Why is this patient on warfarin?" This is the key initial question. Patients may be on warfarin for many different indications and may have markedly different risks for adverse thrombotic events during warfarin cessation (Box 101-2). For patients with a history of VTE, the duration of time from the most recent thrombotic event is the most important risk factor for recurrence during warfarin cessation. Estimates of the *daily* recurrence rate during the first month (first 4 weeks) after an index event range from 0.3%–1.3%.[1-3] Over the next 2 months (4–12 weeks), the rate may drop to 0.03–0.2%.[1,2] Beyond 12 weeks from the index event, the rate is <0.05%.[1,2] The daily thrombosis rate during cessation of warfarin may be somewhat higher for idiopathic VTE as compared with illness-associated VTE.[4,5]

For patients with atrial fibrillation, the following factors increase the risk for cardioembolism: advanced age, diabetes, or hypertension, especially when poorly controlled; prior cardioembolic stroke; rheumatic heart disease, coronary artery disease, or structural heart disease such as congestive heart failure; or possibly female gender.[6-8]

Although the oft-quoted average annual stroke rate of 4–5% in patients with atrial fibrillation not receiving anticoagulation is accurate, estimated annual stroke rates for individual patients may range from about 1% to >10%. Where any individual patient falls in this range depends on the above risk factors. Patients with none of these risk factors have "lone" atrial fibrillation and a very low risk for cardioembolism without warfarin—<1–2% annually. Since this risk is comparable to that of age-matched patients who do not have atrial fibrillation, anticoagulation with warfarin for these patients is not recommended. Patients with only one risk factor fall into a low risk for thromboembolism category and hence do not need "bridging" therapy, but those with major risk factors for stroke, particularly rheumatic heart disease, prior cardioembolic stroke, or multiple risks listed above are at relatively high risk for cardioembolism. Bridging anticoagulation may be considered in these patients with atrial fibrillation to minimize the risk of perioperative cardioembolism.

For patients with newer mechanical heart valves, the risk of stroke while off warfarin is comparable to that of patients with atrial fibrillation. Not all patients with mechanical heart valves are at high risk for cardioembolism, particularly those with newer model valves (e.g., St. Jude valves) in the aortic position.[9] Patients with mechanical valves in the mitral position have a risk of cardioembolism about twice as high as those with valves in the aortic position.[9] Older valve models (such as ball-in-cage valves) may be associated with a high risk of cardioembolism during anticoagulation cessation.[9]

Type of Surgery

Although there is no recognized relationship between the type of surgery and the risk of cardioembolism, the type of surgery does contribute significantly to the risk of postoperative VTE. Surgeries associated with moderate or high risk for VTE include: knee and hip arthroplasty, surgery for long-bone fractures, major abdominopelvic surgery, and intracranial surgery.

The type of surgery also determines the risk of serious postoperative bleeding. Avoid full-dose anticoagulation, or use it with extreme caution in patients undergoing surgeries associated with a high risk of major bleeding. Prophylactic doses of anticoagulation following such surgeries may be better tolerated. The Johns Hopkins Surgical Bleeding Classification[10] categorizes surgeries by risk of bleeding, ranging from low-risk Category 1 to high-risk Category 5 procedures, as shown in Table 101-1.

In addition to the type of surgery, the type of anesthesia can also affect perioperative anticoagulation management. In general, avoid placing and removing epidural or spinal catheters

Box 101-1 Surgeries That Can Be Performed on Warfarin

Dental

Restorations

Endodontics

Prosthetics

Uncomplicated extractions

Dental hygiene treatment

Periodontal therapy

GI

Upper endoscopy with or without biopsy

Flexible sigmoidoscopy with or without biopsy

Colonoscopy with or without biopsy

ERCP without sphincterotomy

Biliary stent insertion without sphincterotomy

Endosonography without fine-needle aspiration

Push enteroscopy of the small bowel

Ophthalmologic

Cataract extractions

Trabeculectomies

Dermatologic

Mohs micrographic surgery

Simple excisions and repairs

Orthopedic

Joint aspiration

Soft tissue injections

Minor podiatric procedures

GI—gastrointestinal; ERCP—endoscopic retrograde cholangiopancreatogram

Table 101-1 Johns Hopkins Surgical Bleeding Classification

Category 1	Minimally invasive, minimal risk, with little or no blood loss. Examples: breast biopsy, cystoscopy.
Category 2	Minimally to moderately invasive, with estimated blood loss <500 cc. Examples: arthroscopy, hernia repair, laparoscopic cholecystectomy
Category 3	Moderately to significantly invasive, with blood loss potential 500–1,000 cc. Examples: thyroidectomy, laminectomy, hip or knee replacement
Category 4	Highly invasive procedure, with expected blood loss >1500 cc. Examples: major spinal reconstruction, Whipple procedure
Category 5	Highly invasive procedure with expected blood loss >1500 cc and often associated with anticipated post-operative ICU stay. Examples: intracranial surgery, major oropharyngeal procedure, major vascular surgery, open-heart surgery

when a patient is fully anticoagulated with warfarin or heparin products.

Preoperative Evaluation and Risk Stratification

There are no randomized clinical trials to guide which patients must receive bridging therapy. The best decision to use bridging therapy requires a detailed review of the patient's risk for both thromboembolism and for bleeding. In determining the risks and benefits of bridging therapy, be sure to consider the patient's preferences as well.

Thromboembolic Risk

Thromboembolic risk, discussed above, is also summarized in Box 101-2. Patients who should receive pre- and postoperative bridging anticoagulation include those at high and moderate thromboembolic risk. Restart bridging therapy postoperatively as soon as hemostasis is secured. Low thromboembolic risk patients do

not require bridging therapy, but just as with high- and moderate-risk patients, restart warfarin as soon as possible postoperatively. In conjunction with bridging therapy, provide postoperative VTE prophylaxis as indicated.

Bleeding Risk

The medical consultant can begin to estimate the risk of bleeding by reviewing the Johns Hopkin's Surgical Bleeding Classification outlined in Table 101-1. For any individual patient, it is important to know the time at which hemostasis can be predicted or actually secured. In many instances, this is not known until after the procedure, so communication from the surgeon or proceduralist is important. This information will help direct management of warfarin postoperatively.

In general, patients undergoing Category 3 procedures or higher should not resume full-dose bridging therapy until hemostasis is secured. This may take up to 2–3 days. These patients may, however, require VTE prophylaxis with heparin or LMWH at appropriate doses.

WARFARIN DISCONTINUATION

Usually, surgery can be safely performed with minimal risk of bleeding at an INR of <1.5. However, in neurosurgical procedures and certain major noncardiac surgeries, near-normal INRs (INR <1.2) may be desirable. If this is the goal, White et al.[11] have shown that for almost all patients with a steady-state INR of 2–3, the INR falls to less than 1.5 within 115 hours (4.8 days) after the last dose of warfarin. Thus, it is recommended that patients take their last dose of warfarin 5 days before surgery. If the steady-state INR is >3 and/or the patient is elderly, it may take longer to achieve a goal INR <1.5. Therefore, it is important to check an INR immediately before surgery in all patients stopping warfarin

Box 101-2 Risk of Thrombotic Complications of Selected Conditions in the Absence of Anticoagulant Therapy

High risk: bridging advised
- Venous or arterial thromboembolism within the preceding 3 months
- Mechanical heart valve
  - In the mitral position
  - Any position with placement in the preceding 3 months
  - Older valves (tilting disk, cage ball)
- History of thromboembolism and known hypercoagulable state
  - Antiphospholipid antibody
  - Homozygous factor V Leiden
  - Multiple genetic defects
  - Protein C or S deficiency
- Acute intracardiac thrombus
- Atrial fibrillation
  - With history of stroke, TIA, or systemic embolism
  - Associated with rheumatic valve disease
  - With mechanical valve
  - With multiple risk factors for stroke (see text)

Moderate risk: bridging on a case-by-case basis
- Newer mechanical aortic valve (bi-leaflet)
- Atrial fibrillation with risk factors
- Venous thromboembolism
  - Within the past 3–6 months
  - Idiopathic

Low risk: bridging not recommended
- Venous thromboembolism
  - >6 months ago
  - Heterozygous factor V Leiden
- Atrial fibrillation without risk factors

Box 101-3 Protocol for Bridging Therapy with Low-Molecular-Weight Heparin (LMWH)

Pre-Procedure Protocol:
- If INR 2–3, stop warfarin 5 days (4 doses) before procedure.
- If INR 3–4.5, stop warfarin 6 days (5 doses) before procedure.
- Start LMWH 36 hours after last warfarin dose.
- Give last dose of LMWH 24 hours before procedure.
- Ensure patient is thoroughly educated in self injection, including providing written instructions and contact phone number for questions or problems.
- Confer with surgeon and anesthesiologist to plan treatment.
- Check INR on morning of procedure.

Post-Procedure Protocol:
- Restart LMWH approximately 24 hours post-procedure, or consider using a thromboprophylaxis dose of LMWH on post-procedure days 1 to 3 if patient is high risk for bleeding.
- Confer with the surgeon to ensure he or she is comfortable with the planned start time for anticoagulant therapy.
- Start warfarin at patient's preop dose on post-op day 1.
- Daily PT/INR until patient is discharged and periodically thereafter until INR therapeutic.
- Daily telephone contact with pharmacist on discharge.
- CBC with platelets at day 3 and day 7.
- Discontinue LMWH when INR is 2–3 for two consecutive days.
- *Enoxaparin 1 mg/kg SQ q12h or 1.5 mg/kg SQ 24 hr*
- *or Dalteparin 120 units/kg q12h or Dalteparin 200 units/kg SQ q24h*
- For patients with creatinine clearance <30 mL/min consider using UFH or enoxaparin 1 mg/kg SQ q24h if full dose LWMH is desired or use 30 mg SQ q24h if prophylactic dose of LMWH is desired

INCLUSION CRITERIA:
- Age >18 years, needing to undergo therapy with LMWH.
- Treating physician thinks patient needs bridge therapy.
- Medically and hemodynamically stable.
- Scheduled for elective procedure or surgery.

EXCLUSION CRITERIA
- Allergy to UFH or LMWH.
- Weight >150 kg
- Pregnant woman with a mechanical valve.
- History of bleeding disorder or intracranial hemorrhage.
- GI bleeding within the last 10 days.
- Major trauma or stroke within the past 2 weeks.
- History of HIT or severe thrombocytopenia.
- Language barriers.
- Potential for medication noncompliance.
- Unsuitable home environment to support therapy.
- Severe liver disease.

INR—international normalized ratio; LMWH—low molecular weight heparin; PT—prothrombin time; UFH—unfractionated heparin; GI—gastrointestinal; HIT—heparin induced thrombocytoperin

preoperatively to ensure that anticoagulation has been adequately reversed.

If an emergency procedure must be performed while a patient's INR is therapeutic, immediate reversal of anticoagulation is required. This can be achieved with fresh frozen plasma (FFP), intravenous vitamin K, or recombinant activated factor VII (NovoSeven). FFP will lead to immediate reversal without any resistance to postoperative anticoagulation. Check an INR after initial FFP administration and every few hours thereafter if there is ongoing bleeding or a high risk for bleeding. The use of FFP carries the known risks of transfusion, and the effects of FFP are short lived.

In semi-urgent situations—surgery or procedure within 24–96 hours—oral vitamin K alone can be used. Doses of vitamin K in excess of 5 mg can cause postoperative resistance to anticoagulation. Doses of vitamin K as low as 1–2.5 mg are preferred and can achieve timely reversal of warfarin anticoagulation.

BRIDGING THERAPY

Both LMWH and UFH are suitable for use as bridging therapy. Because of its bioavailability and predictable pharmacokinetics, subcutaneous LMWH can be used as outpatient treatment and decreases the cost of hospitalization associated with bridging therapy with UFH.

If UFH is necessary, patients should be admitted to begin infusion approximately 2 days after warfarin is stopped. In most cases, this means at least 2 days of inpatient hospitalization before the surgery or procedure. A suitable heparin nomogram is recommended, for example one starting with an 80 units per kilogram bolus followed by an 18 unit per kilogram per hour infusion, with a goal PTT of 60–80 seconds. In patients with normal renal function, stop the heparin drip at least 4 hours before the procedure and sometimes up to 6 hours before the procedure in patients with renal insufficiency.

When LMWH is used for outpatient bridging therapy, the protocol[12] outlined in Box 101-3 can be used.

CONCLUSIONS

An understanding of the patient's thromboembolic risk is fundamental to the management of warfarin in the perioperative setting. The patient's bleeding risk and timing of hemostasis affect the schedule for resuming anticoagulation safely. Warfarin can be stopped 5 days prior to most procedures, and, when indicated, bridging anticoagulation can be performed in a safe and cost-effective manner. For many minor procedures, warfarin can be continued as outlined in Box 101-1. Communicating perioperative anticoagulation plans with the surgeon is essential to ensure maximum patient safety.

Key Points

- Contrary to popular belief, warfarin can be safely continued for minor procedures without dose alteration.

- Discontinuing warfarin 5 days before surgery is usually adequate to allow the INR to fall below therapeutic levels.

- Provide bridging therapy for patients at high risk for thromboembolic events, and for those at moderate risk on a case-by-case basis.

- Both LMWH and UFH are suitable for use as bridging therapy.

- **Be certain that hemostasis is secured before resuming full dose bridging therapy postoperatively.**

SUGGESTED READING

Kearon C, Hirsh J. Management of anticoagulation before and after elective surgery. N Engl J Med 1997; 336(21):1506–1511.

White RH, McKittrick T, Hutchinson R, et al. Temporary discontinuation of warfarin therapy: changes in the international normalized ratio. Ann Intern Med 1995; 122(1):40–42.

Jaffer AK, Brotman DJ, Chukwumerije N. When patients on warfarin need surgery. Cleve Clin J Med 2003; 70(11):973–984.

Horlocker TT, Wedel DJ, Benzon H, et al. Regional anesthesia in the anticoagulated patient: defining the risks (the second ASRA Consensus Conference on Neuraxial Anesthesia and Anticoagulation). Reg Anesth Pain Med 2003; 28(3):172–197.

CHAPTER ONE HUNDRED AND TWO

Cardiovascular Preoperative Risk Assessment and Evaluation

Steven L. Cohn, MD, FACP, and Dennis M. Manning, MD, FACP, FACC

BACKGROUND

Each year in the United States, over 27 million patients, approximately one third of who have coronary artery disease (CAD) or risk factors for cardiovascular (CV) disease, undergo surgery. One million will have a cardiac complication, including 50,000 perioperative myocardial infarctions (PMI).[1-3] Hospitalists are often consulted preoperatively to discern and minimize cardiovascular risk. Risk stratification strategies evolved over two decades[4] from the seminal work of Goldman, Detsky, Lee, and others[5-7] to the most recent guidelines published in 2002 from the ACC/AHA[1] (Fig. 102-1). Several other experts have rendered well-organized opinions[2,9-11] that will also be incorporated into this chapter, as will primary-source studies published in the last few years.

The purpose of this chapter is to present a succinct, evidence-based approach to the following questions:

1. What is the preoperative patient's CV risk?
2. Is any specialized testing and/or CV referral indicated?
3. What, if any, intervention or medical management will reduce CV risk?

PATHOPHYSIOLOGY

Perioperative CV events: The important CV complications of surgery (*see* Chapter 110 for details) include acute coronary syndromes (including PMI for which mortality may be as high as 40%), congestive heart failure (CHF), and arrhythmias. The aggregate risk can range from a low of <1% for minor procedures to >30% in vascular surgery patients who have both coronary artery disease (CAD) and inducible ischemia on stress testing.[12]

The primary mechanism of PMI is usually coronary atheromatous plaque disruption. Other contributing mechanisms may include ischemia mediated by activation of neurohumoral (catecholamine) pathways, tachycardia increasing myocardial oxygen demand, platelet activation, and coronary artery spasm.[13]

CLINICAL ASSESSMENT/EVALUATION

Questions to Be Answered

The hospitalist should consider the viewpoint of each stakeholder:

1. Patient and family: "Will my heart make it through, without a hitch?"
2. Surgeon: "Cleared for surgery?" Personal conversations concerning risk/benefit help transcend falsely dichotomous mental models of Red Light ("No—Can't allow surgery") versus Green Light ("Proceed—Clear sailing guaranteed").
3. Anesthesiologist: Is CAD, aortic valve stenosis (AS), or arrhythmia present? If an exercise or dobutamine stress test has been done, what is the ischemic threshold (double product = heart rate × systolic blood pressure)?

Preoperative Risk Stratification

Of the various tools available to aid the clinician in assessing risk, we prefer a combination of the ACC/AHA Guidelines[1] and the Lee Revised Cardiac Risk Index.[7] Components to be considered include surgery-specific risk, clinical risk factors and exercise capacity, and previous workup or treatment (revascularization).

The Surgical Procedure: Context, Timing, and Inherent Risk

The hospitalist should first consider the patient's overall general condition, any recent illness prompting surgery (including the urgency of the procedure), and risk category of the procedure itself according to the risk stratification in the ACC/AHA guidelines (Table 102-1). **High-risk procedures** include emergent major operations, aortic and peripheral vascular surgery, and anticipated prolonged surgical procedures associated with large fluid shifts/blood loss. **Intermediate-risk procedures** include carotid endarterectomy, intraperitoneal and intrathoracic surgery, and major orthopedic surgery. **Low-risk procedures** include endoscopies, superficial procedures, cataract surgery, and breast surgery. We tend to include the hip fracture population, whose postoperative CV complication risk is 8%, in the high-risk group.[14]

Patient Risk Factors

The hospitalist should be keen to detect clinically important cardiac disease and CV risk factors by performing a thorough history *and* physical in order to properly apply the guidelines. Such an evaluation, as described in the following, will ensure

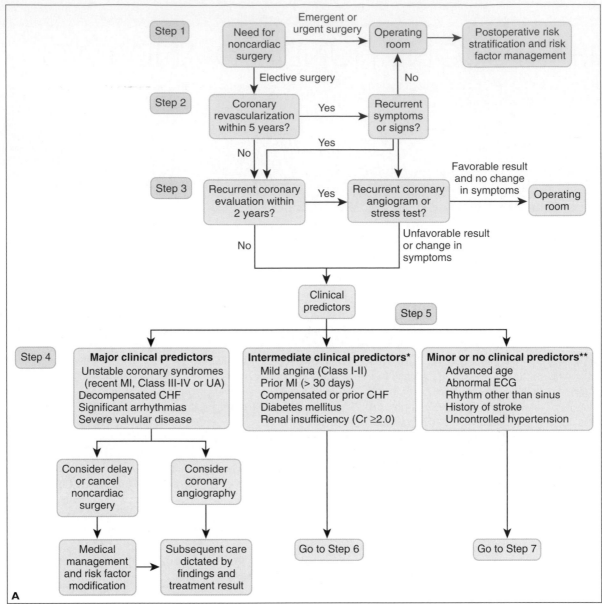

Figure 102-1 • ACC-AHA Algorithm for Preoperative Cardiac Risk Evaluation. Reprinted from: Cohn SL, Goldman L. Med Clin North Am 2003; 87(1):111–136; with permission from Elsevier. (Adapted from Eagle et al., ACC/AHA Guidelines, 2002; with permission.) MI—myocardial infarction; CHF—congestive heart failure; ECG—electrocardiogram; UA—unstable angina

that no additional or burdensome tests are requested unless the result will affect treatment decisions.

Patient-Supplied Past Medical History (PMH): Ask about a history of cardiac disease and cardiovascular risk factors (or CAD equivalents)—CAD (myocardial infarction [MI] or angina), CHF, arrhythmias, valvular disease or murmurs, hypertension, diabetes mellitus, hyperlipidemia, cerebrovascular accident (CVA), peripheral arterial disease (PAD), and tobacco use. Clinicians often wonder about the accuracy of a patient's past medical history. A recent population-based study found that a patient's denial of MI or CAD was generally reliable (>85% negative predictive value). A positive notation, though highly reliable when present, had poor sensitivity (60%) for the presence of a previously diagnosed heart condition.[15] Inquire about any previous cardiac work-up or interventions. Results of past stress tests, echocardiograms, angiograms, and hospital summaries are

helpful. Significant information gaps may warrant a diligent search for any special cardiac records.

Functional Capacity: Self-reported exercise capacity is emphasized as an important factor (for consideration of stress testing) in the ACC/AHA Guidelines. Low functional capacity is below 4 METs (inability to climb a flight of stairs, walk up a grade, or do heavy housework, etc.) and may lead to preoperative stress testing to unmask important CAD. Ask open-ended questions: "Tell me about your most recent strenuous physical activity. How often? How do you feel during the exertion? How many blocks can you walk without stopping? Why do you stop?"

Atypical Symptoms of Ischemia: Individuals who regularly avoid walking up grades or stairs in recent months or who must cease during such exertion to rest are somewhat worrisome. Angina is Greek for "strangling," connoting the sensation of suffocation, not "pain." Ischemia in the elderly may manifest as

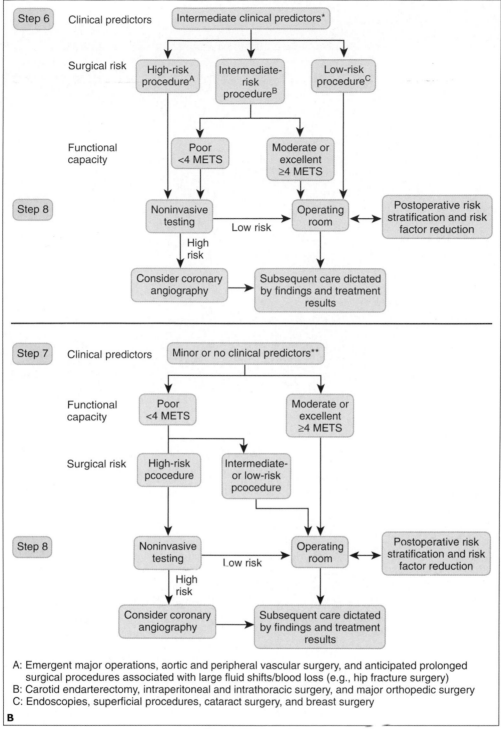

Step 6   Clinical predictors   **Intermediate clinical predictors***

Figure 102-1, cont'd

A: Emergent major operations, aortic and peripheral vascular surgery, and anticipated prolonged surgical procedures associated with large fluid shifts/blood loss (e.g., hip fracture surgery)
B: Carotid endarterectomy, intraperitoneal and intrathoracic surgery, and major orthopedic surgery
C: Endoscopies, superficial procedures, cataract surgery, and breast surgery

dyspnea or recurring idiosyncratic exertional discomfort in thorax, arms, or neck. The most reliable features are not location or intensity, but consistency of exertional-provocation, worsening with further exertion, and relief with rest. Some patients may rationalize and discount symptoms.

Auscultation: Heart Murmurs. Important aortic stenosis is the most significant valvular lesion associated with perioperative complications. The examiner should listen for a systolic ejection murmur (>Grade 2/6) at the base radiating to the clavicles and neck with a *late systolic peak*. The latter is a key feature distin-guishing significant (moderate or severe) AS from both mild AS and the aortic sclerosis murmurs commonly found in the elderly. The finding of *tardus et parvus* pulse and left ventricular hyper-trophy (LVH) with strain—though helpful—are neither sensitive nor specific for important AS. These auscultatory findings, espe-cially if associated with chest pain, dyspnea, or syncope, should prompt further assessment by echocardiography. Mitral stenosis may be associated with perioperative cardiac complications but usually when accompanied by established heart failure or arrhythmias (AF).

Table 102-1 Recommendations for Patients to Include in Beta-Blocker Therapy (BBT) by Surgery Type and Clinical Risk Factors[1,2,4,8,9,10]

Surgery type	High risk:	Intermediate Risk:	Low Risk:
	Aortic Vascular Emergent Hip fracture	Orthopedic Major head/neck Radical Prostatectomy Carotid Endarterectomy Intrathoracic Abdominal	Cystoscopy Endoscopy Cataract Breast
1.1.1 Risk Factors			
Any of the following "compelling indications": Known CAD Prior MI Ischemic heart disease Uncontrolled BP Chronic BBT	Yes	Yes	Yes
Other RCRI Risk factors: Diabetes Creatinine >2.0 CVA	Yes, if any RCRI factor	Yes, if 2 or more RCRI factors	Yes if >2 RCRI factors
Minor risk factors: (age >65, current smoker, cholesterol >240, male)	No, if no Risk factors	No, if 0–1 risk factors	No, if ≤2 risk factors

MI—myocardial infarction; BP—blood pressure; CAD—coronary artery disease; BBT—beta-blocker theraphy; CVA—cerebrovascular accident; RCRI—revised cardiac risk index

Other Issues of Importance

- **Heart failure:** Patients with clinical symptoms and signs of heart failure (PND, bilateral rales, elevated jugular venous pressure (JVP), S_3) have increased risk of perioperative events. Routine echocardiography does not appreciably add to the risk discrimination.[16]
- **Ischemic cardiomyopathy:** Patients with known ischemic cardiomyopathies with low (<35%) left ventricular ejection function (LVEF) are at risk for perioperative MI, arrhythmias, and CHF. When such patients face higher-risk surgery, consider CV consultation and/or dobutamine stress echocardiography (in which ischemic threshold can be discerned with prognostic importance).[17]
- **Advanced age:** By itself, advanced age is at best a minor predictor of complications and most likely represents decreased cardiac reserve. Age ≥70 is a powerful (and often neglected) risk factor for the presence of CAD (which may be asymptomatic and without ECG manifestations). Likewise, 30% of octogenarians have mild cognitive impairment, and their history may be incomplete or lack detail. Verification and clarification from caregiving family members can be helpful.
- **Hypertension:** Although hypertension has not been found to be a significant risk factor in any of the cardiac indices (unless the BP is extremely high), it is a common problem leading to cancellation of surgery. The risk with hypertension relates more to the etiology (e.g., pheochromocytoma), end organ damage (CHF, chronic renal insufficiency [CRI], MI, CVA), and intra- or postoperative hypotension than to the preoperative blood pressure per se. In general, there is no need to postpone surgery if the blood pressure is <200 mmHg systolic and 110 mm Hg diastolic, unless the patient has significant ischemic heart disease.[18] If necessary, additional antihypertensive medications can be administered on the morning of surgery and in the operating room to control BP.

Diagnostic Tests: Electrocardiogram

Patients undergoing intermediate or high-risk surgery, especially men over age 45 and women over age 55, and those with CAD should have a preoperative resting 12-lead ECG. The following ECG abnormalities may impact management decisions.

- **Silent or age-indeterminate MI** might prompt noninvasive testing in an otherwise asymptomatic patient undergoing high-risk surgery.
- **Unexplained left bundle branch block (LBBB),** especially if new or of uncertain duration, should be understood as a sign of organic heart disease (CAD and/or LV dysfunction) until proven otherwise. Asymptomatic bifascicular block rarely progresses to complete heart block perioperatively and therefore does not warrant placement of a temporary pacemaker.
- **Hemodynamically significant arrhythmias** such as supraventricular tachycardia (SVT), atrial fibrillation with a rapid ventricular response, and runs of ventricular tachycardia require therapy prior to any elective surgery.

Blood Tests: Serum Electrolytes

- Check serum potassium, blood urea nitrogen (BUN), and creatinine in patients on diuretics, angiotensin converting enzyme (ACE) inhibitor, or ARBs. Correct any hypokalemia, especially in the presence of CAD, CHF, or digoxin use.

Table 102-2 Lee Revised Cardiac Risk Index (RCRI)

- High-risk surgery
- History of ischemic heart disease
- Congestive heart failure
- Cerebrovascular disease
- Diabetes mellitus requiring treatment with insulin
- Preoperative serum creatinine >2.0 mg/dL.

Risk Factors	Complication Rates
0 or 1	0.4–1.3%
2	4–7%
3 or more	9–11%

Who Needs A Stress Test? And If So, Which One?

- Which patients require preoperative specialized cardiac tests is still a matter of debate. If a patient is asymptomatic or has stable symptoms with adequate exercise capacity, noninvasive testing is probably not indicated and will rarely change management. As stated in the ACC Guidelines, "in general, indications for further cardiac testing and treatment are the same as those in the non-operative setting" and "coronary revascularization before noncardiac surgery to enable the patient to 'get through' the noncardiac procedure is appropriate only for a small subset of patients at very high risk." On the other hand, if the patient is facing intermediate- to high-risk surgery and is suspected of having critical or severe CAD based on significant or low-threshold ischemic symptoms, the risk-benefit balance is thrown into question. If further risk stratification will possibly make a difference to management, then a provocative stress test may be indicated.

- In general, results from either dipyridamole (Persantine) or adenosine nuclear tests or dobutamine stress echocardiography are comparable in predicting postoperative cardiac complications. The negative predictive values are usually above 95%; however, positive predictive values are low at 15–20%. Dobutamine testing is preferred in patients with asthma or COPD because dipyridamole may cause bronchospasm. On the other hand, dipyridamole testing is preferred for patients with LBBB because false positive reversible septal defects may occur with exercise or dobutamine.

- If surgery is urgent or emergent, time does not permit further evaluation. These patients must be optimized medically in the limited time available before surgery.

- Patients who have undergone coronary artery bypass grafting (CABG) or percutaneous coronary intervention (PCI) in the last few years (up to 5 years) and remain asymptomatic do not require further testing. However, if they are symptomatic, re-evaluation may be indicated preoperatively.

- Patients with recent (within 2 years) noninvasive tests with satisfactory results and no new symptoms require no further testing. Alternatively, those with new symptoms may warrant repeat testing.

The **Lee Revised Cardiac Risk Index (RCRI)**[7] identified six independent predictors of postoperative cardiac complications—high-risk surgery, history of ischemic heart disease, CHF, cerebrovascular disease, diabetes mellitus requiring treatment with

insulin, and preoperative serum creatinine >2.0 mg/dl. Patients with 0–1 risk factors had complication rates of 0.4–1.3%; with 2 factors, 4–7%; and with 3 or more factors, 9–11% (Table 102-2). Using a variation of these risk factors, Boersma[19] analyzed data from 1,351 patients undergoing vascular surgery to decide when dobutamine stress echocardiography and/or beta-blockers would be helpful. With 0–2 risk factors, the patients did well, regardless of the dobutamine stress echocardiography (DSE) results; on the other hand, patients with three or more risk factors were at increased risk that was further stratified by DSE results but significantly reduced by beta-blockers in all subgroups, except those with new wall motion abnormalities in >4 segments. This latter group might benefit from revascularization.

RECOMMENDATIONS/MANAGEMENT

Revascularization: CABG/PCI

- A retrospective analysis of patients randomized to CABG in the coronary artery surgery study (CASS) who subsequently had a high-risk noncardiac surgical procedure reported a lower perioperative MI and mortality rate than those treated medically. There was no difference for low-risk procedures. Similarly, data for patients with previous percutaneous transluminal coronary angioplasty (PTCA) undergoing noncardiac surgery reported morbidity and mortality less than expected, compared with historical controls.

- On the other hand, the recent landmark study (Coronary Artery Revascularization Prophylaxis—CARP) reported that stable CAD patients, without AS or LV failure, undergoing elective vascular surgery did not benefit from preoperative cardiac catheterization and prophylactic revascularization (PCI stent or CABG);[70] however, *both the control group and the revascularization group received aggressive medical therapy.* Procedural complications of prophylactic revascularization included 1.7% mortality, 5.8% perioperative MI, and 2.5% reoperation. After vascular surgery, the 30-day mortality rate was 3% in both groups, and the perioperative MI rates were comparable (12% vs. 14% using elevated troponin). The primary endpoint of long-term death (an average of 2.7 years after randomization) was not different between the groups (22% vs. 23%). Therefore, routine stress testing and cardiac catheterization in patients with stable CAD are probably unwarranted, and preoperative prophylactic revascularization is rarely indicated for the purpose of getting a patient through surgery.

Based on this information, the risks and benefits of cardiac testing and possible revascularization need to be evaluated on an individual basis. If they are indicated, the consultant must be aware of several caveats pertaining to the timing of subsequent noncardiac surgery.

- The risk of perioperative complications is increased if the noncardiac surgery is performed within 30 days of the CABG, as opposed to after 30 days.

- If necessary, noncardiac surgery can be performed reasonably safely on an average of 7–14 days after PTCA without stenting;[21,22,23] however, after stent placement, surgery should probably be postponed for at least 4 weeks, preferably 6 weeks.[24] This period will allow for dual antiplatelet therapy to minimize the chance of in-stent thrombosis while having a short "washout interval" to minimize the risk of perioperative bleeding.

Depending on the type of stent (bare metal vs. drug-eluting stent [DES]), even longer treatment with antiplatelet agents prior to elective noncardiac surgery may be warranted. Uninterrupted dual antiplatelet therapy is recommended for a minimum of 2–3 months following placement of a sirolimus DES and for at least 6 months after a paclitaxel DES. Several studies have reported complication rates greater than expected if shorter durations are used or dual antiplatelet therapy is continued through the noncardiac surgery.

- If time does not permit postponing surgery for these intervals, the consultant should consider optimizing medical therapy as the primary option to reduce perioperative risk or consider PTCA without stenting.

Prophylactic Medical Therapy

Beta-adrenergic blocking medications: Studies indicate that beta-adrenergic blockade affords higher-risk patients some cardio protection,[3,12,19,25] reducing perioperative ischemia in the DECREASE study,[12] and lowering the risk of perioperative MI or cardiac death in patients undergoing vascular surgery. However, closer inspection and meta-analysis[26] of the data reveal that this lowering of risk just reached statistical significance for MI and cardiac death. Additionally, more recent studies (POBBLE, MaVS, DIPOM)[27–29] have failed to show a benefit in postoperative CV events. A large trial (POISE) is currently underway and hopefully will answer the question of who will benefit from prophylactic beta-blockade. In the interim, we agree with both Auerbach and Goldman[9] and Fleisher and Eagle[2] that there should be liberal application of beta-blocker therapy (BBT) to patients in the higher risk groups. This is in accord with the ACC/AHA Guidelines[30] regarding BBT, including both Class I (general agreement) and by Class IIa recommendations (favoring treatment, despite some remaining controversy in the evidence).

Lindenauer et al.[31] and Siddiqui et al.[32] noted that perioperative beta-blockers are underutilized. However, a retrospective cohort study[33] of over 600,000 patients using the revised Cardiac Risk Index (RCRI) revealed a benefit of perioperative beta-blocker therapy in reducing inhospital death only in high-risk (RCRI > 2) patients; with two risk factors, benefit was equivocal, but in low-risk patients with RCRI of 0–1, treatment was associated with no benefit and possible harm.

Our recommendations for BBT by surgical procedure risk and clinical risk are outlined in Table 102-1. We include all patients with known CAD or prior MI, as well as patients with a strong CAD risk profile who face an intermediate or high-risk procedure. Based on recent studies, however, we do not include minor risk factors from the Mangano study as being equal to those in the RCRI.

- The target resting heart rate for both groups is <70 beats/minute, and ideally the BBT should be started prior to the day of surgery to achieve this goal. Tight heart rate control has been shown to be associated with fewer postoperative cardiac complications and may obviate the need for non-invasive testing in some patients.[34]
- Continue BBT perioperatively (including on the morning of surgery) in any patient already taking them. New BBT patients should probably continue BBT for at least 30 days postoperatively.

- Start either metoprolol 25–50 mg PO BID, metoprolol LA 50 mg PO once daily, or atenolol 50 mg PO once daily, preferably at least 7 days prior to surgery, and continuing for at least 30 days. Many patients do not achieve goal heart rate in short preoperative windows[35] and need intraoperative and postop (upward) titration.
- Use of a hospital order set to "follow" the postoperative patient through the various care venues and provision of the option for IV alternative beta-blocker for patients unable to take oral medications increases use.
- Educate hospital staff and patients to ensure the morning dose of beta-blocker is administered to avoid tachycardia (BBT withdrawal syndrome) even if "NPO after midnight." Such a strategy resulted in an increase (from 38 to 62%) in the proportion of high-risk patients having a resting preoperative heart rate of <70 beats/min at one center.[36]

Alpha-agonists (clonidine): No definitive answer is available on the cardioprotective effects of the alpha-2 agonist clonidine (oral or transdermal), but pooled data from several small studies suggest a protective effect against perioperative ischemia.[37,38] A more recent double-blinded clinical trial demonstrated that clonidine reduced the incidence of perioperative ischemia and subsequent postoperative cardiac death.[39] In a meta-analysis comparing alpha-agonists to beta-blockers, it appears that the protective effect of the latter drugs is greater.[40] The alpha-agonists require further study but may prove to be helpful, especially in patients with contraindications or intolerance to beta-blockers.

Antiplatelet medications (aspirin, clopidogrel): The potential benefit of these medications must be balanced with the potential increased risk of bleeding, and perioperative management should be discussed with the surgical team.

- There is evidence to support stopping clopidogrel 5 days before CABG to minimize bleeding and perioperative morbidity;[41] conversely, there is also evidence demonstrating that patients on aspirin within 48 hours of CABG (postoperatively) as well as within 5 days preoperatively had fewer deaths and myocardial infarctions.[42]
- Premature discontinuation of dual antiplatelet therapy after coronary stent placement has been associated with in-stent thrombosis, myocardial infarction, and death.
- If antiplatelet agents are stopped temporarily, they should be restarted as soon as hemostasis permits.

Statin medications: All patients with CAD, significant hypercholesterolemia, or diabetes mellitus should be taking one of these medications, and despite recommendations to the contrary in the package inserts, we recommend that they remain on the drugs during the perioperative period without hiatus, for plaque stabilization. Several studies demonstrated improved perioperative outcomes for patients on a statin either preoperatively or postoperatively.[43–46]

Postoperative Monitoring

Pulmonary Artery Catheters: In ASA class III and IV patients (over age 60), a large randomized study of almost 2,000 patients showed that the PA catheter (and goal-directed therapy based on the data obtained from the PA catheter) provided no survival advantage beyond that of routine postoperative management.[47] In another retrospective analysis of over 4,000 patients, those who received a PA catheter also failed to show any benefit on outcome.[48]

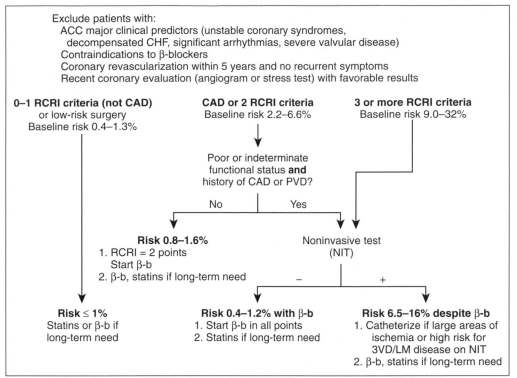

Figure 102-2 • Algorithm for patient selection for cardioprotective agents and cardiac testing before elective major noncardiac surgery. Modified from: Auerbach A, Goldman L. Cire 2006; 113:1361–1376.

Surveillance for Perioperative MI

ECG: Routine ECGs obtained at baseline, immediately after surgery, and on the first 2 days after surgery appear to be cost effective in patients with known or suspected CAD who are undergoing high-risk procedures.[1] An ECG done immediately postoperatively has also been found to be helpful in updating risk stratification of all patient groups after major noncardiac surgery.[49]

Cardiac Enzymes: Use of cardiac biomarkers is best reserved for patients at high risk and those with clinical, ECG, or hemodynamic evidence of cardiovascular dysfunction.[1]

SUMMARY

We recommend an approach to preoperative cardiac evaluation, testing, and therapy that individualizes decisions but combines elements of the ACC Guidelines, Lee Revised Cardiac Risk Index (RCRI), and beta-blocker and statin data (Fig. 102-2). Assuming patients have no contraindications to beta-blockers, have not been revascularized, and have not had a recent noninvasive stress test:

- Patients with 0–1 RCRI factors are at low risk and require no further workup or beta-blockers.
- Patients with three or more RCRI factors are at high risk and are potential candidates for further tests or revascularization in select cases and for intensive medical therapy including beta-blockers and statins.
- Patients with two factors are at intermediate risk and may warrant further evaluation if they have poor functional capacity, angina, or PAD and are scheduled for intermediate- to high-risk surgery. In any case, beta-blockers are indicated, and statins may also be beneficial.

Key Points

- The history and physical examination are the most important components in evaluating preoperative cardiac risk.

- Consider the clinical risk factors, procedural risk, and patient's functional capacity in your decision-making.

- No test should be performed unless the result will alter management.

- The positive predictive value of noninvasive testing is low, but the negative predictive value is high.

- Prophylactic revascularization is rarely necessary just to get a patient through surgery.

- Consider intensive prophylactic medical therapy for patients deemed to be at high risk.

- If beta-blocker therapy is to be helpful, it should be started far enough in advance to achieve a target heart rate of <70 beats/min by the time of surgery.

- Continue most cardiac medications perioperatively.

SUGGESTED READING

Eagle KA, Berger PB, Calkins J, et al. ACC/AHA guideline update for perioperative evaluation for noncardiac surgery—executive summary: a report of the American College of Cardiology/American Heart Association Task Force on Practice Guidelines (Committee to Update the 1996 Guidelines on perioperative cardiovascular examination for noncardiac surgery). J Am Coll Cardiol 2002; 39:542–553.

Fleisher LA, Eagle KA. Lowering cardiac risk in noncardiac surgery. N Engl J Med 2001; 345:1677–1682.

Mangano DT, Layug EL, Wallace A, et al. Effect of atenolol on mortality and cardiovascular morbidity after noncardiac surgery. N Engl J Med 1996; 335:1713.

Cohn SL, Goldman L. Preoperative risk evaluation and perioperative management of patients with coronary artery disease. Med Clin North Am 2003; 87:111–136.

Lee T, Marciantonio ER, Mangione CM, et al. Derivation and prospective validation of a simple index for prediction of cardiac risk of major noncardiac surgery. Circulation 1999; 100:1043–1049.

Auerbach AD, Goldman L. Beta-blockers and reduction of cardiac events in noncardiac surgery: scientific review. JAMA 2002; 287:1435–1444.

Poldermans D, Boersma E, Bax JJ, et al. The effect of bisoprolol on perioperative mortality and myocardial infarction in high-risk patients undergoing vascular surgery. N Engl J Med 1999; 341:1789–1794.

Das MK, Pellika PA, Mahoney DW, et al. Assessment of cardiac risk before nonvascular surgery. J Am Coll Card 2000; 35:1647–1653.

Boersma E, Poldermans D, Bax JJ, et al. Predictors of cardiac events after major vascular surgery: role of clinical characteristics dobutamine echocardiography, and beta-blocker therapy. JAMA 2001; 285:1865–1873.

McFalls EO, Ward HB, Moritz TE, et al. Coronary-artery revascularization before elective major vascular surgery. N Engl J Med 2004; 351:2795–2804.

Wilson SH, Fasseas P, Orford JL, et al. Clinical outcome of patients undergoing non-cardiac surgery in the two months following coronary stenting. J Am Coll Cardiol 2003; 42(2):234–240.

CHAPTER ONE HUNDRED AND THREE

Pulmonary Preoperative Risk Assessment and Evaluation

Rendell W. Ashton, MD, Ognjen Gajic, MD, MSc, FCCP, and Gerald W. Smetana, MD

BACKGROUND

Postoperative pulmonary complications, defined as any lung-related complications that lead to increased morbidity, mortality, or longer hospital stay, are very common in medical practice. As more and more patients with preexisting pulmonary conditions or other risk factors undergo surgical procedures, pulmonary complications will continue to be an important consideration in the care of surgical patients. The reported incidence of pulmonary complications after nonthoracic surgery varies between 2–10%.[1–3]

Even using a conservative estimate of 2–3%, of the approximately 45 million North Americans who will undergo nonthoracic surgery in the next year, over 1 million will experience a postoperative pulmonary complication.[3] Box 103-1 lists the most important postoperative pulmonary complications.

Although postoperative pulmonary complications are more common than postoperative cardiac complications,[2] they are less well studied. In fact, until recently, there have been no validated models for predicting pulmonary complications and no widely accepted algorithms for managing them. This chapter will review the pathophysiology of common and severe postoperative pulmonary complications. We will also provide the hospital-based internist with tools to assess and minimize risk for postoperative pulmonary complications through targeted evaluation and interventions in the preoperative period.

PATHOPHYSIOLOGY

A variety of factors contribute to the development of postoperative pulmonary complications. These relate to preexisting conditions, anesthesia and surgery itself, and pain and other postoperative conditions. The most important changes result from anesthesia-induced chest wall dysfunction and subsequent development of atelectasis in the dependent regions of the lung.[4] This atelectasis forms within minutes after the induction of anesthesia and is an important cause of intraoperative gas exchange abnormalities. Several other factors may also contribute to postoperative pulmonary complications. Endotracheal intubation and volatile anesthetics inhibit normal mucociliary transport, which is important for the clearance of particles from the lung. Anesthesia and opioid analgesics suppress respiratory drive. Cough inhibition due to medications or pain can lead to atelecta-

sis, derecruitment, and pooling of secretions. Neuromuscular paralysis and use of high concentrations of inspired oxygen also contribute to atelectasis formation.

Numerous insults can lead to acute lung injury (ALI), including infection, inflammation, ischemia-reperfusion injury, blood transfusion (transfusion-associated acute lung injury, or TRALI), stretch injury from mechanical ventilation (baro- or volutrauma), and reinflation injury of the lung collapsed during surgery. Patients with obstructive airways disease, such as asthma or emphysema, can experience exacerbations when any factor upsets the delicate balance of inflammatory mediators in the airways. Potential factors include irritation from inhalational anesthetics or an endotracheal tube and nosocomial infection, including ventilator-associated pneumonia.

Physiologically, these insults may result in decreased functional lung volumes (FRC) and airflow (FEV$_1$), and $\dot{V}/\dot{Q}$ mismatching with impairment of gas exchange. Hypoxic and/or hypercarbic respiratory failure may occur, particularly in the setting of preexisting lung disease. The more severe the preexisting lung disease, the more likely it is that the additional insult of surgery and anesthesia will result in a postoperative pulmonary complication. The preoperative evaluation serves to identify both patient- and procedure-related factors that increase the risk of postoperative pulmonary complications.

CLINICAL ASSESSMENT/EVALUATION

The most important tools for estimating the risk of postoperative pulmonary complications are a careful medical history and physical examination. Table 103-1 summarizes several recent prospective studies of risk factors for perioperative pulmonary complications. While some risk factors, such as smoking, are generally accepted to carry increased risk, the importance of other factors varies in the published literature. As Table 103-1 demonstrates, this results in part from study heterogeneity. Individual studies focus on different complications, types of surgery, and, in some cases, patient populations. The disparity in the findings is not surprising, and this points out the need for clinical judgment in assessing risk, as well as for more systematic research in this area. Here, we indicate the relative strength of recommendation for potential risk factors, based on the strength of the published evidence.

Box 103-1 Common Perioperative Pulmonary Complications

Atelectasis, leading to gas exchange abnormalities and/or respiratory failure

Hypoxic and hypercarbic respiratory failure

Prolonged mechanical ventilation

Acute lung injury, acute respiratory distress syndrome

Pneumonia

Exacerbation of obstructive airway disease (asthma or COPD)

Pneumothorax

Pleural effusion, empyema

Box 103-2 Surgical Factors Associated with Higher Risk of Perioperative Pulmonary Complications

AAA repair and other vascular surgery

Thoracic and upper abdominal surgery

Neurosurgery

Neck surgery

Emergency surgery

General anesthesia (as opposed to spinal or local/regional anesthesia)

Duration of surgery (greater than 2–3 hours)

Placement of a nasogastric tube after abdominal surgery

Pancuronium use

- Cigarette smoking increases the risk of pulmonary complications. A patient who has never smoked has the lowest risk, but former smokers have an intermediate or even increased risk, with respect to current smokers, depending on the timing of their quitting. One study showed that smokers who quit less than 2 months prior to surgery had a four-fold higher rate of complications, compared to quitters of longer than 2 months' duration.[5] However, a recent report has introduced some controversy by finding that recent quitters have similar pulmonary complication rates compared with less recent quitters.[6] Virtually every study looking at pulmonary complications lists smoking as a significant risk factor,[1,3,7,8] even for patients without clinically apparent smoking-related lung disease.

- A history of other pulmonary disease can also influence a patient's risk. Obstructive diseases, such as COPD and asthma, as well as restrictive diseases, such as pulmonary fibrosis, are important risk factors that increase vulnerability to respiratory compromise due to the pathophysiologic mechanisms discussed above. Asthma is a risk factor only when poorly controlled at the time of surgery. It is important to evaluate patients with preexisting lung disease to assess the severity of the disease. Clinical evaluation, including exercise capacity, daily symptoms, and evidence of significant airflow obstruction on physical examination, will identify high-risk patients. Spirometry usually confirms the clinical estimation of risk and only rarely identifies high-risk patients who escape clinical detection. However, consider spirometry if the severity of lung disease is uncertain after clinical evaluation or if it is uncertain whether a patient is at his or her best baseline before surgery.

- Age-related changes in pulmonary function predispose elderly patients to increased risk of pulmonary complications. In multivariate studies that have evaluated the impact of age, the risk of pulmonary complications increases after approximately age 65. Not all studies have found age to be a significant risk factor, and no age cutoff exists above which surgery is automatically too risky. Such a decision must involve other considerations, such as functional status and comorbid conditions.

- Obesity is controversial as a risk factor for pulmonary complications. The majority of studies have not shown an increased risk due to increased weight or body mass index, but some recent studies have reported this to be a risk factor.[1,3] Obesity is a risk factor for obstructive sleep apnea (OSA), which increases the risk of airway management complications in the immediate postoperative period. These include reintubation, hypercapnia, and hypoxemia. The management of these complications falls within the realm of the anesthesiologist. Whether obesity itself directly leads to lung injury, respiratory failure, or other more direct adverse outcomes is less clear. A history of recent weight loss has been associated with increased complication risk as well.

- Decreased exercise capacity increases the risk of postoperative pulmonary and cardiac complications. Poor exercise capacity is defined as the inability to walk four blocks on level ground or climb two flights of stairs without symptoms. The most common underlying causes of decreased exercise capacity are cardiac limitation and deconditioning; but particularly in cases where capacity is limited by problems of gas exchange or respiratory reserve, the risk of adverse pulmonary events after surgery may be high. This distinction between cardiac and pulmonary limitations is usually apparent from the history and physical examination. If diagnostic uncertainty exists, spirometry and formal cardiopulmonary exercise testing may each be helpful.

- Chronic illness, as classified in the American Society of Anesthesiologists (ASA) classification (see Chapter 97) confers increased perioperative risk. This simple scale stratifies patients according to the presence or absence, as well as severity and stability, of chronic disease. Studies have validated the ASA classification as a predictor of risk for perioperative pulmonary complications. The risk increases significantly for patients who are >ASA class 2.[9]

- Selected physical exam findings predict higher risk. Those correlated with perioperative pulmonary complications include positive cough test (repeated coughing after a single voluntary cough), decreased maximal laryngeal height (less than 4 cm), and prolonged forced expiratory time. These findings each suggest hyperinflation and underlying COPD.

- In addition to patient-related risk factors, some aspects of the planned surgery also may contribute to the risk of perioperative pulmonary complications. In general, longer duration procedures and those close to the diaphragm carry the highest risk. Emergency surgery also increases risk. Surgery involving the lung itself, such as lobectomy or lung volume reduction surgery, poses especially high risk and may warrant preoperative consultation with a pulmonary specialist. Box 103-2 sum-

Table 103-1 Comparison of Studies of Risk Factors for Perioperative Pulmonary Complications

Study Author and Date	McAlister 2005[3]	McAlister 2003[1]	Arozullah 2001[8]	Arozullah 2000[7]	Mitchell 1998[11]
Type of surgery	Elective nonthoracic	Nonthoracic	Major noncardiac	Major noncardiac	Elective nonthoracic
Complication studied	Respiratory failure Pneumonia Atelectatis requiring intervention Pneumothorax or pleural effusion requiring intervention	Respiratory failure Pneumonia Atelectasis requiring intervention	Postoperative pneumonia	Postoperative respiratory failure	Acute bronchitis Bronchospasm Atelectasis Pneumonia ARDS Pleural effusion Pneumothorax Prolonged mechanical ventilation Death due to respiratory failure
Patient population (N)	Men and women (1,055)	Men and women (272)	Men and women (160,805)	Men (99,390)	Men and women, age >40 (148)
Overall postoperative pulmonary complication rate (%)	2.7	8	1.5	3.4	11
Significant patient risk factors	Age ≥65 BMI ≥30 Smoked >40 pack-years FEV_1 <1 L Positive cough test* FVC FEV_1/FVC ratio	Age ≥65 Smoked >40 pack-years COPD Decreased exercise capacity BMI ≥30 Positive cough test* Positive wheeze test† Forced expiratory time ≥9 seconds Maximal laryngeal height ≤4 cm FEV_1 <1 L/min FVC <1.5 L/min PCO_2 ≥45 mm Hg PO_2 <75 mm Hg	Increasing age Worsening functional status Recent weight loss COPD Impaired sensorium History or stroke Abnormal BUN Transfusion Steroid dependency Smoking Alcohol >2 drinks/day	Albumin <3.0 mg/dL BUN >30 mg/dL Dependent functional status COPD Increasing age	Preoperative sputum production
Significant surgical risk factors	Duration of surgery ≥2.5 hours Perioperative nasogastric tube Upper abdominal incision	Duration of surgery ≥2.5 hours	AAA repair Thoracic surgery Upper abdominal surgery Neck surgery Neurosurgery Vascular surgery Emergency surgery General anesthesia	AAA repair Thoracic surgery Neurosurgery Upper abdominal surgery Vascular surgery Neck surgery Emergency surgery	Postoperative NG tube Duration of surgery

*A positive cough test is repeated involuntary coughing after a singe voluntary cough.
†A positive wheeze test is the presence of wheezing heard on auscultation between the patient's shoulder blades after 5 deep breaths.
ARDS—acute respiratory distress syndrome; FEV—forced expiratory volume in one second; FVC—forced vital capacity; COPD—chronic obstructive pulmonary disease; BUN—blood urea nitrogen; NG—nasogastric; AAA—abdominal aortic aneurism; BMI—body mass index

marizes the list of surgical procedures and factors associated with higher risk.

- There is considerable debate about the role of laboratory testing and imaging studies. Studies have not shown consistent benefit from any specific test or imaging study, although many tests are routinely ordered or even required by institutional policy. The available literature does not support ordering "routine" preoperative tests unless required to answer a specific question about a patient's condition. This includes routine chest x-ray, spirometry, and blood gas analysis. Reserve testing for situations in

Table 103-2 Preoperative Predictors of Postoperative Respiratory Failure

Risk Factor	Odds Ratio (99% confidence interval)
Type of surgery	
Abdominal aortic aneurysm	14.3 (12.0–16.9)
Thoracic	8.14 (7.17–9.25)
Neurosurgery, upper abdominal or vascular	4.21 (3.80–4.67) 3.10 (2.40–4.01)
Neck	
Other surgery	1.00 (reference)
Emergency surgery	3.12 (2.83–3.43)
Albumin <30 g/L	2.53 (2.28–2.80)
Blood urea nitrogen >30 mg/dL	2.29 (2.04–2.56)
Partially or fully dependent status	1.92 (1.74–2.11)
History of COPD	1.81 (1.66–1.98)
Age in years	
≥70	1.91 (1.71–2.13)
60–69	1.51 (1.36–1.69)
<60	1.00 (reference)

From: Arozullah AM, Daley J, Henderson WG, et al. Multifactorial risk index for predicting postoperative respiratory failure in men after major noncardiac surgery. Ann Surg 2000; 232(2):242–253.

Table 103-3 Postoperative Pneumonia Risk Index

Risk Factor	Point Value
Type of surgery	
Abdominal aortic aneurysm repair	15
Thoracic	14
Upper abdominal	10
Neck	8
Neurosurgery	8
Vascular	3
Age in years	
≥80	17
70–79	13
60–69	9
50–59	4
Functional status	
Totally dependent	10
Partially dependent	6
Weight loss >10% in past 6 months	7
History of COPD	5
General anesthesia	4
Impaired sensorium	4
History of stroke	4
Blood urea nitrogen level	
<8 mg/dL	4
22–30 mg/dL	2
≥30 mg/dL	3
Transfusion >4 units	3
Emergency surgery	3
Steroid use for chronic condition	3
Current smoker within one year	3
Alcohol intake >2 drinks/day in past 2 weeks	2

From: Arozullah AM, Khuri SF, Henderson WG, et al. Development and validation of a multifactorial risk index for predicting postoperative pneumonia after major noncardiac surgery. Ann Intern Med 2001; 135:847–857.

which a diagnosis is uncertain, such as distinguishing between cardiac or pulmonary etiologies for dyspnea, or in which a patient's baseline disease severity is unclear, as in asthma or COPD.

- Consultation with a pulmonologist may be helpful for patients with severe preexisting pulmonary disease or previous lung transplant, and those undergoing thoracic surgery, lung resection, lung volume reduction surgery, or lung transplantation.
- Some recent publications have developed prediction models for estimating the risk of perioperative pulmonary complications (Tables 103-2 and 103-3). When considering these models, it is important to remember that investigators developed and validated these risk indices specifically to predict the risk for postoperative respiratory failure and pneumonia. It is unknown if they equally predict the risk of other postoperative pulmonary complications, such as atelectasis or COPD exacerbation.

RECOMMENDATIONS/MANAGEMENT

Figure 103-1 presents an algorithm outlining a general approach for assessing the risk of perioperative pulmonary complications and strategies to minimize this risk. As with any perioperative complication, prevention of pulmonary complications is much easier and more effective than dealing with complications once they occur.

- Standard preventive strategies are always appropriate, regardless of the risk assessment. The assumption is that all patients will benefit from these interventions, and therefore they should be part of any perioperative routine. These include smoking cessation at least 8 weeks prior to planned surgery and training in incentive spirometry or deep breathing exercises to lower the risk of postoperative atelectasis. Early ambulation after

surgery and postoperative pain management also minimize the risk of pulmonary complications in all patients.

For patients at greater risk of perioperative pulmonary complications, based on patient-related or procedure-related risk factors, more aggressive preventive strategies are appropriate in addition to the standard strategies. These additional measures include:

- Perioperative steroids for patients with evidence of airways inflammation or exacerbated chronic airways disease who are not at their personal best baseline. Often the wisest course is to delay elective surgery for these patients until their inflammatory or chronic disease is in better control. A brief course of perioperative systemic corticosteroids is safe and does not increase the risk of wound infection or respiratory infection.
- Consider spinal or local/regional anesthesia for patients at high risk for pulmonary complications. The hospital medicine consultant may provide valuable input regarding the patient's specific risks of pulmonary complications and risk factors, but should allow the anesthesiologist to make decisions regarding the type and method of anesthesia. Avoid long-acting neuromuscular blocking agents when possible for high risk patients.
- For patients who are hypoxic or expected to be hypoxic following their surgery, postoperative continuous positive airway pressure (CPAP) reduces risk of pulmonary complications.

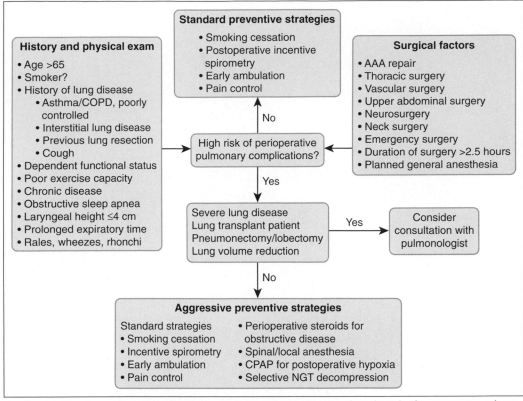

Figure 103-1 • An algorithm for preoperative pulmonary assessment and strategies to reduce the risk of postoperative pulmonary complications.

Establish contingency plans to have the appropriate apparatus ready in case it is required.[10] This may facilitate earlier extubation or prevention of reintubation for hypoxemic respiratory failure.

• Where possible, avoid the use of a routine nasogastric tube after abdominal surgery. Instead, selectively use nasogastric tube decompression based on nausea, abdominal distension, or evidence of postoperative ileus.

Key Points

• Pulmonary complications are more common than cardiac complications and result in significant morbidity and prolonged hospitalization.

• When estimating risk, consider both patient-related and procedure-related risk factors. Risk prediction models exist to stratify the risk of postoperative pneumonia and respiratory failure.

• Preoperative history and physical examination are usually sufficient for risk stratification.

• Key risk-reduction strategies include smoking cessation (probably best if weeks or months before surgery), perioperative steroids for poorly controlled obstructive lung disease, consideration of spinal or local anesthesia, postoperative CPAP for hypoxic patients, and selective use of a nasogastric tube following abdominal surgery.

SUGGESTED READING

Qaseem A, et al. Risk assessment for and strategies to reduce perioperative pulmonary complications for patients undergoing noncardiothoracic surgery: a guideline from the American College of Physicians. Ann Intern Med 2006; 144(8):575–580.

Rehder K, Sessler AD, Marsh HM. General anesthesia and the lung. Am Rev Resp Kis 1975; 112:541–563.

Lawrence VA, Cornell SE, Smetana GW. American College of Physicians. Strategies to reduce postoperative pulmonary complications after noncardiothoracic surgery: systemic review for the American College of Physicians. Ann Intern Med 2006; 144(8):596–608.

Smetana GW, Lawrence VA, Cornell JE. American College of Physicians. Preoperative pulmonary risk stratification for noncardiothoracic surgery: systemic review for the American College of Physicians. Ann Intern Med 2006; 144(8):581–595.

CHAPTER ONE HUNDRED AND FOUR

Perioperative Management of Diabetic Patients

Maged Doss, MD, and Guillermo E. Umpierrez, MD, FACP, FACE

BACKGROUND

Patients with diabetes are more likely to undergo surgery than are people without diabetes. An estimated 25–50% of diabetic subjects will undergo surgery during their lifetime.[1] Maintaining glycemic control in subjects with diabetes presents a challenging problem during the perioperative period. Surgery in patients with diabetes is associated with longer hospital stay, higher health care resource utilization, and greater perioperative mortality than nondiabetic subjects.[2,3] The higher morbidity and mortality relate in part to the heightened incidence of coronary heart disease, hypertension, renal insufficiency, and increased rates of life-threatening postoperative complications.[4,5] Increasing evidence from observational and interventional studies indicates that hyperglycemia by itself is associated with adverse clinical outcomes in surgical and critically ill patients.[6-9] In this chapter, we review the pathophysiology of hyperglycemia during trauma and surgical stress; and we provide practical recommendations for the preoperative, intraoperative, and postoperative care of diabetic patients.

PATHOPHYSIOLOGY

Metabolic Consequences of Surgical Stress and Anesthesia

The stress of surgery and anesthesia results in increased secretion of counter-regulatory hormones (catecholamines, cortisol, glucagons, and growth hormone) and excessive release of inflammatory cytokines, such as tumor necrosis factor-α, and interleukin-6 and 1β.[10] The counter-regulatory response results in a number of alterations in carbohydrate metabolism, including insulin resistance, increased hepatic glucose production, impaired peripheral glucose utilization, and relative insulin deficiency.[2,11,12] Increased counter-regulatory hormones during stress also lead to enhanced lipolysis and increased free fatty acids (FFAs).[10,12-14] Increased FFA levels produce insulin resistance in a dose-dependent fashion in diabetic and nondiabetic individuals[15] and are considered an important factor in the development of stress-induced hyperglycemia. Increased FFA levels inhibit insulin-stimulated glucose uptake, glycogen synthesis, and intracellular signaling in skeletal muscle.

The type of anesthesia may influence the hyperglycemic response during surgery. General anesthesia is associated with higher rates of hyperglycemia and higher catecholamine, cortisol, and glucagon concentrations than local and epidural analgesia.[2,16] Volatile anesthetic agents inhibit insulin secretion[17] and increase hepatic glucose production.[2,16] In contrast, epidural analgesia has minimal effect on carbohydrate metabolism, and levels of counter-regulatory hormones are not significantly elevated. The reduced hyperglycemia associated with epidural analgesia is strictly limited to the operative period; afterward, there is no difference in glycemic control.

Blood Glucose and Perioperative Outcome

Increasing evidence suggests that in hospitalized patients with and without diabetes, the presence of hyperglycemia is associated with poor clinical outcomes,[1,3,13] and aggressive glycemic control reduces morbidity and mortality.[6,8,18] One report showed that a third of patients admitted to general medicine and surgery wards in an urban general hospital had hyperglycemia, defined as an elevated fasting glucose level >126 mg/dL or two or more random blood glucose levels >200 mg/dL; a third of those patients did not have a prior diagnosis of diabetes.[7] Stress or new hyperglycemia was associated with a higher in-hospital mortality rate (16%) compared to those patients with a prior history of diabetes (3%) and subjects with normoglycemia (1.7%).

A strong relationship exists between perioperative glucose control and postoperative infection rate among diabetic patients undergoing elective surgery. A single blood glucose level >220 mg/dL (12.2 mmol/L) on the first postoperative day was a sensitive (87.5%) predictor of postoperative infection in one study of 100 surgical patients with diabetes.[9] Patients with blood glucose values >220 mg/dL had infection rates that were 2.7 times higher than the rate for patients with blood glucose values <220 mg/dL (31.3% vs. 11.5%, respectively). When minor infections were excluded, the relative risk for serious postoperative infection, including sepsis, pneumonia, and wound infections, was 5.7 higher than those with glucose levels less than 220 mg/dL.

Diabetes is recognized as an independent risk factor in hospitalized patients undergoing coronary artery bypass grafting (CABG).[19,20] Perioperative hyperglycemia is associated with a higher risk of deep sternal wound infections and increased mortality,[19,20] and aggressive glucose control improves outcome in subjects undergoing CABG.[1] In a prospective study of 1,499 consecutive patients undergoing CABG, a conservative perioperative insulin infusion protocol aimed at maintaining blood glucose levels between 150–200 mg/dL was associated with a 59% reduction in deep sternal wound infections versus historical controls.[19] Continuous intravenous insulin therapy compared with subcutaneous insulin resulted in lower mortality, 2.5% versus 5.3%, respectively.[20] In this study, the higher the blood glucose level, the greater was the mortality rate (i.e., blood glucose >250 mg/dL resulted in 14.5% mortality, compared with blood glucose <150 mg/dL, which reduced mortality to 0.9%).

In 2001, Van den Berghe[6] published a landmark report of a prospective study of 1,548 intensive care unit (ICU) patients randomized to intensive insulin therapy to maintain target blood glucose between 80 and 110 mg/dL (actual mean daily blood glucose = 103 mg/dL) or conventional therapy to maintain target blood glucose between 180 and 200 mg/dL (actual mean daily blood glucose = 153 mg/dL). Two thirds of these patients had undergone cardiac surgery, and the rest had noncardiac major surgical procedures. In this study, intensive insulin therapy led to a 42% mortality reduction (8.0% vs. 4.6% in conventional group) and reduced overall in-hospital mortality by 34% among patients with more than 5 days of ICU length of stay. It also reduced requirement for antibiotics, red cell transfusions, kidney dialysis, and prolonged ventilatory support.

The reasons for poor outcome when blood glucose levels are high remain unclear. Much of the attention has focused on increased rate of infections and poor wound healing.[22] Hyperglycemia is associated with impaired leukocyte function, including decreased phagocytosis and impaired bacterial killing and chemotaxis.[23] Several prospective and well-designed studies document that patients with postoperative glucose greater than 200 mg/dL have a 17–86% increased risk of infection,[21] and that reduction of blood glucose with insulin therapy improves leukocyte function and lowers the risk of local and systemic infections.[23]

Hyperglycemia also impairs collagen synthesis and wound healing among patients with poorly controlled diabetes.[22] In human and animal models of diabetes, hyperglycemia causes multiple defects in wound healing, including reduced collagen synthesis, reduced wound tensile strength, and reduced neovascularization capillary volume at the site of injury. Advanced glycosylation end products accumulate in diabetes and may adversely affect extracellular matrix production, cell function, and cytokine production and prevent wound healing.[24]

PREOPERATIVE ASSESSMENT OF THE DIABETIC PATIENT: RISK EVALUATION

Comprehensive operative risk assessment is the most important step in the management of the diabetic patient before surgery.[16] The evaluation is oriented to identify underlying cardiac, renal, and pulmonary disease, as well as assessment of antecedent glycemic control, electrolyte disturbances, and presence of macrovascular and microvascular complications. See Chapter 98 for a more detailed review of preoperative assessment.

The risk of coronary artery disease (CAD) is two to four times higher among patients with diabetes compared to the corresponding general population.[25] Patients with proven coronary artery disease and diabetes have poorer long-term outcome after vascular surgery, with an increased probability of cardiac death

or myocardial infarction compared to patients with similar CAD but no diabetes. Thus, a low threshold for cardiac testing is recommended among patients with diabetes, especially those with other risk factors such as age >50 years, obesity, physical inactivity, hypertension, albuminuria, dyslipidemia, and chronically elevated glucose (>200 mg/dL) and A_{1C} levels >7%.[26]

Unfortunately, the preoperative detection of CAD in diabetic patients may not be easy, as many suffer from diabetic autonomic neuropathy characterized by degeneration of afferent and efferent fibers of the sympathetic and parasympathetic nerves of the heart and peripheral vasculature. Cardiac autonomic neuropathy is reported in up to 20–40% of diabetic patients with hypertension and appears to be independent of age, duration of diabetes, or the presence of microvascular complications. Cardiac autonomic neuropathy explains the occurrence of silent myocardial ischemia[16] and may predispose to cardiovascular complications and perioperative hypotension.[29] During the examination, providers should note the presence of resting tachycardia, postural hypotension, and loss of normal respiratory heart rate variability.[28] Additionally, the standard baseline electrocardiogram has a poor value of 25% for predicting cardiac events.

According to the American College of Cardiology (ACC) and American Heart Association (AHA) guidelines on preoperative cardiac risk assessment,[27,28] asymptomatic diabetic patients with multiple risk factors should be investigated by stress testing if they have a low functional capacity, or if they are to undergo major or vascular surgery. The positive predictive value of stress tests is modest (20–30%); however, their negative predictive value is excellent (95–100%).[25] Stress tests with dipyridamole-thallium scintigraphy or dobutamine echocardiography are dynamic investigations with better diagnostic accuracy. Coronary angiography should be reserved for unstable coronary syndromes, high-risk patients undergoing major surgery, or when considering coronary revascularization.[26–28]

Renal failure is the most common major complication in the postoperative period and is associated with increased morbidity, mortality, and in-hospital resource utilization.[28,30] The prevalence of renal dysfunction, defined as a postoperative serum creatinine level of ≥2.0 mg/dL and an increase in serum creatinine level of ≥0.7 mg/dL from preoperative values, is observed in about 7% of patients undergoing major general surgery.[30,31] Risk factors for postoperative renal dysfunction include advanced age, type 1 diabetes mellitus, preoperative hyperglycemia, a history of moderate-to-severe congestive heart failure, a previous coronary artery bypass graft, or preexisting renal disease.[30] A preoperative urinanalysis had been recommended in the past to rule out urinary tract infection[31] and to determine the amount of proteinuria. The presence of proteinuria has been associated with a greater risk of developing acute renal failure in the postoperative period; however, perioperative management is almost never changed by the test results; and, in the absence of urinary symptoms, it is no longer recommended as a preoperative screening test.

GLYCEMIC GOAL DURING THE PERIOPERATIVE PERIOD

In recent years, increasing efforts worldwide aim to improve appropriate glycemic control in critically ill patients and in the perioperative period.[6,8,12,13,32] A recent position statement by the American Association of Clinical Endocrinologists and American

Diabetes Association recommended glycemic targets between 80–110 mg/dL for critical patients in the ICU. For patients with noncritical illness, a pre-prandial blood glucose less than 110 mg/dl (6.1 mmol/L) and a random blood glucose level less than less than 180 mg/dL were recommended.[32] These glucose control parameters should be applied to surgical patients in the surgical ICU, especially after CABG procedures. In surgical patients discharged from the ICU, it is recommended that glucose levels be controlled by intensive subcutaneous insulin therapy.[32] However, several groups have raised objections because these recommendations were based primarily on the findings of one single center study in a surgical ICU and the fact that there were no differences on mortality in patients with an ICU length of stay <5 days or in patients after vascular surgery.[33] Intensive management of diabetes with continuous insulin infusion requires taxing nursing attention, frequent blood glucose monitoring, and insulin-dosing adjustments that may be difficult to implement in the non-ICU settings. Intensive glucose control is associated with increased risk of hypoglycemia, which may increase hospital morbidity.[13]

APPROACHES TO MANAGEMENT: RECOMMENDATIONS

General Principles

Treatment recommendations are generally categorized based on the type of diabetes, nature and extent of the surgical procedure, antecedent pharmacologic therapy, and state of metabolic control prior to surgery. A key factor for success of any regimen requires frequent blood glucose monitoring to allow early detection of any alterations in metabolic control. In general, all patients with type 1 diabetes undergoing minor or major surgical procedures require insulin during the perioperative period. In such patients, the stress of surgery may result in the development of diabetic ketoacidosis or hyperosmolar hyperglycemic nonketotic syndrome, with negative prognostic consequences.[34] Patients with type 2 diabetes undergoing major surgery, especially those already receiving insulin therapy, are also candidates for intensive perioperative diabetes management.[8,13,32]

Insulin, given either intravenously as a continuous infusion or subcutaneously, is currently the only available agent for effectively controlling glycemia in the hospital. The best method of providing insulin during surgery is debatable. There are myriad protocols for the management of this problem, but there is none with clear superiority. Any good regimen should attempt to maintain good glycemic control while avoiding both hyperglycemia and hypoglycemia, should be easy to understand, and should be applicable to different settings (operating room, recovery room, general medicine and surgical wards). Concern about hypoglycemia due to altered nutrition during the perioperative period is the leading limiting factor to maximizing glycemic control in patients with diabetes.[13,35] Fear of hypoglycemia frequently leads to the inappropriate practice of holding a patient's previous outpatient diabetic regimen and initiating "sliding scale" insulin coverage, a practice associated with limited therapeutic success.[36] The use of sliding scale should never be the sole regimen in patients with type 1 diabetes or in patients with type 2 diabetes undergoing major surgical procedures (Table 104-1).

Patients Treated With Diet Alone

Patients whose diabetes is well controlled by a regimen of diet and physical activity may require no special preoperative intervention for diabetes. Measure fasting blood glucose on the morning of surgery, and use small doses of supplemental short-acting insulin to control blood glucose. In contrast, hospitalized patients with poor metabolic control on diet alone (blood glucose >180 mg/dl) require insulin therapy either by a combination of intermediate- and short-acting insulin or with the intravenous infusion of insulin (Box 104-1).

Table 104-1 Supplemental Sliding Scale Insulin

- Type of insulin: rapid-acting (lispro, aspart, glulisine) or regular insulin to be given before each meal and at bedtime.
- Each column represents number of units of insulin to be added to scheduled insulin dose.
  - *"Sensitive" column:* elderly, cachectic, renal and liver failure, and patients with poor oral intake or NPO.
  - *"Usual" column:* for most patients who are expected to eat all or most of their meals.
  - *"Insulin Resistant" column:* for patients not controlled with "usual" column dose, or receiving glucocorticoids, obesity (BMI >30 kg/m^2), or patient with diabetes receiving >80 units/day of insulin.

Blood Glucose (mg/dL)	☐ Insulin Sensitive	☐ Usual	☐ Insulin Resistant
<150	0	0	0
151–180	1	2	3
181–220	2	3	4
221–260	3	4	5
261–300	4	5	6
301–340	5	6	7
341–380	6	7	8
381–420	7	8	9
>421	8	9	10

Check appropriate column below and cross out other columns

Patients Treated with Oral Antidiabetic Agents

Of the three primary categories of oral agents—secretagogues, biguanides, and thiazolidinediones—none has been systematically studied during the perioperative period. In general, oral agents should be discontinued 1 day before surgery. Sulfonylureas increase the risk of hypoglycemia; in addition, a long-standing controversy exists regarding the vascular effects of sulfonylureas in patients with cardiac and cerebral ischemia.[37] Although

metformin has a short half-life of approximately 6 hours, it is prudent to temporarily withhold therapy prior to surgery, especially in patients undergoing procedures that increase the risks for renal hypoperfusion, tissue hypoxia, and lactate accumulation.[38] Thiazolidinediones increase intravascular volume and may precipitate or worsen congestive heart failure and peripheral edema.[39]

In patients with good metabolic control after discontinuation of oral agents, use small subcutaneous doses (4–10 units) of

---

Box 104-1 Perioperative Management of Patients with Diabetes

Inpatient Glycemic Targets:

- ICU: 70–120 mg/dL (3.9–6.6 mmol/L)
- Noncritical care:
  Pre-prandial: 90–130 mg/dL (5–7.2 mmol/L)
  Maximum: 180 mg/dL (10 mmol/L)

Surgery in DM2 Patients Not Treated with Insulin—*Minor surgery:*

- Hold oral agents the day of surgery
- `Patients in "good" control—FBG <180 mg/dL (10 mmol/L)—cover with short-acting insulin (see Table 104-1)
- Patients in "poor" control—FBG >180 mg/dL—start continuous IV Insulin(CII)
- Goal: Avoid excessive hyperglycemia (BG >180 mg/dL) and hypoglycemia (BG <70 mg/dL)

Surgery in DM1 and DM2 Patients Treated with Insulin—*Minor surgery:*

- Discontinue oral agents the day before surgery
- Patients in "good" control—FBG <180 mg/dL (10 mmol/L)
  - Start D5% NS + KCl at 100—150 mL/hr
  - Patient treated with basal (glargine) insulin should receive their usual basal insulin dose. Patients treated with intermediate-acting (NPH) insulin give ½ of insulin dose in the morning of the surgery
  - Restart preadmission insulin therapy once food intake is tolerated
- Patients in "poor" control—FBG >180 mg/dL—start CII

Major Surgery in DM1 and DM2 Patients

- Discontinue oral agents the day of surgery
- Start CII prior to surgery and continue during perioperative period

Transition from Intravenous (CII) to Subcutaneous Insulin

- Start subcutaneous insulin 2 hours prior to discontinuation of CII.
- Calculate the total daily insulin requirement based on insulin rate during the last 4 hours of IV insulin infusion
  - Give half of total daily dose as insulin glargine and half as rapid-acting insulin (lispro, aspart, glulisine).
  - Give insulin glargine once daily, at the same time of the day. NPH insulin twice daily can be used as an alternative to glargine insulin.
  - Give rapid-acting insulin in three equally divided doses before each meal. If a subject is not able to eat, hold prandial insulin. Regular insulin can be used as an alternative to rapid-acting insulin.
- **Insulin adjustment:**
  - If the FBG is >140 mg/dL in the absence of hypoglycemia the previous day, increase daily insulin glargine (or NPH) dose by 20%.
  - If a patient develops hypoglycemia (BG <70 mg/dL), reduce insulin glargine (or NPH) dose by 20%.
- **Blood glucose monitoring:**
  - Measure BG at bedside before each meal and at bedtime (or every 6 hours if NPO). Record all BG readings in blood glucose flow-sheet.

CII—continuous insulin infusion; DM1—type 1 diabetes; DM2—type 2 diabetes; BG—blood glucose; NPO—nothing per oral route, fasting; ICU—intensive care unit. Conversion factors to SI units: serum glucose (mg/dL) × 0.055 mmol/liter.

short acting insulin to control blood glucose. Restart most antidiabetic medications once patients start eating, with the exception of metformin, which should be withheld for 48 hours following surgery or iodinated radiocontrast procedures until documentation of normal renal function. Treat patients with poor metabolic control or those scheduled to undergo major surgery with an intravenous infusion of insulin and dextrose during the perioperative period.

Type 1 or Type 2 Diabetes Treated with Insulin

Minor Surgery

Use conventional subcutaneous insulin therapy to treat most patients who were receiving insulin prior to admission. If the surgery is to be performed in the morning in a patient treated with intermediate-acting (NPH) insulin, administer half of the total morning dose of NPH insulin.[1,13] While a patient remains NPO, infuse a 5% dextrose-potassium solution at a rate of 100 mL/hr. Discontinue the dextrose infusion once oral intake is reinitiated. If necessary, use small doses of supplemental short-acting insulin for better glucose control. For patients treated with basal/bolus insulin combination—glargine and rapid-acting insulin analogs (lispro, aspart, glulisine)—continue the dose of glargine, but hold bolus doses until meals are tolerated. Similarly, for patients treated with continuous insulin infusion therapy (insulin pumps), continue their usual basal infusion rate.

Major Surgery

During the period before admission, carefully monitor insulin-treated patients undergoing major elective surgery. Consider admitting the patient the evening before surgery or at least several hours prior to surgery, especially if glycemic control is suboptimal (hemoglobin A_{1c} >8%). This will allow sufficient time to perform a complete clinical assessment and start an insulin infusion before surgery. Intravenous infusion of insulin is the standard therapy for the perioperative management of diabetes in type 1 diabetic patients and patients with type 2 diabetes undergoing major procedures.[13,40]

Two main methods of insulin delivery have been used: either combining insulin with glucose and potassium in the same bag (GIK regimen), or giving insulin separately with an infusion pump. Initiate a GIK regimen with a solution of 500 mL of 10% dextrose, 10 mmol of potassium, and 15 units of insulin at a rate of 100 mL/hr. Make adjustments in the insulin dose in 5-unit increments according to blood glucose measurements performed at least every 2 hours.[1] Add potassium to prevent hypokalemia, and monitor levels at 6-hour intervals. The combined GIK infusion is efficient, safe, and effective but does not permit selective adjustment of insulin delivery without changing the bag. In the United States, separate continuous glucose and insulin infusions are used more frequently than the glucose-potassium-insulin solution.[6,18] In most insulin infusion protocols, orders to "titrate drip" are given to achieve a target blood glucose range using an established algorithm or by the application of mathematical rules by nursing staff.[13] The duration of insulin (and dextrose) infusions depends on the clinical status of the patient. Continue the infusions postoperatively until oral intake is established, and then resume usual diabetes treatment.

Provide adequate glucose to prevent catabolism, starvation ketosis, and insulin-induced hypoglycemia. The physiologic amount of glucose required to prevent catabolism in an average nondiabetic adult is ~120 g/day (or 5 g/hr). With preoperative fasting, surgical stress, and ongoing insulin therapy, the caloric requirement in most diabetic patients averages 5–10 g/hr glucose. This can be given as 5% or 10% dextrose. An infusion rate of 100 ml/hr with 5% dextrose delivers 5 g/hr glucose. If fluid restriction is necessary, use the more concentrated 10% dextrose. Fluids containing lactate (i.e., Ringer's lactate, Hartmann's solution) cause exacerbation of hyperglycemia.[1]

DISCHARGE RECOMMENDATIONS

Provide diabetes education to all patients with newly diagnosed diabetes, and discuss the outpatient treatment regimen prior to discharge.[38] The patient, or caregiver, should receive appropriate instruction on proper dietary therapy as well as home glucose monitoring techniques. Make arrangements for follow-up with a health care professional who will oversee the patient's diabetes management. Educate the patient on the signs and symptoms of hypoglycemia and hyperglycemia. In addition, review instructions for "sick day" management, including the importance of insulin administration during an illness, blood glucose goals, and the use of supplemental short or rapid-acting insulin. These recommendations to achieve tight control of blood glucose will help minimize the likelihood of infection and hopefully reduce other perioperative complications as well.

> **Key Points**
>
> - Surgery in patients with diabetes is associated with longer hospital stay, higher health care resource utilization, and greater perioperative mortality than those without diabetes.
>
> - The stress of surgery and anesthesia results in increased secretion of counter-regulatory hormones and excessive release of inflammatory cytokines. These changes lead to alterations in carbohydrate metabolism, including insulin resistance, increased hepatic glucose production, impaired peripheral glucose utilization, and relative insulin deficiency
>
> - Hyperglycemia during the perioperative period in patients with and without diabetes is associated with worse clinical outcomes. Aggressive glycemic control reduces morbidity and mortality.
>
> - Practical recommendations for the preoperative, intraoperative, and postoperative care of diabetic patients can be applied to improve care.

SUGGESTED READING

Jacober SJ, Sowers JR An update on perioperative management of diabetes. Arch Intern Med 1999; 159(20):2405–2411.

van den Berghe G, Wouters P, Weekers F, et al. Intensive insulin therapy in the critically ill patients. N Engl J Med 2001; 345(19):1359–1367.

Umpierrez GE, Isaacs SD, Bazargan N, et al. Hyperglycemia: an independent marker of in-hospital mortality in patients with undiagnosed diabetes. J Clin Endocrinol Metab 2002; 87(3):978–982.

Finney SJ, Zekveld C, Elia A, et al. Glucose control and mortality in critically ill patients. JAMA 2003; 290(15): 2041–7.

Mizock BA: Blood glucose management during critical illness. Rev Endocr Metab Disord 2003; 4(2):187–194.

Clement S, Braithwaite SS, Magee MF, et al. Management of diabetes and hyperglycemia in hospitals. Diabetes Care 2004; 27(2):553–597.

Montori VM, Bistrian BR, McMahon MM. Hyperglycemia in acutely ill patients. JAMA 2002; 288(17):2167–2169.

Furnary AP, Zerr KJ, Grunkemeier GL, et al. Continuous intravenous insulin infusion reduces the incidence of deep sternal wound infection in diabetic patients after cardiac surgical procedures. Ann Thorac Surg 1999; 67(2):352–60; discussion 360–362.

Eagle KA, Berger PB, Calkins H, et al. ACC/AHA Guideline update for perioperative cardiovascular evaluation for noncardiac surgery: executive summary. A report of the American College of Cardiology/American Heart Association Task Force on Practice Guidelines (Committee to Update the 1996 Guidelines on Perioperative Cardiovascular Evaluation for Noncardiac Surgery). Anesth Analg 2002; 94(5):1052–1064.

Karnath BM. Preoperative cardiac risk assessment. Am Fam Physician 2002; 66(10):1889–1896.

CHAPTER ONE HUNDRED AND FIVE

Nutrition in the Perioperative Period

Lisa Kirkland MD, FACP, CNSP, MSHA

OVERVIEW

The American Society of Parenteral and Enteral Nutrition defines malnutrition as "a state induced by nutrient deficiency that may be improved solely by administration of nutrients."[1] Diagnosing malnutrition involves clinical intuition drawn from subjective input, such as the patient's history, physical findings, functional assessment, and few, if any, laboratory tests. No single objective measurement or diagnostic test for the presence of malnutrition exists. Interpretation of available literature is challenging, due to inconsistent definitions of malnutrition, resulting in wide differences in reported incidence and high variability in methods and amount of nutrition provided.

The incidence of malnutrition on admission to the hospital ranges from 32–54%.[2–4] In 55–59% of inpatients, malnutrition either develops or worsens during hospitalization.[2,4] Thirty-four percent of surgical patients lose >5% of preoperative body weight.[5] Malnutrition results in problems with wound healing and skin integrity. Impairment of opsonization, complement activity, and cell-mediated immunity from malnutrition increase susceptibility to infection. Malnourished surgical patients have more complications such as sepsis and longer length of stay (LOS),[6,7] and medical patients have longer length of stay and hospital costs up to 50% higher than if they are well nourished.[4] For example, mortality is higher, and hospital readmission occurs more often in malnourished pneumonia patients.[3,4] If nutritional status declines during admission, both surgical and medical patients have longer lengths of stay, higher hospital charges, and more complications, regardless of admission nutritional status. Unfortunately, patients with "normal" nutritional status on admission to the hospital do not seem to undergo additional nutritional screening or assessment, despite up to 38% of these normally nourished patients experiencing a decline in nutritional status during a hospital stay. Thus, nutritional status in all patients hospitalized for >5 days should be reassessed and compared to admission status.

PATHOPHYSIOLOGY

In metabolically unstressed starvation, hormonal responses trigger glycogenolysis, which exhausts liver glycogen stores within 24 hours and stimulates lipolysis. Metabolic rate slows. Fatty acid-derived ketones provide most of the oxidative substrate required for fuel, and catabolism from muscle and other protein stores falls to 10–12 g nitrogen/day to provide the obligatory glucose requirements. In this manner, protein is spared until very late in starvation. Serum protein levels such as albumin remain relatively normal until this point. Catabolism of muscle stores results in diminished skeletal muscle strength, and visceral protein loss causes reduced immune function and wound healing, although exogenous administration of dextrose may attenuate protein breakdown.

Immediately after severe injury or onset of severe illness, before adequate resuscitation, oxygen delivery to tissues may be insufficient to maintain aerobic metabolism, resulting in less efficient anaerobic metabolism and a compensatory reduction in metabolic rate. If this "ebb" or hypometabolic phase persists, byproducts of anaerobic metabolism and oxygen debt accumulate, causing cell injury, multiple organ dysfunction, and eventually death. If the patient is adequately resuscitated, the inflammatory stimulus of severe illness or injury causes the metabolic rate to increase to supranormal, or hypermetabolic, levels. This metabolic stress produces demands for fat, carbohydrate, and protein sources of fuel; the protein sparing seen in unstressed starvation does not occur. Protein and nitrogen losses may be quite high almost immediately, with nitrogen losses of 20–50 g/day. Exogenous nutrients are less effective at attenuating protein catabolism. Hypermetabolism continues until the inflammatory stimulus subsides.[1]

Hypermetabolism in critically injured, hemodynamically stable blunt trauma patients starts by day 3 after the event, peaks around day 10, and continues.[10] Energy imbalance occurs because actual energy expenditure is up to 30% higher than provided. A prolonged hypermetabolic state occurs in critically injured patients, and large skeletal muscle protein loss still occurs, despite careful attention to meeting energy requirements and reducing lipolysis with adequate energy provision from enriched feeding.[9] Diaphragmatic muscle is also depleted in malnutrition,[11] with decreased muscle contractility and altered muscle fatigability, potentially impacting respiratory function.

Box 105-1 Questions to Evaluate Patient's Risk of Malnutrition*

Tell me what you ate for each meal yesterday.

Did you have any snacks?

What did you have to drink?

How has your appetite been for the last 2 weeks?

Have you had any nausea, vomiting, diarrhea, constipation, or abdominal pain over the last 2 weeks? (Malabsorption)

Does someone do your shopping for you, or prepare your meals?

Do you smoke or drink alcohol; if so, how much?

Do you take any over-the-counter dietary supplements?

Are there any foods that don't agree with you? How so? (Specific food allergy/intolerance, malabsorption)

Does food taste and smell good to you?

How is your vision; can you see well enough to eat?

Do you have someone assisting you with eating?

Do you have trouble with choking or swallowing the wrong way? (Dysphagia)

How do your dentures feel? Do you have any mouth, gum, lip, tongue, or tooth pain? (Vitamin B)

Have your gums been bleeding? (Vitamin C, K)

Do you have enough energy to do what you want?

Do you do your own vacuuming, cleaning?

Does your hair feel dry, or does it break or fall out when you brush or comb it? (Biotin, zinc, vitamins E and A)

Does your skin feel dry or chapped? Has it changed color anywhere? (Vitamin A, niacin)

Do your fingernails crack or break easily, or do they look different? (Fungal infection)

How do your clothes fit? Is that a change?

Do you have any cuts or bruises or wounds that are not healing as you think they should? (Vitamin C, zinc)

Do you have acne or pimples? (Vitamin A)

Do you bruise easily? (Vitamin C, K)

Are your feet numb or tingling? (Vitamin B$_{12}$)

Do you ache or are you sore all over? (Vitamin D)

*Parenthetical items specify possible associated deficiency or illness.

CLINICAL ASSESSMENT

History

A careful history can elicit the majority of information needed to diagnose a patient at risk for malnutrition (Box 105-1). Asking the patient to recall a typical single day's oral intake prior to hospitalization may provide insight; however, recognize that many patients cannot accurately recall their intake for more than a few days. A general impression of poor intake for up to 2 weeks should alert the clinician to the possibility of malnutrition. Realize that calorie counts often overestimate intake.[12] Note chronic medical conditions such as gastrointestinal disorders or diabetes, amenorrhea, recent hospitalizations or surgeries, or food intolerances. Taste, smell, vision, fine motor function, chewing, and swallowing often decline in elderly or chronically ill individuals. Elderly patients may also have difficulty accessing adequate food and water. Finally, the circumstances of the current hospitalization are important: recent trauma versus prolonged complicated postoperative course versus acute or chronic medical illness.

Physical Examination

A valid clue to malnutrition, documented weight loss of 5 kg over 3 months or 10% of body weight over 6 months, may not be available to the clinician. Important nutritional changes can occur in much less time in the acutely ill or injured patient. Anthropomorphic measurements of height, weight, or calculated body mass index (BMI) can also be misleading. Age-related height loss may artificially increase BMI, and height may be difficult to accurately measure in a kyphotic, unsteady, or bedridden patient.[12] Arm span may be helpful, but the accuracy of this measurement has not been assessed in elderly patients. Comparing current weight with that previously documented may be helpful, but illnesses that increase total body water will complicate matters. Skinfold thickness and arm circumference have similar limitations, and the accuracy of these measurements has been questioned. Physical findings of interest are listed in Box 105-2. Poor wound healing or dehiscence may be a drastic result of previously unrecognized malnutrition.

Laboratory

Serum albumin is the most commonly used laboratory value in the assessment of nutritional status; however, it is an insensitive indicator of nutritional status when compared to validated clinical assessment tools.[13] Albumin makes up about 40% of a group of proteins synthesized by the liver, often called visceral proteins to distinguish them from muscle proteins. This group also includes prealbumin and transferrin. These "negative acute-phase proteins" decrease in the setting of metabolic stress, especially illness caused by chronic inflammation. Inflammation produces cytokines, which stimulate the production of "positive" acute phase proteins, important in organism response and survival. As the liver produces more positive acute phase proteins, the synthesis of negative acute phase proteins decreases. In addition, cytokine-induced capillary leak causes intravascular proteins to move to the extravascular space, and the subsequent fluid resuscitation of the intravascular space dilutes protein concentration. Increased catecholamine and stress hormone levels cause catabolism of body proteins. The result is a decline in the serum levels of albumin, transferrin, and prealbumin, independent of nutritional status but reflective of the degree of metabolic stress.[1]

As a marker of metabolic stress, albumin has been shown to be predictive of postoperative complications, hospital length of stay, and mortality.[6] Prealbumin and transferrin have not been studied as outcome predictors, although they are also affected by inflam-

Box 105-2 Physical Findings in Malnutrition

1. Musculoskeletal

Absence of subcutaneous fat

Interosseous, temporal, extremity muscle wasting

Diminished muscle strength

2. Cutaneous

Glossitis, cheilosis, angular stomatitis

Dry, bruised, or thin skin

Hyperpigmentation

Folliculitis

Acneiform lesions

Edema, anasarca

Decubitus ulcers

Petechiae

3. Hair

Dry or brittle hair

Alopecia

4. Neurologic

Peripheral neuropathy

5. Mouth

Bleeding or tender gums

Loose teeth

Halitosis

6. Wounds

Poor granulation tissue

Dehiscence, even of previously healed wounds

7. Cardiovascular

Tachycardia

Pulmonary edema

8. Endocrine

Thyromegaly

9. Respiratory

Diminished negative inspiratory force or forced vital capacity

Ineffective cough

Ventilator dependence

mation or illness. Prealbumin has serum half-life of 24-48 hours and is often used to assess adequacy of nutritional replacement after the inflammatory state is resolved. Transferrin's longer half-life of about 9 days reduces its value in nutrition replacement adequacy, and it is adversely affected by serum iron status as well as inflammation.[9]

In summary, use intravascular protein levels as a reflection of the degree of inflammation and as predictors of mortality and postoperative complications. They may also serve as indicators of the patient's inability to maintain protein stores, need for nutritional support, and adequacy of that support once inflammation subsides.

Subjective Assessment Tools

A thorough review assessed 44 nutritional screening and assessment tools and concluded "no one tool satisfied a set of criteria regarding scientific merit."[15] Keeping this in mind, the clinician may wish to use a variety of assessments, including subjective tools, to evaluate a patient's nutritional status. Two tools seem particularly helpful. The Subjective Global Assessment (SGA) has been validated in surgical,[16] medical,[7] and geriatric[17] inpatients (Fig. 105-1 and Chapter 4). It has positive predictive ability for mortality and is more reliable than the body mass index in diagnosing malnutrition.[7] The SGA has been used as a reference method for other tools, although it is suboptimal in certain subgroups, particularly dialysis patients. The Mini Nutritional Assessment (MNA) has also been shown to be predictive of mortality in geriatric patients.[12] However, it may be more useful as a preventive indicator tool, identifying elderly at risk of malnutrition rather than those already malnourished.

Objective Tools

Bioimpedance analysis (BIA) detects changes in cellular membrane integrity and body fluid balance. Comparison with the SGA found little agreement in detecting malnutrition, but BIA was accurate at detecting changes in body composition and may be useful as a monitoring tool in reflecting changing nutritional status.[18,19] Dual-energy x-ray absorptiometry (DEXA) also measures body composition and may be best used in serial measurements to assess changing nutritional status by looking at lean body mass.[19] Further research is necessary to establish these tools as reliable in the clinical setting.

Functional Tools

Efforts to estimate nutritional status by skeletal muscle function have resulted in a number of clinical tests of muscle strength. Handgrip dynamometry is easy to perform, requires little training or patient instruction, and may be an excellent adjunct to clinical examination in determining current nutritional status and risk of inpatient complications. Diminished handgrip strength was predictive of longer length of stay and postoperative complications.[20] Adductor pollicis contraction to electrical ulnar nerve stimulation is a potentially useful clinical tool. Other functional tests, such as respiratory muscle strength, maximum heart rate, and maximum ergonometric work load, are less well studied, difficult to perform, and may require specialized equipment as well as significant patient and clinician time and effort.

Comparing actual caloric expenditure (calorimetry) with caloric intake can indicate the potential for malnutrition. Direct calorimetry is cumbersome and used only in research. Indirect calorimetry, obtained by analyzing oxygen consumption and carbon dioxide production, is possible in the hospital. It requires several measurements at steady metabolic state. Nursing care, patient movement, fever, and fluctuating metabolic state reduce its accuracy; and a skilled interpreter is required. Indirect calorimetry is best used as a monitoring tool rather than in initial assessment.[12]

(Select appropriate category with a checkmark, or enter numerical value where indicated by "#")

A. History
  1. Weight change
      Overall loss in past 6 months: amount = # _____ kg; % loss = # _____
      Change in past 2 weeks: _____ increase,
                               _____ no change,
                               _____ decrease.

  2. Dietary intake change (relative to normal)
       _____ No change
       _____ Change _____ duration = # _____ weeks.
                     _____ type: _____ suboptimal solid diet, _____ full liquid diet
                                   _____ hypocaloric liquids, _____ starvation.

  3. Gastrointestinal symptoms (*that persisted for >2 weeks*)
       _____ none, _____ nausea, _____ vomiting, _____ diarrhea, _____ anorexia.

  4. Functional capacity
       _____ No dysfunction (e.g., full capacity),
       _____ Dysfunction _____ duration = # _____ weeks.
                     _____ type: _____ working suboptimally,
                                   _____ ambulatory,
                                   _____ bedridden.

  5. Disease and its relation to nutritional requirements
      Primary diagnosis (specify) _____
      Metabolic demand (stress): _____ no stress, _____ low stress,
                             _____ moderate stress, _____ high stress.

B. Physical (for each trait specify: 0 = normal, 1+ = mild, 2+ = moderate, 3+ = severe).
   # _____ loss of subcutaneous fat (triceps, chest)
   # _____ muscle wasting (quadriceps, deltoids)
   # _____ ankle edema
   # _____ sacral edema
   # _____ ascites

C. SGA rating (select one)
   _____ A = Well nourished
   _____ B = Moderately (or suspected of being) malnourished
   _____ C = Severely malnourished

Figure 105-1   •   Subjective global assessment

MANAGEMENT

Provide nutrition support for at least 1 week or more prior to surgery to severely malnourished inpatients (as assessed by the SGA) and those with gastrointestinal cancer undergoing elective surgery.[21,22] Other preoperative patients who are anticipated to be nil per os (NPO) for longer than 7 days or to be taking <60% of estimated caloric needs by postoperative day 10, or critically ill patients who are anticipated to be taking less than full oral diet by 72 hours should also receive nutrition support.[23,24] Continue nutritional support postoperatively until inflammatory markers and nutrition levels improve. As discussed in the previous section, traditional measurements of nutritional status are insensitive for short-term assessment and may not improve during hospital admission in all but the most severely malnourished, despite improved clinical outcomes. Attempts to normalize albumin levels by exogenous administration do not improve nutritional status or nitrogen balance; albumin usually leaves the intravascular space within 24 hours if inflammation-induced capillary leak is present. Exogenously administered nitrogen does not reduce muscle protein catabolism either. The only way to reverse protein loss is to reduce inflammation and stop the catabolic state by treating the underlying cause, if possible. Clinical assessment

of wound healing and respiratory muscle strength, presence of infections or other complications and stabilization of vital signs are the best monitors of adequacy of nutritional support at this time.[1]

The enteral route is preferred for administration of nutritional support. With enteral nutrition, all of the following are reduced: inflammatory cytokines, oxidants, acute phase proteins, hyperglycemia, insulin resistance, nosocomial infections, mortality, and cost.[21,22] Unfortunately, enteral nutrition support is underutilized, often because of outdated or poorly documented practices such as measuring gastric residuals, prolonged NPO status prior to diagnostic or surgical procedures, cessation of tube feeding for nursing care activities, or other avoidable causes.[25] Patients intolerant of gastric feeding should receive enteral nutrition via small bowel feeding tubes, which can be placed at the bedside, under fluoroscopy, or in the operating room. Enteral nutrition is not contraindicated in the absence of bowel sounds[25] or passage of stool or gas, if bowel obstruction is excluded.

If abdominal distension, pain, intractable nausea or vomiting develops during enteral nutrition, prescribe parenteral nutrition until symptoms subside. Preoperative total parenteral nutrition (TPN) has been shown to reduce mortality and postoperative complications such as infections in severely malnourished or gastrointestinal cancer patients,[7,22] challenging the landmark Veteran's Administration (VA) study finding that preoperative TPN increased postoperative infections but did not affect mortality in all but the most severely malnourished patients.[23] Reviews of studies of TPN in surgical patients found no overall advantage in preoperative or postoperative TPN in significantly reducing complications or mortality in severely malnourished versus non-malnourished patients.[26] Another meta-analysis of trials comparing early (within 96 hours of admission or surgery) enteral versus parenteral nutrition found infections were more frequent in all patient groups receiving parenteral nutrition. Noninfectious complications were more frequent in the medical patients receiving parenteral nutrition. Mortality was not affected by route of feeding.[27] More prospective, randomized, controlled trials are needed to determine if parenteral nutrition support is better than no support at all at decreasing postoperative infections in severely depleted surgical patients.

Gastrointestinal surgery patients receiving only routine postoperative TPN have no better or even worse outcomes than similar patients receiving no nutrition.[28] Routine postoperative TPN before postoperative day 14 in unselected trauma or major surgery patients did not confer benefits in mortality or complications over dextrose infusions; however, dextrose infusion alone beyond 9 days was associated with higher morbidity and mortality.[29]

In summary, severely malnourished medical or surgical patients benefit from early nutritional support, preferably via the enteral route. One to three weeks of preoperative enteral or parenteral nutrition reduces postoperative complications, LOS, and mortality in severely malnourished elective surgery patients and those with gastrointestinal cancer. Routinely initiating postoperative parenteral nutrition provides no benefit and may increase postoperative complications; most patients do better receiving standard dextrose plus oral supplementation or enteral nutrition support. Withholding enteral feedings for arbitrary gastric resid-

ual volumes or other avoidable causes leads to inadequate caloric intake or inappropriate use of parenteral nutrition. Simultaneous initiation of enteral and parenteral nutrition in patients without absolute indications for parenteral nutrition is not recommended, unless >60% of caloric needs cannot be met by the enteral route alone.[23] (Fig. 105-2).

After the decision is made to provide nutritional repletion, the quantity should be calculated. In general, severe sepsis and trauma patients are believed to require 20–50% more calories than their basal energy expenditure amounts; burn patients may need up to 70% more, while uncomplicated postoperative cases may need only 10% more calories for a few days. The Harris-Benedict and Ireton-Jones equations appear to be reasonably accurate in estimating basal energy expenditure, with total caloric intake increased based on severity of illness as above.[5] However, matching caloric intake to actual energy expenditure may be less important than providing some calories, rather than making a patient NPO for prolonged periods. Empiric caloric intake of 22–25 kcal/kg/day approximates most critically ill patients' resting energy expenditure, although it may not meet the actual expenditure.[10] Deliberate hypocaloric parenteral feeding (up to 20 kcal/kg/day) for limited periods, perhaps by withholding lipids, has not been shown to be deleterious to postoperative or critically ill patients unable to tolerate enteral feeding, and it is better tolerated than hypercaloric feeding.[30]

The Canadian Clinical Practice Guidelines recommend standard enteral tube feeding formulas.[30] Enhancing enteral tube feeding solutions with immunostimulants, antioxidants, or specific proteins or oils may be beneficial in selected patient groups. Solutions with fish or borage oils and antioxidants may improve outcomes in critically ill patients with acute respiratory distress syndrome (ARDS). Glutamine-supplemented tube feeding may reduce infectious complications in burn and trauma patients. Arginine and other specific nutrients do not appear to alter outcomes in critically ill or injured patients. Insufficient data exist to support peptide-

Figure 105-2 • Nutrition management algorithm. Mildly or moderately malnourished patients are characterized by 5% weight loss within 3 months, mild subcutaneous tissue loss, and reduced dietary intake. Severely malnourished patients are characterized by 10% weight loss within 6 months and functional impairment, or their subjective global assessment results indicate that they are severely malnourished. If not severely malnourished, administering no preoperative but only postoperative TPN before POD 10 results in no better or worse outcomes than use of standard dextrose and oral supplements. Initiate nutrition support if expected either NPO for seven days or to be taking <60% caloric needs by POD 10.

GI—gastrointestinal; TF—tube feeding; TPN—total parenteral nutrition; NPO—nil per os; POD—postoperative days

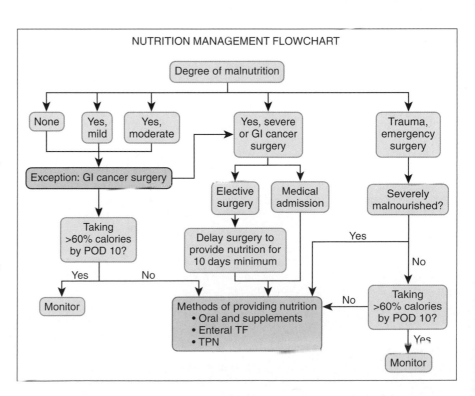

Box 105-3 Recommendations for Nutrition in Critically Ill Patient

Begin enteral nutrition with polymeric full-strength tube feeding solution with 48 hours of admission

Exceptions:

ARDS patient: consider solution with fish oil or borage oil and antioxidants

   Burn patient: consider glutamine supplementation

Start at target feeding rate

Check gastric residuals every 6–8 hours

If residual volumes persistently >250 mL, consider adding prokinetic agent

If residual volumes persistently >500 mL despite prokinetic agent or patient develops vomiting, place small bowel feeding tube and continue feeds

If vomiting continues or abdominal distension develops, discontinue enteral feeding and begin parenteral nutrition

If parenteral nutrition utilized, add parenteral glutamine

If patient is not malnourished and parenteral nutrition duration is anticipated to be <10 days, feed a hypocaloric prescription by withholding lipids.

ARDS—acute respiratory distress syndrome

Table 105-1 Risk Factors for Aspiration and Recommendations for Avoiding Aspiration

Major Risk Factors for Aspiration:	Recommendations:
	All patients:
Documentation of previous aspiration	
Decreased level of consciousness	Elevate head of bed 30–45 degrees
Neuromuscular disease	Good oral care
Structural abnormalities of gastrointestinal tract	Regularly assess feeding tolerance
Endotracheal intubation	Tube position
Vomiting	One major risk factor:
Persistently high gastric residual volumes	
Prolonged duration in supine position	All of the above, plus:
	Tight glycemic control
	Correct electrolyte disorders
	Minimize narcotics
	Continuous enteral feeding

based enteral formulas as the initial choice in patients with absorption difficulties. Critically ill patients who require parenteral nutrition should receive supplemental intravenous glutamine, as mortality is modestly reduced. These enhanced formulas are more expensive than standard formulas.

Methods of initiation and maintenance of nutrition support in non–critically ill inpatients have not been well studied. Studies in the critically ill recommend early initiation, attention to attaining target infusion rate and caloric intake, use of prokinetic agents and small bowel feeding tube placement where indicated rather than cessation of enteral feeding and inappropriate use of parenteral nutrition, and minimizing risk of aspiration by using proper body positioning or other methods (Box 105-3).[30,31] These recommendations appear reasonable and applicable in non–critically ill patients as well.

Tube position depends on patient requirements. For short-term use, a small-bore flexible nasogastric feeding tube is easiest to place and the most comfortable for the patient, as opposed to a large sump tube often used for gastric aspiration. Smaller bore tubes may have a lower risk of reflux by minimizing gastroe-

sophageal junction incompetence. The Canadian Guidelines recommend routine use of small bowel tube placement (nasoduodenal or nasojejunal) where feasible, as risk of pneumonia may be reduced. If routine small bowel tube placement is logistically problematic, limit its use to higher risk patients receiving continuous sedatives, neuromuscular blockers, or who are unable to tolerate adequate enteral formula volumes.[30] The North American Summit Consensus Statement describes the major risk factors for aspiration and recommendations to avoid aspiration (Table 105-1).[31] Place a percutaneous feeding tube (gastrostomy or jejunostomy) only if tube feedings are required for more than 30 days. Surgical jejunostomy may be performed at the time of laparotomy in selected cases, and it has the same complication rate as other small bowel feeding tubes.[21]

In summary, diagnosing malnutrition requires assessment of risk factors and clinical clues in the history and physical examination, rather than by laboratory tests. Severely malnourished patients or those not expected to be or not receiving >60% of estimated caloric need by Hospital Day 10 should receive enteral nutritional support, unless proven to be intolerant.

Key Points

- A patient who has lost either 5 kg over the last 3 months or 10% of his or her body weight over the last 6 months is at risk of being severely malnourished.

- Maintain high clinical suspicion for malnutrition, and make the diagnosis by careful history, physical examination, and validated tools assessing nutritional risk.

- Laboratory testing, including serum albumin, is not specific for malnutrition.

- Periodically reassess nutritional status, as up to 60% of inpatients become malnourished during their hospital stay, increasing their risks of nosocomial infection, poor wound healing, length of stay, and costs.

- In very sick or severely injured patients, a sustained hypermetabolic state causes large muscle and visceral protein losses, despite adequate caloric intake.

- Provide nutrition support for at least 1 week prior to surgery to severely malnourished inpatients and those with gastrointestinal cancer undergoing elective surgery.

- Patients anticipated to be NPO for >7 days, those expected to be or not taking <60% of estimated caloric needs by postoperative day 10, or critically ill patients who are anticipated to be taking less than full oral diet by 72 hours should also receive nutrition support until inflammatory markers and nutrition levels improve.

- Make every effort to provide enteral nutrition rather than parenteral, as routine parenteral nutrition provides no benefit and may increase complications and mortality. Standard enteral formulas are adequate for most inpatients, although selected critically ill patients may benefit from specialized or enhanced formulas.

SUGGESTED READING

Jones JM. The methodology of nutritional screening and assessment tools. J Hum Nutr Dietet 2002; 15:59–71.

McClave SA, Snider HL, Spain DA. Preoperative issues in clinical nutrition. Chest 1999; 115:64S–70S.

Kreymann KG, Berger MM, Deutz NEP, et al. ESPEN guidelines on enteral nutrition: intensive care. Clin Nutr 2006; 25:210–223.

Winawer N, Williams MV. Nutritional support. In: Shojania KG, Duncan BW, McDonald KM, et al., eds.Making Health Care Safer: A Critical Analysis of Patient Safety Practices. Evidence Report/Technology Assessment No. 43, AHRQ Publication No. 01-E058; July 2001. Full report available at http://www.ahrq.gov.

Heyland DK, Dhaliwal R, Drover JW, et al. Canadian Clinical Practice Guidelines for Nutrition Support in Mechanically Ventilated, Critically Ill Adult Patients. JPEN 2003; 27:355–373.

McClave SA, DeMeo MT, DeLegge MH, et al. North American Summit on Aspiration in the Critically Ill Patient: Consensus Statement. JPEN 2002; 26:S80–S85.

Section

Sixteen

Postoperative Evaluation and Care

106 Routine Postoperative Assessment and Management
Norman Egger, Kevin Whitford

107 Perioperative Pain Management
Kevin Whitford, Norman Egger

108 General Wound Care, Postoperative Evaluation and Care
Antonio Ramos-De la Medina, David R. Farley

109 Postoperative Abnormal Signs and Symptoms
Kulsum K. Casey, Jeanne M. Huddleston

110 Postoperative Cardiac Complications
Michael P. Phy, Jeanne M. Huddleston

111 Non-cardiac Postoperative Complications
Kulsum K. Casey, Jeanne M. Huddleston

112 Surgical Site Infection Prophylaxis
James Stone, Jason Stein, James Steinberg

CHAPTER ONE HUNDRED AND SIX

Routine Postoperative Assessment and Management

Norman Egger, MD, MS, and Kevin Whitford, MD

BACKGROUND

Over the last decade, there has been a shift in the postoperative care of the surgical patient. Traditionally, patients remained hospitalized after their surgery for observation and treatment of anesthesia or surgical complications, and they were not discharged until reaching a certain "self-care" level. Advances in anesthesia and surgical techniques, together with new developments in perioperative care, changed the emphasis from inpatient to ambulatory care while at the same time enabling sicker and older patients to undergo more complicated surgery. The current inpatient population includes more complex, older, and acutely ill surgical patients in addition to those requiring emergent operations. Increasingly, their perioperative medical care is being shifted to hospitalists.

This chapter is an overview of the most common general situations encountered by hospitalists while taking care of the postoperative patient after discharge from the postanesthesia care unit (PACU) and transfer to the floor.

PATHOPHYSIOLOGY

Surgery is associated with a stress response that activates a complex pattern of hormonal changes initiated by neuronal activation of the hypothalamic–pituitary–adrenal axis.[1] Secretion of cortisol and catecholamines, an altered carbohydrate and protein homeostasis, and activation of the acute phase response are all important markers. The overall metabolic effect is an increase in catabolic hormones with a reduction in anabolic hormones, which mobilizes substrates to provide energy sources, resulting in increased catabolism and hypermetabolism.

Following surgery, there additionally is a locally triggered tissue response to injury, with increases in cytokine production. These alterations are accompanied by hemodynamic, metabolic, inflammatory, and immunologic changes aimed at maintaining homeostasis and assisting recovery. The magnitude and duration of this response are proportional to the surgical injury and the development of complications. Surgery-related metabolic and endocrine derangements have the potential for adverse systemic effects, including increased myocardial oxygen consumption, increased catabolism, and impaired immune function. Poor postoperative course and clinical outcome have been associated with

these changes in patients who already had suboptimal organ functioning before surgery.

CLINICAL ASSESSMENT/EVALUATION

The use of short-acting volatile and intravenous anesthetics allows for earlier recovery from anesthesia. Patients need close monitoring and documentation of alertness and changes in mental status, as failure to regain alert mental status may herald complications such as cerebral embolism, subarachnoidal hemorrhage, carotid occlusion, or delirium. (See Table 106-1.)

Hospitalists should evaluate and aggressively treat pain, since this will reduce anxiety and provide subjective comfort.[2] Furthermore, when pain is controlled, the autonomic and somatic reflex responses are alleviated, allowing earlier mobilization, reduced postoperative complications, and an accelerated recovery. Chapter 107 provides a more detailed discussion of postoperative pain.

Postoperative nausea and vomiting are among the most common and by patients the most feared complaints[3] that limit speed of recovery and hospital discharge. Predictive factors include a previous history of postoperative vomiting or motion sickness, anxiety, the type of surgery (mainly ophthalmologic, auditory, gynecologic), poorly controlled pain, hypotension, and multiple agents (such as opioids) used intraoperatively. The presence of postoperative gastrointestinal tract dysfunction (such as ileus) should be considered. A more detailed review of nausea and vomiting can be found in Chapter 9.

Postoperative respiratory complications are common. Perform a careful history and focused physical examination, looking for respiratory symptoms and signs such as stridor, tachypnea, dyspnea, bradypnea, rales, and wheezing. Further assess respiratory status via pulse oximetry[4] and, if indicated, arterial blood gas. Consider obtaining a postoperative chest x-ray to determine complications (such as pneumothorax) after chest, upper abdomen, neck, and axillary surgery, as well as for patients who had central vein cannulations if there are concerning symptoms.

Postoperative **hypoxemia** may occur in the early recovery period, as a result of anesthesia-related effects, or several days later. All patients should initially receive supplemental oxygen immediately after surgery. Late postoperative hypoxemia[5] can present as persistent or intermittent desaturations (related to sleep disturbances and rebound rapid eye movement [REM] sleep). The significance of postoperative hypoxemia is its contribution to cardiac ischemia and arrhythmias, cognitive dysfunction, and impaired wound healing and wound infections.

Hypertension and hypotension occur frequently in the postoperative period. Hypotension and tachycardia may indicate hemorrhage with the need for volume repletion and possible surgical intervention. Obtain an urgent hematocrit in this situation. Alternatively, consider the possibility of adrenal insufficiency or pulmonary embolism in certain patients. Postoperative hypotension is a predictor of cardiac morbidity in known hypertensive patients. Early postanesthesia hypertension may be due to uncontrolled pain, fluid overload, or anxiety and can precipitate cardiac ischemia.[6] Late postoperative hypertension may be secondary to the reversal of peripheral vasodilatation from discontinued epidural anesthesia, mobilization of fluid from the extravascular space into the intravascular space, or the effects of inadvertently stopped antihypertensive medication.

Surgical stress can induce **cardiac ischemic events.** Peripheral or superficial procedures, such as eye surgery, have the least risk for MI (<1%) while major emergent surgery and vascular procedures have the greatest risk (>5%). The peak risk for a perioperative myocardial infarction is in the first few postoperative days. With the introduction of β-blockers perioperatively, acute ischemic events have been decreased.[7] Evaluation in the early postoperative period is by symptoms (if the patient is awake) and electrocardiogram (ECG) changes with cardiac enzymes when myocardial damage is suspected. The demonstration of myocardial necrosis in the absence of acute ST-T changes such as non–ST-elevation myocardial infarction (NSTEMI) can be challenging, given the false positive increases in the creatinine phosphokinase (CPK) MB fraction after surgery. In that respect, serum troponin-I and T levels are more specific but less sensitive in the very early phases. More recent research indicates that troponin levels can be falsely elevated in certain noncardiac conditions (e.g., renal insufficiency).[8] Myocardial ischemia often presents silently without pain shortly after surgery and also in patients with diabetes mellitus. Atypical presentations of postoperative myocardial ischemia may include unexplained hemodynamic changes, heart failure, or arrhythmias. **Arrhythmias** are mostly of atrial origin and are often seen in the elderly as well as after cardiopulmonary surgery. These arrhythmias can be secondary to uncontrolled pain, fever, hypovolemia, or hypoxemia. **Early postoperative congestive heart failure** (within the first few hours) can be precipitated by fluid overload during surgery, while late CHF (24–48 hours after surgery) may be due to redistribution of accumulated fluids from the extravascular space. Consider myocardial ischemia as a possible cause in both situations.

Patients at risk for postoperative renal failure, usually from acute tubular necrosis, include those who had vascular surgery, massive blood loss, and inadequate fluid resuscitation. Also consider postrenal causes, such as bladder retention after high doses of opioids, and renal causes after medications, such as after nonsteroidal anti-inflammatory drugs or antibiotics.

Postoperative **neurologic complications** include delirium and cerebral vascular accidents (CVA). The best methodology to assess the presence of delirium is uncertain, but multiple tools, such as the confusion assessment method (CAM), are available.[9]

Obtain additional information about baseline mental status from a caregiver or from the family. Postoperative delirium is multifactorial and is usually associated with older patients with preexisting cognitive impairment, drug reactions, hypoxemia, electrolyte imbalances, infection, cardiac ischemia or arrhythmias, stroke, trauma, uncontrolled pain, sleep deprivation, or isolation. Do not ignore the possibility of withdrawal effects from alcohol, illicit drugs, or certain medications. Postoperative delirium results in more complications, longer hospital stays, and increased need for skilled nursing or rehabilitation after discharge.

The occurrence of a CVA in the postoperative period is heralded by sudden changes in mental status, the presence of focal deficits, or delayed awakening after anesthesia. It is more common in cardiac surgery, and associated risk factors include the presence of carotid artery bruits, atrial arrhythmias, heart failure, and prior CVA. Urgent assessment should include head imaging to distinguish between a hemorrhagic or an ischemic event.

RECOMMENDATIONS/MANAGEMENT

A multidisciplinary approach, with close communication between surgeon, anesthesiologist, internist, physical therapist, nursing, and pharmacy, is an essential component of postoperative care. This interaction should ideally be started in the preoperative phase.

Traditional postoperative care promoted bed rest. Recent perceptions are that bed rest is undesirable since it increases muscle loss, weakness, deconditioning, pulmonary complications with hypoxemia; delays wound healing; and increases risk for thromboembolism.

Oral intake is frequently restricted in the postoperative period, and nasogastric tubes are often placed routinely after elective abdominal surgery. When enteral feedings are started, it is common practice to use a slowly advanced regimen from liquids to more solids. A scientific basis for such a practice is lacking,

Table 106-1 Common Postoperative Complications	
Cardiac	MI, angina, CHF, arrhythmias, hypertension, hypotension
Pulmonary	Respiratory failure, pneumonia, aspiration, COPD/asthma exacerbation, atelectasis, hypoxemia, DVT/PE
Gastrointestinal	Nausea/vomiting, GI bleed, jaundice, constipation/diarrhea, ileus
Renal	Renal failure, UTI, electrolyte abnormalities, urinary retention
Neurologic	CVA, delirium, seizures
Hematologic	Anemia, bleeding, HIT
Fever	Infectious (pneumonia, UTI, wound, hepatitis), postsurgical, drug-induced, malignant hyperthermia

MI—myocardial infarction; CHF—congestive heart failure; COPD—chronic obstructive pulmonary disease

while studies have demonstrated early oral feedings are safe, even after bowel surgery, with placement of anastomoses. Albeit still somewhat controversial, early enteral feedings may reduce gut permeability, prevent bacterial translocation and infections, and, most importantly, improve outcome.

Treat nausea and vomiting with effective pharmacologic interventions such as serotonin-5HT$_3$ antagonists, glucocorticoids, and even rarely droperidol (only to be used if all others fail), while feeding can be initiated. The presence of postoperative paralytic ileus should prompt the use of non- or reduced-opioid analgesia, administration of opioid antagonists if necessary, and provision of continuous epidural local anesthetics. Judicious, but not routine, use of nasogastric tubes for gastric decompression, and correction of fluid imbalance (both dehydration and overhydration) is important. The use of parasympathetic agents (such as neostigmine) or prokinetics (such as erythromycin and metoclopramide) has not been shown to decrease the duration of postoperative ileus. More recent data suggest that the use of epidural bupivacaine significantly shortens the duration of postoperative paralytic ileus.[10]

Many postoperative practices still liberally employ the use of invasive indwelling drains, tubes, or catheters. The routine use of these devices has not been shown to improve outcome, and with few exceptions, is unnecessary and may contribute to complications and delayed recovery.[11]

Treatment of postoperative hypoxemia should include oxygen supplementation for probably all patients in the immediate postoperative period and reevaluation of oxygenation thereafter. Adequately treat pain to avoid sleep disturbances, and encourage early mobilization to avoid the supine position. The most common postoperative respiratory complication is atelectasis. Incentive spirometry is a cost-effective modality for lung expansion and yields similar results to intermittent positive pressure breathing.

Surgical injury acts as a procoagulant, and the risk for deep venous thrombosis and pulmonary thromboembolism in the postoperative period is increased. It is therefore essential to ascertain that patients are on the appropriate prophylactic anticoagulation regimen to prevent postoperative thromboembolism. Chapter 26 covers this in detail.

Treat severe postoperative hypertension with short-acting intravenous antihypertensives, similar to hypertensive emergencies; and simultaneously institute interventions to address pain, diuresis, and oxygenation.

The management of delirium involves treating any underlying condition if found. Multiple triggers are often present. In the postoperative phase, in particular, provide adequate pain control and avoid hypoxemia. Avoid certain analgesics (meperidine and propoxyphene) since better alternatives exist (morphine and oxycodone). Early mobilization after surgery, avoiding certain drugs, avoiding restraints (including Foley catheters), attending to hydration, promoting normal sleep, compensating for sensory disorders, and stimulating daytime activities and reorientation can prevent delirium. Including family members in discussions and merely their presence may be helpful. If the delirious patient is restless, companionship, reassurance, and touch can provide help. For more severe agitation, a brief course of low-dose haldol (starting at 0.5 mg) can be used or, alternatively, olanzapine[12] if longer duration treatment is needed.

Key Points

- Relative to surgical outpatients, hospitalized surgical patients are older, acutely ill, and have more often emergent surgery and complex illnesses.

- Hospitalists are increasingly involved in perioperative care.

- A multidisciplinary approach, started in the preoperative phase, is an essential component of postoperative care.

- Common postoperative symptoms like nausea, vomiting, and inadequate pain control negatively impact speed of recovery and should be treated aggressively.

- Early recognition, assessment, and intervention of postoperative signs, such as hypoxemia, anemia, abnormal volume status, renal failure, and blood pressure deviations, are important to prevent the development of common postoperative complications, such as cardiac ischemia, respiratory failure, thromboembolic events (including cerebral and pulmonary), as well as delirium.

SUGGESTED READING

Wilmore DW. From Cuthbertson to fast-track surgery: 70 years of progress in reducing stress in surgical patients. Ann Surg 2002; 236(5):643–648.

Auerbach A, Goldman L. Beta-blockers and reduction of cardiac events in noncardiac surgery: scientific review. JAMA 2002; 287(11):1435–1444.

CHAPTER ONE HUNDRED AND SEVEN

Perioperative Pain Management

Kevin Whitford, MD, and Norman Egger, MD, MS

BACKGROUND

Despite an increased emphasis on pain control, a majority of patients still experience significant postoperative pain.[1] Because of this, patients may be anxious and may hesitate to proceed with surgery. The responses to pain lead to suffering, dissatisfaction, delayed recovery, and postoperative complications. Postoperative pain impairs mobility, and increases the risk of cardiopulmonary complications, thromboembolic complications, delirium, and agitation. The Joint Commission on Accreditation of Health Care Organizations has emphasized pain as the "fifth vital sign." Health care institutions are required to assess pain in all patients and incorporate management of pain in the plan of care. When pain is identified, it must be treated and reassessed regularly. Hospitals must have criteria in place for follow-up and management of pain, and must assess effectiveness of pain management on an ongoing basis.

Recent developments have increased options available for achieving excellent pain management in the perioperative period. These include preemptive measures to reduce pain after surgery, and specialty pain services that evaluate and use advanced treatments including advances in regional anesthesia and pharmacologic management. The entire health care team must be vigilant in the assessment and ongoing management of perioperative pain and suffering. Transitions in care must be managed so that the patient has an ongoing plan from presurgery to postsurgery to eventual recovery at home or in transitional care. Ongoing evaluation of quality and effectiveness is imperative for continuous improvement of systems for management of postoperative pain.

PATHOPHYSIOLOGY

At the surgical site, tissue injury causes release of mediators of inflammation, including prostaglandins, cytokines, and neuropeptides. The primary transmission of pain signals to the dorsal horn of the spinal cord is via the C nerve fibers and A-sigma nerve fibers. At the dorsal horn of the spinal cord, neurotransmitters and endorphins modulate and transmit signals to higher centers. Complex interactions lead to central sensitization with alterations in pain thresholds and perception of painful stimuli.

Tolerance to pain is variable between individuals and varies with prior painful experiences, prior medications (particularly chronic opioid use), and the context of pain. Despite increasing knowledge of the neuroscience of pain, only direct communication from the patient can measure pain. Hospitals must have common systems for this measurement, such as a numerical pain scale, visual-analog scale, or images. Alternatives to the numerical scale should be available for pediatric patients. The system for recording and tracking pain control must be applied uniformly across the institution.

PREOPERATIVE EVALUATION

During the preoperative evaluation, review allergies, sensitivities, anesthesia history, and medications to plan the optimal strategy for pain management. Consider preemptive treatment with non-steroidal anti-inflammatory drugs (NSAIDS) in patients with normal renal function.[2] In patients with contraindications to NSAIDS, acetaminophen may be used.[3] Avoid selective cyclooxygenase 2 inhibitors in patients undergoing cardiac procedures.[4] The anesthesiologist may offer spinal anesthesia and/or other regional anesthesia procedures to reduce requirements for opioid analgesics and to improve pain control.[5] In partnership with the surgeon and anesthesiologist, the hospitalist must ensure the safest and most effective pain control regimen and consider its impact on risk for complications.

POSTOPERATIVE CARE

Patient-controlled analgesia (PCA) is the mainstay of postoperative pain control. Morphine, hydromorphone, and fentanyl are all effective drugs for use with PCA. Avoid meperidine because of drug interactions and the risk of accumulation of toxic metabolites. Suggested dose ranges for initial PCA use in opioid-naïve patients are shown in Table 107-1. Monitor geriatric patients closely for adverse effects, as they will generally require lower dosages of narcotics.[6] Evaluate patients reaching the lockout dose without adequate pain control for adjustment of the analgesic regimen. Provide orders to address the common side effects of narcotics on the bowel and bladder.

Change to oral medications (Table 107-2) as early as possible to ensure that pain control will be adequate on transition out of hospital. Provide clear instructions regarding use of pain medications, bowel care, resumption of preoperative pain analgesics, and limitations of activity on discharge from the hospital.

Table 107-1 PCA Medication Dose Ranges

Medication	Dose	Frequency	4-Hour Lockout
Morphine	2 mg	10 minutes	24 mg
Hydromorphone	0.2 mg	10 minutes	2.4 mg
Fentanyl	25 mcg	10 minutes	300 mcg

Table 107-2 Oral Pain Medications and Dosing

Medication	Oral Equivalent (mg)	IV Equivalent (mg)
Morphine sulfate	30	10
Hydromorphone	7.5	1.5
Hydrocodone	30	n/a
Oxycodone	15	n/a
Fentanyl	n/a	0.1

IR = immediate release, n/a = nonapplicable

SUMMARY

Surgery triggers a stress response that has the potential for poor postoperative outcomes in patients with suboptimal physiologic reserves. The hospitalist, as a multidisciplinary team member, increasingly provides care to such complex at-risk patients. A thorough understanding of preoperative risk-factor assessment and prevention, early recognition, and intervention of postoperative complications is an important asset of such physicians.

Key Points

- Adequate postoperative pain management is still undervalued, despite the availability of newer and more effective modalities.

- An ongoing plan from presurgery to postsurgery to eventual recovery at home is imperative for management of postoperative pain.

SUGGESTED READING

Apfelbaum JL, Chen C, Mehta S, et al. Postoperative pain experience: results from a national survey suggest postoperative pain continues to be undermanaged. Anesth Analg 2003; 97(2):534–540.

American Society of Anesthesiologists Task Force on Acute Pain. Practice guidelines for acute pain management in the perioperative setting: an updated report by the American Society of Anesthesiologists Task Force on Acute Pain Management. Anesthesiology 2004; 100(6):1573–1581.

CHAPTER ONE HUNDRED AND EIGHT

General Wound Care, Postoperative Evaluation and Care

Antonio Ramos-De la Medina, MD, and David R. Farley, MD

BACKGROUND

Wound healing is the physiologic response of living tissue to injury that encompasses a series of events that attempt to restore the tissue to its original state. Although most surgical wounds closed (sutured or stapled) primarily heal without complications, some wounds are either left open or closed by secondary intention, while others develop complications and require continued care.

PATHOPHYSIOLOGY

Wound Healing Basics

With the exception of bone, all tissues heal with a scar, and the process of wound healing is identical. Acute wound healing can be divided into different interrelated and overlapping stages, described as phases: inflammatory, proliferative, and remodeling (Fig. 108-1).

The **inflammatory phase** of acute wound healing begins immediately following injury with the disruption of blood vessels. Hemostasis ensues by activation of the coagulation cascade, which produces fibrin, an essential element necessary for clot formation and wound healing. After formation of a stable clot, inflammatory cells migrate into the wound, attracted by chemotactic factors generated by the coagulation and activated complement pathways. Macrophages are the most important cell in this phase; they produce growth factors such as platelet-derived growth factor (PDGF) and vascular endothelial growth factor (VEGF), and cytokines, which induce fibroblast and endothelial cell proliferation as well as production of an extracellular matrix. Some evidence suggests that macrophages are the only inflammatory cell type absolutely necessary for tissue repair.[1] Re-epithelialization of the wound begins within hours after injury, and by 48 hours a thin layer of epithelium confers protection against bacteria and foreign bodies, but this layer can easily be disrupted.

The **proliferative phase** is characterized by the formation of granulation tissue. At 72–96 hours post injury, fibroblasts proliferate and populate the wound, stimulated especially by PDGF and transforming growth factor β1 (TGF- β1),[2] and they start synthesizing collagen. Growth factors produced by macrophages induce angiogenesis at this stage.

The **remodeling phase** starts around 2–3 weeks post injury when collagen accumulation reaches its peak, and its synthesis is down-regulated with decreasing cellularity of the wound. Type III collagen is gradually replaced with type I collagen, and the tensile strength increases. At this point, tensile strength of the scar reaches 20–30% when compared to unwounded tissue. After complete healing, the maximal strength of a scar reaches only 70% of the tensile strength of normal skin.[3]

Acute Wounds

An acute wound is defined as the traumatic loss of normal structure and function to recently uninjured tissue after a noxious insult.[4] Postoperative incisions are by definition acute wounds and will be the focus of this chapter.

Clinical Assessment/Evaluation

Accurate wound assessment is a critical component of effective postoperative care[5,6] and should include evaluation for the following:

1. **Approximation/epithelialization of wound margins:** All incisions should be evenly approximated with no separation and epithelialized by postoperative day 3.
2. **Drainage:** Closed incisions should have minimal, if any, drainage.
3. **Signs of infection:** Erythema, purulence, pain, warmth, and swelling.
4. **Palpable healing ridge:** Palpate along the incision looking for a ridge indicative of granulation tissue formation present by postoperative day 5. Absence of a healing ridge by postoperative day 5–9 signals delayed healing and risk for dehiscence.
5. **Factors affecting wound healing:** Malnutrition, immunosuppression, diabetes, smoking, and local edema.

RECOMMENDATIONS/MANAGEMENT

Postoperative Incision Care

The prototypical postoperative care of the surgical wound involves protection from contamination by bacteria, foreign material, and trauma; maintenance of normothermia; adequate perfusion and oxygenation of the tissues; and optimal nutrition.

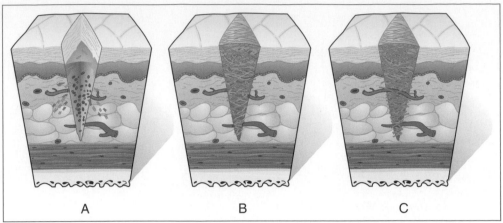

Figure 108-1 • Phases of wound healing. A, inflammatory phase, B, proliferative phase, C, remodeling phase. Mayo Clinic Basic Surgical Skills, DA, Sherris, EB Kern, Mayo Clinic Scientific Press, 1999; page 9. By permission of Mayo Foundation for Medical Education and Research. All right reserved.

The Centers for Disease Control and Prevention (CDC) recommendations regarding postoperative incision care are the following:

1. Postoperatively protect a primarily closed incision with a sterile dressing for 24–48 hours.
2. Wash hands before and after dressing changes or with any contact with the surgical site.
3. When an incision dressing must be changed, use sterile technique.
4. Educate the patient and family regarding proper incision care, symptoms of infection, and the need to report such symptoms.

The CDC guidelines for the prevention of a surgical site infection (SSI) offer no recommendations regarding incisions closed primarily beyond 48 hours, nor on the appropriate time to shower or bathe with an uncovered incision.[7] Our own practice allows patients to shower within several days of the surgical procedure, and sterile dressings are unnecessary after re-epithelialization occurs.

Open Wounds

Acute wounds sometimes need to be left open to heal by secondary intention (i.e., dirty or infected wounds). A chronic wound is an open lesion that fails to heal after 3 months of continued care or one that recurs. In both cases, healing takes place following the same basic process, but the inflammatory, proliferative, and remodeling phases take longer. Open wounds require more care than those closed primarily. Necrotic and devitalized tissue needs to be removed from the wound and desiccation prevented. A warm, clean, sterile, and moist environment is required for healing to occur, and it can be created by packing the wound with normal (0.9%) saline-moistened gauze (Fig. 108-2). The mechanism by which these dressings promote healing is not completely understood, but several factors may be involved. Mechanical debridement with wet-to-dry dressing changes is the standard of care in many places. This method does not discriminate between devitalized tissue and granulation tissue, may theoretically delay healing, and should be used to debride wounds containing necrotic tissue. The alternative of wet-to-wet dressing

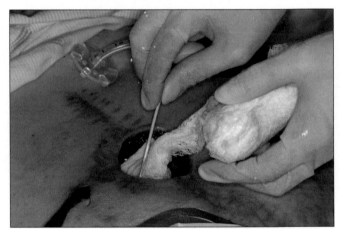

Figure 108-2 • Open wound packing. Open wound packing with sterile normal saline-moistened gauze.

changes disrupts the healing process to a lesser degree and is a good option in clean wounds. Other dressings like hydrogels, hydrocolloids, and alginates have been used with varying degrees of success and are beyond the scope of this chapter. Antibacterial ointments and solutions are also applied, but experimental data have demonstrated that some of these substances are toxic to fibroblasts and can be detrimental to the healing process. As a rule of thumb, one should remember the old adage "never put anything in a wound that you wouldn't put in your eye."

Recently, some mechanical devices have been developed to help promote wound healing. The Vacuum Assisted Closure (V.A.C.®) system is one of the most popular of such devices. It uses a reticulated foam dressing attached to a vacuum tube on the wound, which is then sealed with an occlusive drape. Negative pressure is applied at 50–125 mm Hg. The mechanism of action of this device seems to be related to enhancement of local blood flow, decrease in the edema and bacterial proliferation, and increase in granulation tissue formation and angiogenesis. Encouraging results of the use of this device in terms of rates of healing have been reported in the literature.

Wound Complications

Seroma

A seroma is a subcutaneous serous fluid collection. It is a benign but frequent complication of many surgical wounds, specially those that require extensive subcutaneous dissection and skin flap development like mastectomy, axillary or groin dissection, ventral hernia repair, and abdominoplasty. Clinically significant seroma after breast cancer surgery varies from 5–85%, and some breast surgeons consider it an expected side effect rather that a complication. Furthermore, it can prolong hospital stay, increase costs, and may delay adjuvant treatment. The pathogenesis of seroma formation is not completely known, but it has been suggested that it is an exudate resulting from an acute inflammatory reaction[8] or that it may originate from fat liquefaction or lymph.[9]

A seroma causes discomfort and if left untreated can become infected. Small collections usually need no intervention, as they resorb with time. If symptomatic, our practice is to aspirate the seroma using a 21 G needle + syringe and sterile technique. Large or persistent seromas require management. Repeated needle aspiration, placement of a wound closed-drainage system, or reopening all or part of the wound and healing by secondary intention are all generally successful in treating most cases. Seroma formation can also be a sign of wound infection. Antibiotics may be used to prevent secondary infection of the fluid.

Hematoma

Hematoma is defined as a mass of usually clotted blood that forms in a tissue as a result of a broken blood vessel. The hematoma may result from poor surgical technique, but one should always have in mind that it may be the result of a coagulopathy. Development of a hematoma in a recent incision should trigger consideration of a coagulation disorder and review of the patient's current medications to ensure that anticoagulants or antiplatelet agents are not a contributory factor. Clinically, hematomas present as ecchymotic tumefaction and drainage of dark sanguineous fluid from the wound. Although the management principles are the same as those for seroma, hematomas carry a higher risk of infection than seromas, and the use of antibiotics is recommended in many cases. Ultrasonography can help determine the etiology and assess the extent of subcutaneous fluid collections in complex wounds or when findings are subtle, but we seldom find ultrasonography usage necessary.

Hematomas can be a surgical emergency in some anatomical areas. Postoperative bleeding after neck surgery (thyroidectomy, neck dissection, or carotid surgery) can cause compression of the trachea with suffocation and requires emergent evacuation (Fig. 108-3). Roughly, one in 300 neck operations for thyroid or parathyroid disease require emergent/urgent operative intervention for cervical hematoma.[10]

Dehiscence

Dehiscence is defined as partial or complete separation of a suture line in the early postoperative period. Dehiscence can range from splitting open of the superficial skin layers to complete dehiscence of the fascia (Fig. 108-4). Fascial dehiscence is particularly important after abdominal surgery. When the fascial separation is complete during the first days after an operation, it may lead to evisceration, a complication that carries a mortality of 5–30%[11,12] (Fig. 108-5). Evisceration is a surgical emergency. The

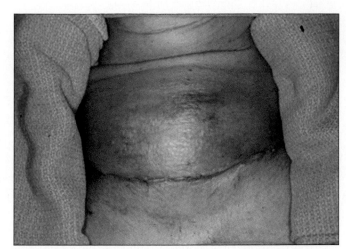

Figure 108-3 • Neck wound hematoma. Postoperative hematoma after thyroidectomy.

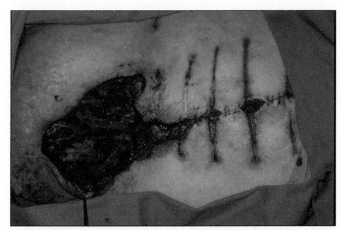

Figure 108-4 • Wound dehiscence. Partial wound dehiscence resulting in open wound healing by secondary intention.

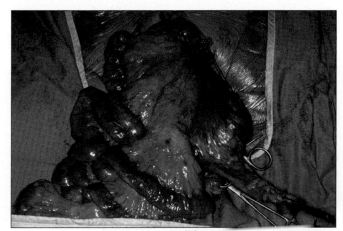

Figure 108-5 • Fascial dehiscence. Evisceration of abdominal contents after a laparotomy.

initial management of evisceration requires covering of the eviscerated abdominal contents with saline-moistened sterile laparotomy pads followed by surgical closure in the operating room.

Most fascial dehiscences occur between postoperative days 5 and 8. Although partial dehiscence of a short segment of the fascia can often be observed, especially if discovered after the first postoperative week, it will invariably lead to an incisional hernia.

Dehiscence usually presents clinically as a sudden increase in the volume of drainage from the wound. If dehiscence is suspected, it is necessary to explore the wound under sterile conditions at the bedside to evaluate the integrity of the fascia.

Risk factors for wound dehiscence include wound infection, enterocutaneous fistula, intra-abdominal sepsis, malnutrition, advanced age, malnutrition, severe coughing, chronic lung disease, prolonged ventilatory support, jaundice, vomiting, prolonged intestinal paralysis, urinary retention, use of steroids, and emergency surgery.[11,13]

Wound Infection

Infection remains a common complication after most types of surgery. The CDC estimates that more than 500,000 SSI occur annually in the United States.[14] Surgical infections are expensive complications in both economic and clinical terms. Patients who develop SSI are two times more likely to die than uninfected patients.[15] Early recognition and treatment are essential in preventing or limiting morbidity. Signs of infection like erythema, pain, or warmth should prompt further evaluation of any surgical incision (Table 108-1). Gently compress the edges of the wound to express any fluid contained in the wound. Evaluate the appearance of the obtained drainage, and send it for culture and a Gram-stained smear. Although the results seldom change wound management, antibiotics may be adjusted accordingly.

Table 108-1 CDC Criteria for Definition of Superficial Surgical Site Infection

Infection occurs within 30 days after the operation *and* infection involves only skin or subcutaneous tissue of the incision *and* at least *one* of the following:

1. Purulent drainage, with or without laboratory confirmation, from the superficial incision
2. Organisms isolated from an aseptically obtained culture of fluid or tissue from the superficial incision
3. At least one of the following signs or symptoms of infection: pain or tenderness, localized swelling, redness, or heat, and superficial incision is deliberately opened by surgeon, unless incision is culture negative
4. Diagnosis of superficial incisional SSI by the surgeon or attending physician

Do *not* report the following conditions as SSI:

1. Stitch abscess (minimal inflammation and discharge confined to the points of suture penetration)
2. Infection of an episiotomy or newborn circumcision site
3. Infected burn wound
4. Incisional SSI that extends into the fascial and muscle layers (deep incisional SSI)

SSI—surgical site infection

From: Mangram AJ, Horan TC, Pearson ML, et al. Guideline for prevention of surgical site infection, 1999. Hospital Infection Control Practices Advisory Committee. Infect Control Hosp Epidemiol 1999; 20:250–278.

Laboratory studies are usually not necessary or contributory. The presence of an abscess requires opening the wound, local care (i.e., removing devitalized tissue) and packing with gauze. The bacteriology of the wound depends on the anatomical location and type of surgical procedure; however, *Staphylococcus aureus* is the most common pathogen followed by *Staphylococcus epidermidis, Entrerococcus,* and *Escherichia coli.* Administer antibiotics if the surrounding tissue shows evidence of infection. Cellulitis requires the administration of antibiotics, and patients who present with fever and systemic sepsis should be admitted to the hospital for blood and wound cultures and intravenous antibiotics. Surgical exploration may be needed in cases that do not improve after adequate management to rule out necrotizing soft tissue infection.

It is important to remember that prophylactic antimicrobials should begin within 60 minutes *before* surgical incision and discontinued within 24 hours in the absence of infection (see Chapter 112).[16]

Necrotizing Infections

Necrotizing infection of the soft tissue can be secondary to clostridial (*Clostridium perfringens*) and nonclostridial organisms (group A β-hemolytic *Streptococcus*). Although rare, these devastating infections can complicate any surgical wound. Necrotizing soft tissue infections are difficult to recognize since the overlying skin can maintain a normal appearance initially while subcutaneous and deep fascial edema or necrosis is present. Systemic signs of toxicity can be present, but some patients (especially if immunocompromised) can be initially asymptomatic. Diagnosis requires a high index of suspicion, and delay in management can result in loss of tissue and life.

Necrotizing fasciitis is characterized by angiothrombotic microbial invasion and necrosis of the fascia and has a mortality that ranges from 6–76%. It is commonly caused by a polymicrobial infection, with streptococcal species being the predominant organisms. *Staphylococcus aureus, Escherichia coli, Pseudomonas, Enterobacter, Klebsiella, Proteus, Bacteroides,* and *Clostridium* have also been isolated and seem to act synergistically to cause this disease. Early in its evolution, a necrotizing infection usually is clinically impossible to differentiate from severe cellulitis. Blisters or bullae are pathognomonic, but they present late in the disease and are imminent signs of skin necrosis (Fig. 108-6). Diagnosis is most commonly made on clinical grounds upon exploration of the wound. The so-called "finger test" is accomplished by infiltrating the skin with a local anesthetic followed by a 2-cm incision extending to the fascia. Lack of bleeding and the presence of

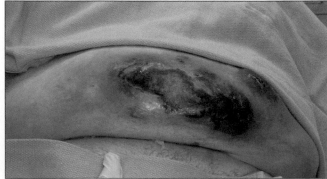

Figure 108-6 • Necrotizing fasciitis. Advanced stage of necrotizing fasciitis showing skin necrosis.

"dishwater fluid" are suggestive of the diagnosis. The fascia is then probed with the finger, and if tissues dissect with minimal effort, the test is considered positive. A positive "finger test" should prompt aggressive surgical debridement and antibiotic management. Send tissue for culture and frozen section.[17,18]

Clostridial myonecrosis (gas gangrene) is commonly caused by *C. perfringens*, although other members of the *Clostridium* genus have been implicated. As with necrotizing fasciitis, diagnosis is complicated by an indolent initial course. The initial symptoms include increase in wound pain, fever, and systemic toxicity. If not treated, they are soon followed by the development of skin gangrene and crepitus. Surgical debridement and early administration of penicillin and clindamycin are essential. Hyperbaric oxygen therapy is also useful but should not be the initial treatment.

Sutures/Staples Removal

Any noninfected wound can be safely closed by several different methods. Sutures and staples have been used for decades with good results, and since their results are equivalent, the choice of the method of wound closure is a matter of personal preference. Our preference at Mayo Clinic is to use an absorbable subcuticular skin closure that avoids the need to remove sutures in follow-up and prevents unsightly scars; leaving external sutures or staples too long generates "railroad track" type wounds.

The time to remove sutures or staples should be individualized according to the characteristics of each patient and the location of the incision (Table 108-2). Skin sutures left in place too long result in poor cosmetic appearance (i.e., more than 5 days for neck incisions); on the other hand, removing sutures prematurely risks wound dehiscence (i.e., over a moving joint), which can lead to wound infection and poor cosmetic results. In tension-free wounds, remove external sutures or staples by 5–7 days. Sutures over a joint or under tension may be best left in place 2 weeks or more.

Skin Adhesives

Skin adhesives have recently surfaced as an option for wound closure. They offer some advantages to both physician and patient since they are easy to apply; take less time; offer no risk of needle-stick injury to the surgeon; there are no sutures to remove; and the infection rates and cosmetic results are at least comparable to sutures, tapes, or staples.[19] However, its use in wounds under tension can be complicated by dehiscence of the tissue, and they are not practical for large incisions.

SUMMARY

For the hospitalist caring for postoperative patients, careful assessment and evaluation of surgical or traumatic wounds should be done daily. Healthy wounds require little care and only timely suture/staple removal. Wounds showing signs of cellulitis, fluid accumulation (hematoma or seroma), or deeper soft tissue infections require immediate intervention: antibiotics and strong consideration for opening the wound. In conjunction with surgical consultation, it remains prudent to "look and find nothing wrong" if your suspicion is high for potentially morbid complications (fasciitis, abscess, and necrosis).

Key Points

- At 2–3 weeks post-injury or surgical incision, tensile strength of the scar reaches 20–30% when compared to unwounded tissue. After complete healing, the maximal strength of a scar reaches only 70% of the tensile strength of normal skin.

- A ridge indicative of granulation tissue formation should be present by postoperative day 5–9; absence of a healing ridge signals delayed healing and risk for dehiscence.

- Development of a hematoma in a recent incision should trigger consideration of a coagulation disorder and review of the patient's current medications to ensure that anticoagulants or antiplatelet agents are not a contributory factor.

- Abdominal surgery wound dehiscence that results in complete fascial separation may lead to evisceration, a surgical emergency that carries a mortality of 5–30%. Dehiscence usually presents clinically as a sudden increase in the volume of drainage from the wound.

- Necrotizing soft tissue infections are difficult to recognize since the overlying skin can maintain a normal appearance initially while subcutaneous and deep fascial edema or necrosis is present. Surgical debridement and early administration of penicillin and clindamycin are essential with clostridial myonecrosis (gas gangrene).

SUGGESTED READING

Singer AJ, Clark RA. Cutaneous wound healing. N Engl J Med 1999; 341:738–746.

Dubay DA, Franz MG. Acute wound healing: the biology of acute wound failure. Surg Clin North Am 2003; 83:463–481.

Bates-Jensen BM. Chronic wound assessment. Nurs Clin North Am 1999; 34:799–845.

Bratzler DW, Houck PM. Surgical Infection Prevention Guidelines Writers Workgroup. Antimicrobial prophylaxis for surgery: an advisory statement from the National Surgical Infection Prevention Project. Clin Infect Dis 2004; 38:1706–1715.

Wong CH, Wang YS. The diagnosis of necrotizing fasciitis. Curr Opin Infect Dis 2005; 18:101–106.

Table 108-2 Time to Removal of Sutures or Staples According to Location*

Location	Time (days)
Face/neck	3–5
Scalp	6–8
Fingers	7–10
Chest/abdomen	7–10
Hand	10–12
Foot	10–14
Back	12–14
Extremities	12–14

*Applies to patients without factors that may delay wound healing.

CHAPTER ONE HUNDRED AND NINE

Postoperative Abnormal Signs and Symptoms

Kulsum K. Casey, DO, and Jeanne M. Huddleston, MD, FACP

BACKGROUND

As a result of improved surgical techniques, many more elderly patients and patients with multiple comorbidities are now undergoing surgery; however, they are often at risk for complications after surgery. Early evaluation of abnormal signs and symptoms after surgery is critical in preventing and treating complications.

This chapter focuses on some of the common signs and symptoms that patients may develop after surgery and current management strategies. Hypoxemia, dyspnea, and chest pain are discussed in other chapters (Anesthesia—Chapter 97, Postoperative Noncardiac Complications—Chapter 111, Postoperative Cardiac Complications—Chapter 110).

FEVER

Risk Factors and Pathophysiology

Fever is a common finding in the first few days following major surgery (25–74% depending on site of surgery),[1-3] but an infectious etiology is infrequent.

The timing of the onset of fever is crucial in determining its origin.

The extent and duration of the fever are related to morbidity. A fever of <38.5C in the first 48 hours (without localizing symptoms or examination findings) is considered part of the normal postoperative recovery and does not warrant any laboratory or other investigative studies. Within the first 48 hours after surgery, fever may result from blood transfusions, localized operative site hematoma or inflammation, or dehydration. Atelectasis, even if present postoperatively, is not a cause of fever. The differential diagnosis for other common postoperative noninfectious etiologies of fever includes pulmonary embolus, myocardial infarction, and inflammatory mono- or polyarthritis.

An *infection-related* fever typically occurs beyond **48–96 hours postsurgery**. The differential diagnosis of the most common postoperative infections is related to the timing of the fever with urinary tract infection (particularly in patients who have been catheterized) as the primary etiology >48 hours following surgery, and pneumonia and wound infection >72 hours following surgery. Patients with advanced age and/or end-stage renal disease may not mount a significant febrile response to an acute inflammatory process. Thus, a rising white count, change

in hemodynamics, or altered mental status should suggest a possible infection and should prompt an evaluation. Despite the wide variety of causes for postoperative fever, it has not been shown to increase mortality in postoperative patients.[3]

Clinical Assessment/Evaluation

A thorough history and physical examination are the most important assessment and evaluative tools for discerning the cause of fever. These findings should guide selection of subsequent laboratory or diagnostic tests. Do not perform routine, nonfocused screening for infection, as it is not cost effective.

Fever beyond 48 hours following surgery associated with leukocytosis is more likely to be infectious in etiology. A urinalysis is a cheap and easy test to rule out a urinary tract infection, particularly in patients who have a bladder catheter. Perform a chest x-ray in patients who develop a productive cough or shortness of breath requiring oxygen 48 hours after surgery, especially those with known pulmonary disease or risk factors (*see* Chapter 103). Blood cultures are likely to be negative unless there are physical signs and symptoms consistent with sepsis. Evaluate patients who have an intravenous catheter for catheter-associated line infection. If the patient appears septic, remove the catheter and send the tip for culture.

Recommendations and Management

Treatment is dependent upon the cause of fever and is identical to the nonoperative setting. Regardless of timing postoperatively, if other vital signs and physical examination findings are consistent with sepsis, stabilize the patient hemodynamically, and treat with broad-spectrum antibiotics until a source is localized. In the first 48 hours, encourage cough and deep-breathing exercises to improve ventilatory mechanics and to decrease atelectasis and risk for developing pneumonia. Observe for changes in the wound appearance including pustular drainage, dehiscence, or evolving hematoma.

Antipyretics may be used in the immediate postoperative setting and may help to decrease narcotic burden as well. Exercise caution when using Toradol immediately postoperatively if the patient is potentially hypovolemic. Patients with abnormal renal function are susceptible to further renal compromise in this setting.

ALTERED MENTAL STATUS

Background

There are many physiologic causes (Table 109-1) for altered mental status after surgery. Immediately after surgery, a change in a patient's mental status is often related to the effects of residual anesthesia and/or narcotics. The patients at highest risk are elderly patients and those with baseline cognitive impairment.[4,5]

Clinical Assessment and Evaluation

Altered mental status after surgery is rarely due to an acute neurologic event such as a stroke. Most often, the development of altered mental status is the result of a vulnerable patient being exposed to a metabolic derangement, unfavorable environmental conditions, or medications resulting in somnolence and/or confusion; however, it is still important in the initial evaluation to assess if an acute event has occurred. Depending on the type of surgery, physical examination, and the patient's overall risks, one should evaluate the patient for acute myocardial infarction, arrhythmia, congestive heart failure, infection (in particular pneumonia and urinary tract), seizure, stroke, hypoglycemia, and/or electrolyte abnormality.

Patients with known cognitive impairment (such as patients with dementia, a history of stroke, or Parkinson's disease) are much more susceptible to confusion after surgery. Patients who are alert should undergo a full neurologic examination including a bedside mental status test.[6] To distinguish dementia from delirium, the *Diagnostic and Statistical Manual of Mental Disorders, Fourth Edition* has defined delirium with distinct features making

it easy to identify. The Glasgow Coma Scale can be used for patients who are obtunded or comatose.

Hyponatremia is the most likely electrolyte abnormality after surgery resulting in an altered mental status. This may be due to infusion of hypotonic fluid during surgery (also absorption of hypotonic glycine buffer irrigating solution during transurethral prostatectomy), secretion of antidiuretic hormone, and/or fluid shifts after surgery. Diabetic patients who are on insulin or have taken oral hypoglycemic agents (especially sulfonylureas) the day of surgery are at risk for developing hypoglycemia, especially after a prolonged fast. Patients with severe liver disease with impaired glycogenolysis may also be at risk.

Management

The management of altered mental status is based on its cause. For stable patients, the initial management is preventing patient harm and minimizing exposure to medications and conditions that may perpetuate cognitive impairment. This includes reducing fall risks, maintaining adequate pain control and a normal sleep-wake cycle, avoiding narcotics and sedatives, and routine assessment of patient's mental status.

Details of management strategies for specific causes of altered mental status are described elsewhere (*see* Chapter 93).

DECREASED URINARY OUTPUT

Decreased urinary output is a common finding in the immediate postoperative period with hypovolemia, urinary retention, and renal failure being the most common causes.

Hypovolemia

Background

Administration of anesthesia (general, spinal, and epidural) causes peripheral vasodilation leading to a relative hypovolemia and possibly secondary hypotension. Inadequate renal perfusion secondary to relative hypovolemia in the immediate postoperative period is the most common cause of decreased urine output.

Risk Factors and Pathophysiology

Hypovolemia and hypotension decrease renal blood flow. Patients with autonomic dysfunction or those taking vasodilating agents for cardiac disease or hypertension may be at increased risk based on the extent of vasodilation. Decreased urine output secondary to hypovolemia signals impending acute renal failure if volume status is not corrected.

Urinary Retention

Background

Urinary retention is a common but usually self-limiting postoperative complication. Inability to void within 6–7 hours after surgery has been reported to occur in less than 1% of low-risk patients[7] and 8–10% of patients undergoing colonic and spinal surgery.[8,9] It may delay discharge following outpatient surgery in 5–19% of the cases.[10] The most common causes include: surgical manipulation, pain, residual effects of spinal or epidural anesthesia, narcotic and excess fluid administration resulting in bladder distention, and urinary tract infection.[7,11]

Table 109-1 Causes of Altered Mental Status Postoperatively

Metabolic causes
Hypoxia
Hypercapnia (often seen in patients with chronic lung disease and obstructive sleep apnea)
Hypotension
Hypoglycemia
Electrolyte disturbances (particularly hyponatremia secondary to hemodilution)
Infection

Organic causes
Cerebrovascular event
Seizures

Medication-induced
Residual anesthetic affects
Sedatives (benzodiazepines, tricyclics)
Anticholinergics
Antihistamines
Barbiturates
Opioids

Other causes
Drug/alcohol withdrawal (narcotic or benzodiazepines)
Exacerbation of psychiatric disease
"Sun-downing," especially in the elderly or in the ICU setting

ICU—intensive care unit.

Risk Factors and Pathophysiology

Risk factors for urinary retention include: history of urinary retention, symptomatic benign prostatic hypertrophy, spinal/epidural anesthesia, pelvic or urologic surgery, and perioperative catheterization.[7,11] Physiologically, postoperative urinary retention is the result of discoordination of the trigone and detrusor muscles and inhibition of the micturition reflex. Often, this resolves on its own postoperatively if given time. However, intermittent catheterization may be needed for patient comfort, but placement of an indwelling catheter should be avoided if at all possible.

Renal Failure

The causes and risk factors of acute renal failure are described elsewhere (see Chapter 49).

Clinical Assessment/Evaluation

Monitor patients for urine output during the entire hospitalization, but most attentively during the first 72 hours after surgery and until the first successful spontaneous void following removal of an indwelling catheter. Most patients should void within 6–8 hours of surgery or removal of an indwelling catheter.

Physical examination should include: assessment for fever, intravascular volume depletion, abdominal tenderness (specifically suprapubic), and costovertebral angle tenderness. Note, given fluid extravasation into the subcutaneous fluids secondary to anesthetic agents, the presence of extremity and sacral edema may not indicate increased intravascular volume. If bedside ultrasound bladder scanners are available, use them proactively to monitor patients at high risk for urinary retention in order to avoid significant bladder distention, which could prolong the rate of bladder function recovery.

Recommendations and Management

Treatment is dependent upon cause. For hypovolemia, restore adequate renal perfusion through volume expansion in order to prevent or minimize the occurrence of prerenal failure and acute tubular necrosis. Repletion with packed red blood cells is the most effective method of restoring intravascular volume if significant anemia is a contributing factor. Isotonic crystalloid including 0.9% sodium chloride, lactated Ringer's, and isotonic sodium bicarbonate solutions will also remain intravascular and increase renal perfusion more than hypotonic solutions. Of note, intravenous dextrose and water will do little or nothing to increase end-organ perfusion.

For urinary retention, intermittent catheterization is indicated for: patients who have not voided within 6–8 hours after surgery, patients with ultrasound-scanned volumes of greater than 200 mL, and every 6–8 hours in patients with ongoing urinary retention (to avoid bladder distention). Do not place indwelling catheters for the sole purpose of treating urinary retention. A study in one high-risk population demonstrated that patients who were randomized to intermittent catheterization every 6–8 hours as opposed to an indwelling urinary catheter had a significant reduction in time to normal urinary voiding with no significant increase in urinary tract infections.[12]

Treatment and prevention of urinary retention include: adequate pain control, judicious use of intravenous fluids, avoiding bladder distention and anticholinergic agents, and minimizing the use of narcotics in high-risk patients. Adjuvant pain control regimens which decrease narcotic use (such as preoperative oral gabapentin for spinal surgery) may decrease the occurrence of postoperative urinary retention.[9]

Management of urinary tract infections and acute renal failure is reviewed in detail in Chapters 35 and 49, respectively

HYPERGLYCEMIA

Background

The development of hyperglycemia is most often due to either a relative deficiency of insulin or insulin resistance (Table 109-2). Hyperglycemia, defined as a random glucose >200 mg/dL or sustained levels >140 mg/dL, may impact morbidity and mortality in critically ill patients in the hospital. In the past, concern for reactive hypoglycemia prevented the liberal use of insulin for

Table 109-2 Risk Factors Associated with Hyperglycemia

Etiology	Mechanism of Hyperglycemia
History of diabetes mellitus	Relative or absolute insulin deficiency, resistance or increased hepatic gluconeogenesis
Iatrogenic catecholamine infusion (epinephrine)	Inhibition of insulin release or insulin deficiency
Elderly	Insulin deficiency
Obesity	Insulin resistance
Increase severity of illness	Excess counterregulatory hormone concentrations
Excess carbohydrate ingestion or (dextrose) infusion	Inadequate uptake of glucose
Glucocorticoids	Insulin resistance
Pancreatitis	Insulin deficiency
Severe inflammation or sepsis	Insulin resistance
Hypothermia	Insulin deficiency
Uremia	Insulin resistance
Cirrhosis	Insulin resistance
Hypoxemia	Insulin deficiency

Adapted from: McCowan KC, Malhoota A, Bistrian BR. Endocrine and metabolic dysfunction syndromes in the critically ill. Crit Care Clin 2001; 17:107–124.

blood glucose levels between 140–180 mg/dL. Recent studies have shown that poor glycemic control (blood glucose levels >140 mg/dL) is associated with worse outcomes in critically ill, hospitalized patients.[13–16] Intensive insulin therapy aimed at lowering glucose to near-normal levels has been shown to reduce mortality in the surgical ICU.[17]

Risk factors associated with hyperglycemia in postsurgical hospitalized patients are listed in Table 109-2. Patients undergoing surgery are particularly at risk due to stress-induced hyperglycemia. The mechanism of stress hyperglycemia is suggested to be the result of counter-regulatory hormones and cytokines that cause gluconeogenesis, hepatic and skeletal glycogenolysis, increased lipolysis, insulin resistance, and direct suppression of insulin secretion.[18] Major concerns of postoperative hyperglycemia are the development of infection, myocardial ischemia/infarction, and acute renal failure (due to excessive osmotic diuresis).

Clinical Assessment and Evaluation

Postoperative hyperglycemia is usually not symptomatic, and it is often recognized incidentally when a fingerstick glucose analysis or a plasma chemistry panel is noted to be abnormal. An evaluation of blood glucose may be prompted due to the patient's symptoms such as excessive diuresis, gastrointestinal complaints, or confusion. In the initial assessment of patients without a history of diabetes, evaluate them for exogenous sources of glucose, prior symptoms suggestive of diabetes, use of systemic steroids, evidence of infection, inflammation or hemorrhage, and other risk factors that may contribute to hyperglycemia (see Table 109-2). Exogenous sources of glucose infusion may include: dextrose infusion with antibiotics or electrolyte replacement, in replacement fluids or total peripheral nutrition (TPN), or in dialysis solutions. Since many patients are unaware that they are diabetic, consider measuring a hemoglobin A_{1c} in patients with newly diagnosed hyperglycemia. Although hemoglobin A_{1c} is not currently recommended as a diagnostic assay for diabetes, patients found to have a level that is >2 SDs above the laboratory mean are considered to have diabetes.

Management

For patients identified as having excessive exogenous glucose, modify their solutions or infusion source. Total peripheral nutrition (TPN) may be given as hypocaloric TPN, or insulin can be admixed to the solution. In addition, consider infusing medications with saline instead of dextrose if possible. In patients expected to have elevated blood sugars due to chronic steroid use or TPN, administer a long-acting insulin preparation to maintain basal levels of insulin and maintain glucose control. Subcutaneous insulin may be given as supplementation for tighter glucose control.

Oral hypoglycemic agents are not recommended for glucose control in nondiabetic patients perioperatively. It is still controversial whether post-surgical patients in general benefit from tight glucose control, but growing evidence supports treatment at least in the critically ill. The benefits of tight glycemic control (blood glucose levels <150 mg/dl) for noncritically ill patients are still unknown.

Using standard insulin infusion protocols can help achieve tight blood glucose control and minimize reactive hypoglycemia. When transitioning to subcutaneous insulin, give a basal dose of insulin prior to stopping the infusion to prevent rebound hyperglycemia. Basal insulin may be given as long acting, divided on an every 12-hour basis or mixed with regular insulin (such as 70/30). Totaling the amount of insulin given in a 24-hour period provides a baseline for basal insulin requirements. We recommend starting with two thirds the amount given in a 24 hour period and adjusting as needed with correction (short-acting) insulin. Patients who are expected to return to normal glucose levels shortly after surgery may be covered with correction insulin only.

Key Points

- A thorough history and clinical assessment are necessary to determine the etiology of abnormal signs and symptoms postoperatively.

- Management of abnormal signs and symptoms should be based on likely cause.

- Routine screening for infection in patients with fever (T <38.5 C) <48 hours after surgery is unnecessary.

- Patients at highest risk for postoperative confusion are those with underlying cognitive impairment.

- Postoperative urinary retention is self-limiting and should not be treated with an indwelling Foley catheter unless necessary.

- Standard insulin infusion therapy may be used to achieve tight blood glucose control in patients with postoperative hyperglycemia.

SUGGESTED READING

Mahon P, Shorten G. Perioperative acute renal failure. Curr Opin Anaesth. 2006; 19(3):332–338.

Strumper-Groves D. Perioperative blood transfusion and outcome. Curr Opin Anaesth. 2006; 19(2):198–206.

Shander A, Goodnough LT. Objectives and limitations of bloodless medical care. Curr Opin Hematol. 2006; 13(6):462–70.

Qaseem A, Snow V, Fitterman N, Hornbake ER, et al. Risk assessment for and strategies to reduce perioperative pulmonary complications for patients undergoing noncardiothoracic surgery: a guideline from the American College of Physicians. Ann Intern Med. 2006; 144(8):575–80.

Smetana G, Lawrence V, Cornell J. Preoperative Pulmonary Risk Stratification for Noncardiothoracic Surgery: Systematic Review for the American College of Physicians. Ann Intern Med. 2006; 144(8):581–595.

Lawrence V, Cornell J, Smetana G. Strategies To Reduce Postoperative Pulmonary Complications after Noncardiothoracic Surgery: Systematic Review for the American College of Physicians. Ann Intern Med. 2006; 144(8):596–608.

Inouye S.K. Current Concepts: Delirium in Older Persons. NEJM. 2006; 354(11):1157–1165.

Perlino C. Postoperative fever. Med Clin North Am 2001; 85:1141–1149.

CHAPTER ONE-HUNDRED AND TEN

Postoperative Cardiac Complications

Michael P. Phy, DO, MSc, and Jeanne M. Huddleston, MD, FACP

MYOCARDIAL INFARCTION AND ISCHEMIA

Background

Postoperative myocardial ischemia or infarctions are the major endpoints in studies evaluating accuracy of preoperative cardiac risk stratification, and their occurrence markedly affects outcomes and length of stay. Studies vary, but the range of postoperative myocardial infarction, ischemia, and unstable angina following noncardiac surgery is 1–10.3%.[1–5] Among patients undergoing abdominal surgery, the highest incidence of postoperative myocardial infarction occurs within 1 day postoperatively.[6] A study completed in the early 1990s utilized continuous cardiac monitoring to assess the postoperative period for signs of ischemia. The most severe ischemia occurred throughout days 1–3, with the most severe electrocardiographic evidence of ischemia on postoperative day 3.[7] Of note, length of hospital stay was longer in patients who experienced postoperative myocardial ischemia (11 days; 95% CI 9–12 days) compared to patients without any complications (4 days; 95% CI 3–4 days), even after adjustment for surgical and medical morbidity.[3]

Risk Factors and Pathophysiology

Perioperative myocardial ischemia arises from increased myocardial oxygen demand, decreased supply, or both. Factors that increase demand include the catecholamine stress response to surgery, tachycardia, hypertension, anemia, or sympathomimetic drugs. Decreased oxygen supply may be due to hypotension, anemia, tachycardia, or hypoxemia. The majority of fatal perioperative myocardial infarctions (MI) are related to disruption of an atherosclerotic plaque leading to coronary thrombosis; however, many of these MIs occur in areas without a critical fixed coronary stenosis. Therefore, even coronary artery bypass grafting (CABG) or percutaneous coronary intervention (PCI) may not necessarily prevent perioperative MIs.

The most common and thoroughly reviewed evidence-based approach to preoperative cardiovascular evaluation is the Guideline for Perioperative Cardiovascular Evaluation for Noncardiac Surgery published jointly by the American College of Cardiology (ACC) and the American Heart Association (AHA).[8] In this guideline, there are both surgery-specific and patient-specific risk factors for postoperative adverse cardiac events (see Chapter 102, Cardiovascular Preoperative Risk Assessment and Evaluation for full explanation). Specific surgical and patient specific risk factors are delineated in Box 110-1.

Patients with known coronary artery disease whose ischemic threshold is <60% of age-predicted maximal heart rate during a noninvasive cardiac stress test are at highest risk (odds ratio 7.002; 95% CI 2.79–17.61).[9] New regional wall motion abnormalities (RWMA) in preoperative stress echocardiography increase the risk of cardiac death, nonfatal MI, or unstable angina. After multivariate analysis, noncardiac vascular surgery patients with extensive (>3 segments) stress-induced RWMA had a 6.5-fold elevated risk of adverse cardiac events.[1]

Aortic stenosis is an important, underestimated risk factor for perioperative complications. Patients with severe aortic stenosis have a significantly higher postoperative rate of myocardial infarction and death as compared to those with moderate and no aortic stenosis (31%, 11%, and 2% respectively).[10]

Additional Factors in Postoperative Myocardial Ischemia

Pain Management

Effective pain management, with epidural and patient-controlled analgesia, leads to a reduction in postoperative catecholamine surges and hypercoagulability. Appropriate use of epidural analgesia has been shown to decrease postoperative myocardial infarctions.[11–13]

Anemia

A paucity of data explicates the role of anemia in postoperative MI. Theoretically, a reduction of oxygen-carrying capacity on top of the known increase in myocardial workload in the perioperative period would increase the risk of suffering a significant adverse cardiac event. One study suggests that patients with a hematocrit <28% had a significantly higher incidence of MIs as compared to those whose hematocrit was >28% (10 out of 13 vs. 2 out of 14 with MIs, respectively).[14]

Box 110-1 Specific Risk Factors for Postoperative Myocardial Ischemia

Surgical:

- Type of surgery
- Blood loss
- Fluid shifts
- Length of anesthesia
  - The type of anesthesia (general or spinal) does not appear to have a significant effect on rates of postoperative adverse myocardial events.

Patient-specific (ACC/AHA preoperative evaluation consensus guideline)

- Past medical morbidity
  - History of myocardial infarction
  - Unstable angina
  - Diabetes
  - Renal insufficiency
  - Advanced age
  - Congestive heart failure
  - Peripheral vascular disease
  - Poor functional status

Core Body Temperature

One prospective, double blind study of 300 noncardiac surgery patients found hypothermia to be an independent predictor of adverse cardiac events (RR, 2.2; 95% CI, 1.1-4.7; P = 0.04). There was a 55% reduction in adverse cardiac events when normothermia was maintained.[15]

Despite even optimal perioperative management, some patients will have a perioperative MI, which is associated with a 40–70% mortality rate.[16]

Clinical Assessment/Evaluation

The constellation of indicators includes clinical symptoms, intraoperative or postoperative ECG changes, and elevation of the creatine kinase, MB fraction (CK-MB) or troponin. However, many patients will not have chest pain because of postoperative narcotic pain control, hence making the diagnosis challenging. Besides chest pain, other presentations of perioperative MIs include shortness of breath, arrhythmias, syncope, unexplained hypotension, and mental status changes (confusion).

Routine surveillance for a perioperative MI should be reserved for patients who develop signs of cardiac ischemia or hemodynamic compromise intraoperatively or for those who are considered high risk by patient- or surgery-specific risk factors.[8] Screening methods include:

- *ECG:* Preoperatively, immediately postoperatively, and daily for 2 days. Patients with new ischemic changes on a 12-lead ECG immediately following surgery have a higher risk of cardiac complications (including MI) (OR 2.2, 95% CI 1.2–3.9, p < 0.01).[17]
- *Cardiac enzymes:* Immediately postoperatively (and possibly day 4 or prior to discharge if earlier) and when there are signs or symptoms of myocardial ischemia or significant changes in hemodynamics.
- *Cardiac telemetry monitoring:* Routine use in the absence of documented myocardial ischemia or hemodynamic compromise is controversial. One study comparing telemetry monitoring and 12-lead ECG for the detection of postoperative ischemia post aortic vascular surgery found that routine intensive care unit surveillance has low sensitivity for detecting myocardial ischemia compared with frequent 12-lead electrocardiograms.[18]

In the evaluation of patients with symptoms consistent with possible acute postoperative myocardial ischemia, the first principle is to ensure the patient is hemodynamically stable. Then, obtain an ECG and cardiac enzymes, looking for evidence of decreased myocardial perfusion. See Recommendations/Management below for immediate treatment.

- *Obtain a directed clinical history for ischemia related symptoms:* Chest pain severity, quality, radiation and duration, nausea, diaphoresis, dyspnea, palpitations, and mental status. Evaluate pulse, blood pressure, evidence of peripheral perfusion, presence or absence of arrhythmias, and signs of congestive heart failure. Review recent medical history for any suggestion of early congestive heart failure in the immediate postoperative setting.[4]
- Obtain documentation of left ventricular function, prior electrocardiograms, and assessments of myocardial function, if available. Review the operative record for evidence of intraoperative hemodynamic instability including hypotension, requiring vasopressor support, or tachycardia. Search for infectious, pulmonary, or electrolyte abnormalities. Determine level of oxygenation and severity of postoperative anemia.
- Troponin T may be elevated (>0.1 ng/mL) in the absence of obvious MI. In one study, Troponin T was elevated from baseline in 87% of patients who had clinically evident myocardial ischemia and in 16% of those without.[5] Troponin T has a similar receiver-operating curve as CK-MB in the diagnosis of postoperative MI; however, it is a much better marker of other cardiac-related complications without definitive MI.

Recommendations/Management

As a preventive measure for those patients on β-blockers preoperatively, continue them for the duration of hospitalization and potentially beyond. (For a more thorough discussion of β-blocker therapy, see Chapter 102, Cardiovascular Preoperative Risk Assessment and Evaluation). In the setting of an evolving postoperative myocardial ischemic event, start pharmacologic therapy with aspirin as soon as possible. Give β-blocker therapy (if not already on it) to minimize myocardial oxygen demand by slowing heart rate. An angiotensin-converting enzyme (ACE) inhibitor may also be helpful. Transfer the patient to a telemetry monitoring setting.

Use of anticoagulants and antiplatelet therapy beyond aspirin obviously raises concern in the setting of surgery. Weigh the risks and benefits of blood loss versus the potential of incompletely treated myocardial ischemia. The site of the surgical procedure and duration of time since surgery are the determining factors. This decision should be made in conjunction with the surgeon.

In the setting of documented symptomatic ST segment elevation MI, strongly consider coronary angiography with PCI.[19]

At the time of discharge, ensure that appropriate medical follow-up is arranged. Patients may need functional cardiac evaluation or interventional procedures once they have recovered from surgery. Elevated troponin T in the first 3 days after surgery is a prospective marker for both major and minor cardiac complications in the following 3 months,[20] as well as a predictor of 6-month survival.[21] If β-blockers cannot be tolerated, diltiazem may be a reasonable alternative to decrease risk of postoperative myocardial ischemia and death.[22] For secondary risk reduction, ensure that patients with postoperative MIs are discharged on a β-blocker, aspirin, statin, and an ACE-inhibitor or angiotensin receptor blocker (as per Joint Commission on Accreditation of Healthcare Organizations (JCAHO) and Centers for Medicare and Medicaid Services (CMS) recommendations). If one or more of these is contraindicated or not tolerated by a patient, then documentation of this is necessary.

HEART FAILURE

Background

Heart failure (HF) is the most frequently encountered postoperative cardiac complication of noncardiac surgery,[23,24] occurring in 1–6% of patients after major surgery. In patients with existing coronary artery disease, prior HF, or valvular heart disease, the risk of HF is 6–25%.[25-27] Other risk factors include diabetes mellitus, renal insufficiency, high-risk surgery such as vascular surgery,[26] or excessive fluid administration intraoperatively.[28]

Pathophysiology: Etiology and Timing

Heart failure (HF) is a complex clinical syndrome that can result from any structural or functional cardiac disorder that impairs the ability of the ventricle to fill with or eject blood. (Heart failure is reviewed in detail in Chapter 21.) Postoperative HF can be due to systolic dysfunction, diastolic dysfunction, or left ventricular volume overload.

Systolic dysfunction refers to a decrease in myocardial contractility. This leads to a reduction in cardiac output and a subsequent increase in sympathetic activity in an effort to restore cardiac output by increasing heart rate and contractility. As systolic heart failure progresses, there is a progressive decline in cardiac output for any given cardiac filling pressures or increase in positive inotropic agents. Postoperative systolic dysfunction is most often due to ischemia, tachyarrhythmias, and hypertension.

Diastolic dysfunction is an increase in ventricular stiffness with reduced compliance that impairs ventricular filling during diastole. Postoperative causes include ischemia and hypertensive crisis.

Left ventricular volume overload refers to heart failure when a normal heart is suddenly presented with a load that exceeds its capacity. This may occur when a large volume of intravenous fluid or blood is infused into the intravascular volume, resulting in an acute increase in left ventricular volume, with subsequent elevation of left ventricular end-diastolic and left atrial pressures and pulmonary edema.

The occurrence of postoperative heart failure has biphasic peaks with somewhat different causes: *early* (in the recovery room or first 24 hours) due to intraoperative fluid overload, myocardial ischemia or infarction, hypertension or hypotension, sympathetic stimulation, hypoxia, and cessation of positive-pressure breathing; and *later* (24–72 hours) due to reabsorption of fluid that was third-spaced during surgery, myocardial ischemia or infarction, and failure to restart a patient's usual medications for HF. Other cardiac causes of postoperative heart failure include valvular heart disease, cardiomyopathy, pericardial disease, and arrhythmias. Noncardiac causes include anemia, hypoxia, and fever.

Clinical Assessment/Evaluation

General Assessment—The approach to the patient with postoperative HF uses the history and physical examination, review of intraoperative and immediate postoperative records with particular attention to the volume infused perioperatively, chest x-ray, and a series of diagnostic tests to establish the diagnosis and determine the cause.

History

There are two major symptom groups in HF—those due to excess fluid accumulation (dyspnea, edema, hepatic congestion, and ascites) and those due to a reduction in cardiac output (fatigue, weakness) that is more pronounced with exertion.

Regardless of symptoms, evaluate all postoperative patients found to be in heart failure for new or unstable myocardial ischemia.

Physical Examination

Check vital signs. Note any acute changes or trends in blood pressure levels. Assess rate and compare pre- and postoperative heart rate. Assess for tachypnea and need for oxygen supplementation (based on O_2 saturation). Look for signs of volume overload—pulmonary edema, peripheral edema, elevated jugular venous distention. Signs of decreased cardiac output may include sinus tachycardia, diaphoresis, and peripheral vasoconstriction (cool, pale, and sometimes cyanotic extremities).

Blood Tests

Recommended initial blood tests for patients with signs or symptoms of HF include a complete blood count (since postoperative anemia can exacerbate HF), serum electrolytes and creatinine (baseline to follow when initiating therapy with diuretics and/or ACE inhibitors), liver function tests (which may be affected by hepatic congestion), and plasma brain natriuretic peptide (BNP).

Measurement of plasma BNP is useful for distinguishing between HF due to systolic and/or diastolic dysfunction and a pulmonary cause of dyspnea. Plasma concentrations of BNP are markedly higher in patients with clinically diagnosed HF (including patients with right heart failure due to cor pulmonale) compared to those without HF.[29] A consistent finding in most studies is a high negative predictive value of low BNP concentrations, suggesting that BNP may have particular value in ruling out HF and eliminating the need to perform additional costly tests.

Chest X-Ray

Findings suggestive of heart failure include cardiomegaly (cardiac-to-thoracic width ratio above 50%), pulmonary vascular congestion (cephalization of the pulmonary vessels), Kerley B-lines, and pleural effusions. A systematic review of the utility of the chest x-ray to diagnose LV dysfunction concluded that redistribution and cardiomegaly were the best predictors of increased preload and reduced ejection fraction, respectively.[30]

Electrocardiogram

Obtain an electrocardiogram to diagnose frequent conditions that contribute to postoperative heart failure, including acute ischemia or injury, tachyarrhythmias (atrial fibrillation, atrial flutter, persistent sinus tachycardia), or complete heart block.

Echocardiography

Consider echocardiography in all patients with new-onset postoperative heart failure. It allows for evaluation of left ventricular systolic function, valvular abnormalities, presence of diastolic dysfunction, regional wall motion abnormalities, pericardial thickening in constrictive pericarditis, right ventricular size and function in right heart failure, and cardiac output.

Management

Treating underlying conditions—Since the most frequent causes of postoperative heart failure are ischemia, volume overload, tachyarrhythmias, hypertension, and anemia, treatment strategies should focus on improvement or correction of these conditions.

Ischemic heart failure—See Chapters 19 and 20 for management of ACS. Consult with the surgical service before starting any type of anticoagulation. Consider consultation with cardiology for further recommendations on noninvasive or possible invasive strategies

Volume Overload—Use diuretics. Consider addition of β-blockers (not acutely) and ACE inhibitors in patients with decreased left ventricular systolic function.

Tachyarrhythmias—See management of postoperative arrhythmias below.

Hypertension—Initiate or augment diuretic therapy. Consider initiation or increasing dose of ACE inhibitors or β-blockers.

Postoperative Anemia—Cautiously transfuse if necessary to alleviate symptoms.

ARRHYTHMIAS

Background

Cardiac arrhythmias are common in the postoperative period, but most are clinically benign. A study using continuous telemetry for postoperative patients revealed that more than 80% of patients may have postoperative arrhythmias, but only 5% were deemed to be clinically important.[31]

Supraventricular arrhythmias—A prospective cohort study of 4,181 patients undergoing major noncardiac surgery found that 6.1% had a sustained supraventricular arrhythmia in the postoperative setting, of which 87% required specific therapy.[32] The development of supraventricular arrhythmias is associated with an increased risk of an acute cardiac event (congestive heart failure, MI, unstable angina), infection, or cerebrovascular acci-

dent. These arrhythmias were associated with a 33% increase in the length of hospital stay.

Ventricular arrhythmias—Sustained, malignant ventricular arrhythmias occur in up to 2% of patients after open cardiac procedures but are very infrequent after noncardiac surgery.[33] In a study of 230 male patients with or at high risk for coronary artery disease undergoing major noncardiac surgery, 36% experienced significant ventricular arrhythmias (defined as the presence of >30 ventricular premature contractions per hour or ventricular tachycardia); however, sustained ventricular tachycardia and ventricular fibrillation did not occur.[34]

Risk Factors and Pathophysiology

Patient-specific risk factors for arrhythmias include advancing age (>50 year or older), personal history of arrhythmias, congestive heart failure, and certain preoperative ECG abnormalities.[32,33,35,36]

In one study, atrial abnormalities and intra-atrial conduction delay on baseline 12-lead ECG increased the risk for postoperative atrial fibrillation or atrial flutter.[37] A second, large prospective cohort study found that premature atrial complexes on a preoperative baseline ECG were associated with an increased chance of developing a postoperative supraventricular arrhythmia (OR 2.1, CI 1.3–3.4).[32]

The presence of bundle branch block does not appear to increase risk of postoperative arrhythmia.[38,39] Multiple small studies have failed to show an increase in the incidence of new high-grade heart block in patients with preoperative bifascicular block.[40-42]

Postoperative stress predisposes patients to development of arrhythmias. Precipitating factors include hypoxemia, hypercarbia, myocardial ischemia, endogenous or exogenous catecholamines, electrolyte or acid-base imbalances, and drug effects, as well as mechanical factors, such as instrumentation.[43]

Clinical Assessment/Evaluation

In the evaluation of a new postoperative arrhythmia, the first principle is to treat the patient rather than the electrocardiogram. Clinical assessment includes evaluation of pulse, blood pressure, peripheral perfusion, and the presence of myocardial ischemia and congestive heart failure.

If the patient is hemodynamically stable, obtain a12-lead ECG, focused history, and examination. If not, see treatment below. Obtain documentation of left ventricular function, if available. Search for infectious, pulmonary, or electrolyte abnormalities.

Recommendations/Management

Hemodynamically unstable patients—If the patient loses consciousness or becomes hemodynamically unstable in the presence of a tachyarrhythmia other than sinus tachycardia, prompt electrical cardioversion is indicated. Initiate strict ACLS protocol for patients with hemodynamically unstable tachyarrhythmias or bradyarrhythmias.[44]

Stable patients—There is more time to establish the diagnosis and decide on the most appropriate course of treatment (Table 110-1).

Table 110-1 Treatment of Newly Diagnosed Postoperative Arrhythmias

Arrhythmia	Recommendations
Atrial/ventricular ectopy	Evaluate and correct electrolyte abnormalities if applicable; no treatment indicated.
Sinus tachycardia	Evaluate and treat specific conditions such as, pain, anxiety, occult hypovolemia, infection, hypoxia, hypercarbia, alcohol withdrawal, CHF; rate control is rarely indicated.
Atrial fibrillation	Initiate rate control with β-blocking or calcium-channel blocking drugs; give digoxin to patients with (relative) hypotension.
	If surgical bleeding risk is acceptable and atrial fibrillation lasts >48 hr, start anticoagulation with heparin followed by warfarin.
	Cardioversion indicated if hemodynamically unstable, severe symptoms, or contraindications to anticoagulation.
	Consider drug conversion with amiodarone.
Atrial flutter	Initiate rate control, as with atrial fibrillation.
	Anticoagulate if no conversion to NSR in 48 hours, if surgically acceptable bleeding risk.
	Cardioversion indicated if hemodynamically unstable, severe symptoms, or contraindications to anticoagulation.
	Give ibutilide, 1 mg IV, for drug cardioversion.
Reentrant supraventricular arrhythmias: AV nodal reentrant tachycardia, and AV reentrant tachycardia	Treat initially with vagal maneuvers (carotid sinus massage). If unsuccessful, try adenosine, β-blockers, or calcium-channel blockers.
	If hemodynamically unstable perform DCCV. For recurrent arrhythmias, initiate chronic β-blocker or calcium-channel blocker therapy.
Multifocal atrial tachycardia	Evaluate and treat any underlying pulmonary complications.
	Use β-blockers or calcium-channel blockers for rate control. Consider trial of amiodarone. DCCV is ineffective.
Ectopic atrial tachycardia	Evaluate and treat any underlying pulmonary complications. Consider digitalis intoxication If associated with AV block (e.g., 2 : 1 AV block).
	Use β-blockers or calcium-channel blockers for rate control. Consider trial of amiodarone.
Nonsustained ventricular tachycardia	Evaluate for secondary causes, such as electrolyte abnormalities or myocardial ischemia.
	Use β-blockers to reduce episodes of NSVT.
	No specific therapy is indicated for patients with hemodynamically insignificant NSVT.
Sustained wide complex tachycardias	Consider all wide complex tachycardias to be ventricular in origin, in absence of convincing evidence to the contrary.
	Obtain a 12-lead ECG in all hemodynamically tolerated, wide complex tachycardias.
	Perform DCCV in all hemodynamically unstable, wide complex tachycardias.
	Use epinephrine or vasopressin for initial hemodynamic.
	Give IV amiodarone or lidocaine after cardioversion for arrhythmia suppression.
Sinus node dysfunction, AV Wenckebach, and junctional rhythms	No specific therapy if hemodynamically stable.
	Identify initiators, such as laryngoscopy, endotracheal suctioning, pain, drugs, and spinal anesthetics.
	Give IV atropine if hemodynamically unstable.
New left or right bundle branch block	Evaluate for occult myocardial ischemia with serial enzymes and ECG.
	If sinus tachycardia or atrial fibrillation with rapid ventricular response is present, control rate with AV nodal drugs; often new bundle branch block is rate related.
High-grade or complete heart block	Discontinue negative chronotropic (rate slowing) drugs.
	Give IV atropine.
	Initiate transcutaneous pacing immediately if hypotension is present and atropine is unsuccessful.

AV—atrioventricular; CABG—coronary artery bypass graft; DCCV—direct current cardioversion; ECG—electrocardiogram; NSR—normal sinus rhythm; NSVT—nonsustained ventricular tachycardia; CHF—congestive heart failure.

Adapted from: McClennen S, Zimetbaum J. Perioperative Management of Rhythm and Conduction Disorders. http://pier.acponline.org/physicians/diseases/periopr877/periop877.html. Accessed: 2005 March 14. In: PIER (online database). Philadelphia: American College of Physicians, 2005.

Key Points

- The majority of fatal perioperative MIs are related to disruption of an atherosclerotic plaque in areas without a critical fixed coronary stenosis. Therefore, preoperative CABG or PCI may not necessarily prevent perioperative MIs.

- The presence of new RWMA in preoperative stress echocardiography increases the risk of perioperative cardiac death, nonfatal MI, or unstable angina.

- Routine surveillance for a perioperative MI should be reserved for patients who develop signs of cardiac ischemia or hemodynamic compromise intraoperatively or for those who are considered high risk by patient- or surgery-specific risk factors.

- HF is the most frequently encountered postoperative cardiac complication of noncardiac surgery.

- Cardiac arrhythmias are common in the postoperative period, but most are clinically benign.

- In the evaluation of a new postoperative arrhythmia, the first principle is to treat the patient rather than the ECG.

SUGGESTED READING

Poldermans D, Arnese M, Fioretti PM, et al. Sustained prognostic value of dobutamine stress echocardiography for late cardiac events after major noncardiac vascular surgery. Circulation 1997; 95:53–58.

Eagle KA, Berger PB, Calkins H, et al. Guideline Update for Perioperative Cardiovascular Evaluation for Noncardiac Surgery-Executive Summary: A Report of the American College of Cardiology/American Heart Association Task Force on Practice Guidelines (Committee to Update the 1996 Guidelines on Perioperative Cardiovascular Evaluation for Noncardiac Surgery). Anesth Analg 2002; 94:1052–1064.

Das MK, Pellikka PA, Mahoney DW, et al. Assessment of cardiac risk before nonvascular surgery: dobutamine stress echocardiography in 530 patients. J Am Coll Cardiol 2000; 35:1647–1653.

Maisel AS, Krishnaswamy P, Nowak RM, et al. Breathing Not Properly Multinational Study Investigators. Rapid measurement of B-type natriuretic peptide in the emergency diagnosis of heart failure. N Engl J Med 2002; 347:161–167.

CHAPTER ONE HUNDRED AND ELEVEN

Non-cardiac Postoperative Complications

Kulsum K. Casey, DO, and Jeanne M. Huddleston, MD, FACP

PULMONARY

Pulmonary complications significantly contribute to postoperative morbidity and mortality. Postoperative mortality is higher in patients who have experienced pulmonary complications; approximately 25% of deaths occurring within 6 days of surgery are related to postoperative pulmonary complications.[1] The clinically important postoperative pulmonary complications include pneumonia, acute respiratory distress syndrome, respiratory failure, and atelectasis requiring bronchoscopy. Variable definition of what constitutes a postoperative pulmonary complication makes interpreting the medical literature difficult. Microatelectasis and mild episodes of bronchospasm rarely prolong hospitalization or result in mortality.

Respiratory Failure

Background

The most concerning postoperative pulmonary complication is respiratory failure defined as mechanical ventilation for >48 hours after surgery or reintubation and mechanical ventilation after postoperative extubation. In an evaluation of Medicare patients in Pennsylvania, respiratory compromise was associated with a 7.2-fold increase in the odds of dying (95% CI 4.5–11.6).[2]

Risk Factors and Pathophysiology

The development of respiratory failure postoperatively is associated with patient-specific preoperative markers and surgery-specific factors as noted in Chapter 103.[1,3–5] These are very similar to the risk factors for developing postoperative pneumonia. The main mechanisms and differential diagnosis for respiratory failure are the same as in the nonoperative setting. However, the likelihood of some diagnoses, such as pulmonary emboli or hypoventilation from oversedation, is increased in the postoperative setting (Table 111-1).

Mechanisms of Postoperative Respiratory Failure

- *Hypoventilation:* Inadequate ventilation to meet the body's requirements for removal of carbon dioxide.
- *Ventilation/Perfusion ($\dot{V}/\dot{Q}$) mismatching:* This is the most common cause of hypoxemia. For hypoxemia to occur, mismatch must happen in areas of the lung where ventilation is decreased out of proportion to perfusion.
- *Shunt:* This is a situation of extreme $\dot{V}/\dot{Q}$ mismatch. Shunt is distinguished from $\dot{V}/\dot{Q}$ mismatch by the magnitude of the increased FiO_2 required to provide adequate arterial oxygenation. In an area of shunt, added O_2 cannot reach alveoli since there is no ventilation exchange, and blood flowing past these areas of filled or collapsed alveoli has pO_2 tensions equal to that of mixed venous blood.

Clinical Assessment/Evaluation

The clinical assessment and evaluation of a patient with potential respiratory failure in the surgical setting is identical to that in the nonoperative setting.

Recommendations/Management

- *Initial treatment:* Immediately establish an open airway, and provide oxygen supplementation. For clinically unstable patients, implement advanced cardiac life support (ACLS) protocol immediately, and transfer the patient to the appropriate level of intensive care.
- Subsequent treatment is dependent upon cause:
- *Hypoventilation:* The goal is to increase alveolar ventilation. Oxygen supplementation will not improve respiratory acidosis that may have developed. If the cause of hypoventilation is oversedation with pain medication or sedatives, reverse narcotics with Narcan and provide ventilatory support as needed. Treat any components of airflow obstruction with bronchodilators.
- *$\dot{V}/\dot{Q}$ mismatching:* Hypoxemia will be corrected with relatively little oxygen supplementation. The definitive treatment is the reversal or treatment of the cause (asthma, pulmonary emboli, emphysema) similar to that in the nonoperative setting. The only caution would be if the $\dot{V}/\dot{Q}$ mismatch were secondary to a pulmonary embolus, since anticoagulation poses risks of excessive bleeding in the immediate postoperative course.
- *Shunt:* Hypoxemia will not be completely corrected in this setting, even with high levels of oxygen supplementation. Treatment is dependent on the cause and parallels the nonoperative setting (pneumonia with significant pulmonary consolidation, lobar collapse, acute lung injury, cardiogenic pulmonary edema, large pulmonary emboli).
- Instruct every patient, ideally before surgery, on deep breathing exercises and/or incentive spirometry.

Table III-I Risk Factors for Postoperative Pulmonary Complications

Patient-specific risk factors	Nutritional	Weight loss >10% 6 months preceding surgery
		Low albumin
	Social	Smoking (>40 pack-years)
		Alcohol use
	Comorbidities	Impaired sensorium
		Chronic obstructive pulmonary disease
		Cerebrovascular accidents
		Long-term steroid use
		Elevated blood urea nitrogen levels
		Obstructive sleep apnea
	Functional status	High ASA classification
		Dependent for any activities of daily living
		Unable to climb one flight of stairs
Surgery-specific risk factors	Anesthetic	General anesthesia
	Time	Longer preoperative hospitalization
		Longer operative procedures

Postoperative Pneumonia

Nosocomial pneumonias in surgical patients are characterized by the high frequency of early-onset infections and the high proportion of gram-negative and staphylococci bacteria isolates. In an evaluation of Pennsylvania Medicare patients, pneumonia was associated with a 5-fold increase in the odds of dying within the first 60 postoperative days (95% CI 2.1–12.1).[2]

Risk Factors and Pathophysiology

The development of postoperative pneumonia is associated with patient-specific preoperative markers and surgery-specific factors as detailed in Chapter 103,[1,3,4] which are similar to those for developing postoperative respiratory failure. The majority of cases of postoperative pneumonia are detected and diagnosed between postoperative day 4 and 5, but it may occur up to 9 days after surgery.

Clinical Assessment

If you suspect the patient has pneumonia postoperatively, ensure the patient is hemodynamically stable, and document assessment of oxygenation. Also document a directed clinical history for pneumonia-related symptoms: shortness of breath, cough, pleuritic chest pain severity, fever, chills or rigors, diaphoresis, and mental status. Perform a chest examination for signs of pneumonia auscultating for crackles, diminished breath sounds, bronchial breath sounds in the periphery, and presence or absence of egophony. Percuss for areas of decreased tympany.

Review recent medical history for prior pulmonary infections, risk factors for aspiration, immunization status, and preexisting pulmonary disease. Review the operative record for evidence of difficulty at the time of intubation or extubation that may signal aspiration. Obtain laboratory studies, including complete blood count with white blood cell count differential and electrolyte panel. If the patient has not been on antibiotics for other reasons, a set of blood cultures may be helpful. If there is evidence of new tachycardia or irregularity of heartbeat, obtain an electrocardiogram to rule out concomitant development of a new arrhythmia or myocardial ischemia. Examine for new signs of congestive heart failure or pulmonary edema as well. Obtain chest x-ray. Ideally, this should be taken in the radiology department with both posterior to anterior (PA) and lateral views; however, this may not be possible, depending on the time since surgery. Compare the x-ray to any available prior chest x-rays.

Recommendations/Management

Transfer hemodynamically unstable patients secondary to sepsis to the appropriate care unit for aggressive resuscitation. Provide oxygenation support for any level of hypoxemia. Provide ventilatory support in the form of bilateral positive airway pressure (BiPAP) or intubation for significant levels of hypercarbia. Instruct every patient postoperatively on deep breathing exercises and/or incentive spirometry.

Initial antimicrobial therapy of postoperative pneumonia should empirically cover *Enterobacteriaceae,* streptococci, and *Staphylococcus aureus.* Tailor antibiotics to local microbial resistance patterns and bacterial sensitivities once reported. Choice of an oral or intravenous route of antibiotic therapy depends on the severity of the pneumonia and the extent of systemic illness at the time of detection and diagnosis.

If the patient remains significantly febrile after 3 days of antibiotic therapy, repeat a chest x-ray to rule out a parapneumonic effusion that may require a thoracentesis. At the time of discharge, ensure that there is timely medical follow-up with the patient's primary care provider (PCP). Communicate to the PCP that the patient will require clinical evaluation following completion of antibiotic therapy to ensure adequate duration of treatment and a repeat chest x-ray in 6 weeks to verify resolution of a pulmonary infiltrate. Counsel patients regarding smoking cessation, and evaluate for indications for pneumococcal and influenza vaccination. Document each of these in the medical record.

RENAL ABNORMALITIES

Background

Acute renal failure (ARF) is characterized by a rapid decline in glomerular filtration rate (GFR), disruption in extracellular fluid volume, electrolyte and acid-base balance, and accumulation of nitrogenous wastes. The incidence of postoperative acute renal failure (ARF) has been reported to be 1–17%.[6] The development of even mild renal dysfunction is associated with poor outcome.[7]

Blood loss, fluid shifts, surgical manipulation, and anesthesia may place surgical patients at risk for developing ARF postoperatively. Some surgical procedures (cardiothoracic, renal and liver transplantation, urologic, pancreatic, and obstetrical) are more likely to be associated with postoperative ARF.[8]

Pathophysiology

Due to variation in pathophysiology, ARF is traditionally differentiated as prerenal and postrenal azotemia and intrinsic ARF.

Prerenal azotemia. This is the most common form of ARF. Due to numerous causes (Table 111-2) a significant decline in renal arterial blood flow eventually results in a decline in GFR. Initially, decreasing systemic arterial pressure results in a series of responses including the activation of the sympathetic nervous system and the renin-angiotensin-aldosterone system. This autoregulation helps maintain systemic blood pressure. Compensatory mechanisms, such as afferent arteriole dilatation (through prostaglandins) and efferent arteriolar vasoconstriction (induced by angiotensin II), help maintain intraglomerular pressure, thereby preserving tubular integrity. When this balance in overwhelmed and renal tubules become ischemic, acute tubular necrosis develops (ATN).

Intrinsic renal failure. Intrinsic renal failure may be categorized as (1) ATN; (2) acute interstitial nephritis; (3) acute glomerulonephritis or vasculitis; and (4) renal vascular disease. ATN is the most common cause of postoperative intrinsic ARF. As noted above, ATN may result from severe renal hypoperfusion (ischemic ATN) that is not quickly reversed. ATN may also develop as a result of toxins (Table 111-3) damaging renal tubules. The next most common type of postoperative intrinsic renal failure is interstitial nephritis, which results from cell-mediated immune responses to medications or, less often, infections or immunologic disorders.

Postrenal azotemia. Postrenal azotemia results from obstruction of the urethra, bladder neck, or from both ureters leading to the bladder. If both kidneys are present, unilateral ureteral obstruction can lead to ARF only if the other kidney is diseased. Postoperative causes may include blood clots, kidney stones, and bilateral papillary necrosis. Aside from anatomical obstruction, neurogenic bladder (resulting from surgery, anticholinergics) can also lead to renal distention and subsequent failure.

Clinical Assessment and Evaluation

Patients who develop ARF are frequently asymptomatic. Initial recognition is often due to a decline in a patient's urine output or by a routine serum chemistry panel revealing an increase blood urea nitrogen (BUN) and creatinine levels.

Initial assessment includes a careful history and physical examination. Review the perioperative record for evidence of intraop-

Table 111-3 Drugs and Toxins Associated with Renal Failure
Nephrotoxic drugs
ACE inhibitors
Aspirin
NSAIDs
Immunosuppressive agents (cisplatinum, cyclosporine)
Sulfonamides
Radiocontrast agents
Diuretics
Allopurinol
Methotrexate
Antibiotics (aminoglycosides, amphotericin B, ciprofloxacin, cephalosporins)
Endogenous nephrotoxins
Myoglobin
Hemoglobin
Uric acid
Paraproteins

ACE—angiotensin-converting enzyme; NSAIDs—nonsteroidal anti-inflammatory drugs

Table 111-2 Causes of Prerenal Acute Renal Failure

Intravascular Volume Depletion	Decreased Cardiac Output	Systemic Vasodilatation/Change in Renal Vascular Resistance
Massive hemorrhage renal losses (*excessive diuresis, diabetes insipidus*)	Myocardial disease (*infarction, cardiomyopathy*)	Sepsis
Gastrointestinal losses (*vomiting, diarrhea, nasogastric suctioning*)	Valvular disease	Anaphylaxis
Dehydration	Conduction system abnormality (*bradycardia, tachyarrhythmia*)	Medications preventing renal arteriolar vasodilatation (*NSAIDs, anesthetics, high-dose dopamine, epinephrine, norepinephrine*)
Skin and mucous membrane loss (*burns, hyperthermia*)	Cardiac tamponade Pulmonary embolism	Medications preventing efferent renal arteriolar constriction (*ACE inhibitors*)
Extravascular space sequestration (*hypoalbuminemia, pancreatitis, cirrhosis*)	Positive-pressure mechanical ventilation	

ACE—angiotensin-converting enzyme; NSAIDs—nonsteroidal anti-inflammatory drugs

Table 111-4 Laboratory Assessment in the Diagnosis of Acute Renal Failure

Serum and Urine Chemistry	Prerenal Azotemia	Postrenal Azotemia	INTRINSIC ARF	
			ATN	Interstitial Nephritis
Serum BUN/creatinine ratio	>20 : 1	———	<20 : 1	<20 : 1
Urine osmolality (mOsm/kg H2O)	>500	———	<350	———
Urine sodium concentration (mmol/L)	<10–20	———	>20	———
Fractional excretion of sodium (FENa)%	<1	———	>1	———
Urine/plasma creatinine	>40	<20	<20	<20
Urine sediment	Few red or white blood cells or hyaline casts, relatively benign	Often normal	Muddy brown granular casts	White blood cells/casts ± eosinophils (<5%)

*——— denotes variable results.

erative hypotension, significant blood loss, and use of nephrotoxic agents (Table 111-4). Assess the patient for adequacy of blood perfusion, volume status (skin turgor, pulmonary edema), abdominal flank pain, bladder distention and Foley catheter placement, skin changes, and evidence of vascular occlusion. Serum chemistry and urinalysis with microscopy can help determine the type of ARF (see Table 111-4).

If postrenal obstruction is suspected, perform a renal and bladder ultrasound, or attempt catheterization.

Management

Management of ARF depends on the underlying cause. For patients who develop prerenal azotemia due to volume depletion, immediate and aggressive intravenous hydration may reverse renal damage. Isotonic crystalloid including 0.9% sodium chloride, lactated Ringer's, and isotonic bicarbonate solutions can improve renal perfusion by remaining intravascularly compared to hypotonic solutions. Similarly, patients with prerenal azotemia due to significant blood loss would benefit most by immediate resuscitation with packed red blood cell transfusions. For drug-induced renal failure, discontinue the suspected causative medication (see Table 111-4), and monitor renal function. Obtain a nephrology consultation for patients who do not respond to initial efforts.

ANEMIA

Background

Anemia after surgery is due to excessive blood loss during surgery as well as to other contributing factors (Box 111-1) that may lead to bleeding. Hip fracture repair, hip and knee replacements, and cardiothoracic surgery have a high risk for postoperative anemia. Prior to the 1980s, patients who had hemoglobin levels less than 10 g/dL after surgery routinely received a blood transfusion because oxygen delivery was thought to be optimum at this level. Due to the subsequent rise in transfusion-related infections (HIV and hepatitis C), transfusion indications were re-evaluated. Although studies now show that healthy patients can tolerate lower Hb levels, there is evidence that markedly lower levels after surgery are associated with increasing mortality.[9]

Box 111-1 Factors Associated with Post Surgical Bleeding

Inadequate surgical hemostasis

Use of perioperative anticoagulants (unfractionated or low molecular weight heparin, warfarin)

Platelet dysfunction (often due to ASA or NSAIDs)

Clotting factor depletion

Hemodilution, with dilutional thrombocytopenia and coagulopathy

ASA—Aspinal; NSAIDs—nonsteroidal anti-inflammatory drugs

Pathophysiology

The most important physiologic aspect of hemoglobin is its capacity to deliver oxygen to vital tissue. Oxygen delivery at rest is typically four times greater than tissue consumption requirements. By maintaining intravascular volume, significant blood loss may be tolerated. In addition, as hemoglobin levels decline, a number of compensatory mechanisms help maintain tissue oxygen perfusion. These changes include increases in cardiac stroke volume and heart rate, reduction in systemic vascular resistance, and increased extraction of oxygen by the tissues. Complications occur when these mechanisms are inadequate, either due to cardiopulmonary disease or significant blood loss, leading to tissue hypoxemia.

Clinical Assessment and Evaluation

Most patients after surgery only perform low intensity activity. Without exertion, patients with mild-to-moderate anemia may not be symptomatic. Detection of anemia in these patients is often a laboratory finding. Patients with severe anemia (<6 g/dL) are more likely symptomatic. Initial symptoms may be exertional chest pain or shortness of breath and weakness. Physical examination may reveal pallor, tachycardia followed by hypotension, and decreased consciousness. As intravascular volume is depleted, urine output may decrease. It is important to note that many patients (especially young, healthy patients) may not demonstrate any symptoms, even with levels consistent with tissue hypoxia.

Management

The management of anemia not only includes reversing the underlying cause and treating symptoms but also preventing subsequent complications (such as myocardial ischemia in patients with coronary artery disease) from decreased oxygen perfusion. For stable patients with active bleeding, initially withhold medications that inhibit or disrupt coagulation (e.g. heparin, warfarin, aspinal [ASA], nonsteroidal anti-inflammatory drug [NSAID]) until the bleeding is controlled. Consider resuming these medications on a case-by-case basis, weighing risks and benefits. In addition, hold antihypertensive medications if there is a risk of hypotension.

Due to the paucity of large randomized trials, there are no clear guidelines for when to transfuse blood. According to the American Society of Anesthesiology, a "transfusion trigger" should no longer be used, and the decision for transfusion should be based on clinical factors and risks of complications.[10] However, it is generally accepted that patients with Hb levels <6 g/dL should receive a transfusion. Patients with cardiovascular risks should probably be transfused at higher levels (closer to 9 g/dL). Table 111-5 lists the various types of anemia treatment and their indications.

Prevention

Certain measures may be taken for patients who are at risk for postoperative anemia:

- *Iron supplementation*—Iron may be given orally or intravenously (IV). Oral iron requires weeks to build stores, and absorption is decreased in patients who already have normal stores. However, the body can utilize IV iron immediately, which makes erythropoiesis more effective. Asymptomatic patients with low hemoglobin levels (<12 g/dL) prior to emergent surgery may

benefit from the intravenous form. An initial dose (100 mg iron sucrose) can be given on admission and repeated just before surgery.

- *Pre-donation of autologous blood*—This transfusing-saving strategy requires patients to donate their own blood prior to surgery so that it can be used during or after surgery for blood loss or anemia. The benefits include prevention of transfusion-related infection and immune-related complications. To prevent subsequent anemia due to removal of blood, patients are given iron supplementation and may also be given erythropoietin therapy to increase their hemoglobin. Major disadvantages of this procedure are inconvenience for the patients and the high rate of unused blood that is wasted.
- *Surgical and blood-saving techniques*—Acute normovolemic hemodilution (ANH), intraoperative cell salvage, and postoperative reinfusion of blood can minimize the need for postoperative transfusions.
- *Other pharmacologic agents*—Agents that may aid in controlling bleeding include fibrin seal (not yet approved in the United States), antifibrinolytics, desmopressin (increases circulating factor VIII and von Willebrand factor), and aprotinin (inhibits hemostasis through multiple mechanisms). More studies are needed to evaluate efficacy in surgical patients.

NEUROLOGIC COMPLICATIONS

Background

Postoperative neurologic complications may include delirium, seizure, neuroleptic malignant syndrome (NMS), and cerebrovascular disease (CVA). Delirium is by far the most of these complications. Defined as a global impairment that is often transient, DSM-IV (*Diagnostic and Statistical Manual of Mental Disorders, Fourth Edition*) characterizes delirium as: reduced ability to maintain attention to external stimuli, disorganized thinking, reduced consciousness, perceptual disturbances, disturbances of wake cycle, change in psychomotor activity, disorientation, and

Table 111-5 Treatment for Postoperative Anemia

Treatment Options for Postoperative Anemia	Description and Usage	Comments
Packed red blood cells	**Allogenic** Blood donated by persons other than the recipient of the transfusion. Autologous blood removed from patient prior to surgery. Indications for use are the same for allogenic transfusion.	Preferred treatment for acute blood loss and postoperative anemia. Allogenic blood accounts for the vast majority of transfusions Each unit will raise the hematocrit by roughly 3%.
Leukocyte-depleted blood products	Used in patients who are chronically transfused, had previous transfusion related reactions, or may be transplant recipients	Costly
Recombinant human erythropoietin (EPO)	To be used in anemic patients (target level between 10 and 12 g/dL) with reduced erythropoietin levels (renal insufficiency/failure) May also be used in patients undergoing autologous transfusion to build Hb level prior to surgery.	Patients should be hemodynamically stable. Patients should be ruled out for iron deficiency and other causes of anemia. Require adequate iron, folate, and vitamin B_{12} stores.
Oral iron supplementation	Used in stable patients with low risk of anemia-induced complications	Patients often have gastrointestinal intolerance including nausea, vomiting, constipation, and diarrhea

memory impairment. Elderly patients are often at great risk for developing postoperative delirium due to underlying cognitive impairment. In addition, postoperative delirium may lead to functional decline in addition to increased mortality.

Pathophysiology

The pathophysiology of postoperative delirium or cognitive impairment is based on precipitating factors. Medications, most commonly residual anesthetics and medications used for pain or sedation, can often result in postoperative neurologic changes. Typically, these changes resolve once the medication is cleared from the body. Elderly patients with impaired renal function are particularly at risk, due to prolonged plasma levels of medications.

Delirium unrelated to medications is often a result of inadequate cerebral oxygenation due to hypotension, hypoxemia, or hypercapnia (seen in patients with chronic lung disease). Glucose abnormality, electrolyte disturbances (particularly hyponatremia from hemodilution), and infection may also result in delirium.

Clinical Assessment and Evaluation

The initial assessment should include a thorough evaluation of possible precipitating factors. History should include recent medication use (particularly narcotics, benzodiazepines, anticholinergics, and antihistamines), pain level, previous use of hearing and visual aids, sleep/wake cycle, and previous history of delirium (and its cause). Along with vitals and temperature, the physical examination should evaluate for evidence of infection (wound, lung, or urine), bleed or other neurologic symptoms (including speech/swallow disturbances, paresis, and tremors), bowel or bladder obstruction, and dehydration.

Obtain serum chemistries, to evaluate glucose and electrolyte abnormalities, along with a urinalysis for detection of urinary tract infection. There is usually no need for imaging studies such as computed tomography (CT) scan or magnetic resonance imaging (MRI), unless there is suspicion of a cerebrovascular accident (CVA) or mass effect. Perform an electroencephalogram (EEG) if there is concern of seizures.

Management

The management of postoperative neurologic changes depends on the underlying cause. For patients with delirium, early recognition and reversal of underlying cause is crucial.
- Discontinue medications that may contribute to impaired cognitive function.
- Correct glucose and electrolyte abnormalities.
- Treat hypoxemia, hypotension, dehydration, and hypercapnia immediately.
- Minimize agitation (particularly in the elderly), which may also improve cognitive function and prevent further episodes. Such interventions include removal of restraints and Foley catheter, maximizing bowel and bladder function, noise reduction, and improving sleep/wake cycle.

Only use medications such as neuroleptics and benzodiazepine (BZDs) to prevent patient harm. Although BZDs have a rapid onset, they may worsen confusion. Haldol is the most studied neuroleptic for delirium and can be given PO, IV, or IM. Starting dose for IV is typically 2–10 mg repeated every 20–30 minutes for up to 6 hours. Starting dose for IM is 5 mg, and for oral it is 5–10 mg (usually total dose not to exceed 20 mg for sedation). Reduce the dose in elderly patients. Monitor patients receiving IV dosing for QTc prolongation, hypotension, and arrhythmias. Newer atypical antipsychotics (risperidone and olanzapine) are also being used, although they are less well studied.

The development of a CVA is rare after surgery. Patients who do develop a postoperative CVA should be evaluated with CT/MRI or magnetic resonance arteriogram (MRA), carotid Doppler, and echocardiography. There is much debate about treatment for postoperative CVA. The use of tissue type plasminogen activator (tPA) is generally contraindicated in postsurgical patients. Individually assess the risks and benefits of thrombolysis. Consider intra-arterial thrombolytic therapy for patients with proven thrombosis.

The management of seizures depends on the underlying cause. Patients with a history of seizures may have had their antiepileptic medications held perioperatively and may need a loading dose of antiepileptics to achieve a steady state. This is rare, since these medications have a long half-life, and patients who were previously well controlled usually do not develop postoperative seizures. A metabolic abnormality (specifically, electrolyte or glucose) is usually the cause in patients without a history of epilepsy. With prompt correction, further treatment is usually not necessary.

Key Points

- The clinical assessment and evaluation of a patient with potential respiratory failure in the surgical setting is identical to that in the nonoperative setting.

- Initial antimicrobial therapy of postoperative pneumonia should empirically cover *Enterobacteriaceae*, streptococci, and *Staphylococcus aureus*.

- Postoperative acute renal failure is more likely after the following types of surgery: cardiothoracic, renal and liver transplantation, urologic, pancreatic, and obstetric.[8]

- For patients who develop prerenal azotemia due to volume depletion, immediate and aggressive intravenous hydration may reverse renal damage.

- According to the American Society of Anesthesiology, a "transfusion trigger" should no longer be used, and the decision for transfusion should be based on clinical factors and risks of complications.[10]

SUGGESTED READINGS

Reddy VG. Prevention of postoperative acute renal failure. J Postgrad Med 2002; 48:64–70.

Sural S, Sharma RK. Etiology, prognosis and outcome of post-operative acute renal failure. Renal Failure 2000; 22:88–97.

CHAPTER ONE HUNDRED AND TWELVE

Surgical Site Infection Prophylaxis

James Stone, MD, Jason Stein, MD, and James Steinberg, MD

BACKGROUND

Surgical site infections (SSIs) are associated with significant morbidity and high economic costs. Patients who develop an SSI have an average increased hospital length of stay (LOS) of 7 days and are 60% more likely to spend time in the intensive care unit than are patients without an SSI. A patient with an SSI is five times more likely to be readmitted to the hospital and is twice as likely to die. According to CDC's National Nosocomial Infections Surveillance System, SSIs add cost ranging from $2,700 to $26,000 per episode.[1] Given the common involvement of hospitalists in co-management of surgical care, they have an opportunity to work within the system of care delivery to reduce the high morbidity and financial costs of SSIs. This chapter reviews the factors contributing to SSIs and will focus on interventions the hospitalist can make to reduce surgical site infection risk.

PREVALENCE AND ETIOLOGY

Unfortunately, surgical site infections are common. Among health care–acquired infections, SSIs rank second only to urinary tract infections in frequency and above bloodstream infections and nosocomial pneumonia. There are approximately 30 million operations annually in the United States, and an SSI complicates 1–5% of clean extra-abdominal sites. The rate is much higher for complicated intra-abdominal operations, approaching 20%.

Microorganisms that cause SSIs usually gain access to the operative site during the procedure. Consequently, the perioperative period is the most crucial for modifying the risk of SSI. Although hospitalists have little control of events that occur in the operating room, by offering clinical expertise in pre- and postoperative management, hospital medicine programs can help patients and hospital systems lower morbidity, mortality, and costs associated with this complication. Adherence to best practices, and therefore success, requires multidisciplinary cooperation. Host factors also contribute to the development of postoperative infections, including diabetes, advanced age, obesity, tobacco use, malnutrition, other immunosuppression and infection, or colonization at other body sites. Some of these are modifiable.

Several important interventions that have direct impact on decreasing SSI fall under the control of the anesthesia and surgical teams, such as administering perioperative oxygen, ensuring perioperative normothermia, and surgical site preparation.[2] These are reviewed at the end of the chapter.

PREVENTION OF SSI—ANTIMICROBIAL PROPHYLAXIS

Perioperative prophylactic antibiotics effectively reduce the postoperative infection rates following a variety of operative procedures. Timing of the preoperative dose is critical; infection rates are higher if the antibiotic is administered more than 2 hours before surgery or after the incision is made. One preincisional dose is usually sufficient, although a second dose administered during procedures that last more than 3 to 4 hours may be indicated. Some authorities recommend the continued administration of prophylactic antibiotics for 24 hours after surgery. Antibiotics given beyond this time should be considered therapeutic and not prophylactic. Prolonging therapy longer than 48 hours in the absence of established infection should be avoided because of the increased cost and the increased likelihood of colonization and infection with antibiotic resistant bacteria. The use of broad-spectrum agents also exerts selective pressure on the microbiologic flora. These agents, including third-generation cephalosporins, have limited role in perioperative prophylaxis.

In June 2004, the National Surgical Infection Prevention Project (NSIPP) published an advisory statement on antimicrobial prophylaxis in which it outlined three performance measures for quality improvement in prevention of SSIs:

1. The proportion of patients who have parenteral antimicrobial prophylaxis initiated within 1 hour before surgical incision
2. The proportion of patients provided with a prophylactic antimicrobial agent that is consistent with currently published guidelines
3. The proportion of patients whose prophylactic antimicrobial therapy is discontinued within 24 hours after the end of surgery[3]

Fully administering the appropriate antibiotic within 60 minutes of incision ensures that serum and tissue drug levels exceed the minimum inhibitory concentrations (MICs) of the most likely contaminating organisms. Dosing the antibiotic immediately prior to the start of surgery also provides the best opportunity to extend therapeutic levels for the duration of the surgery. The fact that anesthesia and surgical teams are in the most practical time-space positions to apply this measure underscores the multidisciplinary efforts necessary to reduce SSI rates.

Of the three performance measures, hospitalists can have the greatest impact by limiting the duration of antimicrobial prophylaxis, the measure that historically has the lowest compliance rate. Antibiotics are frequently continued for more that 24 hours after the operation for a variety of reasons, including early postoperative fever, the presence of drains, and belief of the surgeon (not supported by randomized controlled trials) that longer antibiotic course will further reduce the infection risk. The temptation to continue the administration of perioperative antibiotics because of early postoperative fever should be balanced by the realization that fever on the first postoperative day is rarely due to infection and by knowledge of the hazards of prolonged antibiotic coverage. Prolonged use of antimicrobial prophylaxis is associated with the emergence of resistant organisms.[4] By ensuring that the duration of prophylaxis does not exceed 24 hours past the end of the operation, hospitalists can make valuable contributions to public health and cost containment.

Hospitalists can also help counter the practice of continuing antibiotics while drains are in place. Surgical drains do confer an increased risk of developing SSI because of local inflammation, and they should be removed as quickly as possible. However, continuing antibiotics does not reduce this risk substantially and can increase the risk of infection caused by antibiotic-resistant pathogens. Although the surgeon generally makes the choice of perioperative antibiotic, there are situations where hospitalists can have valuable impact on appropriate antibiotic selection.[5]

Cephalosporins, because of their spectrum and half-life, are the most commonly used perioperative antibiotics. Alternative agents such as vancomycin are often used when there is a history of penicillin allergy. Before cephalosporins are abandoned, however, the penicillin allergy should be characterized. If the penicillin allergy is mild, such as a delayed rash, cephalosporins can be used perioperatively. A history of an IgE-mediated allergy such as hives, wheezing, or anaphylaxis is grounds for avoiding cephalosporins. The recommendations of the NSIPP advisory statement (summarized in Box 112-1) are a helpful starting point for understanding evidence-based selection of antibiotic prophylaxis. An area of uncertainty is the need to use vancomycin or other agents when there is an increased risk of methicillin-resistant *Staphylococcus aureus* (MRSA). The hospitalist is well positioned to be aware of MRSA colonization. If a patient is colonized with MRSA, attempts to decolonize with intranasal mupirocin with or without systemic antimicrobials and the use of vancomycin perioperatively might be warranted.[6]

Free access to the NSIPP advisory statement is available at www.journals.uchicago.edu/CID/journal/issues/v38n1/33257/33257.html.

OTHER MODIFIABLE FACTORS TO REDUCE SSI

Infections at Remote Sites

Patients with active infections remote to the planned surgical site have a two- to three-fold increased risk of developing a SSI. If possible, the procedure should be postponed until the remote infection is treated. At times, the surgeon may be reluctant to delay the procedure, and it may fall to the hospitalist to weigh the pros and cons of proceeding with the procedure. For many situations, the optimal strategy is not clear. There are data indicating that treating the remote infection for 1–2 days decreases infection risk. However, if the planned surgery is elective, the approach that probably has the lowest risk of subsequent SSI is to complete the treatment course for the remote infection and wait an additional 1–2 weeks with the patient at home off of antibiotics prior to performing the procedure. Management should be individualized, based on the urgency of surgery, type and microbiology of the remote infection, and the planned surgical procedure.

Patients who have furuncles without signs or symptoms of systemic illness would benefit from cleansing with chlorhexidine as well as receiving systemic antibiotics. Ideally, surgery should be postponed until the infection has been successfully treated. The patient should also be tested for nares colonization by *S. aureus*. If this is the case, the patient would benefit from 5 days of intranasal mupirocin treatment.

Bacteriuria

Patients who are undergoing transurethral resection of the prostate or other urologic procedures in which mucosal bleeding is anticipated should have bacteriuria treated, even if it is asymptomatic, and antibiotics should be initiated prior to the procedure. Furthermore, patients should be adequately hydrated to keep the urinary tract flushed.

Dermatitis

In patients with eczema, psoriasis, and other dermatologic disorders in whom the integrity of the skin may be compromised, every effort should be made to treat the skin disease before elective surgery. In so doing, as much as possible of the natural protective barrier of the skin is preserved. Gently cleansing the affected areas with chlorhexidine may also be beneficial when surgery in the setting of active skin disease is unavoidable. Chlorhexidine does reduce skin microbial colony counts but has not necessarily been shown to reduce SSI.

Smoking

Tobacco use increases risk of SSI. Ideally, patients should abstain from smoking for >30 days prior to elective surgery. Patients for

---

Box 112-1 Factors That Reduce Surgical Site Infections

- Avoid shaving of the surgical site
- Surgical skin antisepsis
- Antimicrobial prophylaxis
- Perioperative glycemic control
- Abstain from smoking for >30 days prior to elective surgery
- Treat remote infections prior to elective surgery
- Treat bacteriuria prior to all urologic procedures
- Treat skin disease prior to elective surgery among patients with eczema, psoriasis, and other dermatologic disorders

whom an elective surgery is planned should be aggressively counseled by hospitalists about smoking cessation.

Blood Glucose Control

Hyperglycemia, an established independent risk factor for an array of adverse outcomes in hospitalized patients, is also an independent risk factor for SSIs across a range of surgical patients.[7] Short-term hyperglycemia depresses immune function through nonenzymatic glycosylation of immunoglobulin and by impairing normal leukocyte performance. Among diabetic cardiac surgery patients, reduction of hyperglycemia with an intravenous insulin infusion lowered the incidence of deep sternal wound infection by as much as two thirds. As high-quality studies emerge proving that glycemic control lowers SSIs among noncardiac surgical subpopulations, hospitalists may increasingly be relied upon to achieve strict glycemic targets.

Other Strategies to Reduce SSI Rates

Several other measures also can affect SSI rates. Those that fall outside the domain of the hospitalist and into the direct purview of the operative team include ensuring high levels of inspired oxygen, maintenance of perioperative normothermia, and appropriate hair removal. Hair removal often is not needed but, if performed, should be done just prior to the operation, using clippers, not razors.

The risk of SSIs is directly related to tissue oxygenation. Bacterial infectivity is enhanced and cellular immunity is compromised in hypoperfused, poorly oxygenated tissue. The practice of administering perioperative supplemental oxygen (at least 80% FiO_2 in intubated patients) reduces the risk of SSI by nearly half. For nonintubated patients, oxygen at 12 L/min by nonrebreather facemask applied intraoperatively and for at least 2 hours following surgery leads to similar reductions of SSI rates. Besides being effective, this intervention is inexpensive, has no recognized adverse effects, and carries the added benefit of significantly reducing postoperative nausea and vomiting.

Hypothermia also predisposes the surgical wound to infection. Even mild perioperative hypothermia (i.e., core temperature 35–36.5°C) typically occurs in the absence of specific measures to prevent net heat loss. Perioperative hypothermia is the combined result of exposure and anesthetic-induced thermodysregulation, with redistribution of core body heat to the periphery. Even mild hypothermia causes vasoconstriction, which diminishes perfusion, dropping tissue oxygen tension, which impairs phagocytosis and oxidative killing by neutrophils. Hypothermia also blunts scar formation, which further diminishes wound integrity. Active warming of the patient to maintain a core temperature near 36.5°C constitutes the intraoperative standard of care and is effective at reducing the risk of SSIs by as much as two thirds.

CONCLUSION

By recognizing and coordinating practices known to reduce SSIs, hospitalists can elevate the level of care provided for surgical patients. At the same time, hospitalists can help lower costs and keep the hospital system mindful of public health goals, such as prevention of antimicrobial resistance. While individual hospitalists have key roles to play, the overall approach to SSI reduction calls for a coordinated, multidisciplinary approach with process and system-level efforts.

Key Points

- A multidisciplinary approach can minimize risk for SSIs.
- Antibiotic prophylaxis is for "clean" and "clean-contaminated" wounds.
- Antibiotics should be given prior to surgery according to the NSIPP guidelines for optimal perfusion at the tissue level.
- Prophylactic antibiotics should be stopped no later than 24 hours after surgery, even if drains are used.
- Treat nares colonization by S. aureus with 5 days of intranasal mupirocin treatment prior to elective surgery.

SUGGESTED READING

Auerbach AD. Prevention of surgical site infections. In: Shojania KG, Duncan BW, McDonald KM, et al, eds. Making health care safer: a critical analysis of patient safety practices. Evidence report/technology assessment no. 43. AHRQ publication no. 01-E058. Rockville, MD: Agency for Healthcare Research and Quality, 20 July 2001. 221–244.

Sessler DI, Akca O. Nonpharmacologic prevention of surgical wound infections. Clin Infect Dis 2002; 35:1397–404.

Bratzler D, Houck PM. Antimicrobial prophylaxis for surgery: an advisory statement from the National Surgical Infection Prevention Project. Surgical Infection Prevention Guidelines Writers Workgroup. Clin Infect Dis 2004; 38:1706–1715.

Harbarth S, Samore MH, Lichtenberg D, et al. Prolonged antibiotic prophylaxis after cardiovascular surgery and its effect on surgical site infections and antimicrobial resistance. Circulation 2000; 101:2916–21.

Hecker MT, Aron DC, Patel NP, et al. Unnecessary use of antimicrobials in hospitalized patients: current patterns of misuse with an emphasis on the antianaerobic spectrum of activity. Arch Intern Med 2003; 163:972–978.

Garber AJ, Moghissi ES, Bransome ED Jr, et al. American College of Endocrinology position statement on inpatient diabetes and metabolic control. American College of Endocrinology Task Force on Inpatient Diabetes Metabolic Control. Endocr Pract 2004; 10 (Suppl 2):4–9.

Perl TM, Cullen JJ. Intranasal mupirocin to prevent postoperative staphylococcus aureus infections N Engl J Med 2002; 346:1871–1877.

Section

Seventeen

Medical Complications of Pregnancy

113 Medical Complications of Pregnancy
Lisa Bernstein, Stacy M. Higgins, Anna Kho,
Guillermo E. Umpierrez, Clyde Watkins, Jr.

CHAPTER ONE HUNDRED AND THIRTEEN

Medical Complications of Pregnancy

Lisa Bernstein, MD, Stacy M. Higgins, MD, FACP, Anna Kho, MD, Guillermo E. Umpierrez, MD, FACP, FACE, and Clyde Watkins, Jr., MD

Increasingly, generalists and hospitalists are being asked to assist in the medical management of the pregnant patient. This chapter focuses on the medical care of several conditions that are unique to pregnancy or influenced by the physiologic changes of pregnancy, labor, delivery, and the immediate postpartum period.

PHYSIOLOGIC CHANGES IN PREGNANCY

The cardiovascular, hematologic, pulmonary, and renal systems are all affected by pregnancy. Systemic vascular resistance (SVR) decreases in early pregnancy, due to the low resistance circulation in the uterus and placenta. SVR slowly rises in the second half of pregnancy, normalizing near term. Whereas SVR decreases early on, cardiac output increases by 30–50%. Hematologically, both plasma volume and red cell volume increase, but the plasma volume increases to a greater degree than red cell volume. As a result, a relative anemia develops.

Progesterone from the placenta stimulates central respiratory centers, producing hyperventilation with hypocapnia and creating a sensation of dyspnea. Arterial pCO_2 during pregnancy normally decreases to 28–32 mm Hg, leading to a decreased plasma bicarbonate level, with minimal change in pH, creating a state of compensated respiratory alkalosis. Forced vital capacity (FVC), forced expiratory volume in 1 second (FEV_1), and peak expiratory flow rate (PEFR) remain stable through the physiologic pulmonary changes of pregnancy.

Creatinine clearance increases during pregnancy. This is important when prescribing in pregnancy, since renally cleared medications may need to be dosed more frequently. Table 113-1 summarizes some of the physiological changes that take place during pregnancy.

PRESCRIBING IN THE PREGNANT PATIENT

Prescribing medications to pregnant women with medical disorders can be a daunting task for physicians who do not routinely care for them. The Food and Drug Administration (FDA) classifies each medication into safety classes based on prior studies (Table 113-2), but evaluating the risks and benefits of each medicine in treating your pregnant patient's medical disorder is vital, regardless of its classification. Before prescribing, consider alternatives to medications, such as lifestyle modification. Do not start or discontinue medications unless there are clear indications. The provider must weigh the medication's benefits to the mother against the risks to her and her developing fetus, as well as consider the risks to the mother if she does not take the medication. Very few drugs are absolutely contraindicated. Table 113-3 is by no means all inclusive, but can serve as a quick reference for the preferred pharmacologic agents for common medical problems.

DIAGNOSTIC STUDIES IN PREGNANCY

Physicians may consider ordering radiologic tests in the pregnant patient to assist in their decision-making. Each radiologic study is associated with a set amount of ionizing radiation; however, very few adverse effects occur if the total amount of radiation exposure to the fetus is limited to less than 5 rads (1 rad = 1 roentgen-equivalent man) throughout the entire pregnancy,[1] and the total amount of monthly fetal radiation exposure is limited to <50 mrad.[2] Above the 5-rad limit, the fetus is at an increased risk of developing childhood leukemia (about 1 in 2,000 versus 1 in 3,000 in the general population).

When ordering a diagnostic study in pregnancy: 1) consult with the radiologist about the patient's pregnancy to help choose a study with the least amount of radiation, while still providing the diagnostic information; 2) inform the radiologist and radiology technologist that the patient is pregnant to help limit the number of films taken and the radiation exposure to the fetus; 3) when appropriate, use a lead apron to shield the fetus; 4) limit the amount of iodinated contrast, which can cross the placenta and cause transient fetal thyroid effects; however, brief exposures do not appear to cause any adverse fetal outcome; 5) limit MRI studies until after the first trimester; 6) gadolinium is not yet recommended for use in pregnancy unless the potential benefit justifies the potential risk to the fetus[1]; 7) avoid "radioactive" studies, such as radioactive iodine uptake and scans, during pregnancy; nuclear studies, on the other hand, such as ventilation-perfusion scans, may be obtained during pregnancy.

Table 113-4 lists a number of diagnostic studies that may be ordered during pregnancy and their corresponding amounts of ionizing radiation.

Table 113-1 Physiologic Changes During Pregnancy

Parameter	Physiologic Change
Systemic vascular resistance	↓
Cardiac output	↑
Blood volume	↑
Plasma volume	↑
Red cell volume	↑
Hematocrit	↓
Tidal volume	↑
FVC	No change
FEV_1	No change
pCO_2	↓
HCO_3	↓
Creatinine clearance	↑
BUN	↓
TSH	↓ early, later returns to baseline.
Free T_4	No change
Coagulation factors II, VII, IX, X	↑
Protein S	↓

Table 113-2 FDA Pregnancy Drug Safety Classification

Category	Description
A	Adequate, well-controlled studies in pregnant women have not shown an increased risk of fetal abnormalities.
B	Animal studies have revealed no evidence of harm to the fetus; however, there are no adequate and well-controlled studies in pregnant women. **or** Animal studies have shown an adverse effect, but adequate and well-controlled studies in pregnant women have failed to demonstrate a risk to the fetus.
C	Animal studies have shown an adverse effect, and there are no adequate and well-controlled studies in pregnant women. **or** No animal studies have been conducted, and there are no adequate and well-controlled studies in pregnant women.
D	Studies, adequate well-controlled or observational, in pregnant women have demonstrated a risk to the fetus. However, the benefits of therapy may outweigh the potential risk.
X	Studies, adequate well-controlled or observational, in animals or pregnant women have demonstrated positive evidence of fetal abnormalities. The use of the product is contraindicated in women who are or may become pregnant.

HYPERTENSIVE DISORDERS OF PREGNANCY

Hypertensive disorders are the most common medical complication of pregnancy, occurring in 12–22% of pregnancies,[4] and they carry an increased risk of perinatal morbidity and mortality for both the mother and fetus. The American College of Obstetrics and Gynecology defines four categories of hypertension during pregnancy: preeclampsia, preeclampsia on chronic hypertension, gestational hypertension, and chronic hypertension.

Preeclampsia

Preeclampsia affects 5–8% of pregnancies,[4] occurring most commonly after 36 weeks gestation and rarely before 20 weeks. Box 113-1 lists the risk factors for preeclampsia. Women with a history of preeclampsia in a previous pregnancy are at high risk for recurrence particularly if the disease occurred remote from term.[5]

The clinical features (Box 113-2) of preeclampsia are few, nonspecific, and tend to appear late in the course of the disease. Hypertension may be absent in up to 33% of cases.[6] Proteinuria is the most prominent laboratory abnormality, and its presence should prompt a search for other features of preeclampsia. Edema is common in pregnancy, but facial edema, upper extremity edema, and rapid weight gain are suggestive of preeclampsia.

A high index of suspicion is key to early diagnosis. The presence of a rising blood pressure or new-onset proteinuria should prompt a workup. Confirm hypertension by two blood pressure measurements at least 6 hours apart but no more than 7 days apart. Quantify proteinuria, defined as excretion of ≥300 mg of protein in 24 hours, with a 24-hour collection. Avoid urine dipstick measurements, as they correlate poorly with 24-hour

Box 113-1 Risk Factors for Preeclampsia

First pregnancy

Multiple pregnancies

African American

Diabetes mellitus

Family history of preeclampsia

Obesity

Renal disease

Age

Chronic hypertension

Past obstetrical history

Coagulation disorders

• APA

• Protein C or S deficiency

• Factor V Leiden mutation

• Hyperhomocysteinemia

APA—antiphospholipid antibody syndrome

Table 113-3 Pharmacologic Agents for Common Medical Issues

Medical Issue	Use Justified When Indicated	Use Almost Never Justified or Contraindicated
Dyspepsia	Antacids*—Tums, Mylanta Amphogel, Maalox, Sucralfate (B)* H₂-blockers—ranitidine* (B), famotidine (B), nizatidine (C), cimetidine (B)	Proton pump inhibitors— Omeprazole (B), Lansoprazole (C) Misoprostol (X)
Nasal congestion	Antihistamines diphenhydramine* (B)—avoid first trimester, cetirizine (B), fexofenadine (C), loratadine (B) Pseudoephedrine (C) Nasal steroids (C)	
Analgesics (including for headache)	Acetaminophen* (A) Amitryptiline (B) Codeine (C) Meperidine (C) Morphine (C)	NSAIDS (B/C) Aspirin (D) Sumatriptan (C) Ergotamine (X)
Nausea	Prochlorperazine (C) Dimenhydrinate (B) Metoclopramide (B)	Odansetron (B)—rarely justified
Diarrhea	Loperamide (B) Diphenoxylate/atropine (C)	
Laxatives	Bisacodyl(C) Docusate Lactulose (B) Psyllium Sodium biphosphate enema Magnesium hydroxide	
Depression/anxiety	Amitriptyline (B) Fluoxetine (C)	Lithium (D) Benzodiazepines (D)
Hypertension	*Labetalol (C) *Methyldopa (B) Pindolol (B) Acebutolol (B) All other B-blockers (C) Hydralazine (C) Rarely justified: nifedipine (C) Clonidine (C), prazosin (C) Hydrochlorothiazide (B)	ACE inhibitors (D) Angiotensin II receptor Blockers (D)
Diabetes	Insulin	Oral hypoglycemic agents: glipizide (C), glyburide (B), metformin (B), rosiglitazone, pioglitazone (C)
Thrombosis	Unfractionated or low molecular weight heparin	Warfarin (X)
Asthma	β-Agonists (all C) Inhaled steroids (all C, except triamcinolone D) Systemic steroids (C) Ipratropium (B) Cromolyn sodium (B) Theophylline (C) Aminophylline (C)	
Antimicrobials	Penicillins (B) Erythromycin and azithromycin (B) Cephalosporins (B) Vancomycin (C) Nitrofurantoin (B) Acyclovir (C) AZT (C) Aminoglycosides (D) Metronidazole (B)—OK after first trimester Trimethoprim (C) Sulfonamides (C)—not close to term Fluoroquinolones (C)	Tetracycline (D) Doxycycline (D) Clarithromycin (C)
Seizures	Phenytoin (D) Carbamazepine (C) Phenobarbital (D)	Rarely: Valproic acid (D) and gabapentin (C)

*Indicates preferred agents, drug class included in parentheses
Adapted from: Educational materials developed by Dr. Raymond Powrie for the Women and Infants' Hospital of Rhode Island Obstetric Medicine 2005 Curriculum for Internal Medicine Residents.

Table 113-4 Diagnostic Studies and Their Content of Ionizing Radiation[3,31]

Imaging Study	Radiation Exposure (Rads)
Head CT	<0.001
Chest CT	0.03
Abdominal CT	0.25
Pulmonary angiogram	<0.050 via brachial route 0.2–0.3 via femoral route
Cardiac catheterization	0.5
Intravenous pyelogram	0.8 for complete series 0.2 for limited series
Ventilation-perfusion scan	~0.02 ventilation 0.01–0.03 perfusion
Dental	0.01
Cervical spine x-ray	<0.001
Lumbosacral spine x-ray	0.2–0.6
Hip and femur x-ray	0.1–0.4
Chest x-ray	<0.001
Abdominal x-ray	0.2–0.3
Ultrasound (any kind)	None
MRI/MRA/MRV	None

Box 113-2 Clinical Features of Preeclampsia

Hypertension

Papilledema

• Rare

Proteinuria

• Absent in 20% of eclampsia cases

Retinal disease

• Edema, hemorrhage, detachment

Visual disturbances

• Scotomas, scintillations

Headache

• Frontal, migraine quality

Epigastric discomfort

• Hepatic edema, capsule stretching

Edema

• Unreliable

Table 113-5 Indications for Delivery in Preeclampsia.

Maternal	Fetal
Gestational age ≥38 weeks	Severe fetal growth restriction
Platelet count <100,000 cells/mm³	Nonreassuring fetal testing results
Progressive deterioration in hepatic function	Oligohydramnios
Progressive deterioration in renal function	
Suspected abruptio placentae	
Persistent severe headaches or visual changes	
Persistent severe epigastric pain, nausea, or vomiting	

From: Magee LA, Ornstein MP, vonDadelszen P. Fortnightly review: management of hypertension in pregnancy. BMJ 1999; 318:1332.

collections in pregnant women with hypertension.[7] Order a complete blood count, serum chemistries, and liver function tests to look for the presence of end organ damage. Serum uric acid concentration above 5.5 mg/dL is often found in preeclampsia. Preeclampsia is rare before 20 weeks' gestation, and its presence should prompt suspicion of molar pregnancy, illicit drug use or withdrawal, and chromosomal aneuploidy.[8] Complications of preeclampsia include DIC/HELLP syndrome, eclampsia, cerebral hemorrhage, pulmonary edema, renal failure, abruptio placentae, hepatic failure, and hepatic rupture.

The clinical course of preeclampsia is unpredictable and often deteriorates rapidly. The only cure for preeclampsia is delivery. Table 113-5 lists the current indications for delivery. Maternal and fetal assessment must be continuous, using serial physical examinations, blood pressure monitoring, and laboratory evaluation to ensure that the disorder is not rapidly progressive.[9]

Antihypertensive therapy remains controversial, as there is limited objective evidence to support current established practice patterns.[10] There is agreement that those with severe hypertension (SBP >160 mmHg, DBP >110 mmHg) or hypertensive end organ damage should be treated. Antihypertensive therapy for mild or moderate hypertension has not been shown to improve perinatal outcomes.[10] Currently, the drug of choice for acute hypertension in pregnancy is parenteral labetalol (Table 113-6). Hydralazine, an alternative first-line agent, has a long history of safety and efficacy when used in pregnancy. Potential adverse effects include reflex tachycardia, flushing, and rare reports of neonatal thrombocytopenia.[10] Avoid calcium channel blockers in patients using magnesium, as the combination has been associated with severe hypotension.[10] Sodium nitroprusside is rarely needed to control hypertension in the obstetrical patient but can be used when all other medications have failed. Nitroprusside

crosses the placenta and can result in fetal cyanide poisoning.[11] Do not use nitroprusside for more than 4 hours, and follow maternal thiocyanate levels.

The drug of choice for seizure prophylaxis in pregnancy is magnesium sulfate, which is thought to exert its anticonvulsant effects in preeclampsia through its action as a cerebral vasodilator.[12] It is usually given as an intravenous bolus of 4–6 g followed by a continuous infusion of 1–4 g/hour to attain a therapeutic plasma level of 4–7 mmol/L.[12] In the event that an eclamptic seizure occurs while patient is on magnesium prophylaxis, use an intravenous benzodiazepine to terminate the seizure activity, and add phenytoin to the magnesium regimen.[13]

Preeclampsia and eclampsia may present or worsen during the postpartum period. Continue seizure prophylaxis for up to 48 hours postpartum, and monitor complete blood count and serum chemistries. Continue antihypertensive therapy in women with persistent hypertension postpartum.

Table 113-6 Treatment of Acute Hypertension in Pregnancy

Agent	Dose	Comments
Labetalol	5–10 mg IV bolus. ↑ dose q 10 min PRN to control BP (total bolus 300 mg)	First-line agent
Hydralazine	5–10 mg IV q 20–30 min (total bolus 40 mg) 0.5–10 mg/hr infusion	First-line agent. Flushing, tachycardia, nausea, headache
Calcium channel blockers	Avoid	Reports of severe hypotension when combined with $MgSO_4$
Diuretics	Avoid	Use indicated when pulmonary edema present
Nitroprusside	Start 0.3 mcg/kg/min titrate to max 10 mcg/kg/min	Use antepartum when all else fails; check thiocyanate levels; risk of fetal thiocyanate toxicity

Box 113-3 Diagnosis of Superimposed Preeclampsia

Suspect with:

- New-onset proteinuria in women with hypertension and no proteinuria early in pregnancy (<20 weeks)
- Hypertension and proteinuria before 20 weeks' gestation
- Sudden increase in proteinuria
- Sudden increase in blood pressure where hypertension has previously been well controlled
- Thrombocytopenia (platelet count <100,000 cells/mm³)

Preeclampsia Superimposed on Chronic Hypertension

The greatest risk of chronic hypertension is superimposed preeclampsia. The incidence of superimposed preeclampsia ranges from 10–52%, with the greatest risk occurring in women with renal insufficiency, hypertension for at least 4 years' duration, or preeclampsia in a previous pregnancy.[14] The diagnosis of superimposed preeclampsia is often difficult; therefore, a high index of suspicion is necessary (Box 113-3).

Gestational Hypertension and Chronic Hypertension

Gestational hypertension is a provisional diagnosis given to women with blood pressure elevations for the first time after mid-pregnancy without proteinuria.[14] A final diagnosis is not assigned until the postpartum period. Transient hypertension is diagnosed if preeclampsia has not developed and the blood pressure elevation normalizes by 12 weeks postpartum. Chronic hypertension is diagnosed if the blood pressure elevation does not normalize by 12 weeks postpartum.[14]

Chronic hypertension is defined as either a history of hypertension before pregnancy, repeated blood pressure elevations ≥140/90 mm Hg before 20 weeks' gestation, or hypertension that is diagnosed for the first time during pregnancy and does not normalize postpartum.[14] The perinatal risks associated with chronic hypertension include intrauterine growth retardation, abruptio placentae, prematurity, stillbirth, and superimposed preeclampsia.[15]

Current evidence favors the treatment of severe hypertension. Treatment of mild hypertension does not decrease the frequency of superimposed preeclampsia, preterm delivery, abruptio placentae, or perinatal death; but the data are unclear on whether treatment of mild hypertension prevents progression to severe hypertension.[15] Because of the physiologic decrease in blood pressure during pregnancy, some women are able to discontinue their antihypertensive medications. Reinstitute therapy when blood pressure levels exceed 150 mm Hg systolic or 100 mm Hg diastolic. Since methyldopa has not been associated with any significant short-term or long-term effects on the neonate or infant, it is considered first-line therapy in treating chronic hypertension of pregnancy. β-blockers are generally considered safe for use in pregnancy, although there is a suggestion that β-blockers prescribed early in pregnancy (specifically atenolol) may be associated with growth restriction.[10] The data on the use of calcium channel blockers outside of the third trimester are limited. Angiotensin-converting enzyme (ACE) inhibitor and angiotensin II receptor blocker (ARBs) should be discontinued when pregnancy is diagnosed and are contraindicated in the second and third trimesters. Recent data suggest that diuretic use is safe in women with chronic hypertension when started prior to conception; however, lingering questions around the association of diminished plasma volume expansion and its potential effect on fetal growth suggest that diuretics should not be used as first-line antihypertensive agents.

PERIPARTUM CARDIOMYOPATHY

Peripartum cardiomyopathy is a dilated cardiomyopathy that occurs in approximately 1 per 3,000 to 4,000 live births in the United States. While rare, mortality can be as high as 50%, with most deaths within the first 3 months of diagnosis. Women at increased risk for this disease are older, multiparous, have pregnancies with multiple fetuses, have a history of preeclampsia or gestational hypertension, and are African American.[16]

Peripartum cardiomyopathy is defined as the onset of cardiac failure of unknown etiology that occurs in the last month of pregnancy or within 5 months of delivery in a woman who had no recognizable heart disease earlier in her pregnancy.[16] Echocardiography will confirm left ventricular systolic dysfunction and exclude other causes of heart failure.[17] Several possible causes have been proposed for this rare disorder, with the most evidence found for infectious or autoimmune myocarditis.[18]

Symptoms of early congestive heart failure are identical to those considered common late in pregnancy, such as exertional dyspnea, dependent edema, and fatigue. Paroxysmal nocturnal dyspnea, chest pain, pulmonary rales, or jugular venous distention should lead the provider to pursue the diagnosis of heart failure. If myocarditis is suspected and symptoms persist, obtain viral titers, such as coxsackievirus, and consider performing an endomyocardial biopsy.[19] Management of peripartum cardiomyopathy is a collaborative effort between the internal medicine physician, obstetrician, cardiologist, and perinatologist.

The treatment goals of peripartum cardiomyopathy are preload and afterload reduction with increased inotropic force. Salt should be restricted to less than 4 g per day and water to fewer than 2 L daily. Diuretics may also be used, with caution to avoid dehydration, during pregnancy. ACE inhibitors are contraindicated during the second and third trimesters, but they are the cornerstone of afterload reduction in the postpartum period. If the diagnosis is made during pregnancy, the combination of hydralazine and nitroglycerin or amlodipine may be used instead.[19]

Digoxin can improve contractile function. β-blockers may be best reserved for use in the postpartum period because of the association with low-birth-weight babies, and there are no data specifically supporting their use in peripartum cardiomyopathy. Consider anticoagulation therapy in patients with an ejection fraction <35%, as they are at high risk for thromboembolism. Subcutaneous or low-molecular-weight heparin is preferred until the postpartum period, as warfarin is contraindicated during pregnancy.[16,19] In those patients with biopsy-proven myocarditis, immunosuppressive therapy may be considered.[16,18,19] Patients with severe heart failure may require intravenous therapy, with invasive hemodynamic monitoring best performed by an intensivist or cardiologist. In patients who continue to deteriorate, cardiac transplantation may be an option.[16,19]

Prognosis is better for women with peripartum cardiomyopathy whose left ventricular size and function normalize by 6 months postpartum, while mortality is very high for those women who have persistent cardiomegaly and congestive symptoms.[16,19] Counsel patients with persistent cardiomyopathy to avoid subsequent pregnancies.[20] Recommendations for future pregnancy are not as clearcut in those women who seem to normalize their heart size and function. Counsel these women and refer them to a high-risk perinatal center if they choose to become pregnant again.[16,19,20]

GESTATIONAL DIABETES MELLITUS

Gestational diabetes mellitus (GDM) is defined as "carbohydrate intolerance of variable severity with onset or first recognition during pregnancy" and does not exclude the possibility that unrecognized glucose intolerance may have antedated the pregnancy.[21] Gestational diabetes mellitus complicates ~14% of pregnancies, or 135,000 women a year in the U.S.[22,23] Women at greatest risk of developing GDM are those who are obese, older than 25 years, have a previous history of abnormal glucose metabolism or poor obstetrical outcome, have first-degree relatives with diabetes, or are members of ethnic groups with high prevalence of diabetes.[23]

Gestational diabetes mellitus is characterized in most cases by mild-to-moderate postprandial hyperglycemia, resulting from impaired insulin release and an exaggeration of the insulin resistance seen in normal pregnancies.[26] It is believed that maternal–fetal complications are directly proportional to the degree of maternal carbohydrate intolerance. Macrosomia, hypoglycemia, jaundice, respiratory distress syndrome, polycythemia, and hypocalcemia have been reported with varying frequency in the infants of women with gestational diabetes. Macrosomia results from the delivery of excess glucose to the fetus that leads to fetal hyperglycemia and to an exaggerated fetal insulin response. However, there appears to be a weak positive correlation between the degree of maternal glycemia and birth weight and the frequency of macrosomia.[21,24]

Other maternal factors that may contribute to fetal macrosomia include obesity, high serum concentrations of amino acids, and lipids. Screen all pregnant women between 24 and 28 weeks of gestation by measurement of serum or plasma glucose one hour after a 50-g oral glucose load without regard to the time of day or the time of the last meal.[24] If the plasma glucose 1 hour later is ≥140 mg/dL, perform a full diagnostic 100-g oral glucose tolerance test (GTT).

The physician should follow patients with GDM every 1–2 weeks until 36 weeks' gestation and then weekly until delivery. Dietary therapy is the key element in treating patients with GDM. The caloric prescription is based on the patient's ideal pre-pregnancy body weight, 30 kcal/kg for the average patient and 25 kcal/kg for obese women, and emphasizes the use of complex, high-fiber carbohydrates with the exclusion of concentrated sweets. Encourage patients to exercise at least 3–4 times weekly for 20–30 minutes per session. Exercise involving minimal motion of the abdomen appears to be safe.[23] Regular exercise improves glycemic control by 4 weeks and may lead to normalization of the abnormal glucose challenge test 6 weeks into a training program, without associated adverse fetal outcomes.

Patients should check their fasting glucose and a 1-hour or 2-hour postprandial glucose level after each meal, for a total of four determinations each day. The Fourth International Workshop-Conference on GDM recommended "lowering maternal capillary blood glucose concentrations to ≦95 mg/dL (5.3 mmol/L) in the fasting state, ≦140 mg/dL (7.8 mmol/L) at 1 hr, and/or ≦120 mg/dL (6.7 mmol/L) 2 hr after meals" in order to reduce incidence of fetal macrosomia toward that of the general population.[27] If these goals are not achieved with diet and exercise, initiate insulin therapy. The recommended starting insulin dose is 0.8 units/kg actual body weight per day in the first trimester, 1 units/kg per day in the second trimester, and 1.2 units/kg per day in the third trimester.[24] Divide the total dose and administer two thirds in the fasting state as two thirds NPH and one third rapid-acting insulin, and the remaining one third of the total dose given as half rapid-acting insulin at dinner and half at bedtime as NPH. Regular insulin or insulin lispro may be used.

An alternative to insulin therapy is the oral hypoglycemic agent glyburide. This second-generation sulfonylurea does not cross the placenta, has its onset of action in approximately 4 hours, and has a duration of action of approximately 10 hours. In a study of 404 women conducted by Langer et al.,[28] glyburide was found to be comparable to insulin in improving glucose control, with >10% of patients randomized to glyburide requiring insulin. Although there was no difference noted in maternal complications or neonatal outcomes, the rate of maternal hypoglycemia was significantly lower with glyburide. However, clinical data with glyburide in pregnancy are limited, and insulin is the preferred agent for treatment.

Evaluate the patient postpartum to determine whether she has returned to a state of normal carbohydrate tolerance. Approximately 15% of women who have had GDM will remain glucose intolerant or will demonstrate overt diabetes in the postpartum state. The American Diabetes Association recommends that a 75-g oral GTT administered under the conditions described for the 100-g oral GTT be performed 6–8 weeks after delivery. If the patient's postpartum GTT is normal, check fasting glucoses periodically, but at no longer than 3-year intervals. If glucose intolerance persists in the postpartum period, institute dietary treatment and exercise, and follow up annually. Encourage all patients who have had GDM to exercise and lose weight if they are obese to reduce the likelihood of developing type 2 diabetes mellitus.

VENOUS THROMBOEMBOLISM IN PREGNANCY

Venous thromboembolic disease (VTE) is the leading cause of nonobstetrical maternal mortality in the United States and Canada, complicating 0.5 to 3 of every 1,000 pregnancies.[29]

During pregnancy, a number of physiologic changes occur that predispose the patient to venous thromboembolic disease. First, pregnant women have an increase in blood stasis in the deep veins of the pelvis and legs due to the gravid uterus compressing the pelvic veins. This stasis may be exacerbated by an increase in immobility that may occur in pregnancy (e.g., bed rest). Second, most clotting proteins increase in pregnancy, while clot-inhibiting factors (such as protein S) decrease.[30] As a result, pregnant women are more likely to develop a venous thromboembolic event than the average nonpregnant woman.

VTE in pregnancy may be difficult to diagnose because normal physiologic changes (e.g., dyspnea) or common findings in pregnancy (e.g., leg edema) mirror those of VTE. Nevertheless, one should always consider the possibility of VTE because of its high maternal mortality in pregnancy. Uterine compression of the iliac veins may make interpretation of diagnostic studies difficult in pregnancy.

If a VTE is suspected, ultrasound of the lower extremities is a quick, simple test that confers no radiation exposure to the fetus. On the other hand, if an ultrasound is nondiagnostic and VTE is still suspected, pursue the diagnosis by obtaining a ventilation-perfusion scan, CT angiogram, pulmonary angiogram, MRV, or venogram. Although most of these studies are associated with ionizing radiation, the amount of fetal radiation exposure is well below the 5-rad cumulative limit recommended in pregnancy.

Traditionally, unfractionated heparin (UFH) is used in the treatment of VTE in pregnancy, although use of low molecular weight heparin (LMWH) is increasing. Neither UFH nor LWMH crosses the placenta; however, LMWH is associated with less osteoporosis, thrombocytopenia, and bleeding than UFH. Once a VTE is suspected or diagnosed, begin treatment, assuming no bleeding or other contraindication to anticoagulation. If intravenous UFH is used, initiate treatment in the same manner as in the nonpregnant patient with weight-based protocols and a target PTT of 60–80 sec (see Chapter 26). When therapeutic

levels have been maintained for at least 5 days, intravenous UFH may be converted to subcutaneous twice daily (BID) dosing.[29,31] To do this, first calculate the total number of units of UFH used within a 24-hour period when the PTT was maintained between 60–80 sec, and then divide and administer twice daily. Use mid-interval PTT drawn 6 hours after injection to monitor whether or not the patient is therapeutic on this form of treatment. There is no consensus on the optimal treatment duration for VTE in pregnancy. However, most experts recommend that treatment should be continued for at least 3 months. Some recommend that treatment be continued until the time of delivery, since maternal mortality is high with VTE in pregnancy. If subcutaneous heparin is continued until term, discontinue its administration 24 hours prior to delivery. After delivery, when hemostasis has been established, resume intravenous or subcutaneous heparin. Initiate warfarin, and continue for 4–6 weeks postpartum. If LMWH is used, it is dosed twice daily as in the nonpregnant patient. Monitor mid-interval anti-Xa levels to ensure a therapeutic drug level because of altered drug pharmacokinetics that occur in pregnancy. Discontinue LMWH at least 24 hours before an epidural is performed to minimize the risk of an epidural hematoma.

The use of warfarin during pregnancy is generally avoided. Warfarin crosses the placenta and can cause severe fetal anomalies, including skeletal malformations, intracerebral hemorrhaging, and mental retardation, even if it is used after the first trimester. Postpartum, warfarin may be taken while breastfeeding, since it is not excreted in breast milk.

Should a pregnant patient with a VTE develop a contraindication to anticoagulation, an inferior vena cava filter may be safely placed.

THYROID DISEASE AND PREGNANCY

Interpretation of Thyroid Function Tests in Pregnancy

Pregnancy is associated with significant but reversible changes in thyroid function that are a result of the normal physiologic state. Additionally, certain medications can significantly alter thyroid function studies (Table 113-7). Initially during pregnancy, thyroid-binding globulin (TBG) increases as a direct result of increased levels of estrogen.[32] In response, thyroid-stimulating hormone (TSH) secretion rises and stimulates increased levels of total thyroxine (T_4) and triiodothyronine (T_3), most of which remains bound to TBG. The free, active fraction for both of these hormones generally remains in the normal range, and a new steady state is rapidly achieved.[33] Therefore, do not use total thyroxine levels in isolation when evaluating thyroid function during pregnancy.

Pregnancy also increases clearance of iodine by the kidneys secondary to an increased glomerular filtration rate.[32] Although this does not pose a risk in areas of sufficient iodine intake, a pregnancy-related goiter may develop in areas with low iodine intake. If severe, the mother may also develop hypothyroidism. Iodine supplementation of 100–200 mcg daily has been shown to completely prevent the development of goiter and is recommended in areas where dietary iodine intake is low.[34]

In the first trimester, human chorionic gonadotropin (hCG) can stimulate a substantial increase in thyroid hormone production

Table 113-7 Medication Effects on Thyroid Function

Medication	Effect
Salicylates	Initial transient increase in free T_4 followed by reduction in total T_4 and normal TSH with chronic administration
High-dose IV furosemide	
Heparin	
Phenytoin	Stimulate hepatic metabolism of thyroid hormones
Phenobarbital	
Rifampin	
Carbamazepine	
Amiodarone	Interfere with conversion of T_4 to T_3
High-dose β-blockers	
Glucocorticoids	
Iodine contrast agents	
Ferrous sulfate	Interfere with absorption of exogenous thyroxine therapy
Aluminum hydroxide	
Sucralfate	
Colestipol	
Cholestyramine	

T_4—thyroxine
TSH–thyroid stimulating hormone

from the thyroid gland by cross- reacting with the TSH receptor.[35] This leads to suppression of serum thyrotropin (TSH) concentration in the first trimester, when hCG levels are highest. In cases of hyperemesis gravidarum, hydatidiform mole, or choriocarcinoma, elevations in hCG are much higher and can result in undetectable TSH levels and clinical hyperthyroidism or frank thyrotoxicosis.[36]

Hyperthyroidism and Pregnancy

Hyperthyroidism in pregnancy occurs in up to 0.2% of women. Causes include Graves' disease (85–90%), toxic multinodular goiter, toxic adenoma, and subacute thyroiditis.[34] Many of the symptoms associated with hyperthyroidism—palpitations, sweating, and dyspnea—may be attributed to normal pregnancy, making the suspicion for disease low. Complications include miscarriage, preterm delivery, congestive heart failure, thyroid storm, and preeclampsia.[36]

Graves' disease affects 1% of American women, with peak incidence in the reproductive years. Graves', an autoimmune disease, is caused by circulating antibodies directed toward the TSH receptor that also activates it. It is characterized by diffuse goiter, with or without infiltrative eye signs. Pregnancy generally alters the course of many autoimmune diseases, including Graves' disease, and remission of hyperthyroidism with progression of pregnancy and recurrence in the postpartum period are features of Graves' disease. Check thyroid status frequently for women planning pregnancy to minimize the risk of miscarriage. Patients previously treated for Graves' with antithyroid drugs, surgery, or radioiodine therapy still have a risk of hyperthyroidism in their neonate. Measure TSH receptor antibodies in euthyroid pregnant women previously treated with surgery or radioiodine (not in those treated with medication) to predict fetal thyroid status.

For patients diagnosed with hyperthyroidism during pregnancy, medical therapy is preferred. Propylthiouracil (PTU) has been preferred over methimazole because of less transfer of the drug across the placenta, safety of breastfeeding with PTU, and the rare development of aplasia cutis with methimazole.[34,36] Both drugs are effective and should be given at the lowest possible dose to control the disease. Dose PTU at 100–150 mg three times a day and methimazole at ≤20 mg/day. Once the patient is euthyroid, reduce the medication to the lowest amount to maintain euthyroidism (50–100 mg PTU or 5–10 mg methimazole daily).

Use β-blockers to control the adrenergic manifestations of thyrotoxicosis. Subtotal thyroidectomy is indicated if hyperthyroidism cannot be controlled with medication alone or if the patient has a very large goiter causing anatomical symptoms.

Hypothyroidism and Pregnancy

About 2% of pregnant women are hypothyroid, most antedating the pregnancy. Most cases are the result of Hashimoto's thyroiditis or postablative iodine[131] therapy for Graves' disease. Subclinical hypothyroidism has little effect on the mental development of the offspring; with more advanced hypothyroidism, there is increased risk of fetal and maternal morbidity, including pregnancy-induced hypertension and prematurity. Be aware that many women with hypothyroidism may discontinue thyroid therapy while pregnant (up to 50% in one study).[36]

The dosage of thyroxine increases in 75% of pregnant women with primary hypothyroidism in which control was adequate before pregnancy. It usually must be increased about 50–100 mcg to achieve a normal serum TSH concentration. This is critical to ensure adequate maternal thyroxine levels for delivery to the fetus, especially during the first trimester to prevent impaired neurodevelopment outcome in the child. Assess thyroid function with a serum TSH each trimester in women on thyroxine.

Post-Partum Thyroiditis (PPT)

The incidence of PPT varies from 3–17% worldwide because of differences in diagnostic criteria and hormone assay methodology, as well as the frequency with which thyroid assessment is done postpartum. This autoimmune disorder is a form of Hashimoto's thyroiditis and is caused by lymphocytic infiltration of the thyroid leading to tissue destruction. Women with type I diabetes have a three-fold higher incidence of the disease as compared to nondiabetics, and it is recommended that all women with type 1 diabetes be tested for anti-thyroperoxidase (TPO) at the time of diagnosis of pregnancy. The risk of PPT in subsequent pregnancies in a woman who has had a previous episode is 70%. In woman without prior history, but anti-TPO positive, the risk of PPT in subsequent pregnancies is 25%.[34]

The clinical features of PPT are characterized by three phases: thyrotoxicosis, hypothyroidism, and a recovery phase. The development of transient hyperthyroidism occurs a few months after delivery, lasts <2 months, and is characterized by a low radioactive iodine uptake (RAIU). Hypothyroidism develops about 3–6 months after delivery, occasionally without clinically apparent preceding thyrotoxicosis. Painless goiter is almost always present.

Most women are euthyroid within 1 year after parturition, although hypothyroidism remains permanent in 25–30% of women.

Thyroid antibodies are present in >75% of patients with PPT.[37] The diagnosis of PPT is made by thyroid function testing in anti-TPO positive women, or a classic presentation of transient thyroid dysfunction in an antibody negative woman. TSH is a good screening test, followed by a free thyroxine test if abnormal. The RAIU will distinguish between Graves' (increased uptake) and PPT (low uptake). Treatment is often not required in the thyrotoxic phase of PPT unless symptoms are severe, in which case β-blockers can be used, and thyroxine treatment is not always needed in the hypothyroid phase.

- The drugs of choice for treatment of venous thromboembolic disease in pregnancy are unfractionated heparin and low molecular weight heparin.

- Significant but reversible changes in thyroid function occur in thyroid function tests during pregnancy, and autoimmune diseases of the thyroid may be suppressed during pregnancy, but exacerbate after delivery.

Key Points

- Optimizing the mother's health and wellbeing during pregnancy will ensure that the fetus has the best outcome.

- Although the FDA drug safety classification is helpful in deciding what medications to prescribe during pregnancy, each provider should weigh the risks and benefits of a particular medication before prescribing to a pregnant patient.

- Preeclampsia and peripartum cardiomyopathy symptoms mimic those of a normal pregnancy, so keep a high clinical suspicion, and corroborate your diagnosis with appropriate testing.

- Limit the amount of radiation exposure to less than 5 rads cumulative throughout the entire pregnancy.

- Gestational diabetes mellitus complicates ~14% of pregnancies and if identified in the hospital setting requires close outpatient follow-up.

SUGGESTED READING

ACOG Committee Opinion #299: Guidelines for diagnostic imaging during pregnancy. Obstet Gynecol 2004; 104:647.

Sibai BM, Bedder G, Kupferminc M. Preeclampsia. Lancet 2005; 365:785.

National High Blood Pressure Education Program Working Group Report on High Blood Pressure in Pregnancy. Report of the National High Blood Pressure Education Program Working Group on High Blood Pressure in Pregnancy. NIH Publication # 00–3029, 2000. 1–38.

Pearson GD, Veille JC, Rahimtoola S, et al. Peripartum cardiomyopathy: National Heart, Lung and Blood Institute and Office of Rare Diseases workshop recommendations and review. JAMA 2000; 283:1183–1188.

Brown CS, Bertolet BD. Peripartum cardiomyopathy: a comprehensive review. Am J Obstet Gynecol 1998; 178:409–414.

Buchanan TA, Xiang AH. Gestational diabetes mellitus. JCI 2005; 115(3):485.

Rosene-Montella K, Barbour LA. Thromboembolic disease and hypercoagulable states. In: Lee RV, Rosene-Montella K, Barbour LA, et al. Medical Care of the Pregnant Patient. Philadelphia, PA: American College of Physicians—American Society of Internal Medicine, 2000. 423–448.

Section

Eighteen

Consultation for the Psychiatric Patient

114 Evaluation and Management of Medical Patients
with Psychiatric Disorders
Christopher M. Whinney, Leopoldo Pozuelo, Joseph Locala

115 Preoperative Psychiatric Evaluation and Perioperative
Management of Patients with Psychiatric Disorders
Leopoldo Pozuelo, Christopher M. Whinney, Joseph Locala

CHAPTER ONE HUNDRED AND FOURTEEN

Evaluation and Management of Medical Patients with Psychiatric Disorders

Christopher M. Whinney, MD, Leopoldo Pozuelo, MD, FACP, and Joseph Locala, MD

BACKGROUND

Psychiatric disorders are quite common in general medical settings and may significantly affect the course of comorbid medical illnesses. In addition to increased morbidity and mortality,[1-4] patients with untreated or undertreated psychiatric illnesses may experience a delay in rehabilitation,[5,6] increased rates of adverse drug reactions,[7] increased hospital lengths of stay,[8] and increased resource utilization.[6] Unfortunately, the majority of these disorders are unrecognized and/or not addressed in medical inpatients.[9,10] The inpatient physician faces a more complex picture in these patients, as psychiatric conditions such as depression, anxiety, psychosis, or mania, may be exacerbated or even caused by medical conditions. The hospitalist must have or develop the skills to recognize and treat these psychiatric conditions in the medical patient, especially when formal consultation-liaison psychiatry services are not available.

The relationship between medical illness and psychiatric conditions is well characterized in terms of occult medical illnesses presenting with psychiatric symptoms, as well as psychiatric illnesses complicating or worsening medical conditions. Table 114-1 outlines psychiatric conditions that are influenced by medical disease states.

Mental illness can show a stronger association with disability than the severity of physical illness.[10] The Global Burden of Disease Study by the World Health Organization indicates that major depression is the fourth leading cause of early death and disability worldwide, and by the year 2020 it is projected to be the second leading cause of disability, outranked only by ischemic heart disease.[11,12] One or more chronic medical conditions raise the incidence of depression, and medical illness severity correlates with severity of depressive symptoms.[13] The comorbidity of depression and cardiac disease is well established, to the extent that depression is regarded as an independent risk factor of morbidity and mortality in the setting of coronary artery disease.[14-16]

There is less evidence regarding the effect on morbidity and mortality from psychosis and mania in the general medical population, but these disorders can create significant problems with medication and treatment compliance and with comprehension of treatment plans. For the purposes of this chapter, we will review clinical pictures of depression, anxiety, mania, and psychosis not necessarily associated with delirium. Although it is beyond the scope of this chapter, delirium, a syndrome of altered mental status secondary to medical condition, presents with the above varied psychiatric symptoms and may increase length of hospital stay as well as cause increased morbidity and mortality in the medically ill hospitalized patient.[17-19] Delirium is reviewed in more detail in Chapter 93.

CLINICAL ASSESSMENT AND EVALUATION

Make the Diagnosis

It is essential that hospital-based clinicians consider the presence of psychiatric conditions in medical inpatients. Depression is found more frequently in general medical inpatients than in the general population[20] and has a significant effect on morbidity and mortality in association with acute and chronic illnesses, but it is markedly under diagnosed and undertreated. This is often due to the mistaken concept that a "reactive" depression (in the setting of difficult medical or environmental circumstances; i.e., "no wonder he/she is depressed") does not require assessment or treatment.[21]

Anxiety disorders may occur in 10–30% of medical-surgical inpatients, and patients with chronic medical conditions have a higher adjusted prevalence of anxiety disorders than the general population. An evaluation of 1,020 inpatients found 22% suffer significant anxiety, which was associated with longer length of hospital stay and higher costs for the index hospitalization.[22]

Psychotic disorders may present with a predominance of harmful symptoms (social and emotional withdrawal, indifference, apathy, poor hygiene) that can affect inpatient and post-discharge compliance if not recognized and addressed.[23]

Rule Out An Organic Etiology

After diagnosing a comorbid psychiatric condition, determine whether an organic etiology is present. For example, when a patient fulfills the Diagnostic and Statistical Manual of Mental Disorders, Fourth Edition (DSM-IV) criteria for major depression, rule out hypothyroidism, adrenal insufficiency, or other treatable medical conditions in the appropriate clinical situations. Exclude various common conditions, medications, and intoxication and/or withdrawal from substances of abuse (see Tables 114-1 and 114-2).

Table 114-1 Medical Conditions Causing Psychiatric Symptoms

DEPRESSION

Endocrine and Metabolic Disorders
  Hypo- and hyperthyroidism
  Hypercortisolism
  Adrenal insufficiency
  Hypo- and hyperparathyroidism
  Electrolyte disturbances of Na, K, calcium, glucose

Neurological Disorders
  Parkinson's disease
  Stroke
  Dementias (Alzheimer's, vascular)
  Subdural hematomas
  Normal pressure hydrocephalus
  Amyotrophic lateral sclerosis
  Multiple sclerosis
  Seizure disorders
  Traumatic brain injuries
  Huntington's disease

Malignancy
  CNS tumors (primary or secondary)
  Leukemia
  Pancreatic and other GI tract tumors
  Lung tumors
Other
  Chronic obstructive lung disease
  Renal failure
  Hepatic failure
  Systemic lupus erythematosus
  Infections (CNS and systemic, including HIV)
  Vitamin deficiencies (B_{12}, thiamine, folic acid)
  Hypoxia
  Obstructive sleep apnea
Cardiovascular Disorders
  Myocardial infarction
  Congestive heart failure

ANXIETY

Endocrine and Metabolic Disorders
  Hypo- and hyperthyroidism
  Hypo- and hypercortisolism
  Electrolyte disturbances
  Hypoglycemia
  Porphyria
  Vitamin deficiencies (B_{12}, folate)
Neurological Disorders
  Early dementias
  Seizure disorders
  Strokes
  Transient ischemic attacks
  Pulmonary infections
  Traumatic brain injuries
  CNS infections
  CNS tumors
  Parkinson's disease

Cardiovascular Disorders
  Myocardial infarction
  Angina pectoris
  Paroxysmal atrial tachycardia
  Arrhythmias
  Congestive heart failure
  Valvular heart disease
  Cardiomyopathy
Respiratory
  Chronic obstructive lung disease
  Asthma
  Pulmonary embolism
  Pulmonary infections
Other
  Anemia
  Systemic lupus erythematosus
  Chronic pain

PSYCHOSIS

Neurological Disorders
  Parkinson's disease
  Dementias
  Seizure disorders
  Strokes
  CNS tumors infection, and vasculitis
  Paraneoplastic encephalitis
  HIV encephalopathy
  Wilson's disease
  Huntington's disease
  Encephalitis
Endocrine and Metabolic Disorders
  Hypo- and hyperthyroidism
  Hypo- and hyperparathyroidism
  Hypoglycemia
  Hyponatremia
  Cushing's syndrome
  Acute intermittent porphyria
Other Disorders
  Systemic lupus erythematosus
  Temporal arteritis
  Uremia
  Hepatic encephalopathy
  Vitamin deficiencies (B_{12}, thiamine, folate)

MANIA

Neurological Conditions
  CNS tumors, infections, and vasculits
  Stroke
  Seizure disorders
  Neurosyphilis
  Traumatic brain injuries
  Multiple sclerosis
  Wilson's disease
  Huntington's disease
  HIV encephalopathy
  Kleine-Levin syndrome
  Encephalitis
Other Conditions
  Cushing's syndrome
  Hyperthyroidism
  Vitamin deficiencies (B_{12}, niacin)

Data from: Marsh CM. Psychiatric presentations of medical illness. Psychiatric Clinics of North America 1997; 20(1):189–195; and Goff DC, Freudenreich O. Psychotic patients. In: Stern TA, Fricchione GL, Cassem NH, et al., eds. Massachusetts General Hospital Handbook of General Psychiatry, (5th Edition). Philadelphia: Mosby, 2004. 156; and Pollack MH, Otto MW, Bernstein JG, et al. Anxious patients. In: Stern TA, Fricchione GL, Cassem NH, et al., eds. Massachusetts General Hospital Handbook of General Psychiatry, (5th Edition). Philadelphia: Mosby, 2004. 183; and Fricchione GL, Huffman JC, Stern TA, et al. Catatonia, neuroleptic malignant syndrome, and serotonin syndrome. In: Stern TA, Fricchione GL, Cassem NH, et al., eds. Massachusetts General Hospital Handbook of General Psychiatry, (5th Edition). Philadelphia: Mosby, 2004; and Masand PS, Christopher EJ, et al. Mania, catatonia and psychosis. In: Levenson JL, ed. Textbook of Psychosomatic Medicine, (1st Edition). Washington, DC: American Psychiatric Publishing,, 2005. 237, 244.

Table 114-2 Medications Causing Psychiatric Symptoms

DEPRESSION

Antihypertensives
- Methyldopa
- Clonidine
- Calcium channel blockers
- Hydralazine
- Guanethidine
- Reserpine; thiazides

CNS Depressants
- Alcohol
- Opiates
- Barbiturates
- Benzodiazepines
- Hypnotic agents

Others
- Isotretinoin
- Chemotherapy drugs (asparaginase procarbazine, vincristine, vinblastine)
- Interferon
- Indomethacin
- Corticosteroids
- Statins
- Estrogen
- Amantadine
- Antimicrobials (amphotericin, metronidazole)

ANXIETY

Intoxication or Side Effect
- Antidepressants
- SSRIs, TCAs, bupropion
- Psychostimulants
- Interferon
- Caffeine
- Alcohol
- Antipsychotic agents and antiemetics (akathisia)
- Anticholinergic drugs
- Steroids
- Decongestants
- Bronchodilators
- Theophylline
- Histamine H_2 blockers
- Digoxin

Withdrawal Syndromes
- Alcohol
- Narcotic drugs
- Sedative hypnotic agents
- Benzodiazepines

PSYCHOSIS
- Antiarrhythmics
- Antiparkinsonian drugs
- Anticholinergic drugs
- Antihistamines
- Digoxin
- Antiarrhythmic drugs
- Corticosteroids
- Disulfiram
- Symapthomimetics
- Anticonvulsants
- Opioid
- Ciprofloxacin
- Antineoplastics
- Antivirals (acyclovir, interferon, vidarabine, zidovudine)
- Immunosupressants (cyclosporine, tacrolimus)

MANIA
- Anabolic steroids
- Corticosteroids
- Levodopa, amantadine
- Antidepressants
- Sympathomimetics amines
- Decongestants (with phenylephrine)
- Cimetidine
- Cocaine
- Amphetamines
- Dextromethorphan
- Benzodiazepines
- Methylphenidate and other stimulants
- Bromocriptine
- Isoniazid

Data from: Marsh CM. Psychiatric presentations of medical illness. Psychiatr Clin North Am 1997; 20(1): 189–195; and Cassem NH, Murray GB, Lafayette JM, et al. Delirious patient. In: Stern TA, Fricchione GL, Cassem NH, et al., eds. Massachusetts General Hospital Handbook of General Psychiatry, (5th Edition). Philadelphia: Mosby, 2004. 126; and Goff DC, Freudenreich O. Psychotic patients. In: Stern TA, Fricchione GL, Cassem NH, et al., eds. Massachusetts General Hospital Handbook of General Psychiatry, (5th Edition). Philadelphia: Mosby, 2004. 157; and Pollack MH, Otto MW, Bernstein JG, et al. Anxious patients. In: Stern TA, Fricchione GL, Cassem NH, et al., eds. Massachusetts General Hospital Handbook of General Psychiatry, (5th Edition). Philadelphia: Mosby, 2004. 183; and Fricchione GL, Huffman JC, Stern TA, et al. Catatonia, neuroleptic malignant syndrome, and serotonin syndrome. In: Stern TA, Fricchione GL, Cassem NH, et al., eds. Massachusetts General Hospital Handbook of General Psychiatry, (5th Edition). Philadelphia: Mosby, 2004. 516; and Rodin GM, Nolan RP, Katz MR. Depression. In: Levenson JL, ed. Textbook of Psychosomatic Medicine, 1st ed. Washington, DC: American Psychiatric Publishing, 2005. 205; and Masand PS, et al. Mania, catatonia and psychosis. In: Levenson JL, ed. Textbook of Psychosomatic Medicine, (1st Edition). Washington, DC: American Psychiatric Publishing, 2005. 237, 245; and Epstein SA, Hicks D. Anxiety disorders. In: Levenson JL, ed. Textbook of Psychosomatic Medicine, 1st ed. Washington, DC: American Psychiatric Publishing, 2005. 257–258.

TREATMENT

Pharmacologic Treatment

If symptoms are severe enough, begin pharmacologic treatment. Tables 114-3, 114-4, 114-5, and 114-6 highlight the most common psychiatric medications of benefit. Given that some of these agents may require days to weeks to manifest a clinical response, ensure continuity of care to the outpatient or rehabilitation setting to monitor treatment response and side effects.

Nonpharmacologic Treatment

An important step in management of comorbid psychiatric disorders is to initiate nonpharmacologic treatment. Allowing patients to express feelings of guilt, isolation, or loss of control

TABLE 114-3 Medications for Depression

	Trade Name	Initial Dose Range	Target Dose Range	Side Effects	Comments
Tricyclics					
Imipramine	Tofranil	10–75 mg qHS	100–300 mg/day	Anticholinergic symptoms (dry mouth, constipation, tachycardia, urinary retention); diaphoresis, tremor, sedation, weight gain; postural hypotension, cardiac conduction effects (can prolong PR, QRS, QTc)	Typically dosed HS; overdose can be lethal
Desipramine	Norpramin	10–75 mg qHS	100–200 mg/day		
Amitriptyline	Elavil	10–50 mg qHS	100–300 mg/day		Nortriptyline and desipramine less hypotensive and anticholinergic, preferred in the elderly
Nortriptyline	Pamelor	10–25 mg qHS	75–150 mg/day		
Protriptyline	Vivactil	5–10 mg qHS	20–50 mg/day		
Doxepin	Sinequan	25–75 mg qHS	100–300 mg/day		Must check serial ECGs
Clomipramine	Anafranil	25 mg qHS	150–300 mg/day		Blood levels available
Selective Serotonin Reuptake Inhibitors					
Fluoxetine	Prozac	10–20 mg/day	10–80 mg/day	Nervousness, insomnia, tremor, agitation, headache, weight loss, weight gain (more with paroxetine), weight loss	Fluoxetine has a long half-life; only one that will not cause discontinuation syndrome
Sertraline (*)	Zoloft	50 mg/day	50–200 mg/day		
Paroxetine	Paxil	20 mg/day	20–50 mg/day		
Fluvoxamine	Luvox	50 mg/day	50–300 mg/day		Least drug-drug interactions are Zoloft, Celexa, Lexapro
Citalopram (*)	Celexa	10 mg/day	10–40 mg/day		
Escitalopram (*)	Lexapro	10 mg/day	10–20 mg/day		
Serotonin Norepinephrine Reuptake Inhibitors					
Venlafaxine (*)	Effexor XR	37.5 mg XR/day	150–225 mg XR/day	Hypertension (diastolic) nausea, jitteriness, dry mouth	Measure blood pressure: has minimal drug-drug interaction, effective in pain syndromes
Duloxetine	Cymbalta	20, 30 mg/day	60 mg/day	Nausea, jitteriness	Approved for diabetic neuropathy, measure blood pressure, check liver function tests, some moderate drug-drug interaction
Novel Dual-Acting Antidepressants					
Mirtazepine (*)	Remeron	15 mg/day	30–45 mg/day	Somnolence, weight gain	Available in dissolvable tablets, antiemetic (blocks same nausea receptor as ondansetron)
Monoamine Oxidase Inhibitors					
Phenelzine	Nardil	15 mg tid	60–90 mg/day in divided dosages	Hypertensive crises with medications (i.e., SSRI, meperidine) and foods (cheese, aged meats); Must follow tyramine-free diet	Patients taking these drugs must be on a tyramine-free diet
Tranylcypromine	Parnate	10–20 mg	60 mg/day in divided dosages	Other side effects are sedation, tremor, insomnia, hypotension, anorgasmia, weight gain	Multiple drug drug interactions
					Rarely used as front-line antiderpressant due to significant interactions
					Need 14 day washout before starting new antidepressant
Selegiline	Emsam (patch)	6 mg/24 hr patch		Topical reaction, insomnia, hypotension	Dose >6 mg/24 hr must observe tryamine free diet

Data from Goldberg RJ "Antidepressants" in Practical Guide to the Care of the Psychiatric Patient, (2nd Edition). Edited by Goldberg RJ St. Louis, Mosby, 1998, pp. 89–119 and Cassem NH, Papakostas GI, Fava M. "Mood-Disordered Patients" in Massachusetts General Hospital Handbook of General Hospital Psychiatry (5th Edition). Edited by Stern TA, Fricchione GL, Cassem NH, et al. Philadelphia, Mosby, 2004, pp. 75–81 and Wise MG, Rundell JR "Depression" in Clinical Manual of Psychosomatic Medicine: A Guide to Consultation-Liaison Psychiatry. (1st Edition). Washington DC, American Psychiatric Publishing, 2005, pp. 75–77.

HS—bedtime

TABLE 114-3 Medications for Depression—Cont'd

	Trade Name	Initial Dose Range	Target Dose Range	Side Effects	Comments
Atypical or Nontricyclics Antidepressants					
Amoxapine	Asendin	25–75 mg	100–300 mg	Can cause EPS	Seizure risk
Trazodone	Desyrel	25–75 mg/day in divided doses	300 mg/day in divided doses	Priapism: Use with caution in patients with ventricular arrhytmias?	Helpful as second drug for sleep disturbance, at dosages of 25-50 mg at HS
Bupropion (*)	Wellbutrin SR Wellbutrin XL	100 mg SR bid 150 mg XL daily	300 mg/day	Jitteriness, activation; lowers seizure threshold at higher dosages	Indication also for smoking cessation: **not** front-line antidepressant for anxiety disorders
Psychostimulants					
Dextroamphetamine	Dexedrine	2.5 mg daily	5–10 mg	Can be used in the medically ill, help with fatigue; actually may stimulate appetite	Abuse potential must be considered, monitor HR, BP
Methylphenidate	Ritalin	2.5 mg bid	5–20 mg	Can be used in the medically ill; May help with fatigue and stimulates appetite	Abuse potential must be considered, monitor HR, BP

*Medications recommended for medical inpatients.

EPS—extrapyramidail symptoms

and providing reassurance can reduce anxiety or depression and potentially augment medical therapy. Identifying and addressing psychosocial issues often involve family assistance, social service or case management, occupational therapy, or even a psychologist or psychiatrist evaluation.

DEPRESSION

Background

The term "depressive disorder" describes a syndrome of mood fluctuations of varying severity with accompanying clinical symptoms; it does not refer to a simple emotional reaction of sadness or distress. The prevalence of depression in general medical inpatients has been estimated to be 10–14%, but it is significantly underdiagnosed and undertreated.

Hospitalists should not miss depression in medically ill patients. Untreated depression in elderly inpatients is associated with increased morbidity and mortality, higher rates of adverse drug reactions,[7] diminished rates of recovery, and poorer functional status after hospital discharge.[24–27] Morbidity of depression is strongly correlated in cardiac disease; neurologic illness such as strokes, dementia, and Parkinson's disease, and in diabetes mellitus. Mortality is increased in depressed patients with myocardial infarction and stroke.[28–31]

Clinical Assessment and Evaluation

The Diagnostic and Statistical Manual for Mental Disorders, Fourth Edition (DSM-IV)[32] criteria for major depressive disorder requires one of the following:

- Depressed mood, subjective or observed, most of the day, particularly in the morning

- Markedly diminished interest or pleasure (subjective or observed) in almost all activities nearly every day (anhedonia) and at least four of the following seven symptoms to be present for most of the day, nearly every day, for at least 2 weeks:
  - Significant weight loss or gain (more than 5% of body weight per month)
  - Insomnia or hypersomnia
  - Psychomotor agitation or retardation (observed)
  - Fatigue or loss of energy
  - Feelings of worthlessness or excessive or inappropriate guilt
  - Impaired concentration or indecisiveness
  - Recurring thoughts of death or suicidal ideation (with or without a plan) or suicide attempt

Clinicians can use the mnemonic "SIG-E-CAPS" to remember these symptoms (Sleep disturbance, diminished Interest, Guilt, Energy, Concentration, Appetite, Psychomotor agitation or retardation, Suicidal ideation) that accompany depressed mood. Because medically ill patients can be physically fatigued and show disruptions of sleep and appetite, it useful to use the following substitution items: withdrawal, anhedonia, rumination, and tearfulness. The mnemonic "WART" places more emphasis on psychological symptoms rather than physical.

The diagnosis of major depressive disorder in the general medical patient requires a detailed assessment for conditions affecting the central nervous system (CNS). Perform a thorough history and physical examination with attention to past medical and psychiatric history, psychosocial factors, medications (including over-the-counter and herbal preparations), substance use, and neurologic and mental status examinations. Depression can be the initial manifestation of medical illnesses such as pancreatic cancer, Huntington's disease, and adrenal and thyroid dysfunction.[33,34] Delirium and dementia may superficially present as reticence, flat affect, and indifference, which may be perceived

Table 114-4 Antianxiety Medications

Drug	Trade Name	Initial Dose	Target Dose Range	Side Effects	Comments
SSRI (Useful for long-term management of anxiety disorders) (see SSRI in "Medications for Depression")					
BENZODIAZEPINES (used in acute and short-term management of anxiety disorders)					
Lorazepam	Ativan	0.25 mg– 0.5 mg, bid	2–6 mg total dosage, given bid, tid	Sedation	No active metabolites, best suited for hepatic impairment
Oxazepam	Serax	10 mg bid, tid	60–120 mg/day	Less sedating	No active metabolites; best suited for hepatic impairment
Temazepam	Restoril	7.5 mg HS	15–30 mg/day	Moderate sedation, given at HS. Used as sedative hypnotic	No active metabolites; best suited for hepatic impairment
Diazepam	Valium	5 mg bid	10–30 mg/day	Sedation; rapid onset, high addictive potential	Active metabolites
Chlordiazepoxide	Librium	5–10 mg bid	15–50 mg/day	Moderate sedation, used in alcohol detoxification regiments; use only PO	Active metabolites; for alcohol detoxification with liver impairment, lorazepam preferred
Alprazolam	Xanax	0.25 mg tid	2–6 mg/day	Ataxia, drowsiness, tolerance and dependence, less tolerance	Active metabolites; short half-life, can cause rebound phenomenon
Clonazepam	Klonopin	0.25 mg daily	1–3 mg/day	Sedation, ataxia	Long duration of action permits bid dosing
β-Blockers					
Propranolol	Inderal	10 mg bid	Individualize 40–120 mg/day	Bradycardia, hypotentsion, fatigue	Controls the sympathetic response of anxiety (palpitations, sweating). Does not block the psychologic (fear) component of anxiety or panic
Other					
Buspirone	BuSpar	5 mg bid	30–60 mg/day	Nervousness, headache; nonsedating	No dependence with prolonged use; not effective for panic attacks, neeeds 7–10 days to efficacy
Hypnotics (treating insomnia only)					
zaleplon	Sonata	5 mg HS	10–15 mg/day	Habituation, drowsiness, used as sedative hypnotic	Most useful on an as-needed basis
Zolpidem	Ambien	5–10 mg HS	10 mg/day	Habituation, drowsiness, used as sedative hypnotic	Most useful on an as-needed basis
Eszopiclone	Lunesta	1–2 mg HS	2–3 mg/day	Somnolence, dizziness, used as sedative hypnotic	Most useful on an as-needed basis

Data from Goldberg RJ "Treatment of Anxiety" in Practical Guide to the Care of the Psychiatric Patient, 2nd Edition. Edited by Goldberg RJ St Louis, Mosby 1998, pg 154–165 and Pollack MH, Otto MW, Bernstein JG, et al. "Anxious Patients" in Massachusetts General Hospital Handbook of General Hospital Psychiatry 5th Edition. Edited by Stern TA, Fricchione GL, Cassem NH, et al. Philadelphia, Mosby 2004, pg 191–197 and Wise MG, Rundell JR "Anxiety and Insomnia" in Clinical Manual of Psychosomatic Medicine; A Guide to Consultation-Liaison Psychiatry 1st edition. Washington DC, American Psychiatric Publishing 2005, pg 111.

Table 114-5 Medications for Psychosis

Class	Generic Name	Trade Name	Acute Dose per 24 hr	Maintenance Dose	Side Effects
Typical Antipsychotics					
Low potency	Chlorpromazine	Thorazine	25–50 mg	200–600 mg/day	High anticholinergic profile, very sedating, low eps. Check QTc internal
	Thioridazine	Mellaril	25–50 mg	200–600 mg/day	High anticholinergic profile, very sedating, low eps, retinal pigmentation at high dosages, severe risk of QTc interval prolongation
Medium potency	Perphenazine	Trilafon	4–8 mg	16–32 mg/day	Mild anticholinergic, mild eps Check QTc interval
High potency	Haloperidol	Haldol	5–10 mg bid	20–30 mg/day	Extrapyramidal symptoms, less with IV than PO, IM Haldol: must monitor QTc interval
	Haloperidol	Haldol Decanoate	25–50 mg im q month	100–200 mg monthly maintenance dose	Confirm no eps first with oral dose before giving im monthly decanoate
	Fluphenazine	Prolixin	5–10 mg bid	20–30 mg/day	Same considerations as Haldol Decanoate IM maintenance form available, given q 2 wk
Atypical Antipsychotics					
	Clozapine	Clozaril	50–100 mg bid	300–600 mg/day	Risk agranulocytosis, requiring weekly CBC: sedation, anticholinergic, weight gain, seizure risk
	Olanzapine	Zyprexa	5–10 mg dialy	20–30 mg/day	Sedating, weight gain; oral dissolvable form available
	Risperidone	Risperdal	1–2 mg daily	4–6 mg/day	EPS can be seen at dosages 4 mg or above; elevates prolactin titrate dose due to orthostatic hypotension; Risperdal Consta IM maintenance dose available, bimonthly injections
	Quetiapine	Seroquel	100 mg bid	400–600 mg/day	Very low incidence of extrapyramidal effects, can cause sedation
	Ziprasidone	Geodon	40–80 mg bid to be given with food	160–240 mg/day	Check ECG for QTc prolongation
	Aripiprazole	Abilify	10, 15 mg daily	30–45 mg	Nausea, akathisia at higher dosages

Data from Goldberg RJ "Psychotic Symptoms, Schizophrenia, and Neuroleptic agents" in Practical Guide to the Care of the Psychiatric Patient, 2nd Edtion. Edited by Goldberg RJ St Louis, Mosby 1998, pg 186–208 and Goff DC, Freudenreich O, Henderson DC. "Psychotic Patients" in Massachusetts General Hospital Handbook of General Hospital Psychiatry 5th Edition. Edited by Stern TA, Fricchione GL, Cassem NH, et al. Philadelphia, Mosby 2004, pg 162–167 and Wise MG, Rundell JR "Mania" in Clinical Manual of Psychosomatic Medicine; A Guide to Consultation-Liaison Psychiatry 1st edition. Washington DC, American Psychiatric Publishing 2005, pg 94–95 and Adapted from Marder SR; "Antipsychotic Medication" in Essentials of Clinical Psychopharmacology 1st Edition. Edited by Schatzberg AF, Nemeroff CB. Washington DC, American Psychiatric Publishing, 2001, pg 112.

Table 114-6 Antimanic Medications

	Trade Name	Initial Dose Range	Target Dose Range	Side Effects	Comments
Lithium	Eskalith	300 mg daily	300–1200 mg daily; serum level 0.6-1.2 mEq/L	Tremor, nausea, vomiting, diarrhea, polyuria, polydipsia; nephrogenic diabetes insipidus;	Impaired clearance with renal failure, thiazides, NSAIDs; CNS toxicity at high levels (ataxia, dysarthria, nystagmus, coma)
Carbamazepine	Tegretol	200 mg bid	400–1,200 mg daily	Transient leukopenia; aplastic crisis; elevated liver enzymes	Monitor liver function: inducer of hepatic enzymes, can lower concentration of co-administered medications
Valproic acid	Depakote, Depakene	250 mg bid	500–1,500 mg daily	Nausea, hepatitis, pancreatitis, thrombocytopenia	Monitor liver function
Lamotrigine	Lamictal	25 mg daily	100–150 mg daily	Skin rash, serious reaction Stevens-Johnson syndrome	Follow titration guidelines
Gabapentin	Neurontin	300 mg daily	600–1,800 mg dialy	Somnolence, dizziness, ataxia	Renal clearance: second-line mood stabilizer: used also for adjuvant anxiety control as alternative to benzodiazepine
Clonazepam	Klonopin	0.5 mg–1 mg bid	1 mg–3 mg daily	CNS depression, disinhibition, respiratory suppression	Longer half-life, used short term for control of symptoms of mania: not primary treatment
Lorazepam	Ativan	0.5 mg–1 mg bid	1–6 mg daily	CNS depression, disinhibition, respiratory suppression	Shorter half-life, no hepatic metabolites, used short term for control of symptoms of mania
Typical antipsychotics		see "Medications for Psychosis" chart	Haldol is used short term for PO, IM, IV for control of symtoms of mania, especially with psychotic symptmoms		Extrapyramidal symptoms, less with IV than PO, IM Haldol: must monitor QTc interval
Atypical antipsychotics		see "Medications for Psychosis" chart	Zyprexa, risperidone, Seroquel, Geodon, Abilify are used manic phase of bipolar disorder, can exert mood stabilization		Weight gain with atypical antipsychotics, predispose metabolic syndrome

Data from Goldberg RJ "Bipolar Disorder and Mood Stabilizing Drugs" in Practical Guide to the Care of the Psychiatric Patient, 2nd Edition. Edited by Goldberg RJ St Louis, Mosby 1998, pg 121–134 and Alpert JE, Fava M, Rosenbaum JF. "Psychopharmacologic Issues in Medical Setting" in Massachusetts General Hospital Handbook of General Hospital Psychiatry 5th Edition. Edited by Stern TA, Fricchione GL, Cassem NH, et al. Philadelphia, Mosby 2004, pg 247–251 and Adapted from Wise MG, Rundell JR "Mania" in Clinical Manual of Psychosomatic Medicine; A Guide to Consultation-Liaison Psychiatry 1st edition. Washington DC, American Psychiatric Publishing 2005, pg 94–95.

IV—intravenous; IM—intramuscular; PO—oral

as depression unless further explored. Promptly address and treat abuse of depressants such as alcohol or benzodiazepines and withdrawal from stimulants such as cocaine or amphetamines, as they are potential contributors to depressive symptoms.

Laboratory studies should begin with a complete blood count, routine chemistries, thyroid function assessment, and toxicology screening. Neuroimaging is not warranted in the routine evaluation of depression, but should be considered with any unexplained focal neurologic deficit, or with disorders such as malignancy or HIV that can affect the CNS.

Assess medical patients with significant depression for the risk for suicide. Inquiring about suicidal thoughts and intentions does not increase suicide risk; rather, not inquiring may increase patient mortality and, potentially, physician liability. Risk factors for suicide in medical inpatients include older age, male gender, cancer, chronic renal failure, AIDS, preexisting mood disorder, alcoholism or substance abuse, bipolar disorder, schizophrenia, and prior suicide attempts.[35] Goldberg recommends several fundamental steps in the evaluation of a suicidal patient[36] (Table 114-7).

Treatment

Treatment of depression in medical inpatients should first focus on the underlying medical disorders, whether previously established or discovered by the above evaluations. Psychosocial support is critical to the depressed medical inpatient. Medical inpatients may perceive several kinds of losses: health, privacy, physical autonomy, productivity, and self-esteem. Allowing the patient a forum to express his or her feelings and "vent" frustrations regarding the above life changes, however brief they may be, can be quite therapeutic. Explore and develop coping strategies. However, with diminishing length of stay and frequent procedures and studies, there is limited time to provide this support;

Table 114-7 Fundamentals of Suicide Assessment

1. Determine whether delirium, psychosis, or depression is present.
2. Elicit the patient's statements about his or her suicidality.
3. Elicit the patient's ideas about what would help to mitigate his or her suicidality.
4. Confirm the patient's story with a third party.
5. Make a global formulation that includes acute and chronic management suggestions.
6. Ask a series of escalating questions addressing suicidality in medically ill hospitalized patients:

    Are you discouraged about your medical condition?
    Are there times when you think about your situation and feel like crying?
    When you feel that way, what sort of thoughts go through your mind?
    Did you ever feel that if your life were to go on like this, it would not be worth living?
    Have you gotten to the point at which you've actually thought of a specific plan to end your life?
    You say you've thought of shooting yourself. Do you have a gun?

Data from: Goldberg RJ. The Assessment of Suicide Risk in the General Hospital. *General Hospital Psychiatry* 1987; 9:446-452. Copyright 1987. Elsevier Science. Used with permission.

thus, the clinician must be concise and focus on the most pertinent issues.

Acute treatment of a suicidal patient requires a secure environment and a sitter for constant observation. **Seek psychiatric consultation immediately.** Consider physical or chemical means of restraining the patient if he or she is an imminent danger to self or others. Transfer to a psychiatric facility is appropriate in the presence of poor impulse control, psychosis, or established suicide plan and intent, independent and specific psychiatric diagnosis.

Despite good efficacy, pharmacotherapy for depression in medical patients is often withheld due to concerns about drug and disease interactions, such as tricyclic agents in the setting of cardiac disease. Numerous agents in various drug classes are available, with the most commonly used agents highlighted in Table 114-3. Newer agents such as the selective serotonin reuptake inhibitors (SSRI) and serotonin–norepinephrine reuptake inhibitors (SNRI) offer distinct advantages in overdose safety, side-effect profile, and decreased drug–drug interactions.

Choosing an antidepressant often starts with an assessment of patient symptoms, side-effect profile, other medications, and prior antidepressant treatment. Side effects include orthostatic hypotension, anticholinergic side effects, gastrointestinal and cardiac conduction effects, as well as potential drug-drug interactions. Tricyclic antidepressants (TCA) are more associated with side effects of hypotension and anticholinergic symptoms, and thus not well suited for patients with conduction abnormalities. The anticholinergic symptoms of dry mouth, blurred vision, tachycardia, constipation, urinary retention, and the predisposition for delirium can be detrimental in the medically ill patient. Monoamine oxidase inhibitors (MAOIs) are much less commonly encountered in clinical practice and require a tyramine-free diet, observance of multiple drug–drug interactions, and a washout period when changing from and to another antidepressant.

SSRIs, on the other hand, have been very well studied and deemed safe in cardiac patients.[37,38] SNRI (e.g., venlafaxine, duloxetine); a novel dual-acting serotonin and norepinephrine antidepressant, mirtazapine; and the primary enhancing dopamine antidepressant bupropion also do not cause cardiac conduction abnormalities and appear to be safe to use in the setting of cardiac disease.

Actual pharmacologic effect takes at least 10 days, and an adequate trial of antidepressant treatment requires at least 4–6 weeks of uninterrupted dosing at maximal dosage. Stimulants like methylphenidate take just 2–3 days to increase mood and energy and can be very useful as an adjuvant therapy in the depressed and medically ill patient with psychomotor retardation.[39]

ANXIETY DISORDERS

Background

Anxiety disorders are the most common class of psychiatric disorders in the general population, with lifetime prevalence estimated at 29%.[40] In hospitalized patients, anxiety disorders are found with similar frequency; however, this does not discern whether the anxiety disorder is a preexisting condition, a reaction to current stressors, or a manifestation of medical illness. Illness, uncertain prognosis, pain, potential loss of one's vitality or ability to work, foreign surroundings, and lack of privacy can all increase the distress and fear felt by medical inpatients. Hospitalists benefit patients through early recognition and treatment of these primary and secondary anxiety syndromes, as their cost is quite high, due to continued suffering, prolonged length of stay, and increased utilization of resources.

Clinical Assessment and Evaluation

Anxiety presents with physical, affective, cognitive, and behavioral signs and symptoms. The most common physical symptoms reflect autonomic arousal, such as palpitations, chest pain, dyspnea, lightheadedness, diaphoresis, and tremor. Affective symptoms may range from mild uncertainty or nervousness to outright terror and panic. Patients experience worries, apprehension, obsessions, and may have persistent thoughts about physical or emotional destruction. Behavioral changes may include compulsions and avoidance of people, places, and objects that provoke the described symptoms.

While anxiety is often considered a normal response to stress and helps to facilitate adaptation and coping, excessive or pathologic anxiety is counterproductive and must be distinguished from normal anxiety. Four criteria help to provide this distinction:

- Pathologic anxiety is *autonomous* and has little basis in external stimuli.
- It is of such *intensity* and severity that the patient is seeking relief.
- The *duration* of symptoms is much greater than would be expected—symptoms persist over time.
- Patient *behavior* becomes pathologic, in that normal function and coping skills are disrupted, often resulting in social withdrawal and avoidance.

Anxiety disorders in hospitalized medical patients may have diverse origins. Most medical patients manage the "threats" of hospitalization with various coping strategies such as rationalization, minimization, and reliance on social support. Sometimes, these strategies fail, such as when social support is not present, when the perceived danger is significant, or when personality factors lead to regression and passivity. Helping the patient augment or change these strategies or providing support can help reduce anxiety in this setting; pharmacologic therapy is not always necessary.

Another source of anxiety for inpatients is invasive procedures. Post-traumatic stress disorder (PTSD) symptoms can occur after major surgery, such as coronary bypass grafting[41] and after treatment for breast cancer.[42] Symptoms of PTSD have been noted among patients after surgery under inadequate anesthesia, resulting in the frightening experience of surgical pain while paralyzed. Ask postoperative patients about awareness during surgery to enable them to verbalize their memories and allow for prompt assessment and treatment if they manifest symptoms of anxiety or trauma.

Underlying medical illnesses (including intoxication and withdrawal from substances of abuse) may be responsible for anxiety and depressive symptoms in up to 40% of patients referred for psychiatric treatment. Although the list of conditions and medications leading to anxiety symptoms is extensive, consider contributing factors (Tables 114-1 and 114-2) that may cause anxiety.

Some characteristic features of primary anxiety disorders help differentiate them from disorders with an organic etiology. Patients with organic anxiety syndromes more typically have:
- Onset of symptoms >35 years of age
- No personal or family history of anxiety disorders
- No childhood history of anxiety symptoms
- No significant life events antecedent to symptoms
- No avoidance behavior
- Poor response to antianxiety agents

Treatment

Treatment of anxiety disorders should first address any medical or toxic causes. Concomitant treatment of distressing symptoms is appropriate, with medications, psychotherapy, or cognitive-behavioral therapy. Anxiolytic medications are listed in Table 114-4.

Benzodiazepines are the most commonly used agents for anxiety in the acute medical setting. They have a comparatively rapid onset of action of hours compared to days with the antidepressants, are easy to administer, and come in a wide spectrum of duration of action. They can cause oversedation, confusion, incoordination, and diminish the central respiratory drive in very high doses, so use caution in patients with respiratory impairments. Consider combination therapy with an antidepressant if the anxiety disorder becomes chronic and/or depressive symptoms become prominent.

Antidepressants in the SSRI class are first-line agents in treating panic disorder, obsessive-compulsive disorder, generalized anxiety disorder, and social phobia due to their broad spectrum of efficacy and minimal side effects and toxicities. Use lower starting doses than those for depression, and raise the dose as tolerated over 1–2 weeks. Since onset of benefit occurs after 2–3 weeks, this is a disadvantage compared with benzodiazepines when acute treatment is needed. SNRI, tricyclic agents, and monoamine oxidase inhibitors are also effective, but the two latter classes have more side effects and should be used as second-line treatment.

Other agents used in anxiety disorders include low doses of atypical neuroleptics, β-adrenergic antagonists (whose long-held association with depression has not been validated in recent metananalyis of clinical trials),[43] and buspirone, which is useful in chronic anxiety states but is not effective for acute anxiety or panic disorder (*see* Table 114-4).

PSYCHOSIS

Background

Psychosis refers to impairment of reality-testing in perceptual or cognitive domains. Symptoms of psychosis may take the form of hallucinations or illusions (sensory perceptions in the absence of an external source), delusions (false beliefs held to be true), and formal thought disorders (disorganization of thinking). Patients with disorganized thinking may be incoherent or unable to communicate, making this difficult to differentiate from delirium.

Clinical Assessment and Evaluation

Evaluation of psychosis in medical inpatients must initially rule out medical or toxic etiologies. Impaired memory or orientation as well as waxing and waning course make delirium or dementia more likely as a cause of symptoms. Obtain a complete medication history, including substance use and abuse. Collateral history from family or friends helps establish the time course of psychotic symptoms (acute, intermittent, chronic, and/or recurrent) and identify causative factors. Past hospitalization experiences of illnesses and medication exposure can be very helpful collateral history as well.

A thorough history and physical examination, including mental status and neurologic examination, can identify most secondary causes of psychosis. Obtain routine chemistries for renal, hepatic and thyroid function, electrolytes, complete blood counts, and toxicology screening. Neuroimaging is likely to be low yield if no focal deficits are found, but this is typically standard for first-onset psychosis.

Key diagnostic questions[44] to ask during evaluation of psychosis include:
- Have reversible organic causes been ruled out?
- Are deficits in cognition present?
- Are psychotic symptoms continuous or episodic?
- Is there evidence of a decline in functioning?
- Are mood episodes prominent? (i.e., depression or mania; do psychotic symptoms occur during mood symptoms?)

Primary psychosis (i.e., schizophrenia) will have relatively normal level of consciousness, with a predominance of auditory hallucination and complex delusions. Secondary psychosis will often have abnormal level of consciousness and can be accompanied by visual or tactile olfactory hallucinations. Table 114-8 lists the common primary psychiatric diagnostic categories for psychotic disorders. Tables 114-1 and 114-2 list secondary psychosis caused by medical illnesses, toxic states, and medications. Psychiatric consultation, if available, should be obtained to clarify specific diagnosis and establish a long-term care plan.

Treatment

Treatment of psychotic symptoms must first address any underlying causes determined by the previously described evaluations. A primary psychiatric psychotic disorder will require mainte-nance treatment with antipsychotic medication throughout the hospitalization. In the treatment of secondary psychosis, most psychotic symptoms will improve with the use of antipsychotic medication. Table 114-5 highlights the most commonly used antipsychotic agents.

As all antipsychotic agents have established efficacy, choice of medication is guided by side-effect profile. Conventional antipsychotic agents (also referred to as typical neuroleptics) are stratified into low-, mid-, and high-potency agents, with decreasing sedation and anticholinergic properties and increasing extrapyramidal side effects as potency increases. Longterm use of antipsychotics carries risk of tardive dyskinesia.

Newer "atypical" antipsychotic agents seem to have superior efficacy compared with conventional agents in treating both positive symptoms (auditory and visual hallucinations) as well as the negative symptoms of schizophrenia (such as lack of initiative and cognitive dulling). Although the atypical antipsychotic can lead to orthostasis, sedation, and weight gain, they have significantly fewer extrapyramidal side effects, which makes their use quite favorable on the inpatient medical service. Predisposition for a metabolic syndrome has been a recent concern of the atypical antipsychotics and does require monitoring of weight gain, hyperglycemia, and dyslipidemia after discharge.[45,46] Patients taking clozapine require frequent white blood count monitoring for chronic therapy, as agranulocytosis can occur in 1%.

Other symptoms to heed when initiating antipsychotic therapy are acute dystonic reactions during the first week of medication, which can include laryngeal spasm, akathisia (motor restlessness in the lower extremities), and parkinsonism. Benztropine, 1–2 mg BID, may help alleviate symptoms. The risk of tardive dyskinesia (drug-induced involuntary movements) is lower with the atypical antipsychotics than with the typical ones.

The neuroleptic malignant syndrome (NMS) is a rare but potentially lethal complication of antipsychotic therapy characterized by accelerated hyperthermia, rigidity, confusion, autonomic dysfunction, leukocytosis, and elevated creatine kinase. These findings should prompt immediate discontinuation of the medication; hospitalize the patient for intravenous fluids, antipyretics, and supportive care.

Benzodiazepines can be used synergistically with antipsychotics to improve control of acute agitation in the setting of psychosis. Lorazepam, 1–2 mg, may be given IV or IM in conjunction with haloperidol, and may be continued orally as required for agitation. Benzodiazepines will require a taper to discontinue if used regularly for longer than 10–14 days.

MANIA

Background

The term mania refers to a persistent elevated, expansive, or irritable mood, over at least 1 week. It must be severe enough to cause impairment in social or occupational functioning. Mania may present as a phase of primary bipolar disorder or may be secondary to medical or toxic causes. Secondary mania is more likely to be accompanied by cognitive dysfunction than primary mania, and can be attributed to varied etiologies, including substance abuse and medications, CNS injury, epilepsy, infections, and metabolic causes.[47]

Table 114-8 Psychiatric Disorders That Manifest with Psychosis

Continuous psychosis
  Schizophrenia
  Schizoaffective disorder, bipolar type (prominent episodes of mania)
  Schizoaffective disorder, depressed type (with prominent episodes of depression)
  Delusional disorder (nonbizarre, fixed delusions)
  Shared psychotic disorder

Episodic psychosis
  Depression with psychotic features
  Bipolar disorder (manic or depressed)
  Schizophreniform disorder (<6 month duration)
  Brief psychotic disorder (<1 month duration)

From: American Psychiatric Association: Diagnostic and Statistical Manual of Mental Disorders, (4th edition). Washington, DC: American Psychiatric Association, 1994.

Clinical Assessment and Evaluation

To differentiate primary from secondary mania, one must understand the risk factors and demographics of primary bipolar disorder:

- Mean age of onset 30 years
- Increased duration of episodes with age
- Initial episodes of mania rare after 50 years of age
- Positive family history of bipolar disorder

Tables 114-1 and 114-2 list the most common secondary causes of mania. Sleep deprivation can precipitate primary mania, while steroid exposure can aggravate primary mania and precipitate secondary mania in the vulnerable patient.

To evaluate mania, obtain a detailed history including medications, drugs of abuse, prior psychiatric disorders and reaction to medications, family history of psychiatric disorders, recent infections, and illnesses. Many neurologic conditions such as head trauma, epilepsy, movement disorders, multiple sclerosis, and strokes can present with manic symptoms.[48] Even though right hemispheric lesions have been reported to predispose to manic symptoms, no discrete location for a CNS lesion has been distinctly proven in secondary neurologic mania.[49]

Treatment

Patients with primary mania should be on their maintenance treatment regimen through the hospitalization, protecting the sleep pattern as much as possible. Treatment of secondary mania should focus on the underlying etiology, using pharmacologic intervention to control symptoms in the acute setting. The classic mood stabilizers lithium, valproic acid, and carbamazepine take 5–7 days to reach therapeutic effect,[50] so adjunctive medications such as the typical antipsychotic haloperidol or the atypical antipsychotics can by used during this lag period in the treatment of acute mania. Table 114-6 highlights these agents. Finally, benzodiazepines can be used as adjuvant treatment with consideration to not cause further disinhibition or confusion in patients with neurologic injury.

Key Points

- Depression in general medical inpatients is significantly underdiagnosed and undertreated. Mortality is increased in depressed patients with myocardial infarction and stroke.

- The prevalence of anxiety disorders in medical-surgical inpatients (up to 30% and higher in patients with chronic medical conditions) exceeds that in the general population.

- Inquiring about suicidal thoughts and intentions does not increase suicide risk; rather, not inquiring may increase patient mortality, and potentially, physician liability. Acute treatment of a suicidal patient requires a secure environment and a sitter for constant observation. **Seek psychiatric consultation immediately.**

- Newer agents such as the SSRI and SNRI offer distinct advantages in overdose safety, side-effect profile, and decreased drug–drug interactions.

- Stimulants like methylphenidate can be very useful as an adjuvant therapy in the psychomotor-retarded depressed and medically ill patient.

- Compared to patients with primary anxiety disorders, those with organic anxiety syndromes more typically have onset of symptoms >35 years of age and no personal or family history of anxiety disorders.

- Consider combination therapy with an antidepressant if the anxiety disorder becomes chronic and/or depressive symptoms become prominent.

- The NMS is a rare but potentially lethal complication of antipsychotic therapy characterized by accelerated hyperthermia, rigidity, confusion, autonomic dysfunction, leukocytosis, and elevated creatine kinase.

- Patients with primary mania should continue their maintenance treatment regimen through the hospitalization, protecting the sleep pattern as much as possible.

SUGGESTED READING

Friederich HC, Hartmann M, Bergmann G, et al. Psychiatric comorbidity in medical inpatients: Prevalence and effect on the length of stay. Psychother Psychosom Med Psychol 2002; 52(7):323–328.

Iouye SK, Bogardus ST Jr, Charpentier PA, et al. A multicomponent intervention to prevent delirium in hospitalized older patients. N Engl J Med 1999; 340(9):669–676.

Frasure-Smith N, Lesperance F, Talajic M. Depression following myocardial infarction: Impact on 6 month survival. JAMA 1993; 270:1819–1825.

Goldberg, RJ. The assessment of suicide risk in the general hospital. Gen Hosp Psychiatry 1987; 9:446–452.

Glassman AH, O'Connor CM, Califf RM, et al. Sertraline treatment of major depression in patients with acute MI or unstable angina. JAMA 2002; 288:701–709.

Masand PS, Tesar GE. Use of stimulants in the medically ill. Psychiatr Clin North Am 1996; 19:515–547.

Consensus Development Conference on Antipsychotic Drugs and Obesity and Diabetes. Diabetes Care 2004; 27:596–601.

CHAPTER ONE HUNDRED AND FIFTEEN

Preoperative Psychiatric Evaluation and Perioperative Management of Patients with Psychiatric Disorders

Leopoldo Pozuelo, MD, FACP, Christopher M. Whinney, MD, and Joseph Locala, MD

PREOPERATIVE EVALUATION

Background

Preoperative evaluation of patients with psychiatric disorders includes assessment of capacity and consent, baseline psychiatric disorder and how it can be exacerbated with the surgical procedure, and patients' fears of the upcoming surgery. Timely preoperative psychiatric screening can help elicit vital information such as previous coping with surgical fears, which perioperative medications have been most effective in treating the psychiatric disorder, and the expected psychologic recovery after surgery based on the patient's personality and previous surgical experience. This chapter focuses on identification and management of some psychiatric risk factors that can impact on the surgical procedure.

Clinical Assessment

Preoperative risk factors for psychiatric decompensation include substance abuse, depression, psychosis, anxiety, and delirium. The detection of these disorders, preferably prior to the surgical procedure, can help with the perioperative management.

Alcohol abuse is very common in the surgical patient, with up to 50% of all trauma beds involving patients who are under the influence of alcohol.[1,2] An alcohol history is essential, and the CAGE questionnaire can serve as a good screening instrument.[3] Laboratory findings seen with alcohol abuse include elevated aspartate aminotransferase (AST), alanine aminotransferase (ALT), lactate dehydrogenase (LDH), gamma glutamyl transpeptidase (GGT), prolonged prothrombin time (PT), and increased serum carbohydrate-deficient transferrin level.[4] It is also important to obtain a **chemical dependency** history and, when indicated, to use a screening instrument such as blood and urinary toxicology.

Depression is common in patients undergoing surgery, with up to 35% of them taking antidepressants.[5] Screening SIGECAPS as described in Chapter 114 as well as instruments such as the Beck Depression Inventory allow quick assessment. Patients can experience some degree of **anxiety** prior to a surgical procedure, specifically regarding anesthesia,[6] or fear of needles—affecting up to 8–10% of adults.[7] For patients who have experienced a pre-

vious trauma, the prospect of upcoming surgery may rekindle the anxiety disorder of post-traumatic stress disorder (PTSD).

Psychotic disorders present a challenge in the preoperative phase of surgery, as patients subject to paranoid delusion may not consent to the surgery. Concrete reasoning and cognitive impairment in the patient with schizophrenia pose challenges in the consent process and in the alliance to cooperate fully with the surgical process.[8] Finally, **delirium** is associated with preoperative factors such as older age; alcohol use; preexisting cognitive impairment; severe comorbid medical illnesses; and medication exposure, such as anticholinergics, opiates, and benzodiazepines.[9]

Management

In general, antidepressants should not be discontinued prior to general anesthesia.[10] The only exception is the monoamine oxidase inhibitors (MAOIs), due to their drug–drug interaction profile, and a washout period of 14 days is recommended prior to surgery. If the MAOI cannot be discontinued, surgery has been cautiously performed on MAOI patients by avoiding meperidine, indirect sympathomimetics, and anticholinergics.[11] The stress of surgery can destabilize bipolar disorder as well as schizophrenia, so mood stabilizers such lithium and anticonvulsants, as well as antipsychotics, should not be discontinued prior to surgery.

Benzodiazepines have been given for preoperative anxiety and do not appear to delay discharge after outpatient adult surgery.[12] Exposure techniques and other behavioral strategies are used for decreasing needle phobia and its vasovagal response.[13]

The dispensing of timely and empathic information about the procedure and mobilizing good social support should be guiding principles for the hospitalist in curbing preoperative anxiety.

As far as chemical dependency, certain elective or high-risk procedures (i.e., transplants) will require detoxification and recovery programs prior to surgery. It is advisable for the alcohol abuse patient to cut down alcohol consumption and abstain from alcohol well in advance of surgery, minimizing postoperative occurrence of alcohol withdrawal and delirium. Opiate-dependent patients should also be considered for detoxification prior to elective surgery. Patients maintained on opioids, such as those on methadone, should have their methadone dose continued preoperatively and postoperatively.[14]

PERIOPERATIVE MANAGEMENT

Background

Even with optimal preoperative assessment, breakthrough and/or exacerbation of the psychiatric illness can occur during the perioperative period. An added difficulty facing the hospitalist is how to continue the patient's home psychiatric medications through an extended surgical period of time when the patient is "NPO."

Clinical Assessment

The hospitalist should develop a heightened clinical acumen in the assessment of the essential psychiatric disorders reviewed in Chapter 114. Pharmacologic management is often necessary in acute and escalating psychiatric episodes. Patients can decompensate when they are exposed to the stress of surgery, further aggravated when the patient is off his or her maintenance medications. We will first review a limited set of available parenteral psychiatric medications (Table 115-1) and then discuss practical management techniques.

Parenteral Medication Management

Antidepressants

For the depressed patient in the perioperative period, there are currently few options for parenteral antidepressants available in the United States. In Europe, intravenous tricyclic antidepressants (TCA) such as clomipramine and imipramine have been studied as well as the intravenous SSRI citalopram[15] and the dual-acting mirtazapine.[16] Parenteral amitriptyline and imipramine are FDA approved for intramuscular use but are not commercially available. No antidepressants have been marketed for rectal preparation; however, a transdermal preparation of selegiline,[17] MAO-B (monoamine oxidase type B), has received FDA approval, and further studies are expected in the medically ill patient.

Currently, the hospitalist does have the option of dispensing the SSRIs in liquid preparation form, and the use of the dissolvable oral tablet mirtazapine (Sol-tab) is an option in the nothing by mouth (NPO) patient.

Benzodiazepines

Intravenous (IV) midazolam, lorazepam, and diazepam are available as well as intramuscular (IM) midazolam and lorazeapm. Chlordiazepoxide and diazepam are not recommended for IM use due to erratic absorption, but diazepam can be administered rectally if needed. Lorazeapm is available sublingually and more rapidly absorbed than via the oral route. A conversion chart is provided in Table 115-2 for commonly used benzodiazepines, and a good rule of thumb is that intravenous (IV) preparations are twice as potent as oral preparations (PO).

Antipsychotics

Many of the **typical antipsychotics** are available in short-acting IM form, with the high-potency agents more likely to cause extrapyramidal effects compared to low-potency agents' side effects of hypotension and sedation. Both haloperidol decanoate and fluphenazine decanoate are long-acting depot preparations that are given monthly and every 2 weeks, respec-

tively. Intravenous haloperidol, although not approved by the FDA for IV use, is the most common intravenous antipsychotic used in the hospital setting. It has minimal hemodynamic or extrapyramidal side effects,[18] and progressive dosing guidelines have been published for the agitated patient.[19,20]

Of the **atypical antipsychotics,** several parenteral forms have emerged. Short-acting forms of IM olanzapine and ziprasidone are available. A long-acting preparation risperidone (Consta) is used as a maintenance treatment. Olanzapine does have an oral dissolvable tablet form (Zydis), as well as risperidone (M-Tab), which can be used for the NPO patient in need of an antipsychotic.

Mood Stabilizers

The only FDA-approved parenteral mood stabilizer is a preparation of valproic sodium (Depacon) that can be given IV. Case reports in the psychiatric literature suggest both tolerability and efficacy.[21,22]

Perioperative Management Techniques

Depression

For patients with major depression, continue their antidepressant medication through the entire hospitalization course, reinstating the medication as soon as possible postoperatively. The discontinuation syndrome, including minor symptoms of dizziness, tremors, and jitteriness, will resolve with resumption of the antidepressant. If a prolonged NPO status is to be observed, consider using the Sol-Tab dissolving antidepressant mirtazapine; hopefully, other parenteral antidepressants will soon be available in the United States.

Anxiety Disorders

Patients with preexisting anxiety disorders should continue their anxiolytic medication, antidepressants, or benzodiazepines, through the hospital course. If NPO status applies, IV administration of a benzodiazepine at the equivalent PO dose should be instituted, with the two-fold purpose of treating the underlying anxiety disorder and preventing benzodiazepine withdrawal.

The distinct anxiety disorder of PTSD, discussed in Chapter 114 should be recognized by the hospitalist. At least 20% of burn patients experience PTSD,[23] and the disorder can also be seen after trauma, motor vehicle accidents, and even in patients after cardiac, neuro-, or cancer surgery. Combinations of psychotherapeutic techniques and medications are employed, including antidepressants, benzodiazepines, and antipsychotics.

Anxiety and the Ventilator Patient

Certain psychologic parameters have been identified to facilitate successful discontinuation of ventilator support. These include orientation to person, place, and date, having a positive mental attitude, and being at relative mental ease.[24–26] Biofeedback, relaxation techniques, and cognitive reinforcement have all been used to facilitate weaning in the anxious patient. To assist psychological readiness in the setting of high anxiety and agitation, some pharmacologic agents can be used with minimal effect on central nervous depression.[27] These agents include:

- Haloperidol, low dose, 0.5–1 mg IV, mindful of extrapyramidal side effects
- TCAs such as nortriptyline at 10 mg TID with mild anxiolytic effect and anticholinergic effect helpful in drying up secretions

Table 115-1 Parenteral and Alternative Modes of Psychotropic Administration

Generic Name	Trade Name	Alternative Delivery Mode	Initial Dose Range	Target Dose Range	Side Effects	Comments
Tricyclic Antidepressants						
Amitriptyline	Elavil	IM, IV	10–50 mg	100–300 mg	Same side effects as oral form. For IM, IV must use test dose, monitor for blood pressure drop, check serum levels at 4–5 days, monitor closely for side effects during infusion	Amitriptyline, imipramine, clomipramine not approved by the FDA for IV use, limited IM availability
Imipramine	Tofranil	IM, IV	10–75 mg	100–300 mg		
Clomipramine	Anafranil	IV	25 mg	100–250 mg		
Doxepin	Sinequan	liquid PO	25–75 mg	75–300 mg		
SSRI						
Fluoxetine	Prozac	Liquid PO	10 mg	20–40	Same side effects as with the SSRI	May use dropper and titrate up slowly every few days in sensitive patient, i.e., 2 mg, 4 mg, 6 mg, to reach 10 mg of fluoxetine
Setraline	Zoloft	Liquid PO	50 mg	50–200		
Paroxetine	Paxil	Liquid PO	10 mg	20–40		
Citalopram	Celexa	Liquid PO	10 mg	20–40		
Escitalopram	Lexapro	Liquid PO	10 mg	20–40		
Novel Dual-Acting Antidepressant						
Mirtazapine	Remeron Sol-Tab	PO dissolvable tablets	15 mg	30–45	Sedation main side effect, can promote weight gain. Has antiemetic effects, helpful in GI patients	Available in 15, 30, 45 mg tab. Place tab on tongue immediately after opening blister pack, handle with dry hands to avoid dissolving
Monoamine Oxidase Inhibitor	Emsam	Patch	6mg/24hr	9–12mg/24hr	Topical reaction, insomnia, hypotension	Tyramine free diet needed at >6 mg/24hr dose Drug-drug interoption
Mood Stabilizer						
Valproate sodium	Depacon	IV	1 g added to 500 mL of solution, infused at 20 mg/min	1–2 g for adults	Nausea, hepatitis, pancreatitis, thrombocytopenia	Monitor liver function
Benzodiazepines						
Lorazepam	Ativan	IM, IV, sublingual	0.25 mg–0.5 mg, bid	2–6 mg total dosage, given bid, tid	Sedation	No active metabolites, best suited for hepatic impairment.
Diazepam	Valium	IV, (IM erratic absorption)	5 mg bid	10–30 mg daily	Sedation; rapid onset, high addictive potential	Active metabolites;
Midazolam	Versed	IV, IM, syrup	1 mg IV slowly q 2–3 min, for procedural sedation	Max 5 mg for procedural sedation	Used also for preoperative sedation, anesthesia induction.	Quick action IV in 1–5 minutes and IM in 5–15 mintues, action lasts <2 hours

Data from Belles KE "Alternative Routes of Administration of Psychotropic Agents" in Psychiatric Care of the Medical Patient 2nd Edition. Edited by Stoudemire A, Fogel BS, Greenberg DB. New York, Oxford University Press, 2000, pg 393–403 and Robinson MJ, Owen JA "Psychopharmacology" in Textbook of Psychosomatic Medicine 1st Edition. Edited by Levenson JL. Washington DC, American Psychiatric Publishing, 2005, pg 894–898.

Table 115-1 Parenteral and Alternative Mode of Psychotropic Adminstration—cont'd

Class	Generic Name	Alternative Delivery Mode	Trade Name	Acute Dose per 24 hr	Maintenance Dose	Side Effects
Typical Antipsychotics						
Low potency	Chlorpromazine	IM, pr (for nausea, vomiting), liquid	Thorazine	25–50 mg	200–600 mg/daily	High anticholinergic profile, very sedating, low EPS. Check QTc
	Thioridazine	IM, liquid	Mellaril	25–50 mg	200–600 mg/daily	High anticholinergic profile, very sedating, low EPS, retinal pigmentation at high dosages, **severe risk** of QTc prolongation
Medium potency	Perphenazine	IM	Trilafon	4–8 mg	16–32	Mild anticholinergic, mild eps Check QTc
High potency	Haloperidol	IM, IV, liquid	Haldol	5–10 mg	10–20 mg daily	Extrapyramidal symptoms, less with IV than PO, IM Haldol: must monitor QTc
	Haloperidol	IM decanoate	Haldol Decanoate	25–50 mg IM q month	100–200 mg monthly maintenance dose	Confirm no eps first with PO dose before giving im monthly decanoate
	Fluphenazine	IM	Prolixin	5–10 mg	20–30 mg mg daily	Same considerations as Haldol. Decanoate im maintenance form available, given q 2 wk
Atypical Antipsychotics						
	Olanzapine	PO dissolvable tablets	Zyprexa Zydis	5–10 mg dissolve on top of tongue	10–20 mg daily	Sedation, can be favorable effect, titrate effect
	Olanzapine	IM (for acute agitation)	Zyprexa	10 mg IM × I. Repeat in 2 hr and 6 h prn, max 30 mg/24 hour period	30 mg daily	sedation, can be favorable effect, titrate effect, monitor for hypotension
	Risperidone	PO dissolvable tablets	Risperdal M-tab	I mg/day	4–6 mg/day do not	EPS can be seen at dosages 4 mg or above. Elevates
		PO solution	Risperdal		mix oral solutin with cola or tea	prolactin; titrate dose due to orthostatic hypotension;
	Ziprasidone	IM (for acute agitation)	Geodon	10 mg IM, q 2 hr prn, max 40 mg/24 hr period, max 3 days	40 mg/day for 3 days	activation; Check ECG for QTc prolongation
	Aripiprazole	PO solution	Abilify	10, 15 mg daily tablets equivalent to solution up to 25 mg, then 30 mg = 25 mg solution	30–45 mg	Nausea, activation

Table 115-2 Benzodiazepine Conversion Chart

Generic Name	Trade Name	Equivalent Oral (mg) Dose
Chlordiazepoxide	Librium	10
Diazepam	Valium	5
Lorazepam	Ativan	1
Clonazeapm	Klonopin	0.5
Alprazolam	Xanax	0.25

Adapted from Goldberg RJ "Alcohol and Substance abuse" in Practical Guide to the Care of the Psychiatric Patient, 2nd Edtion. Edited by Goldberg RJ St Louis, Mosby 1998, pg 247 and Renner JA, Gastfriend DR "Drug-Addicted Patients" in Massachusetts General Hospital Handbook of General Hospital Psychiatry 5th Edition. Edited by Stern TA, Fricchione GL, Cassem NH, et al. Philadelphia, Mosby 2004, pg 128–129, 224–228 and Pollack MH, Otto MW, Bernstein JG, et al "Anxious Patients" in Massachusetts General Hospital Handbook of General Hospital Psychiatry 5th Edition. Edited by Stern TA, Fricchione GL, Cassem NH, et al. Philadelphia, Mosby 2004, pg 196.

- Psychostimulants (methylphenidate) for patients with apathy and low activity.[28]
- Buspirone, with its delayed action, in the chronic setting for anxiety and when weaning takes place over weeks.
- Benzodiazepines, preferably those with a short half-life such as lorazepam 0.5 mg, can be used with great care for potential of respiratory suppression.[29]

Bipolar Disorder

As with all psychiatric disorders, resumption of the patient's home medications is the key goal. Parenteral antipsychotics, such as IM or IV haloperidol, as well as IM olanzapine and ziprazidone and the dissolvable olanzapine, Zydis, can be used to curb any manic or psychotic phase of the bipolar illness. They can also be used temporarily to control mood lability until NPO status resolves and the patient's usual medications can be resumed. Many of the atypical antipsychotics confer mood stabilization properties and thus can be used briefly as a monotherapy substitute in the perioperative period of the bipolar patient, especially if NPO. Usually, this will suffice, and the physician will not need to resort to IV valproate sodium (Depacon).

Psychosis and Delirium

Again, typical and atypical antipsychotic medications are available in parenteral formulation, facilitating the management of premorbid psychotic illness in the perioperative stage. Likewise, antipsychotics are the front-line psychotropics used in the symptomatic treatment of delirium. A parenteral approach using IV haloperidol is outlined in Table 115-3. Clinicians can also use lorazepam IV 0.5–1 mg concurrently or alternating with the haloperidol when initial response with haloperidol is not adequate in controlling the agitated patient.[30] The concern with benzodiazepines in delirium, except in alcohol withdrawal, is that prolonged use can actually potentiate the delirium itself.

Olanzapine in dosages of 5–15 mg a day has also been helpful in the management of delirium,[31,32] and the oral dissolving Zydis formulations is used frequently on our consultation services. Less data are available for newer IM olanzapine and ziprasidone in the medically ill patient. All antipsychotics should be monitored for prolongation of QTc, especially greater than 450 msec.[33] In April

Table 115-3 Guidelines for Use of IV Haloperidol in the Agitated Patient

Halperidol can precipitate phenytoin and heparin, flush line before administration.

Check pre-haloperidol QTc interval, if QTc >450 ms proceed with caution, if QTC >500 ms, use other options.

Check and correct potassium and magnesium.

Give first dose of haloperidol based on level of agitation, age, and size.

> Mild agitation use 0.5 mg–2 mg IV starting dose
> Moderate agitation use 2–5 mg IV starting dose
> Severe agitation use 5–10 mg IV starting dose

Wait 20–30 minutes, if patient remains agitated, double dose.

Follow QTc, if increases by 25 % or >500, consider other options.

Once goal of having patient calm and awake, consider the total dose needed and may distribute over next 24 hours, in divided dosages q 6 hr, then reducing the dose 50 % every next 24 hours.

Alternatively, may use effective dose as needed for agitation.

Adapted from Huffman JC, Stern TA, Januzzi JL "The psychiatric management of patients with cardiac disease" in Massachusetts General Hospital Handbook of General Hospital Psychiatry 5th Edition. Edited by Stern TA, Fricchione GL, Cassem NH, et al. Philadelphia, Mosby 2004, pg 562–564.

of 2005, the FDA issued a black box warning for all atypical antipsychotics, due to increased cardiovascular events in elderly patients with dementia related psychosis.[34] The clinical implications of this labeling are still being evaluated, but the hospitalist may elect to avoid the atypical agents in the elderly demented patient with recent heart attack or stroke.

The concept of "ICU psychosis,"[35] referring to postoperative delirium, brought about environmental interventions to the intensive care unit (ICU) such as natural light exposure, use of clocks, and reorientation from staff in the perioperative period. One must not, however, desist in looking for the underlying physiologic causes of delirium that cause the "ICU psychosis."

Behavioral interventions addressing cognitive impairment, sleep deprivation, immobility, visual and hearing impairment, and dehydration appear to decrease the frequency and duration of delirium,[36] although it appears to be a more robust effect in the index hospitalization than in the subsequent recovery.[37]

Alcohol Withdrawal

Benzodiazepines are the treatment of choice for prevention and active management of alcohol withdrawal. A fixed detoxification regimen (instead of "as needed" if properly educated nursing staff is not available) should be applied to alcoholic patients with histories of delirium tremens, alcohol withdrawal seizures, and comorbid medical illnesses.[38] Two such protocols using chlordiazepoxide and lorazepam are outlined in Table 115-4. Chapter 89 provides a detailed exploration of the management of alcohol withdrawal in the hospital setting.

Chlordiazepoxide has a long half-life with long acting metabolites. In patients with liver disease, lorazepam is preferred with its

Table 115-4 Use of Benzodiazepine in Alcohol Withdrawal

Benzodiazepine	**LIBRIUM** (chlordiazepoxide) only use PO chlordiazepoxide will safe taper	50 mg PO every 6 hours first 24 hours 25 mg PO every 6 hours second 24 hours 10 mg PO every 6 hours third 24 hours
	ATIVAN (lorazepam) can give PO, IM, IV IV lorazepam twice as potent as PO or IM lorazepam preferred in liver impairment	2 mg PO every 6–8 hours first 24 hours 1 mg PO every 6–8 hours second 24 hours 0.5 mg every 6–8 hours third 24 hours taper 25–50% per day

Above recommendations vary by individual patient, need to monitor correct medication dosage and correlate with withdrawal signs (elevated BP, HR, hyperefelxia,) as well as monitor for excess sedation.

Adapted from Goldberg RJ "Alcohol and Substance abuse" in Practical Guide to the Care of the Psychiatric Patient, 2nd Edition. Edited by Goldberg RJ St Louis, Mosby 1998, pg 244–249 and Gastfriend DR, Renner JA, Hackett TP. "Alcoholic Patients—Acute and Chronic" in Massachusetts General Hospital Handbook of General Hospital Psychiatry 5th Edition. Edited by Stern TA, Fricchione GL, Cassem NH, et al. Philadelphia, Mosby 2004, pg 206.

renal excretion and safer metabolization in the liver via conjugation instead of oxidation. Lorazepam can be given PO, IM, or IV, again with the caveat that IV is twice as potent as PO, and its short half-life provides no self-tapering effect.

Thiamine 100 mg/day (can be given IM or IV if unable to give PO) must be given to the patient withdrawing from alcohol, especially prior to glucose infusion to avoid precipitating Wernicke's encephalopathy. Folic acid 1 mg/day and multivitamins round out other essential nutrients for the alcoholic patient. Finally, for uncomplicated alcohol withdrawal, adding an anticonvulsant is not usually necessary,[39] although it is recommended with any patient having a known history of seizures unrelated to alcohol withdrawal.

ECT CONSULTATION.

Background

Electroconvulsive therapy (ECT) still holds a place in the modern psychiatry armamentarium and is very safe, with death rates due to treatment of 1 per 10,000 patients treated.[40] Indications for ECT range from mood disorders (major depression, bipolar depression, and mania) to psychotic disorders (schizophrenia catatonic subtype, and schizoaffective disorders) and some mental disorders due to medical conditions (catatonic states). Substantial clinical improvement can occur after the first few treatments, and an initial therapy regimen of ECT typically entails 6–8 treatments, usually given three times per week on an alternate-day schedule (e.g., Monday, Wednesday, Friday). ECT can be performed in both the inpatient and outpatient settings, depending on the severity of the patient's psychiatric and medical conditions.

The technique of ECT is quite straightforward, with the objective of inducing a controlled and monitored seizure. The procedure is done in a typical postanesthesia care unit setting, with anesthesia presence as well cardiac, hemodynamic, and respiratory monitoring. The patient is put to sleep (e.g., IV methohexital) and once asleep is given a muscle relaxant (e.g., IV succinylcholine) to minimize muscle response to the seizure. The anesthetist will ventilate the patient with an Ambu bag, monitor respiratory status with oximetry, and insert a bite block to avoid

oral injury. Once the patient is asleep and fully paralyzed, an electrical stimulus is delivered via electrodes placed in the bifrontal or bitemporal areas. Unilateral stimulation can also be used. The induced seizure usually lasts 20–60 seconds. Once the seizure is completed, the patient recovers in 5–15 minutes, with amnesia for the treatment episode.

Interventions for the hospitalist in the care of the ECT patient revolve around careful pretreatment assessment and stabilization of medical comorbidities, as well as continued assessment of the patient's medical status along the treatment course.

Clinical Assessment

According to the American Psychiatric Association Task Force report on ECT (2001),[40] the pre-ECT assessment should include the following:
- Psychiatric history and examination, assessing the indications for ECT and current mental status examination as part of the ECT psychiatric consultation.
- Medical examination, including general medical history, physical examination, and presence of medical risk factors.
- Suggested laboratory studies, including CBC, electrolytes, renal function, and ECG. Routine neuroimaging, CXR, or spine films are not warranted unless clinically indicated.
- Pre-ECT anesthesia consult to address anesthetic risk, modification of medications, and anesthetic technique related to any cardiac, pulmonary, or other medical risk factors.
- Informed consent.

There are no "absolute" medical contraindications to ECT. That being said, there are specific conditions that have substantial increased risk associated with ECT, and these include[40]:
- Increased intracranial pressure, as may occur with some brain tumors or space occupying cerebral lesions
- Aneurysm or vascular malformation that might be susceptible to increased blood pressure
- Unstable or severe cardiovascular conditions such as recent muocardial infarction (MI), unstable angina, unstable congestive heart failure (CHF), or severe valvular disease
- Recent cerebral infarction
- Pulmonary conditions such as severe COPD, asthma, or pneumonia

- Patient status of American Society of Anesthesiologists (ASA) level 4 or 5

Careful risk/benefit assessment must be carried out in the above settings as well as considering any potential modification in patient management of ECT technique that can decrease the level of medical risk.

Cardiac considerations of ECT include the physiologic observation of initial parasympathetic stimulation followed by sympathetic stimulation with corresponding effects on heart rate, blood pressure, rate pressure product (which increases several-fold), and temporary increase (up to 81%) in cardiac output.[41] Patients with chronic atrial fibrillation can have the ECT procedure done safely, and therapeutic anticoagulation should be continued. Newly identified atrial fibrillation should be evaluated by a cardiologist for proper management before ECT.[42] A cardiology consultation is also recommended for patients with pacemakers and/or implantable defibrillators; these patients can safely undergo ECT. Depending on the pacemaker type, some patients will require adjustment of the pacemaker (changing to pacing only mode with sensing function turned off), especially if they are pacemaker dependent. ICD patients require turning off the ICD device immediately prior to the ECT, monitoring on the ECG monitor during the ECT stimulus and procedure, and then turning on the ICD when the treatment is complete.

Some **neurologic considerations** include the use of antihypertensives to mitigate the ECT-related increase in blood pressure in patients at risk with known aneurysms or vascular malformations. Stroke patients should have good control of their blood pressure pre-ECT. Consider using short-acting antihypertensives in stroke patients to avoid a later drop in blood pressure in this patient population with impaired autoregulation of blood pressure.[43] ECT can actually improve, albeit briefly, the motor symptoms of patients with Parkinson's disease. ECT can also be safely administered in epilepsy patients, whose anticonvulsant regimen is continued through the ECT treatments. The ECT treatments do not increase the incidence of spontaneous seizure frequency in the epilepsy patient. Finally, patients with dementia who are taking cholinesterase inhibitors (e.g., donepezil) could pose a theoretical interaction with succinylcholine (which is metabolized by plasma cholinesterase): however, ECT has been administered safely to patients taking these medications.[44]

Pulmonary considerations involve careful attention to airway management and instructing COPD or asthma patients to use their inhalers right before ECT. Theophylline has been reported to increase the risk of prolonged seizures and should be discontinued before ECT. **Diabetes mellitus** patients should receive half of their morning insulin, receive prompt ECT treatment, and then post-ECT, be fed breakfast and given the remaining insulin dose.[42] Oral hypoglycemic agents should be held in the AM of ECT and in patients prone to hypoglycemia, consider holding AM insulin and use regular coverage only. **Glaucoma patients** can experience a limited increase of intraocular pressure after the ECT treatment, so patients should receive their medication in the morning of treatment, except for anticholinesterase medications, which could theoretically prolong the effect of succinylcholine.[45]

Management

The hospitalist's role in the ongoing management of the ECT patient should include optimal control of hemodynamic, cardiac,

respiratory, and other medical conditions as well as screening for treatment complications. Patient medications that should be continued prior to each treatment include antihypertensives, antianginals, antiarrhythmics (except lidocaine which could negatively affect seizure threshold), antireflux agents, bronchodilators (except theophylline), and corticosteroids. Medications can be given with sips of water in the morning of ECT.

The APA Task Force report on ECT (2001) made recommendations of medications that should be discontinued prior to and during the course of ECT.[40] They include theophylline, lithium (can predispose to delirium and prolonged seizures), and benzodiazepines, which can interfere with seizure elicitation. If benzodiazepines are needed, the dosage should be minimal and with agents of short half-life (e.g., lorazepam). Anticonvulsant medication also should be discontinued prior to the start of ECT, except if used for the treatment of an underlying seizure disorder. Finally, psychiatric medications such as antipsychotic medications, which can exert synergistic therapeutic effects, as well as antidepressants should be continued during ECT.

Key Points

- A timely preoperative psychiatric screening can help elicit vital information such as previous coping with surgical fears, which perioperative medications have been most effective in treating the psychiatric disorder, and the expected psychologic recovery after surgery based on the patient's personality and previous surgical experience.

- For treatment of depression, SSRIs in liquid preparation form and the dissolvable oral tablet mirtazapine (Sol-Tab) can be used in the NPO patient.

- Parenteral antipsychotics such as IM or IV haloperidol, as well as IM olanzapine and ziprasidone and the dissolvable olanzapine, Zydis, dissolvable and rispendone, M-Tab, can be used to curb any manic or psychotic phase of the bipolar illness.

- All antipsychotics should be monitored for prolongation of QTc, especially greater than 450 msec.

- There are no "absolute" medical contraindications to ECT, although increased intracranial pressure from brain tumors, aneurysms or vascular malformations, recent MI, unstable angina, decompensated CHF, recent stroke, and severe pulmonary conditions are associated with increased risk.

- Short-term cardiovascular effects associated with ECT include increased heart rate, blood pressure, rate pressure product, and cardiac output.

SUGGESTED READING

Inouye SK, Bogardus ST, Charpentier PA, et al. A multicomponent intervention to prevent delirium in hospitalized older patients. N Engl J Med 1999; 340:669–676.

Tesar GE, Stern TA. Evaluation and treatment of agitation in the intensive care unit. Intens Care Med 1986; 1:137–148.

Powers PS, Santana CA. Surgery. In: Levenson JL, ed. Textbook of Psychosomatic Medicine. 1st Edition. Washington, DC: American Psychiatric Publishing, 2005. 654.

Inouye SK, Bogardus ST, Williams CS, et al. The role of adherence on the effectiveness of non-pharmacological interventions: evidence from the Delirium Prevention Trial. Arch Intern Med 2003; 163:958–964.

Weiner RD, ed. American Psychiatric Association, Committee on electroconvulsive therapy: The Practice of Electroconvulsive Therapy, 2nd Edition. Washington, DC: American Psychiatric Association, 2001. 30, 59, 79, 94–95.

Section

Nineteen

Hospitalist Program Operations

116 Developing the Financial Plan and Establishing Workforce
Needs for a Hospital Medicine Program
Leslie Flores, Winthrop F. Whitcomb, John R. Nelson

117 Structuring a Hospital Medicine Program: An Overview
of Contracting Options, Operating Procedures, and
Recruitment Strategies
Leslie Flores, John R. Nelson

118 Scheduling and Staff Deployment for Hospital
Medicine Programs
Bipinchandra Mistry, Winthrop F. Whitcomb

119 Communication in Hospitalist Systems
Winthrop F. Whitcomb, Russell Holman, John R. Nelson

120 Compensation Principles and Practices
Russell Holman, Winthrop F. Whitcomb, John R. Nelson

121 Documentation, Coding, Billing, and Compliance in Hospital
Medicine
M. Tray Dunaway, Beth B. Golden, Steven T. Liu

122 Measuring Value of a Hospital Medicine Program
Ron Greeno

CHAPTER ONE HUNDRED AND SIXTEEN

Developing the Financial Plan and Establishing Workforce Needs for a Hospital Medicine Program

Leslie Flores, MHA, Winthrop F. Whitcomb, MD, and John R. Nelson, MD, FACP

INTRODUCTION

The successful start-up of a new hospital medicine program depends on having sound financial and implementation plans. This chapter describes a process for projecting workload and staffing requirements for a new hospital medicine program, and for developing a financial plan. Each of these planning components is crucial in generating support for the program and in designing it so that appropriate resources can be allocated from the outset.

Projecting workload and professional fee revenue for a new hospital medicine practice is a difficult proposition: Numerous variables must be taken into consideration, and most cannot be predicted with a high degree of certainty. However, a structured, stepwise approach can go a long way toward minimizing the uncertainty. Also, a thorough, organized, and well-documented process for projecting workload and revenues can enhance both credibility and negotiating leverage when it comes time to establish a budget and hospitalist recruitment plan with the sponsoring organization.

PROGRAM DRIVERS AND SCOPE OF SERVICE

The starting point for the financial plan of any hospital medicine practice is to determine what types of services the practice will provide and the source of business. This requires an understanding of the factors driving program development. This may include:

- Primary care physicians' desire to limit practice to the outpatient setting, whether due to the increasing complexity of inpatient care, the inconvenience of rounding on a small number of patients, or for financial reasons
- Unwillingness of physicians to take calls for the emergency department unassigned patients
- Hospitals' goals to reduce variability, improve clinical quality and patient safety, and manage inpatient costs
- Code blue, rapid-response team, inhouse intensive care unit (ICU) coverage, or other full-time hospital-based services
- Provision of medical coverage for specialty units such as psychiatry, acute rehabilitation, or skilled nursing
- Medical comanagement of surgical patients

- Hospital market share growth by attracting referrals from outlying communities

ESTABLISHING REFERRAL ASSUMPTIONS

Once the key program drivers have been identified, they can be used to articulate an initial scope of service for the practice, which in turn will suggest potential sources of referrals and other service demands. This analysis may be divided into two categories:

- Referrals for inpatient admissions that will be managed by the hospitalists
- Other services that the hospitalists may be asked to provide

Inpatient Admissions

Inpatient admissions represent the core of the hospital medicine practice, and they typically account for the vast majority of the workload. When projecting inpatient referrals, it is helpful to consider separately each of three potential sources listed in Box 116-1.

Most hospital medicine programs are expected to provide all or a portion of the emergency department (ED) call coverage by admitting unassigned medical patients (i.e., those with no primary care physician or whose primary physician does not have admitting privileges). Unfortunately, few hospitals have a formal system for tracking unassigned admissions, and estimates of the number of unassigned admissions may be biased. Thus, the best way to determine the volume of potential admissions from providing ED call coverage is to track such admissions prospectively for a period of time. Ideally, this should be done at different times of the year to account for seasonal variations. If time does not allow, then a 1-month study that is annualized based on variations in ED admission volume from month to month will suffice. In other words, if during the study month unassigned medical admissions accounted for 20% of total emergency department admissions, then total annual unassigned medical admissions can be estimated by taking 20% of the previous year's total ED admissions.

In order to project the volume of referrals by primary care physicians (PCPs), obtain a report from the hospital of the number of admissions and total patient days for the previous year for each PCP on staff. Then, either ideally through a formal survey

> ## Box 116-1 Three Major Referral Sources for a Hospital Medicine Practice
>
> Emergency department—unassigned patients
>
> Referrals from primary care physicians
>
> Referrals from medical subspecialists, surgeons, and specialty units

> ## Box 116-2 Projecting Initial Number of Referrals
>
> Quantify—prospectively, if possible—the number of ED unassigned needing admission
>
> Query the medical staff—PCPs and specialists—as to how many wish to refer to the program
>
> Estimate volume of referrals from specialty units if included in the scope of service

> ## Box 116-3 How Hospitalists Add Value Beyond Billings
>
> Treating unassigned patients
>
> Leading hospital medical staff
>
> Improving physician practices
>
> Providing extraordinary availability
>
> Maximizing throughput and improving patient flow
>
> Educating through formal and informal learning processes
>
> Improving patient safety and quality of care
>
> From: Miller JM. The hospitalist. Official Publication of the Society of Hospital Medicine 2005; 9(Suppl 1):6.

process or by educated guess, the PCPs who will initially refer patients can be assessed, yielding a patient volume figure. Be sure to subtract anticipated ED unassigned admissions from the total estimate of PCP referrals, so that they are not counted twice.

Finally, potential referrals from other sources should be considered. These include medical subspecialists, surgeons, and overflow from residency programs coping with resident work hour restrictions. Also, consider specialty unit populations such as psychiatry, acute rehabilitation, and skilled nursing facility that may require medical management. Box 116-2 summarizes steps for projecting the initial number of referrals to the hospital medicine practice.

It is important to consider each of these referral sources separately, in order to account for differing average length of stay (ALOS) depending on the source. Once the number of annual referrals from each source is identified, the unique characteristics of each population should be considered to estimate an ALOS for each. It may be appropriate to build in a modest (5–10 %) reduction in ALOS upon implementation of the hospital medicine program.[1] Based on the anticipated volume of inpatient referrals and a projected composite average length of stay, a projected annual number of patient days can be derived. NOTE: Because hospitals typically count length of stay by the number of midnights a patient is in the hospital, there will be an additional billable day for the physician. For example, for a 5-day LOS, there will be an admission and a discharge day, and 4 days in between. A 5-day hospitalization as counted by the hospital (i.e., 5 midnights) will yield six billable patient contacts.

Other Hospitalist Services

Other common sources of hospitalist workload include observation unit admissions, procedures, responding to code blues or to unstable patients in or out of the ICU, providing "tuck-in" services for other attending physicians, or operating a preoperative assessment clinic or outpatient indigent follow-up clinic. The volume of observation admissions and procedures is sometimes estimated as a percent of inpatient admissions. These percentages will vary,

based on local practice patterns. It may be possible to obtain information from the hospital or local private practices to assist in projecting the volumes of these services. When in doubt, estimate on the high side rather than the low side, as these are areas in which demand is often underestimated.

Nonbillable Hospitalist Activities

There will often be significant nonbillable service expectations of the hospital medicine program as well, such as medical staff committee membership, resident teaching, participation in system improvement work, or other hospital "citizenship" activities. Box 116-3 provides a framework for categorizing nonbillable activities. (NOTE: Although treating unassigned patients may be partially a billable activity, it also confers benefits to the hospital system above the associated billings.) Each nonbillable activity should be carefully delineated with a corresponding hourly workload or other mutually agreed upon metric assigned. Then, nonbillable workload should be added to billable workload to arrive at overall workload for the program. Failure to account for nonbillable activities is one of the most common pitfalls leading to an underestimate in projecting hospitalist workload.

PROJECTING WORKLOAD BY ENCOUNTER TYPE

Once referrals and ALOS have been projected, one can project the types and quantities of encounters to be provided. For example, for each inpatient admission, there will be one initial hospital care encounter and one discharge care encounter. The number of continuing care encounters from inpatient admissions is equal to the total number of projected patient days minus the number of initial encounters. Occasionally, there will be more than one continuing care encounter per hospital day, but this number is small enough to be omitted from the initial projection.

The number of continuing care encounters arising from consults must also be projected. It is not unusual for each initial consult to result in almost as many continuing care encounters as an average admission; however, this ratio will vary, based on local practice patterns. It is important to consider whether the majority of hospital medicine consults will be one-time visits such as preoperative medical management, or whether they will likely involve multiple visits to manage comorbidities for subspecialists.

For observation admissions, the vast majority will have a separate initial care and discharge encounter. The rest are admitted and discharged in the same calendar day, for which there is a single CPT code. Finally, the performance of procedures should be assessed, but the volume undertaken by hospitalists is highly variable. Projections should be based on local patterns and medical staff needs.

PROJECTING FULL-TIME EQUIVALENT (FTE) REQUIREMENTS

The hospitalist staffing plan must take into consideration both the projected workload and the coverage expectations of the sponsoring organization. A number of methods can be used to arrive at a projected FTE requirement, each relying on a set of assumptions. Box 116-4 lists the key assumptions in FTE projections, regardless of the method used. Below is one method that may be employed to arrive at a projected FTE requirement.

Frequently, the number of FTE hospitalists required to do the projected work will not be adequate to provide the level of 24/7 coverage expected, due to the fact that the workload is not spread evenly between days and nights, nor over the days of the week. For this reason, it is best to start with basic coverage requirements. Is a hospitalist expected to be physically inhouse 24 hours a day, 7 days a week? Or can an acceptable level of service be obtained by providing daytime inhouse coverage with on-call coverage for nights? The answer to this question will depend on expected daily encounter volume, how that volume is distributed throughout the day, and service expectations such as code blue management.

Based on the coverage requirements, it is possible to calculate the number of work days (or shifts) needed to ensure at least one hospitalist is on site during the times of required coverage. A typical hospitalist work day may be anything from 8 to 14 hours long, but usually 2 hospitalist work days are required to provide basic coverage for a 24-hour period (e.g., a 7a.m.–7p.m. shift and a 7p.m.–7a.m. shift). The required number of FTEs for basic coverage can then be calculated by dividing the total number of work days needed to provide the basic coverage for a year by roughly 220, which is a reasonable number of work days per FTE hospitalist per year. (NOTE: there is no standard number of annual days worked for a hospitalist. If working very long shifts, many nights and weekends, or providing significant on-call coverage, the number of work days per year will likely be lower than 220. A common staffing pattern is 7 on/7 off, or 182.5 days/year.)

Once the number of FTEs needed to provide basic coverage has been determined, it is necessary to look at daily workload. The total number of annual encounters projected above is divided by

365 to arrive at an average daily encounter volume. For the first example below, it is assumed that 90% of total encounters will occur during the day, with the rest occurring at night. This figure is purely an assumption and will vary based on locale and how "night" is defined. An adjustment to the base number of FTEs needed for coverage can be determined by dividing the projected average daytime encounters by a production target per hospitalist work day.

A single hospitalist usually averages 12–18 encounters in a work day, though this is highly variable and dependent on the mix of encounter types. For example, if a hospitalist is assigned to do mostly admissions on a given day, he or she will be able to see far fewer total encounters. It is also important to consider the potential for workload variability from day to day. If an average production target of 17 or 18 encounters per work day is established, it is likely that there will be a number of days (especially in the winter months) when the hospitalist must see 25 or more encounters. While managing more than 20 encounters on an occasional basis is acceptable, to do so on a regular basis will likely result in overwork, burnout, and a potential for medical errors. In programs with a high degree of workload variability, establishing a lower average production target of 13 or 14 encounters per day may be more appropriate.[2–4]

Examples

FTE Requirement for 24/7 Inhospital Coverage

If the program requires 24/7 coverage, the minimum number of FTEs required to provide the necessary coverage is calculated at 3.3 if plans include an expectation of 220 work days.

365 days/year × 2 hospitalist work days/day/220 work days/FTE = 3.3 FTEs

However, with only 3.3 FTE hospitalists, each physician will be working many nights and weekends; so it may be more appropriate to reduce the expected number of work days per FTE. If the requirement is recalculated at 190 work days per FTE, the base number of FTEs becomes 3.8:

365 days/year × 2 hospitalist work days/day/190 work days/FTE = 3.8 FTEs

Assuming average daily encounter volume of around 30, of which 10% or 3 encounters occur on the night shift, the average daytime encounter volume will be 27. Typically, two daytime hospitalists will be required for an encounter volume of 27, so the base number of FTEs needs to be adjusted to add another hospitalist work day or shift, each day of the year:

365 days/year/190 work days/FTE − 1.9 FTEs

Based on this set of assumptions, then, the estimated total number of required FTEs is 5.7:

3.8 coverage FTEs + 1.9 FTEs to provide a second rounding physician = 5.7 FTEs

Daytime Only Inhospital Coverage

For a program with the same volume but not requiring 24/7 inhospital coverage, one could assume each full-time hospitalist works 200 days per year (plus providing a share of the night call coverage). Then the FTE requirement is 3.7:

$$365 \text{ days/year} \times 2 \text{ daytime hospitalists/day/200 work days/FTE} = 3.7 \text{ FTEs}$$

Typically, the FTE requirement is rounded up to the nearest full (or sometimes half) FTE, since there will often be unanticipated needs for additional coverage.

The number of FTEs needed is clearly related to the hospitalists' work schedule. While the specifics of scheduling are discussed in the Chapter 118, it is instructive to point out that hospitalists in a program that uses a 7 days on/7 days off work schedule (a common schedule) work 182 days per year, compared to a more typical 210–230 worked days per year. With a 7on/7off schedule, either more FTEs will be required to provide the necessary coverage, or fewer hospitalists will be scheduled to work each day, resulting in each hospitalist needing to see more patients and work much harder each day that he or she works.

Using Productivity Benchmarks

Some programs utilize national benchmark surveys such as those published by the Society of Hospital Medicine (SHM)[4] or the Medical Group Management Association (MGMA)[5] to establish productivity expectations for individual hospitalists, which then drives the definition of how many FTEs are needed. While such benchmarks are a useful as a reference point, they have significant limitations. They do not distinguish between 24/7 inhouse coverage models and on-call coverage models. Further, they do not recognize the scaling of productivity typical in 24/7 inhouse programs based on the size of the program and the proportion of staffing dedicated to low-productivity inhouse night shifts. For example, the night hospitalist in a 24/7 inhouse program with 1,500 annual admissions will be substantially less productive than in a program with 5,000 annual admissions—the benchmarks do not differentiate the two.

The SHM survey data include a significant proportion (about 15%) of academic practices, which tend to have very different staffing and productivity; the MGMA respondents, on the other hand, represent a much smaller sample size and consist of around 90% multispecialty medical groups (some of which may be academic faculty practices). Based on the MGMA survey results, it appears that many of the included hospitalists may provide inpatient coverage strictly for their own multispecialty medical groups, perhaps even on a daytime coverage basis only. For these reasons, planners must be cautious when interpreting the results of such surveys.

PROJECTING PRACTICE REVENUE

In order to develop a realistic financial plan and garner sponsoring organization support, it is necessary to understand both the projected practice revenue (usually from professional services fees billed to third party payors) and the projected practice costs.

The sponsoring organization should be able to provide reports indicating overall payor mix by financial class or major payor category [e.g., health maintenance organization (HMO), preferred provider organization (PPO), commercial, self-pay, etc.] for various anticipated referral sources. Based on the various payor mixes of the potential referral sources, one can estimate an overall payor mix for the hospital medicine practice. A hospital medicine practice's payor mix will usually be weighted more toward Medicaid, Medicare, and uninsured patients than the average private physician or even the hospital's overall payor mix.

Professional fee reimbursement is one of the most difficult components for a new practice to project, especially if it is not affiliated with (or able to obtain reimbursement information from) private practices in the community. If the sponsoring organization employs other types of physicians and has a physician billing department or contracted service, this is a good resource for estimating reimbursement. Also, the Medicare fee schedule is available on the Center for Medicare and Medicaid Services website (http://www.cms.hhs.gov/physicians/mpfsapp/default.asp), and many states post their Medicaid fee schedules on line.

Because retail charges for physician fees are extremely variable from practice to practice, it is not usually helpful to estimate reimbursement by various payors as a percent of charges. The most common method for representing reimbursement levels is to estimate the percent of the Medicare fee schedule paid by each financial class.

A worksheet should be developed that lists the CPT codes commonly billed in a hospitalist practice along the left-hand side, and the major payor categories across the top. The distribution of CPT codes should be estimated, so that a calculation of the number of times each CPT code will be billed by the practice over the course of a year can be made and added to the worksheet. The best way to project the distribution of CPT codes for the practice is to use historical information from existing community practitioners, if available. If not, it may be possible to work with the sponsoring organization's physician billing department or a third-party billing service to develop some estimates. Then the total number of units for each CPT code should be distributed across financial classes, based on the projected payor mix.

Expected reimbursement by CPT code should then be entered into the worksheet, so that a calculation can be performed multiplying the expected frequency of each CPT code for each financial class by the expected reimbursement for that CPT code for that financial class. The sum of this reimbursement will be the projected professional fee revenue for the practice (Table 116-1).

It is common to see average reimbursement in the range of $60–$70 per encounter, though in areas with an excellent payor mix, this number is sometimes in the $80 range.

ANTICIPATING HOSPITAL MEDICINE PROGRAM COSTS

Direct Hospitalist Compensation

Hospital medicine program costs typically include cost of direct compensation and benefits for the hospitalists, and a variety of practice management costs. Direct compensation per FTE hospitalist should be projected based on an assessment of fair market value for hospitalist services. The range of fair market value can be determined by considering a number of factors, including:

- Published compensation surveys, such as those conducted by the SHM, the MGMA, and others
- What other hospitalists are earning in the local and regional market
- What doctors with the same training as the hospitalists (e.g., internists or pediatricians) typically earn in traditional office practice in the local and regional market

Table 116-1 Hospital Medicine Program Revenue Model Revenue Projection

CPT Code	Description	Annual Units of Service per CPT Code	Annual Net Revenue per CPT Code	Total Annual Net Revenue
Inpatient Care				
Initial Hospital Care				
99221	H&P low	57	$3,481.42	
99222	H&P moderate	511	$51,737.10	
99223	H&P high	2,270	$319,854.72	
			Subtotal Initial Hospital Care	*$375,073*
Subsequent Hospital Care				
99231	F/U low	1,833	$56,021.44	
99232	F/U mod	2,723	$135,544.82	
99233	F/U high	628	$44,512.81	
99356	Prolonged svc 1st hr.	209	$17,031.87	
99357	Prolonged svc add'l. 30 min.	26	$2,150.82	
99291	Critical care svc 1st hr.	52	$9,785.90	
99292	Critical care svc add'l. 30 min.	26	$2,444.13	
			Subtotal Subsequent Hospital Care	*$267,492*
Discharge Care				
99238	D/C	1,987	$125,449.20	
99239	D/C, ext	851	$73,352.65	
			Subtotal Discharge Care	*$198,802*
Other Encounters				
Inpatient Consults				
99251	Consult limited	0	$0.00	
99252	Consult low	2	$124.51	
99253	Consult moderate	42	$3,712.36	
99254	Consult mod/high (80 min)	48	$6,072.05	
99255	Consult mod/high (110 min)	28	$4,897.68	
			Subtotal Inpatient Consults	*$14,807*
Observation Management				
99217	OBV D/C	473	$29,977.93	
99218	OBV admit low	59	$3,579.03	
99219	OBV admit mod	148	$14,883.90	
99220	OBV admit high	325	$46,002.93	
99235	OBV/Hosp same day	59	$9,493.86	
			Subtotal Observation Management	*$103,938*
Procedures				
20605	Arthrocentesis	0	$0.00	
31500	Intubation	0	$0.00	
32000	Thoracentesis	9	$675.75	
36000	Periph IV	0	$0.00	
36140	Femoral line	0	$0.00	
36410	Venipuncture	0	$0.00	
36489	Central line	0	$0.00	
36620	Arterial line	0	$0.00	
49080	Paracentesis	0	$0.00	
62270	Lumbar puncture	9	$564.02	
91100	NG tube	0	$0.00	
92950	CPR	10	$1,668.20	
			Subtotal Procedures	*$2,908*
			Total Annual Net Revenue	$963,019
			Total Encounters	12,386
			Net Revenue per Encounter	$77.75

H&P—history and physical, F/V—follow up; D/C—discharge; OBV—observation; NG—nosogastric; CPR—cardiopulmonary resuscitation

A detailed discussion of legal and regulatory issues affecting the determination of fair market value for hospitalist compensation is included in Chapter 134. Ultimately, however, fair market value for any given practice is the amount of compensation generally required to recruit and retain competent hospitalists to that practice.

Hospitalist Benefits

Consideration must be given to the types of benefits to be provided. This may include health insurance, a retirement contribution, continuing medical education reimbursement, malpractice insurance, plus statutory benefits (typically around 10–12% of

Table 116-2 Hospital Medicine Program High Level *Pro Forma*

	# FTEs	Unit Cost	Total
Revenue			
Net Annual Revenue (per "Revenue Projection" worksheet)			$963,019
Less: Billing Expense @ 9%			86,672
Net Annual Revenue after Billing Expense			$876,347
Expenses			
Salaries and Benefits			
Physician Salaries—Clinical	5.25	$175,000	$918,750
Health Insurance @ Family Rate	5.50	9,500	52,250
Retirement Benefit @ 5% of Salaries	5.50	8,750	48,125
Malpractice Insurance	5.50	12,000	66,000
Payroll Tax, Unemployment, W/C @ 10% of Salary	5.50	17,500	96,250
Subtotal Salaries and Benefits		222,750	1,181,375
Medical Director Fee	0.25	165,000	41,250
Practice Support Staff Salaries	0.50	42,000	21,000
Support Staff Benefits @ 28% of Salaries	0.50	11,760	5,880
			68,130
Other Operating Expenses (@15% of direct provider comp.)			144,000
Total Annual Expenses			$1,393,505
Projected Hospital Financial Support			$517,158

direct compensation) such as Social Security and Medicare contributions, unemployment, and workers' compensation costs.

Practice Management Costs

Practice management expenses must be planned for, including:
- Professional fee billing and collection costs
- Physician licenses, dues, and CME costs
- Recruitment and relocation expenses
- Practice administrative support (consisting of full- or part-time practice administrator with clerical assistance)
- Other practice overhead, such as stationery, postage, pagers, etc.

Professional fee billing and collection costs will typically run from 6–10% of net collections. Other practice management costs usually will run between 12–18% of total physician direct compensation. Practice requirements such as a small amount of office space, computers, and telephones are often provided by the sponsoring organization as part of the service agreement.

DEVELOPING THE FINANCIAL PLAN

Hospital medicine program professional fee revenue is rarely adequate to cover the cost of employing hospitalists and providing basic practice management services. Almost all hospital medicine programs require a significant degree of financial support from a sponsoring organization, such as a hospital, multispecialty medical group, or health plan.[4]

It is imperative to create a financial plan *pro forma* statement that shows projected annual practice revenues (net of billing and collection costs), projected annual practice costs, and the projected bottom line practice profit or loss. Since this is almost always a loss, this number becomes the basis for negotiating financial support with the sponsoring organization (Table 116-2). It is useful to create a multiyear financial plan that projects revenues and costs at various workload levels, so that it is understood how the financial dynamics of the practice will change with different levels of growth.

CONCLUSION

This chapter reviews important considerations during the initial stages of creating a hospital medicine program. Defining the program's scope of service is critical, after which staffing needs may be defined. From this, a financial plan can be developed, based on projected program revenues and costs. Frequently, revenue in addition to that from professional fee billings is required to support a program. Despite inherent uncertainty in each of these planning steps, a structured process based on the program's financial plan will create a strong foundation for sustainable short- and long-term growth, thereby maximizing the chances for success.

Key Points

- The starting point for the establishment of a hospital medicine program is a sound financial plan.

- Initial scope of service for a program can be obtained from understanding the factors driving program development.

- Referrals generally come from PCPs, specialists, and unassigned patients from the ED.

- Billable and nonbillable workload must be systematically projected.

- The number of hospitalists required to staff a program depends on the number of annual days or hours worked, the number of expected daily encounters per hospitalist, nonbillable service expectations, and whether 24/7 inhouse coverage is needed.

- Most hospital medicine programs will require financial support from the sponsoring entity in addition to professional fee revenues.

SUGGESTED READING

Dichter JR, Cowan LE, eds. The Hospitalist Program Management Guide. Marblehead, MA: HCPro, Inc., 2003.

Geehr EC, Nelson JR. Hospitalist Program Essentials, 2nd edition. Newport Beach, CA: Acute Care Partners, 2003.

Miller JA, ed. How hospitalists add value. A supplement to the Hospitalist. The official publication of the Society of Hospital Medicine 2005; 9(Suppl 1).

Nelson JR, Whitcomb WF. Organizing a hospitalist program: an overview of fundamental concepts. Med Clin North Am 2002; 86(4):887–909.

CHAPTER ONE-HUNDRED AND SEVENTEEN

Structuring a Hospital Medicine Program: An Overview of Contracting Options, Operating Procedures, and Recruitment Strategies

Leslie Flores, MHA, and John R. Nelson, MD, FACP

INTRODUCTION

The previous chapter addressed the development of a financial plan and workforce needs for a hospital medicine program. This chapter will address the following operational issues:
- Organizational structure options
- Operating standards and procedures
- Practice management
- Hospitalist recruitment

ORGANIZATIONAL STRUCTURE

Once a hospital or medical group commits to developing a hospital medicine program, a key decision must be made regarding the organizational structure under which the professional services will be provided. Will the sponsoring organization employ the hospitalists, or will it contract with another entity for the provision of hospitalist services? A wide variety of employment and contracting alternatives are available, each with its advantages and disadvantages. In many organizations, this may be the most difficult aspect of implementation, as it may raise political concerns related to issues of control and perceived favoritism.

Sponsoring organizations for a hospital medicine program such as an organized medical group or integrated delivery system can provide a vehicle for employing hospitalists. Thus, the organizational structure question is usually easily answered, since it already exists in this situation. However, if the sponsoring organization is a hospital or health plan, the decision may be more complicated. The various options available to most sponsoring organizations are delineated below.

Employment of Hospitalists by the Sponsoring Organization

One of the most common models for organizing hospitalist practices is for the physicians to be employed by the sponsoring organization, in states where it is legal for these entities to do so. According to the 2005–2006 Society of Hospital Medicine compensation and productivity survey, 34% of hospitalists are employed by hospitals, with another 20% employed by academic institutions. The remainder of hospitalists are employed by medical groups or staffing companies.[1]

The advantages and disadvantages of the employment model (versus a contracted model) are listed in Table 117-1.

Contracting for Hospitalist Services

If the sponsoring organization chooses not to employ its hospitalists, a variety of contractual alternatives exists.
- *Contracting with a Local Medical Group*
  The sponsoring organization may identify an existing medical group in its local medical community to serve as the employment vehicle for the hospitalists. This is an attractive option if there is an existing, well-respected physician in the group who has both the interest and the aptitude to serve as the initial hospitalist and hospital medicine program practice leader. The greatest concern with this model would be the potential for political backlash from other community physicians who might perceive favoritism or be concerned about losing their patients postdischarge, or losing inpatient consults, to other nonhospitalist members of the contracting group.
- *Facilitating Formation of a Hospitalist Group*
  The sponsoring organization might opt to recruit a hospitalist from outside the community or work with an existing independent physician in the community to facilitate the formation of a new hospitalist-only medical group specifically for the purposes of contracting with the sponsoring organization. This new group would presumably be seen as being more independent than an existing group with office practices and existing community loyalties, thus minimizing concerns about favoritism and loss of patients. However, it can be time consuming and expensive to facilitate the start-up of a new group, especially for a sponsoring organization that does not have any physician practice management resources at its disposal. In addition, it is critical that the selected lead physician be not only clinically excellent but also someone with strong leadership, administrative and interpersonal skills—not an easy individual to find.
- *Contracting with a Local or Regional Hospitalist Group*
  In many parts of the country, there are independent local or regional hospitalist-only medical groups that already cover more than one hospital. It may be possible to contract with such a group to expand its coverage to meet the needs of the sponsoring organization. The primary advantages of this option are that these groups typically have an effective practice management infrastructure in place, and they may be more

Table 117-1 Assessment of the Employment Model for a Hospital Medicine Program (In Comparison to a Contracted Model)

Advantages	Disadvantages
Sponsoring organization may more directly influence alignment of goals and incentives, and exert more direct control over physician performance, than in a contractual relationship model.	Many hospitals and integrated delivery systems have had negative experiences in the past with employing physicians and may be reluctant to do so again.
Rapid and relatively simple implementation, assuming the sponsoring organization already has administrative infrastructure in place for recruiting and employing staff.	Sponsoring organizations that do not employ other types of physicians may not have an adequate practice management infrastructure in place.
For recruitment, hospitalist candidates may see employment by a large entity such as a hospital as more stable and secure than employment by a contracting medical group.	Other stakeholders, such as potential referring physicians, may perceive the hospitalists as being too closely aligned with the sponsoring organization's interests, or they may perceive that the hospitalists are "getting a sweet deal" from the sponsoring organization, resulting in distrust or resentment and lack of referrals.

flexible in their ability to provide coverage by rotating physicians among multiple hospitals. Potential disadvantages are that the contracting group's primary allegiance may be elsewhere, and the sponsoring organization may not be able to exert as much control or influence over the practice as it might in the models discussed above.

- *Contracting with a National Hospitalist Management Company*
There are at least a dozen competent, qualified hospitalist staffing and practice management companies operating on a regional or national basis with which an organization might contract for hospitalist services. These companies bring hospital medicine experience and expertise not usually available with any other model, including comprehensive practice management infrastructure and substantial corporate resources directed at enhancing practice performance in areas such as clinical quality, patient safety, resource utilization, and customer satisfaction. In addition, the implementation time is often lowest with this model because these companies bring well-honed operating procedures and physician recruitment capabilities to the table. Finally, because these companies have strong administrative and performance reporting capabilities, this model usually requires much less administrative effort by the sponsoring organization than other models. However, the cost (at least in terms of up-front dollars) of contracting with a national staffing company is usually higher than with other models. Although these companies usually advertise that their higher operating cost is offset by institutional savings related to reduced length of stay and similar metrics, in practice these savings can be difficult to accurately capture and attribute to the hospital medicine program. In addition, the sponsoring organization may find that it has less influence over the priorities and operating practices of these large companies than with a smaller local entity.

There is no right or best organizational model for a hospital medicine program. Each sponsoring organization should carefully consider the organizational options available to it and select the one best suited for its specific situation and needs.

Contract Considerations

If the sponsoring organization employs the hospitalists, it will need to develop a standard employment agreement. If the sponsor contracts for hospitalist services, the most common form for doing so is a Professional Services Agreement. This discussion is directed at Professional Services Agreements, but many of the comments will apply to employment contracts as well.

Performance Expectations

The agreement should specify overall program goals, as well as coverage, service requirements, and other performance expectations. Sometimes, the agreement may define different service levels over time, allowing for a ramp-up as program volume grows.

Medical Director

The agreement should designate a medical director or practice leader and, in most cases, provide for dedicated time and compensation for medical director duties.

Remuneration

In exchange for services rendered, the sponsoring organization agrees to make certain payments to the hospitalist entity. These payments are usually intended to cover the shortfall between practice revenues and costs, and may be structured as fixed monthly payments, as payments that vary based on volume or as the actual difference between program costs and collections. The sponsoring organization may also provide other remuneration, such as performance bonuses or assistance with hospitalist recruitment by paying search fees and interview/relocation expenses.

When sponsoring organizations, particularly hospitals, are providing financial support that helps pay hospitalist salaries, a variety of legal and regulatory limitations come into play when considering the methodology and amount of compensation to be paid by the hospital to the hospitalist group (or individual hospitalists). Chapter 134, "Legal Issues in Hospitalist–Hospital Relationships," addresses these issues in detail. Hospitals are generally restricted in their business relationships with physicians by:

- The provisions of 42 U.S.C. §1320(a)-7(b), the so-called Medicare and Medicaid Anti-Fraud and Abuse Act ("Anti-Kickback Statute"), which prohibits the offering or acceptance of anything of value for the referral of patients where payment for such services is made by a Federal payment program such as Medicare or Medicaid.

- The Federal self-referral prohibitions of 42 U.S.C. 1395nn (Stark I and Stark II, collectively "Stark"), which prohibit referrals by physicians for certain specified health care services when such physicians maintain an ownership interest in or other financial relationship with the provider receiving the referral.

In addition, nonprofit hospitals must comply with Internal Revenue Code requirements prohibiting hospitals from providing "excess benefits" to a "disqualified person" (an individual who is "in a position to exercise substantial influence over the affairs of that organization"). Disqualified persons might include, for example, physicians who are members of the hospital's board of directors, who hold leadership positions in the organized medical staff, or who are investors with the hospital in a joint venture initiative. An excess benefit exists when the economic value to the disqualified person of a given transaction exceeds the value of the services received by the hospital in return. If, for example, the owner of the hospital medicine group also happened to be the president of the medical staff, the hospital would need to be able to demonstrate that its payments to the group did not exceed the value of the services provided by the group, or it could face IRS sanctions.

This IRS requirement is separate and distinct from the "fair market value" requirements of Stark, and involves separate potential sanctions. In the event the IRS determines that a transaction between a hospital and a physician or physician group resulted in an excess benefit to a disqualified person, it may impose significant penalties ("intermediate sanctions") on both the physician or group, *and* the individual organization manager who participated in the transaction.[2]

No agreement between a hospital and a physician or group should be entered into without the review and approval of the agreement by experienced health care legal counsel for both parties.

In-Kind Payments. Some remuneration may be in the form of in-kind support, such as the provision of rent-free office space, furnishings, and supplies or the provision of program clerical or clinical support staff employed by the sponsoring organization. Such in-kind payments are considered part of the overall remuneration and should be taken into account when evaluating whether the relationship is consistent with fair market value.

Professional Fee Revenue. The agreement should address whether professional fee collections are retained by the contracting group or turned over to the sponsoring organization.

The agreement entered into between the sponsoring organization and the entity employing the hospitalists can make or break a hospital medicine program. The most common problems with professional services agreements are listed in Box 117-1.

Professional services agreements should be carefully drafted with the assistance of an experienced health care attorney, and with due consideration for a wide variety of possible consequences, circumstances, and interpretations.

OPERATING STANDARDS AND PROCEDURES

In addition to assessing the preferred organizational structure for the hospital medicine program, the sponsoring organization and its hospitalists should have an operational plan that addresses *how* the program will operate, including service requirements, performance expectations, and policies and procedures.

Box 117-1 Common Problems with Professional Services Agreements

- Unforeseen and unintended consequences of a provision
- Lack of clarity resulting in differing interpretations
- Changed circumstances not contemplated in the agreement
- Failure of the agreement to address key performance expectations

---

Program Oversight

It is important to identify clearly to whom the hospitalists, and specifically the practice leader, will be accountable. Typically, there will be a representative of the sponsoring organization who is administratively responsible for the smooth and effective operation of the hospital medicine program. In addition, the hospitalists may also be accountable to a medical staff department chair or committee, particularly for clinical performance. It is often desirable to convene a hospital medicine program Oversight Committee to monitor program start-up, to help define operating expectations and procedures, and to address unforeseen problems as they arise. This committee can include representation by multiple stakeholders, including referring physicians and medical consultants. This may go a long way toward allaying any medical staff political issues or concerns, and will create a forum for administration, medical staff, and the hospitalists themselves to discuss openly the program's goals and operation.

Service Requirements and Performance Expectations

The obligations of the hospital medicine program in terms of coverage, response times, sources and types of patients accepted, and scope of practice should be clearly delineated. It should be clear to all parties whether referral of patients to the hospital medicine service will be mandatory or voluntary (it should almost always be strictly voluntary, except in the case of certain programs designed specifically to support managed care initiatives, such as in a staff model setting). Expectations may also be articulated with regard to issues such as whether the hospitalists must accept all clinically appropriate referrals without regard to insurance or ability to pay, utilization of preferred medical consultants, communication expectations (*see* Chapter 119, "Communication in Hospitalist Systems" for details), and expected participation in activities such as medical staff committees or organizational performance improvement initiatives. In addition, performance standards should be negotiated in areas such as physician productivity, clinical quality, resource utilization, medical record documentation, and customer satisfaction.

Operating Policies and Procedures

The mechanisms by which the hospital medicine program will operate should be defined in written operating procedures. These will document the service requirements and performance expectations discussed above, as well as day-to-day operations of the program. For example, written procedures should be developed to include:

- How to refer a patient to the hospital medicine program
- What floor(s) hospital medicine patients will be aggregated on and how case management/discharge planning will be integrated with hospitalist care
- How communication will occur between hospitalist and referring physician
- Protocols for posthospitalization care of unattached patients
- Forms, order sets, reports, and other documents that are specific to the hospital medicine program
- How problems and concerns with the program should be raised and addressed
- How program performance will be monitored and reported to stakeholders (*see* Chapter 122, "Measuring Value in Hospital Medicine Programs")

PRACTICE MANAGEMENT

Like any medical practice, hospital medicine programs require careful oversight, whether provided by a single practice manager or multiple individuals who oversee the day-to-day administrative functions of the program. Box 117-2 outlines the management roles for a hospital medicine program.

If the hospitalists are employed by a large medical group, existing practice management infrastructure may be utilized for some of these functions. However, an important consideration for hospitalists employed by a large medical group is that a hospitalist's practice overhead is typically much lower than that of office-based physicians because hospitalists do not have rent, utilities, office staff, etc. Thus, it is not usually appropriate to assess a hospitalist the same overhead rate that office-based physicians are assessed by the medical group.

If the hospitalists are employed by a hospital, health plan, or newly formed hospitalist-only group, the challenge of providing effective practice management often becomes much greater. Competent resources must be allocated, either internally or via outsourcing, to ensure that the hospitalists are appropriately credentialed with all applicable hospitals and managed care plans, that charges are being accurately captured and coded, and that professional fee bills are being effectively submitted and collected. In addition, resources are needed to administer hospitalist payroll and benefits, to maintain malpractice and other insurance contracts, and to manage other aspects of the hospitalist practice such as physician license, DEA and dues/subscriptions renewals, pagers, answering services, etc.

Finally, it is critical that an appropriate corporate compliance plan be developed and administered. This will include provisions for periodic hospitalist coding and documentation training, as well as periodic independent coding and billing audits. (*See* Chapter 121, "Documentation, Coding, Billing, and Compliance in Hospital Medicine.")

Facilities, Equipment, and Hospital Systems

The hospital medicine program will need facilities and equipment within the hospital, including a small hospitalist office with phone, fax, computer, and Internet access, as well as access to sleep rooms. In addition, if possible, the hospital should provide stat transcription of hospitalist dictations (at least the admitting history and physical (H&P) and discharge summary), and auto-faxing of admission and discharge dictations to the referring physician. Clerical or administrative support will be required for answering the hospital medicine program phone line, taking messages and communicating with the hospitalists and referring physicians, distributing the hospitalist schedule, managing mail and paperwork, etc. The sponsoring organization may also consider providing dedicated case management support (Box 117-3).

Communication Plan

A communication and marketing plan should be developed (Box 117-4). The purpose of this communication is to make physicians, hospital staff, and patients aware of the hospital medicine program and how it works, and to alleviate any concerns these constituencies may have. The communication plan may include letters to physicians (both those affiliated with the sponsoring organization, and unaffiliated community physicians and clinics, if appropriate), orientation meetings and fact sheets for

---

Box 117-2 Management Functions for a Hospital Medicine Program

- Hospitalist recruitment and orientation
- Human resources and payroll functions
- Health plan contracting and provider credentialing
- Negotiation/administration of the professional services agreement
- Staffing and scheduling
- Malpractice and other insurance contract administration
- Professional fee billing and collections company
- Corporate compliance
- Financial management, including budgeting, banking, accounts payable, and financial reporting
- Performance monitoring (individual and group)
- Practice marketing, communications and customer relations
- Day-to-day operational oversight and problem-solving

Box 117-3 Facilities, Equipment, and Systems Requirements

- Office space
- Access to sleep rooms, locker rooms, and shower facilities, if a 24/7 on-site program
- Computer and Internet access
- Phone and fax
- Access to medical library or other information resources
- Stat transcription of hospitalist admission and discharge dictations, with auto-faxing to referring physician
- Clerical or administrative support
- Case management and/or other clinical support

Box 117-4 Communication Plan Components

- Introductory letters to physicians
- Orientation meetings
- Fact sheet for hospital staff
- Hospital medicine program brochures

Box 117-5 Recruiting Strategies Involving Residency Programs

- Consider whether any of a hospital medicine program's existing hospitalists have relationships with a residency program that could be utilized to market to residents.
- Program representatives (including existing hospitalists) should visit residency programs at least annually. A dinner for second- and third-year residents can be hosted in order to build relationships and talk with them about practice opportunities. Contact should be made through the chief resident whenever possible, rather than the program director or program office.
- Offer to have hospitalists who are effective speakers give didactic lectures to residents on hospital medicine-related topics.
- The sponsoring organization may offer a hospital medicine residency elective, which is likely to provide a different perspective than that at the university medical center. The residents will gain exposure to the community and the practice, and increase the potential for recruiting them later.

Box 117-6 Common Mid-level Provider Activities

- Rounding on patients
- Writing prescriptions
- Performing histories and physicals
- Communicating with primary care physicians
- Acting as initial responder
- Participating in discharge planning

From: Society of Hospital Medicine. 2005–2006 Survey: The Authoritative Source on the State of Hospital Medicine. Society of Hospital Medicine, 2006. Philadelphia, PA.

hospital staff, and a hospital medicine program brochure for patients.

HOSPITALIST RECRUITMENT

One of the most significant challenges facing any hospital medicine program, whether new or established, is the recruitment of hospitalists to the practice. When queried about their professional concerns, 35% of hospital medicine group leaders cited recruitment[1] as one of their top 10 concerns, second only to concerns about work hours/work–life balance.

Turnover may be higher in hospital medicine programs than in other types of medical practices because hospital medicine is a new and evolving field, the barriers to entry and exit are quite low, and demand for hospitalists greatly exceeds supply. For this reason, programs should consider recruiting on a continuous basis, even when all current positions are filled. Unanticipated turnover and/or rapid growth in demand for hospitalist services often require programs to remain constantly on the lookout for qualified candidates.

The best place to look for hospitalists is usually within the sponsoring organization's existing medical community. It is often pos-

sible to find local physicians who are interested in giving up the stress of private office practice to work as a hospitalist.

An effective method for recruiting hospitalists from outside the community is to establish strong ties with nearby medical schools and residency programs. See Box 117-5 for explanation.

Classified advertising in medical journals is part of an overall recruitment strategy for many programs. Finally, the use of search firms experienced in hospitalist recruitment may be considered.

It may not always be possible to recruit enough dedicated, full-time hospitalists who are committed to settling in the community and becoming part of the core hospitalist group. In this case, the practice may recruit physicians to work as hospitalists for a period of time, such as 2 years, before they go on to a fellowship or other plans. Sometimes doctors become disenchanted with fellowships and decide to work as hospitalists for a longer term. While not ideal, having 2-year hospitalists can be a valuable way to address critical manpower shortages, and will be much less expensive than locum tenens physicians.

Another approach to address temporary manpower shortages or to increase scheduling flexibility is to utilize moonlighters. These may be fellows from nearby training programs, or they might be existing community physicians who are willing to work a few nights or weekends a month for extra income.

Finally, programs facing manpower shortages should consider whether mid-level providers such as nurse practitioners or physician assistants might supplement the physician hospitalists and provide additional capacity. Functions commonly filled by mid-level providers are listed in Box 117-6.

CONCLUSION

This chapter provides an overview of key structural issues for a hospital medicine program. Whether to employ or contract with a hospital medicine program is an important early step in an implementation plan. Service requirements should be specified in an operational plan. Provision must be made for effective management of the hospital medicine program. Finally, recruitment is a challenge and requires a carefully considered strategy to be successful. This discussion is designed to give individuals responsible for planning a new program or improving an existing one a clear idea of the types of issues that may be encountered and some useful suggestions for addressing them.

Key Points

- There is no single best organizational model for hospital medicine programs. Each institution must choose the option that best meets its specific needs from the wide variety of employment and contracting options available.

- When the selected organizational model involves a contractual relationship between the sponsoring organization and the entity employing the hospitalists, a carefully crafted professional services agreement will be a critical component of the program's success.

- Successful hospital medicine program operations require clearly defined performance expectations, supporting policies and procedures, and effective program oversight.

- Internal practice management for hospital medicine programs requires a solid infrastructure for functions such as human resources management, financial management (including professional fee billing and collections), practice marketing, and performance monitoring.

- One of the most significant challenges facing any hospital medicine program is recruitment of an adequate number of qualified hospitalists. Programs should develop robust, multifaceted recruitment plans, and should not stop recruiting, even when all current positions are filled.

SUGGESTED READING

Society of Hospital Medicine. 2005–2006 Survey: The Authoritative source on the State of Hospital Medicine. Society of Hospital Medicine, 2006. Philadelphia, PA.

26 U.S.C. §4958(a)

Dichter JR, Cowan LE, eds.The Hospitalist Program Management Guide. Marblehead, MA: HCPro, Inc., 2003.

Geehr EC, Nelson JR. Hospitalist Program Essentials. Second Edition. Acute Care Partners, 2003. Newport Beach, CA.

Nelson JR, Whitcomb WF. Organizing a hospitalist program: an overview of fundamental concepts. Med Clin North Am 2002; 86(4):887–909.

CHAPTER ONE HUNDRED AND EIGHTEEN

Scheduling and Staff Deployment for Hospital Medicine Programs

Bipinchandra Mistry, MD, MRCP(Ireland), and Winthrop F. Whitcomb, MD

INTRODUCTION

Scheduling for a hospital medicine program is a complex task that requires consideration of numerous factors. Several scheduling models exist, driven by varying service needs of different programs, each with merits and drawbacks. This chapter outlines important factors in developing an appropriate schedule, and examines the major scheduling models, identifying their strengths and weaknesses. Important considerations in scheduling such as in-hospital continuity of care, weekends, nights, vacation, sick call, and the use of part-time hospitalists are reviewed. Ultimately, a given hospital medicine program schedule will be a unique reflection of the service demands of the program combined with the preferences of the hospitalists themselves. Despite each program's unique features, the following fundamental elements must be considered in the creation of any hospital medicine program's schedule:

- Patient volume
- Peak hours for admissions and other services such as discharges and consultations
- Nighttime, weekend, holiday, and back-up coverage needs
- Hospitalist career sustainability

MAJOR SCHEDULING MODELS

Shift-Based versus Call-Based Schedules

The critical initial decision in scheduling for a hospital medicine program is whether to provide staff on site during nighttime hours. If there is insufficient volume and lack of other service requirements (e.g., code blue or rapid response team coverage), then coverage may be accomplished off site via beeper, using a call-based schedule. In this case, hospitalists work on site in the hospital during the day while admitting, rounding on, and discharging patients. Once work is done, coverage may be accomplished via beeper call, with the hospitalist returning when necessary based on demand for service. This is known as a *call-based schedule*, and it is often seen in small-volume or young programs, academic programs with residents on site in the hospital, and groups covering more than one hospital. In contrast, the *shift-based schedule* provides on-site physician staffing 24 hours a day. Single institution programs most often use this

model, and typically hospital employed, although multihospital groups may employ this approach if volume and service needs support it. According to the 2006 Society of Hospital Medicine Productivity[1] and Compensation Survey, 40% of programs used shift-based staffing and 25% used a call-based system, while 35% used "mixed-model staffing," defined as a combination of shift- and call-based staffing models (Table 118-1). Examples of call-based and shift-based schedules are provided in Tables 118-2 A and B.

A chief advantage of a call-based schedule is that in-hospital continuity of care—characterized as the percentage of patients seeing a single hospitalist during a hospitalization—is easier to achieve, since the hospitalist tends to work more days in a row. On the negative side, the day after night call may be impaired by fatigue and negatively affect patient care and physician well-being.

Over the last several years, more hospital medicine programs have transitioned to shift-based schedules as their programs have grown.[1] With increased program size and volume of night admissions, it is more difficult to cover via beeper call when, in effect, the hospitalist is on site much of the night. While a major advantage of a shift-based model is hospitalist presence regardless of time of day, there are drawbacks. These include a tendency toward less continuity of care if shifts are filled without regard to number of hospitalists a patient sees throughout the stay. In such a scenario, a patient may readily see three different physicians during a stay (e.g., one doctor admits the patient in the evening; another sees the patient the following day, and then a third might discharge the patient with change in coverage). Patient satisfaction may suffer, given the lack of continuity. Additionally, consultants may be frustrated if there is hospitalist discontinuity, if they must deal with hospitalists unfamiliar with the details of the case.

At What Point Should a Program Transition from Call-Based to Shift-Based Scheduling?

In most cases, this is determined by the number of nighttime admissions and other service requirements. As a guide, once the average number of night admissions exceeds 4–6, it is time to consider 24 hour on-site staffing. Other important considerations when considering moving to shift-based scheduling include:

Table 118-1 Comparison of Shift-Based versus Call-Based Hospitalist Schedules

	Call-Based	Shift-Based
Used commonly for	Small or young programs; academic programs with resident coverage; programs covering multiple hospitals	Large programs; single institution programs; programs providing code blue or rapid response team coverage; programs providing "house doctor" coverage for traditional (nonhospitalist) medical staff
Cost of program	Relatively low, due to the fact that physicians are not being paid to be on site when not clinically productive	Tends to be high, since physician must be on site regardless of demand for services; nights are typically 10–40% less productive than days in terms of billings
In-hospital continuity of care (i.e., percentage of patients seeing a single hospitalist during stay)	Usually good, with a single physician following a group of patients throughout hospitalization	Can be challenging, with a tendency to "plug shifts" without regard to continuity of physicians
Effect on hospital throughput	During off hours, can be problematic, since physician less available to see patient	Can be ideal, since physician available to see patient as condition demands, regardless of hour
Ease of recruiting for	More difficult due to unpredictability of beeper call	Less difficult, due to predictability of work and boundary around work (i.e., typically no call from home)
Effect on hospitalist group cohesiveness	May be less favorable than shift-based if there is lack of shift change sign out, thus not affording an occasion for frequent meetings and exchange of ideas	Favorable—programs usually have a sign out conference at change of shifts, allowing for frequent, open communication

- Does the program's subsidy appropriately support and recognize the added value of 24-hour on-site staffing? For most programs, the added expense of moving to 24-hour on-site staffing involves hiring 1 or 2 more full-time hospitalists.
- With increasing focus on patient safety, does the hospital wish to have a hospitalist on site 24 hours a day to run the rapid response and code blue teams?
- Are there other service lines the hospitalists are expected to cover during the night? This might include:
  - Admissions or cross-coverage for nonhospitalist patients
  - Intensive care unit coverage
  - Managing capitated patients and/or transfers from out of network hospitals
  - Nonurgent medical consultations
  - Procedures
  - Resident supervision and support

The Block Schedule

Perhaps the most popular schedule is the "block schedule," which has hospitalists working a number of consecutive days or nights, usually 5–7, followed by a similar period of days off. Other examples include 21 days on with 6–8 days off, or 10 days on and 4 days off. Shifts are typically 12 hours in length, utilizing a 24-hour on-site approach (a form of a shift-based schedule). The main advantage of this schedule is ease of administration and initial attractiveness to candidates for the hospitalist position, who like the idea of an equal number of days off as days worked (e.g., a typical block schedule may have hospitalists working 183 days a year and off 182 days a year). Table 118-3 outlines advantages and disadvantages of this approach. While some have observed that physician acceptance of this schedule wanes over time for the reasons listed, it is unclear whether it will ulti-

mately have the durability of more customized approaches to scheduling.

Block scheduling can also be used in a "pod" system. If the hospitalist group is large enough, such a system allows subgroups of physicians to be assigned to weekends and night shifts. It is then up to each subgroup to provide a physician for the allocated shift. Such an approach can make a large group easier to administer and may confer scheduling autonomy to individual hospitalists.

Matching Staff to Peak Admission Times and Other Service Demands

A key challenge to hospitalist scheduling is deployment of staff to mirror work demands over the course of the day. Demand for hospitalist services will fluctuate substantially throughout a 24-hour period, a week, and seasonally. Reviewing peak admission and discharge times is important and should indicate appropriate staffing. A pitfall in hospitalist scheduling is failing to account for diurnal, weekly, and seasonal variation in volumes. Table 118-4 describes techniques to address varying work volume based on demand.

Quantifying in-Hospital Continuity of Care

Because many feel that in-hospital continuity of care is an overriding concern in scheduling, it is worth examining how the number of consecutive days worked (regardless of shift-based or call-based models) affects number of different hospitalists a patient sees during a hospital stay. The following example illustrates this:

A hospitalist group employing a 5-days-on and 5-days-off schedule is compared to another group that uses a 21-days-on and 8-days-

Table 118-2A Call-Based* Schedule. Weekdays Are Covered by Hospitalists with Off-Hours and Weekends Covered by Combination of Hospitalists and PCPs

	Weekdays	Sat	Sun
Daytime	Hospitalist A and B	Hospitalist A, PCP (hospitalist B and other PCPs cover subsequent weekends)	Hospitalist A, PCP (hospitalist B and other PCPs cover subsequent weekends)
Nighttime	Rotation of hospitalists and PCPs	Rotation of hospitalists and PCPs	Rotation of hospitalists and PCPs

NOTE: As in all hospitalist schedules, customization based on local factors will be required. The following examples are meant to outline general concepts.

Notes:

• Designed for small or young program with average daily census of no more than 24–28, often less.

• Not enough volume to justify self-contained hospitalist group.

• PCPs agree to cover either for a limited time until program becomes self-contained or because they see benefit in being office-focused during weekdays and/or want to maintain hospital skills/presence.

• Frequency of weekend and night call for both hospitalists and PCPs is determined by number providing coverage (e.g., for two hospitalists and six PCPs doing equal call coverage, frequency would be split into every 8th weeknight and every 4th weekend if two MDs are rounding on weekend days).

*"Call-Base" refers to off hours being covered via beeper, off site. In such a schedule, off-hours may be covered solely by hospitalists or a combination of hospitalists and PCPs covering.

Table 118-2B Shift-Based Schedule: For Programs Providing 24-Hour on-Site Coverage

	Mon	Tues	Wed	Thurs	Fri	Sat	Sun
Week 1							
Day	A, E	A, E	A, E	A, E	A, E	A, ML	A, ML
Night	C	C	C	C	C	C	C
Week 2							
Day	A, B	A, B	A, B	A, B	A, B	B, ML	B, ML
Night	D	D	D	D	D	D	D
Week 3							
Day	B, C	B, C	B, C	B, C	B, C	C, ML	C, ML
Night	E	E	E	E	E	E	E
Week 4							
Day	C, D	C, D	C, D	C, D	C, D	D, ML	D, ML
Night	A	A	A	A	A	A	A
Week 5							
Day	D, E	D, E	D, E	D, E	D, E	E, ML	E, ML
Night	B	B	B	B	B	B	B

NOTE: As in all hospitalist schedules, customization based on local factors will be required. The following examples are meant to outline general concepts.

Notes: A, B, C, D, and E denote hospitalists. ML denotes moonlighter, or part-time hospitalist.

• Cycle: Each hospitalist works 12 consecutive days, then has 9 days off, then works 7 consecutive nights, then 7 days off.

• There can be overlap of day and night shifts in order to accommodate high demand.

• One of the day hospitalists may leave early if work is done, in order to allow for recuperation during long stretches of workdays. Duration of the day and night shifts is to be determined locally.

• Each hospitalist is contracted to work a certain number of hours each year, allowing for week-to-week fluctuations in hours.

• Number of consecutive days worked can be made shorter, based on hospitalist preference. In-hospital continuity will then be less.

• Moonlighters are utilized in order to decrease weekend frequency for full-time hospitalists. If pool of moonlighters is smaller than in this sample, A–E fills in weekends. With present scheme, hospitalists work one in three weekends.

• Average daily census is 30. With this schedule, five full-time hospitalists and a part-time position comprised of several moonlighters are needed.

• Cycles for hospitalists will be altered due to additional time off.

off schedule. Assuming the average length of stay is 4 days, the dynamics of the first group will be that patients admitted on days 1 and 2 of the 5-day stretch would be discharged before the end of that block. However, patients admitted on day 4 or 5 will be transferred to another physician prior to discharge. Therefore, approximately 40% (2 of 5) of the patients will be seen by one physician only and 60% (3 of 5) by two physicians. When observing the second group, patients admitted on days 19, 20, and 21 will be carried over to the next physician. This means that 85% of patients will be seen by one physician (18 of 21) and 15% of patients by two physicians.

Table 118-3 The Block Schedule: Advantages and Disadvantages

Advantages	Disadvantages
Straightforward to administer	Work days are long, making day-to-day work–life balance difficult
Defined, predictable time off	Because of relatively few days worked annually (a block schedule may provide for 183 days worked, compared to around 230 in a typical non-block hospitalist schedule), hospitalists are relatively unproductive from a billings standpoint, despite a perception of being very busy during work days
Large number of days off	Long stretches of days off may pose a threat to work–life balance
May offer a recruiting advantage	Abundant time off may erode a hospitalist's ability to regularly and consistently collaborate with the hospital team to improve systems of care
In hospital provider continuity of care good	Puts hospitalist out of phase with family or friends with traditional work schedules

Table 118-4 Common Approaches to Hospitalist Staffing Based on Fluctuating Volumes

Time Period	Approach
Day–night	Extra staff for morning discharges Extra staff for afternoon and evening admissions and consultations Consider a separate "admission shift" where a single hospitalist performs admissions while the others can focus on rounding/discharges
Season to season	Extra staff during high-volume season—tends to be winter (summer in some resort areas) Flex staffing by: using part-time hospitalists during high-volume periods; encourage utilization of vacation time during low-volume periods; add mid-level providers during high-volume periods; provide incentives such as more hourly pay or reward for billings during high-volume periods

Box 118-1 Strategies for Staffing a Hospital Medicine Program during Off-Hours Such as Weekends, Nights, and Holidays

- Employ physician extenders such as physician assistants or nurse practitioners.
- Utilize a "rounding assistant" who can help gather data and coordinate care.
- Provide an incentive to work off-hours—higher pay, a larger year-end bonus, more vacation time, or more desirable vacation time.
- Be willing to "skeleton staff" weekends and holidays, trading higher patient loads for lower frequency of these workdays.
- Utilize part-time hospitalists, or moonlighters.

While increasing the number of consecutive days worked enhances continuity, the trade-off is physician fatigue. One approach to combating this is to shorten the workday. In such a scenario, the hospitalist may be able to have a short day, perhaps leaving the hospital at 3 p.m. followed by a longer day (such as when performing admitting responsibilities).

Determining Shift Duration

This is dependent on workload and personal preference. For hospitalists with high workloads and patient acuity, shorter shifts, such as those 8 to 10 hours in duration, may be most appropriate. If workload and patient throughput is lower, then longer shifts, such as 12–16 hours, may be acceptable and produce manageable fatigue. In general, shifts over 16 hours in length should be reserved for low workload situations. There is evidence that working 24-hour shifts, and in cases of multiple consecutive

days worked with shorter shifts such as 12 hours, may impair cognition and adversely affect patient safety.[3,4]

Techniques for Staffing Nights, Weekends, and Other Off-Hours

Providing appropriate staff for nights, weekends, and holidays ranks among the biggest scheduling challenges. Because hospital medicine demands greater off-hours staffing than, for example, a primary care practice, a major source of work stress for hospitalists is the proportion of off-hours worked. Box 118-1 lists a number of strategies that can help alleviate the burden on full-time staff in providing this coverage, and thus help to mitigate this reality.

Vacation, Sick Time, and Other Critical Times of Year

Scheduling vacation time requires foresight, especially with a large group. A clearly defined approach to prioritizing vacation requests alleviates potential strife. It might factor in previous peak vacation times worked and seniority, or be on a first-come first-serve basis. Certain critical times of the year, such as high vacation demand times, require careful forethought (*see* Box 118-1 for staffing strategies during these periods).

Because of the unpredictability of sick time, a system providing backup for illness and other sudden work absences must be devised. Options include:

- Create a back-up on-call schedule, where there is someone on call in the event of sudden absence.
- For small programs, the medical director may be the *de facto* back-up call system.
- The group collectively agrees to cover with less staffing for short periods of work absence (e.g., 1–2 days) instead of having a back-up call system. For longer absences, definitive staffing solutions must be quickly devised.

SCHEDULING FOR SMALL OR YOUNG PROGRAMS

With small or young hospital medicine programs, the average daily census may be too low to support a schedule that is fully covered by hospitalists. In this case, often the hospitalist(s) cover(s) weekdays, while nights and weekends are covered by a combination of hospitalists and primary care physicians (PCPs). (*See* "sample hospitalist schedules" above for an example of this with further explanation.)

SCHEDULING FOR CIRCADIAN RHYTHMS

Hospitalists who ignore research from shift workers outside of and within health care risk excess fatigue and increased medical errors. This data should inform approaches to scheduling. Research demonstrates that shifts should be rotated in a clockwise manner, with days rotated to evenings, evenings to nights, and nights to days, even when there are days off in between. Such an approach attenuates the disruptive effect night work has on circadian rhythms and associated fatigue.[5] (*See* Box 118-2 for more explanation of the effect of night and prolonged periods of shift work on workers.)

CONCLUSION

This chapter reviewed fundamental concepts in scheduling for a hospital medicine program. Because of the need to consider numerous factors in creating a schedule, no one template is applicable to all programs. A critical first step is deciding whether 24-hour on-site coverage is feasible. Schedules must be geared to provide work capacity during times of peak demand. For any schedule, in-hospital continuity of care should be a priority. As hospital medicine schedules must provide for substantial night and weekend coverage, specific approaches to address these times must be devised—including dedicated night hospitalists ("nocturnists"), part-time hospitalists, mid-level providers, and added incentives such as differential pay. Finally, prior research on shift workers demonstrates that attention to circadian rhythms, shift duration, and number of consecutive days worked is critical for the long-term effectiveness and satisfaction of hospitalists.

Box 118-2 Important Issues Regarding Work Hours[6]

Hours of work

- Sleep deprivation lasting 24 hours has a measurable, negative impact on performance. The same level of impairment occurs after being awake 17–19 hours as having a blood alcohol level at the legal limit for driving.
- Working (during the day) more than 55–60 hours per week over an extended period is likely to lead to significant health effects.
- Hours of work limits for day work will be different from those for night work.

Night work

- The effects of working nights and extended hours are interactive.
- Shiftworkers lose, on average, 1–1.5 hours sleep each 24 hour period, resulting in a sleep debt of 6 hours after 4 nights and with significant consequences for health and safety.

Effect of extended hours or night work

- *Sleep deprivation,* coupled with long hours of work over a prolonged period (approximately 12 months) has both a short-term impact on performance and, in the long term, will lead to cardiovascular, mental health, behavioral (safety), and productivity decrements.

Opportunities for recuperation

- In the long term, the average sleep period required for health and alertness is between 7–9 hours.
- A minimum of 6 hours of consecutive sleep in a 24-hour period is the minimum needed to maintain alertness for the next 24 hours, but assumes a zero sleep debt.
- Two consecutive nights' sleep, with a normal day pattern, are required after 3–4 nights' work.

Key Points

- A critical initial step in hospitalist scheduling is to determine whether to provide on-site staffing during nighttime hours.

- A hospitalist schedule must seek to match staffing with peak admission hours and other service demands, such as patient discharges.

- A major pitfall in scheduling is failure to attain in-hospital continuity of care, where a minimum number of hospitalists care for a patient during the hospital stay.

- Night and weekend staffing—one of the major challenges in scheduling—may be supplemented with the use of part-time physicians, mid-level providers (physician assistants and nurse practitioners), and increased pay for staff during these times.

- Attention to fatigue, adequate time off, and circadian rhythms when scheduling is essential to the long-term well-being and career satisfaction of hospitalists.

Comprehensive Hospital Medicine: An Evidence Based and Systems Approach

SUGGESTED READING

Nelson JR, Whitcomb WF. Organizing a hospitalist program: an overview of fundamental concepts. Med Clin North Am 2002; 86(4):887–909.

Geehr EC, Nelson JR. Hospitalist Program Essentials. Second Edition. New port Beach, CA: Acute Care Partners, 2002.

Nelson JR Resource Center. Hospital Medicine Program Scheduling. www.hospitalmedicine.org. Accessed March 12, 2006.

Dichter JR, Cowan LE. The Hospitalist Program Management Guide. Marblehead, MA: HCPro Inc., 2003.

CHAPTER ONE HUNDRED AND NINETEEN

Communication in Hospitalist Systems

Winthrop F. Whitcomb, MD, Russell Holman, MD, and John R. Nelson, MD FACP

BACKGROUND

Effective communication is essential to managing the vast number of relationships within hospital medicine systems. The hospitalist model itself creates additional communication challenges, as patient care is transferred from outpatient physician to hospitalist when a patient enters the hospital. Further, multiple hospitalists may be involved in a patient's care throughout the course of the hospitalization. Experience from other countries with well-established "hospitalist" systems points to the potential for poor hospitalist–referring physician communication—in this case, outpatient physicians were frequently unaware that their patients were admitted or discharged from the hospital. However, a recent observation in the United States found that hospitalists value communication highly, with 24% of total work time devoted to communication activities.[2] The importance of high-quality communication is reflected in JCAHO's 2006 National Patient Safety Goal to "Implement a standardized approach to 'hands off' communications, including an opportunity to ask and respond to questions."[3]

Hospitalist communication may be divided into four major areas. Each brings new challenges and opportunities as a result of the hospitalist model itself. These include communication:

- Between hospitalist and referring (or other involved) physicians
- Between the hospitalist and patient, family, and significant others
- Among members of the hospital multidisciplinary team
- Within the hospitalist group (i.e., between hospitalists)

COMMUNICATION WITH REFERRING AND OTHER PHYSICIANS

An effective system for communication with referring physicians and other physicians involved in a patient's care is the cornerstone of a successful hospitalist program and should be among the first systems put in place when setting up a new program. The most common communication gaps occur between the hospitalist and referring physician in failing to notify the referring physician of his or her patient's hospital admission, discharge, death, or major changes in clinical status.[4] Of note, the referring physician has a responsibility to communicate with the hospitalist on important issues, such as responding to requests from the hospital for office information.

The reliable, timely transmission of discharge summary, history and physical examination, and consultation documents to referring physicians is an important starting point for a communication plan. The transcription and facsimile of these documents should be performed in real time or as close as possible, such as within 6–24 hours (Box 119-1). In some cases, an electronic connection between the hospitalist and referring physician exists, allowing for very rapid communication of information. Such a system requires an alert, such as e-mail, to the referring physician notifying him or her of a patient's admission to or discharge from the hospital. The discharge summary itself should be succinct, with appropriate and uniform format and content (Box 119-2).

The transfer of office information by the referring physician to the hospital at time of admission is of equal importance to the hospitalist sending a timely discharge summary to the primary physician. Also, securing prior hospital records is essential to patient care. A number of approaches may be employed, with the goal being that the hospitalist have appropriate information regarding a patient's medical history, including key diagnostic studies and a medication list. One approach is to create a protocol for obtaining records. After authorization from the patient, this is faxed to the referring physician's office. It requests specific office chart information such as key diagnostics and office notes that will inform the hospitalist's evaluation and management. A sample "request for records" form is shown in Figure 119-1. Another approach is to have referring physician office staff trained to fax key office documents any time an history and physical (H & P) is received from the hospitalist, thus eliminating the step of having the hospitalist request records. Perhaps the ideal mechanism is for the hospital and referring physician to share an electronic medical record (see Fig. 119-1).

Other communication practices for hospitalists to consider include:

- A phone call to the referring physician at discharge for complex patients, those with intensive postdischarge needs, or those at high risk for complications or readmission
- A phone call to the referring physician for serious changes in patient condition while in the hospital
- A "continuity" or "social" visit or phone call to the hospitalized patient by the referring physician when appropriate

---

Box 119-1 Elements of Effective Transmission of Discharge Summary and History and Physical Documents to Referring Physician

- Real-time transcription capabilities. Either manual transcription or voice recognition technology.

- Facsimile (manual or automated) or electronic means of sending documents. If facsimile technology is used, a directory of referring physician numbers may be created.

- A requirement that each hospitalist dictate or create the discharge summary and H & P documents at or soon after the time the patient is seen.

- Clerical support or "rounding assistant" to assist with document and information management.

Box 119-2 Key Elements of the Hospital Discharge Summary

List of discharge diagnoses

Discharge medications

Follow-up

Tests performed

Pending test results (which require follow-up)

History of present illness and hospital course—includes detailed yet concise summary of events, with appropriate paragraph breaks for visual accessibility

Diet and activity

Consultants

Box 119-3 Components of Effective Patient Communication for Hospitalists

Describe the hospitalist-referring physician partnership

Provide a hospitalist group brochure, which contains:

> Pictures of the hospitalists with brief biosketches, including training background
>
> How to contact the hospitalist
>
> The relationship between hospitalist and referring physician, including how the two communicate
>
> Why the patient is under the care of a hospitalist instead of his or her personal physician (i.e., advantages of the hospitalist model)
>
> What the patient and family can do to maximize the chances of a good outcome from the hospital stay (e.g., follow-up with referring physician, comply with prescribed treatments)

Outline expectations regarding daily visits, availability for family meetings, status updates, and timely discussion of test results and management decisions

Use lay terms and language that fosters patients' understanding of their condition.

Coordinate and/or provide complete patient education regarding the plan of care upon transition from the hospital.

Consider calling patients after discharge to review discharge instructions, medications, and follow-up.

Consider providing a copy of the discharge summary (and other relevant documents) to the patient at the time of discharge (often possible if stat transcription is available) or later via mail.

COMMUNICATION WITH CONSULTING PHYSICIANS

A uniform approach to communicating with consulting physicians is important. An in-depth discussion of this may be found in Chapter 96, The Hospitalist as Consultant. Hospitalists requesting consultation from other physicians should articulate the reason for the request, specify the urgency of services needed, and set expectations with the consultant for communication of findings and recommendations. The process for requesting consultation from the hospitalist should be clearly conveyed to both the hospital medical staff and to the nursing staff. Often, a mechanism for engaging consultants is documented in the medical staff bylaws and may include requirements for a direct phone request to the consultant by the requesting physician. Also, the consultant and requesting physician should agree on a process for communicating findings and recommendations to the patient and significant others.

COMMUNICATION WITH PATIENTS AND SIGNIFICANT OTHERS

The referring physician should apprise the patient of the hospitalist's role and the nature of the hospitalist-referring physician partnership prior to hospitalization if possible. The hospitalist should reinforce this by describing his or her role to the patient and loved ones. This can be aided by a brochure outlining important aspects of the function of the hospitalists and how they work with the referring physician. A major pitfall can occur when the patient feels abandoned by the referring physician during the hospitalization or does not understand the hospitalist's role in the care team. Box 119-3 outlines the components of effective patient communication for hospitalists.

A significant area of concern for hospitalist–patient communication is during the period from hospital discharge until the first visit with the primary physician. Often, patients are confused as to what follow-up plans are arranged, which medicines they should be taking, and whom they should contact—hospitalist or primary physician—should a problem arise. After discharge, a phone call to patients in which medications and postdischarge plans are reviewed can be effective in bridging the gap between hospitalist and referring physician.[5] One study indicated that having a pharmacist perform postdischarge telephone follow-up reduces return visits to the emergency department, improves medication compliance, and improves patient satisfaction.[6]

COMMUNICATION WITH NURSES AND OTHER HEALTH CARE STAFF

The hospitalist model affords frequent opportunities for contact with nurses and other members of the hospital team. As a result, communication is often enhanced between the parties, compared to the traditional primary physician model of hospital care. However, new challenges have arisen due to the large number of patients hospitalists may care for on a given nursing unit, for example, and due to the growing numbers of hospitalists within

To:

From: Doctor's name here
Hospitalist Practice
XYZ Hospital Medical Center
1234 Any St.
Your Town, ST 12345
Phone: 555-555-1234   Fax: 555-555-4321

Fax: _____

Pages: _____ (# of pages including cover sheet)

Phone: _____

Date: _____

Re: _____
      (Patient name)

(Additional identifying information, e.g., DOB, SSN)

Records needed _____   _____

☐ All records since _____   ☐ Medication list
             (Date)

☐ Discharge summaries: ☐ All since _____   ☐ Most recent history and physical examination
                      Date

☐ Most recent

☐ Test reports of particular interest

☐ Cardiac cath	☐ PT/PTT	☐ Thyroid test	☐ B_{12}
☐ Echocardiogram	☐ CBC	☐ Ferritan	☐ Folate
☐ Chest X-ray	☐ BUN/Creatinine	☐ ANA	☐ Other _____

                                                                   Specify

Records requested from the following institution or office:

_____

_____

_____

Authorization for release of medical information:

_____ , Authorize _____
Name   Institution, office or physician

To release to XYZ Hospital Medical Center any and all information they possess regarding my medical condition. This authorization includes the release of medical records and/or information concerning drug abuse or drug-related condtions and/or alcoholism and/or psychological and/or psychiatric conditions and/or HIV or other communicable diseases. This authorization will expire 60 (sixty) days from the date below.

_____   _____
Date   Signature of patient

_____   _____
Witness   Other person legally authorized to give consent

• **Comments:** This message is intended for the use of the individual entity to which it is transmitted and may contain information that is privileged, confidential and exempt from disclosure under applicable laws. If the reader of this communication is not the intended recipient, you are hereby notified that any dissemination, distribution, or copying of this communication is strictly prohibited. If you have received this communication in error, please notify us immediately by telephone and return the original communication to us at the address above via the U.S. Postal Service. We will reimburse you for the mailing expense. Thank you.

Figure 119-1 • Example of a Records Requests Form.

hospitals. One such challenge is how a nurse, or other member of the hospital team, contacts the appropriate hospitalist at any point in time, especially when several hospitalists are on duty each day and night. Solutions to contacting the appropriate hospitalist include:

- Create a daily listing of hospitalists on duty, corresponding beeper numbers, and which patients each is following. Distribute this to all nursing units, the hospital operator, and any other party who may need to know, such as the hospitalist practice manager or rounding assistant.
- Ensure that the hospital chart clearly indicates which hospitalist is seeing the patient daily. This requires an entry in the physician orders and/or progress notes section when there is a change in hospitalist seeing the patient.
- Designate teams of hospitalists, and label charts accordingly. Then one pager number can be assigned to each team, simplifying the mechanism of contacting the appropriate hospitalist.
- Display the hospitalist monthly schedule at nursing units and at the hospital operator switchboard.

Formal communication among members of the hospital team is important for careful oversight of discharge planning and other processes of care. Multidisciplinary rounds, held on a regular basis, are an ideal forum for promoting communication among the hospital team members. For such meetings to be successful, there must be allotted time and space and a clear set of goals and objectives. Chapter 128 provides a complete discussion of teamwork in the hospital setting.

HOSPITALIST–HOSPITALIST COMMUNICATION

Important clinical and nonclinical matters must be addressed in a successful approach to communication between hospitalists. Clinical issues should be discussed in scheduled sign-out sessions, often at the conclusion of a shift. Hospitalists may congregate at the outset of the workday to receive sign-out, discuss important clinical matters, and go over minor administrative concerns confronting the group. Sign-out is most effective when there is a standardized template for clinical, demographic, and pertinent social information, such as code status (Box 119-4). This tactic embraces the aforementioned JCAHO 2006 National Patient Safety Goal of implementing "a standardized approach to 'hand

---

Box 119-4 Essential Elements for Successful Handoffs

Team information
Patient identification
Active problems/medical history
Active medications and allergies
Venous access status and contingencies
Pertinent laboratory data
Concerns for next 18–24 hours
Psychosocial status and long-term plans
Code Status

From: Solet D, Norvell L, Rutan, et al. Lost in translations Challenges and apportunities in physician-to-physician communication during patient handoffs. Acad Med 2005; 80(12):1094–1099.

---

off' communications, including an opportunity to ask and respond to questions."[3]

Management of the individual and group hospitalist patient census is a critical communication challenge. Which patients are on the hospitalist service? Which hospitalist is caring for which patient? How many patients is each hospitalist caring for at one time? Much of this can be managed electronically with the use of personal computers and a shared database, with each hospitalist's patient list available to the entire group.

Administrative matters should be addressed in regular—monthly or quarterly—hospitalist group meetings. This is a structured forum for disseminating business and policy information of importance to the group, discussing political issues confronting the group, and generating consensus and solidarity among group members.

MEASURING EFFECTIVENESS

Monitoring how well communication is occurring can by done by means of referring physician, patient or other stakeholder surveys, postacute setting chart review looking for key documents sent from the hospital, and outcome analysis, such as compliance with prescribed postdischarge treatments and follow-up. Specific steps to consider:

- Survey key stakeholders in the communication process, including:
  - Patients: *Did the hospitalist and nurse outline follow-up instructions? Were discharge medications discussed with you and written down for you? Were you pleased with the level of communication with your hospital physician? Would you recommend your hospitalist to others? (See Chapter 131 on Patient Satisfaction.)*
  - Referring and aftercare physicians: *Did you receive discharge summaries in a timely manner? Were you satisfied with the overall level of communication?*
  - Nurses: *Was beeper response time appropriate? Did the hospitalist write his or her orders legibly (for traditional order entry)?*
- Review "downstream" medical records, such as at the skilled nursing facility, for completeness of documentation. This may be done easily for hospitalists with posthospital clinical responsibilities, such as at the rehabilitation facility.
- Review logs of facsimile transmissions to referring physicians compared with lists of patient discharges.
- Examine outcomes that are dependent on communication, such as correct discharge medications or appropriate post discharge follow-up.
- Review time lapse between requests for consultation and performance of consult visit.

SUMMARY

Effective communication in hospitalist systems is the cornerstone of optimal patient care and program operations. With the advent of new vulnerabilities created by the "hand-off" between referring physician and hospitalist, a focus on flow of needed information between hospital and other sites of care is essential. The hospitalist model allows for more effective collaboration with the hospital team, and mechanisms for this to occur must be devised. Finally, the perspective of the patient and significant others must be kept at the forefront, and ideal communication with these parties must be accomplished.

Key Points

- Hospitalists need excellent communication skills focused on four separate areas:

  (1) Between hospitalist and referring (or other involved) physicians
  (2) Between the hospitalist and patients, family, and significant others
  (3) Among members of the hospital multidisciplinary team
  (4) Between the hospitalists themselves

- Upon patient transition into and out of the hospital, there must be prompt preparation and real-time transmission of the history and physical examination, discharge summary, and other necessary documents to those responsible for continuity of care, including the referring physician (e.g., primary care provider), specialists, and skilled nursing/rehabilitation facilities.

- Discussion with the referring physician at hospital admission and discharge may improve information transfer, especially for complex patients.

- A systematized approach for retrieval of patient records from outpatient sites, skilled nursing facilities, and other hospitals is required.

- Communication with patients and significant others includes: description of hospitalist's role, provision of an explanatory hospitalist brochure or card, how to contact the hospitalist, family meeting if appropriate, and a postdischarge call to the patient if appropriate.

- Hospitalist–hospitalist communication should include: sign-out of patients when going off-duty, face-to-face meetings to discuss patient care and administrative issues as appropriate, and notification of new admission/consultations.

- When serving as a consultant or requesting the services of a consultant, hospitalists should follow a set of communication standards to facilitate appropriate collaboration and care coordination.

- Communication with the hospital multidisciplinary team is most effective when it occurs both in regularly scheduled meetings and informally in the course of patient care.

- Some kind of formal meeting with key members of the hospital team, such as case managers, social workers, pharmacists, therapists, etc., should be held regularly to define roles in individual patient management and system improvements.

- For nurses, physicians, other health professionals, and family to be able to contact the appropriate hospitalist on a given day, an updated listing of which hospitalist is caring for which patients should be accessible to the hospital operator and all nursing units. All individual charts need clear, updated physician labeling.

SUGGESTED READING

Pantilat SZ, Lindenauer PK, Katz PP, et al. Primary care physician attitudes regarding communication with hospitalists. Am J Med 2001; 111(9B):15S–20S.

Dudas V, Bookwalter T, Kerr KM, et al. The impact of follow-up telephone calls to patients after hospitalization. Am J Med 2001; 111(9B):26S–30S.

Goldman L, Pantilat SZ, Whitcomb WF. Passing the clinical baton: 6 principles to guide the hospitalist. Am J Med 2001; 111(9B):36S–39S.

Nelson JR. The importance of postdischarge telephone follow-up for hospitalists: a view from the trenches. Am J Med 2001; 111(9B):43S–44S.

Wachter RM, Pantilat SZ. The "continuity visit" and the hospitalist model of care. Am J Med 2001; 111(9B):40S–42S.

Solet D, Norvell L, Rutan G, et al. Essential elements for successful handoffs. Acad Med 2005; 80(12):1094–1099.

O'Leary JK, Liebovitz DM, Baker DW. How hospitalists spend their time: insights on efficiency and safety. J Hosp Med 2006; 1:88–93.

CHAPTER ONE HUNDRED AND TWENTY

Compensation Principles and Practices

Russell Holman, MD, Winthrop F. Whitcomb, MD, and John R. Nelson, MD, FACP

INTRODUCTION

Compensation is one of the most tangible expressions of the mission, vision, and values of a hospital medicine group and its associated institutions. The way a group pays its hospitalists serves to reinforce the core priorities and preferences of the group, and may provide a meaningful basis for incentives to help attain specific goals. During the recruitment phase of hiring physicians into the group, compensation (in addition to location and the characteristics of the practice itself) serves as one of the fundamental elements of attracting excellent candidates, in terms of both the total financial opportunity as well as the model in which dollars are allocated. Allocation, or *distribution*, of monies is important to distinguish from *funding* sources since these two processes may—and often should—be designed very differently from one another. As such, the topic of compensation is often an "emotionally charged" discussion and process for two primary reasons. First, the model itself directly affects the livelihood of group members, and therefore it is vital that constituents be involved in the development process. Second, group revenues such as professional service collections and graduate medical education teaching dollars often do not meet the direct expenses of the practice, therefore requiring the group to receive support dollars from a sponsoring entity. Since physician compensation comprises the vast majority of direct expenses in a hospital medicine group, a sponsoring entity may impose ongoing pressure for the group to demonstrate its value for the compensation being distributed.

As we will discuss below, compensation for hospitalists has evolved in recent years, reflecting a trend toward rewarding performance in productivity and quality of care. This phenomenon has posed an interesting challenge to group leaders who may feel compelled to preferentially offer guaranteed compensation packages, given that demand for hospitalists far exceeds supply and the demographic preferences of this young work force. Society of Hospital Medicine (SHM) survey data from 2005 show the average age of a hospitalist in the United States as 37 years old, and younger physicians tend to be more security minded and risk averse than older postwar baby boomers. This chapter will discuss recent SHM benchmark data and review several compensation methodologies in hospital medicine.

SHM SURVEY RESULTS: COMPENSATION AND PRODUCTIVITY

SHM received survey responses from over 2,100 hospitalists in late 2005 assessing compensation and productivity. This revealed that hospitalists have an annual median salary of $171,000 for hospitalists who care only for adults. It is important to keep in mind that this reflects *total* salary, so it includes both base salary *and* incentive compensation (e.g., bonuses based on quality or productivity). This finding reflects a 3–5% increase compared to 2 years previously.

Figure 120-1 shows historical salary trends, but interpretation needs to consider that the population of hospitalists has changed a great deal from previous surveys, so any variation in survey results may be due to changing demographics (e.g., different portions of academic and community hospitalists in the survey) in addition to real changes in the way hospitalists work and are paid. In addition to their salary, hospitalists received median benefits of $26,000. Benefits include federal payroll taxes, employer contributions for insurance (disability, health, life, workers comp), retirement programs, etc.

The survey shows that hospitalists see a median 2,328 encounters and generate a median 3,213 work relative valve units (wRVUs) annually. Since the prior SHM survey conducted in 2003, median encounters have increased 3%, and wRVUs 7%. Thus, a sizable portion of the salary increase over the last 2 years may be explained by increases in productivity. Combined with enhanced productivity, another likely factor contributing to escalating levels of compensation in hospital medicine is the demand for hospitalists far exceeding supply in today's marketplace. With new hospital medicine programs frequently being created while existing groups are increasing in size and scope of services, competition for recruiting qualified physicians is significant.

Taken together, the survey figures for productivity and compensation can provide a picture of the typical hospitalist, as summarized in Table 120-1. Of note, these compensation and productivity figures vary significantly with:

• Employment type: Local multispecialty groups have higher productivity and compensation than hospitalists who are hospital-employed

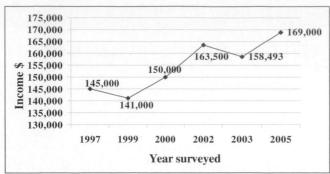

Figure 120-1 • Average hospitalist incomes over time.

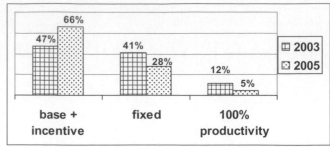

Figure 120-2 • Percentage of hospitalists compensated by each method.

Table 120–1 Survey Medians for Financial Performance of an Individual Hospitalist	
Collected professional fee revenue	$200,000
Additional revenue	$65,000
Total revenue	**$265,000**
Overhead (estimated 18.8%)	$(–48,880)
Net revenue	**$211,120**
Hospitalist salary	$168,000
Benefits	$26,000

- Geographic region: Those in the South typically have higher productivity and compensation than other regions
- Method of compensation: Those who have some portion of salary based on productivity earn more than those who have a fixed ("straight") salary

When thinking about one's own practice, it is important to review the complete survey results to ensure an appropriate comparison group.[1] In our experience, a common mistake is to assume that the aggregate survey results, such as medians or means for the whole survey population, reflect the "right" numbers for a practice. Some make the serious mistake of assuming that the aggregate survey results reflect the SHM's position on the correct or optimal productivity and compensation for hospitalists. Instead, the survey can only serve as a starting point for analyzing an individual practice, and it is vital to consider local factors that might explain why a particular practice is, or should be expected to be, different from the survey mean or median. Another common judgment error is failing to consider productivity (workload) when thinking about compensation. Variations in productivity appear to explain a significant portion of differences in compensation.

COMPENSATION METHODOLOGY

The characteristics of an effective compensation program are listed in Box 120-1 and may be applied to the methodologies described below.

Box 120-1 Characteristics of an Effective Compensation Program

- Aligned and consistent with group vision and goals.
- Model is easily understood by constituents and stakeholders.
- Program is simple to administer.
- Measures and process withstand public scrutiny.
- Meets regulatory compliance guidelines.
- Flexible; straightforward to change over time.
- Limited number of performance measures to avoid "dilution effect."
- Supported by adequate funding pool to meaningfully incentivize behavior.
- Measures are relevant, accurate, and timely relative to behavior.
- Linked to a comprehensive performance management system.
- Rewards desired performance of the group.

Hospitalists are paid via a multitude of compensation schemes that can be grouped into three general types: straight (fixed) salary, 100% productivity-based salary (e.g., one based on wRVUs or charges, etc.), and some combination of a fixed and variable incentive components. Figure 120-2 shows how common each of these compensation methods was in 2003 and 2005.

Straight Salary

A straight salary was the most common way hospitalists were paid in all surveys prior to 2003. Its popularity is likely due to its simplicity for both understanding and budgeting, and its ability to facilitate recruiting because the hospitalist has no risk of making less than the guarantee. However, its inflexibility does not provide a financial reward for good citizenship (e.g., high productivity, organizational contributions, or performing well on quality measures), which has led the majority of practices to move toward a compensation method that incorporates an incentive component.

100% Production-Based Salary

A salary based entirely on productivity may be a reasonable way to compensate hospitalists, but has always been uncommon. It is often based on easy-to-measure metrics of workload such as wRVUs or billable patient encounters. The benefits are that it is usually simple to administer and it allows hospitalists a great deal of flexibility in deciding their optimal workload and staffing and to accept, or "own," the economic consequences of their decisions. Additionally, it provides a financial incentive for the provider to attend to optimal coding and charge capture. Most physicians in all specialties in the United States are essentially paid a 100% production-based salary, and thus this mechanism generally seems reasonable to hospitalists' fellow physicians.

Hospitalists often view a productivity-based income as very risky because they have little control over day-to-day variations in practice volume which would impact their income (i.e., they cannot "schedule" hospital admissions). However, based on their staffing decisions and choices regarding scope of practice, hospitalists have substantial control over their patient volume, especially considering lengthy intervals such as a year. Some express concern that it causes hospitalists to work excessively, to compete with one another for referrals, to damage group culture, or to keep patients in the hospital longer. While these are legitimate concerns, they are rarely a significant problem if there is appropriate management and oversight of other performance metrics (such as length of stay, physician satisfaction, and turnover) of the group. In fact, because a salary based solely on productivity encourages hospitalists to think of themselves more as owners of the practice (even if they are not owners and are employed by a hospital), they may often be happier and feel more in control of daily activities. It also provides a means for some hospitalists in a group to work less and accept a lower income, while others can work and make more, or additional doctors can be added to the practice.

If the group leader or funding sponsors are concerned that basing compensation exclusively on wRVUs productivity provides an excessive incentive for the hospitalist to keep patients in the hospital longer, this can be managed through the method of case-rate payment. With this approach, the hospitalist is paid a case rate for each new patient (admission or consult) accepted to the service. The case rate remains the same, regardless of whether the patient stays in the hospital 1 or many days.

Implementing a 100% production salary requires agreement on the measure of productivity to use, such as wRVUs, and the dollar amount of salary tied to each unit. One such scheme could mean the hospitalist is paid $52.29 per wRVU. Based on the SHM median wRVUs of 3,213 per year, her salary would be $168,000.

Salary That Combines Fixed ("Base") and Incentive Components

In 2005, 66% of hospitalists were paid through a combination of a base salary and a variable, or incentive, component. Eighty-two percent of such groups base some or the entire incentive portion on a measure of productivity such as wRVUs, charges, or number of admissions. Another 60% use quality metrics (e.g., Medicare core measures) as the basis for the incentive. Anecdotal experi-

---

Box 120-2 2006 Quality Bonus. Mercy Medical Center, Springfield, MA

50% of bonus: Medication reconciliation at admission. Target = 90% compliance

50% of bonus: Medicare Core Measure performance. Target = 90% compliance

- For pneumonia: Pneumococcal and influenza vaccine, appropriate antibiotic selection

- For heart failure: Assessment of LV function, ACE or ARB for LV systolic dysfunction

- For myocardial infarction: Aspirin and beta-blocker on discharge, ACE or ARB for LV systolic dysfunction

LV—left ventricular; ACE—angiotensin converting enzyme; ARB—angiotensin receptor blocker

---

ence shows that providing a base salary is helpful for recruiting, and the incentive component can help reward good citizenship in the practice.

Common mistakes in developing a base salary plus incentive program include choosing a metric that is unreasonably difficult to measure accurately, or linking the incentive pay to so many metrics so that each one is connected to an extremely small percentage of the physician's income. And perhaps the most common mistake is making the metric too easy to achieve, which is essentially the same as guaranteeing the providers the incentive payment and removing any potential that it will influence behavior.

Another reasonable alternative is to develop a compensation scheme that combines a fixed base salary, a productivity component, and an incentive payment based on metrics like quality performance. The main drawback to this approach is that dividing the salary into so many portions means the percent of salary tied to each may be relatively small. An example of a quality bonus metric system can be found in Box 120–2.

Issues related to the fixed and production-based components of the salary are discussed above. Important aspects of creating a quality incentive include the following.

- Decide on how much money to allocate for the bonus. Money may come from payers that have pay-for-performance programs or other sources available to hospitals.
- Decide on quality indicators that the hospitalists can readily influence, such as percentage of myocardial infarction patients receiving aspirin on discharge, and avoid indicators over which they have little influence, such as antibiotic timing in the emergency department.
- Choose indicators that are already being measured by the hospital, so no additional administrative effort is required for measurement.
- Set targets that are attainable, yet "stretch" the hospitalists to perform at a high level. Previous hospitalist performance and relevant national benchmarks may guide the setting of the target. If the target is reached, the bonus is paid.
- Pay the bonus out frequently enough to influence behavior change, such as every 3 or 6 months. If longer intervals are used, the incentive can still affect behavior, as long as regular feedback on the metrics is provided to the physicians

Table 120–2 Advantages and Disadvantages of Group versus Individual Compensation Measures

Measure Type	Advantages	Disadvantages
Group	Reinforces teamwork Ease of administration May improve accuracy of data	May allow individuals to "hide" poor performance May not recognize positive differential performance of individuals Counterintuitive to physician training and expectations
Individual	Consistent with general expectations of physicians Enables unique ability to achieve personal compensation targets Allows management to better understand intragroup performance differences	Reinforces individualism May be more difficult to obtain accurate data Complexity of administration

- Since patients are shared by the hospitalist group, it might be most appropriate for the bonus to be paid out equally to all group members. The group's culture will determine whether this leads to some diffusion of responsibility for good performance, or whether each member of the group encourages and assists his or her colleagues in achieving the goals. Advantages and disadvantages of group versus individual performance measures are listed in Table 120–2.

COMMON PITFALLS OF COMPENSATION PROGRAMS

Barriers to an effective compensation program can be categorized into three main areas: planning, modeling, and expectations.

Planning

Sharp focus on the vision and strategic direction of the group or organization should guide creation of the compensation program. This provides tangible evidence of the support for the vision and links it to daily activities. When compensation models are derived in the absence of the group vision, trust in the group's espoused values and vision may be undermined or regarded with skepticism. Furthermore, planning that takes place without meaningful involvement of constituents or sponsors is less likely to produce desired results. Instead of using compensation planning as an opportunity to build a cohesive, engaged team, planning that occurs "behind closed doors" will fail at achieving group buy-in. Planning must also consider available benchmarks for compensation targets and specific measures. These include national survey data from Society of Hospital Medicine (SHM), Medical Group Management Association (MGMA), and others, as well as local and regional marketplace assessments.

Modeling

Keep in mind that the *funding* of a compensation program may— and often should—differ from the *distribution* of dollars. For example, if a group receives no institutional support monies and the only source of revenues (funding) to the group comes from professional service fees, then a conscious choice must be made to tie all performance-based compensation to productivity or to include other metrics such as quality or satisfaction. Performance-based models must also consider the actual amount of funding allocated for variable/bonus compensation. Insufficient dollars tied to bonus measures will fail to drive desired behaviors, and physicians will commonly ignore the performance measures outlined by the plan. A variation on this theme occurs when the model includes too many performance measures so that dilution of available dollars renders the goals meaningless. Finally, the specified measures must be relevant to the work of the hospital medicine group, be supported by good data and reporting systems, and be timely related to the physicians' or group's behaviors.

Expectations

Often, sponsors and constituents alike regard compensation as being the most important means by which to effect behavioral changes in the hospital medicine group. Ignoring all the other elements of a performance management system—recruiting the right people, setting clear expectations, measuring actual performance, providing regular feedback, managing poor performance—will render a compensation model far less effective and lead to frustration of all stakeholders. Managers should expect that compensation programs in general will drive behaviors that are rewarded and discourage behaviors that are not. A model is equally powerful in *what it does not include,* as well as what measures are actually employed.

SUMMARY

Compensation should reflect the vision of the group or organization, and serve a prominent role in the tangible expression of its strategic direction and goals. Both hospitalist compensation and productivity have risen since 2003 and depend in part on employment type, geographic region, method of compensation, and medical specialty. Compensation programs may be devised according to either a straight salary or some variation of a performance-based system that rewards individual or group achievement of specified goals. Through appropriate planning, modeling, and alignment of expectations for the program, a compensation program will optimally support a more comprehensive performance management system. A hospital medicine group that regularly assesses the efficacy of its method of paying physicians will further ensure its ability to recruit and retain qualified team members.

Key Points

- The basis for an effective compensation program is the vision and goals of the hospital medicine group and/or sponsoring institution.

- Society of Hospital Medicine (SHM) national survey data collected in 2005 show that hospitalist incomes and productivity are increasing.

- Hospitalist salaries and productivity vary significantly, depending on many variables such as differences in practice locale, employment status, and method of compensation.

- Performance-based compensation models, including productivity or quality metrics, have become increasingly prevalent.

- Compensation may help to drive desired behaviors if it is part of a comprehensive performance management system.

- Hospital medicine groups should review their compensation methodology on a regular basis to ensure it supports organizational objectives and strategy.

SUGGESTED READING

Committee on Quality of Health Care in America, Institute of Medicine. Crossing the Quality Chasm: A New Health System for the 21st Century. Washington, DC: National Academy Press, 2001.

American College of Physician Executives. Managing Physician Performance in Organizations. Ongoing courses offered through www.acpe.org

Savavi K. Paying for efficiency. Journal of Healthcare Management 2006; 51(2):77–80.

Safavi K. Aligning financial incentives. J Health Manag 2006; 51(3):146–151.

CHAPTER ONE HUNDRED AND TWENTY-ONE

Documentation, Coding, Billing, and Compliance in Hospital Medicine

M. Tray Dunaway, MD, FACS, CSP, CHCO, CHCC, Beth B. Golden, CPC, and Steven T. Liu, MD

BACKGROUND

The triad of compliance, correct physician documentation, and coding and billing increases the likelihood of economic success while minimizing risk of third-party payer audits and reviews, as well as potential fines and penalties. Education about reimbursement-based medical documentation, coding, and subsequent medical billing for services is limited or nonexistent during training, leaving new physicians to fend for themselves in the "real world" of clinical medicine. Physicians typically choose to focus on patient care in practice and neglect the lifetime practice benefits acquired through education in reimbursement-based documentation, coding, and billing.

When physicians decline to play an active role in optimizing documentation, compliance, and reimbursement, they leave money on the table to the benefit of third-party payers, and they inadvertently expose themselves to unfavorable regulatory audits.

This chapter serves as an overview of the documentation, coding, billing, and compliance process. Intended as a primer in common terminology, it is designed as a starting point for further self-education.

DOCUMENTATION

Documentation serves a variety of purposes, each requiring key phrases to meet the needs of the specific type of documentation. We document for patient care, for medical-legal reasons, for disease research, for hospital benefit, and for physician benefit for reimbursement, quality, and credit/recognition. Some key phrases serve only one element of documentation; other phrases may serve all elements. The summation of all of these documentation elements creates what is termed the *medical record.*

Hospital and physician documentation serves two basic functions:

Financial element (reimbursement)
Credit/recognition element (quality/regulatory)

Aspects of documentation in the medical record that determine financial reimbursement for physicians are generally separate from those influencing hospital reimbursement. However, hospitalists who understand key hospital documentation issues can reap substantial benefit. By appropriately documenting the correct information determining a patient's diagnosis, which gets converted into a diagnosis-related group (DRG) payment, the hospital will more likely receive reimbursement owed for care delivered. Additionally, providing appropriate documentation for the optimal DRG determines the expected length of stay (LOS). Under documenting will negatively impact both physician and hospital reimbursement while also underestimating expected LOS. For hospitalists who receive support from the hospital, knowing the rules of documentation is simply good business. Rather than being entirely separate issues, the credit/recognition component that physicians document fortunately overlaps with the quality and regulatory aspects that hospitals seek.

The most important concept physicians must understand is **there is no substitute for physician documentation.** Unless a physician writes a diagnosis in a chart, the diagnosis does not exist for subsequent coding and billing and therefore will not generate reimbursement or give credit and recognition to hospital or physician. Documentation in a medical record by *anyone other than a physician* simply does not count. If a nurse documents "anemia" on an inpatient chart, it does not count. In the same chart, if a laboratory report demonstrates a hematocrit of 24, it does not count. Only when the word "anemia" is documented by a physician does it count. The next most important concept physicians must understand is that documentation does not justify subsequent coding or billing. Documentation *supports* coding and billing, but *medical necessity* (described below) justifies coding and billing.

Hospital-Driven Physician Documentation

For Medicare beneficiary reimbursement, hospitals derive payment from the DRG payment system. DRG coding basics are covered in this chapter's Coding section, but the DRG codes are determined by ICD-9-CM (a reference book) diagnosis codes. Other third-party payers may have technically different payment schedules, but the broad concepts of Medicare are usually related and applicable.

Based on *physician-documented diagnoses* on inpatients, a set amount of reimbursement is provided to hospitals for financial compensation of care. (NOTE: An entirely different classification for hospital outpatient care has been developed with Medicare APC—Ambulatory Patient Classification—systems.)

There are two key components in determining what the actual Medicare payment amount is: the actual calculated DRG score and the blended rate of the particular hospital where the patient is admitted.

A DRG score is calculated by taking into consideration the primary diagnosis a patient is determined to have. According to Medicare, the primary diagnosis is the diagnosis determined, after study, to be chiefly responsible for the admission of the patient to the hospital for care. *"After study"* is critical. It may be the same as the admitting diagnosis, but it could be technically determined even after discharge when studies become available to the physician. Whatever the primary diagnosis is determined to be is the basis of the DRG calculation. Depending on the *physician-documented* secondary diagnoses the patient may have had during the admission, the ultimate DRG score is determined. Certain secondary diagnoses (also called additional diagnoses), may allow a higher weighed final DRG score.

Secondary diagnoses that increase DRG scores are called CCs. CC is short for Comorbid Conditions and/or Complications. A basic DRG *with* a CC is worth more in terms of both reimbursement and credit/recognition to a hospital than an identical basic DRG *without* a CC. Often, these key additional diagnoses that determine a CC seem insignificant to physicians. For instance, a patient with a diagnosis of "gastroenteritis" results in a DRG payment that is significantly less than the DRG payment of a patient with the diagnosis of "gastroenteritis with dehydration." Documentation of "dehydration" (an additional diagnosis) makes a critical difference. Many CCs go undocumented because as clinicians, we do not bother to write down words we think of as superfluous that would indicate "obvious" conditions. Most physicians are surprised to learn that the difference in reimbursement between *gastroenteritis with dehydration* and simply *gastroenteritis* to most hospitals is around $1,200.

The actual amount of reimbursement is determined by not only the ultimate DRG score (with or without a CC), but also by the specific hospital blended rate, a functional dollar conversion factor determined by the government for individual hospitals. The actual payment to a particular hospital is determined by multiplying the blended rate by the DRG score. Physicians do not share in the reimbursement that is determined by hospital DRGs, but they do share elements of credit/recognition.

The Severity of Illness Index (SI index) is also determined by the hospitalized patient DRG score. Think of the SI index as a measure of how "sick a patient is." A *high* patient SI Index means the patient is *sicker* than a patient with a *low* SI Index. It's easy to see that the DRG payment would therefore be greater for higher SI indexed patients because it is essentially measured in the same way a DRG score is calculated. Therefore, hospitals with high SI Indexes are taking care of sicker patients and are reimbursed at a higher rate. Hospitals with low SI Indexes are taking care of patients who are not as sick. The fact of the matter is that the assessment of how sick a hospital's patients are depends on physician documentation, not actual severity of illness.

While the SI Index may appear to be a "hospital value," it is also a physician value. A hospital's SI Index is merely a summation of the individual SI Indexes of admitting physicians in a given hospital. The reality is that third-party payers track SI Indexes of physicians and hospitals. So hospitals *and* physicians demonstrating high SI Indexes are judged to be taking care of sicker patients.

Finally, no discussion of hospital documentation would be complete without a discussion of Case Mix Index (CMI). CMI is best described as the sum of all of a hospital's Medicare DRG scores divided by the total number of Medicare admissions. The higher the CMI, the better. Hospitals and physicians, with regard to credit/recognition, find a high CMI more desirable, as it reflects that they took care of "sicker" patients. Similarly, higher CMIs are of great importance to hospitals because they translate into higher reimbursement of services. That's why hospital administrators are concerned about the CMI. If improved accuracy of physician documentation moves the CMI higher, hospitals are happy. SI and CMI are essentially the same qualitative measurements. When SI, or CMI, valuation increases, it's a positive value for hospitals. They are credited for taking care of more acutely ill patients, and thus they are reimbursed at a higher rate.

CODING

Coding is clinical documentation translated into numeric codes. These numeric codes represent clinical information in a format that is transmitted, electronically or with hard copy, to third-party payers for payment as well as giving information to interested parties, about quality and credit/recognition elements of patient care. If the translation is incorrect, we suffer consequences, including loss of credit/recognition from insufficient documentation of actual work, audits by third-party payers that might determine that the billed service was not performed, and potential accusations of error or fraud.

If documentation fails to support billed E&M (Evaluation & Management) services in audits, third-party payers can deny payment or request refunds. Passage of the Kennedy-Kassebaum bill allows *all* third-party payers to levy criminal charges against physicians with E&M documentation guidelines variances for "fraud and abuse."

Coding accuracy is the critical element that moves physician clinical documentation along the reimbursement and credit/recognition pathway. If there is no coded translation for a clinical description (e.g., "↓hct"), no reimbursement or credit/recognition is received. If the clinical word we use (e.g., "urosepsis") does not correctly state the clinical description we actually mean (such as "septicemia from a urinary source"), the translation may be relegated to a lower-paying DRG (like urinary tract infection), and reimbursement and credit/recognition are less. A book titled *ICD-9-CM* lists all the currently approved diagnosis codes that accompany both hospital and physician billing for reimbursement. The ICD-9-CM codes come from a long pedigree and will be replaced in the future by ICD-10-CM codes.

The rules for selecting diagnosis codes for physician services are in the front of the *ICD-9-CM* and are different from the system hospitals must use. Although the coding rules are extensive, there are two keys:

1. List first the ICD-9-CM code for the diagnosis, condition, problem, or other reason for the visit shown to be chiefly responsible for the services provided; then list additional codes that describe any coexisting conditions.
2. Do not code diagnoses documented as "probable," "suspected," "questionable," "rule out" or "working diagnosis." Rather, code the condition(s) to the highest degree of certainty for that visit, such as symptoms, signs, abnormal test results,

or other reason for the visit. The entire set of diagnostic coding guidelines is available at *http://www.cdc.gov/nchs/data/icd9/icdguide.pdf.*

The American Medical Association has its own codes, (for which they own a copyright; they must be licensed for use by publishers and businesses of health care that use the codes). These codes are the physician CPT codes.

CPT stands for Current Procedural Terminology, and as the name suggests, codes are listed in the *CPT* book that describes procedures conducted by physicians. There are two sets of codes in *CPT*. E&M codes describe the activity of physicians when we evaluate patients and manage subsequent care. Described activities include office visits, hospital visits and admissions (including observation encounters), nursing home visits, ER visits, home visits, a wide variety of consultative encounters, and even boarding home visits! They are listed numerically, sequentially, by location; and some are further divided by distinctions between new and established patients, initial or subsequent visits, and even day of discharge from hospital. The common characteristic of E&M codes is that they are 5-digit numbers that initiate with a 99 sequence (99XXX).

E&M codes have seven components of documentation, but all share the three key components that include a history, a physical examination, and a component called "Medical Decision Making" (MDM). In the authors' opinion, MDM could more accurately be described as "medical *billing* decision-making"; it is composed of three factors: the medical risk the patient presents with to the physician as determined by AMA/CMS standards; the amount/complexity of data that are ordered or reviewed by the physician at the time of service; and finally, the number of diagnoses or management options related to the patient. These three factors, risk, data, and diagnoses, together determine MDM. Putting it all together, documentation of MDM, (and its key components), the documented history, and the documented physical examination determine the correct E&M code (depending on the location of the visit). To add to the complexity, various modifiers describing variances of services may be added to an E&M code as suffixes (99xxx-xx) to change payments when the code is billed out. Under certain circumstances, various components required can be collective or individual and if you use certain rules concerning the time spent with patients, further differentiated between "critical care" versus "prolonged services," you may be able to skip the history, physical, MDM components entirely, but you then must account for how time was spent on the patient's care. Table 121-1 presents an example of a summary of documentation to be considered when generating E&M codes.

The pages devoted to E&M codes in the published CPT codebooks are few in comparison to the other group of codes, referred to as procedural codes. Procedural codes refer to a wide variety of codes devoted to surgical, laboratory, x-ray, and other procedures. They are listed in groupings roughly according to systems (e.g., appendectomies are located near EGDs). The procedural codes are easier in some ways than E&M codes; however, they also can become very arcane in determining which is the most accurate code to describe all the procedures that we do in medicine.

Despite the complexities of E&M coding, these are the most commonly used codes for physicians, often making up more than 85% of billed physician services. Downcoding refers to the practice of choosing a lower code than would be legitimately possible because of either: 1) inadequate documentation to support the code, or 2) fear of an audit by third-party payers to avoid possible payment of refunds if the documentation fails to support the code. Upcoding is use of a code to bill when the 1) service was not performed (this is fraud), or 2) the service was performed and billed for, but was not documented. If the case can be proven that there was criminal intent to defraud the third-party payer, fines and even jail time can be meted out. Furthermore, physicians, hospitals, and others who bill Medicare for beneficiary care who are convicted of fraud can be temporarily or permanently suspended from Medicare and are prohibited from working for entities that bill Medicare. Fraud has serious consequences. The desired goal is correct coding.

Because it is complex, there are specialists—called coders—who do nothing but coding. Physicians often run two separate functions together and call it "billing and coding." But there is a fundamental difference between billers and coders. Coders have received an education not only on "coding," how to use the myriad of code references to secure the most accurate code for the work performed, but also have a background that includes instruction in anatomy, physiology, pharmacology, and other clinical areas. A coder is a professional who serves as the interface between physician clinical documentation and identifying the right code to send out for billing purposes. Understandably, with this knowledge of both clinical and coding worlds, the coder is a very important person.

BILLING

Billing consists of submitting a bill to a patient for payment or, in most cases, submitting a claim to a third-party payer. Claim forms are becoming more standardized, and the gold standard is the HCFA/CMS 1500 form. Healthcare Finance Administration (HCFA) changed their name in July of 2001 to Center for Medicare and Medicaid Services (CMS). Information about the patient (beneficiary), the provider (doctor or other healthcare provider), and the encoded diagnosis and procedural information is submitted for payment to an insurer.

The information is submitted either as a paper claim or electronically for payment. An electronic version gets to the third-party payer more quickly since a paper claim must be entered into an electronic database manually by the insurer. If all the information is correct, payment is sent to the provider. However, if there are errors or mismatch among diagnosis/procedural codes, or if the claim fails to meet medical necessity criteria, the claim will be rejected, and no payment follows. One distinct advantage of electronic claim submission is the rapid discovery of rejected claims that may be resubmitted after an error is fixed or supplemental information is provided.

Medical necessity is a term often misunderstood by physicians. Although "medical necessity" sounds clinical, it is not. The presence or absence of medical necessity determines if a submitted claim will be paid by a third-party payer. Medical necessity is a contractual agreement between an insurance company and the beneficiary (the insured). If documentation and subsequent coding support medical necessity, payment is made. If medical necessity is not met, the bill is rejected, and no payment is made. Medical necessity also refers to *appropriateness* of medical claim submission. If a patient presents with a minor problem and a physician submits a high-level code that is supported by only a voluminous history and physical, technically the rules regulating

Table 121-1 ADMITTING H&Ps: 3 of 3 Key Components (History, Examination, MDM) Required For Code Level

	HISTORY			Exam	MEDICAL DECISION MAKING (MDM)		
	HPI	ROS	P/F/S		#DX/MGMT options	Amount of DATA (laboratory/x-ray)	Risk Level
99221	4+	2–9+	1+ of 3	5–7+ area/systems	1–2	0–2	Min.—low.
99222	4+	10+	3 of 3	8+ organ/systems	3	3	Moderate
99223	4+	10+	3 of 3	8+ organ/systems	4+	4+	High

SUBSEQUENT HOSPITAL CARE: 2 OF 3 Key components (history, examination, MDM) required for code

	Interval History	Examination	Medical Decision Making
99231	Pt. is stable	1 area/system	Straightforward—Low
99232	Pt. not responding or developed a Minor complication	2–4 area/system	Moderate
99233	Pt. is unstable or developed a Major complication	5–7+ area/system	High

HOSPITAL DISCHARGE INCLUDES: Final exam, discussion of stay, instructions, prep of discharge records.

99238 Inpatient discharge: 30 minutes or less.
99239 Inpatient discharge: more than 30 minutes (Document time in record)

ELEMENTS OF HPI:
Location Duration Severity Quality
Timing   Context   Modifying factors
Associated signs/symptoms

REVIEW OF SYMPTOMS
Constitutional   Musculoskeletal
Eyes   Gastrointestinal
Cardiovascular   Genitourinary
Respiratory   Endocrine
Neurologic   Psychiatric
Ears, nose, mouth, throat   Hematologic/Lymphatic
Integumentary   Allergic/Immunologic

PAST/FAMILY/SOCIAL HISTORY:
PAST: Prior/current illness/injuries, current.
                                        Medications, prior surgeries/hospitalizations/allergies, diet, exercise.
FAMILY: Parents/siblings ages and health or cause of death.
SOCIAL: Marital status, occupation, education, living situation, drugs/alcohol/tobacco.

PHYSICAL EXAMINATION:

BODY AREAS:
Head/face   Genital/Groin/Buttocks
Neck   Back/Spine
Chest/Breast/Axilla   Each extremity
Abdomen

ORGAN SYSTEMS:
Constitutional   Respiratory   Integumentary
Eyes   Muscle   Neuro
ENMT   Psych   GI
Cardiovasc   Heme/Lymph/IMM GU

TEACHING PHYSICIAN NOTES:

When performed with a resident the code level is determined by a combination of the resident's and teaching physicians (TP) notes.

The TP must see the patient, perform critical portions of the service, and agree with the residents note or revise it.

EX. "I saw and evaluated the patient. Reviewed resident's note. Agree with plan as written.

EX: "I saw and evaluated the patient. Agree with resident's note but . . ."

payment may be met. But if medical necessity does not justify the billed claim, audits may be triggered. A pattern of abusive billing practices (the "abuse" of "fraud and abuse") may result in investigations by third-party payers. If investigations discover a willful intent to deceive a payer, charges of fraud (the "fraud" of "fraud and abuse") may be brought against the physician.

It is the biller's job to ensure that claims are successfully submitted and accurate payment is made. A coder can also be a biller, but typically, a biller will not be a coder. You do not need a coder or a biller in your practice, but then you will be doing your own coding and billing or relegating this duty to someone who is not trained for the job.

Table 121-2 Optimal Coding and Compliance Plan

Learn the rules	There are several resources that contain coding rules every hospitalist should know. Look up the definitions for codes you most commonly use, such as admissions, consults, subsequent hospital care, and critical care. Refer to Appendix C in the CPT manual; it lists clinical examples for each category and evel of code.
	The evaluation and management (E/M) documentation guidelines, developed by the AMA and CMS, provide explicit instructions about the complexity of the encounter and amount of documentation that must be done in order to charge any E/M CPT code. There are two sets: 1995 guidelines and 1997. The full text of both is available on the CMS website: www.cms.hhs.gov/medlearn/emdoc.asp. (See Appendix A, for more details on these guideline sets.)
	If you work in an academic medical center, presence and documentation requirements for teaching physicians are available here: www.cms.hhs.gov/manuals/pm_trans/R1780B3.pdf.
	If your practice employs physician assistants or nurse practitioners, Medicare's rules for split/shared billing in the inpatient setting are available here: www.cms.hhs.gov/manuals/104_claims/clm104c12.pdf (see section 30.6.1).
Apply the rules	Templates can be helpful tools, especially for higher level E/M codes that require the greatest amount of documentation, and are acceptable to Medicare. But you cannot just document your way to the highest code levels. The overarching criterion to bill any CPT code is medical necessity; then the expected amount of documentation must be in place.
	Carrying written or electronic handheld summaries of the documentation guidelines is also helpful.
Check yourself	Two of the main ways to audit your coding and documentation practices include code utilization analysis and chart review.
	Medicare's data about E/M code utilization by specialty is publicly available, here: www.cms.hhs.gov/statistics/feeforservice/default.asp. This database shows how often physicians bill Medicare for all E/M code levels in all categories. Compare how often you bill most-used code categories against your peers nationally. With that, due to variations in the complexity of your patients, your practice may differ from these utilization rates. Only a review of chart documentation, described in detail below, will tell if appropriate codes were used
	The second part of the self-audit process is chart review. Select a variety of services, including H&Ps, consults, subsequent hospital care and critical care, and audit the documentation for coding accuracy.
Stay informed	It's ultimately your responsibility to become informed about coding compliance and stay informed. If you designate part of this responsibility, make sure the designee is knowledgeable and has the correct tools, minimally including the current CPT and ICD-9-CM, access to official coding instruction including CPT Assistant and Coding Clinic, Medicare's Correct Coding Initiative (CCI), and payer-specific information, especially local Medicare carrier and state Medicaid rules.
Integrate compliance into your practice	If you are in a large organization and have access to a compliance department, use them. Ask questions, solicit help with chart review. If you are in a smaller group, the Department of Health and Human Services has advice on setting up an effective compliance program: http://oig.hhs.gov/fraud/complianceguidance.html.

COMPLIANCE

Because third-party payers, (federal, state, and private) are increasing their scrutiny of medical claims, all physicians should have a compliance program for their practices. At a minimum, a compliance program is defined as a PROCESS that every medical practice should have to achieve stated goals of the practice and encompass all areas of regulation applicable to the specific practice. A compliance program is a dynamic entity using a "compliance plan document" that spells out how the practice will maintain compliance with complex and changing rules and regulations, but also directs how it is administered to all the professional and clerical elements in a medical practice. Typically, an office employee is designated a compliance officer. Additional outside training for the employee is typically needed and may result in a certification.

Some of a compliance officer's responsibilities include developing a compliance program that will review all relevant documents and compliance practices of the organization. Audits and reviews are carried out to look for areas of noncompliance in the practice. Developing and coordinating/conducting necessary training programs as well as developing policies and programs for reporting noncompliance issues are critical elements. A system must be in place to initiate and/or coordinate corrective/preventive action for noncompliance. And of course, maintaining files of all areas of the compliance program, developing a budget, and reporting to the managing partners of a practice are also central to the process.

Table 121-2 provides a step-by-step plan to picking the correct codes for every patient encounter: learn the rules, apply them to every code you choose, check yourself periodically, stay informed of regulatory changes, and integrate compliance into your daily practice.

CONCLUSION

The development of a systematic approach to meeting the ever-changing demands of reimbursement and compliance is essential in the current era. This chapter provided tools for billing and coding that may be used to develop a strategy to address each practice's unique needs. As expert as physicians are at patient care, they must also become expert at the "business of medicine" in order to sustain effective care. The chapter highlighted the critical role physician documentation plays in E&M reimbursement and hospital DRG reimbursement. The time and effort physicians can devote to their own education about effective documentation, coding, and subsequent billing will result in significant return on investment over the long term (Box 121-1).

Box 121-1 A Tale of Two Guidelines

The major difference between the 1995 and 1997 AMA guidelines lies in the specificity of the examination.

In the 1995 guidelines, the level of examination is determined by the number of body areas and/or organ systems examined and documented.

The 1997 rules are much more prescriptive: there is a strict counting system, and the elements of the examination that must be performed and documented for any given code level is explicitly defined.

Generally, the perceived advantage of using the 1995 guidelines is that they require less documentation, but the disadvantage is that the difference between the two mid-level types of examinations (expanded problem focused and detailed) is not well defined. The difference between these two examination types is quite clear in the 1997 guidelines, but more explicit documentation is required. Currently, Medicare allows physicians to use either the 1995 or the 1997 version of the guidelines.

Key Points

• The majority of hospitalist income is usually generated through evaluation and management (E&M) codes.

• Understanding how to document, code, and bill for E&M services is essential to the survival of a hospitalist practice.

• The time you invest developing a workable approach to accurate and efficient documentation and coding will pay dividends.

• Optimal physician documentation connects E&M coding (physician services) to DRG coding (hospital services), creating a mutually beneficial hospital–physician relationship.

• Compliance is an integral part of long-term financial success and should be incorporated into all processes related to physician reimbursement.

SUGGESTED READING

CPT 2005 Standard Edition. AMA Press: Chicago, 2006.

ICD-9-CM Professional for Physicians, Volumes 1 & 2, Medicode. Ingenix: Eden Prairie, MN, 2006.

Batte JR, Criser TL, Dunaway MT. Doctors are from Jupiter and Compliance is from a Galaxy Far . . . Far. . . . Away. Rebel Records: Camden, SC, 2004.

www.cms.hhs.gov/medlearn/emdoc.asp. 1997 Documentation Guidelines for E&M Services.

Dunaway MT. Pocket Guide to Clinical Coding and Risk Based Coding Manual. Rebel Records: Camden, SC, 2005. (components of the Dunaway Documentation System).

COMPLIANCE. www.HealthcareComplianceResources.com

http://www.aapc.com. Gives information from the certifying organization about becoming a CPC, (Certified Professional Coder).

http://www.ahima.com. Website of the American Health Information Management Association for a broad range of documentation issues as well as information about becoming a CCS, (Certified Coding Specialist).

http://www.ama-assn.org. The AMA website link to Professional Resources has information for a wide variety of coding resources including CPT, ICD-9-CM references and a helpful Q&A section.

http://www.cms.hhs.gov. The mother lode of rules and regulations. This immense website has everything you'd every want to know about Medicare regulations and is a window into the bureaucratic soul.

http://www.complianceresources.com. Certification courses for training of medical office compliance officers.

http://www.healthcarevalueinc.com. A physician designed E&M documentation system to streamline and simplify the process.

http://www.ingeniousmed.com. A physician designed PDA platform to identify and capture all legitimate charges for billing.

Trites, P. Compliance guide for the medical practice: how to attain and maintain a compliant medical practice. AMA Press: Chicago, 2006.

CHAPTER ONE HUNDRED AND TWENTY-TWO

Measuring Value of a Hospital Medicine Program

Ron Greeno, MD, FACP

INTRODUCTION

The concept of value created by a hospitalist program for a hospital and for the health care system is a topic of great interest to hospitalists and hospitals alike. Leaders recognized early in the history of hospital medicine that programs could not be supported financially by physician billing and collections alone, especially if a program were designed to align with hospital goals of quality and efficiency. Increasingly, hospitals realized that investing in hospital medicine programs made strategic sense, as this new model provided solutions to problems such as emergency department (ED) coverage, community physician preference not to manage inpatients, overnight hospital coverage, and lack of standardized approaches to care. Despite this, most hospital chief financial officers (CFOs) still view their program as a cost center and look to limit resources available for program improvement. Those in our field with more experience in managing programs that are properly resourced and intelligently designed realize that a highly functioning program can create significant return on investment for a hospital and should instead be viewed as a revenue opportunity. This chapter will attempt to serve as a framework that can be used by hospitals and hospitalists to quantify the value being created by their program, or in the case of a hospital that has yet to build a program, to understand the potential value of a program.

It is vitally important to be able to demonstrate and attempt to quantify this value. From the hospital perspective, it allows the members of the institution to understand to what extent they can justify investing in the program. After all, demonstrating value may become the financial justification that allows the hospital to properly resource what may be the most important program in their institution. This exercise also allows the hospital leaders to recognize the key role that a well-resourced, intelligently designed hospital medicine program can play in their overall strategic plan. It directs the hospital administrators to identify what resources will be required from their existing infrastructure to maximize the performance of this new program. Common examples of this include information technology (IT), case management, and an existing billing and collections department.

Importantly, hospitalists should also understand the value they and their program create so that they can emphasize the facets of the program creating the most value for the hospital. In addition, these value components can be utilized by the group to create incentives for each physician to reach the goals that the hospital administration has identified for the program. It will also allow the group to justify the kind of physician compensation required to recruit successfully in an increasingly competitive environment.

Keep in mind several factors that influence the interpretation of metrics. Some of the value metrics reviewed are easily measured and quantified, and they thus represent "hard" ("green") dollars, especially when being considered by a hospital CFO. Other metrics are considered to be "softer" and may therefore be discounted by hospital financial analysis. Similarly, you will see that some performance metrics will create more value for some hospitals than they will for others because of differences in the respective hospital and marketplace economic drivers. In order to quantify some value elements, the group will need access to the hospital institutional electronic data set while other dimensions of value can only be quantified if data are derived from within the hospitalist program itself.

In general, there are three categories in which a hospitalist program can create value for the hospital: cost reduction, cost avoidance, and revenue generation. While these categories have predominantly monetary connotations, quality improvement and risk management reduction are clearly important and essential components that also can generate monetary return.

COST REDUCTION

Cost reduction may be defined as a decrease in direct variable cost per case (DVC/case), and quantification requires information from the hospital cost accounting system. Because it is a direct cost reduction, it is considered an example of a "hard" value by the hospital finance department and administration. Ideally, the DVC/case for hospitalists and nonhospitalists will be adjusted for severity and stratified by diagnosis related group (DRG) and payer. Many times, it is also beneficial to limit the analysis to the highest-volume 20–50 DRGs seen by the hospital medicine group so that it focuses on cases that are common and actionable. The calculation, regardless of adjustment or stratification, is as follows:

(Average Hospitalist DVC/case) minus (Average Nonhospitalist DVC/case) multiplied by (number of hospitalist cases)
= Total Cost Reduction Value

An even more useful aggregate or specific DRG measure is margin per case, which is defined as:

(Average Revenue/case) minus (Average Cost/case)
= Average Margin/case

The difference between the average margin/case for hospitalist-managed patients and nonhospitalist-managed patients multiplied by the total number of hospitalist cases is a powerful measure of value creation. This assessment not only assigns recognition for cost savings, but it also factors in the additional revenue per case that can be achieved by a hospitalist team that has been trained in appropriate DRG documentation (to be discussed below in greater detail).

REVENUE GENERATION

Despite the fact that generation of new revenue can be one of the most substantial performance improvements for a hospital, it is a potential opportunity that is often overlooked when assessing the value of a hospitalist program. Increased hospital revenue can be created from multiple sources, as outlined in Box 122-1.

Increased Capacity Resulting from Decreased Average Length of Stay (ALOS)

As the US population ages and grows, hospital capacity will become more and more of an issue, and in some areas of the country it is already a major problem. A hospital without bed availability for patient admissions (especially for certain high-margin cases like elective surgeries) is placed at a huge financial disadvantage in addition to creating barriers in patient access to necessary care. The following formula can be used to calculate the *potential* revenue that can be generated by a program that is successful in decreasing hospital ALOS:

Box 122-1 Sources of Increased Hospital Revenue

Increased inpatient bed capacity

Improved patient throughput and reduced ED diversions

Improved market share

Improved satisfaction of patients and community physicians

Appropriate documentation

Quality measures and pay for performance initiatives

(Nonhospitalist ALOS) minus (Hospitalist ALOS) = $\triangle$ ALOS

($\triangle$ALOS) multiplied by (# of cases managed by hospitalists per year) = # of open bed days created/year

(# open bed days/yr) divided by (Nonhospitalist ALOS)
= Potential new admissions created/year

(Potential admissions/yr) multiplied by (Average revenue per case) = Total Potential Revenue/year

The incredible value opportunity is apparent as one works through the calculations. A hospitalist program that has an ALOS of 4.0 days compared to an ALOS of 5.0 on 5000 hospitalist cases creates 5000 open-bed days and capacity for 1,000 additional yearly admissions (1,250 if they are filled with hospitalist admissions). If the average admission generates $8500 in revenues, this newfound capacity creates the potential for $8.5 million in revenue for the hospital. Of course, for many hospitals those open beds may not be filled entirely, and the actual revenue may not reach the full potential. Understanding the opportunity in any number of scenarios is very helpful for hospital strategic and financial planning and can be constructed using the following actual example developed for a high-performing program (Table 122-1).

Improved Inpatient Flow and Decreased ED Diversion Time

Additional capacity can be created by the hospitalist program without actually decreasing ALOS. Efforts that use hospitalists as the physician component of an inpatient "flow" initiative have proved to benefit hospitals in both increasing admissions and in decreasing the amount of time their ED is on diversion. Such projects can utilize the organized physician component of a hospital medicine program to schedule discharges, predict capacity, and coordinate discharge planning. The contribution of hospitalists to this type of multidisciplinary project makes an actual calculation of value challenging, but the participation of, and leadership by, an organized and willing physician group to this effort cannot be overlooked.

Most hospitals track the percent of time that the ED is on diversion. Comparing that number before and after the start of the hospital medicine program (or between any two periods in the history of the program) allows one to estimate impact on admission revenue based on historical controls. For instance, if an ED

Table 122-1 Potential Capacity and Revenue Improvements Based on Improved ALOS

Annual Bed Days	ANNUAL ADMITS		Incremental Capacity	$K REVENUE OPPORTUNITY		
	5.5 ALOS	3.9 ALOS		@ 100%	@ 50%	@ 25%
16,500	3,000	4,231	1,231	10,462	5,231	2,615
27,500	5,000	7,051	2,051	17,436	8,718	4,359
38,500	7,000	9,872	2,872	24,410	12,205	6,103
49,500	9,000	12,692	3,692	31,385	15,692	7,846
60,500	11,000	15,513	4,513	38,359	19,179	9,590
71,500	13,000	18,333	5,333	45,333	22,667	11,333

historically has been on diversion 4% of the time and decreases to 2% with the help of a responsive hospitalist team, the impact on both ED visit revenue and admissions through the ED can be calculated or projected. If the ED admits 2,500 patients a year, this seemingly small decrease in diversion time could result in an additional 50 admissions and $425,000 in revenue (assuming $8,500/admission). One may use a similar methodology to calculate revenue generated from the additional ED visits that do not lead to an admission.

Creating a New Service Line That the Hospital Can Market to the Community

Hospitals are discovering that if they possess a hospital medicine program that delivers high-quality care and is extremely service oriented, they can market the program to the physician community as a new service line, resulting in the capture of new admissions and increased market share. The hospitalists themselves can assist the hospital in this effort by educating community physicians on the program benefits to patients and referring physicians. If systems are in place to track sources of patient admissions by referring physician, the value of the program in attracting these new patients can be quantified and value attributed accordingly. Surprisingly small numbers of new primary care physician (PCP) sources of patients can lead to remarkable revenue for the hospital. For instance, if only 10 new PCPs start admitting their patients to a hospital and each PCP is the source of only one patient admission a month, new revenue of $1.02 million (again using revenue/case of $8,500) can be attributed to the programs attraction as a service line. This is a good example of data that typically are not attainable from a hospital data system; the hospital medicine program itself will need the capability to track new sources of patients in order to quantify the revenues and the improved perception of the hospital by the medical community.

Improved PCP and Patient Satisfaction

Additionally, it is important for the program to track both PCP and patient satisfaction, especially if a program wishes to demonstrate the value of an adequately resourced, high-performing program as compared to one of lesser quality. A program that satisfies the needs of 85% of its referring PCPs, although seemingly doing well in this regard, actually risks losing the admissions of 10% of its referral base to another hospital when compared to a program creating 95% satisfaction. If the program has a referral base of 40 PCPs, and again each PCP is the source of only one admission a month, the value at risk from the lower-performing program can be calculated as follows:

(40 PCPs) multiplied by (10% dissatisfied) = 4 PCPs

(4 PCPs) multiplied by (12 admits/yr each) = 48 admits

(48 admits) multiplied by ($8500 revenue/admit)
= $408,000 of revenue at risk

Improved Documentation

Sophisticated hospitals and other managers of hospital medicine programs have recognized that their programs give them a unique opportunity to educate physicians regarding accurate documentation of care. Hospitals recognize that inadequate documentation by physicians can result in under-representation of a patient's severity of illness, inaccurate DRG coding, and subsequent reimbursement shortfalls. Since a busy hospitalist manages a high volume of inpatients, training to ensure accurate physician documentation can result in significant financial benefit to the institution in the form of optimized revenues—accurate and appropriate payment for services delivered. Hospitals achieving improvements in case mix index (CMI) of even a 10th of a point can recognize a several hundred thousand dollar improvement in hospital reimbursement for a modestly sized hospital medicine program.

Leading Quality and Pay for Performance Initiatives

In the very near future, one of the most important ways that a hospitalist program will create revenue for a hospital will be through payor-sponsored pay-for-performance initiatives. Hospitals that plan to attain the highest level of Medicare reimbursement may be successful if they have a high-performing hospital medicine program caring for a significant portion of their inpatient population. The stakes are high when one considers a hospital being able to increase by one or two percentage points their annual total payment from Medicare. The details of how the Centers for Medicare and Medicaid Services (CMS) will structure their pay-for-performance programs are unclear, yet many progressive hospitals have identified their team of hospitalists as a key mechanism to improve health care quality. These hospitals are already designing, resourcing, and building hospital medicine programs to serve as the centerpiece of their strategy to compete.

Cost Avoidance

Of all of the categories of value creation, cost avoidance proposes the "softest" value in the eyes of financial analysts and is therefore most likely to be discounted when program value is being quantified. Nevertheless, one must consider at least two dimensions of cost avoidance—payor mix and malpractice liability—in a comprehensive description of program value.

Decreased Readmissions of Unfunded Patients and Its Impact on Payor Mix

Hospital medicine programs with design features that result in improvement in readmission rates can have dramatic impact on hospital finances for obvious reasons. Since many programs serve as the admitting service for all or most of the unfunded admissions through the hospital ED, it creates an opportunity to put processes in place to minimize preventable readmissions. Programs have created capabilities to insure reliable outpatient follow-up, improve medicine reconciliation, ensure patient compliance to discharge plans, and other interventions to minimize the likelihood of readmission. The value that can be created by such programs can be quantified using readmission data as follows.

(Readmission rate of unfunded patients prior to hospitalist program) multiplied by (number of unfunded admissions/yr)

$$= X$$

(Readmission rate of unfunded patients after start of program) multiplied by (number of unfunded admissions/yr)

$$= Y$$

$$X - Y = \text{number of avoided unfunded readmissions}$$

(Number of avoided unfunded readmissions) multiplied by (cost of average unfunded patient care episode)

$$= \text{Total cost avoidance}$$

If the cost to a hospital of an episode of care for an unfunded patient is $7,000 and the program can avoid 50 readmissions per year, the cost avoidance for the hospital is $350,000. Furthermore, the ability of a program to apply evidence-based protocols and admission criteria to avoid unnecessary *admissions*, especially unnecessary admissions of unfunded patients, adds further to the value created.

Decreased Medical-Legal Liability

The impact on medical-legal risk is significant for hospitals that design and resource a hospital medicine program to facilitate improved physician–patient communication, improve discharge communication to primary physicians, use evidence-based protocols to guide patient care decisions, and create a team-based approach to inpatient care. For a hospital that is self-insured, the positive financial impact of preventing even one legal action a year can be easily quantified by assuming an average settlement cost per malpractice case. The value of any program that takes care of large volumes of sick patients while avoiding significant numbers of malpractice actions can justifiably claim to be creating value for an institution, even if more specific financial impact information is not available.

Even Small Increments of Performance Improvement Create Substantial Value

One of the most important concepts to understand when articulating the benefits of high-performing hospital medicine program is that *even small increments of performance improvement can result in tremendous value*. There are several reasons for this. One is that a hospitalist service can affect a large number of patients, and therefore the opportunity to have an impact on quality and efficiency is likely much larger than any other program in the hospital. Another reason is that the cost of care in the hospital is high, and anything that eliminates even small percentages of waste creates substantial value. The third reason, as outlined above, is that a well-designed and resourced program can create value in many ways, some of which have gone unrecognized. To demonstrate how relatively small improvements in a handful of areas can create significant quantifiable value, a comparison table (Table 122-2) using some basic assumptions and spreading them across several levels of performance can be generated.

In this example, one may observe the impact to the hospital bottom line (including the impact on hospital margin) with very modest reductions in only cost/case and ALOS. Furthermore, the additional impact becomes evident when the program performs at slightly higher levels for these two metrics. This kind of analysis, along with a discussion about the potential of all other areas of value outlined in this chapter, can be used to justify requests for additional program resources. Using this kind of analysis, more and more hospital administrators are recognizing that the most important consideration in designing and building any program should be on maximizing performance rather than on minimizing cost, as the return on investment with a high-performing program can be extraordinary.

Table 122-2 How Incremental Improvements Create Value

Example			
Assumptions			
Annual admissions through program		4,000	
DVC of admission		$ 4,000	
Revenue per admission		$ 8,500	
Margin on incremental patient		50%	
Incremental DVC savings per day saved		$ 350	
Program LOS of program A		4.25	
Incremental performance (program A vs. B)			
Resource management improvement (DVC/case)	5.0%	10.0%	20.0%
LOS improvement (days)	0.25	0.50	1.00
Patient capacity created from LOS improvement	235	471	941
Incremental value generated by program A			
Resource management	$ 800,000	$ 1,600,000	$ 3,200,000
Margin on incremental patient	$ 1,000,000	$ 2,000,000	$ 4,000,000
Impact to bottom line	$ 1,800,000	$ 3,600,000	$ 7,200,000
Impact on pretax margin	5%	11%	21%

SOME FINAL CONSIDERATIONS AND CONCLUSION

Hospital leaders are identifying other less quantifiable ways that their hospital medicine programs are helping them, especially when it comes to quality initiatives. Several of these fall into what has been labeled the "coordination value," often attributed to site-based specialists including hospitalists. A perfect example of this is seen with the group that provides the physician component of the hospital's participation in the Institute of Healthcare Improvement's "flow" collaborative. Another is the hospital medicine team that leads the hospital's attempts at meeting Joint Commission for the Accreditation of Healthcare Organizations (JACHO) guidelines. Hospitalist teams have led quality initiatives by serving as the institution's physician champions in implementing computerized physician order entry systems and in leading committees that oversee quality, utilization, and even medical executive functions. Hospital executives across the country are recognizing the competitive advantage brought by a hospital medicine program designed to drive new quality initiatives. These hospitals have demonstrated the foresight to embrace quality as a business strategy and have the vision to see that their hospitalists can provide them the best chance of achieving their goals.

Key Points

- Measuring the value of a hospitalist program may be considered in three broad categories: cost reduction, cost avoidance, and revenue generation. Two major values, risk management and quality improvement, can be categorized as cost avoidance and revenue generation, respectively.

- Cost-reduction efforts focus on the effect of a program on the direct variable cost per inpatient case.

- Cost avoidance includes the institutional benefits resulting from decreased readmission rates, shifting payor mix, and improved risk profiles in medical-legal liability.

- Revenue opportunities can be potentially quantified by outlining the performance expectations related to increased inpatient bed capacity, new or enhanced service line development, satisfaction of patients and referring physicians, and quality improvement activities.

SUGGESTED READING

Savavi K. Paying for efficiency. J Health Manag 2006; 51(2):77–80.

Safavi K. Aligning financial incentives. J Health Manag 2006;51(3):146–151.

Committee on Quality of Health Care in America, Institute of Medicine. Crossing the Quality Chasm: A New Health System for the 21st Century. Washington, DC: National Academy Press, 2001.

Society of Hospital Medicine. How hospitalists add value. Hospitalist 2005; 9(suppl 1):3–35.

SHM Benchmarks Committee. Value added by hospitalists: providing inpatient care to unassigned and underinsured patients. Hospitalist 2004; 8(1):10–12.

SHM Benchmarks Committee. Systems support work. Hospitalist 2004; 8(2):9–10,26.

Thomas T. "Maximizing the Value of a Hospitalist Program; American Association of Integrated Healthcare Delivery Systems Spring Managed Care Forum. San Diego, May 2006.

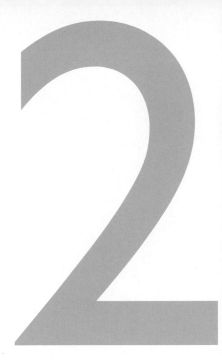

Section

Twenty

Hospital Performance Improvement

123 *Managing Physician Performance in Hospital Medicine*
Russell Holman

124 *Leadership in Hospital Medicine*
Russell Holman

125 *Quality Improvement in the Hospital:*
Theory, Tools, and Trends
Norbert Goldfield

126 *Quality Improvement in the Hospital*
Jason Stein, Grey Maynard

127 *An Overiew of Patient Safety for the Hospitalist*
Lakshmi K. Halasyamani, Saul N. Weingart

128 *Establishing a Teamwork Model of Care*
for Inpatient Medicine
Joseph A. Miller, Joseph L. Dorsey, Jody Hoffer Gittell

129 *Patient Flow and Hospital Throughput*
Burke T. Kealey

130 *Strategies for Standardizing Care and Applying Evidence*
to Practice
Scott Weingarten

131 *Assessing Patient Satisfaction in the Hospital Setting*
Woodruff English, Deirdre E. Mylod

CHAPTER ONE HUNDRED AND TWENTY-THREE

Managing Physician Performance in Hospital Medicine

Russell Holman, MD

INTRODUCTION

Joel Barker, a futurist who popularized the concept of paradigm shifts, describes leadership as "the ability to take people where they otherwise would not go." In other words, leadership is about creating change in something that exists today. Management, on the other hand, may be considered a series of steps to ensure that things happen the desired and consistent way. Although this chapter is not dedicated to exploring the differences between management and leadership, it will address a domain in which the two intimately intersect. Managing people relies upon many foundations of leadership, such as establishing the group's vision and setting key strategic goals. In like manner, successful leadership in stimulating change is dependent on the effective management of personnel to ensure that the culture, work habits, outcomes, and behaviors are consistent with the change efforts. This chapter will focus on the management of physicians in hospital medicine groups. The steps outlined are applicable, regardless of employer type, group size, or mission. Most all of the skills necessary to effectively implement a performance management system can be learned, and the group leader may develop competency by continuous application of the management steps.

DEFINING YOUR GROUP

Before you can manage performance, you must know the parameters by which the group is defined. That is, the prerequisites for performance management include salient statements of mission, vision, and values. The **mission** defines the purpose for the group and reflects the key interests of the hospital and/or group employer. The mission statement should be able to answer the questions, "*Why does our hospital medicine group exist? What purpose does it serve? In very broad terms, what scope of services do we provide?*" The **vision** is a concise summary of what the group would like to be or achieve in the future; and it may relate to growth, range of services, outcomes or other dimensions of performance. Most often, the vision is the leader's platform for change in order to articulate the rationale for creating a better future. **Values** are those standards and principles that guide decision-making and provide parameters for the expected behaviors and conduct in the group. Values can be thought of as the "lens" through which the vision is carried out and the mission upheld.

From the mission, vision, and values come strategies for achieving successful change and the more specific goals that the group is to attain. In some cases, the group may have undertaken a formal strategic planning process that rendered a series of goals, objectives, and/or programs to be carried out in the immediate to intermediate term. We now reach the vital area in which a well-structured and supported performance management system can play a pivotal role in ensuring the successful implementation of strategic thinking. Until now, the thought and planning process had focused on the right thing to *do*. From here, the focus becomes doing things *right*. Once the group confidently understands its purpose and direction, the management steps that follow will support the group achieving its desired level of performance. Figure 123-1 represents the pyramid of performance management, a prioritized and concurrent approach to serve as a framework for the group leader's relationship with team members.

RECRUITING THE RIGHT PEOPLE

The reality in hospital medicine today is that demand for physicians far exceeds the available supply. This "seller's market" places a challenging dynamic for new or growing hospital medicine groups in order to recruit the top candidates. The stakes are higher when one considers hospital medicine as a new specialty in hospitals where the medical staff is skeptical or apprehensive in accepting the new group, and one bad hire can undermine the group's chances of success. Furthermore, there may not be adequate experience or expertise in recruiting new physicians or correctly identifying those who would be a proper fit for the group. What constitutes an excellent physician in one group may not be the case in another. So how does one go about recruiting the *right* people?

Planning begins with having defined the group in terms of the mission and values. Knowing the vision and specific strategies to be employed lends insight into what type of individual would best fit with the needs and culture of the group. It is important to list the desired qualities on paper and to plan for assessing each one, knowing that there is no perfect candidate and these characteristics must therefore be prioritized. Remember, what makes a good physician somewhere else does not mean the candidate will be good in your group—be sure you define very clearly what exactly

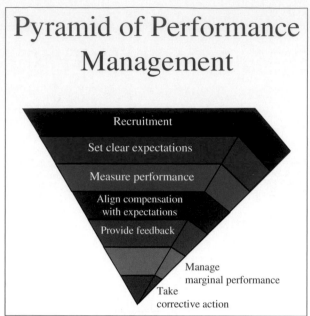

Pyramid of Performance Management

Recruitment

Set clear expectations

Measure performance

Align compensation with expectations

Provide feedback

Manage marginal performance

Take corrective action

Figure 123-1 • Pyramid of Performance Management. Adapted from: The American College of Physician Executives.

candidate, so you must prioritize those qualities you want most from an applicant. If you wait for perfection, the delay will cause you to overlook many very good physicians. Finally, take another look at the performance management pyramid (*see* Fig. 123-1). The area for recruitment is so large because this is the disproportionate amount of time you should invest in recruitment processes. Hiring the right people up front will make the rest of the steps below far easier and minimize the likelihood of your being drawn into the nadir of the pyramid.

SETTING CLEAR EXPECTATIONS

Do you have a job description? When you read it, does it adequately describe what it is you expect from your physicians? Do you have an orientation for new members to your group? How long does it last? Is there additional training you offer? Are there outcomes you expect from this training? And once you have oriented, trained, and offered a job description, does the actual work environment support or negate your efforts (i.e., does culture trump your formal process)? Do your physicians agree with the expectations you have discussed?

The cycle of setting clear expectations about work performance begins during the recruitment phase. Being absolutely forthcoming about what it is like to work in your group and what you expect from each and every member is paramount to allow both you and the candidate to determine a good fit. Once the physician has joined your group, orientation and training should hardly be a one-, two-, or three-day exercise. These are continuous and ongoing processes, given our rapidly changing practice environment. In fact, change is one of the only reliable characteristics of working in health care. Extending the welcome *"The job you take today is unlikely to be the job you will have next year"* to new hires is hardly inappropriate. Be mindful that setting clear expectations with all of your physicians is the bedrock of a functional performance management system. Defining expectations alone will often improve performance, vis-à-vis the Hawthorne effect.

Expectations should always be depersonalized and focus on behavior. Behavior itself may be regarded in two distinct domains: those behaviors that are observed, and those outcomes that are measurable. Examples of observable behaviors include interpersonal interactions with nurses and consultants, pager response times, and attendance at monthly team meetings. Measurable outcomes include work RVU (resource value unit) productivity, patient satisfaction, readmission rates, and compliance with coding and documentation guidelines. Categories of performance expectations may be found in Box 123-1. There are many ways to organize the dimensions of performance you may expect from your physicians—the six aims of quality (safe, timely, effective, efficient, equitable, patient-centered care as outlined in the IOM report *Crossing the Quality Chasm*), maintaining a healthy workplace, citizenship, relationships with others, etc.—yet the key is to define and communicate them, then check often for understanding. Codifying and frequently updating a written job description (Box 123-2) will serve as a durable reference for the existing group members and new physicians alike.

MEASURING ACTUAL PERFORMANCE

There are many inherent problems in measuring actual performance, and the data may never be perfect. As an exercise, try

"good" means. At the same time, it is also critical to outline the three major selling points of potentially joining your group—the practice itself, compensation, and location.

The next step consists of preparing a slate of candidates for interviews. There are many methods of finding (i.e., sourcing) strong candidates, one of the best of which is to ask members of your current group or other trusted colleagues for referrals. If you are interested in filling a position with a more specific skill set such as information technology, palliative care, or clinical teaching, then a "make or buy" decision needs to be made to either recruit for the individual already in possession of such credentials, or to hire more generically and then train accordingly. Once candidates are identified, then a deliberate process of reviewing their written materials and interviewing them by telephone will determine appropriateness for an in-person interview. Speaking with references can occur at any time, and some advocate for this to occur prior to bringing people out for formal interviews as another mechanism of screening and to focus interview questions on site. The formal interview itself should be well structured and enable your key stakeholders to meet with the candidate and submit an immediate assessment. The shorter the turnaround time to extend an offer, the more decisive and committed to the candidate you will appear. Likewise, if you have a diverse composition of interviewers who weigh in with their perspectives, then there should be little to delay a hiring decision.

There are three additional points to remember when looking to hire an additional physician into your group. First, on the whole, a significant percentage of physicians who leave a job cite spousal discontent as the primary cause. To mitigate this possibility, invite the spouse to accompany the candidate to the interview location and assemble a parallel agenda for him or her as well. The group leader also needs to continue nurturing the candidate and family well into the first year of employment to ensure a good transition. Second, be realistic about your expectations. There is no perfect

---

Box 123-1 Categories of Performance Expectations

Productivity

• Professional services—cognitive and procedural

• Other—teaching, research, administrative

Clinical Excellence and Technical Skill

• Quality measures

• Board certification

Interpersonal Skills

• Patients and families

• Hospital and medical staff

• Referring physicians

• Other team members

• Effective use of communication methods

Professionalism

• Medical record and dictation completion

• Credentialing and privileging

• Ethics

• Compliance with regulatory requirements

• Documentation skills

• Meeting attendance

• General work habits

Resource Management

• Efficiency measures

• Referral practices

Hospital Citizenship

• Committee participation

• Departmental involvement

Community Involvement

• Charitable organizations

• Religious, volunteer medical, school groups

Teaching

• Residency programs

• Medical students

• Medical or lay community

Research

• Funding or grant expectations

Management

• Group or project leadership

Box 123-2 Recommended Elements of a Physician Job Description

Position title

Reporting relationships

General purpose of the position

Personal attributes

Required qualifications and skills

Preferred skills and experience

Clinical service expectations

"Other" work expectations (teaching, research, management)

Administrative duties

Key relationships (referring physicians, case management, Emergency Department [ED], ICU, etc.)

---

exercise worth undertaking. In like manner, behavioral observation data are potentially fraught with conflict if the data are focused on judgment of character traits (*I believe this physician doesn't care about quality improvement*) rather than on observable behaviors (*This physician always/sometimes/never comes to meetings on time*). Measures are best when they are objective, relevant to the position, and are interpretable. Remember: all measures are flawed; some are useful.

There are many sources of measuring actual performance. Data systems managed by the hospital or group may provide productivity measures such as work RVUs, quality metrics including readmission rates, and efficiency parameters like severity-adjusted length of stay. Survey data are also useful to determine physician satisfaction by patients (*see* Chapter 131 for further discussion), nursing staff, case management personnel, other members of the medical staff, and referring physicians. Patient complaint rates channeled through the hospital patient representative's office is another complementary resource, as are patient letters of appreciation. Retrospective or real-time chart reviews targeting coding compliance regulations, completeness of documentation practices, and handwriting legibility may be performed in a structured manner. Physician self-assessment tools are useful to track committee participation, awards, publications, and community service activities. Hospital medical records will often generate reports on outstanding and delinquent chart completion. The hospital medicine group itself may elect to administer surveys directed toward other team members, to track meeting attendance, and to record pager response times and effectiveness of patient sign-outs and hand-offs.

assigning individual readmission rates within your group, and you will find that, because of hand-offs within the group and lack of precision in identifying who actually discharged the patient, there will be many arguments over whether the data are valid. However, in most circumstances, if the data are flawed, it still may serve a strong purpose to highlight the relative variation within the group since the same limitations on absolute accuracy apply equally to all group members. Searching for quantifiable systemic data and being transparent about their limitations will be an

ALIGNING COMPENSATION WITH EXPECTATIONS

Conventional wisdom states that people will do more if there are incentives. A compensation system serves as tangible reinforcement for behaviors and outcomes that meet or exceed expectations. Ultimately, compensation must reflect the mission of the group, and great care must be taken to ensure that the construct is consistent with the desired vision and goals. Compensation is only one component of a performance management program and is not a method of successfully making up for inadequate attention to recruitment and or failure to set strong expectations up front.

Here are a few points to consider as you integrate your compensation system into the rest of the steps in the pyramid (*see* Chapter 120 for a detailed explanation of compensation):

1. A straight salary with or without a "guaranteed" bonus is unlikely to reward or motivate any new behaviors.
2. For a performance-based compensation plan to have sufficient impact, I recommend at least 20–30% of compensation should be tied to performance.
3. Consider having both group and individual measures as part of your plan to engender a sense of teamwork and collective effort in performing well.
4. Limit the number of variables in the plan to 3–5; otherwise, measures are too diluted to carry meaningful weight.
5. Perform a local market comparison for benchmarking your goal median compensation.
6. The process of constructing or evolving your plan, being inclusive of members of your group as well as any group sponsors, ends up being far more valuable than the final plan itself.

PROVIDING REGULAR FEEDBACK

In the circles of quality improvement efforts, there is a common saying that "what gets measured gets improved." The direct implication of this statement is that measurement is accompanied by effective feedback of the respective behaviors or outcomes. Feedback is the mechanism for communicating results and making a connection between the results and performance expectations. Actual performance that meets or exceeds expectations can be articulated in terms of appreciation, reward, recognition, and reinforcement. Behavior that is inconsistent with desired results represents an opportunity to restate expectations and make appropriate plans for follow-up. There are a number of venues for providing feedback to group members (Box 123-3).

Feedback to physicians must be both formal and informal. The annual performance review is a common example of the former, but it is in no way meant to be the only feedback they should receive, nor is it the most powerful. The annual review should be well structured, can outline longer term goals and ideas for self-improvement, and may serve in some key administrative functions like compensation and promotion. Informal, regular feedback, however, may serve you much better in driving performance because it is timelier, more relevant to daily work, and more specific to the individual. Individuals also respond much more constructively to positive feedback, and some experts in behavioral psychology believe the ratio of positive to negative feedback should be on the order of 9 to 1. Be sure that feedback is done in a coaching, supportive manner and focuses on the behavior (*When interacting with nurses, ask for their ideas, include them in daily care planning, and review new orders together as opposed to handing the chart to them and walking away*") rather than on the persons themselves ("*You really rub people the wrong way*"). A list of characteristics of effective feedback can be found in Box 123-4.

MANAGING POOR PERFORMANCE

Poor performance can be defined as observed behaviors or measured outcomes that significantly deviate from what is expected, and often represents a pattern over time in spite of having in place all the other elements of a performance management system. Examples of poor or marginal performance include low attendance at group meetings, resistance to assisting colleagues during peak patient volumes, tardiness, low patient satisfaction ratings, failure to submit E & M codes, or chronic rudeness with nursing staff. In order to improve such variances, the following methodology (*see* also Fig. 123-2) can be exercised by the group leader:

1. Ensure there is sufficient and accurate documentation of the variance, as well as the desired behaviors or outcomes.
2. Provide the physician a written outline of the relevant performance issues.
3. Arrange a private meeting to discuss performance.
4. Articulate the variances clearly and succinctly, emphasizing the expected behaviors as the desired result.

Box 123-3 Mechanisms of Providing Periodic Feedback

Routinely on hospital floors; "manage by walking around"

Regularly scheduled group meetings

- Daily "sign-in" meetings
- Weekly/monthly group operational meetings

Distribution of performance reports, including commentary

Personal letter

Privately scheduled meetings

Annual performance review

E-mail of limited value

- Reinforcement of verbal agreements
- Distribution of data not requiring significant commentary

Box 123-4 Characteristics of Effective Feedback

Timely

Specific

Regular and ongoing

Focus on behavior, not the person; nonjudgmental

Includes observable behaviors and measurable outcomes

Provided face-to-face when possible

Nonverbal communication and tone of voice support the intended content

Optimal ratio of positive to negative feedback is 9:1

Managing Poor Performance

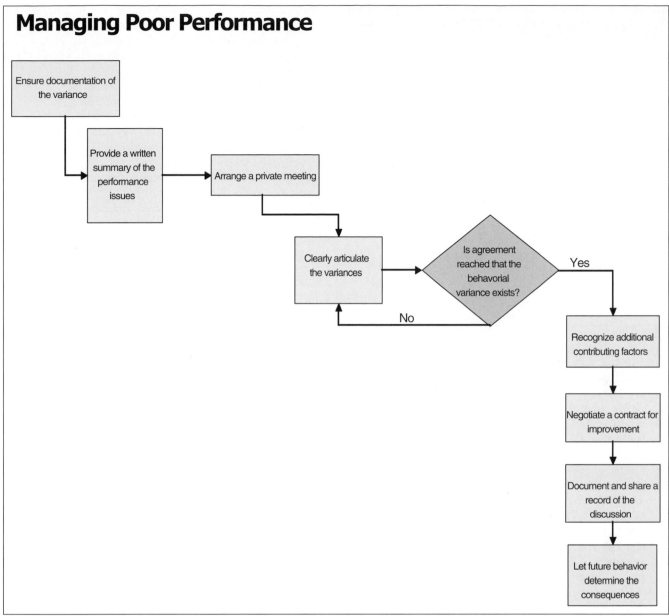

Figure 123-2 • Steps of Managing Poor Performance.

5. Reach agreement with the physician that the variance exists. This is a critical step in moving forward; without acknowledgment from the physician that a problem exists, further steps in managing the behavior cannot take place.
6. Recognize additional factors that may contribute to the variance, yet do not lose focus on the individual's responsibility to improve his or her own behavior.
7. Negotiate a contract for improvement.
8. Adopt a coaching attitude, offering assistance, support, and necessary resources to enable improvement.
9. Document and share a record of the discussion, which includes an outline of the variance, expectations for improvement, timelines, and subsequent actions for failure to improve.
10. Let the future behavior determine the consequences.

Taking Corrective Action

Corrective action can be defined as action taken to remediate or abruptly halt behaviors that are unacceptable for the given organization, including but not limited to suspension or termination. Conduct of a physician that becomes detrimental to patient safety, staff safety, quality patient care, is disruptive to the organization, or is otherwise chronically aberrant may require intervention of this nature. A critical step in skillfully applying corrective action is to have fully documented: a) the variances from expected behavior; b) the communication with the affected physician regarding the variance and potential consequences; and c) actions conducted to date to support improvement. Before proceeding with suspension or termination, it is advisable to consult with a human resources manager and/or employment

Box 123-5 Events Requiring Disclosure to the National Practitioner Data Bank

1. Medical malpractice payments
2. Adverse licensure actions
3. Adverse clinical privileging actions
4. Adverse professional society membership actions
5. Exclusions from Medicare/Medicaid

attorney to avoid problems with inadequate documentation, to maintain reporting and regulatory requirements, and to ensure employee rights. Depending on the nature of the behavior at hand, there may be requirements to report actions to state agencies and the National Practitioner Data Bank (Box 123-5) in compliance with the Healthcare Quality Improvement Act of 1986.

Specific Implementation Steps for Managing Performance

1. Define the group's vision, values, and goals.
2. Structure a recruitment process that thoroughly assesses a candidate's "fit" for the group.
3. Create a physician job description that accurately reflects work requirements.
4. Establish other expectations for performance that may not be appropriate for an actual job description; make this a group exercise, and write them down.
5. Outline a measurement system for individual and group performance measures that include data from the hospital (e.g., readmission rates, patient satisfaction) as well as input from other sources (e.g., complaint rates sent to the group leader, internally created survey tools to nursing or referring physicians).
6. Provide regular feedback both formally and informally.
7. Conduct an annual performance review for each physician.
8. Develop a performance-based compensation system with 3–5 variables that reflect important expectations.
9. Ensure that there is a mechanism to regularly assess and update the compensation model and metrics to adapt to group performance imperatives.
10. Generate other noncompensation opportunities for reward and recognition of group members.
11. Prepare for instances of poor performance; and use a disciplined, firm, coaching approach to optimize chances of improvement.
12. In the event of recalcitrant or egregious behavior, plan for corrective action.

Measuring Effectiveness of a Performance Management System

- Having a codified vision and goals for the group that is agreed upon by its members (yes/no)
- A written, comprehensive job description is regularly updated to reflect current activities (yes/no)
- Subjectively, the job description accurately reflects the actual work expected of your physicians. (yes/no)

- Ratio of positions offered to positions accepted during the recruitment process
- Physician turnover rates
- Physician satisfaction with understanding expectations and receiving feedback
- The compensation system is based, at least in part, on performance elements consistent with the group vision (yes/no)
- Group performance metrics such as efficiency measures, quality and safety indicators, satisfaction ratings from patients and hospital staff, and physician productivity
- Patient and hospital staff complaint rates
- Referral volumes from primary care and subspecialty physicians
- Quality of teaching activities (where applicable)
- Productivity and quality of research efforts (where applicable)

Common Pitfalls in Performance Management

- Regarding the exercise of determining vision and values of the group as a wasteful or meaningless activity
- Once values and vision are reached, not linking them to the rest of the steps in performance management
- Not enough time and resources devoted to recruitment efforts
- Thinking that recruitment ends when the hired physician begins working
- Incongruence between written expectations/job description and what really happens on the job (values are espoused, not enforced)
- Expectations are not clearly defined and not effectively communicated or understood by group members
- The group has inadequate means of measuring performance
- Insufficient or ineffective feedback in terms of frequency, specificity, timeliness, or the ratio of positive to constructive comments
- Compensation not tied to important expectations
- Compensation diluted by too many variables
- Over-reliance on compensation to drive behavior
- Lack of substantive consequences for unwanted behavior
- Inadequate documentation of behavior variances
- Failure of the group leader to confront those behaviors that need to be confronted
- Falling victim to complaining; commiserating instead of holding oneself and others accountable for expected behaviors

SUMMARY

Managing physician performance in hospital medicine requires a structured and disciplined approach by the group leader. The process begins with an understanding of the purpose and goals of the group, followed by recruiting physicians who possess compatibility with those goals. While hiring good people is an enormously important step, the leader must follow this with setting clear expectations of behaviors and outcomes and provide effective feedback about actual performance. By investing disproportionate time and resources to ensure these steps occur proficiently, the likelihood of needing to address poor performance or egregious behaviors is greatly lessened while greatly increasing the probability of the group meeting its intended aspirations.

Key Points

- The goal of a performance management system is to synchronize performance expectations with actual results.

- Managing performance is best achieved with an integrated, systematic approach that considers the behaviors of the individual, the characteristics of the group, and the environment in which they practice.

- No performance management system can be established without first knowing the purpose of the group (the mission), the desired future (the vision), and the specific goals the group is striving to achieve.

- The most critical step in a performance management system is recruiting personnel who are a strong organizational "fit" for the group.

- During the recruitment process and after hiring is complete, the leader of the group must set clear and explicit expectations of desired performance. Such expectations must be based on measurable and observable behaviors.

- A system of periodic feedback of actual performance serves to reinforce positive behaviors and provides an opportunity to coach behaviors that require change.

- Poor performance can successfully be addressed with a structured process that may include corrective action.

SUGGESTED READING

Ury W, Fisher R. Getting to Yes: Negotiating Agreement Without Giving In, 2nd Edition. New York: Penguin Books, 1991.

Reinertsen J. Physicians as leaders in the improvement of health care systems. Ann Int Med 1998; 128(10):833–838.

Crossing the Quality Chasm: A New Health System for the 21st Century. Committee on Quality of Health Care in America, Institute of Medicine. Washington, DC: National Academy Press, 2001.

American College of Physician Executives, Managing Physician Performance in Organizations. ongoing courses offered through: www.acpe.org

National Practitioner Data Bank. http://www.npdb-hipdb.hrsa.gov/

Fernandez-Arroz C. Hiring without firing. HBR 1999; 77:109–120.

Mintzberg H. Covert leadership: notes on managing professionals. HBR 1998; 76:140–147.

Schoenbaum S. Feedback of clinical performance information. HMO Practice 1993; 7(1):5–11.

CHAPTER ONE HUNDRED AND TWENTY-FOUR

Leadership in Hospital Medicine

Russell Holman, MD

INTRODUCTION

Within hospital medicine exists a "perfect storm" of factors leading to a tremendous interest in more effective leadership capabilities. First, the imperative to improve quality and safety of care is at an unprecedented level, requiring collaborative, system-level leadership from physicians. Second, most of this attention is directed toward care within the hospital. Third, the field of hospital medicine is itself new and in a dynamic state of defining its competencies and unique scope within the broader health care system. Finally, leaders of hospital medicine groups are relatively young (Society of Hospital Medicine survey results from 2005 reveal the average age of a group leader is 41 years) and have little differential in age from the typical full-time clinical hospitalist (age 37). Indeed, the Society of Hospital Medicine (SHM) identified leadership as a core area of focus for its educational mission and subsequently charged a standing committee to oversee activities in leadership development for the medical society. This chapter is designed to outline the most prominent attributes of effective leaders, and then to describe their core responsibilities in fulfilling this high profile role.

ATTITUDES AND PERSONAL ATTRIBUTES OF HOSPITAL MEDICINE LEADERS

Leaders in hospital medicine:
- *Have a positive disposition.* In the context of busy clinical demands, conflicts, disappointments and system failures, the leader remains unwaveringly positive and optimistic.
- *Are accessible and available.* Team members, customers, and stakeholders can easily contact the leader and are not made to feel like it is an intrusion.
- *Are fair.* Leaders do not try to have everyone like them or try to please everyone all the time; fairness drives decision-making.
- *Act as stewards of the group.* They understand that the needs of the group—and organization—take priority over their personal desires.
- *Respect others.* They seek to understand the reality of other people and treat them as they would like to be treated.
- *Flex to the dynamic environment.* Leaders know they must amend their style when interacting with different people, as well as adapt their overall leadership approach in different situations.

- *Demonstrate integrity.* Leaders are honest, and they follow through on promises and build trust with others.
- *Are ethical.* The standards of conduct for the group and the overall medical profession are upheld.
- *Show patience.* Change, particularly in health care, can be notoriously slow. Patience for change in people, systems, and culture does not mean complacency but rather an understanding that change takes time.
- *Embrace scholarship.* They are life-long students of leadership principles and are "learning organisms" of their own abilities.
- *Demonstrate humility.* Arrogance and self-interest take a back seat to learning, improvement, and valuing others' contributions to teamwork.
- *Seek vicarious rewards.* Leaders understand their greatest achievements will be accomplished through other people, not themselves.
- *Are visionary.* The desired future of the group is articulated in inspiring, candid terms.

ROLES, RESPONSIBILITIES, AND THE "WORK" OF LEADERSHIP

Mentorship and Coaching

Leading others does not simply mean that one is responsible for group performance outcomes or goals. A leader who is goal oriented is admirable, yet an excessive or imbalanced focus on the goals themselves may result in an over-zealous approach that may alienate one's constituents. Perhaps worse, in more egregious circumstances the force with which the leader emphasizes specific outcomes can engender a culture of blame or of personal judgment of individuals within the group. A leader must not only guide others toward a goal, he or she must appreciate the actual *process* by which the goal is reached. To mentor and coach is to provide others with a unique service, a service that places the leader in a supportive role to align resources and remove barriers. Coaching another person assumes first that the individual can be successful, provided he or she is given reasonable assistance and fair parameters for his or her performance. Typical questions of adopting a coaching style are, "How can I help you attain these goals?" or "What can I do for you to make you/this project a success?" Being a mentor requires the leader to be patient with others, available for frequent reflection and feedback,

Box 124-1 Process for Self-Evaluation

1. Self-evaluation is most formally conducted by a standardized personality test as a structured evaluation tool.

2. Select an evaluation tool designed for developmental purposes (as opposed to hiring or other situations).

3. Ensure that the tool has both reliability and validity data provided by the vendor.

4. Assessment results should indicate general strengths, weaknesses, and guidance for working with other personality types.

5. Optimal results can be achieved when personality types of others are known via the same test, as opposed to making guesses or assumptions about their style.

6. In addition to personality testing, surveys of the leader's peer group, direct reports, and direct supervisor offer others' perspectives on behavior and interpersonal interactions (sometimes known as a 360-degree review).

7. Surveys are ideally performed on a regular basis as a means of ongoing feedback and monitoring improvements.

8. In select cases, a professional coach may be engaged to perform additional assessments (such as targeted interviews), administer personality testing, conduct surveys, interpret results, and plot a development plan.

Table 124-1 Conflict Handling Styles

1. Avoidance
   - Issues are trivial, there is no chance of "winning," or the disruption of confrontation outweighs the benefits of resolution

2. Accommodation
   - Motivated by harmony; helps to build "political equity" with others

3. Compromise
   - Often seen in time-urgent situations or as a stop-gap for complex issues

4. Competition
   - Seen as a "win/lose" approach, where issues are important enough to warrant maximal assertiveness

5. Collaboration
   - Seen as a "win/win" approach, where consensus is a means to resolve differing views and issues are too important to compromise

Adapted from: Fisher R, Ury W, Patton B. Getting to Yes: Negotiating Agreement Without Giving In. New York: Penguin, 1991.

Box 124-2 Dimensions of Principled Negotiations

1. Depersonalize: distinguish the problem from the person

2. Focus on your and the other parties' interests rather than on a fixed position

3. Create new options where both parties mutually gain from the solution

4. Use criteria for resolution that are objective and based on fair standards

5. Make decisions that are based on merit, not on popularity or politics

Adapted from: Fisher R, Ury W, Patton B. Getting to Yes: Negotiating Agreement Without Giving In. New York: Penguin, 1991.

and accessible in times of crisis. A service orientation to one's group will not only build stronger interpersonal relationships and trust, but will increase the likelihood of meeting desired goals as well.

Self-Evaluation

Self-evaluation is the foundation upon which solid managerial skills are built. Understanding one's own approach to various situations and one's manner of interacting with other people has tremendous impact on the ability to effectively communicate, negotiate, resolve conflict, and a host of other leadership activities. There are many ways to complete a self-evaluation process, including various tools that are both reliable and valid, and ways to seek input from others about the leader's style and behaviors (Box 124-1). Leaders will need to appreciate the impact of cross-generational and cross-cultural influences on personal behavior and management style. Because hospital medicine leaders are often working in dynamic team environments, understanding their own personality style, adapting to crisis and conflict, varying their approach to different audiences, and developing political savvy are critical skills to master.

Negotiation and Conflict Resolution

Negotiation is the art and science of securing agreement between two or more interdependent parties who are seeking to maximize their outcomes. In hospital medicine, it is commonplace for leaders to negotiate for precious resources such as physical office space, administrative office support, financial remuneration to cover direct practice expenses, policy change, and cooperation from other specialties in designing new patient care models. The leader's responsibility is to bring forward and fairly represent the interests of the group or particular initiative and to reconcile them with the interests of the other parties. An effective negotiator is clear on the priorities of those at the other end of the table, and he or she is creative in presenting viable alternatives for meeting those interests. Likewise, being in a position of negotiation means you yourself must sometimes be creative and flexible in what options you are willing to accept.

The ability to adeptly resolve conflict is one of the most acutely perceived needs of leadership in hospital medicine. The complex, high acuity environment within the hospital presents a layered challenge to resolve conflicts that may arise with nursing personnel, ancillary staff, other specialists, hospital administration, families, patients, and within one's own team. The experienced leader understands that conflict is inevitable and is not always unwanted. Methods to resolve conflict need to vary with the situation and include compromise, competition, collaboration, and other approaches outlined in Table 124-1. Like negotiation, effective resolution techniques rely on identification of the interests of the affected parties and the ability to adapt the style of approach based on the personality traits of other people (Box 124-2).

Effective Communication

The vehicle through which all leadership occurs is communication, and as important as it is, communication breakdown is also the likely source of most leadership failures. Effective communication depends a great deal on knowing one's own interactive style and reconciling it with (and adapting to) the style of others. Hence, self-evaluation described above is a key prerequisite. In spoken messages, the leader understands that his or her most important role is in effective listening to others and ensuring that comprehension of the message is achieved. When speaking, effective leaders know that the key portions of a message (in ascending order) are the words used, the tone of voice, and the nonverbal behaviors. Because we are often unaware of the various components of our personal communication styles, mastery is highly dependent on broad and regular feedback from others about what messages others are actually receiving.

In hospital medicine, communication also occurs through the written form, whether it is in a business proposal, a letter to the CEO, an e-mail to his or her group, or a response to a patient complaint. Effective business writing skills and understanding one's audience are practical applications of the leader's communication role. Furthermore, the combination of verbal and written communication skills is most acutely demonstrated in conducting group meetings or presentations. The leader, once again, must account for the nuances of the audience and the key components (words, tone, nonverbals) of the message and apply his or her own conviction and enthusiasm in order to engage the group to work toward the intended outcome.

Leading Change

Given the dynamic health care environment in which we work, change is an inevitable characteristic of our daily lives. Imperatives to change current systems, processes, drugs, devices, or procedures are driven by a multitude of forces, including economic demands, regulatory pressures, workforce issues, and patients themselves. The goal of change, ideally, is to transform something today into another entity tomorrow that represents some type of an *improvement*. The challenge for leaders is to distinguish a mere change from an actual improvement, to build a sound case for improvement, to influence others to take part in the effort, and to create a durable mechanism for sustaining the implemented change.

Leading change, according to Jack Silversin, can be approached by three concurrent principles: leadership beyond advocacy, creating a shared vision, and developing a compact aligned with imperatives. Advocacy is a common expectation group members have of their physician leader, including "protection" of the group against outside forces, arguing for group needs/wants, serving as a messenger to/from hospital administration, and preserving group autonomy and independence. In order to sponsor meaningful change, leadership must also embrace organizational needs and system-level improvements that may clash with group or individual interests. Moving beyond advocacy means holding oneself and others accountable for meeting those larger interests. In creating a shared vision, the leader is able to articulate the future desired state of the group. Implied in the "future state" is

not only an improvement over the status quo; this also represents a stretch from the present, is inspiring to others, and is reached through candid, explicit conversations within the group over a period of time. The compact, or psychological agreement among members of the group, is a mechanism of solidifying the vision and the relationship the leader will have with the group. It includes those things the group members will need to give of themselves and should expect to receive in return. The compact not only involves cognitive expectations but includes specific behaviors and measurable outcomes as well.

Accountability

Accountability is holding oneself and others to expected standards of performance and behavior. Accountability in leadership refers to the fundamental understanding of mutual expectations or the compact that exists between leader and stakeholders (e.g., supervisor, constituents, organization, and patients). It is inherent in some of the classic elements of performance management such as (a) setting goals and expectations; (b) measuring actual performance; (c) providing feedback; and (d) designing reward and recognition programs, as well as the establishment of clear consequences of not meeting certain expectations. The concept of accountability outlines how leaders are answerable to others, as well as how group members are answerable to the leader. Accountability ensures that leaders will follow through and deliver on promises, accept responsibility for their own mistakes, and own decisions once they are made.

Ownership of decisions refers to the practice of eliminating blame ("it is someone else's fault") or victimhood ("look what they are doing to me") from the role of leadership. It involves a belief that there is a responsibility to the welfare of the group and a need to make or communicate unpopular choices at times without the undercurrent of blame. A leader must have the ability to present a unified front in public settings, not seceding from decisions once they are made or saying, "This is not what *I* wanted to do, but we have to because someone else is making us." Owning decisions functionally eliminates "us vs. them" language and attitudes. It is also important for leaders to understand how victimhood and blame lead to undermining one's own leadership effectiveness. By assigning responsibility to another person or group for not getting the results you want, you have automatically pronounced to your team that you lack authority, power, and influence to get things done.

Succession Planning

Perhaps one of the most overlooked obligations of leaders, effective succession planning will help to provide consistent direction and stability for the group in anticipation of an impending or potential future change in leadership position (Table 124-2). This notion of stability is particularly important to stakeholders (the medical staff, nursing staff, hospital administration) within the hospital or health care organization, to members of the hospital medicine group itself, as well as to prospective candidates during the recruitment process. Succession planning implies the identification and development of someone *internal* to the group or organization who will likely assume the leadership position once

Table 124-2 Steps of Effective Succession Planning

In advance

1. Engage the group in rationale for, benefits of, and input toward succession planning.
2. Make the decision-making process for succession clear to the group.
3. Assess the viability of internal candidates.
4. Evaluate the intended candidates' strengths and weaknesses.
5. Create an ongoing development plan for the candidates.
6. Evaluate and update job description and position requirements.

During transition

7. Use the process to reinforce group vision and goals.
8. Identify and leverage successor's new or unique skill sets in the position.
9. Develop a timeline of anticipated events once transition is decided.
10. Communicate the succession plan itself to the group and key stakeholders.

Post-transition

11. Debrief with supervisor or governing body regarding key challenges at 30 to 90 days.

it is vacated. Although some may find the process unsettling when the existing leader is relatively new himself or herself or has no intentions of leaving the group, it is nonetheless a tangible acknowledgement that turnover of the position is ultimately inevitable.

With any change in personnel, much like the "handoff" in the clinical care of patients, the effectiveness of succession planning is based on balancing two dichotomous principles: preservation of continuity and the potential benefits of introducing a new skill set. Using succession planning as a platform to reinforce the group's vision, values, and goals will reassure constituents that the strategic direction (i.e., continuity) of the program will be preserved with the new leader. By the same token, a new leader will ideally bring new skills and apply them to help promote the group's achieving its goals and improve overall performance. The transition plan will need to be accompanied by a general timeline of events and a communication process that keeps stakeholders informed of the process. Once the new leader is in place and has sufficient experience within the group—perhaps at the 30- to 90-day point—a post-transition assessment can be made in conjunction with the group leader's supervisor or governing body to discuss key challenges and resources needed for success.

Healthy Workplace

The leadership role provides a unique opportunity to affect the overall work environment that promotes professional satisfaction of those in the group and creates a workplace in which every individual looks forward to being a member. Consider those characteristics that make teachers, mentors, and leaders so popular; and then stimulate learning, growth, and interest in the subject at hand. Certainly, some of the personal attributes listed at the

beginning of the chapter come into play, such as having a positive attitude, having respect for others, and demonstrating patience. But what about enthusiasm? Humor? Having fun? Encouraging group members to enjoy work/life balance? Sponsoring social activities outside the hospital? Role modeling the behaviors that the leader himself or herself expects of others? Publicly recognizing others for a job well done? Building trust with the group and throughout the hospital? In addition, there are other, more formalized, principles that the leader must reinforce in all daily team interactions, including avoidance of harassment (sexual or otherwise) and discrimination. While the institutional human resources department can serve as a key resource, the leader has line-level responsibility for ensuring these potential corruptions do not occur.

Strategic Planning

Hospital medicine is a young, rapidly evolving specialty. The scope of services provided by different groups can vary considerably by institution, employer type, geography, and financing. Each group must be able to define its own meaning of "success," given the business drivers and marketplace forces affecting the practice. Furthermore, in order to move from defining success to actually *achieving* it, the leader must have working knowledge and applied skill in conducting strategic planning.

Strategic planning serves as a structured framework for making key decisions and allocating limited resources, and it is the basis for more detailed planning. In this regard, strategic planning differs from business or operational plans in that the former is a higher-level, conceptual activity. The process begins with clearly identifying the mission, vision, and values of the group. In other words, the group (or organization) must know its purpose for existence, its preferred future state, and the principles and standards of behavior that guide the actions of the team. The leader must also review past performance of the group as a means of retrospectively determining the causes of historical successes and failures. A useful tool for codifying internal and external factors regarding the group's current status is the SWOT analysis, in which strengths and opportunities may be exploited, while weaknesses and threats are mitigated (Table 124-3). Once strategies that support the mission and vision are developed, specific goals can be formulated according to the SMART guideline (Table 124-4). Throughout the strategic planning process, the group leader will need to involve appropriate stakeholders in order to achieve sufficient buy-in to the strategies, to secure expertise and resources to support the goals, and to engage constituents so there is a sentiment of ownership over the outcomes.

The Health Care Environment

The fund of knowledge required of leaders in hospital medicine incorporates multiple dimensions of the health care environment. Below is a representative sample of those areas:

a. Business drivers—those environmental elements that drive the development and evolution of health care (especially hospital) organizations, such as the aging population, declining reimbursement for professional services, technological advances, and the health care workforce.

b. Quality and safety—not only on the radar screen of clinicians and health care management, quality and safety of care are

Table 124-3. SWOT Analysis

INTERNAL TO THE GROUP OR ORGANIZATION

Element	Factors to Consider	Strategic Objective
STRENGTHS	• Marketing—promotion, support, recruitment • Management—systems, expertise, resources • Operations—efficiency, capacity, processes, schedule • Services—quality, costs, scope • Finances—resources, performance • Costs—productivity, satisfaction, turnover • Systems—organization, structure • Personnel—expertise, experience, abilities	**Build** on strengths
WEAKNESSES	Same	**Resolve** weaknesses

EXTERNAL TO THE GROUP OR ORGANIZATION

Element	Factors to Consider	Strategic Objective
OPPORTUNITIES	• The field of hospital medicine (size, segmentation, maturity, growth, standards, niches, attractiveness) • The health care marketplace changing (patient demands, payors, employers, demographics, shortage of specialists) • New technologies or innovations (information management, staffing models, tools for quality/safety)	**Exploit** opportunities
THREATS	• Competition • Reimbursement models • Lack of hospital understanding value proposition of hospital medicine	**Avoid** threats

Table 124-4. Building a SMART Goal

Specific	Describe exactly what is to be accomplished and how
Measurable	Objective criteria to measure progress
Attainable	Can be achieved within the specified timeframe using available resources
Results-oriented	Focus on the results, as well as activities that must be done to attain the results.
Timed	Specify the completion date for attaining the goal

also top priorities for consumers. To be successful as a hospital medicine leader, one must have knowledge of the current state of health care quality on a national level, the efforts to improve quality at an organizational level, and the common methodologies that are employed in the hospital to improve quality and safety.

c. The Hospital Medicine movement—at just over 10 years of age, hospital medicine as a specialty has evolved and grown rapidly. The leader should know the milestones of his or her own field, the forces affecting its ongoing development, and the current and future challenges involved in moving forward.

d. Regulatory standards—to practice effectively, mitigate risk, and meet performance standards, the leader should have strong familiarity with the regulatory issues set forth by agencies such as the Joint Commission (previously known as the Joint Commission on Accreditation of Healthcare Organizations; JCAHO) and the Office of the Inspector General (OIG).

Management Skills

Strong managerial skills serve to reinforce the effectiveness of leadership. The most visionary leader is unlikely to achieve his or her objectives if he or she is unable to adeptly manage the group. Here are some of the more prominent management competencies that will support the hospital medicine leader:

a. *Running an effective meeting.* The leader is responsible for establishing the purpose of the meeting(s) and determining its size, composition, and frequency, and identifying the roles of each member. Ground rules for conducting the meeting must be reinforced through skilled facilitation. Finally, keen organizational skills are required to assemble the agenda and supporting documents and distribute them in advance, and to ensure the meeting minutes/summary reflects action items and responsible parties, and outlines the agenda for the next meeting.

b. *Financial decision-making.* The leader must understand the basics of budgeting, consequences of capital or personnel investments, clinical productivity, and articulating a return on investment.

c. *Managing physician performance.* (See Chapter 123 for details).

d. *Compensation methods.* (See Chapter 120 for details).

e. *Marketing and promotion.* To promote growth and extend breadth of services provided, the hospital medicine leader will need to engage in and coordinate a marketing and promotional effort that serves to educate community physicians on the capabilities of the group, engages subspecialists in the shared care of patients, describes to hospital administration the value proposition for hospital medicine, and partners with patients on how the care itself will be provided.

f. *Time management.* The balance between administrative and clinical duties for the hospital medicine leader requires excellent time-management skills. A potential pitfall here is the gap between the group's expectation of the clinical load carried by the leader and that which the leader realistically can carry. Part of time management, then, becomes being transparent about how the leader's time will be allocated and being clear with the group about how the team will work together to meet the demands of clinical and administrative work.

g. *Customer service.* "Customer" may be defined as patients, families, referring physicians, consultants, nurses, and a cast of thousands. To demonstrate, engender, and manage a culture of customer service will serve the leader well in building teamwork with the larger organization and to deliver on the promise of true patient-centered care.

SUMMARY

Leadership in hospital medicine encompasses many of the classic roles of leadership in medicine as well as other industries, and it adds the demands of working in a highly complex environment. Given the imperatives to improve quality and safety of health care in the United States, the need for effective leadership could not be greater. Leaders themselves must look toward their own professional development to meet these challenges. Leading change, effectively communicating with others, resolving conflict, successfully negotiating, creating a healthy workplace, holding oneself and others accountable, and other leadership responsibilities all require a commitment to life-long learning.

Key Points

• Leadership calls for a number of core attributes of the individual; these attributes serve as a baseline construct for conducting leadership behaviors.

• Leaders conduct practically all of their activities through communication with others, and as such they must have keen self-knowledge of their own personality style.

• Coaching and mentoring the members of one's group are effective means to improve group performance, lead change, and help foster a healthy workplace.

• Negotiation and conflict resolution are essential skills in securing resources and fostering teamwork to reach desired goals.

• A leader is an adept planner, and holds himself or herself and others accountable for results.

• Leaders understand the health care environment and apply specific managerial skills to support their activities.

SUGGESTED READING

Pistoria MJ, et al. The core competencies in hospital medicine. J Hosp Med 2006; 1(suppl 1):76–77.

Connors R, Smith T, Hickman C. The Oz Principle. New York: Prentice Hall Press, 1994.

Heifetz R. Leadership Without Easy Answers. Cambridge, MA: Belknap, 1994.

Kouzes J, Posner B. The Leadership Challenge: How to Get Extraordinary Things Done in Organizations. Jossey-Bass, San Francisco, CA 1987.

Clemmer J. Pathways to Performance: A Guide to Transforming Yourself, Your Team, and Your Organization. Rocklin, CA: Prima, 1995.

Lebos R, Spitzer R. Accountability. Berrett-Koehler, San Francisco, CA 2002.

Miller J. QBQ! The Question Behind the Question. Denver: Denver Press, 2001.

Silversin J, Kornacki MJ. Leading Physicians Through Change. ACPE Press, Philadelphia, PA 2000.

Kotter J. Leading Change. Cambridge, MA: Harvard Business School Press, 1996.

Fisher R, Ury W, Patton B. Getting to Yes: Negotiating Agreement Without Giving In. New York: Penguin, 1991.

Reinertsen J. Physicians as leaders in the improvement of health care systems. Ann Intern Med 1998; 128(10):833–838.

Collins J. Good to Great: Why Some Companies Make the Leap and Others Don't. Harper Business, New York, NY 2001.

CHAPTER ONE HUNDRED AND TWENTY-FIVE

Quality Improvement in the Hospital: Theory, Tools, and Trends

Norbert Goldfield, MD

INTRODUCTION

Quality and price are the two key components in measuring the value of health care.

$$\text{Value} = Quality/Payment$$

The price of health care dominates over quality, especially given the rapidly rising price of health care throughout the world. Countries differ in how they approach this challenge. While the American health care system lurches forward at a frenetic pace of change, an increasing number of Americans have inadequate access to health care because the United States is the only industrialized country that does not have universal health insurance coverage. Other countries try to address the cost challenge of universal coverage by encouraging a lower volume and unit cost of services.[1] As the cost of health care in the United States spirals upward, this approach is being applied in our hospitals. The entire hospitalist movement evolved from recognition that physicians specializing in hospital care delivery can provide high-quality care and, just as importantly, at a lower cost.[2]

This chapter will describe quality improvement in the hospital setting, discuss how health care financing trends influence this, and cover the following key areas that are leading to improved hospital care quality:

- Internal organizational trends
- Innovative methods/tools of measuring hospital quality improvement opportunities—beginning with the *plan-do-study-act* approach and then moving to new trends: patient-derived information, administrative data, and data abstracted from medical records
- External incentives—financial, accreditation, and consumer pressure/public disclosure

PRINCIPLES FOR THE UTILIZATION OF QI TOOLS

Development of tools to improve health care quality has undergone significant changes during the past decade. Yet this panoply of new tools and approaches are necessary but insufficient. The tools are helpful in deciding how to divide up the pie of payment and to report quality of care. The size (private or public monies) of the budgetary pie for health services together with the leadership (or more precisely absence of it[3]) needed to demand a focus on quality represent political challenges. This chapter is guided by three essential principles for the effective utilization of the quality improvement tools discussed in this section. The first principle is the need for universal coverage for health services. While there is significant controversy on how to achieve this goal, researchers have demonstrated conclusively that lack of health insurance leads to significantly poorer outcomes and processes of care for hospitalized patients.[4] This fact is one that all hospitalists confront every day in their practice.

The second principle relates to the fact that the health care system, like all other organizations, revolves around issues of payment. It is important to place the quality improvement work that hospitalists do within the context of payment—otherwise payers will not appreciate the value (quality/payment) of the services being provided. As will be discussed below, hospitalists need to be able to link the work they are doing to the payment systems that they are part of. Thus, the second principle states that it is important to implement tools that can be used to link payment and quality—even if the initial emphasis is on payment.

Health professionals and the rest of the health care team need to have "actionable" information for every type of health care encounter—hospital stays combined with the immediate pre/post hospital period represent one of the four types of health care encounters (the others are ambulatory visits, year-long episodes of illness, and post acute or long-term care). This is the essence of quality improvement. In contrast, clinical research seeks to answer more basic medical questions that may not have immediate and direct application for improving the value of care. Actionable information should be based on the tools derived from the second principle; that is, the health care provider (and team) realizes that the tool either has a direct or, at least, indirect connection with payment. The health care team includes, at a minimum, the patient (most important), health care providers, purchasers such as employers, and payers such as health insurers or managed care organizations. The information needed pertains to data that tie quality and payment together. Without this type of information and without purchasers using this type of information in their payment decisions, all the increasingly cacophonous calls for leadership to improve quality will result in marginal change.

The third principle is that the health care system must be patient-centric. This means not only measuring patient satisfaction, but also empowering patients, if they so desire, to be equal partners on the health care team.[5] A key aspect of, for example, decreasing hospital readmissions (approximately 10% of all discharges result in a readmission within 30 days, reflecting poor quality) is to engage patients/consumers to be a key part of the health care team consisting of the inpatient clinical group, the discharge planning staff, and the receiving outpatient team.

THE KEY CONCEPTS OF QUALITY IMPROVEMENT—PLAN, DO, STUDY, ACT (PDSA)

The PDSA cycle operationalizes three critical Continuous Quality Improvement (CQI) principles:

- Quality is a process of never-ending improvement.
- Data on the process and the results must be collected simultaneously and acted on in an organized manner.
- Action should be taken only after the sources of variation in the process of health care delivery are discovered.

Plan to improve your operations first by finding out what things are going wrong (i.e., identify the problems faced), and come up with ideas for solving these problems.

Do implement changes designed to solve the problems on a small scale first. This minimizes disruption to routine activity while testing whether the changes result in improvement.

Study (or check) to see if the small-scale changes are achieving the desired result and if there are any new problems. In this phase, the data from the preceding step are examined for reliability and validity. The data are also compared to the information gathered in the first phase to determine why differences, if any, exist.

Act to implement changes on a larger scale if the experiment is successful. This means making the changes a routine part of your activity. Also **Act** to involve other persons (other departments, suppliers, or customers) affected by the changes and whose cooperation you need to implement them on a larger scale (you may already have involved these people in the **Do** or trial stage).[6]

A second component of key quality improvement concepts—structure, process, and outcome—is discussed below. Before analyzing this second component, however, one should understand the critical role of "case mix" and how it affects both the payment system and assessment of quality (*see* Box 125-1). Additionally, internal organizational trends should be recognized for their effect on decisions directing quality improvement focus (*see* Box 125-2).

INNOVATIVE METHODS/TOOLS OF MEASURING HOSPITAL QUALITY IMPROVEMENT: STRUCTURE, PROCESS, AND OUTCOMES

The Institute of Medicine defines health care quality as: *The degree to which health services for individuals and populations increase the likelihood of desired health outcomes and are consistent with current*

Box 125-1 Importance of Case Mix

Diagnosis-related groups (DRGs), the archetypal example of a case mix measure, had a "revolutionary" impact, not only on payment but also on the measurement and management of hospital quality.[7] Without attention to case mix or risk adjustment, all we have is adverse risk selection or managed risk (as opposed to managed care)—that is, choosing patients on the basis of their financial risk to the organization. Case mix is used here to denote stratification of cases (diagnostic and procedural) into clinically meaningful categories, while risk adjustment is typically used to refer to the use of case mix for purposes of predicting future costs. The validity of the classification system depends on whether it is applied to payment, quality improvement, or both. In the final analysis, users (individual consumers, purchasers, hospital administrators) are trying to compare providers for selected variables—severity of illness, risk of mortality, readmissions, and the like. Case-mix adjustment ensures that we are comparing apples to apples for the variable in question and for the type of health care encounter we want to examine.

Case-mix measurement began with the development of diagnosis-related groups or DRGs (for hospital management, NOT payment) at Yale University in the late sixties and early seventies. The federal government's implementation of DRGs in the early eighties led to dramatic changes in medical practice, despite the fact that Center for Medicare and Medicaid Services (CMS) has never used DRGs for physician payment. Researchers have developed numerous versions of the DRGs.

There are a number of new developments in case-mix research that build on the new movement termed **Pay for Performance** (P4P), which applies appropriate and/or bonus payment for higher quality care. These are:

- The development of new methods of measuring severity of illness using information drawn from claims from the medical record.
- Rewards for hospitals for not having potentially avoidable complications.
- Rewards for hospitals that coordinate hospital services with immediate postdischarge outpatient services (the time most likely to lead to readmission), thus lowering rates of 15-, 30-, and 60-day readmissions.
- Encouraging hospitals and physicians to coordinate their inhospital care by combining hospital and physician payment together.

professional knowledge.[9] Quality of care must address both individuals and groups of individuals. In addition, while all of us would like to focus on outcomes (what the end results of particular health care practices and interventions on any dimension of care are), we are not able to perfectly measure outcomes and thus need to keep in mind structural (conditions that underlie the care process with such aspects as professionalism, safety, accessibility, and integration) and process (the way in which care is provided on the aspects of attitude, method, continuity, and accountability) measures, both of which examine professional knowledge.

Utilizing the time-honored Donabedian[10] paradigm of structure, process, and outcome, recent developments in QI methods and tools are described.

Box 125-2 Internal Organizational Trends

All hospitals must be accredited by the Joint Commission (previously the Joint Commission for the Accreditation of Health Care Organizations, JCAHO) to receive Medicare reimbursement. However, the Joint Commission has attempted to make significant improvements in its accreditation, including:

- Using administrative data to identify opportunities for improvement that, in turn, become a significant part of the accreditation process
- Allowing individuals to look up quality reports on hospitals that deal with a small number of largely process measures pertaining to best hospital care[8]

Under the current trend toward P4P, the hospital quality improvement department has become more important and more data oriented, resulting in information that is richer in clinical detail. Managers of the quality improvement department, together with other allies, particularly hospitalists, must balance several internal organizational pressures that simultaneously demand attention:

- The requirement to maintain Joint Commission accreditation
- The need to be knowledgeable about current quality improvement tools (many of which are summarized below), the Plan-Do-Study-Act Cycle (PDSA) cycle, and other affiliated tools such as statistical process control
- The need to balance a commitment to quality while understanding that payment issues are often paramount. Knowledge of one's institutional politics along with a grasp of the manifold external organizational pressures is required to advocate effectively for quality improvement.

However, the trend toward the increased importance of hospitalists, in particular, and the quality improvement department in general, will become firmly established only if P4P is implemented with serious attention to quality management goals affecting the operations of the entire hospital. Unless P4P integrates quality and efficiency as described later in this chapter, one will continue to hear statements such as "If my CEO did not have this public report card hanging around his neck, he would rather put me and the rest of quality management into the basement."

Structure

A plethora of organizations provide accreditation services from either legal or political pressures. Clearly, the Joint Commission is the first among equals, as it has significant legal authority. Many state and local governments have also exercised their legal authority to regulate hospital behavior. In contrast, several new organizations, including business and medical society coalitions (e.g., Washington Business Group on Health,[11] Leapfrog,[12] or National Quality Forum[13]) have recently emerged, using "corporate clout" to encourage adoption of structural measures, such as the recommendation that board-certified intensivists staff intensive care units.

As already stated, the Joint Commission together with federal/state/local agencies and medical boards, have legal authority to regulate hospitals' accreditation. Other organizations, such as the National Quality Forum and Leapfrog, have developed "legs" out of corporate frustration with the rising costs of health care. It is not completely clear why or how they have

achieved their political clout or, for that matter, how long it will last. In any event, until now, most of these organizations have provided a range of recommendations for quality measurement that have contributed to an interest in the phrase P4P without having changed the culture, which is still very much focused on payment.[14]

Process

- Joint Commission Core Measures include process measures for myocardial infarction, pneumonia, heart failure, and more recently for surgical infection prevention.
- CMS/Premier Demonstration: This federal waiver demonstration project is probably the most visible at a national level, linking extra payment to hospitals in return for improved performance on a number of largely process indicators for a few conditions.[15]
- Collections of well-validated quality measurement tools are easily available on the Internet and include: the Niagara Health Care Quality Report,[16] a collection of indicators from the RAND Corporation which is an excellent index of quality measurement tools, again largely process measures.[17]

Outcome—Ranging from Morbidity/Mortality to Patient Satisfaction

- Mortality—AHRQ/HCUP: Perhaps of greatest significance, the Agency for Health Care Research and Quality (AHRQ) has recently published a new set of hospital quality indicators (HCUP). There are three different types of indicators:
  - Provider-level Volume Indicators. The HCUP empirical results confirm that hospital volume is an important correlate of quality of care. However, prior studies demonstrate that volume is at best an imperfect reflection of true quality or performance differences.
  - Provider-level Mortality Indicators. The recommended hospital mortality indicators are all associated with large differences in hospital performance; that is, differences in mortality between lower and higher performing hospitals are often several percentage points or larger. Thus, the mortality indicators may be helpful in identifying opportunities for large improvements in outcomes.
  - Area Indicators. There are two types of area indicators assessed:
  - *Utilization indicators* include procedures for which use has been shown to vary widely across relatively similar geographic areas, with (in most cases) substantial inappropriate utilization.
  - *Avoidable hospitalizations/Ambulatory care sensitive condition (ACSC) indicators* involve admissions that evidence suggests could have been avoided, at least in part, through better access to high-quality outpatient care.
- Readmissions: Researchers have attempted to understand varying aspects of readmissions as they try to correlate quality and readmission rate. Carol Ashton provided the largest meta-analysis supporting the relationship between quality of care and readmissions.[18] She concluded that early readmission is significantly associated with the process of inpatient care.
- Hospital Errors/Infection Rates: Bowing to consumer pressure, Illinois, Pennsylvania, Missouri, and Florida have passed laws

Table 125-1 QI Measures and Organizations

Measure	CMS	AHRQ	JCAHO	NQF	Leapfrog
Structure	Premier project		Correct patient identification	Detailed discharge instructions (heart failure)	Intensivist training; Computerized physician order entry
Process		Primary C-section rate	Beta-blockers after an MI	Aspirin prescribed at discharge for AMI	Adapted from NQF safety practices
Outcome	Readmission following knee replacement	Hospital quality indicators	MI mortality	CABG mortality indicator	Adapted from NQF safety practices
		CAHPS survey			

MI—myocardial infarction; NQF—national quality forum; CAHPS—consumer assessment of healthcare providers and systems

forcing hospitals to publicly report infections related to health care. Another 30 states are moving to mandatory release of such information.[19] Additionally, CMS seeks authority to lower reimbursement for cases in which patients develop hospital-acquired infections.

- Potentially preventable hospital complications: Several studies have linked poorer quality care with inhospital complications.[20] Unfortunately, it is difficult to easily identify these complications, as routinely (i.e., administrative) collected data does not specify whether the secondary diagnosis was present on admission (the principal diagnosis almost always is present on admission). Several states, including California, New York, and Florida, mandate the collection of the diagnoses present on admission indicator. It is anticipated that this indicator will be required nationwide in 2009.
- If we knew whether or not the secondary diagnosis was present on admission, we could specify whether the secondary diagnoses that occurred after admission were preventable together with an understanding of the admission severity of illness. The latter is key to knowing the probability with which a hospital-acquired complication will occur.
- Patient satisfaction: An important patient-centric measure that may or may not correlate with quality of care relative to measures such as mortality. Chapter 131 covers this topic in detail.

Table 125-1 provides a summary of organizations involved in hospital quality improvement, together with examples of the measures they are including.

EXTERNAL INCENTIVES

Hospitalists appreciate the high quality of care they deliver and would value its recognition by not just a focus on efficiency as is largely done today, but by a focus on the value (quality/payment) of the services they provide. Continued increases in health care costs have led to experimentation with many forms of external incentives to try and rein in costs. Recognition that opportunities for quality improvement represent an important part of cost

increases has led to a growing link between cost and quality incentives. However, there are a number of overarching tensions—needs versus desires—in this link between cost and quality, as delineated in Table 125-2.

Only a redoubling of customer commitment to the key principles of CQI will resolve the conflicts between these needs and desires. Public disclosure of comparative information represents an important recent trend. The following types of information are typically selected:

- Risk-adjusted mortality using AHRQ HCUP indicators
- Patient satisfaction results
- Accreditation by national organizations such as Joint Commission
- Information from other, more process-oriented, efforts such as the CMS-Premier Demonstration project

What is the impact of the release of this information? Hibbard has recently documented a positive impact[21] while a recent *Journal of the American Medical Association (JAMA)* review summarized the challenges to public disclosure.[22] Public disclosure of the value of hospital care is very important but not nearly as key as the financial incentives described below.

Pay for Performance (P4P)

P4P is generating a great deal of ferment in the United States, in particular, on challenges of implementation. Efforts overseas also aim to move their health care systems in this direction.[23] One way P4P is being accomplished for hospitals is through tiered-hospital contracts, which typically place hospitals into two or more categories, primarily based on the cost of services and to a lesser extent aspects of quality of care. There are many flavors of this effort, with organizations adopting variations on the tiered-hospital strategy.[24] Paying a bonus if certain process (and occasionally an outcome measure such as readmissions) measures are achieved constitutes another P4P technique. The CMS-Premier Demonstration project for hospitals is an example of such an effort.[25] Additionally, a number of payers are giving incentive payments to physicians if they meet certain targets, for mostly process measures such as mammography rates.[26] Unfortunately,

Table 125-2 Needs versus Desires Driving Tensions Between Cost and Quality

Needs	Desires
Improvement over time	Protect public and immediately identify poorly performing providers
Empower the public through education and information	Give out information and hope for the best
Provide case-mix–adjusted information based on universally accepted statistical measures that are, in turn, explained to the public	Avoid all statistical manipulations and trust that an unbiased third party will take care of any problem
Provide information based on clinically reliable and valid methodologies	Provide at least some information to the public
Emphasize both the process and outcome of care	Pay attention primarily to outcomes
Focus greater attention on low-income or uninsured individuals	Political need to satisfy the wants of middle- and upper-income individuals

it is likely that these incentive payments are too small, relatively easily gamed, and provide significant incentives to select healthier patients (e.g., diabetics at lower levels of severity).

The tiered approach as currently implemented is too crude, as there will often be a very small differential in quality and cost between two hospitals that may lead the two institutions to be placed into different tiers. Rather than two tiers, we will likely evolve toward a point system that incentivizes institutions to pursue quality improvement and thus move into one of many higher tiers.[27] In addition, currently available tiering systems are based on tools that have, at best, modest relevance for quality improvement, patient empowerment, or, most important, hospital cost control over a sustained period of time. If a hospital is at the bottom of a two-tier payment system, it is very difficult to move into the top tier, as virtually the only information that is fed back by the payer to the provider is the crude cost for the Medicare DRG with no adjustment for severity and/or quality of the service provided.

The necessary tools to assess severity of illness and quality of care are a combination of well-validated case-mix measures for each type of health care encounter, such as severity adjusted DRGs, together with quality measures endorsed by national organizations such as the AHRQ. Payers need to use these tools as the underpinning of a P4P system that in turn could relentlessly control costs and narrow variations in care. The Alliance in Wisconsin is beginning to attempt the outlines of such an approach.[28]

With respect to hospitals, payers (governmental or private) have used CMS/Medicare DRGs and/or per diems in an effort to control hospital costs. Initially, the Medicare DRG system had a dramatic impact on hospital costs and delivery of care.[29] Unfortunately, the current Medicare DRG system contains several problems that seriously hamper the implementation of an effective P4P system. A number of European countries use either this same system (e.g., Italy) or variations on the same theme (Germany and the United Kingdom). Only Belgium, for example, uses a payment system that is truly severity adjusted.

Most importantly, the Medicare DRGs are not adequately severity adjusted, which continues to provide a perverse incentive for hospitals to select, for example, "healthier" or lower risk patients for procedures and encouraging the "complicated" individuals to go elsewhere.[30] In addition, the Medicare classification system only applies to the elderly and thus misclassifies (thereby leading to difficulties in implementing the quality improvement process) many patients under age 65. Currently, researchers are examining the possibility of switching from the current Medicare DRGs to a system, the All Patient Refined-DRGs (APR-DRG), that is not only severity adjusted but covers all ages.[31] Using, in part, this research work, CMS recently proposed that CMS DRGs be switched to a consolidated, severity-adjusted DRG system.[32]

Lastly, Medicare DRGs perversely reward hospitals with extra payment if avoidable complications occur during the hospital stay and pay hospitals for an entire readmission stay that could have been avoided if coordinated outpatient care were provided. Thus, if hospitals (and hospitalists) wish to avoid the "penalty" inherent in the current CMS DRG structure, Medicare should issue a bundled payment for both outpatient and inpatient services and not pay extra for avoidable complications that occur in the hospital. The tools exist today to implement such incentive payment/pay for performance programs that would recognize the high-quality care that hospitalists provide.

CONCLUSIONS

This chapter outlines the latest developments in quality measurement and management, ALL of which could be utilized in a pay-for-performance system. For it to be successful, pay for performance should have built-in incentives that are significant enough from a financial perspective to compel providers to focus relentlessly on quality improvement. Health care is at a crossroads—it either will become progressively more effective, or it will increasingly limit services (not a compassionate approach). System rewards can drive use of effective evidence-based interventions or continue to force decisions based on financial reimbursement. Hospitalists, with work that almost always improves the overall value of hospital care, will play a key role in this decision-making process, a process that has both individual patient and national ramifications.

Comprehensive Hospital Medicine: An Evidence Based and Systems Approach

Key Points

- Hospitalists must be equipped with adequate tools to engage in quality improvement within their institutions.

- The Plan/Do/Study/Act Cycle provides the foundation of continuous quality improvement.

- Current approaches to quality measurement include all three elements of quality: structure, process, and outcomes of care.

- For pay-for-performance to succeed, it must appropriately reimburse for value in health care (defined as quality—both administrative and clinical—divided by payment).

- Hospitalists should understand potentially preventable complications of hospitalization and the potential to prevent readmissions. Preventable readmissions are those readmissions that can be avoided with a combination of excellent quality care in the initial hospitalization and/or best possible coordinated care between the inpatient and outpatient sectors.

- Patients should be at the center of QI efforts and partners on the health care team.

SUGGESTED READING

Donabedian A. An Introduction to Quality Assurance in Health Care. New York, NY: Oxford University Press. 2002.

Hibbard JH, Stockard J, Tusler M. Hospital performance reports: impact on quality, market share, and reputation. Health Aff (Millwood) 2005; 24(4):1150–1160.

Smith PC, York N. Quality incentives: the case of U.K. general practitioners Health Affairs 2004; 23(3):112–118.

Leape LL, Berwick DM. Five years after To Err Is Human: what have we learned? JAMA 2005; 293(19):2384–2390.

Ashton CM, Del Junco DJ, Souchek J, et al. The association between the quality of inpatient care and early readmission: a meta-analysis of the evidence. Med Care 1997; 35(10):1044–1059.

Werner RM, Asch DA. The unintended consequences of publicly reporting quality information. JAMA 2005; 293(10):1239–1244.

Hibbard JH, Stockard J, Mahoney ER, et al. Development of the Patient Activation Measure (PAM): conceptualizing and measuring activation in patients and consumers. Health Serv Res 2004; 39(4 Pt 1):1005–1026.

CHAPTER ONE HUNDRED TWENTY-SIX

Quality Improvement in the Hospital

Jason Stein, MD, Greg Maynard, MD, MSc

BACKGROUND

Hospitals are complex systems. Over time, each hospital accumulates its own set of care processes—some coordinated, some autonomous—which directly affect inpatient outcomes. As systems, hospitals are perfectly designed to achieve exactly what they do, so improving the output of a hospital requires change. Ideas for what to change, how to change, and how to manage change successfully over time should come from a local improvement team, ideally a group of frontline caregivers with complementary insights. Such a multidisciplinary team should include members familiar with current processes, those who know which evidence to translate into practice or who hold positions of credibility and leadership among the clinical staff. In a growing number of hospital systems, hospitalists are prime candidates to lead such improvement teams

Not all change results in improvement, however, and the same skills most critical for driving actual improvement in the hospital—designing, managing, and leading change successfully over time—are also the ones commonly missing from clinician skill sets.

The realities of the practice of hospital medicine today are not to be overlooked. Excessive patient loads and financial pressures can be overwhelming. Yet hospitalists who find the traction to lead a successful improvement effort may also trigger a cascade of resources, including protected time and dedicated support staff. The successful stewardship of hospital care delivery—and its improvement—is hospital medicine's largely untapped value to the health care system.

ASSESSMENT

Support for change must come from the highest levels in a medical center. Real support should confer the authority and resources needed for the improvement team to design and manage change. A number of forces may fuel administrative will to improve, including public reporting of hospital performance, cost savings from more efficient care, risk aversion, favorable payments for better performance, nursing and medical staff retention, and even quality for quality's sake.[1] Since the right value proposition may be the key to securing executive support, improvement efforts that work in concert with existing institutional goals should find the strongest backing.

As members of the improvement team, hospitalists bring both a hands-on appreciation of care processes and a strong understanding of the clinical topic. Regardless of the clinical focus, hospitalists should strive to command the evidence base supporting clinical decisions, even in subspecialty areas. What may distinguish hospitalists, however, are more experience with the system of hospital care delivery and potential competence with leading an effective, sustained quality improvement effort. The published *Core Competencies in Hospital Medicine* confirms quality improvement as fundamental to the specialty.[2] Curricula have already been developed to help hospitalists learn this skill set.[3]

This chapter, which draws from a model for improvement set forth by others,[4] uses the clinical example of hospital-acquired venous thromboembolism (VTE) to illustrate a framework that hospitalists can use to lead quality improvement.

THREE FUNDAMENTALS FOR QUALITY IMPROVEMENT IN THE HOSPITAL: EMPIRIC, ITERATIVE, AND MEASUREMENT SYSTEM

No two hospitals have the same infrastructure, personnel, resources, or culture. In fact, no two nursing units in a given hospital share all these features, either. Thus, nobody knows how a changed process will perform until it is tested in the local environment. For this simple reason, quality improvement efforts must be both empiric and iterative. Efforts are *empiric* in the sense that effective changes are confirmed only through trying something new and learning from the trial. Efforts must be *iterative* in the sense that it is only through several generations of changes that a new process can be perfected. The evolution of living species may be a useful metaphor: incremental quality improvement proceeds by combining selective pressures with reassortment and replication.

The third fundamental element of quality improvement is a *measurement system*. Without a defined and tracked set of metrics, an improvement team cannot compare new performance with a baseline. It makes no sense to design, test, and spread changes without knowing whether the net effect is better or worse.

Quality improvement leaders from industry have devised a model for improvement that expands on these three fundamental elements, including a step for analysis: the Plan-Do-Study-Act model (Fig. 126-1).

This framework can be adapted to health care systems, giving a hospital improvement team the model it needs to visualize cyclical phases of its efforts. Using a quality improvement initiative to improve rates of VTE prophylaxis, Figure 126-2 is a schematic of how PDSA cycles over time might look.

The many advantages of the PDSA model—and principles for success—are depicted in Table 126-1.

SELECTING SPECIFIC AIMS AND A MEANINGFUL SET OF METRICS

Establishing an ambitious general aim is essential to motivating the team undertaking a QI initiative. Using hospital-acquired VTE as an illustration, the team might decide on the following general aim: reduce by half the rate of hospital-acquired VTE in the medical center. While instrumental in setting the focus and scope of an improvement effort, general aims should also be aggressive enough to force process redesign. The power of changing common hospital processes is what sets quality improvement apart from traditional "quality assurance," itself a practice of applying resources to prevent statistical outliers. Only by changing common processes can the care quality improve for a wider population of inpatients (Fig. 126-3).

The improvement team should make rational choices when deciding which steps in a process to change and which to measure. Ultimately, patients and providers care most about outcome measures, such as the most common preventable cause of hospital death, "hospital-acquired VTE." But detecting clinical endpoints during hospitalization can be impractical, especially for

infrequent events or those with delayed onset or prolonged subclinical periods. For this reason, meaningful intermediate outcomes (also called "process measures") usually represent a more efficient way to measure performance of care delivery. The use of a conceptual flow diagram, as depicted in Figure 126-4, is a valuable way to map a process while also identifying meaningful intermediate outcomes. In the VTE example, a key intermediate outcome (i.e., process measure) is the rate at which physicians order appropriate VTE prophylaxis when the patient is admitted

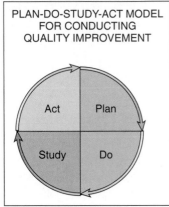

Figure 126-1 • PDSA Model for Conducting Quality Improvement. Adapted from: James, BC. M.Stat. Pragmatic Science. Accessed 12/29/05 at: http://intermountainhealthcare.org/xp/public/documents/institute/prag_science.ppt#256,1, Slide 47.

Figure 126-2 • Cycles of PDSA for VTE Prophylaxis. Kicking off an improvement effort with a decision support tool, the VTE risk assessment in this example is a rational first intervention. A pilot period should allow the tool to be refined, simplified, and integrated into the clinical workflow, in this case as part of the preprinted order set. A stand-alone VTE risk assessment form may not be as available as one that is nested within existing order sets. Similarly, a perfectly crafted and nested VTE risk assessment may not be used if they are not stocked or immediately available where physicians need them in the clinical workflow. These potential barriers can best be addressed by the action-oriented learning that characterizes cycles of PDSA. Adapted from: James BC. M.Stat. Pragmatic Science. Accessed 12/29/05 at: http://intermountainhealthcare.org/xp/public/documents/institute/prag_science.ppt#256,1, Slide 48.

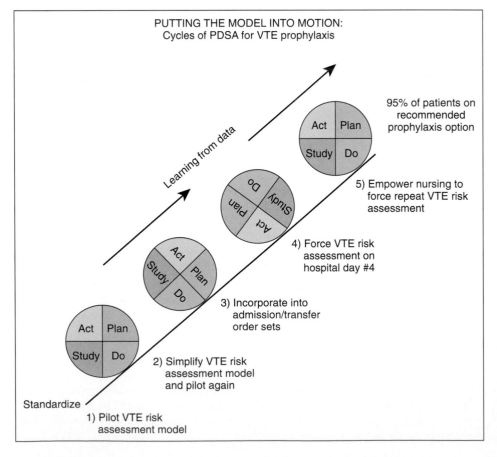

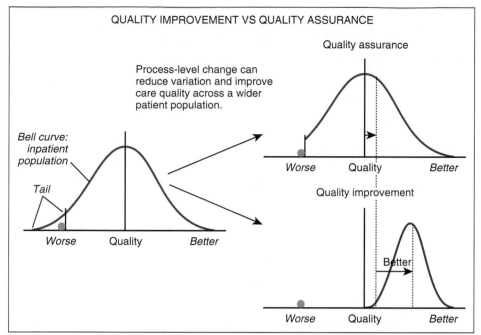

Figure 126-3 • Quality Improvement versus Quality Assurance. If the improvement team identifies a performance gap applicable to a wider patient population, the team may design changes in *processes* with the potential for dramatic effect: standardization in processes can reduce variation (narrowing the curve) and raise quality of care for more patients (shifting *entire* curve toward better care). This potential for radical change is what sets quality improvement (QI) apart from quality assurance (QA). In contrast, traditional QA focuses on fixing the root causes of statistical outliers in the "tail" of a population. Using a QA approach can be very useful within the context of a larger QI effort if a system's SPC chart demonstrates exceptional (or "special cause") variation. In fact, QA tools such as Root Cause Analysis should be used to rid such a system of detrimental assignable causes before any QI can proceed effectively. Adapted from: James BC. M.Stat. Three Methods to Manage Clinical Care. Accessed 12/29/05 at: http://intermountainhealthcare.org/xp/public/documents/institute/3methods.ppt#256,1, Slide 1.

Table 126-1 Advantages of PDSA and Principles for Success

Advantages of PDSA
Allows for valuable modifications to improve effectiveness or preserve productivity
Allows "failures" to come to light without undermining performance and momentum
Identifies areas of resistance that might undermine spread to other units
Allows costs and side effects of the change to be assessed
Increases certainty that change will result in improvement
Allows for detailed documentation of improvement

Principles for Success
Start new changes on the smallest possible scale (e.g., one patient, one nurse, one doctor)
Run just as many PDSA cycles as necessary to gain confidence in a change, then spread incrementally
Spread incrementally to more patients, then more nurses, then doctors, and finally units
Balance changes within overall system to ensure other processes not adversely stressed
Pay special attention to preserving productivity and workflow

to the hospital. As seen in Figure 126-4, that metric itself may be a variable that is dependent on several contributing steps. To enhance the value of this diagram, the improvement team can use local data to annotate performance rates for each step in the outcomes chain, thereby spotlighting high-leverage points that can be targeted for both change and measurement.

After meaningful process measures are selected, the improvement team can craft a more specific aim statement. Good aim statements are specific, measurable, time limited, and applicable to a particular population of patients. Based on the ambitious general goal above and the outcomes chain in Figure 126-4, a

VTE improvement team could select two metrics and incorporate them into these specific aim statements:

1. Of all patients admitted to our general medical units, 95% will be on **appropriate VTE prophylaxis** as defined by our protocol within 6 months.
2. We will reduce the rate of **hospital-acquired VTE** from the baseline of X events per 1,000 patient days to X/2 events per 1,000 patient days within 12 months.

At every team meeting, these specific aims should be reviewed. The performance rates for these metrics should be graphically plotted and presented to the group. In order to do this, strict def-

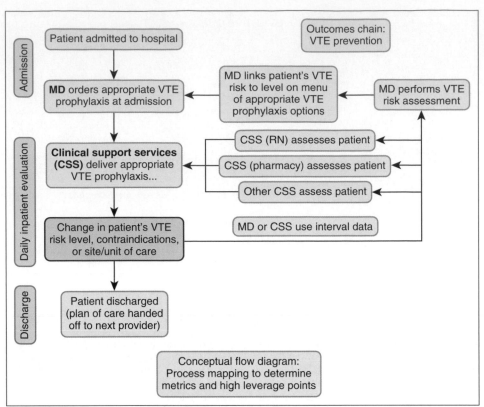

Figure 126-4 • Outcomes Chain for Hospital Care Delivery. This conceptual flow diagram can be used to identify the key metrics to chart and follow in an effort to reduce rates of hospital-acquired VTE. In this example, it is clear that a physician's admission order for appropriate VTE prophylaxis is a prerequisite to the patient receiving it early in the hospital stay. As a meaningful metric, an improvement team might decide to measure the percent of patients with admission orders that include appropriate VTE prophylaxis. By collecting data about the relative performance of each step in this flow diagram, additional key metrics may be discovered by the improvement team. By annotating such a flow diagram with performance rates, "high leverage" points can be identified for closer attention.

initions are needed to perform chart audits or database queries. The team must decide how to define potentially vague elements of each metric (the bolded words in the example above). What will the team consider "appropriate VTE prophylaxis" for a given patient? Auditors must have explicit directions when reviewing medical records to classify patients accurately and consistently; in this case a method to assign a VTE risk level and then check it against an agreed-upon menu of appropriate prophylaxis options.

For the outcome measure, how will the team define and case-find "hospital-acquired VTE"? A common definition for "hospital-acquired" would be a clot first discovered during the course of hospitalization, or discovered within 30 days of a prior hospitalization.

Note that the first and second goals in the VTE example above represent a *process measure* and an *outcome measure*, respectively. It is often useful to include one or more *balancing measures*. Balancing measures account for the reality that any new process in a hospital can introduce potentially detrimental effects. In the case of VTE, these could include incidence of heparin-induced thrombocytopenia, serious bleeding episodes, or the cost of using more pharmacologic prophylaxis.

Additional subjective or objective data about the intervention are also likely to be valuable. For instance, subjective feedback about the usability of a new order form, patient feedback about

receiving more shots, or discordant staff duties could prove vital to spreading the changed process to successive units in the hospital. The impact on hospital costs or length of stay from the new VTE prophylaxis protocol also could be invaluable when the time comes to assess the full value of the initiative.

CREATING A MEASUREMENT SYSTEM FOR COLLECTING DATA AND PLOTTING METRICS

Once metrics are clearly defined, the team has a formula to audit charts precisely, accurately, and with reproducibility. While data collection can be costly in terms of time and money, team effort and focus should always remain on improvement rather than measurement. A sampling strategy that uses 20 randomly selected patient charts per month can be statistically appropriate as well as relatively quick and easy. To advance PDSA cycles, the team needs just enough data to know whether changes are leading to improvement.[4]

The team should articulate who collects, collates, plots, and manages the data and should choose between sampling active inpatients or recent discharges. The former approach may offer several real-time advantages. Providers can be alerted to process oversights, which might create moments to improve care as well as educate. In addition, sampling active inpatients may allow

Table 126-2 Methods for Defining Hospital-Acquired VTE

Method 1	Track total # DVT and PE diagnosis codes in your medical center.*
Method 2	Method 1, then pull charts post-discharge and retrospectively determine if hospital or community acquired.
Method 3	Method 2, then retrospectively determine if patients with hospital-acquired VTE were on appropriate prophylaxis when VTE developed.
Method 4	Prospectively capture new cases of DVT or PE as they occur by setting up reporting system with radiology departments.

*Then divide by 2 to estimate the fraction that are hospital-acquired. The literature suggests that approximately half of all cases of DVT and PE diagnosed in the hospital are hospital-acquired.[6]

Adapted from: Maynard G, Stein J. Workbook for Improvement: Optimize Prevention of Venous Thromboembolism at Your Medical Center. Accessed 12/29/05 at: http://www.hospitalmedicine.org/AM/Template.cfm?Section=Quality_Improvement_Resource_Rooms&Template=/CM/ContentDisplay.cfm&ContentID=6092.

insights into process barriers and valid reasons to amend the new process to emerge more readily. Techniques for minimizing the resource utilization and error inherent in chart abstraction and data entry include the use of self-coding and scanable forms. When feasible, the use of database queries to generate automatic lists of useful data can be very valuable.

Using the example of hospital-acquired VTE (Table 126-2), there are various methods for trying to capture this metric in a useful way, each with its own advantages in terms of accuracy and efficiency.

Available data collection resources may dictate methods and definitions in any given medical center. Whatever method is chosen, consistency and usefulness are critical. It is usually helpful to pilot the metric definitions as well as the steps in data collection to uncover and solve stumbling blocks.

There are two ways to plot improvement data in context to follow trends over time, the run chart and the statistical process control (SPC) chart, and the relative advantages of each are described.

Run Charts

These simply plot data over time. Compared to tables of data, run charts offer our brains a quicker picture of how an intervention is working relative to a baseline.[5] Since run charts can be annotated by superimposing events along the timeline, it can be easier to see the effects of different stages of an intervention and to subtract the effect of known secular trends. For run charts, software such as Excel or any of several free online run chart applications are widely available, and no statistical expertise is needed.

Statistical Process Control

A more powerful alternative to the simple run chart is the SPC chart. Also called "process behavior charts," SPC charts offer all the functionality of run charts but have a significant added advantage; they reveal otherwise hidden information about the stability and reproducibility of the existing process. Such insight could have significant implications on how the improvement team decides to proceed.

An SPC chart has two parts: (1) a series of measurements plotted over time and (2) a three-horizontal line template. The centerline typically represents the mean of all the measurements.

The other two lines are placed on either side of the mean line, typically at values 3 standard deviations away.[6] These two lines, the upper control limit (UCL) and lower control limit (LCL), are what make the SPC chart special. Where data points fall relative to the UCL and LCL communicates whether variation in measurements is routine or exceptional. Routine variation is normal, is expected whenever something is being measured, and can be confirmed visually whenever data points fall between the UCL and LCL. But exceptional (or "special cause") variation—easy to see when measurements continue to fall outside the UCL or LCL—is not only statistically significant but also likely to have an assignable cause, either detrimental or beneficial. When assignable cause is detrimental to system performance, the team should uncover the contributing reasons and take steps to prevent them from recurring in the future. When assignable cause is beneficial, it might be smart to incorporate the root cause formally into the process.[6]

FOCUSING ON CHANGES TO DRIVE RELIABLY BETTER CARE

A contingent from the improvement team should identify the best evidence to translate into practice. The team as a whole, on the other hand, should concentrate on how to integrate the changes successfully into the workflow. Several published systematic reviews have tried to assess the effectiveness of QI strategies, including direction of effect, effect size, and relative effectiveness.[8–11] Most strategies demonstrate wide variations in effect size; the main conclusion that can be drawn from the existing literature is that we still cannot predict which strategies will work.[12] One of these reviews advanced a strong taxonomy for classifying the known quality improvement strategies (Table 126-3).[11] The taxonomy may prove useful for improvement teams wishing to rationally layer multifaceted interventions.

For example, if local data demonstrate that two thirds of VTE prophylaxis failures derive from the combined failures of two related medical decision-making steps (see the marked boxes in the conceptual flow diagram in Figure 126-4), a logical choice for the first improvement change would be a "Provider Reminder"—for example, a decision support tool integrated into admission order sets. Such a provision would ensure the existence of a workflow tool to help clinicians perform an accurate VTE risk assess-

Table 126-3 Common Quality Improvement Strategies and Effectiveness

QI Strategies (Effectiveness)	Examples of Substrategies
Provider education *Generally ineffective if judged on the basis of improving patient outcomes; if judged in terms of increasing provider knowledge can be effective.*	• Conferences and workshops • Educational outreach visits (e.g., academic detailing) • Distributed educational materials
Provider reminder systems *Reminders often effective if well integrated into clinical workflow. Decision support sometimes effective, but less so for the more complex situations in which it would be most desirable.*	• Reminders in charts for providers • Computer-based reminders for providers • Computer-based decision support
Facilitated relay of clinical data to providers	• Transmission of clinical data from data source to hospital physician by means other than medical record (e.g., page, email, phone call)
Audit and feedback of performance to providers *At best, small to modest benefits for various forms of audit and feedback (such as report cards or benchmarking).* *Variations in format may explain some of the observed variations in effectiveness, in addition to providers' attitudes to the accuracy or credibility of the reports.*	• Feedback of performance to individual providers • Quality indicators and reports • National/state quality report cards • Publicly released performance data • Benchmarking—provision of outcomes data from top performers for comparison with provider's own data
Patient education *Modest to large effects for some conditions and patient populations.* *Mixed results for total quality management and continuous quality improvement.*	• Classes • Parent and family education • Patient pamphlets • Intensive education strategies promoting self-management of chronic conditions
Organizational change *Mostly positive results for case management and disease management programs.*	• Case management, disease management • TQM, CQI techniques • Multidisciplinary teams • Change from paper to computer-based records • Increased staffing • Skill mix changes
Financial incentives, regulation, and policy *Some evidence of achieving target goals but also concerning for decreases in access and conflicts of interest in physician–patient relationships.*	**Provider-directed:** • Financial incentives based on achievement of performance goals • Alternative reimbursement systems (e.g., fee-for-service, capitated payments) • Licensure requirements **Health system-directed:** • Initiatives by accreditation bodies (e.g., residency work hour limits) • Changes in reimbursement schemes (e.g., capitation, prospective payment, salaried providers)

Adapted from: Shojania KG, et al. Closing the Quality Gap: A Critical Analysis of Quality Improvement Strategies, Volume 1-Series Overview and Methodology, 2004, http://www.ahrq.gov/downloads/pub/evidence/pdf/qualgap1/qualgap1.pdf.

ment and then link it to an evidence-based menu of appropriate prophylaxis options. Of note, the mere existence of such a tool does *not* ensure its availability at the point of care, its usability, or its actual use. To make such a tool useful, it must be stocked in order-writing locations and be used by admitting physicians. A secondary, logical improvement change may take the form of "Facilitated Relay of Clinical Information," where a pharmacist or nurse notifies the attending physician when a mismatch is discovered between a patient's VTE risk level and the type of prophylaxis ordered.

What is missing from the discipline of quality improvement is a predictive tool—a rational framework to direct decision about what changes to implement, how to sequence them, and how to ensure that they reliably drive desired care.[13] Until such a theoretical base exists, the improvement team must resort to ingenuity, luck, and what experience they can tap from other teams tackling similar problems in similar settings. It also makes sense that, when designing improvement changes, the team should try to include at least one, if not more, of the high reliability strategies in Box 126-1.

Box 126-1 High Reliability Mechanisms

- Desired action is the **default** action (not doing the desired action requires opting out)
- Desired action is **scheduled** to occur at known intervals or events
- Desired action is **standardized** into a process (take advantage of work habits or patterns of behavior so that deviation feels abnormal)
- Desired action is **prompted** by a "decision aide," or reminder
- Responsibilities for desired action are **redundant**

Adapted from: Reason J. Human Error. Cambridge, England: Cambridge University Press, 1990.

Key Points

- Every hospital system is perfectly designed to achieve the results it does; improvement requires change.

- Changes to hospital processes should incorporate high reliability mechanisms while also preserving workflow productivity.

- A multidisciplinary improvement team should integrate the best scientific evidence into the clinical workflow.

- A measurement system must be activated to collect and display data on meaningful metrics.

- The multidisciplinary team should test workflow changes, using a framework for action oriented learning such as the Plan-Do-Study-Act model.

QUALITY IMPROVEMENT LEADERSHIP

Current evidence corroborates what most clinicians may feel instinctively—that we get it "right" in health care only about half the time.[14] Acknowledging this performance gap, accrediting agencies are fostering workforce developmental change by promoting practice-based learning and improvement and systems-based care as core competencies.[15] With hospitalists already recognized as superior teachers on general medicine wards, it seems natural that hospitalists will become the teachers of quality improvement to physicians in training.[16]

The promise of hospital medicine includes advancing hospital care beyond its "state of nature," the unimproved state where care delivery is still not standardized or dependable. Introducing shared baselines or protocols will promote standardization, and using high reliability mechanisms in the clinical workflow should improve dependability. Such changes will require real leadership from real clinicians skilled in the conduct of quality improvement and in demonstrating that higher quality care can indeed control costs. Such changes will also require leaders to have situational awareness—to preserve overall balance while being mindful of the potential pitfalls of "suboptimizing" the hospital system. Multiple improvement efforts can drain resources and ultimately worsen patient safety and quality indicators.[17,18] Careful sequencing and support of multiple quality improvement interventions may prove critical.

The good news is that those of us who sought health care as a career did so for a reason—an inner spark that keeps us caring for those who are sick. The best news is that fanning those intrinsic flames is easy. Leaders of quality improvement will witness dramatic demonstrations of that energy and enthusiasm in many moments: when they sit down with their improvement team, when they communicate a vision, when they supply the tools, when they coordinate across teams, when they remove institutional barriers, and when they celebrate success. Quality improvement leadership is about engaging front-line workers, tapping their fundamental knowledge, and empowering them to improve in their own work assignments and to share that learning with each other.[19]

SUGGESTED READING

Pistoria M, Amin A, Dressler D, et al. Core competencies in hospital medicine. J Hosp Med 2006; 1(S1):92.

Langley GJ, Nolan KM, Norman CL, et al. The Improvement Guide: A Practical Approach to Enhancing Organizational Performance. New York, NY: Jossey-Bass, Inc., 1996.

Wheeler DJ. Understanding Variation: the Key to Managing Chaos. Knoxville, TN: SPC Press, 2000.

Benneyan JC, Lloyd RC, Plsek PE. Statistical process control as a tool for research and healthcare improvement. Qual Saf Health Care 2003; 12:458–464.

Effectiveness and efficiency of guideline dissemination and implementation strategies. Health Technol Assess 2004; 8(6):iii–iv, 1–72. Review.

Shojania KG, McDonald KM, Wachter RM, et al. Closing the quality gap: a critical analysis of quality improvement strategies, volume 1—series overview and methodology, 2004. www.ahrq.gov/downloads/pub/evidence/pdf/qualgapl/quadgap1.pdf. (Accessed January 2007).

Shojania KJ, Grimshaw JM. Evidence-based quality improvement: the state of the science. Health Aff (Millwood) 2005; 24(1):138–150.

Grimshaw J, Eccles M, Tetroe J. Implementing clinical guidelines: current evidence and future implications. J Contin Educ Health Prof. 2004; 24(Suppl 1):S31–7. Review.

McGlynn EA, Asch SM, Adams J, et al. The quality of health care delivered to adults in the United States. N Engl J Med 2003; 348:2635–2645.

Batalden P, Leach D, Swing S, et al. General competencies and accreditation in graduate medical education. Health Aff (Millwood) 2002; 21(5):103–111.

Weiner BJ, Alexander JA, Baker LC, et al. Quality improvement implementation and hospital performance on patient safety indicators. Med Care Res Rev 2006; 63(1):29–57.

Weiner BJ, Alexander JA, Shortell SM, et al. Quality improvement implementation and hospital performance on quality indicators. Health Serv Res 2006; 41(2):307–334.

CHAPTER ONE HUNDRED AND TWENTY-SEVEN

An Overview of Patient Safety for the Hospitalist

Lakshmi K. Halasyamani, MD, and Saul N. Weingart, MD, PhD

BACKGROUND

Medical error became a topic of intense public interest in the United States with the November 1999 release of an Institute of Medicine (IOM) report entitled, *To Err Is Human.*[1] The report summarized existing research, emphasizing the results of several large epidemiologic studies of medical errors in US hospitals.[2-4] Extrapolating from these hospital-based chart review studies, the IOM Committee estimated that 44,000–98,000 Americans per year died in acute care hospitals as a result of medical errors. The report's authors recommended a series of sweeping changes in the way that errors in medicine are reported, analyzed, and prevented. They relied heavily on lessons learned from aviation, manufacturing, and nuclear power; known as "high reliability organizations"[1,5-15] that employ strategies to minimize the rate of mishaps.

Federal and state agencies, regulatory and accreditation organizations, professional associations, and many health care organizations subsequently developed, adopted, and disseminated a variety of improvements and innovations to make health care safer. Spurred on by organizations like the Joint Commission (previously known as Joint Commission on Accreditation of Healthcare Organizations; JCAHO) and the Leapfrog Group (a group of Fortune 500 corporations organized through the Business Roundtable), hospitals were asked to implement a variety of safe practices based on varying degrees of scientific evidence.[16-20]

Recent interest in patient safety has deep historical roots. The Hippocratic injunction of *primum non nocere* (first do no harm) warns physicians about the risk of injury caused by medical care. However, Sharpe and Faden argued that medical error was a taboo subject through much of the late nineteenth and early twentieth centuries. Clinicians and their professional organizations attributed lapses in care to unskilled charlatans with poor qualification to practice medicine.[21] In the 1950s, some clinicians portrayed iatrogenic injury as an unfortunate consequence of advances in medical technology. These "diseases of medical progress" reflected the collateral damage associated with powerful new therapies.[22] Over the subsequent two decades, a series of studies described patients who presented to the hospital as a result of complications associated with their medical care.[23-30]

The current era in patient safety research was ushered in by the Harvard Medical Practice study, a retrospective chart review of over 30,000 admissions to New York State hospitals in 1984. The results of the study showed that injuries due to medical care affected 3.7% of hospitalized patients.[2,31,32] One percent of patients experienced injuries that were due to negligence—care that fell below community standards of practice. In addition to describing the magnitude of patients at risk, this study also highlighted the significant contribution of adverse events due to medications. Adverse events due to medications (adverse drug events) accounted for a large group of adverse events among medical patients. Few demographic characteristics were associated with adverse events, signaling that virtually all hospitalized patients are susceptible to medical injury.

DEFINING ERROR AND ADVERSE EVENTS

Unfortunately, studies of medical error can be difficult to compare if they use different definitions of error and injury. Medical Practice Study investigators defined an adverse event as an injury due to medical care rather than the patient's underlying illness. They set the bar high by requiring that patients suffer a disability, prolonged hospitalization, or death. The Medical Practice Study has been replicated with data from Colorado and Utah, Australia, the United Kingdom, and Canada—all with similar findings.[3,33-35] Subsequent investigators often use a less strict definition of adverse event, qualifying any injury due to medical care as an adverse event. For example, a rash due to penicillin in a patient naïve to penicillin would constitute an adverse (drug) event; it is also an adverse drug reaction. The term adverse drug event does not connote error. However, a subset of adverse events, called *preventable* adverse events are, by definition, injuries due to errors in medical care. For example, the development of a rash in a penicillin-allergic patient whose physician prescribed penicillin constitutes a preventable adverse event.

Investigators have also developed terminology for mistakes that occur but do not result in patient harm. A *potential* adverse event, also called a *close call* or *near miss* error, is a mistake in care that does not result in harm. Some near miss errors are intercepted, for example, when a pharmacist refuses to prescribe penicillin to the penicillin-allergic patient. Other near misses are not intercepted but, by good fortune, result in no injury. Near miss errors are thought to provide important information about possible sources of harm in health care organizations, and have been incorporated into many incident reporting systems.

SYSTEMS AND HUMAN FACTORS

An important breakthrough in understanding medical errors was the appreciation in the 1990s that most errors and injuries are due to problems with the systems of care in health care organizations.[5] In contrast to a traditional view that errors result from poorly trained or poorly performing individuals, the "systems view" identified complexity and poor process design as critical features of error-prone organizations. Rather than training and punishing providers, this perspective directed reformers' attention to complex systems that permit and perpetuate errors.[6–7]

Error theorists have distinguished between *active failures* and *latent conditions*. Active failures are errors that are performed by people (e.g., physicians, nurses) at the point of a service delivery (i.e. patient care). Active failures by professionals at the front lines of patient care can have an immediate impact on safety. In contrast, latent conditions are weaknesses in the organization that can increase the likelihood of active failures and may also affect the magnitude of the consequences of active failures. Examples of latent conditions include poor working conditions, long work hours, complicated processes and procedures, and ambiguous and unpredictable communication expectations and practices. An appreciation for the role of systems and processes in medical error in turn introduced the language of cognitive psychology and human factors science into health care.

When errors and injuries in health care are examined, latent conditions and active failures combine to yield unfortunate but familiar results. For example, when an incorrect medication is administered to a patient, the active failure of drug administration exists within the "medication use system" that may include complex processes of ordering and delivering the medication. In a study of adverse drug events in two academic hospitals, Leape, Bates, and colleagues demonstrated that defects in the system of care accounted for most adverse events.[36]

SAFETY HAZARDS IN ACUTE CARE HOSPITALS

Since the original studies that described the nature and extent of adverse events among hospitalized patients, additional studies characterized vulnerabilities in the care of adult hospitalized patients. Significant attention has focused on injuries due to medications. Studies of adverse drug events have been completed in the acute care hospital, using methods such as clinician surveys and chart reviews. Bates et al. showed that injuries due to medications among hospitalized patients affected 7.3% of patients, and an additional 6.7% of patients experienced near misses.[4]

Another area of vulnerability involves communication among clinicians. Studies by Petersen et al.[37] showed that cross-covering house officer teams make more errors in care than the teams with primary responsibility for the patient. The lapses were attributable to faulty communication among providers, because an enhanced sign-out system eliminated the differences.[38]

The role of sleep deprivation and duty schedules on clinical care is also an area of active investigation. Early studies showed decrements in performance by fatigued house officers on formal pencil-and-paper tests of performance, and in clinical settings that required attention to detail, such as ECG reading and anesthesia monitoring. In a study by Landrigan et al.[38] the research team demonstrated a nearly 36% reduction in serious medical errors

when resident physicians in the intensive care unit went from an every-third-night to an every-fourth-night call schedule, the latter also with shorter shifts.

Technology has been promoted as a solution to diminish errors. Studies by Bates et al.[39] have shown the salutary effect of computerized physician order entry systems on medical errors and adverse drug events among hospitalized patients. This recommendation has been widely embraced. However, electronic order-entry systems that are awkwardly designed or that lack decision support features may provide a false sense of security and introduce new opportunities to make mistakes. Common acute safety hazards in the hospital are summarized in Table 127-1.

Finally, several studies have shown that care transitions increase patients' vulnerability to adverse events.[40,45] Recent work by Rozich and Resar[41] and by Pronovost et al.[42] demonstrated that substantial improvements in the rate of adverse drug events can be attained if clinicians reconcile medications at each transition of care, including admission to the hospital, transfer within the hospital, and discharge to home. This finding resulted in a best practice recommendation adopted by JCAHO.[16] Causes of postdischarge adverse events are not fully understood, although a study by investigators at Columbia University indicated problems with follow-up of inpatient recommendations by primary care physicians. In a study at two academic tertiary-care medical centers, Roy et al.[43] found that more than 60% of test results pending at the time of discharge were not followed up by the physician to whom care was transferred. This occurred primarily because the physician was unaware of the pending test result. In fact, more than 12% of pending test results were identified as requiring "urgent action."[43] Table 127-2 summarizes discharge transition safety issues.

INCIDENT REPORTING

In order to identify targets for improvement, health care organizations must identify and characterize problematic incidents that occur within their walls. To gather this information, hospitals are required by regulators and accreditation bodies to collect reports of specific incidents from front-line staff. These reports may be filled out on paper forms, submitted by telephone, or collected electronically. They are peer-review protected documents collated and analyzed in each hospital's quality or risk management department for trends and patterns.

Some incidents constitute "critical events" or "sentinel events" that the state health department or Joint Commission require to be reported. The Joint Commission, for example, issues alerts when they detect worrisome patterns or hazards. The federal Food and Drug Administration also collects alerts about adverse drug events and incidents related to medical devices and procedures.

Unfortunately, many clinicians fail to report critical incidents.[44] In fact, a study by Cullen et al.[45] showed that incident reporting systems rarely detect the adverse events that are collected using standard research methods. Reasons for low reporting rates are not entirely clear, although some clinicians may fear that reporting errors will result in punishment, stigma, or litigation.[46] In addition to these individual ramifications of reporting critical incidents, some clinicians may stop reporting critical incidents because they were discouraged by the lack of a meaningful institutional response to identified safety issues. A supportive envi-

Table 127-1 Common Inpatient Safety Hazards

Safety Hazard	Examples	Possible Interventions
Medications	• Handwritten orders for medications may lead to inaccurate medications and or dosages dispensed. • Patient may be prescribed and have administered medications he or she is allergic to. • Patients may receive medications that when given together have significant risk for adverse events.	• Implementation of CPOE can decrease errors caused by handwriting medication names and dosages. • Pharmacy checks of medication orders and or computerized alerts can identify important medication allergies and interactions.
Communication among clinicians	• Hand-offs between providers within a hospitalization can lead to loss of information. • Lack of congruent care goals among care providers may lead to ineffective patient care delivery and coordination. • Untimely notification about critical laboratory or diagnostic test results can lead to delays in care.	• Development of standardized care transition templates may improve information transfer and highlight important data. • Use of daily goal sheets may help to coordinate care among providers. • Implementation of web-based paging systems to alert appropriate clinicians of abnormal test results may decrease care delays.
Sleep deprivation and fatigue	• Physician fatigue from lack of sleep can contribute to the number and types of medical errors that occur.	• Enforcement of work hour restrictions decreases the number of errors committed.
Patient identification	• Patients with similar sounding or spelled names may receive interventions or medications meant for another patient.	• Use patient verification strategies that are more unique to an individual—such as birthdate or Social Security number. • Alerts in the unit may help to increase awareness that patients with the same or similar spelled names are on the unit.

CPOE—Computerized Physician Order Entry

ronment on the work unit is associated with higher rates of reporting.[47]

As health leaders recognize the value of incident reports for informing quality improvement, many organizations have begun to develop novel approaches to safety reporting. Near misses or close call reporting systems modeled on NASA's Aviation Safety Reporting System have attracted attention as opportunities to learn from incidents where there was no injury and hence no liability. The US Veterans Health Administration implemented a near-miss reporting system based on the NASA model.

Health care organizations can use incident reports to understand safety hazards and to develop improvements in care. Organizations often use techniques such as root cause analysis (RCA) or failure mode and effects analysis (FEMA) to analyze events, uncovering the latent conditions that made them possible.[48,49] RCA and FMEA methodologies can be educational for the participants and lead to improvement projects. Incorporating input and feedback from front-line staff is useful for identifying safety issues and can also lead to the development and successful implementation of meaningful interventions.

ROOT CAUSE ANALYSIS

Root cause analysis (RCA) provides a systematic method for analyzing critical incidents and near misses with a high potential for harm in a manner that focuses on the system-based root causes and contributing factors and not on the individuals involved in the event. Root cause analyses are conducted as part of a peer-review protected process and involve assembling all of the individuals involved in the incident under review. Effective RCAs identify underlying human and system factors that contributed

to an unsafe incident. Hospitalists may participate in RCA discussions and may help to identify gaps in existing care delivery as well as propose remedies that may lead to improved safety.

FAILURE MODES AND EFFECTS ANALYSIS

Failure Modes and Effects Analysis (FMEA) is another tool adapted from other industries and used in health care to identify gaps and problems in care delivery and then determine corrective action steps. Similar to RCA, FMEA is conducted by an interdisciplinary team familiar with the issue being analyzed. In contrast to RCAs, which are conducted retrospectively, an FMEA is usually undertaken before an adverse event occurs.

After a high-risk process is selected, the team identifies potential "failure modes" and for each failure mode describes possible effects on the outputs of the process. The group then identifies the "root causes" of the failure modes determined by the group to be most critical to the process outcome. The group goes on to examine current process controls in place, redesigns the process to minimize the risk of that failure mode, tests and implements the redesigned process, and ultimately implements measures of effectiveness and a strategy for maintaining the effectiveness of the redesigned process over time. RCA and FMEA are complementary analytic tools used to improve patient safety; Table 127-3 summarizes their similarities and differences.

PATIENT SAFETY REGULATION AND ACCREDITATION

As patient safety has become recognized as a major health policy problem in the United States and abroad, state regulators and

Table 127-2 Best Practices for Transitions in Care

1.1 Clinician Handoffs
- The literature does not endorse any particular method or style of communication.
- Pantilat et al. surveyed clinicians to determine communication preferences and satisfaction with interactions with hospitalists.*
  - Of 1,030 respondents, 77% of receiving MDs stated they would "very much prefer" to communicate by phone at both admission (73%) and at discharge (78%).
  - The second most preferred method of communication was face-to-face communication, followed by email, which was relatively unpopular.

1.2 Discharge Summary
- The emerging expert consensus is that a clear and uniform format for discharge summaries should be implemented after being agreed upon by key hospital staff members.
- In Pantilat's study, the majority of respondents rated the following elements as very important to include in discharge summaries:
  - Discharge medications (94% rated it very important)
  - Discharge diagnosis (93%)
  - Results of procedures (80%)
  - Scheduled follow-up with primary care MD (76%)
  - Results of laboratory tests (73%)

1.2.1.1.1 Continuity Visits
- A continuity visit is defined as either:
  - a) an inpatient visit of the patient by his/her primary care MD
  - b) the first postdischarge visit by the MD that coordinated the inpatient care, rather that the primary care MD
    - A clinical encounter between PCP and hospitalized patient allows the primary care MD to:†
    - Learn first hand the details of the hospitalization
    - Provide insights to the hospital team about aspects of the patient's history that may be relevant to inpatient care
- A second type of continuity visit is one that occurs when the inpatient provider of record conducts the first outpatient visit, rather than the PCP.
  - Van Walraven et al. studied a cohort of adults who were seen after discharge either by the physician who cared for them as an inpatient, their community doctor, or a specialist.‡
  - The authors found that *with each postdischarge visit by a hospital physician, the adjusted relative risk of death or readmission decreased by 5%* as compared to a postdischarge visit with either community doctor or specialist.

1.2.2 Follow-up Telephone Calls After Discharge
- Follow-up telephone calls by nurses have a positive effect on patient satisfaction and adherence to follow-up appointments and discharge instructions.
  - Dudas et al. conducted a randomized trial in which patients received follow-up telephone calls by a pharmacist 2 days after discharge. Patients who spoke with a pharmacist reported greater satisfaction with discharge medication instructions than controls (86% versus 61%, P = 0.007).§
  - *Patients who received a follow-up telephone call from a pharmacist were less likely to have subsequent emergency department visits (10% versus 24%, P = 0.005).*

*Pantilat S, Lindenauer P, Katz P, et al. Primary care physician attitudes regarding communication with hospitalists. Am J Med 2001; 111:15S–20S.

†Wachter R, Pantilat S. The "continuity visit" and the hospitalist method of care. Am J Med 2001; 111:40S–43S.

‡Van Walraven C, Mamdani M, Fang J, et al. Continuity of care and patient outcomes after hospital discharge. J Gen Intern Med 2004; 19(6):624–631.

§Dudas V, Bookwalter T, Kerr K, et al. The impact of follow-up telephone calls to patients after hospitalization. Am J Med 2001; 111:26S–30S.

Table 127-3 Summary of Similarities and Differences between RCA and FMEA

Similarities	Differences
- Focus on system issues - Involve interdisciplinary teams - Use a variety of QI tools such as brainstorming, flow diagrams, cause and effect diagrams and scoring systems - Lead to development of action steps - Lead to the development of measurable outcomes	- RCA emphasizes fundamental conditions or processes that exist and contribute to the incident, rather than generating a list of ways the process can fail (both real and theoretical). - RCA flowcharts are primarily used to document chronology of events rather than processes. - FMEA emphasizes testing interventions more than RCA.

QI = Quality Improvement; RCA = Root Cause Analysis; FMEA = Failure Modes and Effects Analysis

accreditation agencies have taken increased interest in this area. Many state health departments have developed incident reporting systems and coalitions with hospitals, health professional organizations, and other stakeholders in building safer systems of care. However, state health departments have to balance the tension between the development of an open, sharing environment that promotes the identification of critical incidents and their legal responsibility to ensure the public accountability of health care organizations. As a result of this tension, the regulatory approach, often punitive in nature, is difficult to reconcile with the nonpunitive, systems-based approach to understanding and preventing medical error. State health departments and boards of registration in medicine, nursing, and pharmacy continue to play an important role in the licensing of health facilities and health professionals, and in ensuring standards of organizational and professional competence.

The Joint Commission has played a major role in driving patient safety improvements in the United States.[1] Their accreditation standards and national patient safety goals outline requirements in communication of critical results, safe use of medications, and accurate patient identification (e.g., to require health care organizations to implement a variety of safe practices and to monitor their own performance in this regard) (Table 127-4). In a recent survey, health administrators reported that the Joint Commission was the major impetus to patient safety improvement in their organizations.[50] The Joint Commission has been increasingly interested in care transitions and improving medication safety with their emphasis on medication reconciliation and information transfer across the continuum of care.

Other organizations have also played an important advocacy role for the development and implementation of patient safety improvements. The Accreditation Council on Graduate Medical Education (ACGME) has identified core competencies for all graduates of residency training programs. These include competencies in practice-based learning and systems-based improvement, areas linked to quality improvement in patient safety.[51] In addition to including education about error prevention and analysis in the residency curriculum, the ACGME has mandated work-hour restrictions to reduce errors related to fatigue and sleep deprivation.

The transparency advocated by state and federal regulatory organizations is in stark contrast to the possible medicolegal ramifications of disclosing medical errors. Legal theorists argue that the threat of litigation encourages doctors to practice safely, since individuals (persons or institutions) are held accountable for negligent injuries. In contrast, patient safety leaders argue that negligence plays little role in clinical practice. They argue that we should focus on understanding systems of care so that vulnerabilities (i.e., latent conditions that increase the risk of harm) can be identified and re-engineered. The physician is in an awkward position—interested in improving the systems that make care safer, but at the same time recognizing that

Table 127-4 Selected Patient Safety Goals

Organizations	Description	Selected Goals
The Joint Commission (previously know as the Joint Commission on Accreditation of Healthcare Organizations or JCAHO)	Selected items from the 2006 JCAHO Patient Safety Goals www.jointcommission.org/PatientSafety/NationalPatientSafetyGoals/	Standardize list of abbreviations, acronyms, and symbols that are not to be used throughout the organization Implement a standardized approach to "hand off" communications, including an opportunity to ask and respond to questions Implement a process for obtaining and documenting a complete list of the patient's current medications upon the patient's admission to the organization and with the involvement of the patient A complete list of the patient's medications is communicated to the next provider of service when a patient is referred or transferred to another setting, service, practitioner, or level of care within or outside the organization
Leapfrog Group	The Leapfrog Group is a coalition of large employers who encourage public reporting of health care quality and outcomes so that consumers and purchasing organizations can make more informed health care choices. www.leapfroggroup.org/	Computer physician order entry Evidence-based hospital referral Intensive care unit (ICU) staffing by physicians experienced in critical care medicine Ensure that written documentation of the patient's preference for life-sustaining treatments is prominently displayed in his or her chart Ensure that care information, especially changes in orders and new diagnostic information, is transmitted in a timely and clearly understandable form to all of the patient's current healthcare providers who need that information to provide care
100K Lives Campaign	This Campaign, sponsored by the nonprofit Institute for Healthcare Improvement, enlists hospitals across the country in an effort to implement changes in care that have been proven to prevent avoidable deaths. www.ihi.org/IHI/Programs/Campaign	Deploy rapid response team at the first sign of patient decline Deliver reliable, evidence-based care for acute myocardial infarction . . . to prevent deaths from heart attack Prevent central line infections by implementing "central line bundle" Prevent ventilator-associated pneumonia by implementing "ventilator bundle" Prevent adverse drug events by implementing medication reconciliation

reporting of errors may make him or her vulnerable to malpractice litigation.

Brennan and others have advocated for compensation of patients and families harmed by unsafe systems of care, by rectifying systems rather than punishing individuals.[54] However, until these reforms or reforms like these occur, a focus on transparency may increase litigation. Although the advocates of transparency have reported that disclosure decreases the probability of litigation, there has been no rigorous analysis of its effect on litigation rates or malpractice awards.[55,56]

CONCLUSION

Hospitalists have a potentially important role to play at the nexus of providing clinical care while working to improve the systems within which they work. In addition to focusing on the individualized clinical care they provide, hospitalists have an opportunity to lead efforts to improve care and patient safety. By understanding the nature and causes of medical error, hospitalists can help incorporate clinical advances in the safe and effective delivery of care at the bedside.

EXAMPLE CASE STUDY

LG is a 76-year-old man who was admitted in the middle of the night through the emergency department (ED) with shortness of breath. He has a history of chronic obstructive pulmonary disease (COPD) and heart failure (HF) and was evaluated for a possible myocardial infarction. The patient's primary care physician, Dr. Jones, admits his patients to the Academic Internal Medicine (AIM) Hospitalist Service. The night float resident evaluates the patient, enters orders, and then goes to see another admission.

The patient's family who accompanied the patient to the ED has gone home and did not meet the night float resident. They know that LG's primary care physician is Dr. Jones, so they expect that Dr. Jones will be the one caring for their family member in the hospital.

The night float resident speaks to the incoming resident, Dr. Smith, at 7 a.m. about the patient and then goes home to get some sleep. At 7:15 a.m., the patient becomes acutely short of breath and is hypoxic. Initially, the night float resident is paged, but does not answer because his shift is over. The patient becomes more dyspneic, and a respiratory code is called. The code team rushes in to see the patient. However, no one in the room is familiar with LG's clinical issues.

Dr. Smith, the team resident, comes into the room and realizes that LG was a patient who had been handed off to him earlier that morning. He looks at his sign-out paper and sees that LG has multiple medical issues. The nurse reports that his labs from midnight had revealed a large myocardial infarction, but no one had checked the results. The resident sees that the labs are not listed on the patient's sign-out.

The patient is moved to the Coronary Care Unit (CCU), where a new medical team takes over the patient's care, and the CCU resident, Dr. Thomas, begins his evaluation of the patient. In the CCU, the patient's daughter has arrived and is visibly upset by the events that have occurred overnight. After evaluating the patient,

Dr. Thomas calls the cardiology attending, who sends the patient to the cardiac catheterization laboratory for intervention.

Meanwhile, the patient's daughter waits at her father's bedside and is not clear about all of the doctors involved in her father's care. She is still wondering where her father's Primary Care Provider (PCP)—Dr. Jones—is and whether he knows what is going on with her father (see Box 127-1 for case analysis).

Box 127-1 Case Analysis

Critical Incident	Delay in diagnosis
Latent conditions	Multiple admissions throughout the night (work load)
	No notification from the laboratory or nurse about abnormal test result (processes of information transfer)
	Discontinuous care with hand-offs between providers (processes of information transfer)
	Ambiguity about roles of clinicians involved in care (role clarification)
	Gaps in identifying the correct physician currently caring for the patient (procedures to identify covering physician)
Active Failure	Failure to check pending laboratory results
Possible Interventions Identified through FMEA	Development of workload standards and triggers for the deployment of additional support and resources.
	Development of policies and procedures for communication of abnormal test results
	Development of sign-out templates and checklists to decrease information loss and decay at points of care transfer
	Implementation of communication systems that facilitate the prompt identification of the correct covering physician.

Key Points

- Understanding errors may lead to improvement in inpatient safety.

- Increasing federal and state regulations focus on improving patient safety and decreasing medical errors.

- Hospitalists can lead patient safety efforts and participate in processes to improve clinical care delivery.

SUGGESTED READING

Bates DW, Cullen DJ, Laird N, et al. Incidence of adverse drug events and potential adverse drug events. JAMA 1995; 274:29–34.

Devers KJ, Pham HH, Liu G. What is driving hospitals' patient-safety efforts? Health Affairs 2004; 23:103–115.

Gaba D, Structural and organizational issues in patient safety: A comparison of health care to other high-hazard industries. California Management Rev 2000; 43:83–102.

Leape LL. Error in Medicine. JAMA 1994; 272:1851–1857.

Leape LL, Bates DW, Cullen DJ, Cooper J, Demonaco HJ, Gallivan T, et al. Systems analysis of adverse drug events. JAMA 1995; 274:35–43.

Leape LL, Berwick DM. Five years after To Err Is Human: what have we learned? JAMA 2005; 293:2384–2390.

CHAPTER ONE HUNDRED AND TWENTY-EIGHT

Establishing a Teamwork Model of Care for Inpatient Medicine

Joseph A. Miller, MS, Joseph L. Dorsey, MD, MPH, and Jody Hoffer Gittell, PhD

INTRODUCTION

Many organizations have staff whose tasks are highly interdependent, but who, due to functional or disciplinary boundaries between them, achieve only low levels of coordination, with negative effects on both quality and efficiency performance. Health care organizations tend to fall into this category. According to one observer, "Coordination of [health] care, for which personnel are constantly striving but know they are not often attaining, is something of a mirage except for the most standardized of trajectories. Its attainment is something of a miracle when it actually does occur."[1] A recent Institute of Medicine report (2003) identified poor coordination as a key weakness of the current health care system, while a recent Commonwealth Fund report[2] documented lack of care coordination as one of the most common concerns cited by physicians.

WHAT IS COORDINATION?

Coordination, the management of task interdependence,[3] has long been argued to be critical for organizational performance. Indeed, economists and others proclaim that one of the reasons that organizations exist is to facilitate the coordination of work.[4,5] Researchers have found that coordination enables organizations to improve performance along multiple dimensions simultaneously. In particular, improved coordination enables high-quality outcomes to be achieved simultaneously with the efficient use of resources. This phenomenon, labeled "lean production," has been demonstrated in automobile design and assembly,[6] in the design of mainframe computers,[7] in steel production,[8] in apparel production,[9] in air travel,[10] and in health care delivery.[11-14]

The type of coordination needed to achieve these desirable outcomes depends on the type of *task interdependence.*[15] See Figure 128-1 for an illustration of the three principal types of task interdependence. The most complex form of task interdependence—reciprocal interdependence—occurs when there are feedback loops between the tasks being performed by different people. Information that results from the performance of one task needs to be incorporated into the performance of another task, and vice versa. This reciprocal form of task interdependence depends on frequent and high-quality communication among the people who are assigned to perform the tasks at hand.

Much organizational research verifies the importance of communication for coordinating work. For example, Ancona and Caldwell[16] and Keller[17] found that communication by team members was positively related with team performance; and Gant, Ichniowski, and Shaw[18] found stronger, denser communication ties in higher performing steel production plants. Although important, communication by itself may not be sufficient for coordinating work. The people whose tasks are most interdependent often have different areas of functional specialization, as in the case of doctors, nurses, physical therapists, and social workers who are working with the same patient. Organizational scholars have shown that people in different functions tend to be divided in several essential ways. They are often focused on different goals;[19] they often live in different "thought worlds,"[20] and they tend to be part of a pecking order in which they compete for status and respect.[21,22] As a result, their "relationships" are often characterized by the *lack* of shared goals, shared knowledge, and mutual respect.

These relationships can be a problem for coordination[20,23] Even frequent, timely information may not be heard or acted upon if the recipient lacks shared knowledge or shared goals with the source and therefore misunderstands or is not motivated to act upon the information. With shared goals and shared knowledge about the process, participants are better able to react to changing circumstances in a concerted fashion, without the need to discuss each detail. With mutual respect, participants are more likely to account for the impact of their actions on those who are engaged in a different part of the process. For successful coordination to occur, frequent, high-quality communication needs to be reinforced by high-quality relationships.

The *theory of relational coordination* argues that effective coordination is based on frequent, timely, accurate, problem-solving communication, *underpinned and reinforced by* relationships of shared goals, shared knowledge, and mutual respect.[24] Figure 128-2 illustrates how these relationships reinforce communication and how communication in turn helps to reinforce these relationships. As seen in Figure 128-2, this self-reinforcing cycle of relational coordination can result in either high or low levels of relational coordination. Relational coordination in turn is associated with significant improvements in efficiency and quality outcomes in both air travel[10,25] and in health care delivery.[13]

The critical question to be answered is, how can organizations increase levels of relational coordination? Coordinating mecha-

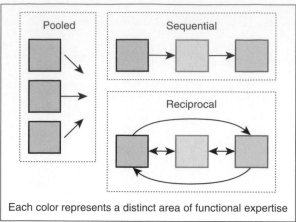

Figure 128-1 • Types of Task Interdependence. Each color represents a distinct area of functional expertise.

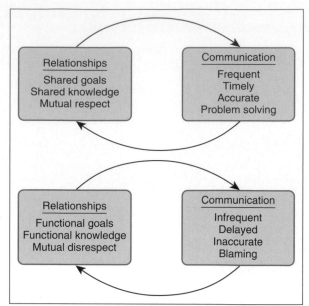

Figure 128-2 • High versus Low Levels of Relational Coordination.

nisms have been identified that play this role (*see* Fig. 128-2). *Routines* or protocols facilitate coordinated action by prespecifying the tasks to be performed and the sequence in which to perform them. Routines capture the lessons learned from previous experiences, enabling a process to be replicated without reinventing the wheel.[26] They also serve as a source of connections among people who work together.[27] Clinical pathways play this role in health care organizations. *Boundary spanners*, also known as cross-functional liaisons, are individuals whose primary task is to integrate the work of other people.[28,29] They integrate work that crosses functional boundaries. Case managers play this role in health care organizations. *Team meetings* give participants the opportunity to coordinate tasks directly with one another. According to organization design theory, team meetings increase performance of interdependent work processes by facilitating interaction among participants, and they are increasingly effective under conditions of high uncertainty.[29,30] Interdisciplinary rounds play this role in health care organizations.

A nine-hospital study showed significant positive effects of these three coordinating mechanisms on the level of relational coordination found between doctors, nurses, physical therapists, social workers, and case managers.[31] Both higher levels of relational coordination and superior quality and efficiency outcomes were found on units that had invested in more inclusive clinical pathways, more inclusive interdisciplinary rounds, and in smaller caseloads for case managers, enabling them to play a more proactive role in coordinating patient care.

RESEARCH RESULTS

The recent growth of hospitalist programs prompts the question, "What is the impact of this physician staffing model on levels of relational coordination among members of the patient care team?" A recent study of the hospitalist program at Newton-Wellesley Hospital in Massachusetts found two interesting results.[32] First, patients whose attending physician was a hospitalist had significantly better risk-adjusted outcomes, including shorter lengths of stay, lower total costs per admission, and lower readmissions in 7 and 30 days. These results are more comprehensive than those found by other studies of hospitalist perfor-

mance, but they are largely consistent with previous findings. The second result is more interesting, in some ways, given that it sheds light on the *reason* for the hospitalist advantage. Hospital staff members assigned to patients attended by hospitalists *reported significantly higher levels of relational coordination with each other, and particularly with the physician on the team*. These hospitalist-led teams reported higher scores on every dimension of relational coordination: higher frequency of communication with each other regarding the patient; greater timeliness of communication; greater accuracy of communication; more problem-solving communication; as well as higher levels of shared goals, shared knowledge, and mutual respect.

THE HOSPITALIST CHALLENGE

What is the basis of this apparent hospitalist advantage? We should start by understanding what a hospitalist does. Inpatient medicine can be defined by the following activities: admitting, diagnosing, treating, managing, coordinating, and discharging hospitalized patients. Inpatient medicine is often complex due to multiple factors.

- The *patient care process* involves many health care providers (e.g., physician specialists, nurses, case managers, physical therapists, etc.) and departments (e.g., intensive care, laboratory, radiology, dietary, social work, etc.).
- *Clinical knowledge* (e.g., disease states, diagnostic tools, medications, therapeutic interventions, best practices, etc.) is specialized and constantly changing; an attending physician must be current on clinical information in many specialty fields.
- The variability and primitive nature of many *communication systems* make it difficult to get information about, get information from, communicate information to, and make decisions with patients and their families.
- *Hospital operating systems* (e.g., procedures, information systems, protocols, reviews, etc.) are often unique, such that a physician's learning about them cannot be readily transferred from one hospital to another.

Table 128-1 How the Hospitalist Model Fosters Teamwork

Unique Characteristics of Hospitalists	How the Characteristic Fosters Teamwork
Consistent presence in a specific hospital	Familiarity with the hospital's providers, departments, systems, procedures, and pressures Opportunity to interact frequently and easily with other team members at key decision points
"Single-minded" focus on managing inpatients	Greater inpatient clinical knowledge and stronger inpatient clinical skills Familiarity with postdischarge options, health plan rules and regulations, etc. Respect of other team members
Organization as a cohesive group	Implementation of consistent practices, structured schedules, and formal communication schemes Shared work load, frustrations, and world view leading to empathy, mutual support, and opportunity to speak with a unified voice

- Physicians who practice inpatient medicine must be familiar with the broad range of *post-discharge alternatives* (e.g., rehabilitation hospitals, skilled nursing facilities, extended care facilities, home health care, community services, etc.).
- There are many *hospital-specific pressures* with regard to financial performance, nursing shortages, throughput, uncompensated care, outdated equipment and facilities, and the quest for improved electronic information systems.
- There is a need to address *environmental pressures* such as at-risk contracts, health plan utilization review, patient safety, and patient privacy.
- At academic hospitals, physicians must also be aware of and aligned with the *teaching* and *research missions* of the institution.

The work of inpatient medicine is clearly arduous and complex. Teamwork or relational coordination might therefore be particularly important in the hospital setting to increase job satisfaction and to protect individual hospitalists from the occasional onslaughts of work that can lead to burnout.

DOES THE HOSPITALIST MODEL FOSTER RELATIONAL COORDINATION, AND IF SO HOW?

The research cited above suggests that the hospitalist model results in higher levels of relational coordination among members of the patient care team, and that these higher levels of relational coordination may be the explanatory factor behind greater efficiency and higher quality outcomes. How does the hospitalist model work, and which aspects of it are likely to foster teamwork and relational coordination?

In the past 10–15 years, the hospitalist model evolved as an alternative to the community physician as the attending physician responsible for hospital care of patients. The hospitalist model has three distinguishing characteristics (Table 128-1):

- Hospitalists have a consistent and intense presence in a specific hospital.
- The work of hospitalists is, for the most part, treating inpatients.
- Hospitalists are part of a cohesive physician group.

A strong theoretical case could be made that these *three characteristics innately lead to a higher degree of teamwork for hospitalists,* as compared to community physicians that see their patients in the hospital. And greater teamwork could result in superior performance.

- *The hospitalist's consistent presence in a specific hospital* is likely to result in a high degree of familiarity with the health care providers, departments, systems, procedures, and pressures particular to the specific institution. A hospitalist is on site throughout the day, allowing for multiple points of decision and the opportunity to interact frequently and easily with other members of the patient's care team.
- *A hospitalist's "single-minded" focus on managing inpatients* means that he or she is likely to have greater inpatient clinical knowledge and stronger inpatient clinical skills ("practice makes perfect"). Also, hospitalists are likely to be more familiar with postdischarge options, health plan rules and regulations, and other issues that surround the patient care process for inpatients. As a result, the members of the health care team may look to the hospitalist as a knowledgeable, competent team leader.
- *The organization of hospitalists as a cohesive group* increases the likelihood that they will work closely with each other and with other hospital-based staff. A hospitalist group is likely to implement consistent practices, structured schedules, and formal communication schemes. Perhaps more importantly, as members of a group, hospitalists "live" together professionally, sharing the workload, and combating the same inefficiencies and frustrations. This can lead to empathy and support of their "teammates" and the realization that to get things changed, it helps to speak with a single, unified voice (i.e., to truly be a team).

HOW HOSPITALISTS CREATE A CULTURE OF TEAMWORK

This theoretical case for greater coordination and teamwork by hospitalists is reinforced by the actions and practices of hospitalist programs around the country. At conferences and in publications, the efforts of hospitalists to create a team-oriented and coordinated process of treating patients in the hospital have been widely presented and documented. Examples include the following:

- When he was President of the Society of Hospital Medicine, Jeff Dichter, MD, wrote a column in the SHM newsletter entitled "The Culture of Teamwork."[33] He described how hospitalists create this culture by developing a shared set of values—values related to standards of care, expectations for professional conduct, common goals, a bias toward evidence-based decision making, mentoring, and the measurement of individual and group performance. Dr. Dichter referred to hospitalists creating "a group culture that places the health of the team as a first priority . . . team members that have confidence and faith in each other." When there is a culture of teamwork, hospitalists are willing to speak out if there are "wrong-minded" (non-teamwork) attitudes.

- Many hospitalists develop, implement, and/or employ clinical protocols and guidelines in their day-to-day responsibilities of managing inpatient care. These protocols and guidelines are a good example of the "routines" previously referenced in this paper (prespecified, sequenced tasks built to ensure conformance with best practices). Routines are another vehicle that facilitate coordination and teamwork, by clarifying roles and responsibilities.

- Although the models vary significantly from program to program, hospitalists formally implement a variety of strategies to maximize inpatient team communication. One particularly effective strategy (although often not feasible at many hospitals) is to physically locate the hospitalists and an assigned team of nurses, case managers, and other providers on a specific unit of the hospital. Another effective communication strategy used by some hospitalist programs is the daily meeting with case management, reviewing each case and agreeing on goals for the inpatient stay. Other hospitalist programs round with other members of the provider team, coordinating a multidisciplinary effort to treating the patient.

- It is critical that hospitalists and primary care physicians (PCPs) have a sense of teamwork. This can be fostered by conveying the cooperative relationship of hospitalists and PCPs in verbal communications to patients and in written materials that describe the hospital medicine program. Furthermore, hospitalist–PCP teamwork will be maximized when there are structured communication processes and expected standards for timely communication at critical milestones during the inpatient stay, most specifically on admission and discharge.

- Hospitalists are increasingly becoming leaders of the medical staffs at their hospitals. They participate in and often chair key (cross-functional) hospital committees, including those related to utilization review, patient safety, and pharmacy. Hospitalists also often participate in or lead hospital projects—projects such as information system implementation, throughput analysis, and JCAHO reviews. In these leadership roles, hospitalists must be team players, getting members of their committees and/or projects to work together.

- At hospitals with house staff, hospitalists often create another level of team-oriented behavior. The house staff can handle much of the time-consuming work of organizing and carrying out patient care. In exchange, the hospitalist can serve as a mentor, providing clinical knowledge, disseminating practical advice, and serving as a role model. Many hospitalists find this a gratifying aspect of their work, as ideas are exchanged on

---

Box 128-1 Teamwork Toolkit for Hospitalists

- Create a culture of teamwork within the hospital medicine group by establishing:
  - Shared values related to standards of care
  - Common expectations for professional conduct
  - Team goals
  - General but clear workload expectations
  - A bias toward evidence-based decision making
  - Mentoring
  - Measurement of individual and group performance
- Implement clinical protocols and guidelines that clarify the roles and responsibilities of the inpatient team
- Devise strategies to maximize inpatient team communication
  - If possible, physically locate the hospitalists and an assigned team of other providers on a specific unit of the hospital
  - Conduct daily meetings with case management, reviewing each case and agreeing on goals for the inpatient stay
  - Round with other members of the provider team, coordinating a multidisciplinary effort to treating the patient
- Ensure there is teamwork between the hospitalist and the PCP
  - Convey the cooperative relationship of hospitalists and PCPs in written materials and in verbal communications to patients
  - Implement structured communication processes and expected standards for timely communication between the hospitalist and the PCP
- Become leaders of the hospital medical staff and get key inpatient "players" to work together
  - Participate in and chair key (cross-functional) hospital committees (e.g., utilization review, patient safety, and pharmacy)
  - Participate in or lead hospital projects (e.g., information system implementation, throughput analysis, and JCAHO reviews)
- Engage house staff in the team approach
  - The house staff can handle much of the time consuming work of organizing and carrying out patient care
  - The hospitalist can serve as a mentor, providing clinical knowledge, disseminating practical advice, and serving as a role model.

how to evaluate cases and how to communicate with patients and their families. Hospitalists can guide the trainees in addressing the most difficult situations.

CONCLUSION

Fostering teamwork (relational coordination) is very much a part of the hospitalist model. The intrinsic nature of hospitalist staffing seems to foster teamwork through a small group of physicians attached to a single hospital for an extended period of time with a single-minded focus on inpatient medicine. Furthermore, hospitalists often take the initiative to reinforce teamwork through a variety of mechanisms, tools, strategies, and roles/responsibilities.

These factors together help to explain the above-cited results from the Newton-Wellesley Hospital study, in which hospital staff members assigned to patients attended by hospitalists reported significantly higher levels of relational coordination with each other, and particularly with the hospitalist leading the team. As noted above, these hospitalist-led teams reported higher scores on every dimension of relational coordination: higher frequency of communication with each other; greater timeliness of communication; greater accuracy of communication; more problem-solving communication; as well as higher levels of shared goals, shared knowledge, and mutual respect. We expect to see these results duplicated for other hospitalist programs around the country.

Key Points

- Teamwork, or relational coordination, has been shown across multiple industries to positively affect performance.

- Hospitalists achieve superior performance with regard to resource utilization, and some studies indicate hospitalists deliver higher quality of care.

- A theoretical argument can be made that the unique characteristics of the hospitalist model innately lead to a higher degree of teamwork.

- By implementing the mechanisms, tools, strategies, and roles/responsibilities outlined in the "Teamwork Toolkit," hospitalists can achieve higher degrees of teamwork and improved performance outcomes (Box 128-1).

SUGGESTED READING

Dichter J. Teamwork and hospital medicine: a vision for the future. The Hospitalist 2003; 7(3):4–5.

The culture of teamwork. The Hospitalist 2003; 7(4):4–6.

Teamwork: experiences from "the front lines." The Hospitalist 2004; 8(1):4–5.

Gittell JH. The Southwest Airlines Way: Using the Power of Relationships to Achieve High Performance. New York: McGraw-Hill, 2003.

Miller JA. How Hospitalists Add Value. The Hospitalist 2005; 9(Supp1):3–35.

Audet AJ, Doty MM, Shamasdin J, et al. Physicians views on quality of care: Findings from the Commonwealth Fund National Survey of Physicians and Quality of Care. The Commonwealth Fund, 2005, 1–108.

Feldman MS, Rafaeli A. Organizational routines as sources of connections and understandings. J Manage Stud 2002; 393:309–331.

Gittell JH. Relational coordination: coordinating work through relationships of shared knowledge, shared goals and mutual respect. In: Kyriakidou O, Ozbilgin M, eds. Relational Perspectives in Organization Studies. Oxfordshire, U.K.: Edward Elgar Publishers, 2005.

Fairfield K, Bierbaum B, et al. Impact of relational coordination on the quality of care, post-operative pain and functioning, and the length of stay: a nine-hospital study of surgical patients. Med Care 2000; 38(8):807–819.

Institute of Medicine. Crossing the Quality Chasm: A New Health System for the 21st Century. Washington, DC: National Academies Press, 2001.

Young G, Charns M, et al. Patterns of coordination and clinical outcomes: study of surgical services. Health Services Research 2000; 33:1211–1236.

CHAPTER ONE HUNDRED AND TWENTY-NINE

Patient Flow and Hospital Throughput

Burke T. Kealey, MD

BACKGROUND

The days of excess hospital capacity and empty beds are over. Competition for space is intense in almost every hospital in the country. High-revenue elective procedural cases vie with unscheduled medical care of the indigent for health care's most precious resource—the hospital bed.

Since 1990, the number of general hospitals has shrunk 12% to 4,862, while the number of total hospitals has followed a similar trend, declining more than 12% to 5,810.[8] All current demographic data point to a sharp rise in the average age of the population well into the 21st century. If we look at current days of hospital care by age-group, we see those aged 65–74 years have a 96% higher utilization rate than those aged 55–64 years. Those aged 55–64 years have a 67% higher utilization rate than those aged 45–54 years.[9] This combination of falling bed counts with rising numbers of Americans requiring more hospital care indicates that demand for hospital beds may get worse.

Overcrowded emergency departments are the most visible sign of a system breaking down. The March 2003 General Accounting Office (GAO) report focusing specifically on emergency department (ED) crowding points to likely etiologies. The most identified factor was the lack of available inpatient beds, both monitored and unmonitored. Key findings from a 2004 American Hospital Association (AHA) survey show that 50% of hospital EDs perceive they are "at" or "over" operating capacity. The situation was even worse in urban hospitals, where 80% of hospitals reported severe congestion.[3]

Hospitals increasingly "run full," keeping as many beds occupied as possible. While on the surface this may seem healthier for the hospital's bottom line, it is at the expense of the hospital's traditional built-in surge capacity. Loss of this surge capacity markedly affects current imperatives to improve quality, patient safety, and patient satisfaction. Both patient safety and satisfaction suffer when congestion and throughput problems force elective surgery cancellations and admitted patients to receive hospital care on gurneys in the ED. Box 129-1 lists some of the chronic problems and maladaptive behaviors caused by overcrowding in hospitals.

So, the problem is before us, but solving it is no simple matter. Some of the factors involved boil down to how health care and current market forces incentivize behaviors. Other factors involve places in the continuum of care that lie outside the hospital walls,

like clinic and nursing home access and availability. Nevertheless, there are strategies that can be used to impact the situation positively. This chapter will discuss some best practices that are currently being used successfully by hospitals and health care systems across the country. Of note, these are only a sampling of the many solutions being tried. Organizations like the Institute for Healthcare Improvement (IHI) and the Advisory Board are hard at work partnering with hospitals to try innovative approaches to patient flow. The first time, the Joint Commission for Accreditation of Healthcare Organizations (JCAHO) has established standards for patient flow (Box 129-2).

STRATEGIES

Develop a Hospitalist Program

The first way that hospitalists improve flow is simply through the inherent clinical efficiency in the care model itself. As multiple studies document, hospitalists enhance efficiency of care. On average, hospitalists typically reduce length of stay (LOS) by 15%. Hospitalists' efficiencies can be leveraged even further when they co-manage patients with specialists and surgeons, thereby affecting care delivery throughout the hospital. Additionally, some hospital systems (e.g., Kaiser) use hospitalists to facilitate triage in the ED, with resultant decreases in hospital admissions and more appropriate utilization of outpatient resources.

Develop Hospitalist Leaders

A higher-level strategy for hospitals, above merely reaping the benefits of a hospitalist program's better clinical throughput, involves developing strong hospitalist leaders. This expands beyond having a strong lead hospitalist to developing each and every hospitalist physician and/or provider as a leader in overall hospital care.

Hospitalists live at the virtual center of the hospital. They work at the entrance points, at the points of major decision-making, and at the departure points. Dealing with almost every department and specialty in the hospital, experienced hospitalists typically earn the respect of colleagues in all hospital disciplines, including nursing, social services, case management, pharmacy, physical and occupational therapy, as well as their physician colleagues in the ED, intensive care units (ICUs), and surgical floors.

Box 129-1 Sequelae of Congestion

- **Internal Diversion**—Patients are sent to floors/ICUs where the nursing skill set does not match the diagnosis.

- **Internal Delays**—Post-Anesthesia care unit and ED backup waiting for beds to open on the floors

- **External Diversion**—ED's divert patients to other facilities.

- **Staff Overloaded and stressed**—Increased patient mortality and increased staff burnout.

- **Gridlock**—Nobody moves and nobody leaves. LOS rises; overall number of patients cared for drops.

- **Lost Revenue**

Box 129-2 2006 JCAHO Leadership Standards for Managing Patient Flow: Elements of Performance. From the Joint Commission on Accreditation of Healthcare Organizations

1. Leaders assess patient-flow issues within the hospital, the impact on patient safety, and plan to mitigate that impact.

2. Planning encompasses the delivery of appropriate and adequate care to admitted patients who must be held in temporary bed locations, for example, postanesthesia care unit and emergency department areas.

3. Leaders and medical staff share accountability to develop processes that support efficient patient flow.

4. Planning includes the delivery of adequate care, treatment, and services to nonadmitted patients who are placed in overflow locations.

5. Specific indicators are used to measure components of the patient-flow process and address the following:
   - Available supply of patient bed space
   - Efficiency of patient care, treatment, and service areas
   - Safety of patient care, treatment, and service areas
   - Support service processes that impact patient flow

6. Indicator results are available to those individuals who are accountable for processes that support patient flow.

7. Indicator results are reported to leadership on a regular basis to support planning.

8. The hospital improves inefficient or unsafe processes identified by leadership as essential to the efficient movement of patients through the organization.

9. Criteria are defined to guide decisions about initiating diversion.

With essential support from the chief executive officer (CEO) and vice president of medical affairs (VPMA), hospitalists can lead and develop partnerships with the multiple hospital departments to achieve success in any flow initiatives. See Chapter 124 for acomplete discussion of Leadership in Hospital Medicine.

Get Your CEO and VPMA on Board

Is the CEO on board? Does the VPMA understand who must be influenced? Not just a hospital-centric view, but a system-wide view of capacity management with clear lines of responsibility and accountability is critical to improving flow through the hospital. Executive level leadership must be present to effect change in the hospital.

If the hospital CEO has not made capacity management a priority, it will be difficult, if not impossible, to successfully align the resources and secure the support necessary for successful improvement. The CEO is the one individual with the responsibility and influence to cross borders between all departments and successfully encourage necessary change. Hospitalists can help the CEO to understand what role congestion is playing in negating other efforts in the hospital to improve quality, safety, and satisfaction.[1]

The VPMA works with all physician groups, across all specialties in the medical staff, and serves the crucial role of obtaining physician buy-in and cooperation. As a vital partner, the VPMA understands and can interpret the culture, behaviors, and interests of the medical staff to sponsor physician change related to flow activities.

Manage Variability in Demand

There are two types of variability that take place in hospitals. The most visible is called *Natural Variability*—what we might see on a daily or seasonal basis, when there is a surge of emergency department patients during flu season or traumas on a holiday weekend night.

Dr. Eugene Litvak and his colleagues at Boston University School of Management have defined a second more insidious type of variation, called *Artificial Variability*—demand created artificially by conscious human effort (unconsciously causing bottlenecks and congestion). For example, typical scheduling of surgical cases keeps the operating rooms packed early in the week to allow discharge by Friday and diminish weekend rounding

duties. This heavy influx of elective cases often happens at the same time there is a heavy unpredictable (but natural) influx of emergency cases. Hospitals can greatly decrease the risk from a natural surge by not allowing artificial surges to happen. One solution is to create a rational surgical block scheduling system to smooth out the flow of these cases[7] throughout the week.

Create Super Systems-of-Care, Not Super Providers

All too often, things function well in a hospital because of a motivated, knowledgeable, experienced "super-provider." When this high-functioning individual quits or happens to be ill during a surge in volume, operations break down, and often quickly. Systems must be created which allow anyone stepping into a position to function in the highest fashion.[1] Systems should support the overall goal of moving patients effectively through the system, and whenever possible the system should be automated (Box 129-3).

Implement a Discharge Appointment System

A discharge appointment system is one approach to capacity management suggested by the Institute for Healthcare Improvement, based on successful implementation at a number of facili-

Box 129-3 Examples of System Strategies to Improve Patient Flow

- Bedside ED registration
- Advanced triage protocols
- Written nursing reports
- Clinical pathways with enforcement
- Discharge appointments
- Admission and discharge "SWAT" teams
- Inbox messaging across handoffs

ED—emergency department

ties across the country. The physician initially predicts the day of discharge soon after admission, and then, as the discharge day approaches, selects a more exact discharge "appointment" time. Importantly, the rest of the health care team, the patient, and his or her family provide essential input into this decision.

The appointments (think of them as one would a scheduled clinic appointment) are set up by the unit care team based on their known patient mix (surgical patients tend to be more predictable) and optimal spacing for decreased congestion. The primary goal of a system that assigns discharge slots is to reduce large clusters of discharges, especially at times when there is already a lot of activity on the floor, like nursing shift change. The discharge appointments garner the secondary gain of stimulating more discussion of discharge planning and promoting more open sharing of the process, especially with the patient and his or her family.

As more thought is put into each discharge, gains are made in several areas that directly and indirectly affect the flow of patients through the hospital. A certain segment of patients will be identified who can be discharged late in the day, rather than spend the night and go home the next morning. Also, data analysis at most facilities indicates that the historical approach to the discharge process yields a large cluster of discharges in the few hours surrounding nursing shift change. Admissions often peak at this time too! This flux, in and out of a unit, concurrent with nurses switching, results in chaos and inefficiency. Moving some discharge slots either before or after shift change will yield less congestion. Additionally, advanced discharge planning systems can tie known discharges to incoming elective cases.

An initial goal for those setting up a discharge appointment system is to aim for 80% of discharges actually occurring within 60 minutes of the appointment.

But what about "Everyone out by 11 a.m."? This attractive idea has been tried many times before in hospitals throughout the country, mostly based on the familiar lament, "If we could only get the doctors to write the discharge orders early . . ." While historically doctors have not made discharging patients in a timely fashion a priority, "out by 11" ignores the realities that many patients simply cannot be discharged by that time; additional testing and consultation are often needed on the last hospital day. This approach also promotes the antiquated idea of "watching one more night" rather than utilizing the last day in the hospital productively, and then discharging the patient in the late afternoon or evening once all of his or her diagnostic and therapeutic treatments are complete.[1]

Engage the Health Care Community at Large

Looking beyond the hospital itself allows interaction with all aspects of throughput. Just as the ED is often congested by the lack of monitored and floor beds, the hospital as a whole is often overwhelmed by the influx of patients seeking help ("inputs") and also limited by the lack of appropriate facilities to send patients upon discharge ("outputs"). Again, hospital leadership must reach out and engage leaders from other care settings in a dialog to help improve flow both in and out of the hospital.

On the input side of the equation, clinics that refer to a hospital can greatly decrease the number of patients ending up in an emergency department by developing better chronic disease-management programs and aggressively managing "frequent flyers." They can also consider implementing so-called advanced access systems, where clinics guarantee that they can see their own patients on a same-day basis. The end result is that the most familiar provider is seeing and managing the patient's problems before they get out of control, requiring an ED visit and possible hospitalization.

On the outgoing side of the equation, transitional care, skilled nursing facilities, hospice, and home care all must have appropriate capacity to accept patients coming out of the hospital. Agreements may be negotiated whereby capacity is reserved through bed-holds in a given facility. Another possibility is investing in a hospital-owned private facility or home care agency to better handle the demand coming out of the hospital.[1]

MEASUREMENT

Develop a Culture of Routine Measurement

"You can't manage what you don't measure." Nowhere is this more evident than in a modern hospital, especially in regard to hospital throughput and congestion. The only way to know and understand what is happening is to actively measure and monitor all flow processes simultaneously. This must be adopted into the culture of every department, and information must be shared among all groups, particularly the CEO and the board. If you are not measuring performance, you are not serious about solving your capacity problem.[1]

The Hospital Flow Diagnostic

The Hospital Flow Diagnostic put forth by IHI serves as a good place to start measuring. An in-depth discussion of the diagnostic is beyond this chapter, but, simply put, it measures how efficient a hospital is at turning beds around. It can also give information on the types of issues that might be involved in a given hospital's throughput problem.[6] The two measures are:

Adjusted bed turns—The number of times the average bed is turned over in a given year in a hospital. Greater than 90 is a good number. If too low, focus on smoothing surgical scheduling and getting beds ready more quickly for the next patient.

Formula:

Adjusted Bed Turns = {(Admissions × Case Mix Index) + Observation cases} all divided by functional beds in the hospital

Figure 129-1 • Flow diagnostic: adjusted turns versus utilization "Where's my dot?" Source: Institute for Healthcare Improvement. Hospital Flow Diagnostic. Online information retrieved April 4, 2007. http://www.ihi.org/IHI/Topics/Flow/PatientFlow/EmergingContent/Hospital/iagnostic.htm

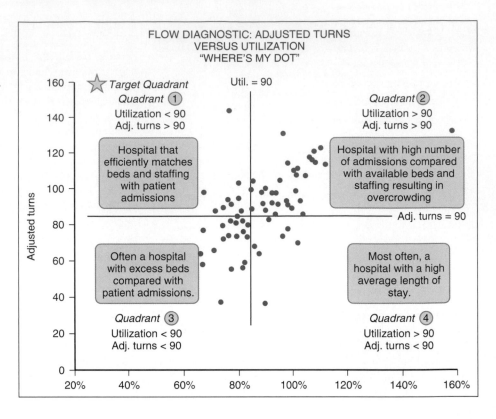

Utilization efficiency—How efficient a hospital is at turning a bed around and filling it again. Less than 90 is a good number. If too high, focus on measures to decrease length of stay.

Formula:

Unadjusted bed turns (same as above, but no CMI adjustment) divided by potential bed turns (365/aggregate length of stay).

Plot the numbers obtained for each measure, and see where your hospital falls (Fig. 129-1). The position on the graph shows what type of flow problems you may have. Figure 129-2 shows strategies on how to move your dot into the most favorable category, Quadrant 1.

SPECIFIC GOALS FOR YOUR HOSPITAL

Analyze your own situation for key bottlenecks or areas that need process improvement and close monitoring. Sample specific goals to consider:
• ED door to MD evaluation <20 minutes for 75% of patients
• Bed request to patient departure from ED <30 minutes
• Inpatient bed turnaround times <60 minutes
• 80% of discharges within 60 minutes of a specific appointment time

These are only a sampling, but they give an idea of the nature of measurement required to try and understand if progress is being made.[1]

COMMON PITFALLS

1. Focusing on the ED's "problem"
   Remember the ED is only a symptom of the rest of the hospi-

tal. Adding ED beds is not the answer. Improving access and flow in the rest of the hospital *is* the answer.
2. Creating a committee to go off and fix flow. The CEO and VPMA are critical to success. This means active management on their part. A regular staff committee will not have the authority or scope necessary to influence all of the areas that must be engaged to solve flow problems.
3. Extreme reverence for sacred cows
   Avoiding problem areas, because some people might get upset is not an excuse. Throughput cannot be improved unless all areas of the hospital step up to improve.
4. Ignoring Artificial Variability in Demand
   Focusing on the obvious problem of natural variation is mostly an exercise in futility. Focusing on variation that we do to ourselves is smart.
5. Not measuring
   Swimming upstream is hard enough. Swimming with blindfolds on is impossible. Measure what you are doing, and then pat yourself on the back as you see the improvement numbers roll in.

SUMMARY

Our population is aging and requiring more health care services every year; at the same time, we are seeing declining numbers of hospital beds in this country. We cannot build ourselves out of this problem, but we must learn to become more efficient stewards of our hospitals.

Active leadership and fearlessness in the face of enormous obstacles are essential to recreate the modern hospital into a safe and highly efficient delivery vehicle of outstanding quality health care.

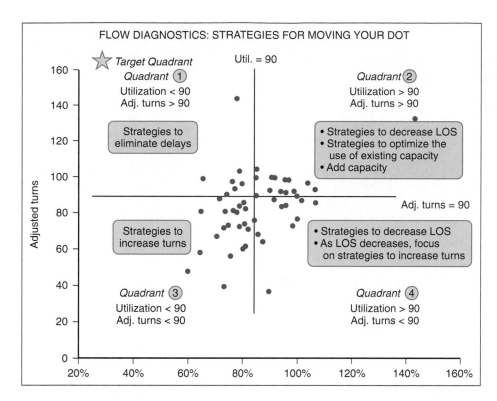

Figure 129-2 • Flow diagnostic: strategies for moving your dot. Source: Institute for Healthcare Improvement. Hospital Flow Diagnostic. Online information retrieved April 4, 2007. http://www.ihi.org/IHI/Topics/Flow/PatientFlow/EmergingContent/Hospital/iagnostic.htm

Box 129-4 List of Other Ideas to Investigate
Occupancy reality audit
Clinical decision units
Electronic bed boards
Preemptive diagnostics
Physician discharge advisor
Day before discharge planning
Difficult discharge team
Ticket home
Multidisciplinary rounds
Preadmission planning for elective surgery
Strict utilization criteria for specialty beds
Eliminate bed-holds
Develop a rapid room cleaning and bed turnaround program
Acuity adjustable beds

Key Points

• Executive Leadership support is crucial for successful improvement of patient flow.

• Focus on planned variation, especially surgical scheduling. It's not just the Emergency Department affecting throughput.

• Develop a hospitalist program with each physician being an engaged leader of improving the system.

• Measure and monitor what you are doing.

• There are lots of ideas out there! Find what fits for your hospital.

Creativity and an unrelenting focus on improvement are needed. New ideas come forth every year from many different organizations (Box 129-4). Pick some, and begin work.

Hospitalists are poised in many ways to help lead the charge as proven stewards of precious resources. They are placed at the center of the hospital and have developed far-reaching influence into many other departments. Lastly, as the field of hospital medicine continues to evolve, so too will hospitalists transition into the natural leaders of hospital systems, teamwork, and improvement efforts.

SUGGESTED READING

Asplin B, Kealey, BT. Throughput and congestion in the modern hospital. The Hospitalist 2004; 8(5):14–17.

General Accounting Office. Hospital Emergency Departments: Crowded Conditions Vary Among Hospitals and Communities. Washington DC: General Accounting Office, 2003.

Hospital Capacity and Emergency Department Diversion: Four Community Case Studies. Hoboken NJ: AHA Survey Results, 2004.

JCAHO's New Leadership Standard on Managing Patient Flow. Washington, DC: JCAHO Leadership Standards, 2005.

Litvak, Long, Cooper, et al. Emergency department diversion causes and solutions. Acad Emerg Med 2001; 8(11):1108–1110.

Nolan, Thomas. The Hospital Flow Diagnostic. Presentation, IHI. 2005.

Program for management of variability in health care delivery. http://management.bu.edu/research/hcmrc/mvp/index.asp.

Recent Trends and Their Impact on Cost and Quality of Care Healthcare Industry Overview. Oakbrook Terrace, IL: White Paper, Porter Research & Solutions, 2003.

U.S. Department of Health and Human Services Centers for Disease Control and Prevention, National Center for Health Statistics. Health, United States. 2002.

CHAPTER ONE HUNDRED AND THIRTY

Strategies for Standardizing Care and Applying Evidence to Practice

Scott Weingarten, MD, MPH

BACKGROUND

Efforts abound to improve the quality, safety, and efficiency of patient care; and many of these initiatives focus on the care of the hospitalized patient (see Chapters 125–127 and 129). Organizations such as the Joint Commission on Accreditation of Healthcare Organizations (JCAHO), the Center for Medicare and Medicaid Services (CMS), the National Quality Forum (NQF), and the Leapfrog Group have been integrally involved with advancing these efforts.[1] As a result, quality measures have proliferated, and clinical information to enable the comparison of hospital performance has become publicly available. The majority of the quality indicators are process of care measures (e.g., use of angiotensin-converting enzyme inhibitors or angiotensin II receptor blockers for heart failure), but a few relate directly to patient outcome (e.g., mortality rate for acute myocardial infarction).[2] Process measures are less dependent on differences in case complexity (e.g., severity of illness) than outcome measures; outcome measures often require adjustment for severity of illness and comorbid conditions to facilitate the meaningful interpretation of this information.

Attempts are often made to ensure that the process measures are "evidence-based," meaning that there is a strong scientific correlation between the process measure and a specific outcome (e.g., ACE inhibitors for patients with heart failure are associated with a lower mortality rate). Often the evidence (Table 130-1) is based on systematic reviews of the literature, meta-analyses, meta-regressions, or randomized controlled trials. However, in certain cases (e.g., early antibiotics for patients hospitalized with community-acquired pneumonia), randomized controlled clinical trials can be either impractical or considered unethical, and the empirical evidence base might be derived from retrospective studies. Furthermore, subspecialty societies may promote guidelines for "best care," and these guidelines may be translated into quality indicators with explicit definitions for numerators and denominators. The development of these measures has enabled the medical, nursing, and quality improvement leadership at many hospitals and health systems to focus their quality improvement efforts in specific areas, and to track their progress longitudinally over time.

"Pay for Performance" programs have also proliferated, which creates a "business case" for hospitals to devote resources toward quality improvement efforts. Hospital executives can estimate the financial benefits and potential "return on investment" for implementing improvements in patient care. For example, the Premier Hospital Quality Incentive Demonstration program enables selected hospitals to increase reimbursement from CMS for selected Medicare patients with predefined medical and surgical conditions by potentially up to 2% per condition. The Leapfrog Group, a coalition of large employer groups, has cataloged "Pay for Performance" programs of payers and purchasers of health care on their website (www.leapfroggroup.org). Many health plans across the United States include "Pay for Performance" reimbursement for physician groups and physicians.

BARRIERS TO THE EFFECTIVENESS OF CINICAL DECISION SUPPORT

As hospitals attempt to demonstrate improvements in care, they have relied on various tools including practice guidelines, clinical pathways, care maps, protocols, and order sets—referred to here generally as clinical decision support. These tools have met with varying degrees of success, ranging from minimal changes in care to significant improvements. Although practice guidelines and clinical pathways were originally felt to hold great promise for improving care, their successful implementation with a heterogeneous group of physicians, nurses, pharmacists, and other clinicians has been difficult. Pathways can be created, but if they are ignored by practicing clinicians, they will result in little measurable benefit. An Institute of Medicine report described this challenge with the axiom that "practice guidelines do not implement themselves." Without successful implementation, there will be no improvements in care or "return on investment" from creating guidelines and pathways.

A number of barriers to the successful implementation of clinical decision support exist. The intended audience for guidelines, order sets, and clinical pathways includes a large and diverse medical, nursing, and clinical staff, which can number in the hundreds to thousands, depending on the size of the hospital or health system. Many physicians hospitalize their patients in more than one hospital and may not feel sufficiently motivated to adopt a hospital's clinical pathway or preprinted order set. Even in cases in which physicians desire to comply with a particular order set or clinical pathway, they might be unfamiliar with the existence or content of an order set or clinical pathway.

Table 130-1 Sample Grading Scheme for Evidence Class

Class of Evidence	Type of Study
M	Meta-analysis
S	Systematic review
A	Randomized controlled trial
B	Nonrandomized prospective study
C	Retrospective study
Q	Cost study (e.g., cost-benefit, cost-effectiveness)
E	Expert opinion

Box 130-1 Important Considerations of a Clinical Decision Support System

- Comprehensiveness (breadth and depth)
- Timeliness (frequency of updates)
- Methodology (e.g., evidence-based)
- Scientific foundation
- Integration with clinical information systems
- Intuitive

This concern may be mitigated by the use of hospitalists, who treat a higher volume of hospitalized patients each year, although there are limited data to support or refute this belief at present. Some hospitalist training programs include educational programs about quality improvement and utilization management, which may contribute to the success of these efforts.

Another challenge to implementing clinical decision support is enabling busy clinicians to remain current about the content of a particular guideline or clinical pathway. Most studies show that continuing medical education programs fail to produce sustained changes in clinical practice. The greatest opportunity to improve care occurs when physicians receive relevant context-specific patient information during the course of caring for patients. For example, if a physician is treating a patient with acute myocardial infarction and a depressed left ventricular ejection fraction, information about the efficacy of ACE inhibitors should be specific to that patient population, rather than information about the efficacy of ACE inhibitors in general.

Even if successful implementation has been accomplished, methodologic challenges can hamper the ability to objectively evaluate the impact of quality improvement programs and clinical decision support. Many published evaluations of quality improvement activities include a time series design or "before and after" studies (comparing the care of patients before and after the introduction of a clinical pathway). In many cases, it is unclear whether an observed change or patient care improvement was associated with a quality improvement program or was consistent with secular changes in patient care that were occurring independently of the quality improvement effort. Understanding the impact of a quality improvement program on patient care is essential for sustaining clinician enthusiasm for the program.

INFORMATION TECHNOLOGY

Information technology has gathered steam as a potential long-term solution for enabling clinically meaningful and sustainable improvements in quality and safety of care.[2-9] A recent study of approximately 4,000 hospitals showed that a majority of hospitals have either implemented computerized physician order entry (CPOE), purchased CPOE, or were planning to purchase CPOE in the future. In the United States, federal programs could make health care information technology more affordable for hospitals and physicians' offices, since price can be an obstacle to the widespread deployment of CPOE.

Studies have shown that clinical information systems and CPOE can improve the quality and safety of patient care in areas such as the reduction of medication errors, improvements in drug dosing, and improvements in preventive care.[2-8] The available research suggests that improvements in the treatment of patients through CPOE and clinical information systems are greater than improvements in the diagnosis of patients with complex conditions.[3] Importantly, much of the research has been conducted in teaching hospitals with faculty members, residents, interns, and medical students. The impact of CPOE in nonteaching community hospitals with physicians in private practice is less well known.

Clinical decision support (Box 130-1) informs decision-making by clinicians for individual patients, by providing relevant information that could influence the care of those patients. Real-time clinical decision support enables context-specific information to be provided at the "point of care." The clinical decision support could be provided as order sets, alerts, structured documentation, and other forms that can be integrated into clinical information systems.[9]

Influencing clinical decisions will be critical to deriving measurable clinical benefits and a "return on investment" from health care information technology. Moreover, clinical decision support must be acceptable to clinicians and perceived as beneficial to their patients for it to be acceptable to physicians and other clinicians. Many individuals are proposing that tools such as order sets and alerts be derived by using the principles of evidence-based medicine to support their scientific validity and credibility with clinicians. If clinical decision support is based on strong scientific evidence, it may be easier to gain clinician acceptance. Also, scientific evidence, quality indicators, and "pay for performance" criteria change over time to reflect advances in the underlying science and the practice of medicine (Table 130-1). Finally, as order sets and alerts are used in day-to-day practice of medicine, physicians, nurses, and pharmacists will provide clinical feedback that can be used to improve these strategies.

Clinical decision alerts (e.g., if a patient with acute myocardial infarction is about to be discharged without aspirin, an alert will appear that reminds the physician about the potential benefits of aspirin for this patient population) can provide significant benefits. Without a sufficient number of alerts, it may be difficult to achieve clinical and economic benefits and a "return-on-investment" from clinical information systems. However, if a large number of alerts interrupt the care of physicians caring for patients, many with a low level of specificity (a high "false positive" rate), some physicians may experience "alert overload" and ignore many of the alerts. It will be important to balance the potential benefits of alerts with potential declines in clinician productivity from "too many" alerts.

More is becoming known about the utility of clinical decision alerts. In a randomized clinical trial, physicians in an intervention group (n = 1,255 eligible patients) were alerted about each patient's risk of deep venous thrombosis, while physicians in the control group (n = 1,251 patients) were not.[6] Physicians were required to acknowledge the alert prior to deciding whether to provide or withhold prophylaxis for deep venous thrombosis. Clinically confirmed deep venous thrombosis occurred more frequently in the control group than the intervention group (8.2% vs. 4.9% of patients) at 90 days, a 41% reduction in the risk of deep venous thrombosis or pulmonary embolism.[6]

In many hospitals, clinical leaders and clinicians will participate in processes to ensure that clinical decision support systems remain scientifically valid and evidence-based (see Table 130-1). These clinicians will also be charged with updating and maintaining these systems, as order sets and alerts contain perishable information that require frequent monitoring. If clinical decision support contains information that is not consistent with the medical literature, or is considered outdated or inaccurate by practicing clinicians, credibility with the clinical staff may be lost. Disciplined processes will be required to ensure that the decision support is vigilantly maintained. Since there are hundreds of medical articles published each day, since new drugs are approved by the Food and Drug Administration (FDA) every year, and since drugs are occasionally withdrawn by the FDA, maintenance of the information can be a daunting task. Efforts to ensure the validity and timeliness of this information will require the involvement of many clinicians.

Summarized below are specific steps in the implementation of an effective clinical decision support system, barriers to implementation, necessary aspects of measurement, and common pitfalls.

SPECIFIC STEPS IN THE IMPLEMENTATION OF EFFECTIVE CLINICAL DECISION SUPPORT SYSTEMS

1. Create an interdisciplinary committee, including physicians, nurses, pharmacists, and other clinicians, to oversee the clinical decision support development and maintenance process.
2. Identify and prioritize clinical conditions for clinical decision support.
3. Inform the creation of clinical decision support, including order sets, alerts, and structured documentation, with relevant scientific information.
4. Work with groups of clinicians to achieve consensus about the content of the clinical decision support.
5. Define the processes to update and maintain content (e.g., how often will the clinical decision support be reviewed and updated?).
6. Identify processes to enable urgent updates if needed (e.g., when a drug is recalled by the Food and Drug Administration).
7. Integrate the clinical decision support with clinical information systems.
8. Deploy the clinical decision support system.
9. Receive feedback from physicians, nurses, pharmacists, and other clinicians.

10. Measure impact on the quality, safety, and efficiency on patient care.
11. Clinician feedback, new scientific literature, and the results of implementing the clinical decision support can be used to update and improve the information.

POTENTIAL BARRIERS TO CLINICAL DECISION SUPPORT IMPLEMENTATION

1. The price of some clinical information systems
2. The performance (e.g., speed) of some clinical information systems
3. Acceptance of clinical information systems by clinician (Clinician acceptance might be greatest if the information system is intuitive and can potentially enhance clinician productivity.)
4. Insufficient resources to update and maintain order sets and alerts
   (Updating and maintaining clinical decision support requires significant dedicated internal resources, including physicians, nurses, pharmacists, and developers, or working with an outside clinical content vendor.)
5. Challenges of integrating clinical decision support into clinical systems, to ensure that the clinical decision support functions as planned in the clinical system (e.g., alerts can fire reliably based on patient-specific information)

MEASUREMENT

Ability to measure components of care with existing information technology:
1. Quality
2. Safety
3. Efficiency

COMMON PITFALLS

1. Insufficient number of order sets, alerts, and other forms of clinical decision support
2. The clinical decision support is based on general clinician consensus, rather than the broader scientific evidence, and therefore the acceptance of the clinical decision support by a diverse clinician base is poor.
3. Failure to plan the integration of preprinted order sets, pathways, and guidelines with clinical information systems
4. Lack of a consistent and systematic process to manage and update order sets and alerts
5. Failure to update order sets and alerts when clinically important results are published in the medical literature

SUMMARY

Clinical leaders within hospitals strive to reduce undesirable variations in care, improve quality of patient care, reduce unnecessary medical costs, and enhance their "pay for performance" reimbursement. Efforts to improve care will require effective strategies that influence the clinical decisions that are made on a daily basis by physicians, nurses, pharmacists, and other clinicians. During the past decade, previous attempts to influence clinical decisions have involved the creation of practice guidelines, protocols, clinical pathways, preprinted order sets, and other forms of paper-based clinical decision support. In many cases, the information contained in these tools was not supported by scientific evidence and not updated in a timely manner. Moreover, some past quality improvement efforts have met with mixed results because ineffective implementation strategies were utilized, and it was unclear whether the quality improvement efforts accelerated changes in clinical care.

With the recent proliferation and adoption of clinical information systems, clinical decision support will become increasingly integrated with clinical systems and expressed as computer-based order sets, alerts, and reminders. Many clinical leaders will be required to develop, customize, maintain, and update clinical decision support in the future. These efforts hold great promise for improving quality, safety, and efficiency of care, and for improving the health of populations of patients.

Key Points

- Many efforts currently underway to improve the quality, safety, and efficiency of patient care focus on reducing undesirable variations in care and ensuring that clinical care is more systematic and consistent with the best available evidence.

- Current approaches to improving quality and efficiency include the use of predeveloped order sets, clinical pathways, alerts, and other forms of clinical decision support, often designed for paper-based medical records.

- The development and adoption of computerized physician order entry (CPOE) and electronic health records (EHRs) promise to converge with these approaches by increasing the effectiveness and sustainability of quality improvement efforts across hospitals and health systems.

- Hospital care has been a major focus of the improvement of quality and efficiency, as many hospitals have the resources, infrastructure, evolving information technology base, and incentives to stimulate these efforts.

- Research and practical experience demonstrate that physician, nursing, and other clinical leadership is essential to the success of attempts to influence clinical practice and improve the quality of care. In the near future, many clinical leaders will be called upon to spearhead efforts to improve the care of hospitalized patients.

SUGGESTED READING

Williams SC, Schmaltz SP, Morton DJ, et al. Quality of care in U.S. hospitals as reflected by standardized measures. N Engl J Med 2005; 353:255–264.

Garg AX, Adhikari NJ, McDonald H, et al. Effects of computerized clinical decision support systems on practitioner performance and patient outcomes: A systematic review. JAMA 2005; 293:1123–1138.

Hunt DL, Haynes RB, Hanna SE, et al. Effects of computer-based clinical decision support systems on clinician performance and patient outcomes: a systematic review. JAMA 1998; 280:1339–1346.

Kaushal R, Shojania KG, Bates DW. Effects of computerized physician order entry and clinical decision support systems on medication safety: a systematic review. Arch Intern Med 2003; 163:1409–1416.

Dexter PR, Perkins S, Overhage JM, et al. A computerized reminder system to increase the use of preventive care for hospitalized patients. N Engl J Med 2001; 345:965–970.

Kucher N, Koo S, Quiroz R, et al. Electronic alerts to prevent venous thromboembolism among hospitalized patients. N Engl J Med 2005; 352:969–977.

Rothschild J. Computerized physician order entry in the critical care and general inpatient setting: a narrative review. J Crit Care 2004; 19:271–278.

Dexter PR, Perkins S, Overhage JM, et al. A computerized reminder system to increase the use of preventive care for hospitalized patients. N Engl J Med 2001; 345:965–970.

Bates DW, Gawande AA. Improving safety with information technology. N Engl J Med 2003; 348:2526–2534.

CHAPTER ONE HUNDRED AND THIRTY-ONE

Assessing Patient Satisfaction in the Hospital Setting

Woodruff English, MD, MMM, and Deirdre E. Mylod, PhD

Hospitalists are expected to be familiar with hospital quality and satisfaction measures. This chapter introduces key concepts for assessing patient satisfaction in the hospital setting. Because external reporting of hospital patient satisfaction is imminent, attention will be given to the standardized written survey.

BACKGROUND FOR INDIVIDUAL KEY CONCEPTS

Know the Difference Between Subject and Function

Quality measures have subject and function. The subject being measured is either a process or an outcome. Almost all patient satisfaction surveys are quality measures of process. All patient surveys are subjective and measure how patients view their care.[1] The function, or purpose, of the measure is either internal or external to the hospital. The critical decision in designing a patient satisfaction survey is to clarify its function (i.e., purpose).

Establish the Function of the Survey

If the purpose of the survey is to improve a clinical or service process, this is a quality improvement function and is internal to the organization. As an internal function, it can also be used for strategic planning and development of new services. When the purpose is to report to parties external to the hospital, this is considered an accountability function. As an external function, the patient satisfaction scores become part of the hospital's "report card" for the consumption of accrediting and regulatory entities, payers, and the general public. Critics of the "report card" function point out that there is no standard scoring system or benchmark among all hospitals at this time.

Choose an Instrument Appropriate to the Function

There are three classes of survey procedures for assessing patient satisfaction: focus group, telephone survey, and written survey. A *focus group* can help you to understand what it is like to be a patient and can probe for beliefs, attitudes, and desires. The focus group is relatively inexpensive. The chief strength is that it allows you to understand the patients' experiences in their own words,

but can lack generalizability, especially if only one focus group is performed. Ideally, three or more should be conducted until repetition of responses occurs.

Telephone surveys can be as valid as written surveys, can provide a personal contact that contributes to the patients' ultimate satisfaction, can follow up on loose ends after discharge, and can allow for branching (i.e., customize the interview by following an algorithm that asks only questions relevant to the interviewee). The chief advantages are a personal touch and a high response rate. The chief weakness is the high expense and the potential for respondents to feel less comfortable offering constructive criticism.

Written surveys can cover a wide range of patients' experiences; they have well-established scientific validity, and they can create a solid database by efficiently sampling a large number of patients. There are two types of written surveys: targeted and standardized. Targeted written surveys for support of quality improvement and other internal purposes are similar to telephone surveys and are not used for external functions and accountability reports. The standardized written survey is more complex than a targeted survey and is a necessary part of hospital management. More discussion is dedicated to standardized survey structure in the "Implementation" section of this chapter. The chief strengths of written surveys are lower cost and anonymity of patient response. The chief weakness is a lower response rate, but they can still yield representative data.

For both telephone and written surveys, the value of statistical inference is dependent upon how representative the sampling frame is and upon the use of appropriate controls. Any survey that will be benchmarked against other institutions will also require adherence to standardized format for data collection. Excellent examples of telephone and simple written survey methods are in the literature.[2-4] Respecting the limited scope of this chapter, we mention the value and application of these methods in Table 131-1, without describing the details of how to conduct such assessments.

Use an Instrument That Is Reliable and Valid

The method of sampling, the design of the questions, and the representation of the data should be reliable and valid. This is especially important for written surveys that have an external function. There are rigorous methods for testing the validity of a

Table 131-1 Characteristics of Survey Methodologies

Type of Survey	Advantages	Limitations	Applications
Focus Group	**Personal** Gives understanding and detail	**Limited topic and participants** **Not standardized** Does not benchmark	**Internal function** Strategic planning for a new or broken product or service
Telephone Survey	**Timely** Rapid turnaround, clarify details (e.g., actual doctor), Can do follow up, fix oversights, create satisfaction	**More Expensive than mail** More costly per the number of returned surveys **Acquiescence bias** Patients do not feel anonymous and may be uncomfortable offering honest criticism	**Internal or external function,** Improve quality, rapid feedback on a changing process, can identify individual hospitalists and respondents
Standardized Written Survey	**Inexpensive, creates large database,** Can assess across all aspects of care, scientific validity, Best tool for benchmarking	**Lower response rate than phone** Smaller proportion of sampled patients return the survey **Must wait for surveys to be mailed back**	**Internal or external function,** Institutional accountability, benchmarking tool, process metric for continuous monitoring

survey instrument.[3] Without the discipline of assessing for validity, you cannot have confidence that your survey process is in fact measuring what you think it is measuring.

The elements of a valid survey instrument include:

- A tested instrument (questionnaire) with appropriate demonstration of reliability and construct validity[3]
- A format with appropriate survey wordings and scale
- Appropriate statistics for reporting and representing data

The method of sampling must fit the situation:[4]

- Adequate sample size (at least 30 responses per subsample of interest (e.g., per month or per physician, etc.)
- Accurate creation of sampling frame (i.e., the universe from which the sample is drawn).

The representation of the data (analysis) must be appropriate:[3]

- Appropriate controls and benchmarks (internal and external)
- Use of appropriate statistics to assess relationships and change over time

HOSPITAL INFORMATION SYSTEMS CAN BE LIMITING

Few hospitals have effective, clinically oriented databases. Often, clinical events cannot be tracked unless the procedure was a billable event. When one physician with a UPIN number (a billing code) is listed for a patient, the hospital's requirement for submitting billable charges has been met. Subsequently, there is no driving incentive to update the record if a new physician takes over the care of the patient. The hospital information system can misidentify the actual treating physician when patient satisfaction data must link with a specific physician.

Be Aware of Scope and Context

Some of the major conceptual areas included in patient surveys include: nursing care, physician care, processes of care (e.g., admission, discharge), and amenities (e.g., physical environment, food service). The hospitalist controls only a few of these areas but can influence many more. It is important to identify what you control and what you can influence. Identify a "summary satisfaction" question that feels right. This taps into a dimension of patient loyalty that can be linked into enhanced reputation and can make your hospital's care something that patients must have and for which they would bypass more convenient institutions because of the perceived added value of yours. One such question is the "likelihood of recommending" your hospital to others. Surveys generate a raw mean score that can be used to measure your own progress from year to year. The hospital's performance can also be represented as percentiles within a group of hospitals matched by common characteristics (e.g., bed size, teaching or nonteaching, urban or rural, etc.). Be aware that the mean score, like a percentile, may be reported on a 0–100 scale; however, the former (raw score) represents the hospital's own performance, and the latter (percentile) tells the proportion of the comparative group that performed lower than your hospital.

Partner with an Expert

Most hospitals conduct patient satisfaction surveys through a professional survey organization with national scope. These organizations have validated their survey instruments and can benchmark the data. Most will profile six or eight aspects of the hospital experience. The Society of Hospital Medicine has encouraged its members to request the vendor who services their hospital to produce reports that are specific to the hospitalists' patients. Some organizations have created a "hospitalist profile."[5,6]

Expectations are Changing Rapidly

Centers for Medicare and Medicaid Services (CMS) plans to encourage all hospitals to publicly report patient satisfaction by means of the HCAHPS initiative. (HCAHPS is the Hospital-CAHPS survey. CAHPS originally stood for the Consumer Assessment of Health Plan Survey, but now is used to represent a family of surveys developed by the Agency for Healthcare Research Quality, AHRQ).[7–9]

The HCAHPS initiative provides a standardized survey instrument and data-collection methodology for measuring and publicly reporting patients' perspectives on hospital care. "The primary purpose of HCAHPS is public reporting. To accomplish that objective, it is critical to have a uniform core set of items to make meaningful comparisons. Hospitals should continue to field items that provide additional information for their internal use, for example, for quality improvement purposes" (www.ahrq.gov/qual/cahps/hcahpfaq.htm).

The HCAHPS survey was developed with the intention of having the minimum number of questions necessary to give consumers information by which to compare hospitals. The final HCAHPS survey consists of 27 questions, 22 of which cover seven key topics: communication with doctors, communication with nurses, responsiveness of hospital staff, cleanliness and noise level of the hospital environment, pain control, communication about medicines, and discharge information. The remaining five questions will be used by CMS to adjust HCAHPS results by patient mix. Participation in HCAHPS is required for a hospital to receive full increases to their reimbursements under the Inpatient Prospective Payment System (IPPS) for FY 2008 HCAHPS results will be publicly reported on the Hospital Compare website (www.hospitalcompare.hhs.gov).

There are three individual items that relate to the domain of communication with doctors that may be of most interest to hospitalists. These questions include:

- During this hospital stay, how often did doctors treat you with courtesy and respect? *(Never, Sometimes, Usually, Always)*
- During this hospital stay, how often did doctors explain things in a way you could understand? *(Never, Sometimes, Usually, Always)*
- During this hospital stay, how often did doctors listen carefully to you? *(Never, Sometimes, Usually, Always)*

Hospitals may be interested in obtaining patient feedback on areas of physician interaction that go beyond these three concepts. Indeed, CMS has noted that HCAHPS is not a stand-alone quality improvement tool; rather, it is a core set of questions that may be combined with a broader set of hospital-specific items. The survey is meant to complement, not replace, the data hospitals currently collect to support quality improvement. For example, HCAHPS has no open-ended questions to collect patient comments and does not measure quality improvement issues such as privacy, emotional support, involvement of family, involvement in decision-making, and coordination of care.

Hospitals that voluntarily participate in the HCAHPS initiative will conduct a straight random sample of patients throughout the year to gather a minimum of 300 returned patient surveys. Hospitals may field the HCAHPS instrument as a stand-alone tool or in conjunction with their current survey efforts. Surveys may be distributed via mail, phone, a combined mail and phone distribution, or through active interactive voice response (IVR).

Accountability in the form of public reporting has already been promoted at the state level (e.g., California and Rhode Island).[10] Within California, public reporting of patient views of care began with the Patient Evaluation of Performance (PEP-C) project. Public reporting of patient perceptions of care in California is now part of the broader CHART program (California Hospital Assessment and Reporting Taskforce) *(see* www.chcf.org/topics/hospitals/index.cfm?itemID=111065). In Rhode Island, public reporting of hospital patient satisfaction measures was prompted by a 1998 law that established the Rhode Island Health Quality Performance Measurement and Reporting Program, whose goal was to promote quality within the state's health

Table 131-2

Overall Assessment of Hospital	Very Poor	Poor	Fair	Good	Very Good
Likelihood of your recommending this hospital to others	1	2	3	4	5

care system through the development of a public reporting program *(see* www.health.ri.gov/chic/performance/satisfaction.php). Rhode Island efforts have led to an assessment of quality of care within the state and subsequent sharing of best practices among hospitals.

Given the increasing momentum and attention to this, hospitalists should anticipate requirements in the United States for measuring, benchmarking, and reporting patient satisfaction.[11,12] However, hospitalists may find that the amount of data available for their patients may be limited if hospitals collect only the minimum of 300 total returned surveys per year.

IMPLEMENTATION: CASE EXAMPLE OF A HOSPITAL USING STANDARDIZED WRITTEN SURVEYS FROM A NATIONAL SURVEY ORGANIZATION

An actual case report is presented and critiqued by the authors using a checklist for illustrating important principles of survey design and application (Table 131-2).

Starting second quarter 2003, this 450-bed community hospital increases its survey intensity from a representative sampling to surveying all patients discharged to home. It uses the same survey instruments and produces a monthly report. Hospital has a strategic objective to be in the 92nd percentile of a distribution of hospitals between 450 and 599 beds for one of the survey's questions, "likelihood of recommending."

Checklist: Is the Survey Instrument Valid?

Has the survey been shown to be reliable, valid, and peer reviewed?
Yes
Are the questions clear and not double barreled?
Yes
Are the questions worded correctly for the response scale?
Yes
Are the questions worded in as neutral a manner as possible?
Yes
Are the appropriate types of statistics being used for the response scale?
Yes

- Likert-type scale allows for parametric statistical analysis (e.g., mean scores, correlations, etc.).

You must be able to consider your data interval quality with the response scale being balanced (having the same number of positive and negative responses) and equidistant (with equal

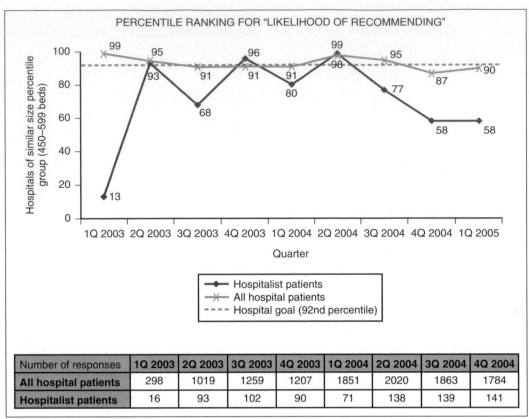

Figure 131-1 • Percentile Ranking for "Likelihood of Recommending."

conceptual space between the anchor points) in order to compute mean scores and other parametric statistics. For the current survey, patients respond on a scale from 1–5 with the following conceptual anchors: Very Poor, Poor, Fair, Good, and Very Good.

Unbalanced scales where there are more positive than negative responses or noninterval spacing between anchor points cannot be considered interval quality data. Such responses are treated only as categories of answers and should be reported as frequency distributions.

The hospital goal to be in the 92nd percentile is to achieve a mean score on the question "likelihood of recommending" that places the hospital better than or equal to 92% of hospitals of equivalent size (between 450 and 599 beds) using the same instrument during the same period of time. You ask the hospital data analyst for the hospitalists' performance on this question, and he produces Figure 131-1.

Checklist: Does the Method of Sampling Fit the Situation?

Are the sample sizes large enough to be stable estimates?
   Yes, but:
   • As a rule of thumb, 30 data points in a cell is a reasonable minimum. The first Quarter 2003 with only 16 responses for hospitalist patients should be interpreted with caution.
Is the measure sensitive enough to reflect forces in the care delivery environment (sample frame)?
   Yes

• Between first quarter 2004 and first quarter 2005, the hospitalists were managing 30% more patient days than prior with the same staffing model. The declining trend in patient evaluations appears to reflect this increased workload. This observation is useful in balancing productivity with other performance objectives.

Is the hospitalist subset of patients (sample frame) well defined?
   No
   • It is known that the hospital information system accurately identifies the attending physician only 80% of the time. How does this impact the data?

Recommendation: Although the scores can be used as a rough measure of quality for the hospitalist group, a more precise process for identifying patients should be implemented before the data are used for accountability reporting.

Checklist: Is the Representation of the Data Appropriate?

Is benchmarking the Hospitalist Patients to all patients appropriate when Hospitalists manage predominantly medical/surgical patients?
   Maybe
   • There are normative differences in the way different patient group experience and evaluate care (Fig. 131-2).
Recommendation: Compare hospitalist patients admitted through the emergency department (ED) to non-hospitalist patients also admitted through the ED.
Can the control group be more accurately defined?
   Yes

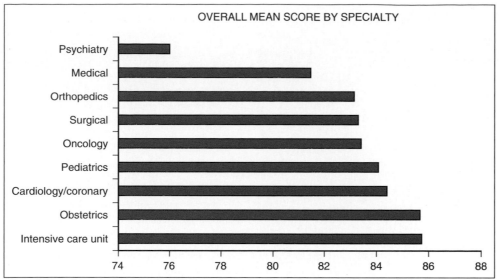

Figure 131-2 • Overall Mean Score by Specialty. © 2005 Press Ganey Associates. Data represent returns inpatient returns from the 1st quarter 2005 including 1,436 hospitals and 565,557 patient responses.

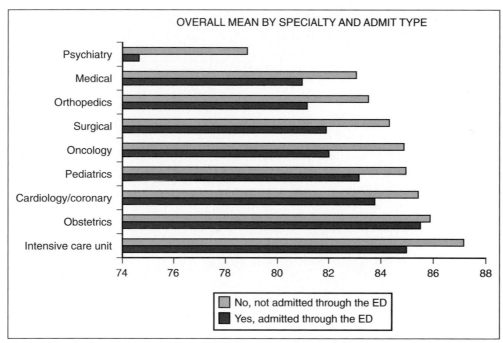

Figure 131-3 • Overall Mean by Specialty and Admit Type. © 2005 Press Ganey Associates. Data represent returns inpatient returns from the 1st quarter 2005 including 1,436 hospitals and 565,557 patient responses.

- 20% of all hospital patients, compared to 75% of all hospitalist patients enter through the ED. Patients admitted through the ED evaluate their hospital stay less favorably. This pattern holds across medical specialties (Fig. 131-3).

Recommendation: Compare hospitalist patients to groups cared for by similar medical specialties.

SUMMARY

The hospitalist needs to know why a patient satisfaction survey should be done and where the survey can benefit the hospitalist practice. If the need is for an internal quality improvement function, often the quick turnaround and simpler design needs are best met by focus groups, telephonic surveys, and simple written surveys. When the need is for an external accountability function, which seems now to be the course for most hospitals in the United States, a well-designed and executed written survey may be the best fit. Hospitalists can benefit from using this survey instrument with little additional cost. Hospitalists should become familiar with the structure and limitations of these survey instruments.

Comprehensive Hospital Medicine: An Evidence Based and Systems Approach

Key Points

- When designing a survey, hospitalists should know the difference between **subject** and **function.**

- The function of the survey must be established.

- An instrument appropriate to the function should be chosen.

- When measuring satisfaction, it is important to use an instrument that is reliable and valid.

- The use of hospital information systems as part of a satisfaction measuring strategy can be limiting, in part because the physician caring for a patient is often misidentified.

- Be aware of scope and context of patient surveys.

- Partner with an expert when assessing hospital patient satisfaction.

- With the push for public reporting and a uniform approach to measuring patient satisfaction, expectations of hospitals are changing rapidly.

SUGGESTED READING

Press I. The measure of quality. Qual Manage Healthc 2004; 13(4):202–209.

Quinn GP, Jacobsen PB, Albrecht TL, et al. Real-time patient satisfaction survey and improvement process. Hospital Topics: Research and Perspectives on Healthcare 2004; 82(3):26–32.

Aday L. Designing and Conducting Health Surveys, 2nd ed. San Francisco, CA: Jossey-Bass, 1996.

The following organizations conduct patient satisfaction surveys and are listed on the Society of Hospital Medicine website:

Avatar International www.avatar-intl.com

The Gallup Organization www.gallup.com

The Jackson Organization www.jacksonorganization.com

National Research Corp + Picker www.nrcpicker.com

Press Ganey www.pressganey.com

Professional Research Consultants www.prconline.com

2006 draft of the HCAHPS Survey. www.cahps.ahrq.gov/content/NCBD/PDF/HCAHPS_Chartbook_2006.pdf

CMS (Centers for Medicare and Medicaid Services). HQI (Hospital Quality Initiative).

www.cms.hhs.gov/quality/hospital/#Patient%20Perspectives%20on%20Care%20HCAHPS

Link to Press Ganey's resources on HCAHPS. www.pressganey.com/news/government_survey/history.php

Link to the official site for HCAHPS. www.cahps.ahrq.gov

Press I. Patient Satisfaction: Defining, Measuring, and Improving the Experience of Care. Chicago: Health Administration Press, 2002.

Baird, K. Customer Service in Health Care: A Grassroots Approach to Creating a Culture of Service Excellence. San Francisco: Jossey-Bass, 2000.

Bell R., Krivich M J. How to Use Patient Satisfaction Data to Improve Healthcare Quality. Milwaukee: American Society for Quality, 2000.

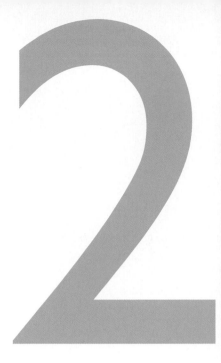

Section

Twenty-one

Legal and Ethical Issues

132 *Ethics in Hospital Medicine*
   Shaun Frost

133 *Medical Malpractice*
   S. Sandy Sanbar

134 *Legal Issues in Hospitalist-Hospital Relationships*
   Andrew M. Knoll

135 *Developing and Maintaining the Physician-Hospital*
   Relationship
   Richard Rohr

CHAPTER ONE HUNDRED AND THIRTY-TWO

Ethics in Hospital Medicine

Shaun Frost, MD, FACP

BACKGROUND

Four major ethical principles apply to the majority of clinical decision-making situations in hospital medicine:

- **Beneficence:** Bringing about or doing good
- **Nonmaleficence:** Doing no harm; or at least ensuring that benefits outweigh any potential harms (principle of double effect)
- **Autonomy:** Respecting people and their right to self-governance and self-determination
- **Justice and fairness:** Distributing benefits and burdens equitably across the health care system

Core ethical issues in hospital medicine include confidentiality, informed consent, advanced directives, competency and decision-making capacity, medical futility, and the limitation or withdrawal of therapy. This chapter reviews these issues, based on a foundation of the major ethical principles.

CORE ETHICAL ISSUES IN HOSPITAL MEDICINE

Confidentiality

Patients expect that discussions with their care providers, and sensitive information about their health and health care, will be kept confidential. The American Hospital Association discusses protection of privacy as a fundamental right in a document entitled "The Patient Care Partnership" (formerly "A Patient's Bill of Rights").[1] The Health Insurance Portability and Accountability Act (HIPAA) of 1996 outlines legal safeguards for the protection of confidential patient identifiable electronic, written, and orally communicated information.[2] Hospitalists should be knowledgeable of these safeguards, as well as specific state laws that may differ from federal legislation.

Hospitalists must also be keenly aware of elements in their workplace that can undermine patient confidentiality (Fig. 132-1).

- ***Nonprivate and semiprivate rooms allow for patient roommate access to privileged discussions.*** To minimize breaches of confidentiality, curtains separating bed-spaces should be closed during interviews and examinations. If necessary, roommates and their visitors should be asked to leave the room temporarily if possible to provide for maximal privacy.

- ***Conversations about patient care should not occur in public places such as hallways, elevators, lobbies, and cafeterias.*** Avoid using telephones in these areas when discussing patient information.

- ***Conversations in semiprivate places such as physician and nurse workstations may be overheard by others.*** Minimize the use of patient-specific identifiers in these settings. Be especially cautious when using speakerphones and dictation services.

- ***Recognize that patients may not want their visitors informed of confidential information.*** Do not assume that it is acceptable to discuss a patient's situation when others are present (including family members). When in the presence of visitors, physicians must seek patient permission prior to discussing or disclosing information.

- ***Computers pose unique challenges to confidentiality.*** Physicians must safeguard access codes and passwords, make a reasonable attempt to shield monitors from the view of others, and log off when work is completed.

- ***Facsimile and electronic mail transmissions may be intercepted by unintended recipients.*** Confidentiality disclaimer statements (Box 132-1) must accompany these transmissions.

Of note, breaching patient confidentiality is appropriate, and may even be legally mandated, in situations where maintaining privacy could be harmful to the patient or others. Examples of when maintaining confidentiality could be harmful to patients includes when they are incapable of making their own medical decisions, are considered "vulnerable adults" due to conditions such as unsafe living environments, or when there is knowledge of homicidal ideation or evidence of physical abuse. Maintaining confidentiality also could be harmful to the public when there is a threat of infectious or communicable disease or when the patient lacks the ability to perform certain activities safely (e.g., operate an automobile).

Informed Consent

Respect for autonomy entails ensuring that patients are fully informed about all aspects of their health care. This is especially relevant to the practice of hospital medicine, given the frequent need for testing, procedures, and treatments having potential

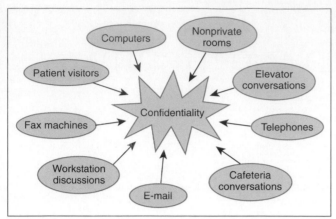

Figure 132-1 • Hospital workplace elements that can create breaches in confidentiality.

Box 132-1 Disclaimer Statement to Accompany Privileged Facsimile Transmissions or Electronic Mail

This e-mail/facsimile transmission and any files transmitted with it are confidential and are intended solely for the use of the individual or entity to which they are addressed. If you are not the intended recipient or the individual responsible for delivering the e-mail/ facsimile transmission to the intended recipient, please be advised that you have received this e-mail/facsimile transmission in error and that any use, dissemination, forwarding, printing, or copying of this e-mail/facsimile transmission is strictly prohibited.

If you have received this e-mail/facsimile transmission in error, please immediately notify _____ by telephone at _____. You will be reimbursed for reasonable costs incurred in notifying us.

significant harms and risks. Hospitalists must recognize that informed consent begins with the decision to hospitalize, and the process of transferring care from a primary physician to a hospitalist should be explicitly discussed. This includes educating patients about the hospital medicine model of care. They should be informed that their primary physician will have a limited role in their hospital care, and also informed about how and when their primary physician will be updated about aspects of their hospitalization.

The goal of informed consent is to provide patients with information to make educated and uncoerced decisions about their medical treatments. This information must be provided in terminology that the patient is able to comprehend. Basic elements of informed consent include[1,3,4] **disclosure** of:

- Nature of the illness, and the reason for the proposed intervention
- Experimental or research-related interventions
- Personal financial liability that could be incurred if the proposed intervention is accepted
- Benefits, risks, uncertainties, and alternatives to the proposed intervention

Informed consent must also **confirm:**

- The patient's decision-making capacity is intact
- The patient understands the information
- Patient's uncoerced acceptance of the proposed intervention

A signed consent form is not a substitute for an in-depth patient discussion about each of these basic elements of the informed consent process. Signed consent forms may, however, result in increased compliance with obtaining proper informed consent.[5] Signed consent forms may also facilitate informed consent discussions. Figure 132-2 presents a sample form and order set for the transfusion of blood products, which includes detailed statistical information about procedural risks that may be used by clinicians to structure accurate discussions with patients.

Advance Directives

Patients have the right when competent to dictate future decision-making about their health care in the event they become incapacitated. This most often takes the form of a written advance directive, a fundamental right recognized by all state govern-

ments. The Patient Self Determination Act of 1990 requires that hospitals participating in Medicare and Medicaid programs inquire about the existence of an advance directive. If patients do not have an advance directive, they must be asked if they would like to complete one.

Variations of advance directives include the living will, the durable power of attorney for health care (DPAHC), and hybrids of these known as "advance care plans." A **living will** is an instructional document outlining for care providers specific medical interventions that patients would accept or refuse in the event they are incapacitated. Although living wills may be highly detailed and specific, they are frequently inadequate, due to limited scope and vagueness about exact instructions. A **DPAHC** is a proxy form authorizing a specific person or people to make health care decisions for an incapable patient. A DPAHC is flexible and expansive, limiting the proxy decision-maker only to the extent specified by the patient.[6] **Advance care plans** are documents that incorporate elements of both living wills and DPAHCs. Advance care plans are generally broad in scope, and they discuss issues beyond medical care such as emotional, spiritual, and personal matters. They thus are potentially more helpful than living wills or DPAHCs in guiding decision-making by proxies and health care providers. In addition to defining desired medical interventions and identifying proxy decision-makers, advance care plans clarify patient goals and values by:

- Describing wishes in specific scenarios
- Defining spiritual beliefs
- Describing important family traditions
- Expressing fears about end-of-life
- Expressing wishes for forgiveness
- Providing instructions for the handling of financial matters
- Providing instructions on how one would like to be remembered and what one would like said to loved ones

Examples of advance care plans include "Caring Conversations" (Fig. 132-3)[7] and the "Five Wishes Document."[8]

Despite attempts to increase awareness about the importance of advance directives, their use is limited and fraught with problems that frequently render them ineffective. These problems have been reviewed by Lo and Steinbrook[9] and include:

- *Limited portability:* Patients, families, and care providers must be aware of state-specific laws governing the use and credibil-

BLOOD TRANSFUSION ORDER FORM

Name:

Medical Rec #   Suffix

DOB

Location

Attending Physician
Name and Code

Medical Necessity Documentation is Required for Regulatory Compliance
DIAGNOSIS CODE(S)
1.   2.

CONSENT OBTAINED FOR TRANSFUSION
☐ Yes   ☐ Emergency

Physician Signature   Date

AUTHORIZATION FOR EMERGENCY RELEASE

The life of the patient is in jeopardy and I hereby authorize the release of

☐ Uncrossmatched - O Negative   ☐ Uncrossmatched Patient Type Specific   ☐ Incompatible Blood per Blood Bank

---

Packed Red Cells - _____ **units**
☐ Acute blood loss anemia
☐ Symptomatic anemia, if no other therapy is likely to correct the anemia.

Transfuse_____ **units at** _____ **over** _____ **hours**

☐ O-negative units

Hemoglobin Value: _____

Platelets - _____ **units (use all ordered)**
☐ Platelet count <20,000/microL
☐ Platelet count <50,000/microL if major surgery is anticipated or life-threatening bleeding is occurring
☐ Platelet count <100,000/microL following cardiopulmonary bypass or neurologic or ophthalmic surgery
☐ Greater than one blood volume replacement with platelet count <100,000/microL
☐ Documented or anticipated platelet dysfunction, if major surgery is anticipated

Transfuse_____ **units over** _____ **hours**

Frozen Plasma - _____ **units**
☐ Coagulopathy with INR >1.5
☐ Anticoagulation therapy in the patient who is deficient in vitamin K-dependent coagulation factors II, VII, IX and X. The patient should be bleeding or require emergency surgery.
☐ Factor XIII deficiency
☐ Plasma exchange for thrombotic thrombocytopenic purpura (TTP) or hemolytic uremic syndrome (HUS)
☐ Other: e.g. anti-thrombin III, protein C, protein S or heparin cofactor II deficiencies.
☐ Active bleeding or prophylactically prior to surgery in a patient with a coagulation factor deficiency (other than factor VIII and factor IX deficiency) when specific concentrates are unavailable.
☐ Major burn

Transfuse_____ **units over** _____ **hours**

Cryoprecipitate - _____ **units (use all ordered)**
☐ Hypofibrinogenemia: consumptive coagulopathy with fibrinogen level below 100 mg/dL
☐ Patients with von Willebrand's disease who are bleeding, or prophylactically before surgery, or who are bleeding and the bleeding is unresponsive to desmopressin (DDVAP).
☐ Fibrin surgical adhesive.
☐ To enhance platelet function in patients with uremia and hemodialysis with active bleeding or prophylactically prior to surgery.

Transfuse_____ **units over** _____ **hours**

Special Blood - (Select Product)
☐ **Irradiated/leukoreduced**
☐ **Leukoreduced**
☐ **Autologous**
☐ **Directed**

Other
Factor VIII Concentrate - _____ units
☐ Factor VIII deficiency
Factor IX Concentrate - _____ units
☐ Factor IX deficiency

Washed red blood cells - _____ **units**
☐ IgA deficiency
☐ Prior severe anaphylactic reactions
☐ Paroxysmal nocturnal hemoglobinuria

Frozen deglycerolized red cells - _____ **units**
☐ Rare patient antigens or antibodies

Other _____

Approved by Pathologist

Name: _____

Tech Initials:_____

Transcriber signature:_____   **Date:**_____

100-800-070 (6/04)   **BLOOD TRANSFUSION ORDER FORM**

Figure 132-2 • Order set and consent form for the transfusion of blood products. Used with permission from Health Partners Medical Group and Clinics, Regions Hospital, St. Paul, MN.

COMPLICATIONS OF TRANSFUSIONS - USA (2003)

INFECTIOUS DISEASE	RISK PER UNIT
Hepatitis C Virus	<1 in 1.0 million
Hepatitis B Virus	1 in 137,000
Human T-Lymphotrophic Virus	1 in 50,000 to 641,000
Human Immunodeficiency Virus	1 in 1.9 million
Fatal Bacterial Sepsis	1 in 1 million
West Nile Virus[†]	<1 in 50,000
Other Infections (Syphilis, Malaria, Chagas', Babesia)	<1 in 1 million

NON-INFECTIOUS COMPLICATION	RISK PER UNIT
Acute Hemolysis	1 in 15,600 to 35,700
Fatal Acute Hemolysis	1 in 630,000
Delayed Hemolysis	1 in 4,000 to 11,600
Fatal Delayed Hemolysis	1 in 3.85 million
Febrile, Non-hemolytic	1 in 50 to 100
Acute Lung Injury	1 in 5,000 to 100,000
Hives	1 in 30 to 100
Severe Anaphylaxis	1 in 18,000 to 170,000
Circulatory Overload	1 in 3,000 to 12,000
Transfusion Associated with Graft vs Host Disease	Unknown

[†]The risk varies by region and season. The numbers given indicate an approximation of average risk in Minnesota using January 2000 data.

DEFINITIONS

Type and hold (same as type and screen)–The patient's ABO and Rh status is determined and the serum is tested against red cells in search of common antibodies. No units are set aside.

Type and cross–The above testing plus an x number of units are tested and set aside for this patient. Done in anticipation of surgery and is particularly important in patients with multiple antibodies.

Suffix: Each time a patient is registered to receive services at Regions Hospital he/she is given a visit specific suffix. On the paperwork the patient receives and on your computer screen you will see their medical record number followed by a four-digit suffix. This suffix drives the appointment/admission, test orders and results and the billing for the patient's account. Each time the patient is registered he/she receives a new suffix. This helps distinguish visits in a patient's history.

RED BLOOD CELLS

Volume:	Approx. 300 mL
Dose:	Per clinical assessment
Expected result:	One unit of red blood cells will increase the hemoglobin approximately 1 g/dL in a 70 kg adult
How to transfuse:	Varies based upon clinical circumstances. In general for chronic anemia, slowly over 2–4 hours piggy backed with normal saline.

PLATELETS

Volume:	Random donor platelet concentrates (from a whole blood donation) 45–65 mL; pheresis platelets from platelet pheresis donation using a cell separator approx. 250 mL
Dose:	1 platelet concentrate unit per 10 kg body weight (up to 6 units or 1 pheresis unit in an adult)
Expected result:	1 unit should increase platelet count by 5–10,000/microL in an average adult, in the absence of consumption. NOTE: For patients not showing adequate response to platelet transfusion, or for indications for Human Leukocyte Antigen matched or crossmatched platelets, consult hematology or the blood bank director.

Platelet transfusions are administered to stop or prevent bleeding associated with deficiencies in platelet number or function.

FROZEN PLASMA

Volume:	250–300 mL
Dose:	10–20 mL/kg body weight
Expected result:	In a 70 kg adult, each unit will increase the activity of all plasma clotting factors by about 4–5%, and fibrinogen by about 10 mg/dL. This should not be used as a replacement for specific clotting factors in hemophilia or Von Willebrand disease.

CRYOPRECIPITATE

Component:	One unit contains 80–120 units Factor VIII and 150–250 mg fibrinogen. Von Willebrand Factor and Factor XIII are also present.
Volume:	Approximately 5–20 mL per unit
Dose:	Per clinical assessment
Expected result:	One unit will increase Factor VIII activity by about 4%, and fibrinogen by about 7–10 mg/dL in a 70 kg adult.

INDICATIONS FOR IRRADIATION
- Allogeneic and autologous bone marrow or peripheral blood progenitor cell recipients
- Patients with congenital immune deficiency syndrome

INDICATIONS FOR LEUKOREDUCTION
- Potential need for a bone marrow transplant (all leukemias: aplastic anemia)
- Prior febrile non hemolytic transfusion reaction

100-800-070 (6/04)

BLOOD TRANSFUSION ORDER FORM

Figure 132-2 • Cont'd

Healthcare Directive

• Take a copy of this with you whenever you go to the hospital or on a trip •

I, _____, SS # _____ want everyone who cares for me to know
  (please print)

what healthcare I want **when I cannot let others know what I want.**

I always expect to be given care and treatment for pain or discomfort even when such care might make me sleepy, make me feel
like not eating, slow down my breathing, or be habit-forming.

I want my doctor to try treatments that may get me back to an acceptable quality of life, with the understanding that treatment will
be withdrawn if my condition does not improve to a quality acceptable to me. By an "acceptable quality of life," I mean living in a
way that lets me do the things that are important and necessary to me.
Those things are

_____

_____

| Examples: the ability to | • recognize family or friends | • make decisions | • communicate |
| | • feed myself | • take care of myself | |

I want to have a natural death; therefore, I direct that no treatment (including food or water by tube) be given just to keep me alive
when I have
  • a condition that will cause me to die soon, or
  • a condition so bad (including substantial brain damage or brain disease) that there is no reasonable hope that I will
    regain a quality of life acceptable to me (as described above).

However, in these conditions, I **would** consent to

_____

Examples:	• resuscitation (CPR)	• dialysis	• ventilator
	• food or water by tube	• chemotherapy	• transfusions
	• surgery	• antibiotics	

I also want _____

_____

| Examples: | • to donate my organs | • hospice care | • to die at home |

☐ Please refer to my *Caring Conversations* Workbook, which is located_____

• Be sure to sign this form on the reverse side of this page •

If you only want to name a Durable Power of Attorney for Healthcare Decisions, draw a large X through this page.

**Talk about this form and your ideas about your healthcare with the person you have chosen to make decisions for
you, your doctor(s), family, friends, and clergy, and give each of them a completed copy.**
You may cancel or change this form at any time. You should review it often.
Each time you review it, put your initials and the date here.

_____

This document is provided as a service by Midwest Bioethics Center, the Kansas City Metropolitan Bar Association, and the
Metropolitan Medical Society of Greater Kansas City.

Figure 132-3 • The Caring Conversations advance care plan. A 7-page workbook allowing for greater in-depth clarification of wishes accompanies
these forms and is downloadable from the website. Center for Practical Bioethics, Kansas City, MO.

ity of advance directives. What is acceptable in one state may not be in others. Furthermore, most states require that advance directives be witnessed or notarized before they are officially recognized.

- *Limited accessibility and availability:* Advance directives are often improperly documented and filed, are inadequately discussed with appropriate individuals (i.e., loved ones, primary physicians, attorneys, clergy), and frequently do not travel with the patient across care sites.

- *Inaccurate proxy decision-making:* Proxies are often unable to convey patients' wishes accurately. Studies suggest that having a general knowledge of a patient's goals and values is not adequate when attempting to identify wishes in specific clinical scenarios.

- *Limited awareness of the consequences of not having an advance directive:* Regulations that specify procedures to be followed in the absence of a written advance directive are often not familiar to patients. For example, most states have laws that specify who will be appointed as decision-maker for an incapacitated patient who has not previously made a proxy designation. Patients must be aware that although this person may not be best positioned to understand and convey their wishes, law dictates that no one else may serve as their proxy in the absence of an advance directive specifying otherwise. Finally, many patients are unaware of certain state laws that allow for proxy decision-making only in specific situations such as terminal illness.

Hospitalists can assist in remedying many of these problems and difficulties. Box 132-2 presents opportunities for hospitalists to educate patients and their loved ones about advance directives.

Box 132-2 How Hospitalists Can Assist in Enhancing the Use of Advance Directives (ADs)

1. Appreciate hospitalization as an opportunity to discuss ADs with every patient.

2. Recognize that the frequent presence of patient visitors affords an excellent opportunity to encourage patients to review life goals and values with loved ones.

3. Consider hospitalization an opportunity to review the challenges of substituted decision-making with proxy decision-makers.

4. Champion the use of standardized forms and processes for education about ADs.

5. Educate patients about state laws governing the use and legitimacy of ADs.

6. Educate patients about state laws that dictate procedure for the appointment of proxy decision-makers in the ABSENCE of ADs.

7. Recognize that ADs are not permanent documents. A change in health condition necessitating hospitalization may prompt a patient to reconsider earlier expressed wishes.

8. Clearly document discussions about advance care planning in medical records and discharge summaries.

Competency and Decision-Making Capacity

A fundamental tenet in the United States is that people have the legal and ethical right to make their own decisions. This right may be denied, however, to incompetent persons who present a harmful risk to themselves or others. Physicians frequently encounter patients having questionable capacity to make their own treatment decisions. These encounters demand an inquiry of a patient's competency. **Competence** is a legal concept dictated by standards that may vary among jurisdictions. What defines competency is thus specific to the legal system in which it is debated. "Incompetence" is therefore a judgment passed by a court of law.

Medical decision-making capacity refers to "a patient's ability to understand information relevant to a treatment decision and to appreciate the reasonably foreseeable consequences of a decision or lack of a decision."[10] Different than "incompetence," "incapacity" to participate in medical decision-making is determined by a physician as opposed to a court. An ethical dilemma is created when physicians must decide how and where to set the threshold at which declining capacity justifies removing a patient's right to act autonomously.

Decision-making capacity is suggested by the presence of four key abilities[11]:

- *Ability to communicate choices:* Capable decision-makers recognize that they have choices, and they have the ability to state a preference. This is clearly demonstrated by the patient who refuses therapy (refusal demonstrates the understanding that treatment may be accepted or declined). The ability to communicate a choice is necessary, but usually not sufficient to indicate capacity.

- *Ability to understand information:* Confirming that patients understand requires that they are able to paraphrase the facts about a diagnosis and the proposed interventions. It is additionally required that patients remember these facts. Physicians must reassess at a later date for understanding, following the initial disclosure of information.

- *The ability to appreciate the situation and its consequences:* Appreciation requires that patients recognize that information and decision-making circumstances apply to their personal situation. It is therefore important to determine patients' beliefs about whether or not they are ill, and the likely effect of treatment on their well-being. In so doing, patients must demonstrate that they have assigned personal value to the facts of the clinical situation.[12]

- *The ability to manipulate information rationally:* Rational manipulation of information requires that patients analyze data to weigh pros and cons in arriving at conclusions that logically follow their starting premises.

Suggested questions to evaluate decision-making capacity are presented in Box 132-3.

Wong and colleagues[13] reviewed various approaches to the evaluation of capacity, such as outcome assessment, status assessment, and functional assessment.

- *Outcome assessment* uses the patient's decision itself to determine capacity, rather than the process by which the decision was arrived at. An individual would be deemed incapable by this criterion if his or her decision were contrary to popular belief or conventional wisdom. This criterion ignores the value of autonomy, and is thus rarely invoked.

Box 132-3 Suggested Questions to Assess for the Abilities of Capable Decision-Makers

Expressing a choice

"Can you tell me what your decision is?"

"Have you decided to accept the suggestions for treatment?"

Understanding

"Why do you think I am giving you all this information?"

"Tell me in your own words what we have discussed about your diagnosis."

"What are the risks and benefits of treating your illness?"

"How likely do you think it is you will experience a complication with the treatment?"

Appreciation

"Do you know why I have recommended this treatment for you?"

"What do you believe is currently wrong with your health?"

"Do you believe that you need treatment?"

"What will happen if you are not treated?"

Rational Manipulation of Information

"How did you reach the decision to accept/reject the treatment?"

"What were the important factors you considered in arriving at your decision?"

"How did you balance these important factors?"

From: Grisso T, Appelbaum P. Assessing Competence to Consent to Treatment. New York: Oxford University Press, 1998.

- *Status assessment* uses the patient's membership in a specific population as the sole means of determining capacity. Patients with illnesses characterized by compromised mental functioning (e.g., delirium, dementia, schizophrenia, depression, retardation, etc.) are globally stereotyped by this criterion as lacking the capacity to decide. This approach fails to recognize that decision-making is both time and task specific. For example, patients with depression may be only temporarily incapacitated until adequately treated, while patients with dementia may be capable of making decisions associated with simplistic issues and risk/benefit analyses. These issues expose the limitation of using global measures of mental functioning such as the Mini Mental Status Exam (MMSE) to determine capacity. While extremely good or extremely poor performance on the MMSE may correlate well with capacity or incapacity in certain situations, performance in between these extremes does not necessarily reflect task-specific capacity.[14]

- A *functional assessment* strives to determine if a patient's personal capacity abilities are sufficient for specific decision-making circumstances. The goal is to "establish the extent to which the person's understanding, knowledge, skills, and abilities meet the demands of the task involved in making a particular decision within a given context."[13] This requires skillful disclosure of information in language appropriate for the patient's educational and cultural background, while carefully

evaluating the patient's cognitive abilities, emotional state, and personal, cultural, and religious values attached to the decision-making situation.[15] The complex nature of such a functional assessment is highlighted by observations that physicians' general impressions about capacity do not correlate well with expert evaluations unless patients are obviously capable or incapable.[14] The MacArthur Competence Assessment Tool[11] and the Aid to Capacity Evaluation[14] provide practical, useful evaluation methods based on a functional assessment approach.

Colleagues who can assist the hospitalist in determining decision-making capacity include psychiatrists, geriatricians, social workers, clergy, and ethicists.[4]

Medical Futility and the Limiting or Withdrawing of Therapy

Hospitalists frequently encounter clinical situations in which the benefit of treatment or further diagnostic investigation is dubious. These situations lead to debate about medical futility and often result in ethical dilemmas about the appropriateness of limiting or withdrawing therapy. Medical futility is difficult to define precisely. Interventions are strictly futile in only three situations[16]:

1. The intervention has been tried and failed.
2. Maximal therapy is failing.
3. There is no pathophysiologic rationale for the intervention to work.

Clinicians often invoke a less precise definition of medical futility, however, to include interventions that they believe are not beneficial because of an inability to result in "meaningful" recovery. Such a definition necessarily makes the assessment of futility more subjective by introducing the value judgments of the physician. Ethical dilemmas and clinical conflict may result if these value judgments differ from those of the patient. Some authors advocate that as long as effective interventions resulting in controversial ends are instituted in support of a patient's values and goals (as elucidated by a capable decision maker), those interventions should be offered.[4] This approach seems reasonable, provided that the interventions in question do not meet the criteria for strict futility as defined above.

Physicians are not obligated to provide therapy that they believe is ineffective or that violates their personal beliefs and values. However, as long as such therapies do not meet criteria for strict futility, transferring the patient's care to another physician or another hospital should be considered.

APPROACHES TO SOLVING ETHICAL DILEMMAS

Ethical dilemmas result when it is difficult or impossible to realize simultaneously and maximally the principles of autonomy, beneficence, nonmaleficence, and justice. Further confusion is introduced when these principles conflict with other interests, such as religious beliefs, legal considerations, societal norms, cultural traditions, and financial obligations. Jonsen et al.[17] described a useful approach to ethical dilemmas that entails a comprehensive review of four topics: medical indications, patient preferences, quality of life, and contextual features. Analyzing the facts of an ethical dilemma in this fashion necessarily considers all of the major ethical principles at play, and therefore usually defines the ethical problem while simultaneously suggesting a solution.[4]

- *Medical indications:* Review of this topic will define the exact nature of the medical problem to include history, diagnosis, and prognosis. Exactly how medical therapy can achieve benefits and avoid harms will be clarified.
- *Patient preferences:* Review of this topic requires assessing decision-making capacity, ensuring the adequate provision of information necessary for patient decision-making, and understanding the patient's values and goals. The objective is to determine if the patient's right to choose is being maximally respected.
- *Quality of life:* Addressing this topic will clarify the patient's chances of returning to a normal life. Analyze the potential deficits a patient might experience due to the illness itself or the therapies proposed to treat the illness. Define the value ascribed by the patient of living a life with these potential deficits. This will clarify available therapy options, including the possibility of palliative care.
- *Contextual features:* Review of this topic will define important extenuating circumstances affecting the ethical issues. Such circumstances include religious, cultural, family, legal, economic, and physician-specific factors that could influence decision-making.

Unfortunately, due to the need to make rapid decisions for patients who are acutely ill, hospitalists often do not have the time and resources needed to apply the four-topic method. In situations in which immediate action is necessary, Iserson suggests the following three-step "rapid approach to ethical problems" (Fig. 132-4).[18]

- Step 1: Apply an approach that has proven successful in resolving similar past ethical dilemmas.
- Step 2: If there is no prior experience to draw from, determine if it is clinically possible to "buy time" to think through the issues more thoroughly, consult with colleagues, or obtain an ethics consultation. If it is possible to delay definitive decision-making, the hospitalist should enact an "ethically reasonable" plan of action that may be modified after further deliberation.

- Step 3: If delay is not possible, immediate action should be guided by application of the impartiality test, the universalizability test, and the interpersonal justifiability test, which requires hospitalists to ask themselves specific questions.
  - *The impartiality test*—"Would I be willing to have my physician act in this manner if I were in this patient's place?"
  - *The universalizability test*—"Would I be comfortable if all clinicians with my background and in these same circumstances act as I am prosing to do?"
  - *The interpersonal justifiability test*—"Am I ready to state openly to my peers, superiors, or to the public my reasons for acting as I propose to do?"

If the answers to the questions posed by these three tests are yes, the proposed action addressing the ethical dilemma is likely acceptable, and the clinician can proceed with plans to clarify further as more time allows. Recognize that this "rapid approach" represents an oversimplification of the issues, and it is intended for guidance only in situations where significant time restraints mandate immediate decision-making. Whenever possible, and as future time allows, hospitalists should employ a more rigorous approach to ethical problem solving.

CONCLUSIONS

Ethical issues addressed in the hospital are defined by elements unique to the practice of hospital medicine. The ethical principles of autonomy, beneficence, nonmaleficence, and justice are core considerations when addressing problem-solving about fundamental ethical issues such as confidentiality, informed consent, advance directives, competency and decision making capacity, and the limitation or withdrawal of therapy. A structured approach to problem-solving will benefit every hospitalist faced with an ethical dilemma.

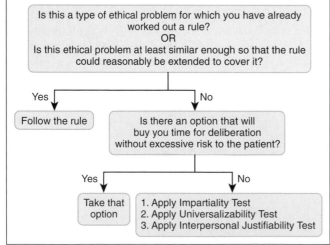

Figure 132-4 • Rapid approach to ethical problem solving. Reproduced with permission. Iserson KV, Sanders AB, Mathieu D. Ethics in Emergency Medicine, (2nd Edition). Tucson, AZ: Galen Press, Ltd., 1995. 45.

Key Points

- Ethical issues encountered in the hospital are shaped by unique factors that define the practice of Hospital Medicine.

- Patients are often most ethically vulnerable when sick.

- Hospitalized patients have few choices. They rarely (or never) have input on decision-making issues ranging from who will provide their care to when they will receive visitors.

- The purposeful discontinuity of care created by the hospital medicine model challenges patients' trust by interfering with the transfer of established doctor–patient relationships from the outpatient to the inpatient setting. Care discontinuity necessitates the need for multiple "hand-offs" of patient information, which creates the potential for ethical problems.

- Medical decision-making in the hospital occurs rapidly, and often with incomplete information.

- A hospital's physical structure (e.g., nonprivate rooms, semiprivate physician and nurse workstations, computerized medical record keeping systems, etc.) contributes to ethical dilemmas.

- A hospitalist's obligations in management of the hospital system related to efficiency and resource utilization may conflict with patient care responsibilities.

SUGGESTED READING

The American Hospital Association. The Patient Care Partnership: Understanding Expectations, Rights, and Responsibilities. 2003. Accessed at: http://www.aha.org/aha/ptcommunication/partnership/index.html on 13 August 2005.

Gostin L. National health information privacy: Regulations under the Health Insurance Portability and Accountability Act. JAMA 2001; 285:3015–3021.

Rajput V, Bekes C. Ethical issues in hospital medicine. Med Clin North Am 2002; 86:869–886.

Mueller P, Hook C, Fleming K. Ethical issues in geriatrics: a guide for clinicians. Mayo Clin Proc 2004; 79:554–562.

Davis N, Pohlman A, Gehlbach B, et al. Improving the process of informed consent in the critically ill. JAMA 2003; 289:1963–1968.

Kirschner K. When written advanced directives are not enough. Clin Geriatr Med 2005; 193–209.

Midwest Bioethics Center. Caring conversations. Accessed at http://www.practicalbioethics.org/mbc-cc.htm on 29 July 2005.

Aging with Dignity. Five wishes. Accessed at http://www.agingwithdignity.org/5wishes.html on 29 July 2005.

Lo B, Steinbrook R. Resuscitating advance directives. Arch Intern Med 2004; 164:1501–1506.

Etchells E, Sharpe G, Elliot C, et al. Bioethics for clinicians. III. Capacity. Can Med Assoc J 1996; 155:657–661.

Grisso T, Appelbaum P. Assessing Competence to Consent to Treatment. New York: Oxford University Press, 1998.

Wong J, Clare C, Gunn M, et al. Capacity to make health care decisions: its importance in clinical practice. Psych Med 1999; 29:437–446.

Etchells E, Darzins P, Siberfeld M, et al. Assessment of patient capacity to consent to treatment. J Gen Intern Med 1999; 14:27–34.

Pantilat S. Ethical issues for hospitalists. Hospitalist 2001; 5:6,21.

Iserson K. Ethical issues in emergency medicine. Emerg Med Clin North Am 1999; 283–306.

CHAPTER ONE HUNDRED AND THIRTY-THREE

Medical Malpractice

S. Sandy Sanbar, MD, PhD, JD, FCLM

BACKGROUND

This chapter provides a brief introduction to the following topics for hospitalists: the medical malpractice crises, the medical malpractice stress syndrome, the etiology (causes of action) of malpractice, the defenses to a claim of malpractice, why patients sue physicians, and malpractice prevention or prophylaxis. Hospitalists generally confront the same causes of malpractice litigation as other practicing physicians. The term *malpractice* refers to any professional misconduct that encompasses an unreasonable lack of skill or unfaithfulness in carrying out professional or fiduciary duties. The term *medical malpractice* is used in this chapter because of the common usage in claims alleging medical negligence by health care professionals.

MEDICAL MALPRACTICE CRISES

The first American malpractice crisis occurred between 1835 and 1865, during which time the courts were inundated with numerous malpractice lawsuits involving fractures and dislocations with imperfect results or deformities such as shortened or crooked limbs. Surprisingly, the attitudes and behaviors of patients, lawyers, physicians, and judges during the first malpractice crisis were similar to those currently held. During the past three decades, there have been three medical malpractice crises in the United States—one in the early 1970s, the second in the mid-1980s, and the third in early 2000s.

In 1956, the number of medical malpractice cases was reportedly 1.5 claims per 100 covered physicians. During the first and second medical malpractice crises, the number of medical malpractice claims per 100 physicians rose sharply. By 1990, the number of medical malpractice claims increased to 15 per 100 covered physicians, a 10-fold increase from 1956. Between 2000 and 2003, the average trends of medical malpractice appear relatively flat nationally, although some states reported a decline in frequency, while other states have experienced a rise in frequency of medical malpractice claims. Louisiana has had the highest number of reported claims for physicians, which is double the national average, approximately 31 claims per 100 physicians. The percentage of patients injured by medical negligence who actually bring suit is very small, with estimates ranging from 1 in 8 to 1 in 10. Of those who sue, only one in three receive any compensation.

MEDICAL MALPRACTICE STRESS SYNDROME

Litigation stress may affect any individual or professional who is involved in litigation. The stress of medical malpractice litigation may directly contribute to physician illness or dissatisfaction with one's medical practice, leading to carrier change, burnout, early retirement or extreme shame and depression, sometimes leading to suicide.

An alleged medical liability suit may be extremely traumatic to the accused physician, and it often causes emotional injury, regardless of whether or not the lawsuit has merit. The emotional turmoil that results from a malpractice lawsuit can be debilitating.

The primary manifestations of medical malpractice stress are psychological symptoms, and the secondary manifestations are physical symptoms, which may precipitate a new disorder or aggravate a preexisting illness. The psychological symptoms generally result from acute or chronic anxiety and from a depressive disorder.

It is often difficult for the physician defendant to acknowledge that he or she may be suffering from medical malpractice stress syndrome. It is more difficult for the physician defendant to formally seek medical attention from a colleague, such as a family physician, internist, or psychiatrist. Where the symptoms are severe, especially if there are thoughts of suicide, the physician should seek prompt psychiatric assistance.

Management and control of the symptoms of litigation stress under the supervision of a treating psychiatrist should never be underestimated. The amelioration of stress will lead to a feeling of well-being, confidence, and behavioral control, thereby reversing the agonizing mental turmoil. Reduction of stress will also allow the physician to think and act with greater objectivity, to remain focused, and to maintain a healthy perspective. Support group/group therapy with other physicians who are or have been through litigation, discussions with family and close friends, meetings with defense counsel, and understanding the legal process are all helpful measures. The physician can derive therapeutic benefit from other measures listed in Box 133-1.

Box 133-1 Measures That Alleviate Litigation Stress

1. Being actively involved with the defense attorney team

2. Participating in official discovery requests

3. Assisting in identifying qualified experts

4. Performing medical literature search to determine nuances of medical care

5. Attending as many depositions and as much of the trial as is feasible

6. Preparing diligently for appearances by thoroughly knowing the medical records and the medical literature

7. Becoming educated and comfortable in dealing with the tactics of the plaintiff's attorney and the time and scheduling difficulties required by legal proceedings

8. Becoming educated about medical malpractice stress and its effects

9. Recognizing that there are inherent conflicts of interest between the insurer and the physician

10. By seeking private counsel

Box 133-2 Malpractice Causes of Action

1. Medical Negligence

2. Wrongful Death

3. Loss of a Chance of Recovery or Survival

4. Res Ipsa Loquitur (The Thing Speaks for Itself)

5. Battery and Assault

6. Lack of Informed Consent

7. Abandonment

8. Breach of Privacy and Confidentiality

9. Breach of Contract or Warranty to Cure

10. Products Liability for Drugs and Medical Devices

11. Vicarious Liability for Acts of Others

12. Negligent Referral

13. False Imprisonment

14. Defamation

15. Failure to Warn or Control

16. Negligent Infliction of Emotional Distress

17. Outrage

18. Failure to Report

19. Fraud and Misrepresentation (Deceit)

20. Loss of Consortium

ETIOLOGY (CAUSES OF ACTION) OF MEDICAL MALPRACTICE

Negligence is the most common basis for a medical malpractice action imposing liability on a physician. However, a medical malpractice lawsuit can be brought simultaneously under several legal theories. If the plaintiff-patient wins under any of these theories, recovery of a monetary award from the defendant-physician may result.

The legal theories, or causes of action, upon which a plaintiff may base a medical malpractice lawsuit are listed in Box 133-2.

DEFENSES TO A CLAIM OF MEDICAL MALPRACTICE

A defendant-physician can defeat a malpractice claim by utilizing one or several legal theories. The defenses available to the physician defendant in a case of medical malpractice are listed in Box 133-3.

SPECIFIC SITUATIONS PERTAINING TO HOSPITALISTS

Medical Negligence

Medical negligence is a breach of the physician's duty to behave reasonably and prudently under the circumstances that causes foreseeable harm to another. In legal terms, to present a cause of action for negligence, an injured patient must prove each of the four essential elements of medical negligence (duty of care, breach of duty or standard of care, causation, and damages) by the preponderance of evidence.

Box 133-3 Malpractice Defense Theories

1. Absence of one of the Four Essential Elements of Negligence:
   i. Absence of Duty
   ii. No Breach of Duty
   iii. Lack of Causation
   iv. No Damages

2. Good Samaritan Laws

3. Agreement with Patient to Exempt Health Care Provider from Liability

4. Statutes of Limitations: Failure to File a Malpractice Claim in a Timely Manner

5. Arbitration Agreement

6. Federal and State Institutional Immunity

7. Charitable Immunity

8. Assumption of the Risk

9. Contributory and Comparative Negligence

10. Last Clear Chance and Avoidable Consequences

11. Prior and Subsequent Negligent Physicians

12. Satisfaction and Release

13. Exculpatory Agreements and Indemnification Contracts

14. Settlement of Malpractice Claim

Vicarious Liability for the Actions of Other Health Care Providers

Physicians usually employ or supervise other less-qualified health care professionals, and consequently owe their patients the duty to properly supervise Physician Assistants, Nurse Practitioners, nurses, technicians, and other subordinates. The duty to supervise may create vicarious liability, whereby one person may be liable for the wrongful acts or omissions of another.

Respondeat Superior, "Captain of the Ship" and "Borrowed Servant" Doctrines

Respondeat superior states that an employer is liable for the negligence of his employees. For example, if a physician's nurse injects a drug into a patient's sciatic nerve, causing injury, that patient may sue the physician for the nurse's negligence.

Hospitalists may be held vicariously liable for the negligence of hospital employees they supervise. For example, surgeons have been sued for errors and omissions by operating room personnel under the "captain of the ship" doctrine, or more commonly the "borrowed servant" doctrine. A surgeon is held liable based on the theory that he has absolute control, much like the captain of a ship at sea, who is responsible for all the wrongs perpetrated by the crew. This doctrine was intended to offer a remedy to persons injured by negligent employees of charitable hospitals, which were otherwise legally immune from suit under the doctrine of charitable immunity.

Negligent Referrals

Physicians frequently request consultations from other physicians, especially regarding hospitalized patients. The referring physician may be liable for the specialist's misdeeds if each physician assumes the other will provide certain care that is omitted by both or if they neglect a common duty (e.g., postoperative care).

Just as physicians generally are not liable for consultants' malpractice, they need not answer for care provided by other physicians who cover their practice. Exceptions include the use of covering physicians who are also partners and the negligent selection of covering physicians.

False Imprisonment

False imprisonment is a tort that protects an individual from restraint of movement, which may occur if an individual is restrained against his or her will in any confined space or area. The plaintiff is entitled to compensation for loss of time, for any inconvenience suffered, and for physical or emotional harm. A physician holding a patient against his will, in absence of a court order, could be held liable for false imprisonment. Such situations arise in cases involving involuntary commitment of a patient with a mental disorder, where a patient is held without compliance with laws governing civil commitments.

Products or Strict Liability for Drugs and Medical Devices

Products or strict liability (i.e., not negligence-based liability) is imposed on manufacturers, sellers, and distributors of unrea-sonably dangerous and defective products for injuries resulting from their use. Such liability is independent of negligence law, and a defendant's degree of care is irrelevant in lawsuits based on the concept of strict liability.

Many medical malpractice suits also include claims for harm caused by the physician's alleged failure to inform and adequately warn the patient of a dangerous or defective product in his role as "learned intermediary."

WHY DO PATIENTS SUE DOCTORS?

The principal reasons why patients sue doctors include:
1. The injured patient's desire to prevent similar incidents from happening in the future
2. The patient's search for an honest and clear explanation as to how and why the injury occurred
3. The injured patients want the staff or organization to be accountable for their actions
4. Most injured patients *do not* sue their physicians because of financial motivation, although this might be another reason why patients or their relatives sue

The most powerful predictor of the likelihood of being sued is probably how well the physician relates to his or her patients. Both juries and judges generally favor physicians in malpractice cases. Physician defendants win approximately two out of three medical malpractice lawsuits that are brought before a jury. What is predictive of the frequency of medical malpractice claims is the number of physicians practicing in the area and not the number of lawyers. According to the General Accounting Office, less than 10% of the time do plaintiffs have injuries that would be regarded as "insignificant." The majority of the plaintiffs who file malpractice lawsuits have serious medical complications, which resulted from medical errors or adverse outcomes.

PROPHYLAXIS OR PREVENTION OF MALPRACTICE BEATS MALPRACTICE LITIGATION

Time-hardened experience has proven that to be forewarned is to be forearmed. This dictum is applicable to medical malpractice prevention. Prophylaxis indeed beats malpractice. Medical malpractice is very often preventable. Prophylactic awareness by physicians of malpractice liability, coupled with the adoption of preventive programs, should minimize allegations of malpractice. Victory is achievable when preventative alertness diminishes the need for aggressive legal defense.

Competently trained, experienced physicians and surgeons are mindful of legal liability. They follow a course of medical and surgical care that is commensurate and consistent with their skill, knowledge, ability, and experience. Such physicians and surgeons, when accused of medical malpractice, rarely lose in a court of law.

On the other hand, medical and surgical errors, mistakes, major judgmental miscalculations, and obvious negligence are difficult to defend. The quintessential physician and surgeon must pursue professional actions that are in the best interests of the patient. This prevails even if it demands personal inconvenience.

SUMMARY

The medical malpractice stress syndrome, etiology of and defenses to a claim alleging malpractice, and the reasons why patients sue physicians were reviewed. The physician should always attempt to relate well to the patient. Good communication skills and collaborative relationships with patients are effective at prevent lawsuits. Medical malpractice is preventable, and prophylaxis beats malpractice. One of the most potent and proven methods of prevention of medical malpractice is to educate physicians about the medical and legal ramifications of medical malpractice lawsuits. Physicians should be educated about malpractice litigation stress, how to react when confronted with a medical malpractice lawsuit, and how to communicate with the defense attorney; and they should have a good grasp of the legal process. Active physician participation in the defense of a medical malpractice lawsuit is the key to a successful outcome.

Key Points

- Medical malpractice crises during the past three decades and current malpractice claims statistics indicate a guarded prognosis for medical malpractice.

- The effects of medical malpractice lawsuits on the alleged negligent physicians are characterized by the "medical malpractice stress syndrome," a variation of litigation stress syndrome.

- Medical malpractice is most commonly due to negligence, is largely preventable, and is usually decided in favor of the physician.

- How well the physician relates to his or her patients is probably the most powerful predictor of the likelihood of being sued.

- Prophylaxis, the prevention of negligence, beats malpractice litigation.

- A most potent method of prevention of medical malpractice is to educate physicians about the medical and legal ramifications of medical malpractice litigation.

- Active physician participation in the defense of a medical malpractice lawsuit is the key to a successful outcome.

SUGGESTED READING

Gibofsky A, Firestone MH, Leblang TR, Liang BA, Snyder JW, Sanbar SS. Legal Medicine, 6th ed. Philadelphia, PA: Mosby, 2004.

Boumil MM, Elias CE, Moes DB. Medical Liability in a Nutshell, 2nd ed. St. Paul, MN: Thomson-West, 2003.

Charles SC, Wilbert JR, Franke KJ. Sued and non-sued physicians' reaction to malpractice litigation. Am J Psychiatry 1985; 142(4):437–440.

Charles SC. How to handle the stress of litigation. Clin Plast Surg 1999; 26(1):69–77.

Andrew LB. Litgation Stress—A Primer. www.acep.org/webportal/PracticeResources/issues/medleg/MedicalLegalACEPNewsOctober1999LitigationStress.htm (Access March 2007.)

Getting Sued. A resident's perspective. www.acep.org/webportal/membercenter/careers/residentsres/profskills/GettingSued.htm (Accessed March 2007.)

Roberts RG. Seven reasons family doctors get sued and how to reduce your risk. Fam Pract Manage 2003; 10(3):29–34.

CHAPTER ONE HUNDRED AND THIRTY-FOUR

Legal Issues in Hospitalist-Hospital Relationships

Andrew M. Knoll, MD, JD, FACP, FCLM

INTRODUCTION

While the practice of medicine is a profession, it is also a business. As a businessperson, the hospitalist must have some understanding of the law as it relates to his or her business. The necessary degree of understanding will vary, depending upon the sophistication of the business model. A hospitalist employed by the Veterans Administration does not require the same knowledge of the law as a hospitalist who is the president of a professional corporation (comprised of many physicians, shareholders, and employees) who has contracts involving more than one hospital. The former needs to primarily know about professional misconduct rules and patient confidentiality (and it does not hurt to know that such a physician is immune from personal medical malpractice liability pursuant to the Federal Tort Claims Act). The latter not only needs to know about these rules but must also have a working knowledge of referral laws (Stark and anti-kickback), Medicare billing rules, antitrust law, basic business law (such as employment laws like the Family Medical Leave Act and Americans with Disabilities Act), and Emergency Medical Treatment and Active Labor Act (EMTALA).

This chapter is designed primarily for the latter hospitalist. Its purpose is to introduce the reader to the federal regulatory scheme that oversees the legal relationship between hospitalists and hospitals. It is not meant to be comprehensive but, rather, a general overview designed to familiarize the hospitalist with the issues and the basic law. Law, like medicine, is fact-specific and nuanced. Moreover, there are exceptions and exceptions to the exception. Legal counsel should be considered whenever entering into contractual relationships with hospitals or other entities to which the hospitalist refers patients, especially where the contractual relationships are complex.

This chapter will discuss five federal statutory/regulatory schemes that are of primary importance to the hospitalist. They are: (1) the Stark Law prohibition against self-referral; (2) the Anti-Kickback Statute (AKS); (3) antitrust law; (4) the Medicare prohibition against gainsharing; and (5) tax-exempt status and not-for-profit law. The reader should be aware that there are also state law equivalents that generally, but not exactly, parallel these federal laws. Hospitalists and hospitals must be compliant with both the federal and state laws.

Failure to comply with these laws can lead to significant sanctions. These include denial and return of payments, Civil Monetary Penalties, False Claims actions, and the professional death sentence of a hospitalist, exclusion from participation in Medicare and Medicaid.[1] Furthermore, while the risk of sanctions against an individual physician is admittedly rare, the hospital also has risk and will not enter into any contract that it believes will increase that risk. Hospitals are extensively regulated and have considerable concern regarding compliance. Hospital medicine, as a distinct field of practice, is also relatively new, and hospitals do not have experience with the business model. A key element of the business model is that the majority of US hospitalist programs require financial support, or a subsidy, from the hospital in which they work.[2] Other and older hospital-based specialties, such as pathology, anesthesiology, radiology, and emergency medicine, rarely, if ever, have required subsidization. Moreover, hospitals (and their attorneys) are conservative in this regard and often erroneously believe that subsidizing hospitalist groups violates the law. A hospitalist must be fully cognizant of these laws when negotiating contracts with the hospital so as to push for permissible and favorable arrangements.

THE STARK LAW

The Stark Law states that a physician (or an immediate family member of such physician) may not make a referral for the furnishing of designated health services to an entity with which he has a financial relationship unless an exception applies.[3]

The law was proposed by Rep. Fortney "Pete" Stark and enacted by Congress in 1992. While the original law only prohibited a physician from referring a patient to a laboratory where that physician had a financial relationship, there have been amendments, as well as additional regulations promulgated by the Secretary of the Department of Health and Human Services (DHHS). The latest revision was promulgated by the Centers for Medicare and Medicaid Services (CMS) on March 26, 2004 as Phase II of Stark II. The new regulations became effective as of July 24, 2004.[4]

In order to understand a statute, one needs to understand the underlying public policy. The ill Congress intended to remedy was over-utilization and increased costs resulting from the financial self-interest inherent in laboratory ownership. Congress was concerned that even a well-intentioned physician may subconsciously increase utilization because of the financial interest, so the law establishes strict liability. Referral for a designated health service (DHS) to an entity with which a physician has a financial relationship, no matter how appropriate the service or fair the price, violates the law. Congress, recognizing that such a prohibition would be unworkable, provided for "exceptions," which, when complied with, permit a physician to refer a patient for DHS to an entity with which he has a financial relationship.

These exceptions are listed either in the statute itself or the accompanying regulations promulgated by CMS and consist of a checklist of conditions that must be satisfied in order to qualify for the exception. Although the federal Stark Law is applicable only to Medicare (and indirectly, Medicaid) patients, most states have their own form of self-referral law, which, like New York, may be applicable to all patients.[5]

DHS is defined to include: (1) clinical laboratory services; (2) physical therapy, occupational therapy, and speech-language pathology services; (3) radiology and certain other imaging services; (4) radiation therapy services and supplies; (5) durable medical equipment and supplies; (6) parenteral and enteral nutrients, equipment, and supplies; (7) prosthetics, orthotics, and prosthetic devices and supplies; (8) home health services; (9) outpatient prescription drugs; and (10) inpatient and outpatient hospital services.[6] Under the Stark Law, a hospitalist who orders a CBC is referring a patient to an entity (the hospital's laboratory) for DHS (the CBC, a "clinical laboratory service"). Stark, therefore, is implicated if the hospitalist has any form of financial relationship with the hospital whatsoever.[7] And Stark is violated if that relationship does not satisfy an express exception.

The common exceptions applicable to a hospitalist are the Employment, Personal Service, and Indirect Compensation Arrangement Exceptions. Certain practices may also implicate the Lease, Fair Market Value, and Recruitment Exceptions. A full recitation of the elements of these exceptions is beyond the scope of this chapter. The elements of the Personal Service Exception, which would be applicable to payments to a hospitalist to provide services as Director of Inpatient Medicine, will be used as an example.

The Personal Service Exception provides that remuneration paid to a physician (or his group practice or immediate family member) for services provided to the DHS entity will not violate Stark so long as the conditions in Box 134-1 are met.

Another potentially important Stark Law exception involves recruitment.[8] This exception would permit a hospital to completely subsidize the compensation package of a new hospitalist so long as certain criteria are met. One important element of the recruitment exception is that the group cannot impose any practice restrictions on the physician.[9] This would preclude enforcing a restrictive covenant (see discussion below).

The other exceptions vary, but there are common points. Generally, any arrangement must be in writing and be a term of at least 1 year; and the remuneration must be set out in advance, be fair market value (FMV), and be calculated in a manner that does not take into account the volume or value of referrals. There is much commentary and nuance regarding these terms. For example, per-unit compensation (e.g., payment per patient admission or consult) is deemed not to take into account the volume or value of referrals so long as the amount and methodology used to calculate the remuneration are set out in advance of execution of the contract, are FMV for services rendered, and do not vary during its term.[10]

Box 134-1 Stark Law Personal Services Exception

- Each arrangement is set out in writing, is signed by the parties, and specifies the services covered by the arrangement.
- The arrangement(s) cover(s) all of the services to be furnished by the physician (or an immediate family member of the physician) to the entity.
- The aggregate services contracted for do not exceed those that are reasonable and necessary for the legitimate business purposes of the arrangement(s).
- The term of each arrangement is for at least 1 year. An arrangement may be terminable, but in that case, the parties may not enter into the same or substantially the same arrangement during the first year of the original term of the arrangement.
- The compensation to be paid over the term of each arrangement is set in advance, does not exceed fair market value, and is not determined in a manner that takes into account the volume or value of any referrals or other business generated between the parties.
- The services to be furnished under each arrangement do not involve the counseling or promotion of a business arrangement or other activity that violates any State or Federal law.[30]

Providing FMV for services rendered is a common requirement, which is included in the Stark Law, the Anti-Kickback Statute (AKS) and not-for-profit law. FMV means the value established in an arms-length transaction, as the result of bona fide bargaining between well-informed parties who are under no compulsion to deal and resulting in terms that would be fair even if there would be no referrals between the parties.[11] There are safe harbors that are deemed to be FMV, such as hourly remuneration that equals that paid to emergency physicians in the area.[12] Safe harbor qualification is not necessary, and any reasonable methodology of establishing FMV (e.g., comparable salaries of other hospitalists in the city, survey data supplied by organizations such as the Society for Hospital Medicine, or independent negotiation between the hospitalist's and the hospital's respective attorneys) would be sufficient.

So long as these criteria are complied with in hospitalist–hospital contracts, the Stark law exception is satisfied, and the hospitalist can refer the patient to the hospital for DHS without either the hospitalist or the hospital running afoul of the law and potentially facing penalties and sanctions.

THE ANTI-KICKBACK STATUTE

The AKS makes it illegal for anyone to receive any remuneration, directly or indirectly, for referring an individual for a service paid by a federal health care program. Violation is a felony, punishable by up to 5 years in prison and a $25,000 fine.[13] Here, the ill Congress intended to remedy was the payment or receipt of bribes in return for referrals. The law, however, is written very broadly, and any remuneration could be considered a potential kickback. Moreover, federal case law holds that the AKS is violated if only one intention of the remuneration is to induce or reward referrals.[14]

Table 134-1 Antitrust Issues

Exclusive contracts	Contract that grants a hospitalist group the sole right to be the hospitalist group at that institution	Held by the U.S. Supreme Court to not violate antitrust law
Sweeps clauses	Contractual provision that terminates hospital privileges of hospitalists when their contract terminates	Permissible because, under the law, are treated as voluntary resignations. Not reportable because no quality issues involved
Restrictive covenants	Restrictions on how far away and for how long a former employee is permitted to compete with his employer	Governed by state law. Generally permissible so long as reasonable
Collective bargaining	Physicians collectively bargaining with third-party payers for rates of reimbursement	Violate antitrust law except in certain circumstances where the physicians are clinically or financially integrated

As with the Stark law, the DHHS has promulgated safe harbors whereby compliance will provide immunity from prosecution. Unlike the Stark law, the AKS is an intent-based statute, and compliance with a safe harbor is not mandatory. Any arrangement that does not exactly comply with a safe harbor is not *per se* illegal but would, if investigated, be evaluated based upon the facts, circumstances, and intentions of the parties. There are safe harbors for employment, personal services arrangements, and leases, which closely parallel the Stark Law exceptions.[15] One noticeable difference is that per-click arrangements (i.e., where payment is made per transaction, and as per admission or consult, and not per month or year) do not qualify for safe harbor treatment because the aggregate amount will change, and the Stark Law special compensation rule stated above is not applicable to the AKS.

The AKS applies both to the giver and recipient of remuneration. This potentially can be beneficial to the hospitalist in negotiating with the hospital. For example, if the Director of Cardiology is typically paid $40,000, the hospital will potentially violate the AKS if it does not pay the Director of Inpatient Medicine $40,000, assuming the provided services are approximately the same.

ANTITRUST LAW

Antitrust law is a highly complex area of law whose purpose is to protect consumers by promoting competition. While physicians typically do not consider their colleagues to be competitors, the Department of Justice and the Federal Trade Commission, who jointly administer and enforce the antitrust laws, do. A new internist, asking an older internist with whom he is not in practice, how much the latter charges for a CPT 99223 admission may be considered by these agencies to have engaged in a horizontal agreement to exchange pricing information in violation of the law. Antitrust issues relevant to the hospitalist are discussed below and include exclusive contracts, sweeps clauses, restrictive covenants, and collective bargaining (Table 134-1).

Hospitalists, like other hospital-based physicians, may be given exclusive contracts. On its face, such a contract would be a restraint of trade, since other hospitalist groups would be precluded from providing services at the hospital or, in antitrust terminology, competitors would be foreclosed from entering the market. Exclusive contracts involving hospital-based physicians were upheld by the Supreme Court in the seminal decision of *Jefferson Parish Hosp. Dist. No. 2 v. Hyde.*[16] *Jefferson Parish* involved an anesthesiologist who was denied privileges because another anesthesiology group held an exclusive contract. The Court held that the arrangement did not violate antitrust law because the hospital did not exert "market power."

Market power is the ability for an actor to raise prices without losing sales. Jefferson Parish is a suburb of New Orleans, where there are a significant number of hospitals. As such, the market for surgery and anesthesia is unaffected by the contractual arrangements between a relatively small number of actors. Since *Jefferson Parish* was decided, courts have uniformly upheld exclusive contracts. A recent case, however, has questioned exclusive contracts in relatively rural areas.

A federal judge denied summary judgment as to whether an exclusive contract for surgical procedures involving the only hospital in Rome, New York would result in impermissible market power.[17] Of note, while Rome Memorial Hospital was the sole hospital in Rome, the court recognized that there were four other hospitals within a 20-mile radius. As this was a motion for summary judgment, a definitive rule of law was not established,[18] and it remains to be seen whether exclusivity will be permissible where the geographic market is serviced by only one hospital. At the time this chapter was written, however, the rule is that exclusive contracts do not violate antitrust law.

Sweeps clauses are the reverse side of exclusive contracts. A sweeps clause provides that should the hospitalist group lose the contract, for whatever reason, the physicians' clinical privileges and membership on the hospital's medical staff will terminate. This permits the hospital to "sweep out" the old hospitalist group to make room for the new.

Like exclusive contracts, on its face, these clauses would appear to be impermissible restraints on trade. Additionally, they would appear to be impermissible adverse credentialing actions rendered without due process. That is not the case because, legally, a sweeps clause is a contractual provision whereby, in consideration of receiving exclusivity, the physicians are contractually agreeing to voluntarily resign should the contract terminate. In effect, a sweeps clause is an undated letter of resignation that will only be executed upon the loss of the exclusive contract. Because the termination of privileges is voluntary (i.e., nothing is forcing a hospitalist to enter into the contract or accept a position with such a clause), due process rights are not implicated.

Other provisions similar to sweeps clauses that result in a permissible restraint of trade are restrictive covenants. These are governed by state law, not federal, and therefore the reader must seek the law of the jurisdiction regarding their enforceability. Generally, restrictive covenants are enforceable, but there are exceptions, such as California, where restrictive covenants are prohibited by statute.[19] The key issue is that a restrictive covenant cannot be punitive but must protect an employer's legitimate business interest. In general, a restrictive covenant must be reasonable with regard to the temporal and geographic scope. As a rule of thumb, 2 years is a reasonable temporal restriction. Geographical restrictions depend upon the catchment area. A geographical restriction reasonable to Manhattan, Kansas is not necessarily reasonable to Manhattan, New York.

The reader should also be aware that payments made to recruit a physician (as discussed more thoroughly above) will only qualify for the Stark Law Recruitment Exception if there is no restraint on the physician. This would preclude a restrictive covenant in that physician's employment agreement.

A final antitrust issue involving hospitalists is collective bargaining. This generally arises in the setting of a Physician-Hospital Organization (PHO) or Physician Organization (PO) that is seeking to collectively bargain with third party payors. PHOs or POs typically offer the full panoply of medical services as a group and compete for contracts with other PHOs and POs in the area. Hospitalists may be asked or required to join these organizations so that inpatient medical services can be included within the offered product.

While a complete discussion of the antitrust rules with regard to these organizations is beyond the scope of this chapter, collective bargaining is only permissible if the organization has achieved financial or clinical integration.[20] Financial integration involves risk sharing, through capitated payments and/or withholds. Clinical integration requires a considerable investment in capital, and physicians must subrogate their individual practices to the network as a whole, through practice protocols and quality improvement indicators. PHOs and POs that are neither financially nor clinically integrated cannot collectively bargain. In those situations, the organization is limited to "messengering" the offer from the third-party payor to the group. The group must then make its own decision to accept or decline the offer.

MEDICARE GAINSHARING PROHIBITION

Section 1128A(b)(1) of the Social Security Act prohibits a hospital from making a payment, directly or indirectly, to induce a physician to reduce or limit services to a Medicare or Medicaid beneficiary.[21] As with many other federal regulatory rules, the prohibition is broad, and no actual reduction in care is required; the hospital's knowledge that remuneration could induce a physician to reduce care is sufficient to violate the law.[22] The quality of patient care need not suffer for the law to be implicated. The financial inducement to reduce benefits is sufficient.

DHHS' concern, and the policy behind the statute, is similar to the Stark Law. Namely, that there exists a high risk of abuse where a physician's financial gain is tied to under-utilizing services, just as with over-utilizing services.

A gainsharing arrangement is implicated where the hospital pays the physician a share of the reduction of its costs that are attributable in part to the physician's efforts. With regard to the hospitalist, the prohibition primarily involves incentive payments for reducing lengths of stay.[23] In a 1999 Special Advisory Bulletin, the OIG noted that reducing unnecessary lengths of stay without compromising quality of care would be laudable. Nevertheless, the OIG prohibited the practice absent legislative amendment because of the clear language of the statute.

Had this chapter been written a year ago, this section would have ended with the sentence above. That is because prior to 2005, the OIG had never issued a favorable Advisory Opinion permitting a gainsharing arrangement. In February of 2005, the OIG issued six favorable Advisory Opinions approving gainsharing arrangements.[24] These opinions all involved proceduralists. The OIG approved gainsharing arrangements where, for example, potentially necessary but often unused surgical packages are not opened unless required or less-expensive stents were used. The arrangements also provided for additional safeguards, such as requiring the medical groups to share the bonus per capita and not based upon an individual physician's reduction in cost. These opinions are not on point with regard to length of stay reductions, but the OIG has opened the door to the possibility. Any group considering length-of-stay bonuses is strongly advised to first obtain an OIG Advisory Opinion.

NOT-FOR-PROFIT LAW

The last issue addressed in this chapter is not-for-profit law. This is a major concern for the hospitalist. A hospital's tax exempt status pursuant to §501(c)(3) of the Internal Revenue Code (IRC) not only permits it to be exempt from paying income tax on any net income, but it also allows the hospital to be exempt from paying sales tax on purchases and permits its donors to take a charitable contribution when making donations. Needless to say, hospitals strongly protect their tax-exempt status and will not enter into any arrangement that may jeopardize this status.

The hospitalist needs to be cognizant of these rules in order to effectively negotiate with the hospital. As a general rule, so long as it is structured fairly and remuneration is FMV, a typical hospitalist–hospital contract will not violate the statutes and regulations of the IRC.

The hospital's primary concern is whether the remuneration paid to the hospitalist will run afoul of the private inurement and excess benefit rules. The prohibition against private inurement provides that net income of a tax-exempt organization cannot inure to the benefit of a private individual.[25] This rule is only applicable to "insiders" (i.e., persons having a personal and private interest in the activities of the organization,[26] which typically include shareholders, directors, officers, major donors and senior management). A hospitalist would rarely, if ever, be an insider.

The more commonly applicable rule is the Excess Benefit Transaction rule that provides for a penalty excise tax for compensation provided to any "disqualified person" in excess of "reasonable compensation."[27] A disqualified person is a person who is in a position to exert substantial influence over the tax-exempt organization.[28] The IRS, in its regulations, gave two examples of physicians, one of whom would be a disqualified person, the other would not.

In those examples, a radiologist who receives both a salary and an incentive bonus from the hospital, but does not have a financial interest in the hospital, does not serve as an officer or on its board, and does not participate in any management decisions affecting either the hospital as a whole or a discrete segment of the hospital that represents a substantial portion of its activities, assets, income, or expenses, was not a disqualified person. In contrast, a salaried cardiologist who is the head of the cardiology department, which is a major source of patients admitted to the hospital and consequently represents a substantial portion of the hospital's income, and is authorized to manage the department, allocate its budget, and distribute bonuses to personnel was a disqualified person.[29] In accordance with those guidelines, the medical director of a hospitalist program that admits a significant number of the hospital's patients would be a disqualified person.

This does not mean that the hospital cannot pay compensation to such an individual. Such compensation must merely be reasonable. This requires that payment be in an amount that ordinarily is paid for like services by like organizations in like circumstances[30] (i.e., FMV). As with the discussion regarding the AKS, typical compensation arrangements between hospitalists and hospitals will not violate the IRS tax-exempt rules. Hospitalists provide a number of essential services to hospitals that further the hospital's charitable mission. So long as compensation is FMV, the hospital's tax exempt status will not be jeopardized, nor will it be subject to excess benefit excise taxes.

to ensure compliance with these complex rules. A hospitalist should be skeptical when told the rules prohibit payment under most circumstances, and a working knowledge of these rules is essential to any hospitalist whose responsibility is to directly negotiate compensation arrangements with the hospital.

Key Points

- The practice of medicine is highly regulated, and contractual relationships between physicians and hospitals must comply with the law.

- The major areas of the law implicated by hospitalist–hospital relations are the Stark Law, AKS, antitrust law, tax-exempt law, and the Medicare gainsharing prohibition.

- Hospitals can permissibly subsidize hospitalists.

- Exclusivity contracts are permissible.

- In order to comply with the law, contracts between hospitalists and hospitals must be written carefully and contain specific regulatory provisions.

CONCLUSION

This chapter has given the reader an introduction to the complex area of regulatory health care law that governs hospitalist–hospital contractual relationships. The bottom line is that hospitals can (and, in fact, legally should) reasonably compensate hospitalists for the services they provide. Legal counsel is required

SUGGESTED READING

Abrams R., Moy D, eds., Legal Manual for New York Physicians. Albany, NY: New York State Bar Association, 2003.

Broccolo BM, et al, eds. Fundamentals of Health Law, 3rd cd. Washington DC: American Health Lawyers Association, 2004.

Sanbar SS, et al, eds. American College of Legal Medicine: Legal Medicine, 6th ed. Philadelphia: Mosby, Inc., 2004.

CHAPTER ONE HUNDRED AND THIRTY-FIVE

Developing and Maintaining the Physician-Hospital Relationship

Richard Rohr MD, MMM

BACKGROUND

The relationship between hospitals and physicians has changed dramatically in recent years. Physicians once placed considerable value upon their affiliation with a hospital. They would concentrate their practice at one hospital, serve on organizational committees, support fund drives, and seek to boost the reputation of the hospital. In recent years, many surgeons and other specialists have chosen to treat patients in specialized facilities other than general hospitals, often facilities in which they have partial ownership. Primary care physicians now focus only on providing ambulatory services in their own offices. This situation promoted development of hospital medicine as a distinct specialty. The hospitalist, often willing to make a significant commitment to the hospital in which he or she works, may nonetheless be frustrated by an obsolete paradigm for hospital–medical staff relations. This chapter outlines a new paradigm for the physician–hospital relationship, based on high-performance partnership concepts developed in other industries.

The predominant driver of the physician–hospital relationship has been the revenue produced for hospitals by the patients referred by physicians. The typical physician in private practice—through patient referral and utilization of ancillary services—generates in excess of one million dollars annually for the hospital; up to 10 times the personal income of the physician.[9] Hospitals have generally sought to receive referrals from as many physicians as possible and have been willing to provide economic incentives in return. Diverting a small portion of the hospital's revenue back to the referring physician can produce a substantially greater effect on the doctor's income. However, the potential for unethical behavior is substantial. This caused the US Congress to enact certain laws restricting the incentives that hospitals can provide to physicians (e.g., the Stark law). These laws, described in greater detail in Chapter 134 (Legal Issues in the Hospital–Hospitalist Relationship), have less relevance to the practice of hospital medicine than is commonly believed, as they do not prevent payments to physicians for defined services provided to the hospital, but the legal requirements must be observed.

The hospitalist occupies a curious position in the paradigm described above. Without a pool of patients available for referral to the hospital, the value of the hospitalist to the hospital could theoretically be zero. However, with private practitioners reducing their involvement while hospitals require even more engagement by physicians, hospitalists may be invaluable. Quality of patient care was once assumed to exist if a certain set of skills and technologies existed within the institution. Doctors provided the skills, and the hospital bought technology with the revenue generated by the doctors. The public now understands that actual performance is more important than the theoretical capabilities of the hospital. CMS (Centers for Medicaid and Medicare Services) increasingly pushes Pay for Performance (P4P—described in more detail in Chapter 125), with proposed adjustments to hospital payments based on certain quality measures. The economic viability of hospitals now depends progressively more upon actual patient outcomes achieved—mandating involvement by those wielding the order pen, physicians.[6,7] Hospital managers find that they have little ability to improve performance among their private medical staffs because the traditional paradigm emphasizes production over quality, and also because the peer review function within the medical staff can only control the most egregious lapses in quality. Hospitalists can assume an important and essential role in changing administrative and clinical processes in hospitals.[1]

A new paradigm for hospital–physician relationships must be based on patient referral volume, resource utilization, and quality of care (Table 135-1). The value of the physician to the hospital must be based on both the ability of the physician to refer or recruit patients and also the contribution of that physician to outcomes of patient care. Financial incentives should be based not solely on the number of patients referred by the physician, but also on the improvement in health that occurs through the physician's efforts and the efficiency with which that is accomplished. Health status is difficult to quantify, and not all outcomes can be ascribed to the doctor. It is reasonable to identify practices shown by scientific evidence to improve health and to provide incentives for the use of these practices (i.e., process measures). This must be done carefully to avoid creating distorted goals, as no incentive plan can reward every aspect of professional performance.[5] Incentives should be linked only to measures fully controlled by physicians and the data used must be accurate. Hospitals must also assign specific value to services performed by physicians that support hospital operations and further the hospital's mission. These services include participation in utilization review, quality improvement, technology assessment, peer review, and care for indigent patients. Physicians once volunteered their services in

Table 135-1 Comparison of Old and New Paradigms for Hospital–Physician Relationships

	Old Paradigm	New Paradigm
Hospital provides	Medical technology	Medical technology
	Financial support for developing practices	Financial support for developing and existing practices
		Information technology
		Quality and financial performance data
Physicians provide	Patient referrals	Patient referrals
	Medical skills	Medical skills
		Responsibility for quality of care
		Responsibility for resource utilization
Interaction between parties	Indirect, generally through medical staff organization	Direct relationships

Table 135-2 Independent Contractors versus Hospital Employee Models

	Independent Contractor	Hospital Employee
Organization specifies	Outcome only	Methods and outcome of work
Income guaranteed by organization	No	Yes
Free to work for multiple organizations	Yes	No
Equipment and supplies provided by organization	No	Yes
Ability to profit	Yes	No
Duration of relationship	Defined, usually by duration of task	Indefinite
Vulnerability to competition	Unlimited	Limited

these areas in return for maintaining an affiliation with the institution. Now that physicians place little value on hospital affiliation, it is necessary for hospitals to pay for those services. Consensus has not emerged on the best methods for compensating these services, but since the time required can be measured, some suggest assigning an hourly rate, as this is permitted by the Stark regulations. This rate should be at least equivalent to the patient care revenues that could be generated in the same period of time and may range up to the average hourly compensation for emergency physicians in the community or the average national compensation for physicians in the same specialty.

The new hospital–physician paradigm must also provide for a different style of interaction. Physicians are socialized to demand complete freedom of action and are reluctant to participate in organizations. When treating patients in the hospital, physicians chafe at requirements to document their actions clearly and to follow standard methods for diagnosis and treatment. However, hospitals can no longer afford to support idiosyncratic approaches to patient care. Effective practice of hospital medicine will require that physicians commit themselves to supporting the goals of the hospital.[11,12] It will also require that hospital managers commit to supporting hospitalists in their aims.[13,14]

While hospitalists may consider themselves to be independent contractors with the hospital, the typical nature of such relationships is not consistent with the new paradigm. The Internal Revenue Service (IRS) has given careful consideration to the distinction between employees and independent contractors (Table 135-2).[8] Their guidelines consider such issues as whether or not the contractor is free to determine the methods used in performing the work; can employ assistants of his or her choosing; uses equipment supplied by the hospital; and is at risk for profit or loss

from the work, along with the permanency of the relationship. Hospitalists working in a single hospital on a long-term basis and receiving financial support from the hospital would be classified as employees under the IRS guidelines. Traditional concepts of employment are also not appropriate for the hospital–hospitalist relationship. Physicians do not fit very well into an organizational chart. While guidelines and policies are suitable as general principles for medical practice, the practitioner must have the ability to modify and override such policies when this is required to meet the needs of an individual patient. This type of discretion is traditionally reserved for senior managers in an organization and is not provided to front-line production workers, but physicians need to function in both roles. They must be allowed to manage themselves, with guidance from top management, not commands.

The hospital–physician relationship must recognize that neither party is fully dependent on the other, but they are not completely independent.[10] The term interdependence was introduced by Covey[2] to describe this type of relationship. Interdependent relationships call for the partners to consider each other's needs and find solutions to problems that advance the interests of both sides. Interdependent relationships employ the strengths of both parties to achieve results that neither could accomplish alone (Box 135-1).

The best models for interdependent business relationships have emerged from the Japanese automobile industry and are being adopted by other businesses worldwide. The Kaiser Foundation Health Plan and the Permanente Medical Groups have interdependent relationships, but these are otherwise rare in health care. The hallmarks of these relationships are joint planning processes, regular discussion about the state of the relationship, willingness to sacrifice advantages that may be enjoyed by one party over the other in order to further the combined enterprise, measurement of joint performance, and a long-term perspective in judging the fairness of the partnership. Lambert and Knemeyer[4] have described a method for establishing high-performance relationships. The legal structure of the relationship may be in the form of an employment agreement or a contract with a corporation established by the physicians; these are the only alternatives until new systems of corporate organization are developed. The choice will be based on legal and financial considerations that are external to the essential nature of an interdependent relationship.

Negotiating the relationship may be difficult for both sides. Physicians may lack business skills, while administrators are not accustomed to approaching physicians as partners. Indeed, the hospital will possess more economic power than any physician or small group. Fisher, Ury, and Patton in their book *Getting to Yes*[3] described an approach to this situation involving four basic principles (Box 135-2). They recommend identifying the best alternative to a negotiated agreement for each party (e.g., terminating the hospitalist service and returning to private practice). If the hospital and hospitalist have an interdependent relationship, neither side will have a satisfactory alternative to negotiated agreement, and they will come to terms. The negotiation process will never be entirely finished and will continue in some form throughout the relationship. As the parties strengthen their relationship, the distinction between doctor and administrator will be blurred, and physicians will come to occupy operational management positions within the hospital.

IMPLEMENTATION OF PRINCIPLED NEGOTIATION

Resources Needed

- Knowledge of the fair-market value for services provided by the hospitalist to the hospital, as indicated by national and regional surveys[18–21]
- Knowledge of the quality and performance measures that determine hospital success (*see* Chapters 125 and 126 on Quality Improvement and Chapter 127 on Patient Safety)
- Listening and relationship skills[15,17]
- Negotiation skills[16]

Specific Steps

- Consider the specific needs that the hospitalist would like to satisfy through a relationship with the hospital, such as income, security, and prestige.
- Determine the types and levels of performance that the hospital requires from its medical staff, such as reduced LOS, improved outcomes, and reduced costs.
- Estimate the level of performance that the hospitalist(s) can achieve in each pertinent area and its potential value to the hospital.
- Identify specific medical services other than direct patient care that can be provided to the hospital and their fair-market value.
- Decide between employment and independent contractor status.
- Negotiate the terms of the relationship with hospital administrators, with the intention of creating a long-term partnership.
- Review the state of the partnership with the administrators regularly and systematically.

Comprehensive Hospital Medicine: An Evidence Based and Systems Approach

Barriers

- Hospital administrators have little experience in establishing partnerships with physicians and may doubt the sincerity of the hospitalist in developing a mutually beneficial relationship.
- Hospitalists may have little or no experience in business negotiation and may require the services of a skilled negotiator.
- When multiple competing hospitalist services exist within a single hospital, it will be difficult for the administration to develop a close relationship with each one.

NEGOTIATION

- Measures of clinical and economic performance should be developed jointly by the hospital and hospitalist.
- Planning processes should be designed to foster the relationship rather than focus on the individual task at hand.
- There should be an explicit plan to meet and review the relationship at regular intervals.
- The focus should be on mutual profitability, rather than each party seeking its own financial advantage.
- Issues should be discussed on a regular basis from a relationship focus, rather than in an isolated fashion as they arise.

Common Pitfalls

- Hospitalists frequently enter negotiations with the idea that they are entitled to a certain level of income by virtue of their status as physicians. Hospitals cannot insulate physicians from external economic forces. Hospitalists must recognize that their incomes will be determined by the sum of their efforts on behalf of patients and the hospital, with value determined by the market at large.
- Hospital administrators have difficulty understanding that they must pay for services that were previously volunteered by the medical staff. They must understand that physicians in private practice have greatly diminished the value that they place on hospital affiliation. Administrators must also recognize that the effort required for control of quality and utilization has increased substantially in recent years.
- Physicians are socialized during training to insist upon total autonomy in practice and do not understand the benefits that may be obtained through teamwork with other professionals.

SUMMARY

A successful relationship between hospitalists and hospital managers is the result of careful planning, cooperative attitudes on both sides, and frequent discussion. The planning process requires an understanding of the factors that will make both the hospital and the hospitalist successful. Both sides need to under-stand that they are each likely to fail without the help of the other party. Hospitalist programs need frequent readjustment in response to changing conditions in the clinical and financial environments.

Key Points

- Hospitalists must develop and maintain strong relationships with the managers of the hospitals in which they practice.

- Hospitalists need financial and organizational support from the hospitals in which they practice, but must demonstrate the value of services provided in return.

- The optimal relationship between hospitalists and hospitals may be described as one of interdependence.

- Both parties in an interdependent relationship must listen and consider carefully the needs of their partners before advancing their own interests.

- Hospitalists will need to understand methods of principled negotiation, including separating the person from the problem and negotiating from interests rather than positions.

SUGGESTED READING

Bernd D. The future role of hospitalists. Hospitalist 2005; 9(Suppl 1):4–5.

Covey S. The Seven Habits of Highly Effective People. New York: Fireside Books, 1989.

Fisher R, Ury W, Patton B. Getting to Yes: Negotiating Agreement Without Giving In. Second Edition. New York: Penguin Books, 1991.

Lambert D, Knemeyer A. We're in this together. Harvard Bus Rev 2004; 82(12): 114–122.

Conway W. Compensation in perspective. In: Silversin J, Kornacki MJ. Leading Physicians Through Change: How to Achieve and Sustain Results. Tampa: American College of Physician Executives, 2000.

Earning hospitals money: How do specialties compare. Am Med News 2004; 47(37):25.

O'Connor E, Annison M. Building trust and collaboration between physicians and administrators. Phys Executive 2002; 28(2):48–52.

Weymier R. The hospital/physician divide: understanding the drivers of their relationships. Phys Executive 2004; 30(3):60–62.

Cohn K, Gill S, Schwartz R. Gaining hospital administrators' attention: ways to improve physician-hospital management dialogue. Surgery 2005; 137(2):132–140.

Conger J. The necessary art of persuasion. Harvard Bus Rev 1998; 76(3):84–95.

Ertel D. Getting past yes: negotiating as if implementation mattered. Harvard Bus Rev 2004; 82(11):60–71.

Katzenbach J, Smith D. The discipline of teams. Harvard Bus Rev 2005; 83(7):162–171.

APPENDIX ONE

NIH Stroke Scale

Score Calculated according to scoring below _____		
1a. Level of consciousness	0	Alert
	1	Not alert, but arousable with minimal stimulation
	2	Not alert, requires repeated stimulation to attend, =Coma
1b. Ask patient the month and their age:	0	Answers both correctly
	1	Answers one correctly
	2	Both incorrect
1c. Ask patient to open and close eyes:	0	Obeys both correctly
	1	Obeys one correctly
	2	Forced deviation
2. Best gaze (only horizontal eye movement):	0	Normal
	1	Partial gaze palsy
	2	Forced deviation
3. Visual field testing	0	No visual loss
	1	Partial hemianopia
	2	Complete hemianopia
	3	Bilateral hemianopia (blind including cortical blindness)
4. Facial paresis (Ask patient to show teeth or raise eyebrows and close eyes tightly):	0	Normal symmetrical movement
	1	Minor paralysis (flattened nasolabial fold, asymmetry on smiling)
	2	Partial paralysis (total or near paralysis of lower face)
	3	Complete paralysis of one or both sides
5r. Motor function—right arm:	0	Normal (extends arm 90(or45) degrees for 10 seconds w/o drift
	1	Drift
	2	Some effort against gravity
	3	No effort against gravity
	4	No movement
	9	Untestable (Joint fused or limb amputated)
5l. Motor function—left arm:	0	Normal (extends arm 90(or45) degrees for 10 seconds w/o drift
	1	Drift
	2	Some effort against gravity
	3	No effort against gravity
	4	No movement
	9	Untestable (Joint fused or limb amputated)
6r. Motor function—right leg:	0	Normal (extends leg 90(or45) degrees for 10 seconds w/o drift
	1	Drift
	2	Some effort against gravity
	3	No effort against gravity
	4	No movement
	9	Untestable (Joint fused or limb amputated)

Score Calculated according to scoring below _____

6l.	Motor function—left leg:	0	Normal (extends leg 90(or45) degrees for 10 seconds w/o drift
		1	Drift
		2	Some effort against gravity
		3	No effort against gravity
		4	No movement
		9	Untestable (Joint fused or limb amputated)
7.	Limb ataxia:	0	No ataxia
		1	Present in one limb
		2	Present in two limbs
		9	Untestable (Joint fused or limb amputated)
8.	Sensory (use pinprick to test arms, legs, truck and face—compare side to side):	0	Normal
		1	Mild to moderate decrease in sensation
		2	Severe to total sensory loss
9.	Best language (describe picture, name items, read sentences):	0	No aphasia
		1	Mild to moderate aphasia
		2	Sever aphasia
		3	Mute
10.	Dysarthria (read several words):	0	Normal articulation
		1	Mild to moderate slurring of words
		2	Near unintelligible or unable to speak
		9	Intubated or other physical barrier
11.	Extinction and inattention:	0	Normal
		1	Inattention or extinction to bilateral stimulation in one modality
		2	Sever hemi-inattention or hemi = inattention to multiple modalities

APPENDIX TWO

Eligibility Criteria Indications for tPA Administration/Treatment

Inclusion criteria
☐ Ischemic stroke with clearly defined time onset <3 hours
☐ Patient has measurable defined neurological deficit on NIH stroke scale

Exclusion criteria
☐ NIH Scale Score of <5 or >22
☐ History of intracranial bleed
☐ Active Internal Bleeding
☐ History of stroke or serious head trauma in preceding 3 months
☐ GI or urinary tract hemorrhage within previous 21 days
☐ Major surgery within 14 days
☐ Arterial puncture in non-compressible site or lumbar puncture within previous 7 days
☐ Symptoms suggestive of subarachnoid hemorrhage
☐ Seizure at time of stroke onset
☐ Rapidly improving neurological deficient or minor symptoms
☐ Hemorrhage in CT scan
☐ Systolic pressure >185 or diastolic >110 on repeated measurement
  or requiring aggressive treatment
☐ Platelet count <100,000
☐ Currently taking anticoagulants or receiving Heparin within 48 hours preceding the stroke (INR > 1.7;
  PTT elevated)
☐ Blood glucose <50 or >400

RELATIVE CONTRAINDICATIONS
- Recent gastrointestinal or genitourinary bleeding
- Recent trauma
- Acute pericarditis
- Subacute bacterial endocarditis
- External cardiac massage (CPR)
- Hemostatic defects including ones caused by severe renal or hepatic dysfunction
- Diabetic hemorrhagic retinopathy or other hemorrhagic ophthalmic condition
- Advanced age (>75 years)
- Patients receiving oral anticoagulants

RASS and CAM–ICU Worksheet

Step One: Sedation Assessment

The Richmond Agitation and Sedation Scale: The RASS*

Score	Term	Description	
+4	Combative	Overtly combative, violent, immediate danger to staff	
+3	Very agitated	Pulls or removes tube(s) or catheter(s); aggressive	
+2	Agitated	Frequent non–purposeful movement, fights ventilator	
+1	Restless	Anxious but movements not aggressive vigorous	
0	Alert and calm		
−1	Drowsy	Not fully alert, but has sustained awakening (eye–opening/eye contact) to *voice* (≥10 seconds)	Verbal Stimulation
−2	Light sedation	Briefly awakens with eye contact to *voice* (<10 seconds)	Verbal Stimulation
−3	Moderate sedation	Movement or eye opening to *voice* (but no eye contact)	Verbal Stimulation
−4	Deep sedation	No response to voice, but movement or eye opening to *physical* stimulation	Physical Stimulation
−5	Unarousable	No response to *voice or physical* stimulation	Physical Stimulation

Procedure for RASS Assessment
1. **Observe patient**
   a. Patient is alert, restless, or agitated.   **(score 0 to +4)**
2. **If not alert, state patient's name and *say* to open eyes and look at speaker**.
   a. Patient awakens with sustained eye opening and eye contact.   **(score −1)**
   b. Patient awakens with eye opening and eye contact, but not sustained. **(score −2)**
   c. Patient has any movement in response to voice but no eye contact.   **(score −3)**
3. **When no response to verbal stimulation, physically stimulate patient by shaking shoulder and/or rubbing sternum.**
   a. Patient has any movement to physical stimulation.   **(score −4)**
   b. Patient has no response to any stimulation.   **(score −5)**

If RASS is −4 or −5, then **Stop** and **Reassess** patient at later time
If RASS is above − 4 (−3 through +4) then **Proceed to Step 2**

*Sessler, et al. AJRCCM 2002; 166:1338–1344. Ely, et al. JAMA 2003; 289:2983–2991

Step Two: Delirium Assessment

Feature 1: Acute onset of mental status changes
or a fluctuating course

And

Feature 2: Inattention

And

Feature 3: Disorganized Thinking   OR   **Feature 4**: Altered Level of Consciousness

= DELIRIUM

Comprehensive Hospital Medicine: An Evidence Based and Systems Approach

CAM-ICU Worksheet

	Positive	Negative
Feature 1: Acute Onset or Fluctuating Course Positive if you answer 'yes' to either 1A or 1B.		
1A: Is the pt different than his/her baseline mental status? Or **1B:** Has the patient had any fluctuation in mental status in the past 24 hours as evidenced by fluctuation on a sedation scale (e.g. RASS), GCS, or previous delirium assessment?	Yes	No
Feature 2: Inattention Positive if either score for 2A or 2B is less than 8. Attempt the ASE letters first. If pt is able to perform this test and the score is clear, record this score and move to Feature 3. If pt is unable to perform this test or the score is unclear, then perform the ASE Pictures. If you perform both tests, use the ASE Pictures' results to score the Feature.	Positive	Negative
2A: ASE Letters: record score (enter NT for not tested) Directions: Say to the patient, *"I am going to read you a series of 10 letters. Whenever you hear the letter'A,' indicate by squeezing my hand."* Read letters from the following letter list in a normal tone. **S A V E A H A A R T** Scoring: Errors are counted when patient fails to squeeze on the letter "A" and when the patient squeezes on any letter other than "A."	Score (out of 10): _____	
2B: ASE Pictures: record score (enter NT for not tested) Directions are included on the picture packets.	Score (out of 10): _____	
Feature 3: Disorganized Thinking Positive if the combined score is less than 4	Positive	Negative
3A: Yes/No Questions (Use either Set A or Set B, alternate on consecutive days if necessary): **Set A** 1. Will a stone float on water? 2. Are there fish in the sea? 3. Does one pound weigh more than two pounds? 4. Can you use a hammer to pound a nail? **Set B** 1. Will a leaf float on water? 2. Are there elephants in the sea? 3. Do two pounds weigh more than one pound? 4. Can you use a hammer to cut wood? **Score** ___(Patient earns 1 point for each correct answer out of 4) **3B:Command** Say to patient: "Hold up this many fingers" (Examiner holds two fingers in front of patient) "Now do the same thing with the other hand" (Not repeating the number of fingers). *If pt is unable to move both arms, for the second part of the command ask patient "Add one more finger) **Score**___(Patient earns 1 point if able to successfully complete the entire command)	**Combined Score (3A+3B):** _____ (out of 5)	
Feature 4: Altered Level of Consciousness Positive if the Actual RASS score is anything other than "0" (zero)	Positive	Negative
Overall CAM-ICU (Features 1 and 2 and either Feature 3 or 4):	Positive	Negative

Index

5-aminosalicylate (5-ASA), 473–474
preparations, usage. *See* Inflammatory bowel disease
5As. *See* Ask Advise Assess Assist Arrange; Assessing asking acquiring appraising applying
5-Fluorouracil (Adrucil), impact. *See* Anticancer agents
6-mercaptopurine (MP), therapy, 474

AASLD. *See* American Association for the Study of Liver Diseases
Abdomen, examination, 757
Abdominal pain, 585. *See also* Acute abdominal pain
history/physical examination, components, 464t
ABGs. *See* Arterial blood gases
ABO compatibility, 574
Aborted sudden cardiac death, 185
Abraxane, usage (approval), 533
Absolute risk reduction (ARR), 504
ACC. *See* American College of Cardiology
Accessory pathways (APs), tachycardias (association), 180f
Accountability. *See* Hospital medicine leadership
ACCP Consensus Conference on Antithrombotic Therapy, recommendations, 542, 765–766
ACCP/SCCM Consensus Conference definitions. *See* Sepsis; Septic shock; Severe sepsis; Systemic inflammatory response syndrome
Accreditation Council for Graduate Medical Education (ACGME), workhour restrictions, 951
ACDRs. *See* Adverse cutaneous drug reactions
ACE. *See* Acute Care for the Elderly; Angiotensin-converting enzyme
Acetaminophen
algorithm, 679
assessment, 679
background, 679
clinical presentation, 679
diagnosis/prognosis, 679
differential diagnosis, 679
disposition, 680
management/treatment, 679–680
toxicity. *See* Acute hepatitis
usage. *See* Critically ill patients
ACGME. *See* Accreditation Council for Graduate Medical Education
Acid-base abnormalities, classification (stepwise approach), 430t
Acid-base case, example, 430t

Acid-base disorders
classification, 429
physiologic compensation data, comparison, 429
reading, 438
Acid-base disturbances, 672
Acidemia, 437
ACIP. *See* Advisory Committee on Immunization Practices
ACLS. *See* Advanced cardiac life support; Advanced Cardiopulmonary Life Support
Acquired hemorrhagic disorders, 594–596
Acquired Immune Deficiency Syndrome (AIDS), 331
assessment, 331–334
background, 331
cryptococcal meningitis, clinical presentation, 333b
diagnosis, 334–335
discharge/follow-up plans, 336
management, 335–336
patients, CNS disorders, 332
prognosis, 335
reading, 336
treatment, resistance, 628
Acquired thrombotic disorders, 597
Acquiring. *See* Assessing asking acquiring appraising applying
ACS. *See* Acute chest syndrome; Acute coronary syndrome
ACSC. *See* Ambulatory care sensitive condition
ACTH. *See* Adrenocorticotropic hormone
Activated partial thromboplastin time (aPTT), 593
monitoring, 212
Activated partial thromboplastin time (aPTT // APTT)
usage, 697
Activated protein C (APC) resistance, 597
Activities, energy requirements (estimation), 757t
Activities of daily living (ADL), 29
function, baseline level, 35
impairments, implication, 37–38
Katz index, 37
list, 38b
Acute abdominal emergencies
assessment, 463
background, 463
CT scanning, clinical evaluation (comparison), 464b
reading, 469–470
types, 463–469
Acute abdominal pain
differential diagnosis, 464t
laboratory evaluation, 464b

Acute aortic dissection
aortography, usage, 230
assessment, 227–232
recommendations, 230–231
background, 227
clinical prediction tool, 231
clinical presentation, 229
CTA, usage, 230
CXR, usage, 229
diagnosis, 229–230
decision tree, 231f
differential diagnosis, 229
drugs, usage, 232t
ECG abnormalities, 229
findings, 229b
follow-up, 233
imaging studies, preference, 230
management, 232–233
mortality, 232
MRA, usage, 230
pathophysiology, 227
prevalence, 227–229
prognosis, 231–232
reading, 233
risk factors, 227–229
TEE, usage, 230
TTE, usage, 229–230
Acute arthritis. *See* Hospitalized patients
causes, development, 604
diagnostic studies, 604b
physical examination findings, 604b
treatment, 606b
Acute asthma exacerbation
discharge checklist, 366b
measurement, 362
Acute bacterial meningitis
adjunctive therapy, 304–305
algorithms, 301
antibiotic therapy/dosages/duration, 304t
assessment, 299–303
associated organisms, empiric antibiotic coverage, 303t
background, 299
clinical presentation, 299
community-acquired cases, 299
corticosteroids, usage, 305
diagnosis, 300–301
differential diagnosis, 300
discharge/follow-up plans, 305
empiric antibiotic therapy, 303t
hospitalization, 302–303
initial management, 303
management, 303–305
mortality rates, 302–303
population-based surveillance study, 302–303
postdischarge, 303

Acute bacterial meningitis (Continued)
  predisposing conditions, empiric antibiotic
      coverage, 303t
  prevention, 305
  prognosis, 302–303
  reading, 306
  studies, preference, 300–301
  subsequent management, 303–304
  therapy, duration, 304
Acute Care for the Elderly (ACE), 37
Acute care hospitals, safety hazards, 949
Acute chest syndrome (ACS), chest pain (sign),
      584
Acute coronary syndrome (ACS), 127, 135,
      149
  antiplatelet/antithrombotic therapy,
      141–144, 154–155
  assessment, 135–140, 149–153
  clinical presentation, 135, 149
  complications, 146t
  diagnostic criteria, 136, 150
  diagnostic studies, 136–139
  differential diagnosis, 136, 150
  discharge/follow-up plans, 146–147,
      156–157
  ECG, usage, 137
  evidence/rationale, 137, 151
  exclusion, absence, 128
  GRACE registry, 139
  hospitalization, medications, 156
  identification, 133
  impact, 267
  management, 140–145, 153–156
  mechanical complication, 146t
  noninvasive testing, 155–156
  options, alternatives, 145, 156
  patient instruction, 156–157
  physical examination, 136
  preferred diagnostic approach, 136,
      150–151
  presenting signs/symptoms, 135–136,
      136t, 149–150
  prevalence, 135–136, 136t, 149–150
  prevention, 145, 156
  prognosis, 139–140, 151
  reading, 148, 157
  representation, signs/symptoms (impact),
      131t, 150t
  risk stratification tools, 140, 152
  treatment, 153–155
Acute decompensated heart failure (ADHF),
      159
  patients, vasodilator/diuretic therapy, 164
Acute diarrhea, imaging (problems), 479–480
Acute diarrheal illnesses, noninfectious causes
      (impact), 479
Acute dissection
  imaging techniques, diagnostic utility
      (comparison), 232t
Acute DVT, 541
  diagnostic approach, 208t
Acute end-organ damage, 264
Acute exacerbations of chronic bronchitis
      (AECB)
  hospital discharge, criteria, 358b
  pathogens, association, 356t
Acute hemolytic transfusion reactions
      (AHTRs), 570
Acute hepatitis
  acetaminophen toxicity, 446
  assessment, 445–447
  background, 445
  care, 448
  clinical presentation, 445
  diagnosis, 446
  diagnosis-specific therapy, availability, 445
  discharge/follow-up plans, 449

Acute hepatitis (Continued)
  etiology-specific therapies, 448t
  laboratory testing, 446
  malignant infiltration, impact, 447
  management, algorithm, 448f
  physical examination, 445
  presenting signs/symptoms, 445
  prevalence, 445
  prognosis, 447
  reading, 449
  treatment, 447–448
Acute hepatitis A, 447
Acute HIV infection, 331, 334
  cutaneous maculopapular eruption,
      association, 332f
Acute hyponatremia, 407
Acute hypotensive transfusion reactions, 573
Acute ICH, antihypertensive medications,
      708t
Acute interstitial nephritis (AIN), 396, 829
Acute limb ischemia (ALI), 255
  clinical categories, 260t
  SVS/ISVS classification, 260t
Acute liver failure (ALF), 445
  complications, 449t
  initial laboratories, 446b
  liver transplantation, King's College Hospital
      Criteria, 447b
  monitoring/management, 449t
Acute lung injury (ALI), 783. See also
      Transfusion-associated ALI; Transfusion-
      related acute lung injury
Acute MI (AMI), 135, 151, 504–505
  antiplatelet/antithrombotic therapy,
      141–144, 154–155
  assessment, 135–140, 149–153
  clinical presentation, 135, 149
  complications, 146t
  diagnostic criteria, 136, 150
  diagnostic studies, 136–139
  differential diagnosis, 136, 150
  discharge/follow-up plans, 146–147,
      156–157
  ECG, usage, 137
  evidence/rationale, 137, 151
  management, 140–145, 153–156
  mechanical complication, 146t
  noninvasive testing, 155–156
  options, alternatives, 145, 156
  physical examination, usage, 136
  preferred diagnostic approach, 136,
      150–151
  preferred treatment, 140, 153–154
  presenting signs/symptoms, 135–136,
      149–150
  prevalence, 135–136, 149–150
  prevention, 145, 156
  prognosis, 139–140, 151
  reading, 148, 157
  risk stratification tools, 140, 151, 155–156
  separation, ECG changes (usage), 250t
  treatment, 140–145, 153–155
Acute neurotoxic complications, 537
Acute normovolemic hemodilution (ANH),
      574, 831
Acute PE
  spiral CT scanning, advantages/limitations,
      221
  symptoms, 218
Acute pericarditis
  assessment, 247–250
  background, 247
  Barcelona Experience Evaluation Protocol,
      253t
  causes, 248b
  clinical presentation, 247–248
  diagnosis, 251

Acute pericarditis (Continued)
  ECG
    changes, 248, 249
    stages, 249t
    usage, 248–249
  laboratory tests, 249–251
  management, 251–253
    flowchart, 252f
  prognosis, 251
  reading, 254
  separation, ECG changes (usage), 250f
  signs, 248
  Stage 3. See Electrocardiogram
  Stage I. See Electrocardiogram
  symptoms, 247–248
Acute Physiology and Chronic Health
      (APACHE) Score
  APACHE II, 646, 711
  APACHE III, 711
  score, 569, 574
  usage, 643
Acute polyarticular arthritis, 603–604
Acute promyelocytic leukemia (APL), 534
Acute pulmonary edema, impact, 267
Acute RA, 325
Acute renal failure (ARF). See Community-
      acquired ARF
  assessment, 391–396
  background, 391
  causes, 559. See also Anuric ARF
  clinical presentation, 391
  diagnosis, 391–392
  diagnostic studies, 392
  discharge/follow-up plans, 397
  etiologies (distinction), urinalysis (usage),
      393
  glomerular disease, impact, 396t
  impact, 267
  initial evaluation, 392
  intrarenal (glomerular) impact, 395–396
  intrarenal (interstitial) impact, 396
  intrarenal (tubular) impact, 396
  intrarenal (vascular) impact, 394–395
  laboratory assessment, 830t
  management, 396–397
  perfusion, decrease (renal response), 393
  physical examination, 392
  post renal (obstructive) causes, 393b
  prevention, 397
  prognosis, 396
  reading, 397
Acute respiratory distress syndrome (ARDS),
      641, 650, 663
Acute respiratory failure
  airway management, 652
  approach, preference, 651–652
  assessment, 649–652
  background, 649
  causes, 651–652
  clinical presentation, 649
  conceptual approach, 652f
  diagnosis, 651
    secondary options, 651
  differential diagnosis, 650
  discharge/follow-up plans, 654
  endotracheal intubation, usage, 653
  hospitalization, 652
  incidence, 649
  laboratory tests, 651
  management, 652–653
  mechanical ventilation, requirement, 653
  NIPPV, availability, 653
  oxygen supplementation, 652–653
  prediction rules, 653
  presenting signs/symptoms, 649–650
  prevention, 654
  prognosis, 652

Acute respiratory failure (Continued)
   reading, 654
   studies, 651
   treatment, 652–653
Acute spinal cord injury, 766t
Acute stroke, testing, 699t
Acute tubular necrosis (ATN), 391
   causes, 394b
   granular cast, phase microscopy, 394f
   treatment options, 396
Acute viral hepatitis, 445
Acute VTE management, 222–223
Acute wounds, 811
   healing
      inflammatory phase, 811
      proliferative phase, 811
      remodeling phase, 811
   opening, 812
ACV. See Assist controlled ventilation
ADA. See Adenosine deaminase
Addison's disease, 549
ADE. See Adverse drug event
Adenosine deaminase (ADA), 253
   elevation, 371
ADH. See Antidiuretic hormone
ADHF. See Acute decompensated heart failure
Adjunctive therapy. See Acute bacterial
      meningitis
Adjusted bed turns, 963
ADL. See Activities of daily living
Admission history, performing, 11
Admission times, staff matching. See Peak
      admission times
Admitting H&P, components, 908t
Adrenal cortical function, inadequacy, 762
Adrenal crisis, 519–520
Adrenal insufficiency. See Hospitalized
      patients
   diagnosis, 518b
Adrenocorticotropic hormone (ACTH)
   ACTH-stimulated plasma cortisol, increase,
      520
   doses, 606
   laboratory assay, 519
   response, 517
   secretion, circadian rhythm, 518
   subnormal response, 518
Adrucil, impact. See Anticancer agents
ADs. See Advance directives
Adult asthma, differential diagnosis, 362t
Adult hospital patients, amino acids/protein
      administration (guidelines), 24
Adult immunization schedule,
      recommendation, 86t, 88t–89t
Adult native joint septic arthritis, empiric
      treatment, 327t
Advance care plan. See Caring Conversations
Advanced age, impact, 778
Advanced cardiac life support (ACLS) protocol,
      implementation, 827
Advanced Cardiopulmonary Life Support
      (ACLS)
   components, 192, 194
   initiation, 192
   pulseless arrest algorithm, 193f
Advanced care plans, 980
Advance directives (ADs)
   ethical issues, 980, 985
   usage (enhancement), hospitalist
      (assistance), 984b
Advanced pulmonary hypertension, CXR,
      385f
Adverse cutaneous drug reactions (ACDRs),
      621
Adverse drug event (ADE), 77
Adverse events, defining, 947
Adverse hemodynamic effects, 746

Advisory Committee on Immunization
      Practices (ACIP), 85
   annual influenza vaccination,
      recommendations, 87b
AECB. See Acute exacerbations of chronic
      bronchitis
Aeromonas, empiric antibiotics (usage), 480
AFI. See Atrial Fibrillation Investigators
Against medical advise (AMA), 116
Age-indeterminate MI, 778
Agency for Healthcare Research and Quality
      (AHRQ), 8, 935
   prevention techniques, indication, 50
Agitated patient, IV haloperidol (usage
      guidelines), 867t
AHA. See American College of
      Cardiology/American Heart Association;
      American Hospital Association
AHRQ. See Agency for Healthcare Research
      and Quality
AHTRs. See Acute hemolytic transfusion
      reactions
AICD. See Automatic implantable cardiac
      defibrillator
AIDS. See Acquired Immune Deficiency
      Syndrome
AIN. See Acute interstitial nephritis
Air embolism, 225
Airflow obstruction, degree, 366
Airway
   breathing, relationship, 191–192
   management. See Acute respiratory failure;
      Intracerebral hemorrhage
   obstruction, diseases, 437
   opening, 191
   oxygen saturation, maintenance, 715
AKS. See Anti-Kickback Statute
Alanine aminotransferase (AST), 113, 586
Alarm symptoms, 53
Alcohol abuse, commonness, 863
Alcohol abuse/dependence
   CAGE questionnaire screen, usage, 756t
   screening tools, 113–114
Alcohol consumption history, 689
Alcohol dehydrogenase, impact, 682
Alcohol history, preoperative health
      assessment, 755–756
Alcoholic hallucinosis, 688
Alcohol use disorders, DSM-IV definition, 756t
Alcohol Use Disorders Identification Test
      (AUDIT), interview version, 114b
Alcohol withdrawal. See Major alcohol
      withdrawal; Minor alcohol withdrawal
   BZDs, usage, 868t
   causes, 688
   differential diagnosis, 689b
   DSM-IV definition, 687
   hospitalization, percentage, 690
   perioperative management techniques,
      867–868
   seizure
      management, 693
      prophylaxis, 693
   symptoms, appearance, 687
   timeline, 689f
   treatment, taper/symptom triggered
      regimens (usage), 692t
Alcohol withdrawal syndrome (AWS)
   assessment, 688–689
   background, 687
   benzodiazepines, impact, 690
   clinical presentation, 687–688
   differential diagnosis, 689
   discharge planning, 693
   drugs, impact, 690–693
   evaluation, 689–690
   fixed dose method, 690

Alcohol withdrawal syndrome (AWS)
      (Continued)
   haloperidol, usage, 692
   management, 690
   nutrition, impact, 690
   pathophysiology, 687
   pharmacotherapies, 690–693
   phenobarbital/propofol, usage, 690, 692
   reading, 694
   summary, 693–694
   symptom triggered methods, 690
   treatment, 690–693
      setting, 690
   vitamins, impact, 690
   volume replacement, impact, 690
Aldesleukin (IL-2), usage. See Anticancer
      agents; Nephrotoxicity
Alemtuzumab (Campath), usage. See Cancer
      management
ALF. See Acute liver failure
ALI. See Acute limb ischemia; Acute lung
      injury
Alkalemia. See Severe alkalemia
Allergic reactions
   assessment, 615–617
   background, 615
   clinical presentation, 615–616
   definition/classification, 615
   differential diagnosis, 616–617
   discharge/follow-up plans, 618
   history, 618
   immunologic/nonimmunologic reactions,
      616t
   management, 617–618
   outpatient physician communication, 618
   pathophysiology, 615
   patient education, 618
   presenting signs/symptoms, 615–616
   prevalence, 615–616
   prevention, 618
   reading, 619
   treatment, 617–618
Allergic (urticarial) transfusion reactions, 571
Allergies, preoperative health assessment, 755
Allogeneic blood transfusion, alternatives,
      574, 576
All-Trans Retinoic Acid (ATRA) (Vesanoid),
      usage. See Pulmonary toxicity
ALOS. See Average length of stay
Alpha-agonists (clonidine), 780
ALT. See Alanine aminotransferase
Alteplase (tPA), 144
Altered mental status (AMS)
   background, 818
   clinical assessment/evaluation, 818
   management, 818
   postoperative causes, 818t
   signs, 459
Alternating pressure mattress overlay,
      illustration, 47f
Alveolar gas equation, 651
AMA. See Against medical advice
Ambulatory care sensitive condition (ACSC),
      935
American Association for the Study of Liver
      Diseases (AASLD), recommendations,
      446
American Association of Clinical
      Endocrinologists, position statement, 505,
      790–791
American College of Cardiology/American
      Heart Association (ACC/AHA)
   algorithm. See Preoperative cardiac risk
      evaluation
   Guideline for Perioperative Cardiovascular
      Evaluation for Noncardiac Surgery,
      821

American College of Cardiology/American Heart Association (ACC/AHA) (*Continued*)
  guidelines, 129. *See also* Preoperative cardiac risk assessment
  recommendation, 759
  risk stratification, 775
American College of Chest Physicians (AACP)
  conference, recommendations. *See* Seventh AACP Conference on Antithrombotic and Thrombolytic Therapy
American College of Chest Physicians consensus conference, usage, 709
American Hospital Association (AHA) survey, 961
American Society of Anesthesiologists (ASA) Physical Status Classification, 759t
American Society on Clinical Oncology (ASCO), 551
Americans with Disabilities Act, 993
AMI. *See* Acute MI
Amino acids/protein
  administration, guidelines. *See* Adult hospital patients
  requirements, estimation, 24–25
Amiodarone
  dosage, 192, 194
  impact, 509
Ammonia lowering strategy. *See* Hepatic encephalopathy
Ammonium (NH_4+), secretion, 433
Amniotic fluid embolism, 224–225
AMS. *See* Altered mental status
ANA. *See* Antinuclear antibody
Analgesia
  inadequacy, 48
  usage. *See* Hospitalized patients
Analgesic agents, usage. *See* Critically ill patients
Analgesic concentration. *See* Minimum effective analgesic concentration
Analgesics (usage), SCCM 2002 Clinical Practice Guidelines Recommendations, 661t
Anaphylactic transfusion reactions (ATRs), 571
Anaphylaxis, 615
  assessment, 622
  diagnosis, 622
  differential diagnosis, 622
  management/treatment, 622
ANCA. *See* Antineutrophil cytoplasmic antibody
Anemia. *See* Hemolytic anemia; Hypochromic microcytic anemia; Macrocytic anemia; Normochromic normocytic anemia; Postoperative anemia; Sickle cell anemia
  assessment, 577–579
  background, 577, 830
  clinical assessment/evaluation, 830–831
  clinical presentation, 577
  diagnosis, 577, 579
  diagnostic algorithm, 579f
  differential diagnosis, 577
  differential diagnosis, marrow response (basis), 578b
  discharge/follow-up plans, 580
  etiology
    kinetic approach, 570f
    morphologic approach, 570b
  hospitalization, 579
  increase, 585
  management, 580, 831
  options, alternatives, 579
  outpatient physician communication, 580

Anemia (*Continued*)
  pathophysiology, 830
  patient instruction, 580
  patients, nontransfusion (risks), 574
  postdischarge, 579–580
  prevention, 831
  reading, 580
  role, 821
  studies, preference, 577
  treatment, 580
Anesthesia. *See* General anesthesia; Regional anesthesia
  cardiovascular complications, 748–749
  cardiovascular effects, 746–747
  complications, 745. *See also* General anesthesia; Neuraxial anesthesia
  consequences. *See* Diabetic patients
  effects, 745–747. *See also* General anesthesia; Neuraxial anesthesia
  gastrointestinal complications, 749–750
  gastrointestinal effects, 747
  neurologic complications, 747–748
  neurologic effects, 745–746
  oversedation, complication, 747
  overview, 745
  postoperative complications, 747–750
  pulmonary complications, 749
  pulmonary effects, 747
  reading, 751
  types, 745
Aneurysm. *See* Patent foramen ovale/atrial septal aneurysm
  function, 609
Angina, CCSC, 150t
Angioedema
  assessment, 615–617, 622
  background, 615
  clinical presentation, 615–616
  deep dermal/subcutaneous tissues, involvement, 622
  definition/classification, 615
  diagnosis, 622
  differential diagnosis, 616–617, 622
  discharge/follow-up plans, 618
  immunologic/nonimmunologic reactions, 616t
  management/treatment, 617–618, 622
  outpatient physician communication, 618
  pathophysiology, 615. *See also* Hereditary angioedema
  patient education, 618
  presenting signs/symptoms, 615–616
  prevalence, 615–616
  prevention, 618
  treatment, 617–618
Angiotensin-converting enzyme (ACE)
  inhibitors, 164, 615
    impact, 391
    usage, 261
  levels, elevation, 377
  usage, 573
Angiotensin receptor blockers (ARBs), 610, 764
ANH. *See* Acute normovolemic hemodilution
Anion gap. *See* Metabolic acidosis
  acidosis, 433. *See also* Normal anion gap acidosis
  list, 683t
Ankle-brachial index (ABI), 255
  method. *See* Peripheral vascular perfusion
  relationship. *See* Resting ABI
Anorexiant-induced valve disorder, 244
Anoxic-ischemic coma
  hypothermia, 716
  neuroprotective agents, 716

Anthracycline impact. *See* Anticancer agents
Anthrax. *See* Cutaneous anthrax; Intentional anthrax
  black eschar, presence, 339f
  clinical presentation, 339–340
  diagnosis, 340
  management, 341
  prognosis, 341
  staging, proposal. *See* Inhalational anthrax
Antianxiety medications, usage. *See* Depression
Antibiotic/antiseptic-impregnated catheters, usage, 121
Antibiotic-associated diarrhea, mechanisms, 496t
Antibiotic overuse, limitation, 281
Antibiotic restriction. *See* Clostridium difficile colitis; Diarrhea
Antibiotics
  discontinuation, hospitalists (impact), 834
  impact. *See* Hepatic encephalopathy
Antibiotic therapy. *See* Sepsis/shock
Anticancer agents, cardiovascular complications, 534–536
  5-Fluorouracil (Adrucil), impact, 536
  Anthracyclines, usage, 535–536
  clinical presentations, 535
  Cyclophosphamide (Cytoxan), usage, 536
  diagnosis, 535
  discharge, 535
  Ifosfamide (Ifex), usage, 536
  Interferon (Intron), usage, 536
  Interleukin-2 (Aldesleukin), usage, 536
  Taxanes, usage, 536
  Trastuzumab, usage, 536
  treatment, 535
Anticardiolipin antibody syndrome, 597
Anticholinergics
  motion sickness/labyrinthine disorders, prevention/treatment, 65
  usage. *See* Asthma
Anticoagulants, usage. *See* Pulmonary hypertension
Anticoagulant therapy
  absence, 773b
  duration guidelines. *See* Venous thromboembolism
Anticoagulation. *See* Cancer patients
  therapy. *See* Ischemic stroke
  usage. *See* Valvular heart disease
Antidepressants, usage. *See* Psychiatric disorders
Antidiarrheals, usage, 72
Antidiuretic hormone (ADH), secretion (decrease), 523
Anti-double-stranded DNA, 377
Antidromic AVRT, 179
Antiemetics, risk/alternatives, 33t
Antiepileptic drugs (AEDs), usage. *See* Convulsive SE; Nonconvulsive SE
Antifibrinolytic agents, 594
Anti-glomerular basement membrane (Anti-GBM), 609
Anti-hepatitis A IgM, sensitivity, 447
Antihistamines
  antiemetic effects, 65
  risk/alternatives, 33t
Antihypertensive drugs, 265–266
Antihypertensive medications. *See* Acute ICH
Antihypertensive therapy, 842
Anti-IgA antibodies, development, 571
Anti-intrinsic factor, 579
Anti-Kickback Statute (AKS), 994–995
Antimanic medications, 858t
Antimicrobial prophylaxis. *See* Infective endocarditis
  usage. *See* Surgical site infection

Antimicrobial-resistant organisms, 282
Antimotility agents, usage, 74, 481
Anti-MPO, 610
Antineutrophil cytoplasmic antibody (ANCA), 385
Antineutrophil cytoplasmic antibody (cANCA), 377, 610
Antinuclear antibody (ANA), 377, 385
  role, absence, 605
Antiparietal cell antibodies, 579
Antiperistaltic agents, usage, 74
Antiphospholipid antibody (APA) syndrome
  diagnosis, 597
  management, 597–598
  presentation, 597
Antiplatelet activity, clinical assessment/evaluation, 762
Antiplatelet medications, 780
  recommendations/management, 762–764
Antiplatelet therapy. See Acute coronary syndrome; Acute MI; Ischemic stroke
Antipsychotics, usage. See Psychiatric disorders
Antiretroviral PEP, usage, 120
Anti-Saccharomyces cerevisiae antibody (ASCA), 473
Antisecretory/adsorbents, usage, 74
Antithrombin deficiency
  diagnosis, 596
  management, 596
  presentation, 596
Antithrombotic therapy. See Acute coronary syndrome; Acute MI
  American College of Chest Physicians guidelines. See Atrial fibrillation
Anti-thyroperoxidase (TPO) test, 846
Antitrust issues, 995t
Antitrust law, 995–996
Antiviral therapy, impact, 628–629
Anuric ARF, causes, 392b
Anuric renal failure, 391
Anxiety
  distinctions, 860
  perioperative management techniques, 864, 867
  symptom management, 734
  syndromes. See Organic anxiety syndromes
  ventilator patient, 864, 867
Anxiety disorders
  background, 859–860
  clinical assessment/evaluation, 860
  perioperative management techniques, 864
  treatment, 860
Aortic coarctation, risk factor, 228
Aortic dissection. See Acute aortic dissection
  classification, composite schema, 228t
  coronal CT angiogram. See Stanford Type I aortic dissection
  CXR. See Proximal aortic dissection
  DeBakey classification system, 228f
  differential diagnosis, 128
  impact, 266–267
  risk factors, 229b
  Stanford classification system, 228
  transverse CT angiogram. See Stanford Type I aortic dissection
  types, 227
Aortic IMH, distinctions, 227
Aortic regurgitation (AR), 241–243
  ascending aorta, prominence, 242
  cardiomegaly, presence, 242
  course/management, 242–243
  CXR, usage, 242
  diagnostic evaluation, 242
  pathophysiology, 242f
  prophylactic intervention, 244

Aortic regurgitation (AR) (Continued)
  signs, physical examination, 242f
  symptoms/signs, 242
Aortic stenosis, 240–241, 777
  carotid pulse, reduction. See Severe aortic stenosis
  course/management, 241
  diagnostic evaluation, 241
  operative mortality, increase, 241
  pathophysiology, 240f
  symptoms/signs, 241
Aortography, usage. See Acute aortic dissection
APA. See Antiphospholipid antibody
APACHE. See Acute Physiology and Chronic Health
APC. See Activated protein C
APIC. See Association of Professionals in Infection Control and Epidemiology
APL. See Acute promyelocytic leukemia
Aplastic crisis, 585
Apnea, 717
Appearance
  Hippocrates, realization, 9
  importance. See Medical professionalism
Appendicitis, 463, 465
  assessment, 463, 465
  clinical presentation, 463
  diagnosis, 463, 465
  discharge/follow-up plans, 465
  management, 465
  operative management, 465
  pain management, 465
  postoperative antibiotics, usage, 465
  prognosis, 465
  respiratory care, 465
Applicability, questions, 3
Applying. See Assessing asking acquiring appraising applying
Appraisal. See Assessing asking acquiring appraising applying
APs. See Accessory pathways
APTT. See Activated partial thromboplastin time
aPTT. See Activated partial thromboplastin time
AR. See Aortic regurgitation
ARA-C. See Cytosine arabinoside
ARBs. See Angiotensin receptor blockers
ARDS. See Acute respiratory distress syndrome
Arca indicators, 935
ARF. See Acute renal failure
Argatroban, infusion rate, 598
Arginine vasopressin, secretion (decrease), 523
ARR. See Absolute risk reduction
Arrhythmias
  agents, 192, 194
  atrial origin, 806
  background, 824
  clinical assessment/evaluation, 824
  impact, 135
  recommendations/management, 824
  risk factors/pathophysiology, 824
Arterial blood gases (ABGs), 194
  analysis
    studies, 683
    usage. See Pulmonary embolism
  evaluation, 651
Arterial cerebral infarctions, 700
Arterial oxygen saturation, maintenance, 715
Arterial oxygen tension (measurement), ABG analysis (usage), 362
Arthritis, recurrence (avoidance), 606
Artificial intelligence (AI), usage. See Cognizant systems
Artificial RBCs, construction, 576

Artificial variability, 962
ASA. See American Society of Anesthesiologists; Atrial septal aneurysm
ASCA. See Anti-Saccharomyces cerevisiae antibody
Ascites, 451
  diagnosis, 452–454
  diuretics, impact, 454
  laboratory testing, 453–454
  large-volume paracentesis, 454
  management, 454–455. See also Refractory ascites
  paracentesis, 452–453, 454
  SBP signs/symptoms, 460b
  serum albumin-ascites gradient classification, 454t
  sodium restriction, 454
  treatment, 454
Ascitic fluid analysis, 459–460
  routine, 460b
Ascitic fluid findings, basis. See Peritonitis
Ascitic fluid PMN count, 455
ASCO. See American Society on Clinical Oncology
Ask Advise Assess Assist Arrange (5As), 94t
Asking. See Assessing asking acquiring appraising applying
Aspartate aminotransferase (AST), 113, 586, 863
  ALT ratio, 446
Aspinal (ASA), withholding, 831
Aspiration
  avoidance, recommendations, 800t
  complication, 749
  risk, 747
    factors, 800t
Aspirin, 780
  impact, 141, 154
Assessing asking acquiring appraising applying (5As), 4–5
Assessment, 549–550. See also Subjective Global Assessment
Assist controlled ventilation (ACV), 669, 670
Association of Professionals in Infection Control and Epidemiology (APIC), 121
AST. See Aspartate aminotransferase
Asthma, 666
  action plan, 367b
  albuterol, administration, 363
  anticholinergics, usage, 364–365
  assessment, 361–363
  atropine, treatment, 364–365
  background, 361
  beta agonists, usage, 363
  clinical presentation, 361
  corticosteroids, usage, 365
  death, risk factors (association), 366b
  diagnosis, 362–363
  differential diagnosis, 361–362. See also Adult asthma
  empiric antimicrobial therapy, 365–366
  exacerbation
    management, 364f
    measurement. See Acute asthma exacerbation
  heliox, impact, 365
  hospital discharge, 368
  hospitalization, indications, 366
  ICU admission, indications, 366–368
  leukotriene antagonists, impact, 365
  magnesium sulfate, usage, 365
  management, 363–365
  mimics, 363t
  oxygen, usage, 363
  physical examination, 361
  reading, 368
  severity, classification, 362t

Asthma (Continued)
  theophylline, usage, 365
  therapeutic considerations, 365–366
Asymptomatic carriage. See Clostridium difficile
    colitis; Diarrhea
ATN. See Acute tubular necrosis
ATRA, usage. See Pulmonary toxicity
Atrial fibrillation, 178t, 690
  antithrombotic therapy, American College of
    Chest Physicians guidelines, 176t
  Wolff-Parkinson-White syndrome, 183f
    relationship, 181
Atrial fibrillation-associated stroke, 702
Atrial Fibrillation Investigators (AFI), 702
Atrial flutter, 175–176
  ECG demonstration, 175f
Atrial premature depolarizations, 173
Atrial septal aneurysm (ASA), 698. See also
    Patent foramen ovale/atrial septal
    aneurysm
Atrioventricular block (AVB), 168
  ECG data. See Second-degree AVB
Atrioventricular dissociation, 167
Atrioventricular nodal reentrant tachycardia
    (AVNRT), 177
Atrioventricular reentrant tachycardia
    (AVRT), 177, 179, 181. See also
    Antidromic AVRT; Orthodromic AVRT
Atropine, dosage, 194
ATRs. See Anaphylactic transfusion reactions
ATS/ERS guidelines. See Chronic obstructive
    pulmonary disease
AUDIT. See Alcohol Use Disorders
    Identification Test
Auscultation, 777
Autoimmune blistering diseases, 636t
Autoimmune hepatitis, 447
Autologous blood
  donation, 574
  pre-donation, 831
Automated peritoneal dialysis, antibiotics
    (intermittent dosing), 405t
Automatic implantable cardiac defibrillator
    (AICD), 145, 165, 204
Autonomy, 979
AutoPEEP, 671–672
AVB. See Atrioventricular block
Average length of stay (ALOS)
  basis. See Capacity; Revenue
  decrease, 912
AVNRT. See Atrioventricular nodal reentrant
    tachycardia
AVRT. See Atrioventricular reentrant
    tachycardia
AWS. See Alcohol withdrawal syndrome

Bacillus anthracis, 339
Bacteremia, 285–286
  assessment, 402
  clinical presentation, 401
  diagnosis/prognosis, 402
  differential diagnosis, 401
  discharge/follow-up plans, 403
  management, –403
Bacteria
  impact. See Gastroenteritis
  presence, 459. See also Invasive bacteria
Bacterial diarrhea, antibiotic therapy, 480t
Bacterial infections, empiric antibiotics
    (usage), 480–481
Bacterial meningitis. See Acute bacterial
    meningitis
  diagnostic evaluation/treatment, algorithm,
    302f
  impact. See Cognitive impairment
  outpatient antibiotic therapy, 305
Bacteriuria, 834

BAL. See Bronchoalveolar lavage
Balloon tamponade, usage. See Variceal
    hemorrhage
Barbiturates, usage. See Critically ill patients
Barcelona experience, 252
Barcelona Experience Evaluation Protocol. See
    Acute pericarditis
Barium enema, usage. See Diverticulitis
Barrier precautions. See Clostridium difficile
    colitis; Diarrhea
Basal energy expenditure (BEE),
    determination, 24
Base/incentive components, combination. See
    Salary
Baseline nutritional assessment, components,
    23b
Basic Life Support (BLS)
  components, 191–192
  initiation, 191
  responsiveness, assessment, 191
BAV. See Bicuspid aortic valve
Bayes' theorem, basis, 209–210
BBB. See Bundle branch block
BBT. See Beta-Blocker Therapy
B-cell chronic lymphocytic leukemia (CLL),
    treatment, 532
Beck's triad, association, 248
BEE. See Basal energy expenditure
Behavioral pain scale, 656t
Beneficence, importance, 979
Benzodiazepines (BZDs)
  antiemetic effect, 68
  conversion chart, 867t
  pharmacokinetics, 692t
  properties, 659t
  risk/alternatives, 33t
  usage, 832. See also Alcohol withdrawal;
    Critically ill patients; Psychiatric
    disorders
Bernard-Souller syndrome, 594
Beta-adrenergic blocking medications, 780
Beta agonists, usage. See Asthma
Beta-blockers
  contraindications, 143
  impact, 142–143
  importance, 692–693
  symptom control, 514
  treatment, 204
  usage, 167, 846
Beta-Blocker Therapy (BBT), patient inclusion,
    778t
Beta-hemolytic streptococcal infections,
    636
BIA. See Bioimpedance analysis
Bicarbonate, usage. See Diabetic ketoacidosis
Bicarbonaturia, 423–424
BiCNU. See Carmustine
Bicuspid aortic valve (BAV), risk factor, 228
Biguanides, usage, 506
Billing. See Hospital medicine
  hospitalist value, addition process, 874b
Biochemical markers, 22–23
Bioimpedance analysis (BIA), 797
Biological agents, potential, 338t
Bioprosthesis, usage, 243
Bioterrorism, 337
  assessment, 337–341
  clinical presentation, 337–340
  management, 341–342
  reading, 342
Bioweapons, 339t
Bipolar disorder
  perioperative management techniques,
    867
  risk factors/demographics, 862
BIS. See Bispectral Index System
Bismuth subsalicylate (Pepto-Bismol), 74

Bispectral Index System (BIS), 657
  impact. See Critically ill patients
Bisphosphonates, impact. See Osteoporosis
Black Death, cause, 340
Black wounds, 43
Bladder obstruction, 832
Bleeding
  disorders, impact, 592t
  risk. See Long-term warfarin management
    assessment, 99
Bleomycin (Blenoxane), usage. See Pulmonary
    toxicity
Blind biopsy, 610
Blistering diseases, 634. See also Autoimmune
    blistering diseases
Blistering drug eruptions
  assessment, 623–624
  clinical presentation, 623
  diagnosis/prognosis, 624
  differential diagnosis, 624
  discharge/follow-up plans, 624
  management/treatment, 624
Block schedule, 888
  advantages/disadvantages, 890t
Blood ammonia, lowering, 457
Blood-borne pathogens, occupational
    exposure, 120
Blood cultures, 605
Blood glucose
  control, 701, 835
  goals, recommendations, 506b
  indication, 759
  perioperative outcome, relationship. See
    Diabetic patients
Blood pressure
  maintenance. See Systolic blood pressure
  outpatient management, 267
  reduction, initial goal, 265
  relationship. See Intracerebral hemorrhage;
    Ischemic stroke
Blood products
  administration, 443
  order set/consent form, 981f–982f
Blood-saving techniques, 831
Bloodstream infection, RRR percentage, 504
Blood-stream infection (BSI), occurrence. See
    Hospital-acquired BSI
Blood tests, 778
Blood urea nitrogen (BUN), 424
  elevation, 395
  level, 261, 829
  studies, 683
  usage, 697, 778
BLS. See Basic Life Support
BMD. See Bone mineral density
BNP. See B-type natriuretic peptide
Body physiology, thyroid disorders (impact),
    512
Body weight history, obtaining, 23b
Boerhaave's syndrome, 62–63
Bone marrow transplants, cure. See Sickle cell
    crises
Bone mineral density (BMD)
  increase, 107
  testing, 105
Bone pain, 585
Bony destruction, radiograph (usage), 293
BOOP. See Bronchiolitis obliterans-organizing
    pneumonia
Borrowed Servant doctrine, 991
Boston University School of Management,
    demand definitions, 962
Botulism
  clinical presentation, 340
  diagnosis, 340
  management, 341–342
  prognosis, 341

Bowel obstruction. *See* Partial small bowel
  obstruction
  assessment, 468
  clinical presentation, 468
  diagnosis/prognosis, 468
  discharge/follow-up plans, 468
  management, 468
  symptom management, 735
Bradyarrhythmias
  physical examination, 167–168
  presentation/diagnosis/treatment,
    167–168
  reading, 171
  specifications, 167–168
  treatment, 168–171
Bradycardia, Cushing's triad, 299
Brain death, 716–717
Brainstem reflexes, absence, 717
Breakthrough pain. *See* Hospitalized patients
BREATH 1 study, 387
Breathing, 192
  relationship. *See* Airway
Bridging therapy. *See* Long-term warfarin
    management
  protocol, LMWH (usage), 773b
Broad-spectrum parenteral antibiotics,
    administration, 402
Bronchiolitis obliterans-organizing pneumonia
    (BOOP), 533
Bronchitis, pathogens (association). *See*
    Acute exacerbations of chronic
    bronchitis
Bronchoalveolar lavage (BAL), 378
Bronchodilators, usage. *See* Chronic
    obstructive pulmonary disease
Bronchoscopy, usage. *See* Interstitial lung
    disease
Brudzinkski's sign, 299
Brugada criteria, usage. *See* Ventricular
    tachycardia
Brugada syndrome, 137
B-type natriuretic peptide (BNP)
  diagnostic characteristic. *See* Heart failure
  level, 160
  impact, 161t
  testing, 651
Bubo, 340
Budd-Chiari syndrome, 445, 447
Bullous pemphigoid
  assessment, 634–635
  diagnosis, 635
  discharge/follow-up plans, 635
  management, 635
Bundle branch block (BBB), 168
Bupropion, impact. *See* Smoking cessation
Busulfan (Myleran), usage. *See* Pulmonary
    toxicity
Butyrophenones
  antiemetic action, 65
  usage. *See* Critically ill patients
BZDs. *See* Benzodiazepines

C677T/A1298C compound heterozygous,
    596–597
C677T homozygous, 596–597
CABG. *See* Coronary artery bypass grating
CAD. *See* Community-acquired diarrhea;
    Coronary artery disease
CAGE. *See* Cut Annoyed Guilty Eye
Calcitonin, impact. *See* Osteoporosis
Calcium channel blockers, usage. *See*
    Pulmonary hypertension
Calcium pyrophosphate crystals, 604–605
Calf pain, intermittent claudication (presence),
    256f
California Hospital Assessment and Reporting
    Taskforce (CHART) program, 973

Call-based schedules
  comparison. *See* Shift-based schedules
  contrast. *See* Shift-based schedules
  weekday hospitalist coverage, 889t
Call-based scheduling, program transition
    (timing), 887–888
Caloric expenditure (calorimetry), comparison,
    797
Calories, overfeeding, 24
CAM. *See* Complementary/alternative
    medicine; Confusion Assessment Method
CAM-ICU. *See* Confusion Assessment Method
    for Intensive Care Unit
Campath, usage. *See* Cancer management
Campylobacter, empiric antibiotics (usage),
    480
CA-MRSA. *See* Community-acquired MRSA;
    Community-associated MRSA
Canadian Cardiovascular Society Classification
    (CCSC), 149. *See also* Angina
Canadian Clinical Practice Guidelines,
    799–800
cANCA. *See* Antineutrophil cytoplasmic
    antibody
Cancer
  DVT treatment, 543b
  Virchow's triad, 542t
Cancer emergencies (elevated intracranial
    pressure)
  assessment, 555
  background, 555
  clinical presentation, 555
  CT scans, usage, 555
  diagnosis, 555
  immediate care, intensity, 556
  medical intervention/therapies, 556
  reading, 556
  symptoms/signs, 555
Cancer emergencies (fever/neutropenia)
  assessment, 545
  background, 545
  clinical presentation, 545
  diagnosis/prognosis, 545
  discharge/follow-up plans, 547
  granulocyte colony-stimulating factors,
    addition, 546
  management, 545–546
  outpatient physician communication,
    547
  patient education, 547
  presenting signs/symptoms, 545
  prevalence, 545
  prevention, 546
  reading, 547
  therapy, 546
  treatment, 545–546
Cancer emergencies (hypercalcemia)
  background, 549
  clinical presentation, 549
  diagnosis, 540–550
  differential diagnosis, 549
  discharge/follow-up plans, 551
  laboratory studies, 550
  management, 550–551
  outpatient physician communication, 551
  patient education, 551
  presenting signs/symptoms, 549
  prevention, 551
  prognosis, 550
  reading, 551–552
  therapy, 550–551
  treatment, 550
Cancer emergencies (hyperviscosity
    syndromes)
  assessment, 553
  background, 553
  discharge/follow-up, 553–554

Cancer emergencies (hyperviscosity
    syndromes) *(Continued)*
  management, 553
  reading, 554
Cancer emergencies (paraneoplastic
    neurologic syndromes)
  assessment, 563–565
  background, 563
  clinical presentation, 563–564
  diagnosis, 564–565
  management/treatment, 565–566
  pathogenesis, 563
  reading, 566
Cancer emergencies (spinal cord compression)
  assessment, 557
  background, 557
  clinical presentation, 557
  diagnosis/prognosis, 557
  differential diagnosis, 557
  management, 557–558
  presenting signs/symptoms, 557
  prevalence, 557
  radiation, impact, 558
  reading, 558
  steroids, impact, 558
  surgery, usage, 558
Cancer emergencies (tumor lysis syndrome)
  assessment, 559–560
  background, 559
  chemotherapy, initiation, 560
  classification, 560
  clinical presentation, 559
  diagnosis/prognosis, 559–560
  differential diagnosis, 559
  discharge/follow-up plans, 560–561
  management, 560
  outpatient physician communication, 561
  patient education, 561
  prevention, 560
  reading, 561
Cancer management, therapeutic agents
    (acute complications)
  agents
    miscellany, 538–539
    usage, 530–533
  Alemtuzumab (Campath), usage, 532–533
  assessment, 529–530
  background, 529
  Cetuximab (Erbitux), usage, 533
  clinical presentation, 529
  diagnosis, 529
  discharge, 530
  Epipodophyllotoxins, usage, 533
  Gemtuzamab ozogamicin (Mylotarg), usage,
    532
  hypersensitivity reactions, 529
  L-Asparaginase, usage, 530–531
  management, 530
  monoclonal antibodies, usage, 531–532
  platinum drugs, impact, 533
  prognosis, 529–530
  pulmonary toxicity, 533–534
  Rituximab (Rituxan), usage, 532
  Taxanes, usage, 533
  Trastuzumab (Herceptin), usage, 532
  treatment, 530
Cancer patients, anticoagulation
  assessment, 541–542
  background, 541
  clinical presentation/diagnosis, 541–542
  diagnosis, 542
  management, 542–544
  pathophysiology, 541
  reading, 544
  treatment, 542–544
Cancer-related VTE, treatment strategies,
    542–543

Cancer treatment (therapeutic agent usage),
    hypersensitivity/cytokine release
    reactions, 530t
Cannabinoids, antiemetic effect, 68
CAP. See Community-acquired pneumonia
Capacity
    improvements, ALOS basis, 912t
    increase. See Hospital medicine program
CAPD. See Continuous ambulatory peritoneal
    dialysis
Captain of the Ship doctrine, 991
Carbamazepine, usage. See Coma
Carbohydrate loads, excess, 25
Carbon monoxide (CO)
    assessment, 685
    background, 684–685
    clinical presentation, 685
    diagnosis/prognosis, 685
    differential diagnosis, 685
    discharge, 685
    management, 685
    poisoning (treatment), hyperbaric oxygen
        (usage), 685
    studies, preference, 586
Carcinoma erysipelatoides, 625
Cardiac arrest
    assessment, 189–191
    clinical presentation, 189–190
    diagnosis, 190
    discharge/follow-up plans, 194
    management, 191–194
    prevention, 194
    prognosis, 190–191
    reading, 195
    resuscitation, pharmacology/interventions,
        192
    treatment, 191–194
Cardiac arrhythmias, 701
Cardiac biomarkers, usage, 137–139, 151. See
    also Pulmonary embolism
Cardiac enzymes, 781
    usage, 822
Cardiac examination, 757
Cardiac ischemic events (induction), surgical
    stress (impact), 806
Cardiac lesions, risk, 307
Cardiac output (CO), 217
Cardiac resynchronization therapy (CRT),
    165
Cardiac telemetry monitoring, 822
Cardiac testing, patient selection (algorithms),
    781f
Cardiogenic pulmonary edema, 665–666
Cardiogenic shock, 139–140
Cardioprotective agents, patient selection
    (algorithms), 781f
Cardiopulmonary resuscitation (CPR) events,
    recording, 190
Cardiovascular preoperative risk
    assessment/evaluation
    background, 775
    blood tests, 778
    clinical assessment/evaluation, 775–779
    diagnostic tests, 778
    issues, importance, 778
    pathophysiology, 775
    questions, 775
    reading, 782
    recommendations/management, 779–781
Cardiovascular stress, 756
Cardiovascular support, medications, 192
Cardiovascular syncope, 204
Care
    improvement, changes (impact), 943–944
    model, shift, 733
    transitions, practices, 950t
Caregiver, role. See Elderly hospitalized patient

Care standardization strategies
    background, 967
    measurement, 969
    pitfalls, 969
    reading, 970
Caring Conversations
    advance care plan, 983f
    example, 980
Carmustine (BiCNU), 534
Case analysis, 952b
Case Mix, importance, 934b
Case Mix Index (CMI), 906
Catheter-associated UTI, 285
Catheter-directed thrombolytic therapy. See
    Venous thromboembolism
Catheterization, duration, 318
Catheter-related bloodstream infection
    (CR-BSI), 317
Catheter-related infections, microbial etiology,
    318t
CBC. See Complete blood count
CBCPD. See Complete blood count with
    platelets and differential
CCSC. See Canadian Cardiovascular Society
    Classification
CD. See Crohn's disease
CDAD. See Clostridium difficile-associated
    diarrhea
CeeNu. See Lomustine
Cell count/differential, usage, 453. See also
    Pleural effusion
Cell lysis, conditions, 420
Cell salvage, 576
Cellulitis, dermatologic mimics, 624
Center for Medicare and Medicaid Services
    (CMS), 8, 122, 907, 967
    Premier Demonstration, 935
    Stark revision, promulgation, 993
Center for Tobacco Research and Intervention,
    97
Centers for Disease Control and Prevention
    (CDC), 85
    annual influenza vaccination,
        recommendations, 87b
    Study of the Efficacy of Nosocomial
        Infection Control, 119
    surveillance system, establishment, 120
Central catheters, aseptic placement, 320
Central diabetes insipidus. See Post-craniotomy
    central diabetes insipidus
Central nervous system (CNS)
    cerebral edema, occurrence, 412
    disorders. See Acquired Immune Deficiency
        Syndrome
    GABA receptor complex-mediated
        inhibition, 659
    infections. See Non-CNS infections
    injury, 669
    malignancy, 543–544
    shunt infection, 305
Central venous catheter (CVC), 317. See also
    Long-term CVC
    infection, 318
Central venous pressure (CVP), elevation,
    248
Cephalosporins, usage, 834
Cerebellum, Purkinje's cells, 563
Cerebral edema, occurrence, 412
Cerebral infarction, mimics, 699t
Cerebral ischemia
    anterior/posterior circulation
        symptoms/signs, contrast, 698t
    cortical/subcortical symptoms/signs,
        contrast, 698t
Cerebral perfusion, maintenance, 715
Cerebral salt wasting, 409
    occurrence, 414

Cerebrospinal fluid (CSF)
    analysis, 564
    Gram stain, usage, 300
    impeding, 555
    inflammatory cells, recruitment/activation,
        299
    penetration, 303, 304. See also Vancomycin
    studies, obtaining, 300t
Cerebrovascular accident (CVA), 776
    development, 832
    occurrence, 806
Cervical spine instability, history, 757
Cetuximab (Erbitux), usage. See Cancer
    management
CHADS. See CHF Hypertension history Age
    Diabetes Stroke history
CHART. See California Hospital Assessment
    and Reporting Taskforce
Chemotherapeutic agents, cardiotoxicity
    profiles, 535t
Chemotherapy-related nausea, prediction, 63
Chest compressions, 192
Chest pain, 127. See also Musculoskeletal chest
    pain; Psychogenic chest pain
    alleviation/exacerbation, factors, 128
    approach, 127
    associated symptoms, 128
    clinical presentation, 127–128
    complication. See Sickle cell crises
    diagnosis, novel approaches, 133–134
    differential diagnosis, 128–129, 136t
        associated characteristics, inclusion, 130t
    ECG, usage, 586
    electrocardiogram, usage, 131
    esophageal causes, 129
    history/physical examination, 129–130
    initial assessment, 129–133
    initial management, 132–133
    location, 127
    myocardial injury markers, 131–132
    onset/duration, 127
    presence, considerations. See Hospitalized
        patients
    reading, 134
    risk stratification, 132–133
Chest radiograph (CXR)
    evaluation, 651
    usage, 160. See also Pulmonary embolism
Chest tubes, placement, 373
CHF Hypertension history Age Diabetes Stroke
    history (CHADS), 702
    index, 702t
Chickenpox, characteristics, 228t
Chief Executive Officer (CEO), involvement,
    962
Cholecystitis, 465–466
    assessment, 465–466
    clinical presentation, 465–466
    diagnosis, 466
    differential diagnosis, 466
    discharge/follow-up plans, 466
    high-risk patients, 4366
    low-risk patients, 466
    management, 466
    prognosis, 466
    treatment, 466
Cholestyramine, usage, 489
Chronic herpes simplex, HIV patient
    (illustration), 630f
Chronic HIV infection, 331, 334
Chronic hypertension, 843
    superimposed preeclampsia, 842
Chronic hypomagnesemia, 427
Chronic hyponatremia, 454
Chronic kidney disease (CKD)
    clinical consequences, 399
    ESRD, relationship, 399

Chronic kidney disease (CKD) (Continued)
incidence, increase, 399
management principles, health care
providers (awareness), 399–400
Chronic limb ischemia (CLI), 255
complications/risk, 259
Chronic liver disease
etiologies/diagnostic tests/treatment, 452t
stigmata, 445
Chronic OAC, 213
Chronic obstructive lung disease, 665
Chronic obstructive pulmonary disease
(COPD), 159, 271
acute exacerbations, treatment, 354
algorithm, 355f
antibiotics, impact, 355–356
assessment, 351–353
asthma, differentiation, 352t
atropine, treatment, 364–365
ATS/ERS guidelines, 354, 354t
background, 351
bronchodilators, usage, 354–355
clinical presentation, 351
corticosteroids, usage, 355
diagnosis, 352–353
differential diagnosis, 351–352
discharge/follow-up plans, 358
exacerbations, 283, 650
hospital assessment/admission,
indications, 353t
ICU admission, indications, 354t
short-acting bronchodilators, impact,
354
GOLD guidelines, 354, 354t
hospitalization, 353
criteria, 353–354
indication, 361
initial treatment, preference, 354–357
management, 353–357
algorithm. See Stable COPD
oxygen, impact, 355
pathogenesis, 351
postdischarge, 353
presenting signs/symptoms, 351
prevalence, 351
prevention, 357–358
pulmonary rehabilitation, 357–358
reading, 359
risk factors, 351
severe exacerbation, 665
spirometric classification, post-
bronchodilator FEV₁ basis, 353t
treatment options, alternatives, 356–357
ventilation, impact, 356
Chronic pain, prevalence, 725
Chronic polyarticular disease, 604
Chronic renal failure
assessment, 401, 402, 404–405
background, 399–400
CHF, impact, 401
dialysis, impact, 399
discharge/follow-up plans, 401, 403–404,
405
inpatient management, 400–401
invasive diagnostic/therapeutic
procedures/surgery, consideration,
400–401
management, 401, 402–403
outpatient physician communication, 401
patient education, 401
presenting disease considerations, 401
reading, 406
volume overload, impact, 401
Chronic renal insufficiency (CRI), 778
Chronic venous insufficiency (CVI), 624
Churg-Strauss, 395
Churg-Strauss syndrome, 610

Chylous ascites, 453
Circadian rhythms, scheduling, 891
Circulation, assessment, 191
Cirrhosis
assessment, 451
background, 451
clinical presentation, 451
complications, 451, 453b
etiologies/diagnostic tests/treatment, 452t
laboratory testing, 451
presenting signs/symptoms, 451
SBP signs/symptoms, 460b
Cisplatin (Platinol), usage. See Nephrotoxicity
CIWA-Ar. See Clinical Institute Withdrawal
Assessment Scale for Alcohol, Revised
CKD. See Chronic kidney disease
CK-MB. See Creatine kinase MB
Class I antiarrhythmic agents, 179t
Class III antiarrhythmic agents, 179t
Claudication, presence. See Calf pain
Cleveland Clinic Foundation (CCF), surgical
cases (distribution), 236f
CLI. See Chronic limb ischemia
Clinical decision alerts, 968–969
Clinical decision support
effectiveness, barriers, 967–968
implementation, barriers, 969
system
considerations, 968b
implementation, steps, 969
Clinical Institute Withdrawal Assessment
Scale for Alcohol, Revised (CIWA-Ar),
691t, 693
Clinical knowledge, importance, 956
Clinical probability scores, usage, 219
Clinical pulmonary infection score (CPIS),
280, 281
Clinical TLS (CTLS), 560
Clinical Trial of Reviparin and Metabolic
Modulation in Acute Myocardial
Infarction Treatment Evaluation
(CREATE), 505
Clinical uremia, 394
CLL. See B-cell chronic lymphocytic leukemia
Clock Draw Test, 41
Clonidine. See Alpha-agonists
Clopidogrel, 780
impact, 141, 154, 763
Clostridium botulism, 340
Clostridium difficile
colonization, prevalence, 486t
transmission, reduction methods, 490t
Clostridium difficile-associated diarrhea
(CDAD), 485, 487
association, strength, 486t
clinical findings, prevalence, 486t
diagnosis (tests), diagnostic capabilities,
488t
initial episodes (oral therapy), randomized
comparative trials (summary), 489t
Clostridium difficile colitis, 123
antibiotic restriction, 489
antibiotics, cessation, 488
antibiotic therapy, 488–489
approach, preference, 488
assessment, 486–488
asymptomatic carriage, 486–487
background, 485
barrier precautions, 489
clinical presentation, 486–487
diagnosis, 487
differential diagnosis, 487
discharge/follow-up plans, 490
hand hygiene, 489
hospitalization, 488
management, 488–489
patient instruction, 490

Clostridium difficile colitis (Continued)
presenting signs/symptoms, 486
prevalence, 486
prevention, 489–490
probiotics, 489–490
prognosis, 488
reading, 490–491
tests, 487–488
treatment, 488–489
Clostridium sp., empiric antibiotics (usage),
480–481
Clot-based phospholipids-dependent
coagulation test, 597
CLOT investigation, 213–214
Clotting factor replacement therapy, 592
Clustered systems, impact, 5
CMI. See Case Mix Index
CMS. See Center for Medicare and Medicaid
Services
CMV. See Controlled mechanical ventilation
CNNA. See Culture-negative neutrocytic
ascites
CO. See Carbon monoxide; Cardiac output
Coaching, 927–928
Coagulation disorders, impact. See Ischemic
stroke
Coagulation studies, 759–760
Cocaine
abuse/dependence screening tools,
114–115
ingestion, risk factor, 228
intoxication/withdrawal, 112
differential diagnosis, 113t
Coding. See Hospital medicine
plan, 909t
Cognitive deficits, revelation, 38, 40
Cognitive impairment. See Geriatric patients
persistence, bacterial meningitis (impact),
303
Cognizant systems, AI (usage), 5
Colitis. See Microscopic colitis;
Pseudomembranous colitis; Ulcerative
colitis
Collagen
diseases, risk factor, 228
synthesis, hyperglycemia (impact),
790
Colles' fractures, 105
Colonoscopy, usage, 480
Coma. See Nontraumatic coma
assessment, 711–712
background, 711
clinical presentation, 711
diagnosis, 711–712
diagnostic scheme, 713
EEG, usage, 712
evaluation, 711–712
evidence, 717
flumazenil, usage. See Drug-induced coma;
Hepatic coma
management/treatment, 715–717
naloxone, usage. See Drug-induced coma;
Opiate-induced coma
neuroprotective agents. See Anoxic-ischemic
coma
neurosurgery consultation, 716
pentobarbital, usage, 715
presenting signs/symptoms, 711
prognosis, 712
prophylactic anticonvulsant/
carbamazepine, usage, 715
reading, 717
traumatic brain injury, impact, 715
Combination immunosuppressive therapy,
612
Combined systems, impact, 5
COMMIT trial, 143

Communication
  ability, 984
  barriers, 12t
  duties. See Physicians
  effectiveness. See Hospital medicine
      leadership
    increase, 16b
    measurement, 896
  plan. See also Hospital medicine program
      components, 885b
  relationship. See Trust
  systems, variability, 956
Community-acquired ARF, 392
Community-acquired bacterial meningitis,
    causes, 300t
Community-acquired diarrhea (CAD), 70, 485
Community-acquired intra-abdominal
    infections, 468
Community-acquired MRSA (CA-MRSA)
  assessment, 625
  background, 625
  diagnosis, 625
  differential diagnosis, 625
  management/treatment, 625
Community-acquired pneumonia (CAP), 666
  antibiotics, delivery, 274
  assessment, 271
  background, 271
  blood cultures, 272
  clinically stable patients, identification
      criteria, 276b
  clinical presentation, 271
  diagnosis, 272–273
  differential diagnosis, 271
  discharge/follow-up plans, 277
  initial treatment, 274–276
  management, 274–276
  options, alternatives, 273
  pathogens, presence, 275t
  patient discharge, identification criteria,
      277b
  physical examination, 271
  plague, possibility, 340–341
  postdischarge, 274
  presence, initial empiric antimicrobial
      therapy. See Immunocompetent
      patients
  presenting signs/symptoms, 271
  prevention, 276–277
  prognosis/admission decision, 273–274
  radiograph, 272f
  reading, 277
  sputum Gram stain, 272
  studies, preference, 272
  treatment, 274–276
Community-associated MRSA (CA-MRSA),
    294
Comorbid DTs, 867
Compatibility testing, 574
Compensation
  expectations, 902
    alignment. See Physician performance
  measures, advantages/disadvantages. See
      Group compensation measures
  methodology, 900–902
  modeling, 902
  planning, 902
  productivity, SHM survey results, 899–900
  programs
    characteristics, 900b
    pitfalls, 902
Compensation principles/practices
  introduction, 899
  reading, 903
Complementary/alternative medicine (CAM)
  discussion, 17
  usage, 15, 17

Complete blood count (CBC)
  inclusion, 577
  level, 261
  usage, 697, 759
Complete blood count with platelets and
    differential (CBCPD), 300
Complete SBO, 473
Compliance. See Hospital medicine
  improvement, 742
  plane, 909t
Computed tomography angiography (CTA),
    156
  usage, 699. See also Acute aortic dissection
Computed tomography (CT) scanning, 272
Computers, confidentiality issue, 979
Confidentiality
  breach. See Hospitals
  ethical issue, 979
Conflict
  handling styles, 928t
  resolution. See Hospital medicine leadership
Confusion Assessment Method (CAM)
  administration, 720–721
  usage. See Delirium
Confusion Assessment Method for Intensive
    Care Unit (CAM-ICU), 721
Congenital disorders, impact. See Valvular
    heart disease
Congestion, sequelae, 962b
Congestive heart failure (CHF), 150. See also
    Decompensated CHF
  assessment, 401
  bilateral effusions, percentage, 372
  diagnosis, 401
  history, 153
  imbalance, 370
  overload/development, 313
  precipitation. See Early postoperative CHF
  pulmonary edema, relationship, 283
Connective tissue disease, impact. See Valvular
    heart disease
Conscious state. See Minimally conscious
    state
Constipation
  assessment, 53–54
  background, 53
  bulk-producing agents, impact, 57
  causes, 54t
  clinical presentation, 53
  diagnosis, 53–54
  diet/physical activity, impact, 55, 57
  differential diagnosis, 53
  discharge/follow-up plans, 59–60
  emollients, impact, 58–59
  enemas, impact, 58–59
  fecal impaction, 59
  lubricants, impact, 58–59
  management, 54–59
    algorithm, 55f
  medications, impact, 54b
  opioid therapy, impact, 59
  options, alternatives, 59
  osmotic laxatives, impact, 57–58
  outpatient physician communication,
      59–60
  patient education, 59–60
  preferred intervention, 55–59
  presenting signs/symptoms, 53
  prevalence, 53
  prevention, 59
  reading, 60
  stimulant laxatives, impact, 58
  studies, preference, 53–54
  suppositories, impact. See Constipation
  symptom management, 735
  therapy, 56t–57t
  treatment, 54–59

Consultation. See Curbside consultation;
    Nonsurgical patients; Surgical patients
  payment, Medicare criteria, 742b
  report, scope, 741
  rules (commandments), 742b
Consulting physicians, communication. See
    Hospitalist systems
Contact dermatitis, 624–625
Context-sensitive systems, clinical context
    awareness, 5
Contextual features, impact, 986
Continuity of Care Task Force, information
    transfer recommendations, 78
Continuous ambulatory peritoneal dialysis
    (CAPD) patients, intraperitoneal
    antibiotic dosing recommendations, 404t
Continuous positive airway pressure (CPAP),
    663
  consideration, 668
  impact. See Postoperative CPAP
  level, 673
  treatment, 747
Continuous renal replacement therapy
    (CRRT), 399
Contractile function, digoxin (impact), 844
Contrast venography, usage, 542
Controlled mechanical ventilation (CMV), 670
Convulsive SE, AEDs (usage), 716
Coordination. See Health care
  definition, 955–956
  theory. See Relational coordination
Co-oximetry, 651
COP. See Cryptogenic organizing pneumonia
COPD. See Chronic obstructive pulmonary
    disease
Core body temperature, adverse cardiac event
    predictor, 822
Coronary artery bypass grating (CABG), 154,
    258, 779–780
  association, 762–763
  impact, possibility, 821
  procedures, 791
  risk factors, 789–790
  surgery, hyperglycemia (impact), 504
Coronary artery disease (CAD), 133, 401, 776
  diagnosis, 129
  differential diagnosis, 128
  impact. See Valvular heart disease
  preoperative detection, 790
Coronary disease, likelihood, 150t
Coronary steal, 266
Corrective action. See Physician performance
Cortical atrophy, 301f
Corticosteroids
  clinical assessment/evaluation, 762
  patients, categories (division), 762
  recommendations/management, 762
  supplementation, duration, 762
  therapy, recommendations, 520
  usage. See Asthma; Sepsis/shock; Septic
      shock
Corticotropin-releasing hormone (CRH),
    secretion, 517
Cost/quality (tensions), needs/desires (impact),
    937t
Cost reduction. See Hospital medicine program
  calculation, 911–912
  definition, 911–912
Coumadin dosing nomogram, 213t
Counter-regulatory hormones, levels, 789
Coupled systems, knowledge linkage, 5
COX-2. See Cyclo-oxygenase-2
CPAP. See Continuous positive airway pressure
CPIS. See Clinical pulmonary infection score
CPK. See Creatinine phosphokinase
CPR. See Cardiopulmonary resuscitation
CPT. See Current Procedural Terminology

CR-BSI. See Catheter-related bloodstream infection
C-reactive protein (CRP)
  elevation, 261, 609
  increase, 22–23
  measures, 326
  test, 249
  usefulness, 605
CREATE. See Clinical Trial of Reviparin and Metabolic Modulation in Acute Myocardial Infarction Treatment Evaluation
Creatine kinase MB (CK-MB), 151
  CK-MB/CK ratio, 136
  information, addition, 139
  isoenzyme, 131
  rise/fall, 139f
Creatinine
  levels, 829
  studies, 683
  usage. See Pleural effusion
Creatinine phosphokinase (CPK)
  MB fraction, 806
  usage, 258
CRH. See Corticotropin-releasing hormone
CRI. See Chronic renal insufficiency
Critical care, prolonged services (contrast), 907
Critical care setting, hyperglycemia (impact), 503–504
Critically ill patients
  nutrition, recommendations, 800b
  specialized enteral/parenteral nutrition support, clinical indications, 24
Critically ill patients, sedation/pain management
  acetaminophen, usage, 658
  analgesic agents, usage, 657–658
  assessment/diagnosis, 655–657
  background, 655
  barbiturates, usage, 660
  benzodiazepines, usage, 659
  BIS, impact, 657
  butyrophenones (Haloperidol), usage, 660
  Dexmedetomidine (Precedex), usage, 660
  Etomidate, usage, 659–660
  management, 657–661
  NSAIDs, impact, 658
  opioids, usage, 657–658
  prevention, 661
  Propofol (Diprivan), usage, 659
  reading, 661–662
  undersedation/oversedation, consideration, 655
Crohn's colitis, 474
Crohn's disease (CD), 471
  diarrhea, presence, 471
  luminal disease, control, 475
  SBO, treatment, 475
  symptoms, 472t
  treatment options, 474–475
Crohn's ileitis, 474–475
Cross-cultural encounters, negotiations (recommendations), 19b
CRP. See C-reactive protein
CRRT. See Continuous renal replacement therapy
CRT. See Cardiac resynchronization therapy
Crush preparation, 632
Cryptococcal meningitis, clinical presentation. See Acquired Immune Deficiency Syndrome
Cryptogenic organizing pneumonia (COP), 377
Cryptosporidium
  empiric antibiotics, usage, 481
  untreatability, 335

Crystal-induced disease, 603
Crystalline arthritis, septic arthritis (coexistence), 603
CSF. See Cerebrospinal fluid
CT. See Computed tomography
CTA. See Computed tomography angiography
CTLS. See Clinical TLS
Cultural competence training, implementation (requirement), 15
Cultural influences. See End-of-life; Patients
Culturally appropriate communication, competence, achievement, 15
Culture-negative IE, diagnostic testing, 311t
Culture-negative neutrocytic ascites (CNNA) diagnosis, 453
Curbside consultation, 743
Current Procedural Terminology (CPT), 907
  codes, billing, 876
Cushing's triad, 299
Cutaneous anthrax, 339
  differential diagnosis, 339–340
Cutaneous candidal infections, 625
Cutaneous candidiasis. See Hospitalized diabetic patient
Cutaneous ecchymoses, inclusion. See Fever
Cutaneous macules/papules, inclusion. See Fever
Cutaneous petechiae, inclusion. See Fever
Cutaneous purpura, inclusion. See Fever
Cutaneous vasculitis
  assessment, 636
  background, 636
  diagnosis/prognosis, 636
  discharge/follow-up plans, 636
  management, 636
Cut Annoyed Guilty Eye (CAGE)
  questionnaire, 863
    screen, usage. See Alcohol abuse/dependence
  questions, 113, 114b
CVA. See Cerebrovascular accident
CVC. See Central venous catheter
CVI. See Chronic venous insufficiency
CVO₂. See Venous oxygen saturation
CVP. See Central venous pressure
CXR. See Chest radiograph
Cyclo-oxygenase-2 (COX-2), impact, 763
Cyclophosphamide (Cytoxan), usage. See Anticancer agents, cardiovascular complications
Cytokines
  release reactions. See Cancer treatment
  release syndrome, 532
  usage, 811
Cytology, usage. See Pleural effusion
Cytomegalovirus (CMV), 332, 333, 630
  disease, 335
  serum PCR, usage, 335
Cytosine arabinoside (ARA-C) (Cytosar), 538
  clinical presentation, 538
  treatment/prognosis, 538
Cytotoxic chemotherapy, 65
Cytotoxin assay, usage, 188
Cytoxan, usage. See Anticancer agents

DAH. See Diffuse alveolar hemorrhage
Darbepoetin, usage, 574
Data collection. See Quality improvement
Data representation, appropriateness, 974–975
DAWN. See Drug Abuse Warning Network
Day care, infectious risks (increase), 479
Daytime only inhospital coverage, example. See Hospital medicine program
DDAVP. See Desmopressin acetate
D-dimer assays, usefulness, 209

D-dimer testing, usage. See Pulmonary embolism
Death. See Good death
  rattle, symptom management, 734
  short-term risk, 132t, 152t
Debridement
  necessity. See Stage IV pressure ulcer techniques, 48t
Decision-makers, abilities (assessment questions), 985b
Decision-making capacity, 984–985
Decompensated CHF, 100, 259
DECREASE study, 780
Deep soft tissue infection, 292
Deep vein thrombosis (DVT)
  acute phase treatment, LMWH/UFH (usage), 210
  algorithms, 209–210
  aPTT range, ACCP recommendations, 211
  assessment, 207–210
  clinical presentation, 207
  diagnosis, 208
    approach, 211f
  diagnostic approach. See Acute DVT
  differential diagnosis, 207–208
  discharge/follow-up plans, 214–215
  evaluation, diagnostic tests (likelihood ratio usage), 210t
  FDA-approved initial therapy, 211t
  finding points, pretest probability (clinical model prediction), 209t
  hospitalization, prognosis, 210
  management, 211–213
    flowchart, 212f
  options, alternatives, 209, 211–213
  outpatient physician communication, 215
  patient education, 214
  postdischarge, 210
  presenting signs/symptoms, 207
  prevalence, 207
  prevention, 214
  prognosis, 210
  prophylaxis, 701–702
  reading, 215–216
  risk factors, surgery (relationship), 766t
  studies, preference, 208–209
  therapy, 213–214
  treatment, 211–213
  usage. See Intracerebral hemorrhage
  VTE risk factors, 207
Deep venous thrombosis (DVT), 625. See also Acute DVT
  prophylaxis, contraindications. See Pharmacologic DVT prophylaxis
  suffering, 99
  treatment. See Cancer
Defibrillation, 192
  employment, 191
Dehiscence. See Fascial dehiscence; Wounds
Dehydration, 832
Delayed hemolytic transfusion reactions (DHTRs), 570–571
Delayed toxicity (production), agents (classification), 678t
Delirium. See Terminal delirium
  assessment, 657, 719–721
  association, 40, 863
  background, 719
  CAM, usage, 720t
  causes, 721b
  clinical presentation, 719–720
  diagnosis, 720–721
  differential diagnosis, 720
  differentiating characteristics, 40t
  discharge/follow-up plans, 722
  DSM-IV criteria, 720b
  hospitalization, 721

Delirium (Continued)
management, 721–722, 807
  goal, 661
measures/screening, 40–41
medication review, 722
options, alternatives, 722
outpatient physician communication, 722
patient/family education, 722
perioperative management techniques, 867
physical examination, 720
post discharge, 721
prediction rules, 721
presenting signs/symptoms, 719–720
prevalence, 719–720
prevention, 722
prognosis, 721
reading, 723
recognition, 719
risk factors/causes, 721
studies, preference, 720–721
symptom management, 734
third-party informants, 719–720
treatment, 721–722
Delirium tremens (DTs), 688–689. See also
    Comorbid DTs
history, 689
management/treatment, 693
risk factors, 688
Demand, variability (management), 962
Dementia, differentiating characteristics, 40t
Department of Health and Human Services
    (DHHS), 996
Depression
antianxiety medications, usage, 856r
assessment, 41
background, 855
clinical assessment/evaluation, 855, 859
commonness, 863
differentiating characteristics, 40t
DSM-IV criteria, 855
medications, 854t–855t
perioperative management techniques, 864
pharmacotherapy, 859
treatment, 859
Dermatitis, 834. See also Contact dermatitis;
    Seborrheic dermatitis; Stasis dermatitis
Dermatologic mimics. See Cellulitis
Dermatology. See Hospitalized patients
Dermatoses. See Human immunodeficiency
    virus
Desmopressin acetate (DDAVP), 592
administration, 594
intravenous dose, 594
testing, 594
Detoxification history, 689
DEXA. See Dual-energy X-ray absorptiometry
Dexmedetomidine, usage. See Critically ill
    patients
DHHS. See Department of Health and Human
    Services
DHTRs. See Delayed hemolytic transfusion
    reactions
Diabetes insipidus (DI)
causes, 415t
disorder, 415–416
presence, probability, 416
principal imbalance, 524t
Diabetes mellitus. See Gestational diabetes
    mellitus
background, 503
management, 503
patients, insulin (reduction), 869
reading, 508
Diabetic ketoacidosis (DKA), 432
adult patients, management protocol, 500f
assessment, 496–499
background, 495–496
bicarbonate, usage, 501

Diabetic ketoacidosis (DKA) (Continued)
causes, 496t
child mortality, 499
classification levels, ADA guidelines, 497
clinical presentation, 496–497
diagnosis, 497–499
diagnostic criteria, 497f
differential diagnosis, 498–499
discharge/follow-up plans, 501
epidemiology, 495
fluid therapy, 499
glucose production, increase, 496f
infectious precipitants, 495
insulin therapy, 499, 501
ketone body production, increase, 497t
leukocytosis, presence, 498
management, 499–501
mental status, variation, 496–497
pathogenesis, 495–496
patients, subcutaneous rapid-acting insulin
    analogs (usage treatment protocol),
    498t
phosphate, usage, 501
potassium, usage, 501
precipitants, 501
precipitating causes, 495
prognosis, 499
reading, 502
subcutaneous insulin, transition, 501
treatment, 499
Diabetic patients, perioperative management
assessment/risk evaluation, 790
background, 789
blood glucose, perioperative outcome
    (relationship), 789–790
diet treatment, 791
discharge recommendations, 793
list, 792b
management, approaches, 791–793
oral antidiabetic agents, treatment,
    792–793
pathophysiology, 789–790
perioperative period, glycemic goal,
    790–791
principles, 791
reading, 793–794
recommendations, 791–793
surgical stress/anesthesia, metabolic
    consequences, 789
Diabetic risk factors. See Foot
    ulceration/infection
Diagnosis Related Group (DRG)
coding, inaccuracy, 913
stratification, 911
Diagnostic and Statistical Manual of Mental
    Disorders, 4th edition (DSM-IV), 719
criteria. See Delirium
definitions. See Alcohol use disorders
Diagnostic paracentesis, indications, 460b
Diagnostic Related Group (DRG)
coding basics, 905
score, 906
Diagnostic tests, 778
Dialysis
antibiotics, intermittent dosing. See
    Automated peritoneal dialysis
impact. See Chronic renal failure
initiation, 401
modality choices, comparison. See
    Hospitalized patients
patients, intraperitoneal antibiotic dosing
    recommendations. See Continuous
    ambulatory peritoneal dialysis
Diarrhea. See Community-acquired diarrhea;
    Hospital-acquired diarrhea
antibiotic restriction, 489
antibiotics, cessation, 488
antibiotic therapy, 480t, 488–489

Diarrhea (Continued)
antimicrobial therapy, 74
assessment, 69–70, 486–488
asymptomatic carriage, 486–487
background, 69, 485
barrier precautions, 489
bismuth therapy, 74
causes, infectious agents (impact), 478b
clinical presentation, 69, 486–487
diagnosis, 487
differential diagnosis, 69–70, 70t, 487
discharge/follow-up plans, 490
evaluation/treatment, 73f
hand hygiene, 489
hospitalization, 488
imaging, problems. See Acute diarrhea
management, 70–74, 488–489
mechanisms. See Antibiotic-associated
    diarrhea
medications, impact, 71t
occurrence. See Hospitalized patients;
    Human immunodeficiency virus
options, alternatives, 74
outpatient physician communication, 75
ova, impact, 479
parasites, impact, 479
patient education, 75
patient instruction, 490
prediction rule, 486
presenting signs/symptoms, 69, 486
prevalence, 69, 486
prevention, 489–490
probiotics, 489–490
reading, 75, 490–491
rehydration/diet, impact, 70–71
studies, preference, 70
symptomatic therapy, 72
symptomatic treatment, 72t
tests, 487–488
three-day rule, 479
treatment, 488–489
Diarrheal infections, causes (antibiotic
    therapy). See Parasitic diarrheal
    infections
Diarrheal pathogens, presence. See Human
    immunodeficiency virus
Diarrheal toxins, presence, 478
Diastolic dysfunction, 823
DIC. See Disseminated intravascular
    coagulation
Dietary intake pattern, determination, 23b
Diffuse alveolar hemorrhage (DAH), 378
Diffusing capacity to carbon monoxide
    (DLCO), 534
DIGAMI study, 504–505
Digit span test, 31b
Digoxin, impact. See Contractile function
Dilaudid, usage. See Hydromorphone
Diphtheria, review, 87, 90
DIPOM study, 780
Diprivan, usage. See Critically ill patients
Direct thrombin inhibitors (DTI), usage,
    212
Direct thrombin inhibitors (DTI), usage
    (approval). See Parenteral DTI
Discharge
appointment system, implementation,
    962–963
appointment time, selection, 963
communications, audits, 77
determination. See Elderly hospitalized
    patient
follow-up arrangements, advice, 80
medications, 147t, 156t
planning. See Geriatric patients
sites, 34b
Disorientation, 688
Disseminated HSV 2, 338–339

Disseminated intravascular coagulation (DIC), 394–395
  evidence, 453
  impact, 700
  syndrome, 842
Diuretics. *See* Potassium-sparing diuretics; Thiazide diuretics
  impact, 391. *See also* Ascites
Diverticulitis, 466–468
  antibiotic choices, 467
  assessment, 466–467
  barium enema, usage, 466
  clinical presentation, 466
  CT scanning, usage, 466
  diagnosis, 466
  differential diagnosis, 466
  elective procedures, pre-operative measures, 467
  emergency procedures, pre-operative measures, 467
  endoscopy, usage, 466
  management, 467
  medical management. *See* Simple diverticulitis
  prognosis, 466–467
  surgery, indications, 467b
  surgical management. *See* Complicated diverticulitis
  water-soluble contrast enema, usage, 466
DKA. *See* Diabetes ketoacidosis; Diabetic ketoacidosis
DLCO. *See* Diffusing capacity to carbon monoxide
Doctors, patient lawsuits (reasons), 991
Documentation. *See* Hospital-driven physician documentation; Hospital medicine improvement, 913
Do Not Intubate advanced directive, 667
Door-to-needle time, 143
Dopamine, impact, 509
Dopamine antagonists, impact, 65
Doppler echocardiography, usage. *See* Mitral stenosis
DPAHC. *See* Durable power of attorney for health care
DPOA-HC. *See* Durable Power of Attorney for Health Care
Dressler's syndrome, 247
DRG. *See* Diagnosis Related Group; Diagnostic Related Group
Drotrecogin alfa, usage. *See* Sepsis/shock
Drug Abuse Warning Network (DAWN), 684
Drug history, preoperative health assessment. *See* Illicit drug history
Drug-induced coma
  flumazenil, usage, 716
  naloxone, usage, 716
Drug overdose
  diagnostic tests, 677
  history/physical examination, 677
  introduction, 677
  reading, 685–686
  treatment, 677–679
Drugs, product/strict liability, 991
DSM-IV. *See* Diagnostic and Statistical Manual of Mental Disorders, 4th edition
DTI. *See* Direct thrombin inhibitors
DTs. *See* Delirium tremens
Dual-energy X-ray absorptiometry (DEXA), 797
Dual x-ray absorptiometry (DXA), 106
Durable power of attorney for health care (DPAHC), 980
Durable Power of Attorney for Health Care (DPOA-HC), existence, 38
DVT. *See* Deep vein thrombosis; Deep venous thrombosis

DXA. *See* Dual x-ray absorptiometry
Dyspnea, pain management, 734

E. coli, empiric antibiotics (usage), 481
EABV. *See* Effective arterial blood volume
Early postoperative CHF, precipitation, 806
Early repolarization (separation), ECG changes (usage), 250t
EBP. *See* Evidence-based practice
ECC. *See* Emergency Cardiovascular Care
ECG. *See* Electrocardiogram
ECHO, usage, 251, 252
Echocardiography
  information, 313
  usage. *See* Pulmonary embolism
Ecstasy. *See* MDMA
ECT. *See* Electroconvulsive therapy
ED diversion time, decrease, 912–913
Education duties. *See* Physicians
Effective arterial blood volume (EABV), 392–393
  decrease, prerenal states, 393
Effects analysis. *See* Failure modes and effects analysis
EGFR. *See* Epidermal growth factor hormone
Ehlers-Danlos, risk factor, 228
Elderly hospitalized patient
  baseline, functional status, 38–41
  caregiver/informant, role, 38
  clinical depression, occurrence. *See* Medically ill hospitalized elderly patients
  discharge determination, 41
  functional assessment, 37
  hospitalization, functional status, 38–41
  mobility assessment, 41
  reading, 42
  sensory assessment, 41
Electrical cardioversion, guidelines, 177b
Electrocardiogram (ECG). *See* Pulmonary hypertension; Signal-averaged ECG
  acute pericarditis
    Stage 3, 250f
    Stage I, 249f
  changes. *See* Acute pericarditis
    usage. *See* Acute MI; Acute pericarditis; Early repolarization
  data. *See* Second-degree AVB; Third-degree AVB
  findings, infarct site basis, 138t
  monitoring. *See* Twenty-four-hour ECG monitoring
  performance/interpretation, 129
  testing. *See* Treadmill exercise stress ECG testing
  usage, 759, 778. *See also* Acute aortic dissection; Acute coronary syndrome; Acute MI; Acute pericarditis; Chest pain; Pulmonary embolism
Electroconvulsive therapy (ECT)
  APA Task Force report, 869
  assessment. *See* Pre-ECT assessment
  cardiac considerations, 869
  neurologic considerations, 869
  pulmonary considerations, 869
Electroconvulsive therapy (ECT) consultation
  background, 868
  clinical assessment, 868–869
  management, 869
Electrolytes
  administration, guidelines. *See* Parenteral nutrient solutions
  disorders, 419
    reading, 427
  initial provision, 25
  usage. *See* Intracerebral hemorrhage
  usefulness, 468

Electronic mail transmissions
  disclaimer statement, accompaniment. *See* Privileged facsimile/electronic mail transmissions
  interruptions, 979
Electrophysiologic studies (EPS), 200
  usage, 564
Electrophysiology studies (EPS), 204
Elevated intracranial pressure. *See* Cancer emergencies
ELISA. *See* Enzyme-linked immunosorbent assay
E&M. *See* Evaluation & Management
Embolic strokes, diagnostic studies, 698
Embolism. *See* Air embolism; Amniotic fluid embolism; Fat embolism; Septic embolism
Emergency Cardiovascular Care (ECC), 189
Emergency Medical Treatment and Active Labor Act (EMTALA), 993
Emollients, impact. *See* Constipation
Empathy, facilitation, 11t
Empiric antibiotic options, 347t
Empiric antibiotic selection. *See* Hospitalized patients
Empiric antimicrobial therapy. *See* Asthma
Empiric system. *See* Quality improvement
Employment Exception, 994
EMTALA. *See* Emergency Medical Treatment and Active Labor Act
EN. *See* Enteral nutrition
Enalaprilat, usage, 266
Encephalitis, antimicrobial therapy, 716
Encounter, interpreter (usage), 16b
Endocarditis, impact. *See* Valvular heart disease
End-of-life
  care, 165
  cultural influences, 17–18
  discussion, 18
End-organ damage, 263
  presence. *See* Acute end-organ damage
Endoscopy, usage. *See* Diverticulitis
Endothelin receptor antagonists, usage. *See* Pulmonary hypertension
Endotracheal aspirates (ETA), sensitivity, 280
Endotracheal intubation
  indications, 653b
  usage. *See* Acute respiratory failure
Endotracheal tube-related complications, 672
End-stage renal disease (ESRD)
  incidence, increase, 399
  management principles, health care providers (awareness), 399–400
  patients
    rigor/fever, development, 402
    vascular access, protection, 400
  relationship. *See* Chronic kidney disease
  usage, 327
End-tidal CO_2 monitoring, 194
Enemas, impact. *See* Constipation
Energy needs, estimation, 23b
Energy requirements, estimation, 24
Enigmatic fever, testing, 345t
Entamoeba histolytica, empiric antibiotics (usage), 481
Enteral access, evaluation. *See* Nutrient delivery
Enteral feeding, initiation, 23
Enteral nutrition (EN)
  receiving, 22
  route, 25
  support, initiation/administration, 26
Enzyme-linked immunosorbent assay (ELISA)
  usage, 209, 340
    combination. *See* Indirect immunofluorescence

Eosinophilic folliculitis (Ofugi disease),
    630–631
  illustration, 631f
EPAP. See Expiratory positive airway
    pressure
Epidermal growth factor hormone (EGFR),
    533
Epidural hematoma, 747–748
Epinephrine, dosage, 192
Epipodophyllotoxins, usage. See Cancer
    management
EPS. See Electrophysiologic studies;
    Electrophysiology studies
Eron classification system. See Skin/soft tissue
    infections
Error, defining, 947
Erythema, presence. See Fever
Erythema multiforme, 632, 634
Erythrocyte sedimentation rate (ESR),
    377
  elevation, 610
Erythropoietin (EPO). See Recombinant
    erythropoietin
  usage, 574
Esmolol, usage, 266
Esophageal causes. See Chest pain
ESR. See Erythrocyte sedimentation rate
ESRD. See End-stage renal disease
ESR measures, 326
Estrogen therapy, impact. See Osteoporosis
ETA. See Endotracheal aspirates
Ethical conflicts, occurrence, 18
Ethical dilemmas, solution. See Hospital
    medicine ethics
Ethical problem solving, approach, 986f
Ethics. See Hospital medicine ethics
Ethylene glycol toxicity, 683
Etomidate, usage. See Critically ill patients
Euvolemic hyponatremia, 409–410
Evaluation & Management (E&M) services,
    906–907
Evidence. See Practice-based evidence
  class, grading scheme (sample), 968t
Evidence-based clinical practice, 3
  reading, 6
Evidence-based information
  cycle, 5As, 4
  systems, usefulness, 3
Evidence-based practice (EBP), 3
  paradigm shift, 6
Evidence-based practitioner, questions. See
    Information
Exanthematous drug reactions, 623f
Exanthematous reactions, 621–622
  assessment, 621
  clinical presentation, 621
  diagnosis, 621
  differential diagnosis, 621
  discharge/follow-up plans, 622
  management, 622
  treatment, 622
Exclusive contracts, 995–996
Exercise-induced tachyarrhythmias, 200
Expectations
  alignment. See Physician performance
  change, rapidity, 972–973
Expiratory positive airway pressure (EPAP),
    663–664
External incentives. See Quality improvement
Extracrainial vessel sources. See Ischemic
    stroke
Extrapyramidal side effects, 861
Extra-thyroidal pathways. See Thyroid
    hormone metabolism
Extremities, gangrene, 344
Extrinsic PEEP (PEEP$_E$), 671–672
Extubation, success (predictors), 674t–675t

FACES Pain Rating Scale. See Wong-Baker
    FACES Pain Rating Scale
Facsimile transmissions
  disclaimer statement, accompaniment. See
      Privileged facsimile/electronic mail
      transmissions
  interruptions, 979
Factor VIII/IX concentrate, dosing, 592
Factor V Leiden, 596–597
Fagerstrom test. See Nicotine dependence
Failure modes and effects analysis (FMEA),
    949
  similarities/differences. See Root cause
      analysis
Fair market value (FMV), 994
Fairness, importance, 979
False imprisonment, 991
Familial hypocalciuric acid, 549
Family conference, usefulness/process, 34b
Family medical history, preoperative health
    assessment, 756
Family Medical Leave Act, 993
Family meeting, conducting, 736t
FARMS. See Fluids/fever air rest prevention
    medications situations
Fascial dehiscence, 813f
Fasting lipid profile, 261
Fat embolism, 224
Febrile non-hemolytic transfusion reactions
    (FNHTRs), 571
Febrile patient, intravascular catheter presence
    (evaluation), 319
Fecal impaction. See Constipation
Fecal leukocytes, tests, 487
Federal Tort Claims Act, 993
Feedback
  characteristics, 922b
  mechanisms, providing, 922b
  providing. See Physician performance
Fenoldopam, usage, 266
FEV$_1$. See Forced expiratory volume in one
    second
  usage. See Time forced expiratory volume
Fever. See Rash/fever
  clinical assessment/evaluation, 817
  cutaneous macules/papules, inclusion, 633t
  cutaneous manifestations, presence, 632b
  cutaneous petechiae/purpura/ecchymoses,
      inclusion, 633t
  emergency. See Cancer emergencies
  erythema, presence, 632t
  impact. See Ischemic stroke
  initial treatment scheme. See Neutropenic
      fever
  occurrence. See Infection-related fever
  pathophysiology, 817
  recommendations/management, 817
  risk factors, 817
  sepsis, proof, 584
  testing. See Enigmatic fever
  vesicles/bullae, presence, 632b
Fever-including bowel ischemia, 344
Fever of unknown origin (FUO), 333–336
FFA. See Free fatty acids
FFP. See Fresh frozen plasma
Fibrillation. See Atrial fibrillation
  sustaining, 185
Fibrinolysis, evidence, 453
Fibrinolytic therapy, 143–144
  choice, 244
Fibrin-specific thrombolytics, 144
Financial plan, development. See Hospital
    medicine program
FIND. See Foundations for Innovations in
    Nicotine Dependence
FiO$_2$, 671
Five Wishes Document, example, 980

Flexible sigmoidoscopy, usefulness. See
    Inflammatory bowel disease
Flow-cycled ventilation, 670–671
  contrast, 669
Flow diagnostic
  adjusted turns, utilization (contrast), 964f
  strategies, 965f
Fluid cultures, diagnostic yield, 646
Fluid leukocytosis, decrease, 604–605
Fluid resuscitation. See Sepsis/shock
Fluids
  replacement. See Post-craniotomy central
      diabetes insipidus
  therapy. See Diabetic ketoacidosis
Fluids/fever air rest prevention medications
    situations (FARMS), usage, 589
Flumazenil, usage. See Drug-induced coma;
    Hepatic coma
FMEA. See Failure modes and effects analysis
FMV. See Fair market value
FNHTRs. See Febrile non-hemolytic
    transfusion reactions
Focus groups
  surveys, 972t
  usage, 971
Folstein Mini-Mental State Examination
    (MMSE), 41
Fondaparinux, impact, 141
Foot ulceration/infection, diabetic risk factors,
    293t
Forced expiratory volume in one second
    (FEV$_1$), stability, 839
Forced vital capacity (FVC), 377
  stability, 839
Foundations for Innovations in Nicotine
    Dependence (FIND), 96–97
Free fatty acids (FFA), 503
  increase, 789
Fresh frozen plasma (FFP), 773
FRISC-II trial, 155
FRV. See Functional lung volume
Full-time equivalent (FTE) requirements,
    875
  projection. See Hospital medicine program
Functional assessment, 985
Functional capacity, 776
Functional decline, risks (reduction), 29
Functional dependency (disability). See
    Geriatric patients
Functional lung volume (FRV), 783
Functional pain, 726f
Functional status, 757
FUO. See Fever of unknown origin
FVC. See Forced vital capacity

GABA. See Gamma-aminobutyric acid
Gabapentin (Neurontin), usage, 728
Gallstones, removal. See Sickle cell crises
Gamma-aminobutyric acid (GABA)
  action, 687
  neurotransmitter system, augmentation,
      745
  receptor complex-mediated inhibition. See
      Central nervous system
Gamma glutamyl transpeptidase (GGT), 863
Gangrene. See Extremities
Gas exchange, failure, 669
Gastric distention, 663
Gastric toxicity/protection issues, 606
Gastroenteritis
  assessment, 477–480
  background, 477
  bacteria, impact, 477–478
  clinical presentation, 477
  complications, 481–482
  diagnosis, 479–480
  differential diagnosis, 477–479

Gastroenteritis *(Continued)*
  discharge/follow-up, 482
  empiric antibiotics, usage, 480–481
  management, 480–481
  presenting signs/symptoms, 477
  prevention, 482
  prognosis, 481–482
  reading, 483
  special cases, 478–479
  studies, preference, 479–480
  treatment, 480–481
  viruses, impact, 477
Gastroesophageal reflux disease (GERD), 129,
    584–585
Gastrointestinal (GI) decontamination,
    677–679
Gastrointestinal (GI) dysmotility, 53
Gastrointestinal (GI) prophylaxis, 757
Gastrointestinal (GI) side effects, 606
Gastrointestinal (GI) surgery patients,
    postoperative TPN (receiving), 799
Gastrointestinal (GI) tract
  function, evaluation, 23b
  impact, 630
GBS. *See* Guillain-Barré syndrome
GCS. *See* Glasgow Coma Scale; Graduated
    compression stockings
G-CSFs. *See* Granulocyte-stimulating factors
GDM. *See* Gestational diabetes mellitus
GDS. *See* Geriatric Depression Scale
Gemtuzumab ozogamicin (Mylotarg), usage.
    See Cancer management
General anesthesia, 745
  effects/complications, 746t
General surgery, risk/prophylaxis, 767t
Genetic thrombophilias, prevalence,
    208t
GERD. *See* Gastroesophageal reflux disease
Geriatric Depression Scale (GDS), 41
Geriatric patients
  approach/background, 29
  cognitive impairment, 31
  discharge planning, 33, 35
  functional dependency (disability), 29
  iatrogenic illness, 32–33
  immobility, 32
  malnutrition, 31–32
  personal preferences, 33
  reading, 25
Geriatric syndromes, 32. *See also* Hospitalized
    patients
  assessment, 29–33
Gestational diabetes mellitus (GDM),
    844–845
Gestational hypertension, 843
GFR. *See* Glomerular filtration rate
GGT. *See* Gamma glutamyl transpeptidase
GI. *See* Gastrointestinal
Giardia, empiric antibiotics (usage), 481
GIK. *See* Glucose insulin-potassium
GIST-UK. *See* United Kingdom Glucose Insulin
    in Stroke Trial
Glanzmann's thrombasthenia, 594
Glasgow Coma Outcome Scale, 715t
Glasgow Coma Scale (GCS), 656–657
  list, 712
  measurement, 711
  score, 712
  usage, 681
Glaucoma patients, intraocular pressure
    (increase), 869
Global assessment. *See* Subjective Global
    Assessment
Global confusion, 688
Glomerular basement membrane (GBM). *See*
    Anti-glomerular basement membrane
Glomerular filtration rate (GFR), 399, 433

Glomerulonephritis (GN), 395, 609. *See also*
    Immune-complex GN;
    Membranoproliferative GN; Postinfection
    GN; Rapidly progressive
    glomerulonephritis
Glucocorticoids, impact, 509, 515
Glucose
  levels. *See* Synovial fluid
  management. *See* Hyperglycemia
  production, increase. *See* Diabetic
    ketoacidosis
  tolerance, impairment, 261
  usage. *See* Intracerebral hemorrhage;
    Pleural effusion
Glucose insulin-potassium (GIK) infusion, 504
  decrease, 505
Glucose tolerance test (GTT), 844
Glycemia (control), insulin (impact), 791
Glycemic goal. *See* Diabetic patients
Glycoprotein IIb/IIIa inhibitors, impact, 142
GN. *See* Glomerulonephritis
GOLD guidelines. *See* Chronic obstructive
    pulmonary disease
Good death, 737
Goodpasture's syndrome, 377, 395
GRACE National Registry. *See* Myocardial
    infarction
GRACE Prediction Score, 140, 142f
GRACE Score, 152–153, 153f
Graduated compression stockings (GCS),
    usage, 100
Gram-negative organisms, IVDA (association),
    327
Gram-positive bacteria, 319
Gram stain. *See* Community-acquired
    pneumonia
  usage. *See* Pleural effusion
Granulational tissue, prolonged intubation
    (bronchoscopic picture), 672f
Granulocyte-stimulating factors (G-CSFs),
    impact, 296
Group compensation measures, individual
    compensation measures
    (advantages/disadvantages), 902t
Group definition, 919
GTT. *See* Glucose tolerance test
G-tube. *See* Percutaneous gastrostomy tube
Guillain-Barré syndrome (GBS), 87, 482
  Miller-Fischer variant, 340
GUSTO-IV trial, 155
Gynecologic surgery, risk/prophylaxis, 767t

HA. *See* Hepatitis A
HAART. *See* Highly active antiretroviral
    therapy
HACEK organisms, 312
HAD. *See* Hospital-acquired diarrhea
Haloperidol
  IV usage guidelines. *See* Agitated patient
  usage. *See* Alcohol withdrawal syndrome;
    Critically ill patients
Hampton's hump, 218
Hand-foot-mouth disease, 632
Hand hygiene. *See Clostridium difficile* colitis;
    Diarrhea
Handling styles. *See* Conflict
Handoffs, success (elements), 896b
Hard (green) dollars, 911
Harris-Benedict equation, usage, 24
Harvard Medical Practice study, 947
HAV. *See* Hepatitis A virus
HB. *See* Hepatitis B
HbA$_1$C levels, change, 505
HBV. *See* Hepatitis B virus
HCAHPS. *See* Hospital Consumer Assessment
    of Healthcare Providers and Systems
HCAP. *See* Health care-associated pneumonia

HCFA. *See* Healthcare Finance Administration
HCUP. *See* Healthcare Cost and Utilization
    Project
HCV. *See* Hepatitis C virus
HDL. *See* High-density lipoprotein
HE. *See* Hepatic encephalopathy
Headache, 585
  indication, 584
Head-up tilt-table (HUTT), 200, 204
Health care
  coordination, 955
  environment, 930–931
  providers, actions (liability), 991
Health care-associated pneumonia (HCAP),
    risk factors, 280b
Healthcare Cost and Utilization Project
    (HCUP), 925
Healthcare Finance Administration (HCFA),
    907
Health care-seeking behaviors, cultural
    aspects, 17
  chest X-ray, 160t
Health care staff, communication. *See*
    Hospitalist systems
Health care system improvement, STEEEP
    (goals), 8b
Health Insurance Portability and
    Accountability Act (HIPAA), 979
Healthy People 2010 (health program), 85
Heart failure (HF), 139–140, 159. *See also*
    Ischemic heart failure
  background, 823
  blood tests, usage, 823
  BNP diagnostic characteristic, 161t
  classifications, 162t
  clinical assessment/evaluation, 823–824
  clinical presentation, 159–160
  CXR, usage, 823
  diagnostic algorithm, 162f
  diagnostic studies, 160–161
  differential diagnosis, 160–162
  discharge/follow-up plans, 165–166
  ECG, usage, 824
  echocardiography, usage, 824
  etiology, 823
  exacerbation (induction), medication
    (usage), 160t
  history, 823
  hospitalization, 163
  impact, 778
  Joint Commission Quality-of-Care
    Indicators, 161t
  Killup classifications, 139t
  low perfusion, congestion at rest (contrast),
    160t
  management, 824
  medications
    avoidance, 165
    impact, 163–164
  mortality, association, 139t
  options, alternatives, 161–162, 165
  outpatient-physician communication,
    165–166
  pathophysiology, 823
  patients
    instruction, 165
    mortality, blood pressure/renal function
      stratification, 162t
    prognostic variables, 163t
  physical examination, 823
  postdischarge, 162–163
  preferred treatment, 163–164
  presenting signs/symptoms, 159–160
  prognosis, 162–163
  reading, 166
  structured discharge program, readmission
    (reduction), 166t

Heart failure (HF) (Continued)
  subsequent treatment, 164–165
  temporary pacing, indications, 170–171
  timing, 823
  treatment, 163–165
  vasodilators, 163t
Heart murmurs, 777
Heel fissure, 256f
Heimlich valves, usage. See Pneumothorax
Helicobacter pylori, antibiotic regimens, 443b
Heliox, impact. See Asthma
HELLP syndrome, 842
HELP. See Hospital Elder Life Program
Hematocrit, usage. See Pleural effusion
Hematologic status, 757
Hematoma. See Epidural hematoma; Neck
    wound hematoma
  complication, 813
  expansion, prevention, 709
Hemodynamically significant arrhythmias,
    778
Hemodynamically unstable patients, 824
Hemodynamic resuscitation/stabilization,
    442–443
Hemoglobin, decrease, 584
Hemolytic anemia, 580
Hemolytic uremic syndrome (HUS), 394–395;
    481–482
Hemophilia A/B
  diagnosis, 591
  follow-up plans, 593
  management, 592–593
  off-label indications, 593
  presentation, 591
  prognosis, 591–592
  ultrasound/CT scanning, 591
Hemophilia C
  clinical presentation, 593
  diagnosis/prognosis, 593
  management, 593
Hemorrhage sites, 706f
Hemorrhagic cystitis, 538–539
  clinical presentation, 538
  diagnosis, 538
  discharge, 539
  treatment, 538–539
Hemorrhagic disorders. See Acquired
    hemorrhagic disorders; Inherited
    hemorrhagic disorders
  background, 591
  reading, 599
Hemostasis, achievement (endoscopic picture),
    443f
Hemostatic abnormalities, association. See
    Liver failure
Hemostatic therapy. See Intracerebral
    hemorrhage
Heparin
  benefit, absence, 701
  impact, 141, 154–155. See also
    Unfractionated heparin
  prophylaxis, summary. See Medical patients
Heparin-induced thrombocytopenia (HIT)
  adverse effect, 223
  cause, 101
  complications, 259
  diagnosis/prognosis, 598
  management, 598–599
  occurrence, 210
  presentation, 598
  recognition. See Rapid-onset HIT pattern
Heparin-induced thrombocytopenia with
    thrombosis (HITT)
  diagnosis/prognosis, 598
  management, 598–599
  presentation, 598
Hepatic coma, flumazenil (usage), 716

Hepatic encephalopathy
  antibiotics, impact, 457
Hepatic encephalopathy (HE), 451
  ammonia lowering strategy, 457
  diagnosis, 456–457
  management, 457
  nutritional management, 457
  suspicion, 456
  treatment, 457f
Hepatic hydrothorax, 451
  management, 458
Hepatitis. See Acute hepatitis; Autoimmune
    hepatitis; Viral hepatitis
Hepatitis A (HA), review, 90
Hepatitis A virus (HAV), impact, 90
Hepatitis B (HB), review, 90
Hepatitis B virus (HBV)
  impact, 90
  risk, 120
Hepatitis C virus (HCV), risk, 120
Hepatopulmonary syndrome (HPS), 451, 458
Hepatorenal syndrome (HRS), 394, 451
  development, risk, 454
  diagnosis, 457
  management, 458
HER2. See Human epidermal growth factor
    receptor 2 proteins
Herceptin, usage. See Cancer management
Hereditary angioedema, pathophysiology, 617f
Herpes simplex virus (HSV), 300, 333
  infections, 630
Herpes zoster, 628–629
  illustration, 629f
HF. See Heart failure
HICPAC. See Hospital Infection Control
    Practices Advisory Committee
High-density lipoprotein (HDL)
  cholesterol concentrations, 512
  level, 261
High-dose ACTH, serum cortisol (response),
    519
Highly active antiretroviral therapy (HAART),
    331
  adverse events, 333t
  discontinuation, 336
  treatment, 334
High-pressure gradients, valvular lesions
    (association), 307
High reliability organizations, 947
High-resolution CT (HRCT)
  appearances, 378b
  lung imaging, 377
  usage. See Interstitial lung disease;
    Pulmonary hypertension
High-risk hospitalized patients, infection risk,
    317
High-risk procedures, 775
High-speed deceleration injury, risk factor, 229
HIPAA. See Health Insurance Portability and
    Accountability Act
Hippocrates, realization. See Appearance
Histamine-1 receptor blockers,
    risk/alternatives, 33t
History. See Admission history
  building, approach (alternatives), 11
History & Physical (H&P). See Admitting H&P
HIT. See Heparin-induced thrombocytopenia
HITT. See Heparin-induced thrombocytopenia
    with thrombosis
HIV. See Human immunodeficiency virus
Hives. See Urticaria
HIV-related dermatoses. See Human
    immunodeficiency virus
HLA. See Human leukocyte antigen
Homeostasis, complications. See Potassium
Homocysteine, 579
HOPE trial, 156

Hormone
  replacement. See Post-craniotomy central
    diabetes insipidus
  therapy, impact. See Osteoporosis
Hospital-acquired BSI, occurrence, 307
Hospital-acquired diarrhea (HAD), 70, 485,
    486
Hospital-acquired fever
  causes, 344t
  diagnosis, approach, 344f
  management, approach, 346f
Hospital-acquired VTE, 941
  methods, 943t
Hospital-based physicians, exclusive contracts,
    995
Hospital Consumer Assessment of Healthcare
    Providers and Systems (HCAHPS) survey,
    8, 972–973
Hospital discharge, 77
  challenges, 77–78
  guidelines, limitation, 78
  medication/reconciliation/education, 79–80
  reading, 81–82
  solutions, 78–81
Hospital-driven physician documentation,
    905–906
Hospital Elder Life Program (HELP), 37
Hospital Flow Diagnostic, usage, 963–964
Hospital Infection Control Practices Advisory
    Committee (HICPAC), 119
Hospitalist
  activities. See Hospital medicine program
  assistance. See Advance directives
  benefits, 877–878
  care responsibilities, 743b
  challenge. See Inpatient medicine
  compensation, percentage, 900f
  contract considerations, 882–883
  coverage. See Call-based schedules
  employment. See Sponsoring organization
  exclusive contracts, 995
  financial performance, survey medians,
    900t
  focus. See Inpatient management
  group
    contracting. See Local hospitalist group;
      Regional hospitalist group
    formation, facilitation, 881
  impact. See Teamwork
  income average, 900f
  interaction. See Patient safety
  leaders, development, 961–962
  management company, contracting. See
    National hospitalist management
    company
  medical director, agreement, 882
  medical malpractice, 990–991
  model, impact. See Relational coordination;
    Teamwork
  organization, cohesiveness, 957
  patient communication, components, 894b
  performance expectations, 882
  presence, consistency, 957
  program, development, 961
  recruiting strategies, residency programs
    (involvement), 885b
  recruitment, 885
  remuneration, 882–883
  services. See Hospital medicine program
    contracting, 881–882
  staffing (approaches), volume fluctuation
    (impact), 890t
  teamwork
    sense, 958
    toolkit, 958b
  value, addition, 874b
    process. See Billing

Hospitalist, consultant role
  background, 741
  discussion, 742–743
  reading, 743
Hospitalist-hospitalist communication, 896
Hospitalist-hospital relationships, legal issues
  introduction, 993
  reading, 997
Hospitalist systems
  background, 893
  consulting physicians, communication, 894
  health care staff, communication, 894, 896
  nurses, communication, 894, 896
  patients, communication, 894
  physicians, communication, 893
  referring, communication, 893
  significant others, communication, 894
Hospitalization, function change (daily query),
    41b
Hospitalized diabetic patient, cutaneous
    candidiasis, 627f
Hospitalized medical patients, VTE
    prophylaxis, 99
  assessment, 99–100
  clinical risk factors, 99–100
  discharge/follow-up plans, 103
  implementation team, leading, 102–103
  monitoring/therapy, 102
  nonpharmacologic options, 101–102
  options, 100
  outpatient physician communication, 103
  patient education, 103
  pharmacologic prophylaxis,
      contraindications, 101–102
  reading, 103
  special situations/dosing adjustments, 102
  studies, 101
Hospitalized patients
  chest pain, presence (considerations), 133
  dialysis modality choices, comparison, 400t
  diarrhea, occurrence, 478
  geriatric syndromes, 30t
  laboratory/radiologic information,
      availability, 343
  short-term indwelling urinary catheter use,
      indications, 289t
  smoking cessation, 93
Hospitalized patients, acute arthritis
  assessment, 603–605
  background, 603
  clinical presentation, 603
  diagnostic studies, preference, 604–605
  differential diagnosis, 603–604
  discharge/follow-up, 606
  management, 605–606
  outpatient communication, 606
  prevention, 606
  reading, 607
  treatment, 605–606
    alternatives, 606
Hospitalized patients, adrenal insufficiency
  assessment, 517–519
  background, 517
  clinical presentation, 517–518
  diagnosis, 517–519
  discharge/follow-up plans, 521
  laboratory testing, 518–519
  management, 519–521
  pathophysiology, 517
  perioperative/pre-procedure treatment, 520
  reading, 521
Hospitalized patients, candidiasis
  assessment, 626–627
  background, 626
  diagnosis/prognosis, 627
  differential diagnosis, 627
  discharge/follow-up plans, 627

Hospitalized patients, candidiasis (Continued)
  management/treatment, 627
  prevention, 627
Hospitalized patients, dermatology
  introduction, 621
  reading, 638
Hospitalized patients, fever (presence)
  assessment, 343–345
  background, 343
  clinical presentation, 343
  diagnosis, clarity (absence), 345
  differential diagnosis, 343–345
  directed studies, 344–345
  empiric antibiotic selection, 346–347
  management, 345–347
  presenting signs/symptoms, 343
  prevalence, 343
  prevention, 347
  prognosis, 345
  reading, 347
  studies, 345
  treatment, 345–346
Hospitalized patients, pain management
  assessment, 725–727
  background, 725
  breakthrough pain, 729–730
  clinical presentation, 725
  diagnosis, 726–727
  differential diagnosis, 725
  discharge/follow-up plans, 730
  management, 727–730
  multimodal analgesia, usage, 730
  nonmedical treatment, 730
  NSAIDs, usage, 727
  opioids, impact, 729
  options, alternatives, 730
  outpatient physician communication, 730
  patient education, 730
  PCA, usage, 730
  presenting signs/symptoms, 725
  reading, 731
Hospitalized patients, substance
    abuse/dependence, 111
  assessment, 111–115
  clinical presentation, 111–112
  diagnosis, 112
  discharge planning, 116–117
  history, 112–113
  inpatient service, medical issues, 116
  laboratory tests, usage, 113
  non-laboratory-based screening, usage,
      113–114
  physical examination, usage, 113
  prognosis, clinical consequences, 115–117
  reading, 117
  treatment, 115–116
Hospital medicine
  background, 905
  billing, 905, 907–908
  coding, 905, 906–907
  compliance, 905, 909
  documentation, 905–906
  guidelines, example, 910b
  physician performance, management,
      919
  reading, 910, 925
Hospital medicine ethics
  background, 979
  dilemmas, solutions, 985–986
  issues, 979–985
  reading, 987
Hospital medicine leadership
  accountability, 929
  change, leading, 929
  communication, effectiveness, 929
  conflict resolution, 928
  introduction, 927

Hospital medicine leadership (Continued)
  management skills, 931–932
  negotiation, 928
  reading, 932
  self-evaluation, 928
  strategic planning, 930
  succession planning, 929–930
Hospital medicine program
  24/7 inhospital coverage, FTE requirement
      (example), 875
  capacity, increase, 912
  communication plan, 884–885
  costs
    anticipation, 876–878
    reduction, 911–912
  daytime only inhospital coverage, example,
      875–876
  employment model, assessment, 882t
  facilities/equipment/systems requirements,
      884b
  financial plan, development, 873, 878
  FTE requirements, projection, 875–876
  high level pro forma, 878t
  hospitalist services, 874
  hospital systems, impact, 884
  inpatient admissions, 873–874
  management functions, 884b
  nonbillable hospitalist activities, 874
  operating policies/procedures, 883–884
  operating standards/procedures, 883–884
  oversight, 883
  performance expectations, 883
  practice
    management, 884–885
    revenue, projection, 876
  productivity benchmarks, usage, 876
  program drivers, 873
  reading, 879, 886, 915
  recruiting strategies, residency programs
      (involvement), 885b
  referral assumptions, establishment,
      873–874
  revenue
    generation, 912–914
    model revenue projection, 877t
  scheduling, 887
    models, 887–891
  service
    requirements, 883
    scope, 873
  staff deployment, 887
  staffing strategies, 890b
  structuring, 881
  value measurement, 911
  workforce needs, establishment, 873
  workload, projection, 874–875
Hospital-physician relationships, paradigms
    (comparison), 1000t
Hospitals
  admission, baseline function (screens), 39b
  care delivery, outcomes chain, 942f
  discharge summary, elements, 894b
  employee models, contrast. See Independent
      contractors
  foreignness, 7
  goals, 964
  information systems
    scope/context, awareness, 972
  information systems, limitations, 972–973
  medicine leaders, attitudes/personal
      attributes, 927
  medicine practice, referral sources, 874b
  operating systems, 956
  quality (measure), vaccination
      (performance), 91
  revenue, increase (sources), 912b
  safety hazards. See Acute care hospitals

Hospitals (Continued)
  service line, creation, 913
  settings, baseline/functional assessment
    (importance), 37
  workplace elements, confidentiality breach,
    980f
  written surveys (usage), case example,
    973–975
Hospital settings, cultural competence
  background, 15
  clinical reference, 15
  communication/culture, 15
    reading, 19
Hospital throughput
  background, 961
  ideas, investigation, 965b
  measurement, 963–964
  pitfalls, 964
  reading, 965–966
  strategies, 961–963
HP. See Hypersensitivity pneumonitis
HPA. See Hypothalamic-pituitary-adrenal
HPS. See Hepatopulmonary syndrome
HRCT. See High-resolution CT
HRS. See Hepatorenal syndrome
HSRs. See Hypersensitivity reactions
HSV. See Herpes simplex virus
Human epidermal growth factor receptor 2
    proteins (HER2), 532
Human factors. See Systems
Human immunodeficiency virus (HIV), 113,
    323
  assessment, 331–334
  background, 331
  clinical presentation, 331
  diagnosis, 334–335
  diarrhea, occurrence, 478–479
  discharge/follow-up plans, 336
  drug interactions, 336
  effusions, impact, 371
  fever, unknown origin, 333, 334–335
    treatment, 336
  gastrointestinal symptoms, 332–333,
    334
    treatment, 335–336
  HIV-associated PAH, 383
  HIV-infected patients, opportunistic
    diarrheal pathogens (presence), 478b
  HIV-related dermatoses, 627–631
    background, 627
  immune status, importance, 331
  impact. See Pleural effusion; Pneumothorax
  infection, 636. See also Acute HIV infection;
    Chronic HIV infection
    conditions, 332t
    recognition, 331
  management, 335–336
  medication-related symptoms, 333–334
  neurologic symptoms, 332, 334
    treatment, 335
  occupational exposure, 336
  prognosis, 335
  reading, 336
  respiratory symptoms, 331–332, 334
    treatment, 335
  risk, 120
    association, CDR count stratification,
    332t
  treatment, 335–336
Human leukocyte antigen (HLA) classes,
    activation, 573
HUS. See Hemolytic uremic syndrome;
    Hemolytic-uremic syndrome
HUTT. See Head-up tilt-table
Hydralazine, usage, 266
Hydromorphone (Dilaudid), usage, 729
Hydroxyurea, usage. See Sickle cell crises

Hyperbaric oxygen, usage. See Carbon
    monoxide
Hypercalcemia
  emergencies. See Cancer emergencies
  treatment algorithm. See Malignancy
Hypercapneic respiratory failure, 649, 650
Hypercapnia, 362–363
Hypercoagulability, emergence, 765
Hyperglycemia. See Postoperative
    hyperglycemia
  background, 503, 819–820
  clinical assessment/evaluation, 820
  correction, impact, 503
  glucose management, 506
  impact. See Collagen; Coronary artery
    bypass grafting; Critical care setting;
    Wounds
  insulin algorithms, usage, 506
  management, 503, 505–507, 820
  pathophysiology. See Stress hyperglycemia
  reading, 508
  risk factors, 819t
  severity, 499
Hyperhomocystinemia, 261
Hyperkalemia, 137. See also Medication-
    induced hyperkalemia; Symptomatic
    hyperkalemia
  adverse electrical cardiac effects, 422
  assessment, 403, 419–421
  causes, 421t
  clinical approach, 421
  clinical presentation, 403, 419
  diagnosis/differential diagnosis, 403,
    419–421
  discharge/follow-up plans, 403–404
  disorders, 422–423
  management, 403, 421–423
  occurrence, 419–420
  sign. See Tumor lysis syndrome
  studies, preference, 421
  treatment, 421–423
Hyperlipidemia, 395
Hypermetabolism, impact, 795
Hypernatremia, 407
  assessment, 414
  background, 414
  calculation, sample, 525t
  causes, 413t
  correction, 525
  diagnosis/differential diagnosis, 414–416
  discharge/follow-up plans, 416
  management, 416
  occurrence, 415
  prevention, 416
  studies, preference, 416
  treatment, 416
Hyperproliferative anemias, 577
Hypersensitive carotid sinus syndrome, 167
Hypersensitivity pneumonitis (HP), 379–380,
    534
Hypersensitivity reactions (HSRs), 616. See
    also Cancer management; Cancer
    treatment
  grading, 530t
  production, 529
  protocol, 531t
Hypertension. See Chronic hypertension;
    Gestational hypertension
  control, absence, 265
  Cushing's triad, 299
  impact, 778, 824
  occurrence, 806
  response, absence, 684
Hypertensive crises
  assessment, 263–265
  background, 263
  clinical presentation, 263

Hypertensive crises (Continued)
  diagnosis, 265
  discharge/follow-up plans, 267
  examples, 264b
  history, 263–264
  laboratory studies, 264–265
  laboratory tests, 264b
  management, 265
  pathophysiology, 263
  physical examination, 264
    focus, 264b
  prognosis, 265
  reading, 268
  targeted historical questions, 264b
Hypertensive emergencies, 265–267
  antihypertensive drugs, usage, 266t
  treatment, 266–267
Hypertensive emergency, drugs (usage), 232t
Hypertensive urgencies, 265, 267
Hyperthyroid clinical/laboratory findings,
    511t
Hyperthyroidism
  beta-blockers, usage, 514
  clinical manifestations, 511
  management, 513–514
  relationship. See Pregnancy
Hyperuricemia, metabolic abnormality, 559
Hyperviscosity syndromes. See Cancer
    emergencies
  pathophysiology, 554f
Hypervolemic hyponatremia, 409, 413–414
Hypervolemic hypo-osmolar hyponatremia,
    409
Hypochromic microcytic anemia, 579, 580
Hypoglycemia. See Severe hypoglycemia
  risk, increase, 792
Hypokalemia
  assessment, 423–424
  background, 423
  causes, 423t
  clinical approach, 424
  correction, potassium chloride (usage), 425
  diagnosis/differential diagnosis, 423–424
  electrocardiographic changes, 423
  insulin/dextrose, administration
    (avoidance), 425
  management, 424–425
  mineralocorticoid excess state, suspicion,
    424
  stepwise approach, 424t
  studies, preference, 424
  symptoms, 423
  treatment, 424–425
Hypomagnesemia. See Chronic
    hypomagnesemia; Iatrogenic
    hypomagnesemia
  assessment, 425–426
  background, 425
  cardiac disease, impact/risk, 427
  causes, 426b
  clinical approach, 426
  clinical presentation, 425–426
  diagnosis/differential diagnosis, 426
  management, 426–427
  oral treatment, 427
  studies, preference, 426
  treatment, 426–427
Hyponatremia. See Chronic hyponatremia;
    Euvolemic hyponatremia; Hypervolemic
    hyponatremia; Hypovolemic
    hyponatremia; Pseudohyponatremia
  assessment, 407–409
  background, 407
  classification, tests (usage/limitations), 411t
  clinical presentation, 407
  considerations, 410, 414
  correction, 412

Hyponatremia *(Continued)*
  diagnosis, 408–409
    stepwise approach, 408t
    tests, usage/limitations, 411t
  differential diagnosis, 408–409
  discharge/follow-up plans, 414
  disorders, clinical management, 407
  electrolyte abnormality, 818
  management, 411–414
    stepwise approach, 411t
  physical examination, 407
  prevention, 414
  prognosis, 411
  reading, 417
  studies, preference, 410–411
  treatment, 411–414
  types, 409–410
Hypoproliferative anemias, 577
  classification, 579
Hypotension
  occurrence, 806
  response, 519
Hypothalamic-pituitary-adrenal (HPA) axis, 517
  regulation, schematic outline, 518f
Hypothalamic-pituitary-thyroid axis, 510f
Hypothermia, 137. *See also* Anoxic-ischemic coma
Hypothyroid clinical/laboratory findings, 511t
Hypothyroidism
  clinical manifestations, 510–511
  management, 512–513
  overtreatment, impact, 512
  relationship. *See* Pregnancy
Hypoventilation, usage, 827
Hypovolemia, 61
  background, 818
  risk factors/pathophysiology, 818
Hypovolemic hyponatremia, 409, 412–413
Hypoxemia. *See* Postoperative hypoxemia
  physiologic causes, 650
Hypoxemic respiratory failure, 649
  studies, 666
Hypoxia, complication, 749

IABP. *See* Intra-aortic balloon counterpulsation pump
IADL. *See* Instrumental ADL
Iatrogenic hypomagnesemia, 426
Iatrogenic illness. *See* Geriatric patients
Iatrogenic injury, risk factor, 229
IBD. *See* Inflammatory bowel disease
ICA. *See* Internal carotid artery
ICD-9-CM. *See* International Classification of Diseases, 9th Revision, Clinical Modification
ICD-10-CM. *See* International Classification of Diseases, 10th Revision, Clinical Modification
ICH. *See* Intracerebral hemorrhage
ICP. *See* Intracranial pressure
Idiopathic pulmonary arterial hypertension (IPAH), 383
  counterparts, 385
Idiopathic pulmonary fibrosis (IPF), 377–378
IDSA, monotherapy guidelines, 546
IE. *See* Infective endocarditis
Ifosfamide (Ifex), 538
  clinical presentation, 538
  treatment/prognosis, 538
  usage. *See* Anticancer agents; Nephrotoxicity
IHI. *See* Institute for Healthcare Improvement
IIF. *See* Indirect immunofluorescence

ILCOR. *See* International Liaison Committee on Resuscitation
ILD. *See* Interstitial lung disease
Illicit drug history, preoperative health assessment, 755–756
Illness-associated VTE, 771
Illnesses, prognostication (ability), 733
Immobility. *See* Geriatric patients
Immune-complex GN, 395
Immune reconstitution inflammatory syndrome (IRIS), 334
Immune reconstitution syndrome, 333–334
Immune response, suppression, 565–566
Immune status, importance. *See* Human immunodeficiency virus
Immunocompetent patients, CAP presence (initial empiric antimicrobial therapy), 275t
Immunocompromised patients, 628
Immunosuppressive medications, recommendations/management, 762
Immunosuppressive therapies, 611. *See also* Combination immunosuppressive therapy
Importance, questions, 3
Imprisonment. *See* False imprisonment
IMV. *See* Intermittent mandatory ventilation
Incident reporting, 948–949
Incremental improvements, impact. *See* Value
Independent contractors, hospital employee models (contrast), 1000t
Indirect Compensation Arrangement Exception, 994
Indirect immunofluorescence (IIF), 610
  ELISA, combination usage, 610
Infection, status, 757
Infection-related fever, occurrence, 817
Infective endocarditis (IE). *See* Subacute IE
  algorithm, 312
  antimicrobial prophylaxis, 315t
  assessment, 307–313
  background, 307
  diagnosis, modified Duke criteria, 310t
  diagnostic cause, clinical clues, 309t
  diagnostic testing. *See* Culture-negative IE
  discharge/follow-up plans, 314–315
  host factors, 308f
  incidence, increase, 308t
  infection, endocardial source (evidence), 311–312
  likelihood, 308f
  management, 313–314
  pathologic/microbiologic/endocardial findings, 310
  physical findings/diagnostic manifestations, 309
  positive echocardiograph, suggestion, 311–312
  reading, 315
  suspicion, initial treatment, 314t
  systemic infection, approach, 312f
Inferior vena cava (IVC)
  dilation, 251
  filter placement, 224
Inflammatory bowel disease (IBD), 325
  assessment, 471–473
  background, 471
  clinical presentation, 471
  diagnosis, 471–473
  discharge/follow-up plans, 475–476
  extraintestinal features, 473t
  flexible sigmoidoscopy, usefulness, 472–473
  laboratory tests, 471–473
  management, 473–476
  presenting signs/symptoms, 471
  prevalence, 471
  reading, 476

Inflammatory bowel disease (IBD) *(Continued)*
  treatment, 473–475
    oral 5-ASA preparations, usage, 474t
Inflammatory pain, 726f
Influenza
  annual vaccination, recommendations, 87b
  characteristics, 339t
  review, 86–87
Informant, role. *See* Elderly hospitalized patient
Information
  convenience/discrimination/integration, 5
  evidence-based practitioner, questions, 3, 6
  manipulation, ability, 984
  systems, integration, 5–6
  transfer/continuity, improvement. *See* Physicians
  understanding, ability, 984
Information technology (IT), 911
  importance, 968–969
Informed consent
  elements, 980
  ethical issue, 979–980
Informed decisions, information/actions (necessity), 3
Ingested toxins/drugs, removal (consideration), 715
Inhalational anthrax
  characteristics, 339t
  staging, proposal, 342t
Inherited hemorrhagic disorders, 591–594
Inherited platelet function defects, 594
  diagnosis/prognosis, 594
  management, 594
  presentation, 594
Inherited proteins C/S
  diagnosis, 596
  management, 596
  presentation, 596
In-hospital continuity of care, quantification, 888–890
Inhospital coverage, FTE requirement. *See* Hospital medicine program
Inhospital mortality, RRR percentage, 504
In-hospital mortality, STEMI patients (relationships), 140f
In-kind payments, usage, 883
Inpatient admissions. *See* Hospital medicine program
Inpatient flow, improvement, 912–913
Inpatient management, hospitalist focus, 957
Inpatient medicine
  hospitalist, challenge, 956–957
  reading, 959
  research results, 956
  teamwork model of care, establishment, 955
Inpatient-outpatient physician
  discharge, information transfer improvement (recommendations), 79b
  discontinuity, 77
Inpatient safety hazards, 949t
Inpatient service, medical issues (addressing), 116
Inpatient setting, thyroid function testing (conditions), 512b
INR. *See* International normalized ratio
Inspiratory positive airway pressure (IPAP), 664
Institute for Healthcare Improvement (IHI)
  development. *See* Sepsis
  recommendations, 643
Institutional information services, time-space borders, 5
Instrumental ADL (IADL), 29
  Lawton/Brody scale, 37
  list, 38b

Insulin. See Supplemental sliding scale insulin
    algorithms, usage. See Hyperglycemia
    delivery, methods, 793
    impact. See Glycemia
    infusion algorithms, 506
    protocol. See Yale Insulin Protocol
    therapy. See Diabetic ketoacidosis;
        Sepsis/shock
    treatment. See Type 1 diabetes; Type 2
        diabetes
Intensive care unit (ICU)
    admission, indications. See Asthma
    medical illness, hospitalization, 504
    pain assessment, 655
    prolongation, 344
    psychosis, concept, 867
    transfer, 530
        result, 79
Intentional anthrax, 339
Interdependent relationships, examples,
    1001b
Interferon (Intron), usage. See Anticancer
    agents
Interleukin-2 (Aldesleukin), usage. See
    Anticancer agents
Intermediate-risk procedures, 775
Intermittent claudication
    differential diagnosis, 257t
    presence. See Calf pain
Intermittent mandatory ventilation (IMV),
    664
Intermittent pneumatic compression (IPC)
    devices, usage, 100
Internal carotid artery (ICA) stenosis, degree,
    699
Internal organizational trends, 935
International Classification of Diseases, 9th
    Revision, Clinical Modification (ICD-9-
    CM), 906
International Classification of Diseases, 10th
    Revision, Clinical Modification (ICD-10-
    CM), 906
International Consensus Conference on
    Cardiopulmonary Resuscitation, 189
International Liaison Committee on
    Resuscitation (ILCOR), 189
International normalized ratio (INR)
    correction, 708
    decline, 679
    elevation, 459, 595
    testing, 702
International Registry of Acute Aortic
    Dissection (IRAD), Marfan syndrome
    (incidence), 228
Interpreters
    selection, guidelines, 16b
    services, language/appropriate use, 15–17
        discussion, 16–17
    usage. See Encounter
Interstitial lung disease (ILD). See Lung-specific
    ILD
    assessment, 375–379
    background, 375
    bronchoscopy, usage, 378
    clinical prevention, 375
    CXR, 377
    data accumulation, 378
    diagnosis, 375
        interim summary, 378
    differential diagnosis, 375
        acute/worrisome diagnoses, 376b
    discharge/follow-up plans, 380
    environmental exposure, 379–380
    etiologies, 376b
    flowchart, 379f
    history, 376–377
    HRCT, usage, 377–378

Interstitial lung disease (ILD) (Continued)
    laboratory data, 377
    management, 379–380
    outpatient physician communication, 380
    patient education, 380
    physical examination, 377
    presenting signs/symptoms, 375
    prevalence, 375
    prevention, 380
    prognosis, 378–379
    pulmonary function testing, 377
    reading, 380–381
    sarcoidosis, impact, 380
    sign/symptom acuity, 376–378
    surgical lung biopsy, 378
    therapies, alternatives, 380
    tobacco smoke, relationship, 379
    treatment, 379–380
Intestinal viral infections, 636
Intimal injury, occurrence, 765
Intra-aortic balloon counterpulsation pump
    (IABP), 165
Intra-articular antibiotics, indication
    (absence), 605–606
Intracerebral hemorrhage (ICH)
    airway management, 707
    anticoagulated patients, 708–709
        management, 708t
    antihypertensive medications. See Acute
        ICH
    assessment, 705–707
    background, 705
    bleed, location, 706
    blood pressure, relationship, 707–708
    clinical presentation, 705
    diagnosis, 706–707
    differential diagnosis, 705–706
    discharge/follow-up plans, 709–710
    DVT, usage, 709
    electrolytes, usage, 707
    etiologies, 706t
    fluid management, goal, 707
    glucose, usage, 707
    hemostatic therapy, 709
    impact, 267
    intravenous fluids, usage, 707
    management/treatment, 707–709
    MRI, usage, 706
    oxygenation, 707
    patient education, 710
    population-based studies, CT verification,
        705
    presenting signs/symptoms, 705
    prevalence, 705
    prognosis, 707
    pulmonary embolism prophylaxis, usage,
        709
    reading, 710
    recombinant activated factor VII, impact,
        709
    score, 707t
    seizures, relationship, 708
    surgical intervention, 709
    volume, 707
Intracranial pressure (ICP)
    elevation. See Cancer emergencies
        treatment, 709
    increase, 555
        intermittent hyperventilation, 715
Intramural hematoma (IMH), distinctions. See
    Aortic IMH
Intramuscular (IM) midazolam/lorazepam,
    864
Intrarenal (glomerular) impact. See Acute
    renal failure
Intrarenal (interstitial) impact. See Acute renal
    failure

Intrarenal (tubular) impact. See Acute renal
    failure
Intrarenal (vascular) impact. See Acute renal
    failure
Intravascular catheter infections
    complication, metastatic infection (impact),
        320
    risk factors, 318t
Intravascular fluid balance, complication,
    748–749
Intravascular ultrasound (IVUS), usage, 222
Intravascular volume status, assessment,
    435–436
Intravenous drug abuse (IVDA), 323
    association. See Gram-negative organisms
Intravenous fluids, usage. See Intracerebral
    hemorrhage
Intravenous trace elements/vitamins, therapy,
    25–26
Intrinsic PEEP, 671–672
Intrinsic renal failure, 829
Intron, usage. See Anticancer agents
Invasive bacteria, presence, 478
Iodinated radiocontrast agent, usage,
    514–515
Iodine solution, usage, 515
Ionizing radiation, diagnostic studies/content,
    842t
IPAH. See Idiopathic pulmonary arterial
    hypertension
IPAP. See Inspiratory positive airway pressure
IPC. See Intermittent pneumatic compression
IPF. See Idiopathic pulmonary fibrosis
IRAC. See International Registry of Acute
    Aortic Dissection
IRIS. See Immune reconstitution inflammatory
    syndrome
Iron supplementation, administration, 831
Irregular respiratory pattern, Cushing's triad,
    299
Ischemia. See Cerebral ischemia
    atypical symptoms, 776–777
    background, 821
    clinical assessment/evaluation, 822
    exercise testing, usage, 200
    factors. See Postoperative MI
    impact, 344
    recommendations/management, 822–823
    risk factors/pathophysiology, 821
Ischemia-related symptoms, directed clinical
    history, 822
Ischemic ATN, 829
Ischemic cardiomyopathy, 778
Ischemic heart failure, 824
Ischemic stroke
    antiplatelet/anticoagulation therapy, 701
    assessment, 697–700
    background, 697
    blood pressure, relationship, 701
    coagulation disorders, impact, 700
    CXR, usage, 697
    differential diagnosis, 698
    discharge/follow-up plans, 702
    ECG, usage, 697
    extracranial vessel sources, 699
    fever, impact, 701
    impact, 267
    large vessel intracranial sources, 699–700
    management, 700–702
    nutrition/mobilization, impact, 703
    outpatient physician communication,
        702
    oxygenation, monitoring, 701
    patient education, 703
    perfusion, monitoring, 701
    prevention, 702
    prognosis, 700

Ischemic stroke (Continued)
    reading, 703
    treatment, 700–702
Isotonic crystalloid, 830
IT. See Information technology
Iterative system. See Quality improvement
IVC. See Inferior vena cava
IVDA. See Intravenous drug abuse
IVUS. See Intravascular ultrasound

Jaundice, increase, 584
Jejunostomy tube (J-tube), usage, 26
Johns Hopkins Surgical Bleeding Classification, 772t
Joint Commission Core Measures, 935
Joint Commission on Accreditation of
        Healthcare Organizations (JCAHO), 725, 967
    hospital infection committees,
            establishment, 119
    Leadership Standards for Managing Patient
            Flow, 962b
    National Patient Safety Goal, 78, 81
    patient safety improvements, impact, 951
    quality measure, 276
    reviews, 958
Joint Commission Quality-of-Care Indicators.
        See Heart failure
Joints
    drainage, 328
    infection, 323. See also Prosthetic joints
    pain, 585
    radiographs, 326
Jugular venous distension (JVD), 162
Jugular venous pressure (JVP), 778
    elevation, 136
Justice, importance, 979

Kaposi's sarcoma (KS), 371
    AIDS-defining skin malignancy, 630
    AIDS patient, illustration, 630f
Katz index. See Activities of daily living
Kawasaki disease, 632
Kernig's sign, 299
Ketoacids, accumulation, 498
Ketone body production, increase. See Diabetic
        ketoacidosis
Ketones, nitroprusside test, 432
Ketosis, disorders, 430, 431t, 432
Kidney disease, 410
Kindling, 688
Kleinman's questions, usage, 16b
Koplik's spots. See Rubeola
KS. See Kaposi's sarcoma
Kussmaul's respiration, 429
Kyphoplasty, 108

Labetalol, usage, 266
Laboratory Response Network for Bioterrorism
        (LRN), 341
Laboratory testing, timing, 760
Laboratory tests. See Acute pericarditis
Laboratory TLS (LTLS), 560
Lactate dehydrogenase (LDH), 605, 863
Lactated Ringer's, 830
Lactate level, studies, 683
Lactic acid accumulation, disorders, 431t
Lactic acidosis, occurrence, 432–433
Lacunar stroke. See Small vessel disease
LAM. See Lymphangioleimyomatosis
Lambert-Eaton myasthenia syndrome (LEMS),
        563
Language
    importance, 16–17
    usage. See Interpreters
Lanoteplase (nTPA), 144
Large vessel arteritis, risk factor, 228

Large vessel intracranial sources. See Ischemic
        stroke
L-Asparaginase, usage. See Cancer
        management
Latex agglutination, usage, 488
Lawton/Brody scale. See Instrumental ADL
LBBB. See Left bundle branch block
LBM. See Lean body mass
LCV. See Leukocytoclastic vasculitis
LDH. See Lactate dehydrogenase
LDUH. See Low-dose unfractionated heparin
Leaders
    attitudes/personal attributes. See Hospitals
    development. See Hospitalist
Leadership. See Hospital medicine leadership;
        Quality improvement
    roles/responsibilities/work, 927–932
Lean body mass (LBM), estimation, 24
Leapfrog Group, 967
Lee Revised Cardiac Risk Index (RCRI), 779
    list, 779t
Left BBB morphologic criteria, 184f
Left bundle branch block (LBBB), 136
    explanation, absence, 778
Left ventricular assist device (LVAD), 165
Left ventricular eject function (LVEF), 778
Left ventricular hypertrophy (LVH), 137, 777
Left ventricular (LV) aneurysm, 137
Left ventricular (LV) dysfunction, 401
Left ventricular volume overload, 823
Legionnaire's disease
    community-acquired cases, 273
    suspicion, 121
LEMS. See Lambert-Eaton myasthenia
        syndrome
LEP. See Limited English proficiency
Lepirudin, infusion rate, 598–599
Leukocytoclastic vasculitis (LCV), 636
    illustration, 637f
    subtypes, 636
Leukocytosis, presence. See Diabetic
        ketoacidosis
Leukotriene antagonists, impact. See Asthma
Libman-Sacks endocarditis, 236
Lidocaine, dosage, 194
Life-threatening drug reaction, features, 622b
Light's criteria, development, 370
Likelihood of Recommending, percentile
        ranking, 974f
Limb ischemia
    etiologies, 258t
Limited English proficiency (LEP), 16–17
Lipid lowering, 702
Liquid medications, sorbitol (presence), 72t
Litigation stress, alleviation measures, 990b
Liver disease
    signs, 453t
    symptoms, 453b
Liver enzyme testing, 760
Liver failure, hemostatic abnormalities
        (association)
    diagnosis, 596
    management, 596
    presentation, 595–596
Liver/kidney/microsome (LKM) type 1
        antibodies, 447
Liver transplantation, 458
    King's College Hospital Criteria. See Acute
            liver failure
LKM. See Liver/kidney/microsome
LMWH. See Low-molecular-weight heparin
Local anesthesia, consideration, 786
Local hospitalist group, contracting, 881–882
Local medical group, contracting, 881
Locked-in syndrome, 711
Lomustine (CeeNu), 534
Long-standing chronic limb ischemia, 257f

Long-term cessation, predictors. See Smoking
        cessation
Long-term CVC, 541
    placement, 543
Long-term indwelling urinary catheters,
        biofilms (usage), 287
Long-term warfarin management. See Surgery
    background, 771
    bleeding risk, 772
    preoperative evaluation, 772
    preoperative history, 771–772
    reading, 774
    risk stratification, 772
    surgery, type, 771–772
    thromboembolic risk, 772
Loop diuretics, usage, 401
Loperamide, CNS action (absence), 74
Lorazepam, administration, 716
Low-dose unfractionated heparin (LDUH),
        usage, 100
Low-molecular-weight heparin (LMWH), 100,
        154–155
    benefit, absence, 701
    discontinuation, 843
    impact, 141
    LDUH, contrast, 101
    placebo, contrast, 101
    preferred option. See Pulmonary embolism
    receiving, 258
    treatment, initiation, 543
    usage, 771. See also Bridging therapy
Low-risk procedures, 775
Low urine osmolality, 409
LRN. See Laboratory Response Network for
        Bioterrorism
LTLS. See Laboratory TLS
Lung-specific ILD, 377
Lupus anticoagulant, 597
LV. See Left ventricular
LVAD. See Left ventricular assist device
LVEF. See Left ventricular eject function
LVH. See Left ventricular hypertrophy
Lyme disease, 300
Lymphangioleimyomatosis (LAM), 377

MAAS. See Motor Activity Assessment Scale
MAC. See Mycobacterium avium complex
Macrocytic anemia, 579, 580
Macronutrients, display, 25t
Maculopapular rash, 615
Magnesium
    balance, disorders, 425
    dosage, 194
    repletion, side effects, 427
Magnesium sulfate, usage. See Asthma
Magnetic resonance angiography (MRA)
    assessment, support (increase), 258
    usage, 699. See also Acute aortic dissection
Magnetic resonance imaging (MRI)
    neuroimaging studies, 564
    sensitivity/specificity, 209
    usage, 542, 586. See also Pulmonary
            embolism
MAHA. See Microangiopathic hemolytic
        anemia
Major alcohol withdrawal, 688–689
Making Healthcare Safer (AHRQ report), 99
Malignancy
    hypercalcemia, treatment algorithm, 550f
    treatment, 565
Malignant hypertension, 394
Malignant infiltration, 445
    impact. See Acute hepatitis
Mallory-Weiss tears, 62–63
Malnutrition. See Geriatric patients; Protein-
        energy malnutrition
    clinical presentation, 21–26

Malnutrition (Continued)
differential diagnosis, usage, 21–22
incidence, 795
physical findings, 797b
presenting signs/symptoms, 21
prevalence, 21
prognosis, 23
risk (evaluation), questions (usage),
796b
treatment, 23–26
Malpractice. See Medical malpractice
causes of action, 990b
defense theories, 990b
litigation, 991
prophylaxis/prevention, 991
Management
costs. See Practice
skills. See Hospital medicine leadership
Mania
background, 861
clinical assessment/evaluation, 862
treatment, 862
MAOIs. See Monoamine oxidase inhibitors
Marfan syndrome, 228
incidence. See International Registry of
Acute Aortic Dissection
Massive PE, 222
treatment considerations, 224
MaVS study, 780
MCV. See Mean corpuscular volume
MDCT. See Multi-detector computed
tomography
MDI. See Metered-dose inhaler
MDM. See Medical Decision Making
MDMA (Ecstasy), 684
MDR. See Multidrug-resistant
MEAC. See Minimum effective analgesic
concentration
Mean corpuscular volume (MCV), 569
calculation, 577
Mean PAP (mPAP), 386
Mean score by specialty. See Overall mean
score by specialty
Measles mumps and rubella (MMR), review,
87
Measurement culture, development, 963
Measurement system. See Quality
improvement
Mechanical prostheses, usage, 243
Mechanical ventilation. See Controlled
mechanical ventilation
assessments, 674t
background, 669
discontinuation, 672–673
indications, 669
initial ventilator settings, recommendations,
670t
initiation, 669
mode, 669–672
monitoring/complications, 672
reading, 675–676
MedEdCME web site, 97
MEDENOX study, impact, 101
Medical Decision Making (MDM), 907
Medical devices, product/strict liability, 991
Medical futility, 985
Medical history, preoperative health
assessment, 755
Medical indications, usage, 986
Medical-legal liability, decrease, 914
Medically ill hospitalized elderly patients,
clinical depression (occurrence), 32
Medical malpractice. See Hospitalist
background, 989
claim, defenses, 990
crises, 989
etiology/causes, 990
stress syndrome, 989

Medical negligence, 990
Medical patients
heparin prophylaxis, summary, 101
VTE risk factors, 100t
Medical patients, psychiatric disorders
(evaluation/management)
background, 851
clinical assessment/evaluation, 851
diagnosis, making, 851
nonpharmacologic treatment, 853, 855
organic etiology, evaluation, 851
pharmacologic treatment, 853
reading, 862
treatment, 853, 855
Medical problems, status, 756–757
Medical professionalism
appearance, importance, 9, 11
charter, 9t
Medical support, providing, 80
Medicare Gainsharing Prohibition, 996
Medication-induced hyperkalemia, 423
Medications
antiplatelet activity, clinical
assessment/evaluation, 762
history (obtaining), optimal strategies
(usage), 80b
intolerances, preoperative health
assessment, 755
preoperative health assessment, 755
reconciliation. See Hospital discharge
evidence, 79–80
process, 79
regimen, changes, 77–78
risk/alternatives, 33t
Medicine leaders, attitudes/personal attributes.
See Hospitals
MELD score, 596
Membranoproliferative GN, 395
Meningitis
antimicrobial therapy, 716
indication, 584
Meningococcal vaccine, review, 90
Mental state examination, 41
Mental status
change, notation, 31
variation. See Diabetic ketoacidosis
Mental status, alteration
assessment, 719–720
background, 719
clinical presentation, 719–720
diagnosis, 720–721
differential diagnosis, 720
discharge/follow-up plans, 722
hospitalization, 721
management/treatment, 721–722
options, alternatives, 722
outpatient physician communication,
722
patient/family education, 722
post discharge, 721
prediction rules, 721
presenting signs/symptoms, 719–720
prevalence, 719–720
prevention, 722
prognosis, 721
reading, 723
risk factors/causes, 721
studies, preference, 720
Mentorship, 927–928
Mercy Medical Center, quality bonus (2006),
901b
Mesenteric ischemia
assessment, 468–469
clinical presentation, 468–469
diagnosis/prognosis, 469
management, 469
treatment, 469
Metabolic aberration, normalization, 715

Metabolic acidosis
anion gap elevation
disorders, 431t
inclusion, 429–433
treatment, 434
assessment, 429–434
background, 429
causes, anion gap (absence), 432t
clinical presentation, 429
differential diagnosis, 429–434
normal anion gap
inclusion, 433–434
treatment, 434–435
renal causes, 432t
studies, preference, 434
Metabolic alkalosis
assessment, 435–437
background, 435
clinical presentation, 435
diagnosis/differential diagnosis, 435–436
etiologic diagnosis, stepwise approach, 436t
generation, 435
iatrogenic cause, absence, 435
mineralocorticoid excess
possibility consideration, 436
state, suspicion, 436
patient, intravascular volume status
(assessment), 435–436
studies, preference, 436–437
treatment, 437
volume depletion, impact, 435
Metered-dose inhaler (MDI), administration,
362
Methamphetamine ingestion, risk factor, 228
Methicillin-resistant Staphylococcus, 645
Methicillin-resistant Staphylococcus aureus
(MRSA), 272, 276, 294. See also
Community-acquired MRSA;
Community-associated MRSA
possibility, consideration, 605–606
prevalence, 327
Methotrexate (Rheumatrex), 538
clinical presentation, 538
prognosis, 538
treatment, 538
usage. See Nephrotoxicity; Pulmonary
toxicity
Methylenetetrahydrofolate reductase
(MTHFR), 596
Methylmalonic acid (MMA), 579
Metrics
plotting. See Quality improvement
set, selection. See Quality improvement
MG. See Myasthenia gravis
MI. See Myocardial infarction
MIC. See Minimal inhibitory concentration
Microangiopathic hemolytic anemia (MAHA),
541
Micronutrients
administration, guidelines. See Parenteral
nutrient solutions
needs, estimation, 23b
Microscopic colitis, 471
Microscopic polyangiitis (MPA), 377, 610
Microsporidia, empiric antibiotics (usage), 481
Mid-level provider activities, 885b
Milk alkali syndrome, 435, 549
Mineralocorticoid excess
possibility, consideration. See Metabolic
alkalosis
state, suspicion, 436. See also Hypokalemia;
Metabolic alkalosis
treatment, 437
Mini-Cog screen
accuracy, 41
usage, 31
Minimal inhibitory concentration (MIC),
adequacy, 304

Minimally conscious state, 716–717
Minimum effective analgesic concentration (MEAC), 730
Mini Nutritional Assessment (MNA), 797
Minor alcohol withdrawal, 687–688
  syndrome, hemodynamic symptoms, 688
Mission, usage, 919
Mitral regurgitation, 238–240
  CXR, usage, 239
  death, relative risk, 239f
  diagnostic evaluation, 239
  management, 239–240
  pathophysiology, 238f
  symptoms/signs, 238–239
Mitral stenosis, 236–238
  diagnostic evaluation, 237
  Doppler echocardiography, usage, 237
  interventions, 239
  management, 237–238
  pathophysiology, 237f
  surgical commissurotomy, 239
  symptoms/signs, 237
Mitral valve prolapse, 240
  diagnosis, 240
  management, 240
MMA. See Methylmalonic acid
MMR. See Measles mumps and rubella
MMSE. See Folstein Mini-Mental State Examination
MNA. See Mini Nutritional Assessment
MNB. See Monomicrobial non-neutrocytic bacterascites
Mobility
  achievement, 32
  assessment. See Elderly hospitalized patient
  improvement, 45
Model of End Stage Liver Disease (MELD), 458
  score, usage. See United Network of Organ Sharing
Modified Duke criteria. See Infective endocarditis
Monoamine oxidase inhibitors (MAOIs), 859, 863
Monoarticular arthritis, 605
Monoarticular flare, 604
Monoclonal antibodies, usage. See Cancer management
Monomicrobial non-neutrocytic bacterascites (MNB), 453
Mononucleosis (petechia), 632
Mood stabilizers, usage. See Psychiatric disorders
Morbidity, outcome, 935–936
Mortality
  indicators. See Provider-level mortality indicators
  outcome, 935–936
Motor Activity Assessment Scale (MAAS), 656–657
Motor disturbance, weakness, 557
MP. See 6-mercaptopurine
MPA. See Microscopic polyangitis
mPAP. See Mean PAP
MRSA. See Methicillin-resistant Staphylococcus aureus
MTHFR. See Methylenetetrahydrofolate reductase
Mucosal candidal infections, 625
Multi-detector computed tomography (MDCT), 134
Multidose charcoal, drug elimination enhancement, 677, 679
Multidrug-resistant (MDR) gram-negative organisms, 645
Multidrug-resistant (MDR) pathogens, risk, 281
Multifocal atrial tachycardia, 175

Multimodal analgesia, usage. See Hospitalized patients
Multiorgan system failure, 587
Musculoskeletal chest pain, 129
Musculoskeletal/extremities examination, 758
Mutations, 596–597
Myasthenia gravis (MG), 563
Mycobacterium avium complex (MAC), occurrence, 331
Myeloperoxidase (MPO), 133. See also Anti-MPO
Myleran, usage. See Pulmonary toxicity
Mylotarg, usage. See Cancer management
Myocardial infarction (MI), 127, 344, 776. See also Acute MI
  background, 821
  clinical assessment/evaluation, 822
  factors. See Postoperative MI
  GRACE National Registry, 135
  history, 153
  pathophysiology, 821
  recommendations/management, 822–823
  risk factors, 821. See also Postoperative MI
  trials, thrombolysis, 152
  ventricular tachyarrhythmias, 185–186
Myocardial injury markers. See Chest pain
Myocardial ischemia, 684
Myocardial ischemia (MI)
  complication, 748
Myocarditis, 137
Myxedema coma, 511
  management, 513
Myxomatous degeneration, impact. See Valvular heart disease

N-acetylcysteine (NAC), 679
Naloxone, usage. See Drug-induced coma; Opiate-induced coma
Narcosis, 649
Narcotic analgesics, risk/alternatives, 33t
Narrow QRS complex. See Tachyarrhythmias
Nasal pillows, usage, 664
National Comprehensive Cancer Network (NCCN), 545, 546
National Health and Nutrition Examination Survey Epidemiologic Follow-up Study, 705
National Hospice and Palliative Care Organization (NHPCO), 734
National Hospital Ambulatory Medical Care Survey, averaging data, 69
National Hospital Discharge Survey, averaging data, 69
National hospitalist management company, contracting, 882
National Institute of Alcohol Abuse and Alcoholism (NIAAA), alcohol use category, 111
National Institute of Health (NIH) Stroke Scale, usage, 697
National Osteoporosis Foundation (NOF), 105
National Practitioner Data Bank, events (disclosure), 924b
National Quality Forum (NQF), 967
  endorsement, 8
National Surgical Infection Prevention Project (NSIPP), 833
National survey organization, impact, 973–975
National Vaccine Advisory Committee (NVAC), adult immunization (status review), 85
Native joint disease, 323–325
Native joint septic arthritis
  diagnostic algorithm, 326f
  empiric treatment. See Adult native joint septic arthritis
  initial treatment, 327f
  signs/symptoms, prevalence, 324t

Nausea. See Postoperative nausea
  antiemetics, 65, 68
  assessment, 61–63
  background, 61
  causes, 62t
  clinical presentation, 61
  CNS, consideration, 62
  diagnosis, 63
  differential diagnosis, usage, 61–63
  evaluation, 64f
  GI obstruction, consideration, 62
  management, 63–68
  medical treatment, 66t–67t
  medications, impact, 63
  metastases, consideration, 62
  options, alternatives, 63
  prediction. See Chemotherapy-related nausea
  rule, 63
  preferred treatment, 64–68
  presenting signs/symptoms, 61
  prevalence, 61
  prevention, 68
  reading, 68
  symptom management, 61, 734–735
  treatment, 63–64, 64f, 807
    guidelines, 64t
NCCN. See National Comprehensive Cancer Network
Nebulizer-induced sputum, examination, 334
Neck wound hematoma, 813f
Necrolysis. See Toxic epidermal necrolysis
Necrotizing fasciitis, 814–815
  illustration, 814f
Necrotizing soft tissue infections, 293–294
  risk factors, 293b
Negligence. See Medical negligence
Negligent referrals, 991
Negotiations. See Hospital medicine leadership; Physician-hospital relationship
  dimensions. See Principled negotiations
Nephrotoxicity, 536–537
  Aldesleukin (IL-2) (Proleukin), usage, 537
  assessment, 537
  Cisplatin (Platinol), usage, 537
  diagnosis, 537
  Ifosfamide (Ifex), usage, 537
  management, 537
  Methotrexate, usage, 537
  risk, 400
Neuraxial anesthesia, effects/complications, 746t
Neuroleptics, usage, 832
Neurologic complications
  background, 831–832
  clinical assessment/evaluation, 832
  management, 832
  pathophysiology, 832
  postoperative, 806
Neurologic syncope, 204
Neuromuscular disorders, impact. See Respiratory acidosis
Neurontin, usage. See Gabapentin
Neuropathic pain, 726f
Neurosurgery, injury, 766t
Neutropenia, emergency. See Cancer emergencies
Neutropenic fever, initial treatment scheme, 546f
Newton-Wellesley Hospital, hospitalist program results, 956
New Zealand SAFE investigators, prospective trial, 644
NHPCO. See National Hospice and Palliative Care Organization
NIAAA. See National Institute of Alcohol Abuse and Alcoholism
Nicardipine, usage, 266

Nicotine dependence, Fagerstrom test, 94t
Nicotine replacement therapy (NRT), 96
Nights/weekends/off-hours, staffing
    techniques, 890
NIH. *See* National Institute of Health
Nil per os (NPO), 798
    status, prolongation, 864
NIPPV. *See* Noninvasive positive-pressure
    ventilation
Nitrogen balance, calculation, 23
Nitroglycerin, usage, 266
Nitroprusside, usage, 265–266
Nitroprusside test. *See* Ketones
Nitrosources, usage. *See* Pulmonary toxicity
NIV. *See* Noninvasive ventilation
NK-I-receptor antagonist, antiemetic effect,
    68
NNT. *See* Number needed to treat
Nociceptive pain, 726f
NOF. *See* National Osteoporosis Foundation
Nomogram, 715f
Nonallergic hypersensitivity reactions,
    occurrence, 617
Nonbillable hospitalist activities. *See* Hospital
    medicine program
Non-cardiac postoperative complications,
    827
    reading, 832
Noncardiac surgery, 781f
Non-CNS infections, 300
Nonconvulsive SE, AEDs (usage), 716
Nondiagnostic V/Q scan, 220
Nonfatal myocardial ischemia, 132t, 152t
Noninfectious causes, impact. *See* Acute
    diarrheal illnesses
Noninfectious phlebitis, 318
Noninvasive positive-pressure ventilation
    (NIPPV), 356
    availability. *See* Acute respiratory failure
    contraindications, 357b
Noninvasive ventilation (NIV)
    acute respiratory conditions,
        appropriateness, 665b
    administration, modes, 663–664
    application, interfaces, 664f
    background, 663
    contraindications, 665
    efficacy, evidence, 665–666
    evaluation, 664–665
    initiation, protocol, 667f
    interfaces, 664
    monitoring, 665b
    rationale, 663
    reading, 668
    response
        monitoring, 667–668
        prediction, 665b
    risks, 663
    therapy, initiation, 667–668
    usage, 283
    weaning, 666–667
Nonischemic cardiomyopathy, ventricular
    arrhythmias (association), 186
Non-laboratory-based screening, usage. *See*
    Hospitalized patients, substance
    abuse/dependence
Nonmaleficence, importance, 979
Nonoliguric renal failure, 391
Non-opioid medications, pharmacologic
    dosing, 728t
Nonpharmacologic therapies. *See* Substance-
    abusing/dependent patients
Nonresectable lung cancer, relationship. *See*
    Syndrome of inappropriate secretion of
    ADH
Non-ST-elevation myocardial infarction
    (NSTEMI), 806

Nonsteroidal anti-inflammatory drugs
    (NSAIDs), 159, 473
    effectiveness, 606
    impact, 391. *See also* Critically ill patients
    inhibition. *See* Platelet function
    side effects, 615
    usage, 251. *See also* Hospitalized patients
    withholding, 831
Non-ST-segment elevation myocardial
    infarction (NSTEMI), 127, 149
    antiplatelet/antithrombotic therapy,
        154–155
    assessment, 149–153
    clinical presentation, 149
    diagnostic criteria, 150
    differential diagnosis, 150
    discharge/follow-up plans, 156–157
    evidence/rationale, 151
    hospitalization, medications, 156
    initial treatment/dosing, recommendation,
        154t
    management, 153–156
    noninvasive testing, 156–157
    options, alternatives, 156
    outpatient physician communication, 157
    patient instruction, 156–157
    preferred diagnostic approach, 150–151
    presenting signs/symptoms, 149–150
    prevalence, 149–150
    prevention, 156
    prognosis, 151
    reading, 157
    risk stratification tools, 151
    treatment, 153–155
Nonsurgical patients, consultation, 743
Nonthrombotic pulmonary emboli, 224–225
Nontraumatic acute abdominal pain,
    approach, 463
Nontraumatic cardiac arrest, causes, 190t
Nontraumatic coma, 715–716
    analysis, 712
    prognosis, data, 714t
Nontraumatic non-drug-induced coma, study,
    712
Normal anion gap acidosis, 433
Normochromic normocytic anemia, 579, 580
Nosocomial infection
    airborne precaution, 120
    contact precaution, 119
    control, 119–120
    droplet precaution, 119–120
    hand hygiene, 120
    isolation guidelines, 119–120
    prevention, 119, 120–123
        reading, 123
    preventive strategies, 122t
    surgical site infection, 121–122
    surveillance, 119
Nosocomial pneumonia, 121
    assessment, 279–280
    background, 279
    bronchoscopic approaches, 279
    clinical approaches, microbiologic
        approaches (combination), 280
    clinical presentation, 279
    diagnosis, 279
    differential diagnosis, 279
    discharge/follow-up plans, 284
    initial treatment, 281
    management, 281–282
    nonbronchoscopic approaches, 280
    options, alternatives, 280
    oxygenation, failure, 282
    pathogens, association, 281t
    prevention, 282–284
        strategies, usage, 283t
    preventive strategies, 282–283

Nosocomial pneumonia (*Continued*)
    prognosis, 282
    reading, 284
    risk factors, 280t
    signs/symptoms, 279
    studies, preference, 279–280
    subsequent treatment, 281–282
    suspicion, management, 282f
    targeted preventive strategies, 283–284
Not-for-profit law, 996–997
Novo VII (recombinant factor VIIa), 592–593
NPO. *See* Nil per os
NQF. *See* National Quality Forum
NRT. *See* Nicotine replacement therapy
NSAIDs. *See* Nonsteroidal anti-inflammatory
    drugs
NSIPP. *See* National Surgical Infection
    Prevention Project
NSTEMI. *See* Non-ST-elevation myocardial
    infarction; Non-ST-segment elevation
    myocardial infarction
Nuclear medicine scans, usage. *See* Skin/soft
    tissue infections
Number needed to treat (NNT), 154, 211
Nurses, communication. *See* Hospitalist
    systems
Nutrient delivery, enteral/parenteral access
    (evaluation), 23b
Nutrition. *See* Malnutrition; Perioperative
    nutrition
    impact. *See* Ischemic stroke
    management. *See* Pressure ulcers; Skin
        integrity
    algorithm, 799f
    support, initiation/maintenance methods,
        800
Nutritional assessment, components. *See*
    Baseline nutritional assessment; Serial
    nutritional assessment
Nutritional assessment/support, 21
    assessment, 21–26
    background, 21
    reading, 26–27
Nutritional management. *See* Hepatic
    encephalopathy
Nutritional repletion, providing, 799
Nutritional risk, diagnosis, 22
Nutritional routes, clinical considerations, 32f
Nutritional status, estimation (efforts), 797
NVAC. *See* National Vaccine Advisory
    Committee
NYHA disease, 386
NYHA heart failure symptoms, 387

OA. *See* Osteoarthritis
Obstructive nephropathy, 392
Occupational Safety and Health
    Administration (OSHA), occupational
    blood exposure surveillance
    standardization, 120
OCPs. *See* Oral contraceptive pills
Office of the Inspector General (OIG), 996
Ofugi disease. *See* Eosinophilic folliculitis
OI. *See* Opportunistic infection
OIG. *See* Office of the Inspector General
Oligoarticular arthritis, 605
Oliguric renal failure, 391
One hundred percent production-based salary,
    compensation, 901
Online continuing education. *See* Smoking
    cessation
OPAT. *See* Outpatient Parenteral Antibiotic
    Therapy
Open wounds, 811
    packing, 812f
Operating standards/procedures. *See* Hospital
    medicine program

Operative risk, assessment, 741–742
Opiate-induced coma, naloxone (usage), 716
Opioids
    abuse/dependence screening tools,
        114–115
    abuse patients, pain management,
        115–116
    algorithms, 682
    assessment, 681–682
    background, 681
    clinical presentation, 681
    diagnosis/prognosis, 682
    differential diagnosis, 681–682
    discharge/follow-up plans, 682
    equianalgesic conversions, 729t
    impact. See Hospitalized patients
    intoxication, 111–112
        differential diagnosis, 113t
    management/treatment, 682
    pharmacologic properties, 658t
    toxicity, diagnosis, 682
    usage. See Critically ill patients
    withdrawal, 115
        clinical manifestations, 112t
        differential diagnosis, 113t
        pharmacotherapies, 116t
Opioid-toxic patients, admission indications,
    682
Opportunistic diarrheal pathogens. See Human
    immunodeficiency virus
Opportunistic infection (OI), 331
ORA. See Osteoporosis risk assessment
Oral 5-ASA preparations, usage. See
    Inflammatory bowel disease
Oral anticoagulation (OAC). See Chronic OAC
Oral contraceptive pills (OCPs), exposure,
    597
Oral cyclophosphamide, dosage, 611
Oral hypoglycemic agents, usage, 820
Oral medications, change, 809
Oral pain medications/dosing, 810t
Oral thiamine, usage, 690
Organic anxiety syndromes, 860
Organic etiology, evaluation. See Medical
    patients
Organizational structure, 881–883
Organizational trends. See Internal
    organizational trends
Organ system-based approach, 264
Orthodromic AVRT, 181f
Orthopedic patients, pharmacologic
    prophylaxis, 768
Orthopedic surgery, risk/prophylaxis, 768t
Orthostatic syncope, 202–203
OSHA. See Occupational Safety and Health
    Administration
Osler, William, 271
Osmolar gap, elevation (disorders), 431t
Osmotic laxatives, impact. See Constipation
Osteoarthritis (OA), 326
Osteoclasts, activity (decrease), 107
Osteomyelitis, 292–293
    antibiotic therapy, summary, 296t
    CT/MRI, usage, 325–326
Osteopenia, 109
    definitions, 106t
Osteoporosis, 105
    assessment, 105–106
    bisphosphonates, impact, 107
    calcitonin, impact, 108
    clinical presentation, 105
    definitions, 106t
    diagnosis, 105
    differential diagnosis, 105
    discharge/follow-up plans, 109
    estrogen/hormone therapy, impact, 107
    hospitalization, 106–107

Osteoporosis (Continued)
    lifestyle modification, 107
    management, 107–108
    measurement, methods, 106
    medical conditions/medications,
        association. See Secondary
        osteoporosis
    monitoring, 109
    outpatient–physician communication,
        109
    patient education, 109
    pharmacologic therapy, 107
    postdischarge, 107
    prediction rule, 106
    prevalence, 105
    prevention, 108–109
    prognosis, 106–107
    PTH, impact, 108
    reading, 109
    risk factors, 106b
    secondary causes, evaluation, 106
    SERM, impact, 107–108
    studies, preference, 105
    surgical management, 108
    treatment, preference, 107
Osteoporosis risk assessment (ORA)
    instrument, scoring system, 107t
Ostwald viscosimeter, measurement,
    553
Outcomes. See Quality improvement
    assessment, 984
    chain. See Hospitals
Outpatient Parenteral Antibiotic Therapy
    (OPAT), 294
Oversedation, complication. See Anesthesia
Oxygen
    impact. See Chronic obstructive pulmonary
        disease
    super-physiologic concentrations,
        maintenance, 671
    supplementation. See Acute respiratory
        failure
    usage. See Asthma
Oxygenation. See Intracerebral hemorrhage
    (ICH)
    monitoring. See Ischemic stroke

P4P. See Pay for Performance
Pacemakers, indications, 169t–170t
PAD. See Peripheral arterial disease
Paget's disease, 549
PAH. See Pulmonary arterial hypertension
Pain. See Functional pain; Inflammatory pain;
    Neuropathic pain; Nociceptive pain
    assessment. See Intensive care unit
    etiologies, 727t
    management, 821. See also Critically ill
        patients; Hospitalized patients;
        Perioperative pain management
    medical management, WHO analgesic
        guide, 727
    medications/dosing. See Oral pain
        medications/dosing
    prevalence. See Chronic pain
    scale. See Behavioral pain scale
    symptom management, 734
    terms, IASP list (usage), 727t
    types, 726f
Palliative hospital care
    background, 733
    care model, contrast, 734f
    communication, 735–737
        phrases, usage, 735t
    helpfulness, 734b
    implementation, 733
    prognostication, 733–734
    reading, 737–738

Palliative hospital care (Continued)
    symptom management, 734–735
        list, 734b
Palms, lesions, 632
pANCA. See Perinuclear anti-neutrophil
    cytoplasmic antibody
Pancreatitis, 113
PAP. See Pulmonary artery pressure
Paracentesis. See Ascites
    indications. See Diagnostic paracentesis
Paraneoplastic antibodies, presence, 564
Paraneoplastic neurologic antibodies,
    pathogenesis, 563
Paraneoplastic neurologic syndromes (PNNS).
    See Cancer emergencies
    antibodies/symptoms, 564t
    clinical features, 563
    electrophysiologic studies, helpfulness,
        564–565
    treatment strategies, syndrome, 565
Paraneoplastic pemphigus, 636
    illustration, 636f
Parapneumonic effusions, 371
Parasites
    empiric antibiotics, usage, 481
    impact. See Diarrhea
    presence, 478
    suspicion, 479
Parasitic diarrheal infections, causes
    (antibiotic therapy), 481t
Parathyroid hormone (PTH), 108
    impact. See Osteoporosis
    level, measurement, 550
Parenteral access, evaluation. See Nutrient
    delivery
Parenteral antibiotic selection. See Skin/soft
    tissue infections
Parenteral DTI, usage (approval), 211
Parenteral feeding, initiation, 23
Parenteral nutrient (PN) solutions,
    electrolyte/micronutrient administration
    (guidelines), 26t
Parenteral nutrition (PN)
    receiving, 22
    route, 25
Parenteral T$_4$, administration, 512
Partial SBO, 63f, 473
Partial thromboplastin time (PTT), 845
Patient safety regulation/accreditation,
    949–952
PARTNERS program-PAD Awareness, 255
Patent foramen ovale/atrial septal aneurysm
    (PFO/ASA), 690
Pathogens, association. See Acute
    exacerbations of chronic bronchitis
Patient-centered approach, 7
    reading, 13
Patient-centered care, 7–8
    principles, 8b
Patient-centered clinical method, 17f
Patient-controlled analgesia (PCA), 586
    medication dose ranges, 810t
    usage. See Hospitalized patients
Patient flow
    background, 961
    ideas, investigation, 965b
    improvement, system strategies (examples),
        963b
    measurement, 963–964
    pitfalls, 964
    reading, 965–966
    strategies, 961–963
Patient-related risk factors. See Venous
    thromboembolism
Patients
    autonomy, cultural influences, 17–18
        discussion, 18

Patients *(Continued)*
  care
    conversations, locations, 979
    process, 956
  communication. *See* Hospitalist systems
    components. *See* Hospitalist
  empowerment, 734
  explanatory model
    elicitation, 16b
    explorations, 17
  input, usefulness, 19
  interaction, 38
  lawsuits, reasons. *See* Doctors
  perceptions, racial differences, 18
  performance status, 733–734
  physician communication,
    problems/solutions, 12t
  preferences, importance, 986
  readmissions, decrease. *See* Unfunded
    patients
  risk factors, 775–777
  specialized enteral/parenteral nutrition
    support, clinical indications. *See*
    Critically ill patients
  surgery, clearing (implications), 741–742
  trust, decrease, 18
  understanding, enhancement (steps),
    12b
Patient safety
  case study, 952
  goals, 951t
  hospitalist interaction, 947
Patient satisfaction, 935–936
  assessment, 971
  concepts, background, 971
  function, instrument selection, 971
  improvement, 913
  instrument, reliability/validity, 971–972
  reading, 976
  subject/function, difference (knowledge),
    971
Patient Self Determination Act of 1990,
  980
Patient-supplied past medical history (PMH),
  776
Patient welfare, primacy (commitment), 8
PAU. *See* Penetrating atherosclerotic ulcer
PAV. *See* Proportional assist ventilation
Pay for Performance (P4P), 936–937
Payor mix, impact, 913–914
PBS. *See* Peripheral blood smear
PCA. *See* Patient-controlled analgesia
PCCs. *See* Prothrombin complex concentrates
PCI. *See* Percutaneous coronary intervention
PCP. *See* Pneumocystis jiroveci pneumonia
PCPs. *See* Primary care physicians
PCR. *See* Polymerase chain reaction
PCWP. *See* Pulmonary capillary wedge
  pressure
PDGF. *See* Platelet-derived growth factor
PDPH. *See* Post-dural puncture headache
PDSA. *See* Plan Do Study Act
PE. *See* Pulmonary embolism
Peabody, Francis W., 7
Peak admission times, staff matching,
  888–890
Peak expiratory flow rate (PEFR), 365–366
  amount, 368
  stability, 839
  usage, 362
Peak flow, 671
PEDIS classification system. *See* Skin/soft
  tissue infections
PEDIS clinical classification system, 293t
PEEP. *See* Positive end-expiratory pressure
PEEP_E. *See* Extrinsic PEEP
PEFR. *See* Peak expiratory flow rate

PEG. *See* Percutaneous endoscopic
    gastrostomy; Percutaneous gastrostomy
    tube; Polyethylene glycol
Pelvis, MRI (usage), 473
PEM. *See* Protein-energy malnutrition
Pemphigus. *See* Paraneoplastic pemphigus
  assessment, 635
  diagnosis, 635
  management/treatment, 635–636
Pemphigus vulgaris, 635f
Penetrating atherosclerotic ulcer (PAU),
    distinctions, 227
Pentobarbital, usage. *See* Coma
Pentoxifyline (Trental), usage, 260
Percutaneous coronary intervention (PCI),
    132–133, 779–780
  fibrinolytic therapy, contrast, 144t
  impact, possibility, 821
Percutaneous endoscopic gastrostomy (PEG)
    tubes, usage, 31
Percutaneous gastrostomy tube (G-tube /
    PEG), usage, 26
Performance. *See* Hospitals
  expectations. *See* Hospitalist; Hospital
    medicine program
    categories, 921b
  initiatives, quality/pay (impact), 913
  interpretation. *See* Electrocardiogram
  management. *See* Physician performance
    pyramid, 920f
    steps, 923f
  measurement. *See* Physician performance
  status. *See* Patients
Perfusion, monitoring. *See* Ischemic stroke
Pericardial effusion, CXR, 251f
Pericardial syndromes, classification, 248b
Pericardiocentesis, indications, 252f
Pericarditis, 137. *See also* Acute pericarditis
  differential diagnosis, 128
  illustration, 253f
  recurrence, 252
Perinuclear anti-neutrophil cytoplasmic
    antibody (pANCA), 610
Perioperative anticoagulation
  background, 765
  discharge recommendations, 768
  follow-up management, 768
  history, 765–766
  laboratory testing, 767
  LMWH, considerations, 769–770
  management, 767
  pathophysiology, 765
  patient education, 768
  physical examination, 766
  postoperative evaluation, 767–768
    clinical assessment, 767
    management, 768
  preoperative evaluation, 765–767
    clinical assessment, 765–767
  reading, 770
Perioperative consultation, 743b
Perioperative CV events, 775
Perioperative management. *See* Diabetic
    patients
Perioperative medication management
  background, 761
  clinical assessment/evaluation, 762
  pathophysiology, 761–762
  principles, 761
  reading, 764
  recommendations/management, 762–764
  summary, 763t
Perioperative medications, 742
Perioperative nutrition
  administration, enteral route, 798
  clinical assessment, 796–797
  functional tools, 797

Perioperative nutrition *(Continued)*
  history, 796
  laboratory tests, 796–797
  management, 798–800
  objective tools, 797
  overview, 795
  pathophysiology, 795
  physical examination, 796
  reading, 801
  subjective assessment tools, 797
  tube position, requirements, 800
Perioperative pain management
  background, 809
  pathophysiology, 809
  postoperative care, 809
  preoperative evaluation, 809
  reading, 810
Perioperative pulmonary complications, 784b
  laboratory testing/imaging studies, role,
    785–786
  patient-related risk factors, 784–785
  physical exam findings, impact, 784
  risk, surgical factors, 784b
  risk factors, studies (comparison), 785t
Perioperative pulmonary risk (increase),
    chronic illness (impact), 784
Perioperative steroids, usage, 786
Peripartum cardiomyopathy, 843–844
  treatment goals, 844
Peripheral arterial disease (PAD), 776
  assessment, 255–256, 258
  background, 255
  clinical presentation, 255
  diagnosis, 257–258
  differential diagnosis, 257
  discharge/follow-up plans, 261
  evaluation, algorithm usage, 259
  handheld Doppler, usage, 256
  hospitalization, 259
  management, 260–261
  outpatient physician communication, 261
  patient care guidelines, 261t
  patient education, 261
  physical examination, 256–257
  postdischarge, 260
  presenting signs/symptoms, 255
  prevention, 261
  prognosis, 259–260
  pulse examination, 256t
  reading, 262
  six Ps, 256b
  supportive tests, 258
  suspicion
    diagnostic options, alternatives, 258
    diagnostic studies, preference, 257–258
  treatment, 260–261
Peripheral blood smear (PBS), 577, 579
Peripheral intravascular (PIV) catheter, usage,
    317
Peripherally inserted central catheter (PICC)
    line
  management, 329
  placement, 284, 294
  usage, 317 542
Peripheral vascular perfusion (evaluation),
    ABI method, 291
Peripheral venous catheter, septic
    thrombophlebitis, 318
Peritoneal cavity, fluid accumulation, 452
Peritoneal dialysis associated peritonitis
  assessment, 404–405
  clinical presentation, 404
  diagnosis, 404
  differential diagnosis, 404
  discharge/follow-up plans, 405
  management, 405
  outpatient physician communication, 405

Peritoneal dialysis associated peritonitis
    (Continued)
  patient education, 405
  prognosis, 404–405
Peritonitis
  assessment, 467
  diagnosis/prognosis, 467
  discharge/follow-up plans, 468
  management, 467–468
  treatment, 467–468
  types, ascitic fluid findings (basis), 460t
Personal Service Exception, 994. See also Stark
    Law
PET. See Positron emission tomography
Petechia. See Mononucleosis
PFO/ASA. See Patent foramen ovale/atrial
    septal aneurysm
PFT. See Pulmonary function testing
PH. See Pulmonary hypertension
pH, usage. See Pleural effusion
Pharmacologic DVT prophylaxis,
    contraindications, 102b
Phenobarbital, usage. See Alcohol withdrawal
    syndrome
Phenothiazines, antiemetic action, 65
Phentolamine, usage, 266
Phenylpropanolamine, 684
PHO. See Physician-Hospital Organization
Phosphate, usage. See Diabetic ketoacidosis
Phosphodiesterase inhibitors, usage. See
    Pulmonary hypertension
Physical examination, 757–760
    performing, 11, 23b
Physician-Hospital Organization (PHO), 996
Physician-hospital relationship,
    maintenance/development
  background, 999–1001
  driver, 999
  negotiation, 1002
  reading, 1002
Physician Organization (PO), 996
Physician performance
  compensation, expectations (alignment),
    921–922
  corrective action, 923–924
  expectations, setting, 920
  feedback, providing, 922
  management, 919
    implementation steps, 924
    pitfalls, 924
    steps, 923f
    system, effectiveness (measurement),
    924
  measurement, 920–921
  poor quality, management, 922–924
  recruitment, impact, 919–920
Physicians
  attire, 10f
  communication. See Hospitalist systems
    duties, 11–12
    problems, 78. See also Patients
    solutions. See Patients
  documentation. See Hospital-driven
    physician documentation
  education, duties, 11–12
  information transfer/continuity,
    improvement, 78–79
  job description, elements (recommendation),
    921b
  patient communication
    effectiveness, increase, 80–81
    ineffectiveness, 78
  physiologic doses, efficacy, 646
PICC. See Peripherally inserted central catheter
PIOPED study, 218, 220
Pituitary hypofunction, 517
PIV. See Peripheral intravascular

Plague
  clinical presentation, 340
  diagnosis, 340–341
  management, 342
  prognosis, 341
Plan Do Study Act (PDSA), 934
  advantages, 941t
  cycles, 940f
  model. See Quality improvement
Plasma renin activity, measurement, 436
Plasma therapy, dosing, 593
Platelet-derived growth factor (PDGF), usage,
    811
Platelet function
  defects. See Inherited platelet function
    defects
  NSAID inhibition, 763
Platinol, usage. See Nephrotoxicity
Platinum drugs, impact. See Cancer
    management
Pleural disease
  assessment, 369–372
  background, 369
  clinical presentation, 369
  diagnosis, 370–372
  discharge/follow-up, 374
  management/treatment, 372–374
  prognosis, 372
  reading, 374
Pleural effusion
  assessment, 369–372
  background, 369
  causes, 370t
  cell count/differential, usage, 370–371
  chest tube placement, indication, 372
  clinical presentation, 369
  creatinine, usage, 371
  CXR, 370
  cytology, usage, 371
  diagnosis, 370–372
    flowchart, 373f
    thoracentesis, usage, 370–371
  discharge/follow-up, 374
  glucose, usage, 371
  Gram stain/culture, usage, 371
  hematocrit, usage, 371
  HIV, impact, 369
  LDH, usage, 370, 371
  management flowchart, 373f
  management/treatment, 372–374
  occurrence, 371
  pH, usage, 371
  physical examination, 370
  prognosis, 372
  reading, 374
  tests, usage, 370–371
  thoracentesis
    complications, 372
    usage, 370–371
  triglyceride levels, usage, 371
  tumor markers, usage, 371
Pleuritis, differential diagnosis, 128
PMC. See Pseudomembranous colitis
PMH. See Patient-supplied past medical
    history
PMI. See Point of maximal impulse
PML. See Progressive multifocal
    leukoencephalopathy
PMN. See Polymorphonuclear
PN. See Parenteral nutrient; Parenteral
    nutrition
Pneumococcal meningitis, CT scans, 301f
Pneumococcal vaccine, review, 85–86
Pneumocystis jiroveci pneumonia (PCP), 331
  conditions, 333t
  interstitial/alveolar infiltrates, 333f
Pneumocystis pneumonia, treatment, 335b

Pneumonia, 663. See also Postoperative
    pneumonia
Pneumonia Severity Index (PSI), 273f
  decision tree, 274f
Pneumothorax
  assessment, 369–372
  background, 369
  clinical presentation, 369
  diagnosis, 370–372
    flowchart, 374f
  discharge/follow-up, 374
  HIV, impact, 369
  management flowchart, 374f
  management/treatment, 372–374
  outpatient management, Heimlich valves
    (usage), 373
  physical examination, 372
  reading, 374
Pneumothorax, differential diagnosis, 129
PNNS. See Paraneoplastic neurologic
    syndromes
PO. See Physician Organization
POBBLE study, 780
POEMS. See Polyneuropathy organomegaly
    endocrinopathy syndrome
Point-of-care information resources,
    categories, 5
Point of maximal impulse (PMI), 160
POISE study, 780
Poisoned patient (treatment), antidotes
    (usage), 678t
Poisonings
  diagnostic tests, 677
  history/physical examination, 677
  introduction, 677
  reading, 685–686
  treatment, 677–679
Polyarteritis nodosa (PRN), 395, 610
  medications, response, 53
Polyethylene glycol (PEG), nonmetabolization,
    58
Polymerase chain reaction (PCR)
  diagnostic value, absence, 605
  requirement. See Quantitative HIV RNA PCR
Polymerase chain reaction (PCR) test, 301
Polymorphonuclear (PMN) count, 453. See
    also Ascitic fluid PMN count
Polymorphonuclear (PMN) predominance,
    300
Polyneuropathy organomegaly
    endocrinopathy syndrome (POEMS), 563
PONV. See Postoperative nausea and vomiting
Portal hypertension, 451–452
Positive airway pressure. See Continuous
    positive airway pressure;
    Expiratory positive airway pressure;
    Inspiratory positive airway pressure
Positive end-expiratory pressure (PEEP), 663.
    See also AutoPEEP; Extrinsic PEEP
Positive pressure, impact, 672
Positive pressure-mask ventilation, usage,
    283
Positron emission tomography (PET)
  scanning. See Whole-body PET scanning
  usage, 564
Post-bronchodilator FEV$_1$, basis. See Chronic
    obstructive pulmonary disease
Post-craniotomy central diabetes insipidus
  assessment, 523–524
  background, 523
  clinical presentation/diagnosis, 523–524
  discharge/follow-up, 526
  fluid replacement, 525
  hormone replacement, 525–526
  management, 524–526
  pathophysiology, 523
  reading, 526

Post-craniotomy central diabetes insipidus
(Continued)
treatment, 524–526
alternatives, 526
flowchart, 524f
triphasic response, 523
Post craniotomy DI management/treatment,
524
Post-dural puncture headache (PDPH),
747–748
recommendations, 748
Postexposure prophylaxis (PEP), 336
usage. See Antiretroviral PEP
Post-hospital discharge, 94
Postinfection GN, 395
Postoperative abnormal signs/symptoms
background, 817
reading, 820
Postoperative anemia, 824
treatment, 831t
Postoperative arrhythmias, treatment, 825t
Postoperative assessment/management
background, 805
clinical assessment/evaluation, 805–806
pathophysiology, 805
reading, 807
recommendations/management, 806–807
Postoperative bleeding, determination, 771
Postoperative cardiac complications, 821
reading, 826
Postoperative complications. See Non-cardiac
postoperative complications
list, 806t
Postoperative CPAP, impact, 786–787
Postoperative hyperglycemia, 820
Postoperative hypoxemia, 805–806
Postoperative incision care. See Wounds
Postoperative MI
factors, 821–822
risk factors, 822b
Postoperative monitoring, 780–781
Postoperative nausea, 61
Postoperative nausea and vomiting (PONV),
63
commonness, 805
complication, 749–750
risk, 747
Postoperative neurological complications, 806
Postoperative pneumonia
antimicrobial therapy, 828
clinical assessment, 828
recommendations/management, 828
risk factors/pathophysiology, 828
risk index, 786t
Postoperative practices, invasive indwelling
drains (usage), 807
Postoperative pulmonary/cardiac
complications (risk increase), exercise
capacity decrease (impact), 784
Postoperative pulmonary complications
risk factors, 828t
risk (reduction), preoperative pulmonary
assessment/strategies algorithm,
787f
Postoperative renal failure, risk, 806
Postoperative respiratory complications, 805
Postoperative respiratory failure
mechanisms, 827
preoperative predictors, 786t
Postoperative TPN, receiving. See
Gastrointestinal surgery patients
Post-partum thyroiditis (PPT), 846–847
Postrenal azotemia, 829
Post surgical bleeding, factors, 830b
Postthrombotic syndrome (PTS), 210
Post-transfusion purpura, 573
Post-traumatic stress disorder (PTSD), 864

Potassium
administration, 414
balance
disorders, 419
perturbations, impact, 420t
cell shifting, factors, 420t
deficiency, treatment, 425
gradient. See Transtubular potassium
gradient
homeostasis, complications, 403
removal methods, 422
renal excretion, disruption, 421
usage. See Diabetic ketoacidosis
Potassium-binding resins, usage, 435
Potassium chloride, usage. See Hypokalemia
Potassium hydroxide preparation, 628
Potassium-sparing diuretics, 421
PPD. See Purified protein derivative
PPT. See Post-partum thyroiditis
PR3-ANCA, sensitivity. See Wegener's
granulomatosis
Practice
evidence, application, 967
management costs, 878
revenue, projection. See Hospital medicine
program
Practice-based evidence, 5–6
support, 5
Practitioners/patients, communication,
735–736
Precedex, usage. See Critically ill patients
Prediction rule. See Nausea; Osteoporosis
Preeclampsia, 840, 842
clinical features, 842b
delivery indications, 842t
diagnosis. See Superimposed preeclampsia
risk factors, 840b
Pre-ECT assessment, 868–869
Preexcitation syndromes, management. See
Tachyarrhythmias
Pregnancy
acute hypertension, treatment, 843t
diagnostic studies, 839
drug safety classification (FDA), 840t
hypertensive disorders, 840–843
hyperthyroidism, relationship, 846
hypothyroidism, relationship, 846
impact, 267
medical complications, 839
medical issues, pharmacologic agents, 841t
physiologic changes, 840t
prescribing, 839
reading, 847
testing, 760
thyroid disease, relationship, 845–847
thyroid function tests, interpretation,
845–846
valvular heart disease, problems, 244
VTE, 845
Premature ventricular depolarizations, 185
Preoperative cardiac risk assessment,
ACC/AHA guidelines, 790
Preoperative cardiac risk evaluation,
ACC/AHA algorithm, 776f–777f
Preoperative evaluation/testing
background, 755–756
history, 755–756
laboratory studies, usage, 758–760
physical examination, usage, 757–760
procedure, issues (focused review),
756–757
reading, 760
Preoperative health assessment. See Alcohol
history; Allergies; Family medical history;
Illicit drug history; Medical history;
Medications; Surgical illness; Tobacco
history

Preoperative risk stratification, 775
Preoperative status (preop status), 758
Preoperative TPN, 798–799
Prerenal acute renal failure, causes,
829t
Prerenal azotemia, 392–394, 829
association, 394
causes, 393
identification, absence, 394
prognosis, 396
treatment, 397
Pressure-cycled ventilation, 669,
670–671
Pressure support ventilation (PSV), 670
Pressure ulcers
assessment, 43–45
clinical algorithms, 50
clinical presentation, 43
debridement, necessity. See Stage IV
pressure ulcer
development, sites, 50f
diagnosis, 44
differential diagnosis, usage, 43
discharge/follow-up plans, 50
evaluation, 45
healing. See Stage IV pressure ulcer
hospitalization, 44
management, 45–49
nutrition management, 45
outpatient physician communication,
50
patient education, 50
postdischarge, 44–45
presenting skin/symptoms, 43
prevalence, 43
prevention, 49–50
keys, 49b
prognosis, 44–45
progression, 44f
reading, 51
stages, management, 46t
staging, 44t
treatment, 45
Prevent Recurrence of Osteoporotic Fractures
(Proof), 108
PREVENT study, 213
Priapism, 584
Primary caregiver, interaction, 38
Primary care physicians (PCPs)
communication, 215
follow-up, 828
improvement, 913
patient, admittance, 77, 80
referrals, 873
teamwork, sense, 958
Primary prophylaxis. See Variceal
hemorrhage
Primary vasculitides, treatment, 611
PRINCE/PRIME studies, 101
Principled negotiations, 1001b
barriers, 1002
dimensions, 928b
implementation, 1001–1002
Privileged facsimile/electronic mail
transmissions, disclaimer statement
(accompaniment), 980b
PRN. See Polyarteritis nodosa
Probiotics. See Clostridium difficile colitis;
Diarrhea
Procedure (plan), issues (focused review),
756–757
Proctitis, risk (increase), 479
Productivity benchmarks, usage. See Hospital
medicine program
Professionalism
charter. See Medical professionalism
impact, 8–11

Professional services agreements, problems, 883
Progressive multifocal leukoencephalopathy (PML), 332
Prokinetics, antiemetic effect, 68
Proleukin, usage, 537
Proof. *See* Prevent Recurrence of Osteoporotic Fractures
Prophylactic medical therapy, 780
Propofol, usage. *See* Alcohol withdrawal syndrome; Critically ill patients
Proportional assist ventilation (PAV), 664
Prostacyclin analogs, usage. *See* Pulmonary hypertension
Prosthetic joints, 328
  infections, 325
    surgical management, 328
Prosthetic valves, usage, 243
Protective mechanisms, failure, 669
Protein
  intake, RDA, 24–25
  needs, estimation, 23b
  requirements, estimation. *See* Amino acids/protein
Protein C/S deficiency, 700
Protein-energy malnutrition (PEM), 31
Proteinuria, dipstick analysis, 392
Prothrombin-complex concentrates, 708
Prothrombin complex concentrates (PCCs), development, 595
Prothrombin gene 20210, 596–597
Prothrombin time (PT)
  prolongation, 679
  usage, 697
Provider-level mortality indicators, 935
Provider-level volume indicators, 935
Proximal aortic dissection, CXR, 230
Prurigo nodularis, 629
  illustration, 629f
Pseudoephedrine, 684
Pseudohyponatremia, 409
Pseudomembranous colitis (PMC), 486, 488
  sigmoidoscopy/colonoscopy, usage, 487f
PSI. *See* Pneumonia Severity Index
Psychiatric consultation, necessity, 859
Psychiatric disorders
  antidepressants, usage, 864
  antipsychotics, usage, 864
  BZDs, usage, 864
  mood stabilizers, usage, 864
  parenteral medication management, 864
  perioperative management, 863–868
    background, 864
    clinical assessment, 864
    techniques, 864, 867–868
  preoperative evaluation, 863
    background, 863
    clinical assessment, 863
    management, 863
  preoperative psychiatric evaluation, 863
  reading, 869–870
Psychiatric disorders, evaluation/management. *See* Medical patients
Psychiatric symptoms, causes (medical conditions), 852t–853t
Psychogenic chest pain, 129
Psychogenic polydipsia, 409
Psychosis
  background, 860
  clinical assessment/evaluation, 860–861
  concept. *See* Intensive care unit
  evaluation, diagnostic questions, 861
  medications, 857t
  perioperative management techniques, 867
  psychiatric disorders, manifestation, 861t
  treatment, 861

Psychotropic administration, parenteral/alternative modes, 865t–866t
PT. *See* Prothrombin time
PTH. *See* Parathyroid hormone
PTS. *See* Postthrombotic syndrome
PTSD. *See* Post-traumatic stress disorder
PTT. *See* Partial thromboplastin time
Pulmonary arterial hypertension (PAH), 383. *See also* Human immunodeficiency virus; Idiopathic pulmonary arterial hypertension
Pulmonary arteriography, usage. *See* Pulmonary embolism
Pulmonary artery catheters, usage, 780–781
Pulmonary artery pressure (PAP), 383. *See also* Mean PAP
Pulmonary capillary wedge pressure (PCWP), increase, 161
Pulmonary complications, 827–828
  cigarette smoking, impact, 784
  obesity, risk factor, 784
  risk factors, 784–786
Pulmonary disease, 243
  history, 784
Pulmonary embolism (PE), 765. *See also* Massive PE
  ABG analysis, usage, 218–219
  assessment, 217–225
  cardiac biomarkers, usage, 220
  clinical presentation, 217–218
  CXR, usage, 218
  D-dimer testing, 219–220
  diagnosis, 218
  differential diagnosis, 128
  discharge/follow-up plans, 225
  ECG, usage, 218
  echocardiography, usage, 222
  FDA-approved thrombolytic regimens, 223b
  heparin, administration, 225
  LMWH preferred option, 223
  management, 222
  MRI, usage, 221–222
  presenting signs/symptoms, 217–218
  pre-test probability, prediction, 218t
  prevalence, 217
  prophylaxis, usage. *See* Intracerebral hemorrhage
  pulmonary arteriography, usage, 220
  reading, 226
  spiral (helical) CT scan angiography, usage, 221
  surgical embolectomy, impact, 224
  suspicion, diagnostic algorithm, 219f
  symptoms. *See* Acute PE
  thrombolytic therapy, 223–224
  UFH, impact, 222–223
  vena cava interruption, 224
  ventilation-perfusion scanning, usage, 220
  VTE, impact, 217
Pulmonary examination, 757
Pulmonary function, age-related changes, 784
Pulmonary function testing (PFT), 534. *See also* Interstitial lung disease
  usage, 759
Pulmonary hypertension
  cardiac examination, usage, 384
  ECG, 385f
  HRCT, usage, 384
Pulmonary hypertension (PH)
  anticoagulants, usage, 387
  assessment, 383–385
  background, 383
  calcium channel blockers, usage, 386
  clinical classification, 384t
  clinical presentation, 383

Pulmonary hypertension (PH) *(Continued)*
  CXR. *See* Advanced pulmonary hypertension
  diagnosis, 384–385
  differential diagnosis, 384
  discharge/follow-up plans, 387
  endothelin receptor antagonists, usage, 387
  epoprostenol, expense, 386
  functional status, WHO classification, 384t
  history, 383
  hospitalization, 387
  invasive testing, 385
  management, 385–387
  medical treatment, comparison, 386t
  options, alternatives, 387
  outpatient physician communication, 388
  pathophysiology, 383
  patient education, 387
  phosphodiesterase inhibitors, usage, 387
  presence, 384
  presenting signs/symptoms, 384
  prevalence, 383
  prognosis, 385
  prostacyclin analogs, usage, 386–387
  reading, 388
  serology, 385
  studies, preference, 384–385
  therapy, 387
Pulmonary preoperative risk assessment/evaluation
  background, 783
  clinical assessment/evaluation, 783–786
  pathophysiology, 783
  preventive strategies, usage, 786
  reading, 787
  recommendations/management, 786–787
Pulmonary status, 756–757
Pulmonary toxicity. *See* Cancer management
  ATRA (Vesanoid), usage, 534
  Bleomycin (Blenoxane), usage, 534
  Busulfan (Myleran), usage, 534
  clinical presentation, 533
  diagnosis, 534
  Methotrexate, usage, 534
  nitrosources, usage, 534
Pulmonary vascular resistance (PVR), 217
Pulmonary veno-occlusive disease (PVOD)
  clinical presentation, 539
  diagnosis, 539
  discharge, 539
  prognosis/treatment, 539
Pulse oximetry, 651
  waveform, 671
Pulse volume recordings (PVRs), usefulness, 257–258
Pupillary light reflex, presence, 712
Pure mitral stenosis, signs (physical examination, usage), 238f
Purified protein derivative (PPD), results, 87
Purkinje's cells. *See* Cerebellum
PVOD. *See* Pulmonary veno-occlusive disease
PVR. *See* Pulmonary vascular resistance; Pulse volume recordings
P waves, relationships/configurations. *See* Supraventricular tachycardia
Pyuria, 286

QI. *See* Quality improvement
QRS complex. *See* Tachyarrhythmias
  escape rhythm, 170
  widening, 419
QRS waves, relationships/configurations. *See* Supraventricular tachycardia
QT interval (prolongation), conditions/medications (impact), 186b

QT prolongation, 559
Quadravalent meningococcal vaccine,
    recommendation, 305
Quality bonus. *See* Mercy Medical Center
Quality improvement (QI)
    aims, selection, 940–942
    assessment, 939
    background, 939
    concepts, 934
    conducting, PDSA model, 940f
    data collection, measurement system
        (creation), 942–943
    empiric system, 939–940
    external incentives, 936–937
    fundamentals, 939–940
    iterative system, 939–940
    leadership, 945
    measurement
        methods/tools, 934–936
        system, 939–940
        system, creation, 942–943
    measures/organizations, 936t
    metrics
        plotting, measurement system (creation),
            942–943
        set, selection, 940–942
    outcomes, 934, 935–936
    process, 934, 935
    quality assurance, contrast, 941f
    run charts, 943
    statistical process control, 943
    strategies/effectiveness, 944t
    structure, 934, 935
    success, principles, 941t
    theory/trends, 933
    tools, 933
        utilization principles, 933–934
Quality of life, importance, 986
Quantitative HIV RNA PCR, requirement,
    334

RA. *See* Rheumatoid arthritis
RAAS. *See* Renin-angiotensin-aldosterone
    system
Racial differences. *See* Patients
Radiation, impact
    See Cancer emergencies
Ramsay Scale (RS), 656–657
Range-of-motion exercises, 32
Rapidly progressive glomerulonephritis
    (RPGN), 395, 610
Rapid-onset HIT pattern, recognition, 598
Rash/fever
    assessment, 631–632
    background, 631
    clinical presentation, 631–632
    diagnosis, 632
    differential diagnosis, 632
    discharge/follow-up plans, 634
    diseases, presence, 634t
    history/physical, components, 631b
    management/treatment, 634
    prognosis, 633
RASS. *See* Richmond Agitation-Sedation Scale
Raynaud's syndrome, 384
RCA. *See* Root cause analysis
RCRI. *See* Lee Revised Cardiac Risk Index
Recombinant activated factor VII, impact. *See*
    Intracerebral hemorrhage
Recombinant erythropoietin (EPO), 574
    initiation, iron studies initiation, 575f
    usage, 575f
Recombinant factor VIIa. *See* Novo VII
Recommended daily allowance (RDA). *See*
    Protein
Records Requests Form, example, 895f
Rectovaginal fistulae, occurrence, 475

Red blood cells (RBCs)
    bacterial contamination, 573
    construction. *See* Artificial RBCs
    mass, maintenance, 576
    sequestration, 587
    substitutes, 576
    transfusion
        algorithm, 571f
        complications, 569
        effectiveness, evaluation, 576
        indications, 569–574
        trigger numbers, 569
Red wounds, 43
Referrals. *See* Negligent referrals
    assumptions, establishment. *See* Hospital
        medicine program
    number, projection, 874b
    sources. *See* Hospitals
Referring, communication. *See* Hospitalist
    systems
Referring physicians, discharge
    summary/history/physical documents
    (transmission elements), 894b
Refractory ascites, management, 454
Regional anesthesia, 745
    consideration, 786
Regional hospitalist group, contracting,
    881–882
Regurgitant orifice area (ROA), 239f
Rehydration, impact. *See* Diarrhea
Relational coordination
    fostering, hospitalist model (impact),
        957
    high levels, low levels (contrast), 956f
    theory, 955
Relative adrenal insufficiency. *See* Septic shock;
    Shock
Relative risk reduction (RRR), 504
Reliability mechanisms, 945b
Remote sites, infections. *See* Surgical site
    infection
Renal abnormalities
    background, 828–829
    clinical assessment/evaluation, 829–830
    management, 830
    pathophysiology, 829
Renal failure. *See* Acute renal failure; Anuric
    renal failure; Intrinsic renal failure;
    Nonoliguric renal failure; Oliguric renal
    failure
    clinical assessment/evaluation, 819
    drugs/toxins, association, 829t
    recommendations/management, 819
Renal function, impairment, 395
Renal replacement therapy, 399–400. *See also*
    Continuous renal replacement therapy
Renal sodium wasting, disorder, 409
Renal tubular acidosis (RTA), 433. *See also*
    Type 4 RTA
    distinction, 433
    occurrence. *See* Type 1 RTA; Type 2 RTA
    types, 432t
Renal vein thrombosis, 394
Renin-angiotensin-aldosterone system
    (RAAS), 419, 421
    impact, 420t
Reperfusion therapy, 143
Report card function, critics, 971
Reset osmostat, 410
Residency programs, involvement. *See*
    Hospitalist; Hospital medicine program
Respiration support, failure, 669
Respiratory acidosis
    assessment, 437
    background, 437
    clinical presentation, 437
    diagnosis/differential diagnosis, 437

Respiratory acidosis (Continued)
    management, 437–438
    neuromuscular disorders, impact, 437
    studies, preference, 437
    treatment, 437–438
Respiratory alkalosis
    assessment, 438
    background, 438
    clinical presentation, 438
    diagnosis/differential diagnosis, 438
    management/treatment, 438
    studies, preferences, 438
Respiratory failure. *See* Acute respiratory
    failure; Hypercapneic respiratory failure;
    Hypoxemic respiratory failure
    background, 827
    causes, 650t
        classification, 669
    clinical assessment/evaluation, 827
    mechanisms. *See* Postoperative respiratory
        failure
    recommendations/management, 827
    risk factors/pathophysiology, 827
Respondeat superior, 991
Rest immobilization ice compression and
    elevation (RICE), 592
Resting ABI, relationship, 258t
Revascularization, 779–780
Revenue
    generation. *See* Hospital medicine program
    improvements, ALOS basis, 912
    increase, sources. *See* Hospitals
RF. *See* Rheumatoid factor
RHC. *See* Right heart catheterization
Rheumatic disease, impact. *See* Valvular heart
    disease
Rheumatoid arthritis (RA), 323. *See also*
    Acute RA
Rheumatoid factor (RF), role (absence),
    605
Rheumatrex. *See* Methotrexate
RICE. *See* Rest immobilization ice compression
    and elevation
Richmond Agitation-Sedation Scale (RASS),
    656–657
Right BBB morphologic criteria, 184f
Right heart catheterization (RHC), 385
Right upper quadrant pain, 584
RITA-3 trial, 155
Rituximab (Rituxan), usage. *See* Cancer
    management
ROA. *See* Regurgitant orifice area
Rocky Mountain spotted fever, 300, 632
Root cause analysis (RCA), 949
    FMEA, similarities/differences, 950t
RPGN. *See* Rapidly progressive
    glomerulonephritis
RRR. *See* Relative risk reduction
RS. *See* Ramsay Scale
RTA. *See* Renal tubular acidosis
Rubeola (Koplik's spots), 87, 632
Rule-out myocardial injury protocol, usage,
    161
Rummack-Mathew nomogram, 680f
Run charts. *See* Quality improvement

SAAG. *See* Serum ascites albumin gradient
Safe Timely Effective Efficient Equitable
    Patient-centered (STEEEP), 8
    goals. *See* Health care system
        improvement
Safety hazards. *See* Acute care hospitals;
    Inpatient safety hazards
SAH. *See* Subarachnoid hemorrhage
Salary
    base/incentive components, combination,
        901–902

Salary (Continued)
compensation. See One hundred percent
production-based salary; Straight
salary
Salicylates
assessment, 681
background, 680–681
clinical presentation, 681
differential diagnosis, 681
discharge/follow-up, 681
intoxication, features, 681
management, 681
prediction rule, 681
therapeutic range. See Serum salicylates
toxicity, hemodialysis indications, 681b
Salmonella, empiric antibiotics (usage), 481
Sampling method, 974
Sapporo diagnostic classification system, 597
Sarcoidosis, impact. See Interstitial lung
disease
SARS. See Severe acute respiratory syndrome
SAS. See Sedation-Agitation Scale
Saturated solution of potassium iodide (SSKI),
515
SBO. See Small bowel obstruction
SBP. See Spontaneous bacterial peritonitis
SBT. See Spontaneous breathing trial
Scarlet fever, 632
SCC. See Spinal cord compression
SCD. See Sudden cardiac death
Schedules. See Block schedule
comparison. See Shift-based schedules
contrast. See Shift-based schedules
Scheduling. See Circadian rhythms; Hospital
medicine program; Small programs;
Young programs
Schistosomiasis, 225
SDD. See Selective digestive decontamination
Seattle Veteran Affairs Medical Center, 289
Seborrheic dermatitis, 627–628
illustration, 628f
Secondary osteoporosis, medical
conditions/medications (associations),
106b
Secondary prophylaxis. See Variceal
hemorrhage
Second-degree AVB, ECG data, 168f
Second-line cytotoxic therapy, 380
Secretagogues, usage, 506
Sedation. See Critically ill patients
agents, usage, 659–660
assessment, 655–656
daily interruption, 660
indications, 656t
scales, 656t
Sedation-Agitation Scale (SAS), 656
Sedatives
choice, preference, 660–661
usage, SCCM 2002 Clinical Practice
Guidelines Recommendations, 661t
Segmental plethysmography, usefulness,
257–258
Seizures, 688
management, 832
prophylaxis. See Alcohol withdrawal
magnesium sulfate, usage, 842
relationship. See Intracerebral hemorrhage
risk factors, 688
Selective digestive decontamination (SDD),
283–284
effectiveness, 284
Selective estrogen receptor modulators
(SERMs), 107–108
impact. See Osteoporosis
Selective serotonin reuptake inhibitors (SSRIs),
859
citalopram, 864

Self-care
promotion, 33, 35
responsibilities, 78
Self-evaluation. See Hospital medicine
leadership
process, 928b
Self-reported exercise capacity, 776
SENIC. See Study of the Efficacy of Nosocomial
Infection Control
Sensory assessment. See Elderly hospitalized
patient
Sepsis
ACCP/SCCM Consensus Conference
definition, 642t
antimicrobial therapy, 716
assessment, 402
bundles, Institute for Health Improvement
development, 643b
clinical presentation, 402
diagnosis/prognosis, 402
diagnostic criteria, 642b
differential diagnosis, 402
discharge/follow-up plans, 403
management, 402–403
steps, 644f
progression, 641
steroid usage, impact, 520
vasoactive agents, usage, 645t
Sepsis/shock
antibiotic therapy, usage, 645–646
background, 641
body response, 641
clinical presentation/diagnosis, 641, 643
considerations, 643
corticosteroids, usage, 646
discharge/follow-up, 646–647
drotrecogin alfa, usage, 646
fluid resuscitation, 643–644
insulin therapy, usage, 646
management, 643–646
prognosis, 643
reading, 647
resuscitation, monitoring, 645
secondary therapy, 646
source control, 645–646
vasoactive agents, usage, 644–645
Septic arthritis
antibiotic selection, 327
assessment, 323–326
background, 323
diagnosis, 325–326
differential diagnosis, 325
discharge/follow-up plans, 329
infection, risk factors, 323
management, 327–328
microbiology, 324t
MRI/tomogram. See Staphylococcus aureus
septic arthritis
outpatient physician communication,
329
patient education, 329
presenting signs/symptoms, 323–325
prevalence, 323–325
prevention, 328
prognosis, 326
reading, 329
signs/symptoms, prevalence. See Native joint
septic arthritis
Septic embolism, 225
Septic shock
ACCP/SCCM Consensus Conference
definition, 642t
corticosteroids, usage, 520b
relative adrenal insufficiency, 520–521
vasoactive agents, usage, 645t
Septic thrombophlebitis, 319. See also
Peripheral venous catheter

Sequential Organ Failure Assessment (SOFA)
score, 643
Sequestration syndromes. See Sickle cell crises
Serial nutritional assessment, components,
23b
SERMs. See Selective estrogen receptor
modulators
Seroma, complication, 813
Serotonin antagonists, impact, 65, 68
Serotonin-norepinephrine reuptake inhibitors
(SNRIs), 859
Serotonin receptors (5-HT3), 65
Serum albumin, half-life, 23
Serum albumin-ascites gradient classification.
See Ascites
Serum aldosterone level, measurement, 436
Serum-ascites albumin gradient, 453
Serum ascites albumin gradient (SAAG), 453
Serum calcium tests, 106
Serum electrolytes
studies, 683
usage, 759, 778
Serum osmolality, studies, 683
Serum potassium
concentrations, reduction (interventions),
422t
reduction, 422
Serum proteins, 22
Serum salicylates, therapeutic range, 681
Serum sodium
correction, requirement, 412
level, raising (clinical interventions), 413t
Serum TSH, reasonability, 53
Serum urate (calcium) levels, 603
Service line, creation. See Hospitals
Seventh AACP Conference on Antithrombotic
and Thrombolytic Therapy,
recommendation, 100
Severe acute respiratory syndrome (SARS),
573
Severe alkalemia, 435
Severe aortic stenosis, carotid pulse
(reduction), 241
Severe hypertension, treatment (evidence),
843
Severe hypoglycemia, AW imitation, 689
Severe sepsis
ACCP/SCCM Consensus Conference
definition, 642t
progression, 641
Severity of Illness (SI) Index, 906
SGA. See Subjective Global Assessment
SHEA. See Society for Healthcare Epidemiology
of America
Shift-based schedules
call-based schedules
comparison, 888t
contrast, 887–888
usage. See Twenty-four-hour on-site
coverage
Shift-based scheduling, program transition
(timing), 887–888
Shift duration, determination, 890
Shigella, empiric antibiotics (usage), 481
SHM. See Society of Hospital Medicine
Shock, relative adrenal insufficiency, 519. See
also Septic shock
Shortness of breath (SOB), 529
Short-term catheter-related line infection, 121
Short-term cessation, predictors. See Smoking
cessation
Short-term indwelling urinary catheter use,
indications. See Hospitalized patients
Shunt
surgery. See Variceal hemorrhage
usage, 827
SI. See Severity of Illness

SIADH. *See* Syndrome of inappropriate
     secretion of ADH
Sick day management, 793
Sickle cell crises
   assessment, 583–586
   background, 583
   bone marrow transplants, cure, 588–589
   chest pain, complication, 584–585
   clinical presentation, 583–584
   CXR, usage, 586
   diagnosis, 585–586
   differential diagnosis, 584–585
   discharge/follow-up plans, 589
   evaluation, 586
   first preventive medication, 588
   gallstones, removal, 588
   hydroxyurea, usage, 588
   inpatient problems, 585t
   management, 586–588
   outpatient-physician communication,
        589
   pain
        episode, 584
        management, 586, 587
   patient education, 589
   preoperative care, 588
   presenting signs/symptoms, 583–584
   prevalence, 583–584
   prevention, 588–589
   prognosis, 586
   psychological support, 588
   reading, 589
   sequestration syndromes, 586
   stem cell transplants, cure, 588–589
   symptoms, laboratory evaluation, 586
   transfusion
        indications, 587b
        role, 587–588
   treatment, 586
        emergence, 589
Sickle cell disease, 580, 583, 700
   clinical manifestations, 583
Sick sinus syndrome, 167
Sick time, scheduling, 890–891
SIG-E-CAPS, mnemonic, 855
Sigmoidoscopy, usage, 480
Signal-averaged ECG, 200
Significant others, communication. *See*
     Hospitalist systems
Silent MI, 778
SIMV. *See* Synchronized intermittent
     mandatory ventilation
Single daily dosing, 770
Single-dose activated charcoal, usage, 677
Sinus bradycardia, 167
Sinus node dysfunction, 167
Sinus pauses/arrest, 167
Sinus tachycardia, 173, 175
SIP. *See* Surgical Infection Prevention
SIRS. *See* Systemic inflammatory response
     syndrome
SIS. *See* Surgical Infection Society
SJS. *See* Stevens-Johnson syndrome
Skin
   adhesives, usage, 815
   biopsy, 632
   examination, 757
Skin Clinical Nurse Specialist, request, 50
Skin integrity
   assessment, 43–45
   clinical algorithms, 50
   clinical presentation, 43
   diagnosis, 44
   differential diagnosis, usage, 43
   discharge/follow-up plans, 50
   hospitalization, 44
   management, 45–49

Skin integrity *(Continued)*
   nutrition management, 45
   outpatient physician communication, 50
   patient education, 50
   postdischarge, 44–45
   presenting signs/symptoms, 43
   prevalence, 43
   prevention, 49–50
   prognosis, 44–45
   reading, 51
   treatment, 45
Skin/soft tissue infections (SSTIs). *See* Deep soft
     tissue infections
   assessment, 291–294
   background, 291
   diagnosis, 291–294
   diagnostic evaluation, elements, 292b
   differential diagnosis, 291
   Eron classification system, 292t
   historical factors, summary, 292b
   management, 294–296
   nuclear medicine scans, usage, 293
   parenteral antibiotic selection, 295t
   pathogens, summary, 294t
   PEDIS classification system, 291
   physical examination findings, 292b
   presenting skin/symptoms, 291
   prevention/follow-up, 296
   reading, 297
   risk factors, 294t
   subsets, 292
   treatment, success, 295
SLE. *See* Systemic lupus erythematosus
Small bowel obstruction (SBO), 473
   causes, 475
   suspicion. *See* Complete SBO; Partial SBO
   treatment. *See* Crohn's disease
Smallpox
   characteristics, 338t
   clinical presentation, 337–339
   diagnosis, 340
   management, 341
   prognosis, 341
   trunk, umbilicated lesions, 338f
   vesicles, development, 338f
Small programs, scheduling, 891
Small vessel disease (lacunar stroke), 700
   classification, 699t
SMART goal, building, 931t
Smoking, impact. *See* Surgical site infection
Smoking cessation. *See* Hospitalized
     patients
   assessment, 93–94
   Bupropion, impact, 96
   counseling, 96
   diagnosis, 93–94
   discharge/follow-up, 96–97
   epidemiology, 93–94
   long-term cessation, predictors, 94
   management, 94–96
   one-week confidence scale, 95b
   online continuing education, 97
   outpatient physician communication,
        97
   patient education, 96
   pharmacologic management, 96
   physician education, 96
   predictors, 94
   prognosis, 94
   reading, 97
   screening, 93
   short-term cessation, predictors, 94
SNRIs. *See* Serotonin-norepinephrine reuptake
     inhibitors
SNS. *See* Specialized Nutritional Support
SOB. *See* Shortness of breath
Social support, 78, 80

Society for Healthcare Epidemiology of
     America (SHEA), 121
Society of Critical Care Medicine (SCCM) 2002
     Clinical Practice Guidelines
     Recommendations. *See* Analgesics;
     Sedatives
Society of Hospital Medicine (SHM)/Society of
     General Internal Medicine Continuity of
     Care Task Force, 78, 79b
Society of Hospital Medicine (SHM) survey
     results. *See* Compensation
Sodium administration, theoretical amount
     (calculation), 413t
Sodium bicarbonate
   alkalinizing agent, 434
   dosage, 194
Sodium nitroprusside, usage (rarity), 842
Sodium restriction. *See* Ascites
SOFA. *See* Sequential Organ Failure
     Assessment
Soft tissue infections. *See* Deep soft tissue
     infection; Necrotizing soft tissue
     infections; Skin/soft tissue infections
Soles, lesions, 632
Somatostatin analogs, usage, 74
Sorbitol, presence. *See* Liquid medications
SPAF. *See* Stroke Prevention in Atrial
     Fibrillation
Specialized enteral/parenteral nutrition
     support, clinical indications. *See* Critically
     ill patients
Specialized Nutritional Support (SNS), 23
   route, 25
Spinal anesthesia, consideration, 786
Spinal cord compression (SCC). *See* Cancer
     emergencies
   diagnosis, 557
   differential diagnosis, 558t
   suspicion, 558
Spinal cord injury, 725
Spiral CT scanning, advantages/limitations.
     See Acute PE
Spiral (helical) CT scan angiography, usage.
     See Pulmonary embolism
Sponsoring organization, hospitalist
     employment, 881
Spontaneous bacterial peritonitis (SBP), 451
   anaerobic organisms, impact, 460
   assessment, 459–461
   clinical presentation, 459
   diagnosis, 455, 459–460
   differential diagnosis, 459
   discharge/follow-up plans, 461
   empiric antibody therapy, options, 461t
   impact, 453
   management, 455, 461
   patient/family education, 461
   prevention, 461
   prognosis, 460–461
   prophylaxis, 455, 461
   reading, 462
   risk factors, 460b
   signs/symptoms, 460b
   susceptibility data, 455
   third-generation cephalosporins, usage,
        461
   treatment, 461
Spontaneous breathing trial (SBT), 673
Spontaneous support ventilation, 670
SSD. *See* Subglottic secretion drainage
SSI. *See* Surgical site infection
SSKI. *See* Saturated solution of potassium
     iodide
SSRIs. *See* Selective serotonin reuptake
     inhibitors
SSTIs. *See* Skin/soft tissue infections
Stable COPD, management algorithm, 357f

Staffing techniques. *See* Nights/weekends/off-hours
Staff matching. *See* Peak admission times
Stage IV pressure ulcer
    debridement, necessity, 47f
    healing, 45f
Stages of Change model, 93–94
    application, 95f
Stanford Type I aortic dissection
    coronal CT angiogram, 228f
    transverse CT angiogram, 228f
Staphylococcal abscess, 626f
Staphylococcus aureus septic arthritis
    intraoperative photograph, 324f
    MRI/tomogram, 324f
Staples, removal, 815
Stark, Fortney "Pete," 993
Stark Law, 993–994
    exceptions, 995
    Personal Service Exception, 994b
Stark prohibitions, 883
Stasis, occurrence, 765
Stasis dermatitis, 625f
Statistical process control. *See* Quality improvement
Status assessment, 985
Status epilepticus (SE), AEDs (usage). *See* Convulsive SE; Nonconvulsive SE
STEEEP. *See* Safe Timely Effective Efficient Equitable Patient-centered
ST elevation, causes, 137–139
ST elevation myocardial infarction (STEMI), 135–138
    angiography/revascularization, necessity, 145f
    diagnosis, 138
    evaluation, 143
    initial treatment/dosing, recommendation, 146t
    patients
        intracerebral hemorrhage, risk, 144t
        30-day mortality prediction), TIMI Risk Score (usage), 141f
    six-month mortality, 139f
Stem cell transplants, cure. *See* Sickle cell crises
Steroids
    antiemetic effect, 68
    impact. *See* Cancer emergencies
Stevens-Johnson syndrome (SJS), 615, 623
    mortality rate, 624
    SJS-TEN overlap, contrast, 624f
Stimulant laxatives, impact. *See* Constipation
Stool character, 69
Stool cultures
    examination, 479
    tests, 487
Stop-order. *See* Urinary tract infections
Straight salary, compensation, 900
Strategic planning, 930. *See also* Hospital medicine leadership
Stress hyperglycemia, pathophysiology, 503
Stress test, identification, 779
Stroke, 505. *See also* Atrial fibrillation-associated stroke; Ischemic stroke; Small vessel disease
    diagnostic studies. *See* Embolic strokes
    etiology, evaluation (tests), 700t
    Framingham Study, 505
    indication, 584
    rate, 771
    testing. *See* Acute stroke
Stroke Prevention in Atrial Fibrillation (SPAF) trials, 702
ST-segment changes, presence, 131
ST segment elevation, examples, 137f, 138f
Studies, point-of-care information resource, 5

Study of the Efficacy of Nosocomial Infection Control (SENIC), 119
Subacute IE, 308
Subarachnoid hemorrhage (SAH)
    cause, 705
    indication, 584
    management, 709
    risk factors, 706
    vasospasm, relationship, 709
Subcutaneous insulin, transition. *See* Diabetic ketoacidosis
Subcutaneous rapid-acting insulin analogs, usage (treatment protocol). *See* Diabetic ketoacidosis
Subdural empyema, 300
Subglottic secretion drainage (SSD), involvement, 283
Subject/function, difference (knowledge). *See* Patient satisfaction
Subjective Global Assessment (SGA), 22t, 797
    advantage, 22
    form, 798f
    score, increase, 24
Substance-abusing/dependent patients, nonpharmacologic therapies, 116
Substance usage, type/route (historical information), 112t
Substance-using patients, background questions, 112b
Substituted benzamides, antiemetic effect, 65
Success, principles. *See* Quality improvement
Succession planning. *See* Hospital medicine leadership
    steps, 930t
Sudden cardiac death (SCD), 189
Suicide assessment, fundamentals, 859t
Superficial surgical site infection, definition (CDC criteria), 814t
Superimposed preeclampsia. *See* Chronic hypertension
    diagnosis, 843b
Supplemental sliding scale insulin, 791t
Support surface/bed, usage, 45
Support surface usage, specialization, 46t
Suppositories, impact. *See* Constipation
Supraventricular arrhythmias, 824
    ventricular rate control, medical treatment, 178t
Supraventricular tachycardia (SVT), 174t, 174f, 184f, 204
Surgery
    long-term warfarin management, 771
    performing, warfarin (usage), 772b
    risk/prophylaxis. *See* General surgery; Gynecologic surgery; Orthopedic surgery; Urologic surgery
Surgical embolectomy, impact. *See* Pulmonary embolism
Surgical illness, preoperative health assessment, 755
Surgical Infection Prevention (SIP) project, 122
Surgical Infection Society (SIS), 121–122
Surgical injury, 807
Surgical lung biopsy. *See* Interstitial lung disease
Surgical patients, consultation, 743
Surgical procedure, context/timing/risk, 775
Surgical site infection prophylaxis
    background, 833
    prevalence/etiology, 833
    reading, 835
Surgical site infection (SSI), 121
    antimicrobial prophylaxis, usage, 833–834
    microorganisms, impact, 833
    prevention, 833–834

Surgical site infection (SSI) (*Continued*)
    rates, reduction strategies, 835
    reduction
        factors, list, 834b
        modifiable factors, impact, 834–835
    remote sites, infections, 834
    risk (increase), smoking (impact), 834–835
Surgical stress
    impact. *See* Cardiac ischemic events
    metabolic consequences. *See* Diabetic patients
Surveys. *See* Focus groups; Telephone surveys; Written surveys
    instrument, validity, 973–974
    methodologies, characteristics, 972t
Surviving Sepsis Campaign, 643b
    Committee, recommendations, 520–521
Sutures, removal, 815
SVT. *See* Supraventricular tachycardia
Sweeps clauses, 995–996
SWOT analysis, 931t
Sympathomimetics
    assessment, 684
    background, 684
    clinical presentation, 684
    diagnosis/prognosis, 684
    differential diagnosis, 684
    discharge, 684
    management/treatment, 684
    studies, preference, 684
Symptomatic hyperkalemia, 403
Symptomatic MI-related pericarditis, 252
Symptom triggered regimen, usage. *See* Alcohol withdrawal
Synchronized intermittent mandatory ventilation (SIMV), 669, 670
    weaning, 673
Syncope. *See* Cardiovascular syncope; Neurologic syncope; Orthostatic syncope; Vasovagal syncope
    algorithms, 200
    assessment, 197–202
    clinical presentation, 197
    diagnosis, 200
    diagnostic modalities, 201t
    differential diagnosis, 197–200
    discharge/follow-up plans, 204
    disorders, mimicking, 198b
    electrocardiography, usefulness, 200
    etiology, 199b
    hospitalization, guideline criteria, 203b
    management, 202–204
    mimics, 199
    patients, evaluation algorithm, 202f
    presenting signs/symptoms, 197
    prognosis, 202
    reading, 205
    seizures, contrast, 199–200
    studies, preference, 200
    treatment, 202–204
Syndrome of inappropriate secretion of ADH (SIADH), 409–411
    medications/conditions, associations, 410t
    nonresectable lung cancer, relationship, 414
    occurrence, 414
Synopses, point-of-care information resource, 5
Synovial fluid
    cell count, 604
    glucose levels, 325
    WBC, 325
Synovial WBC counts, 326
Syntheses, point-of-care information resource, 5

Systemic inflammatory response syndrome (SIRS), 641
   ACCP/SCCM Consensus Conference definition, 642t
Systemic lupus erythematosus (SLE), 605, 610
Systemic mastocytosis, 617
Systemic vasculitis
   assessment, 609–611
   background, 609
   classification, blood vessel size (involvement), 610
   clinical presentation, 609
   diagnosis, 609–610
   differential diagnosis, 609
   discharge/follow-up plans, 612
   drug toxicity, 612t
   management, 611–612
   presenting signs/symptoms, 609
   prognosis, 611
   reading, 612–613
   studies, preference, 610–611
   treatment, 611–612
Systems
   human factors, relationship, 948
   point-of-care information resource, 5
   strategies, examples. See Patient flow
Systems of care, creation, 962
Systolic blood pressure, maintenance, 715
Systolic dysfunction, 823

T_3. See Thiodothyronine
T_4. See Thyroxine
Tachyarrhythmias
   diagnostic studies, 173
      ECG, 183
   differential diagnosis, 173
   ECG evaluation, 173
   ECG studies, 173
   impact, 824
   narrow QRS complex, 173–181
   patient history/physical examination, 173
   pharmacologic therapy, 187
   preexcitation syndromes, management, 182b
   reading, 187
   treatment, 183–184
   wide QRS complex, 181–185
      clinical presentation, 181
      physical examination, 181
Tachycardia, 684
   association. See Accessory pathways
TACO. See Transfusion-associated circulatory overload
TACTICS-TIMI 18 trial, 155
Takayasu's arteritis, 610, 612
Taper regimen, usage. See Alcohol withdrawal
Task interdependence, types, 956f
Taxanes, usage. See Anticancer agents; Cancer management
TBBx. See Transbronchial biopsy
TBI. See Traumatic brain injury
TBW. See Total body water
TCAs. See Tricyclic antidepressants
Teach-back, usage, 12, 13
Team meetings, 956
Teamwork
   culture (creation), hospitalist (impact), 957–959
   fostering, hospitalist model (impact), 957t
   toolkit. See Hospitalist
Telephone surveys, usage, 971
TEN. See Toxic epidermal necrolysis
Tenecteplase (TNK-tPA), 144
Terminal delirium, 721
Tetanus, review, 87, 90
Tetracycline, administration, 635
TGF-B1. See Transforming growth factor Beta1

TH2. See T-helper type 2
Thalassemia, treatment, 580
T-helper type 2 (TH2), 615
Theophylline, usage. See Asthma
Therapy, limitation/withdrawal, 985
Thiazide diuretics, 410
Thiazolidinediones, usage, 506
Thienopyridines, 154
Thiiodothyronine (T_3)
   metabolism (alteration), drugs (impact), 510t
   synthesis, 509
   transport (alteration), drugs (impact), 510t
Third-degree AVB, 169
   ECG data, 169f
Third-generation cephalosporins, usage. See Spontaneous bacterial peritonitis
Third-party payer, 907
   investigations, 908
Third-trimester pregnancy, risk factor, 229
Thoracentesis
   approach, 371–372
   complications. See Pleural effusion
   usage. See Pleural effusion
Thoracic imaging, usage, 651
Three-day rule. See Diarrhea
Thrombotic thrombocytopenic purpura (TTP), 394–395
Thrombocytosis, 700
Thromboembolic risk. See Long-term warfarin management
Thrombolytic therapy. See Pulmonary embolism
   absolute benefit, presentation characteristics, 143
   contraindications, 143t
   eligibility, 701
   usage, 715
Thrombophilia, testing recommendations, 215
Thrombophlebitis, 318
Thromboprophylaxis, 543f
Thrombosis, disorders (impact), 592t
Thrombotic complications, risk, 772b
Thrombotic disorders, 596–599
   background, 591
   reading, 599
Thrombotic microangiopathies, 395
Thrombolysis in Myocardial Infarction (TIMI)
   Risk Score, 140, 152
      usage. See ST elevation myocardial infarction
   trials, score, 152
Thyroid disease. See Pregnancy
Thyroid disorders
   algorithms, 512
   approach, 514f
   assessment, 510–512
   background, 509–510
   clinical assessment, 510–511
   diagnostic studies, 512
   differential diagnosis, 512
   discharge/follow-up plans, 515
   general factors, 512
   impact. See Body physiology
   management, 512–515
   medications, impact, 509
   physiology, 509
   presenting signs/symptoms, 510–511
   prevalence, 510–511
   prevention, 515
   prognosis, 512
   reading, 515
   tests, 512
Thyroidectomy, 513
Thyroid function
   drugs, impact, 510t
   medications, impact, 846t

Thyroid function (Continued)
   testing, conditions. See Inpatient setting
   tests, 513t
Thyroid hormone metabolism, extra-thyroidal pathways, 510f
Thyroid stimulating hormone (TSH)
   secretion, decrease, 509
      drugs, impact, 510t
   secretion, increase, 845
   tests, 106
   usefulness, 385
Thyroid storm, 511
   AW imitation, 689
   management, 5140515
   supportive care, 515
Thyroxine (T_4)
   absorption (decrease), drugs (impact), 509, 510t
   metabolism (alteration), drugs (impact), 510t
   transport (alteration), drugs (impact), 510t
TIA. See Transient ischemic attack
Ticlopidine, impact, 154, 763
Tidal volume, 671
Time forced expiratory volume (FEV_1), 377, 783
   amount, 368
   usage, 362–366
TIMI. See Thrombolysis in Myocardial Infarction
TIPS. See Transjugular intrahepatic portosystemic shunt
TMP-SMZ. See Trimethoprim-sulfamethoxazole
Tobacco history, preoperative health assessment, 755–756
Tobacco use treatment, Public Health Service-sponsored clinical practice guideline, 93
Toe, gangrenous changes, 257f
Topical corticosteroids, treatment, 625
Torsades de pointes, 186–187
Total body water (TBW), 413
Total parenteral nutrition (TPN). See Preoperative TPN
Toxic alcohols
   assessment, 682–683
   background, 682
   clinical presentation, 682
   diagnosis/prognosis, 683
   differential diagnosis, 683
   discharge, 684
   management/treatment, 683–684
   studies, preference, 683
Toxic epidermal necrolysis (TEN), 615, 621, 623
Toxic megacolon, 482
Toxic metabolites, conversion, 682
Toxic shock syndrome, 632
Toxicity, production. See Delayed toxicity
TPO. See Anti-thyroperoxidase
Tracheal erosion, bronchoscopic picture, 672
Tracheal narrowing, prolonged intubation (bronchoscopic picture), 673f
Tracheal stenosis, bronchoscopic picture, 673f
Tracheal wall injury, 672f
TRALI. See Transfusion-associated ALI; Transfusion-related acute lung injury
Transbronchial biopsy (TBBx), 378
Transcranial Doppler ultrasound, usage, 700
Transesophageal echocardiography (TEE), usage, 258, 312. See also Acute aortic dissection
Transforming growth factor Beta1 (TGF-B1), 811

Transfusion
  indications. *See* Sickle cell crises
  reactions, 572t
  role. *See* Sickle cell crises
Transfusion medicine
  background, 569
  reading, 576
Transfusion-associated ALI (TRALI), 783
Transfusion-associated circulatory overload
    (TACO), 573–574
Transfusion-related acute lung injury
    (TRALI), 571, 573
Transfusion-related fatalities, 571
Transfusion-transmitted infectious diseases,
    573
Transient ischemia, mimics, 699t
Transient ischemic attack (TIA), 699
  indications, 587
  symptoms, 258
Transjugular intrahepatic portosystemic shunt
    (TIPS), 454–455
  usage. *See* Variceal hemorrhage
Transthoracic echocardiography (TTE), 161,
    312f, 698
  candidates, proposal, 312
  usage, 312. *See* Acute aortic dissection
Transtubular potassium gradient (TTKG), 421
Transudative effusions, 370
Trastuzumab (Herceptin), usage. *See*
    Anticancer agents; Cancer management
Trauma, 766t
Traumatic brain injury (TBI), 711
  impact. *See* Coma
Treadmill exercise stress ECG testing,
    performing, 133
Tricuspid disease, 243
Tricyclic antidepressants (TCAs)
  IV administration, 864
  risk/alternatives, 33t
  side effects, 859
Triglyceride
  breakdown, 503
  levels, usage. *See* Pleural effusion
Trimethoprim-sulfamethoxazole (TMP-SMZ),
    usage, 74, 457
Troponins
  levels, 140
  rise/fall, 139f, 151f
  T/I, diagnostic performance, 132
Troponin T, elevation, 822
Trust
  communication, relationship, 18–19
  discussion, 18–19
  decrease. *See* Patients
TSH. *See* Thyroid stimulating hormone
TTE. *See* Transthoracic echocardiography
TTKG. *See* Transtubular potassium gradient
TTP. *See* Thrombotic thrombocytopenic
    purpura
Tuberculosis, 300
Tumor lysis syndrome (TLS). *See* Clinical TLS;
    Laboratory TLS
  emergency. *See* Cancer emergencies
  hyperkalemia
    approach, 560
    sign, 559
  hyperphosphatemia, approach, 561f
  hyperuricemia, approach, 561f
  hypocalcemia, approach, 561f
Tumor markers, usage. *See* Pleural effusion
Turner's syndrome, 228
T-wave abnormalities, presence, 131
Twenty-four-hour (Holter) ECG monitoring,
    200
Twenty-four-hour on-site coverage, shift-based
    schedules (usage), 889t
Twice daily dosing, 770

Type 1 diabetes, insulin treatment, 793
Type 1 hypersensitivity reaction,
    pathophysiology, 616f
Type 1 RTA, occurrence, 434
Type 2 diabetes, insulin treatment, 793
Type 2 RTA, occurrence, 433–434
Type 4 RTA, 434

UA. *See* Urinalysis
UC. *See* Ulcerative colitis
UFH. *See* Unfractionated heparin
UIP. *See* Usual interstitial pneumonia
Ulcer, endoscopic picture, 443f
Ulcerative colitis (UC), 471
  luminal disease, control, 475
  physical examination, 471
  symptoms, 472t
  treatment, 474
Ulcer bed color, black yellow red system
    (usage), 43
Uncomplicated pain episodes, impact,
    585–586
Understanding
  barriers, 12t
  enhancement, steps. *See* Patients
Unexplained ischemia, 609
Unfractionated heparin (UFH)
  impact, 141, 154. *See also* Pulmonary
    embolism
  treatment, expense, 543
  usage, 771. *See also* Deep vein thrombosis
Unfractionated heparin (UH), 222
Unfunded patients, readmissions (decrease),
    913–914
United Kingdom Glucose Insulin in Stroke
    Trial (GIST-UK), 505
United Network of Organ Sharing (UNOS),
    MELD score (usage), 458
UNOS. *See* United Network of Organ Sharing
Unstable angina, 132t, 149
  assessment, 149–153
  discharge/follow-up plans, 156–157
  management, 153–156
  outpatient physician communication, 157
  patient instruction, 156–157
  prevention, 156
  reading, 157
UPET. *See* Urokinase Pulmonary Embolism
    Trial
Upper airway occlusion (tongue, impact),
    oral pharyngeal airway device (usage),
    653f
Upper gastrointestinal (GI) bleeding
  assessment, 441–442
  background, 441
  clinical presentation, 441
  diagnosis, 442
  differential diagnosis, 441–442
  discharge/follow-up plans, 443–444
  history, 441
  laboratory studies, 441
  management, 442–443
  mortality rates, 442
  peptic ulcer disease, impact, 443
  physical examination, 441
  presenting symptoms, 442t
  prevalence, 441
  prognosis, 442
  prognosis, factors, 442b
  reading, 444
  treatment, 442–443
  upper endoscopy, diagnostic modality
    (selection), 442
Urinalysis (UA), 261
  usage, 760. *See also* Acute renal failure
Urinary loss, replacement, 525
Urinary output, decrease, 818–819

Urinary retention, 818–819
  background, 818
  risk factors/pathophysiology, 819
Urinary sediment, phase microscopy, 395f
Urinary tract infections (UTIs), 120–121. *See
    also* Catheter-associated UTI
  antibiotic stop-order, 288
  assessment, 285–287
  background, 285
  case-fatality rate, 287
  clinical presentation, 285–286
  diagnosis, 286
  differential diagnosis, 286
  discharge/follow-up plans, 289
  hospitalization, 286–287
  hospitalized patients, empirical treatment
    options, 287t
  management, 287–288
  mortality rate, 286–287
  options, alternatives, 287–288
  outpatient-physician communication, 289
  pathogen isolation, percentage, 286t
  patient education, 289
  postcoital prophylaxis, 288
  presenting signs/symptoms, 285–286
  prevalence, 285–286
  prevention, 288
  prognosis, 286–287
  quantitative urine culture, 286
  reading, 289
  symptoms, 286
  treatment, 288
Urine urea nitrogen (UUN), calculation, 23
Urokinase Pulmonary Embolism Trial (UPET),
    218
Urologic surgery, risk/prophylaxis, 768t
Urticaria (hives)
  assessment, 622
  diagnosis, 622
  differential diagnosis, 622
  discharge/follow-up plans, 622
  management/treatment, 622
  transfusion reactions. *See* Allergic
    transfusion reactions
U.S. Preventive Services Task Force (USPSTF),
    recommendations, 105
USAMRIID, heptavalent product, 341–342
User, information personae (impact), 5–6
Usual interstitial pneumonia (UIP), 377–378
Utilization efficiency, 964
Utilization indicators, 935
UTIs. *See* Urinary tract infections

Vacation, scheduling, 890–891
Vaccination, 85
  performance. *See* Hospital quality
  reading, 91–92
  review, 85–91
Vaccine-preventable diseases, review, 85–91
Validity, questions, 3
Value
  addition. *See* Hospitalist
  creation, incremental improvements
    (impact), 914t
  equation, 933
  standards/principles, 919
Valve prostheses, problems/complications, 243
Valvular heart disease
  anticoagulation, usage, 243–244
  assessment/management, 236
  CAD, impact, 236
  causes, 236
  congenital disorders, impact, 235
  connective tissue disease, impact, 236
  degenerative disease, impact, 236
  endocarditis, impact, 235–236
  etiology, 235–236

Valvular heart disease (Continued)
  iatrogenic causes, 236
  myxomatous degeneration, impact,
    235
  outpatient physician communication/
    patient education, 244
  reading, 244
  rheumatic disease, impact, 236
  secondary involvement, 236
  surgical cases, distribution, 236f
Valvular lesions, 236–243
  association. See High-pressure gradients
Vancomycin, CSF penetration, 305
Vancomycin-resistant enterococci, 645
VAP. See Ventilator-associated pneumonia
Variceal hemorrhage
  balloon tamponade, usage, 456
  endoscopic therapy, 456
  management, 455–456
  pharmacotherapy, 456
  primary prophylaxis, 456
  resuscitation, 455–456
  secondary prophylaxis, 456
  shunt surgery, 456
  TIPS, usage, 456
Varicella, review, 90–91
Varices, 451
Vascular access-related bacteremia/sepsis,
    402
Vascular catheter-related infections
  assessment, 317–319
  background, 317
  clinical presentation, 317–318
  diagnosis, 318–319
  differential diagnosis, 318
  discharge/follow-up plans, 320–321
  management, 319–320
  options, alternatives, 319
  outpatient physician communication,
    321
  patient education, 320
  presenting signs/symptoms, 318
  prevalence/risk factors, 317–318
  prevention, 320
  prognosis, 319
  reading, 321
  risk factors, 319
  studies, preference, 319
  treatment, 319–320
Vascular/embolic phenomena, 312
Vascular endothelial growth factor (VEGF),
    811
Vascular examination, 758
Vasculitic syndromes, patterns, 609
Vasculitis. See Cutaneous vasculitis; Systemic
    vasculitis
  clinical mimics, 610b
  suspicion, 611
Vasoactive agents, usage. See Sepsis;
    Sepsis/shock; Septic shock
Vasopressin, dosage, 192
Vasospasm, relationship. See Subarachnoid
    hemorrhage
Vasovagal syncope, 203–204
VDRL. See Venereal Disease Research
    Laboratory
Vegetative state, 716–717
VEGF. See Vascular endothelial growth
    factor
Vena cava
  dilation. See Inferior vena cava
  interruption. See Pulmonary embolism
  placement. See Inferior vena cava
Venereal Disease Research Laboratory (VDRL)
    slide test, 334
Venous oxygen saturation (CVO₂), monitoring,
    644

Venous thromboembolism (VTE). See Hospital-
    acquired VTE; Illness-associated VTE;
    Pregnancy
  anticoagulant therapy, duration guidelines,
    214t
  catheter-directed thrombolytic therapy,
    212
  development, 541
  management. See Acute VTE management
  patient-related risk factors, 766
  prophylaxis
    agents, 769t
    appropriateness, 941
  recurrence, rate, 213
  risk
    assessment, 99
    categories, 769t
    factors, 208b. See also Deep vein
      thrombosis; Medical patients
    levels, management/prophylaxis, 100
  treatment strategies. See Cancer-related VTE
Venous thromboembolism (VTE) prophylaxis.
    See Hospitalized medical patients
  background, 765
  discharge recommendations, 768
  follow-up management, 768
  history, 765–766
  hospital system integration, 102–103
  laboratory testing, 767
  LMWH, considerations, 769–770
  pathophysiology, 765
  patient education, 768
  physical examination, 766
  postoperative evaluation, 767–768
    clinical assessment, 767
    management, 768
  preoperative evaluation, 765–767
    clinical assessment, 765–767
    management, 767
  reading, 770
Ventilation perfusion (V/Q)
  mismatch, 217, 827
    shunt, viewpoint, 650
  scan. See Nondiagnostic V/Q scan
  scanning, usage. See Pulmonary embolism
Ventilator-associated pneumonia (VAP), 279,
    283–284
Ventilator modes, comparison, 674t–675t
Ventricular arrhythmias, 824
  association. See Nonischemic
    cardiomyopathy
  presentation/diagnosis/treatment/physical
    examination, 185–187
Ventricular fusion, 184f
Ventricular tachycardia (VT), 167, 184f
  distinction, Brugada criteria (usage), 185f
  sustaining, 185
Vertebroplasty, 108
  injection, 108f
Vesanoid, usage. See Pulmonary toxicity
Vibrio, empiric antibiotics (usage), 481
Vice president of medical affairs (VPMA),
    involvement, 962
Viral hepatitis, 446–447. See also Acute viral
    hepatitis
  features, 446t
Virchow's triad, 207. See also Cancer
Viruses, impact. See Gastroenteritis
Vision, usage, 919
Vitamin A/D, excess, 549
Vitamin B₁₂ deficiency, therapy, 580
Vitamin K antagonists (VKA), usage, 213
Vitamin K-depressed factors, 595
VMAC trial, 164
Voltage drop, experience, 78
Volume-cycled respiration, 669–670
  contrast, 669

Volume depletion, impact. See Metabolic
    alkalosis
Volume indicators. See Provider-level volume
    indicators
Volume overload, 401
  clinical presentation, 401
  diagnosis, 401
  differential diagnosis, 401
  discharge/follow-up plans, 401
  impact, 824
  management, 401
  prognosis, 401
Vomiting. See Postoperative nausea and
    vomiting
  causes, 61t
  effects, treatment, 63–64
  evaluation/treatment, 64f
  response, 64–68
  treatment, 807
    guidelines, 64t
Von Reyn/Beth Israel Criteria, usage, 313
Von Willebrand disease
  diagnosis, 593–594
  management, 594
  presentation, 593
  prognosis, 594
VPMA. See Vice president of medical affairs
V/Q. See Ventilation perfusion
VT. See Ventricular tachycardia
VTE. See Venous thromboembolism
Vumon, usage, 533

Warfarin
  discontinuation, 772–774
  management. See Long-term warfarin
    management
  overdose, management, 595
  therapy, duration (selection), 213
  toxicity, management, 595
  usage. See Surgery
  withholding, 831
Water bottle heart, CXR, 251f
Water-soluble contrast enema, usage, 54. See
    also Diverticulitis
WBC. See White blood cell
WBI. See Whole bowel irrigation
WCT. See Wide complex tachycardia
Wegener's granulomatosis (WG), 377, 395,
    609
  PR3-ANCA, 610
Westermark's sign, 218
West Nile virus, 300
WG. See Wegener's granulomatosis
White blood cell count (WBC). See Synovial
    fluid
  effluence, 404
  elevation, 293, 467
  usage, 249
  usefulness, 468
White blood cell (WBC) count
  level, 584
WHO. See World Health Organization
Whole-body PET scanning, 564
Whole bowel irrigation (WBI), 677, 679
Wide complex tachycardia (WCT), 184f
Wide QRS complex. See Tachyarrhythmias
  tachycardias, differential diagnosis, 183
Wilson's disease, 447
Withdrawal. See Cocaine; Opioids
  pharmacotherapies, 115
Wolff-Chaikoff effect, 515
Wolff-Parkinson-White syndrome,
  relationship. See Atrial fibrillation
Women (vaccination), pregnancy/lactation
    contraindication (absence), 90
Wong-Baker FACES Pain Rating Scale, 726f
Woolsorter's disease, 339

Work hours, issues, 891b
Workplace, health, 930
World Health Organization (WHO)
  analgesic
    guide. *See* Pain
      ladder, 728f
  classification. *See* Pulmonary hypertension
  Criteria, 106t
Wounds. *See* Black wounds; Open wounds; Red
    wounds; Yellow wounds
  care, 811
  complications, 813–815
  dehiscence, 813–814
    illustration, 813f
  drainage, 811
  hematoma. *See* Neck wound hematoma

Wounds *(Continued)*
  infection, 814
    signs, 811
  management, 46, 48
  margins, approximation/epithelialization,
    811
  products, 47t
Wounds, healing. *See* Acute wounds
  factors, impact, 811
  hyperglycemia, impact, 790
  phases, 812f
  promotion, mechanical devices (usage),
    812
  ridge, 811
Wounds, postoperative evaluation/care
  background, 811

Wounds, postoperative evaluation/care
  (Continued)
  clinical assessment/evaluation, 811
  pathophysiology, 811
  postoperative incision care, 811–812
  reading, 814
  recommendations/management, 811–814
Written surveys, usage, 971
  example. *See* Hospitals

Yale Insulin Protocol, 507f
Yellow wounds, 43
Yersinia, empiric antibiotics (usage), 481
Young programs, scheduling, 891

Zollinger-Ellison syndrome, 549